KEY TO ESSENTIAL TERMINOLOGY

PATIENT ASSESSMENT DATA BASE

Provides an overview of the more commonly occurring etiology and coexisting factors associated with a specific medical/surgical diagnosis as well as the signs/symptoms and corresponding diagnostic findings.

NURSING PRIORITIES

Establishes a general ranking of needs/concerns on which the Nursing Diagnoses are ordered in constructing the plan of care. This ranking would be altered according to the individual patient situation.

DISCHARGE GOALS

Identifies generalized statements that could be developed into short-term and intermediate goals to be achieved by the patient before being "discharged" from nursing care. They may also provide guidance for creating long-term goals for the patient to work on after discharge.

NURSING DIAGNOSES

The general problem/need (diagnosis) is stated without the distinct cause and signs/symptoms, which would be added to create a patient diagnostic statement when specific patient information is available. For example, when a patient displays increased tension, apprehension, quivering voice, and focus on self, the nursing diagnosis of Anxiety might be stated: Anxiety, severe, related to unconscious conflict, threat to self-concept as evidenced by statements of increased tension, apprehension; observations of quivering voice, focus on self.

In addition, diagnoses identified within these guides for planning care as actual or risk can be changed or deleted and new diagnoses added, depending entirely on the specific patient information.

MAY BE RELATED TO/POSSIBLY EVIDENCED BY

These lists provide the usual/common reasons (etiology) why a particular problem may occur with probable signs/symptoms, which would be used to create the "related to" and "evidenced by" portions of the *patient diagnostic statement* when the specific situation is known.

When a risk diagnosis has been identified, signs/symptoms have not yet developed and therefore are not included in the nursing diagnosis statement. However, interventions are provided to prevent progression to an *actual* problem. The exception to this occurs in the nursing diagnosis *Violence, risk for,* which has possible indicators that reflect the patient's risk status.

DESIRED OUTCOMES/EVALUATION CRITERIA—PATIENT WILL

These give direction to patient care as they identify what the patient or nurse hopes to achieve. They are stated in general terms to permit the practitioner to modify/individualize them by adding time lines and individual patient criteria so they become "measurable." For example, "Patient will appear relaxed and report anxiety is reduced to a manageable level within 24 hours."

In this edition, Nursing Outcomes Classification (NOC) labels have been added. The outcome label is selected from a standardized nursing language and serves as a general header for the outcome indicators that follow.

ACTIONS/INTERVENTIONS

NIC (Nursing Interventions Classification) intervention labels are drawn from a standardized nursing language and serve as a general header for the nursing actions that follow.

Nursing actions are divided into independent (those actions that the nurse performs autonomously) and collaborative (those actions that the nurse performs in conjunction with others, such as implementing physician orders) and are ranked in this book from most to least common. When creating the individual plan of care, interventions would normally be ranked to reflect the patient's specific needs/situation. In addition, the division of independent/collaborative is arbitrary and is actually dependent on the individual nurse's capabilities and hospital/community standards.

RATIONALE

Although not commonly appearing in patient plans of care, rationale has been included here to provide a pathophysiologic basis to assist the nurse in deciding about the relevance of a specific intervention for an individual patient situation.

CLINICAL PATHWAY

This abbreviated plan of care or care map is event- (task-)oriented and provides outcome-based guidelines for goal achievement within a designated length of stay. Several samples have been included to demonstrate alternative planning formats.

NURSING DIAGNOSES
ACCEPTED FOR USE AND RESEARCH (1999–2000)

Activity Intolerance [specify level]†
Activity Intolerance, risk for
Adaptive Capacity: Intracranial, decreased
Adjustment, impaired
Airway Clearance, ineffective
*Anxiety, death
Anxiety [specify level]†
Aspiration, risk for
[Autonomic] Dysreflexia
Autonomic Dysreflexia, risk for
Body Image disturbance
Body Temperature, risk for altered
Bowel Incontinence
Breastfeeding, effective
Breastfeeding, ineffective
Breastfeeding, interrupted
Breathing Pattern, ineffective
Cardiac Output, decreased
Caregiver Role Strain
Caregiver Role Strain, risk for
Communication, impaired verbal
Community Coping, ineffective
Community Coping, potential for enhanced
Confusion, acute
Confusion, chronic
Constipation
Constipation, perceived
*Constipation, risk for
Coping, defensive
Coping, Individual, ineffective
Decisional Conflict (specify)
Denial, ineffective
*Dentition, altered
*Development, risk for altered
Diarrhea
Disuse Syndrome, risk for
Diversional Activity deficit
Energy Field disturbance
Environmental Interpretation Syndrome, impaired
*Failure to Thrive, adult
Family Coping, ineffective: compromised
Family Coping, ineffective: disabling
Family Coping: potential for growth
Family Processes, altered
Family Processes, altered: alcoholism
Fatigue
Fear
Fluid Volume deficit [hyper/hypotonic]†
Fluid Volume deficit [isotonic]
Fluid Volume risk for deficit
*Fluid Volume risk for imbalance
Fluid Volume excess
Gas Exchange, impaired
Grieving, anticipatory
Grieving, dysfunctional

*Growth, risk for altered
Growth & Development, altered
Health Maintenance, altered
Health Seeking Behaviors (specify)
Home Maintenance Management, impaired
Hopelessness
Hyperthermia
Hypothermia
Infant Behavior, disorganized
Infant Behavior, risk for disorganized
Infant Behavior, organized, potential for enhanced
Infant Feeding Pattern, ineffective
Infection, risk for
Injury, risk for
Knowledge deficit [Learning Need]† (specify)
*Latex Allergy
*Latex Allergy, risk for
Loneliness, risk for
Memory, impaired
Mobility, impaired bed
Mobility, impaired physical
*Mobility, impaired wheelchair
*Nausea
Noncompliance, [Compliance, altered]† (specify)
Nutrition: altered, less than body requirements
Nutrition: altered, more than body requirements
Nutrition: altered, risk for more than body requirements
Mucous Membrane, altered
Pain [acute]†
Pain, chronic
Parental Role conflict
Parent/Infant/Child Attachment, risk for altered
Parenting, altered
Parenting, risk for altered
Perioperative Positioning, risk for injury
Peripheral Neurovascular risk for dysfunction
Personal Identity disturbance
Poisoning, risk for
Post-Trauma Syndrome
*Post-Trauma Syndrome, risk for
Powerlessness
Protection, altered
Rape-Trauma Syndrome
Rape-Trauma Syndrome: compound reaction
Rape-Trauma Syndrome: silent reaction
Relocation Stress Syndrome
Role Performance, altered
Self-Care deficit [specify]: feeding, bathing/hygiene, dressing/grooming, toileting

Self-Esteem, chronic low
Self-Esteem disturbance
Self-Esteem, situational low
Self-Mutilation, risk for
Sensory/Perceptual alterations (specify): visual, auditory, kinesthetic, gustatory, tactile, olfactory
Sexual dysfunction
Sexuality Patterns, altered
Skin Integrity, impaired
Skin Integrity, risk for impaired
*Sleep Deprivation
Sleep Pattern disturbance
Social Interaction, impaired
Social Isolation
*Sorrow, chronic
Spiritual Distress (distress of the human spirit)
*Spiritual Distress, risk for
Spiritual Well-Being, potential for enhanced
Spontaneous Ventilation, inability to sustain
Suffocation, risk for
*Surgical Recovery, delayed
Swallowing, impaired
Therapeutic Regimen: Community, ineffective management
Therapeutic Regimen: Families, ineffective management
Therapeutic Regimen: Individual, effective management
Therapeutic Regimen: Individuals, ineffective management
Thermoregulation, ineffective
Thought Processes, altered
Tissue Integrity, impaired
Tissue Perfusion, altered (specify): cerebral, cardiopulmonary, renal, gastrointestinal, peripheral
*Transfer Ability, impaired
Trauma, risk for
Unilateral Neglect
Urinary Elimination, altered
Urinary Incontinence, functional
Urinary Incontinence, reflex
Urinary Incontinence, risk for urge
[Urinary] Incontinence, stress
[Urinary] Incontinence, total
[Urinary] Incontinence, urge
Urinary Retention [acute/chronic]†
Ventilatory Weaning Response, dysfunctional (DVWR)
Violence, [actual]†/risk for directed at others
Violence, [actual]†/risk for self-directed
*Walking, impaired

Permission from North American Nursing Diagnosis Association: Definitions and Classification, 1999–2000. NANDA, Philadelphia, 1999.
*New Diagnoses for 1998
†Author recommendations

NURSING CARE PLANS

GUIDELINES FOR INDIVIDUALIZING PATIENT CARE
EDITION 5

MARILYNN E. DOENGES, RN, BSN, MA, CS
Clinical Specialist
Adult Psychiatric/Mental Health Nursing
Adjunct Faculty
Beth-El College of Nursing and Health Sciences, CU-Springs
Colorado Springs, Colorado

MARY FRANCES MOORHOUSE, RN, CRRN, CLNC
Nurse Consultant
TNT-RN Enterprises
Colorado Springs, Colorado

ALICE C. GEISSLER, RN, BSN, CLNC
Contract Practitioner
Nurse Consultant
Colorado Springs, Colorado

F. A. DAVIS COMPANY • Philadelphia

F. A. Davis Company
1915 Arch Street
Philadelphia, PA 19103

Printed in the United States of America

Last digit indicates print number: 10 9 8 7 6 5 4 3 2 1

Publisher, Nursing: Robert G. Martone
Production Editor: Elena Coler
Cover Designer: Louis J. Forgione

As new scientific information becomes available through basic and clinical research, recommended treatments and drug therapies undergo changes. The authors and publisher have done everything possible to make this book accurate, up to date, and in accord with accepted standards at the time of publication. The authors, editors, and publisher are not responsible for errors or omissions or for consequences from application of the book, and make no warranty, expressed or omissions or for consequences from application of the book, and make no warranty, expressed or implied, in regard to the contents of the book. Any practice described in this book should be applied by the reader in accordance with professional standards of care used in regard to the unique circumstances that may apply in each situation. The reader is advised always to check product information (package inserts) for changes and new information regarding dose and contraindications before administering any drug. Caution is especially urged when using new or infrequently ordered drugs.

Library of Congress Cataloging-in-Publication Data

Doenges, Marilynn E., 1922-
    Nursing care plans: guidelines for individualizing patient care/Marilynn E. Doenges,
Mary Frances Moorhouse, Alice C. Geissler.—Ed. 5.
        p. cm.
    Includes bibliographical references and index.
    ISBN 0-8036-0492-0
    1. Nursing care plans—Handbooks, manuals, etc. I. Moorhouse, Mary Frances, 1947-
II. Geissler, Alice C., 1946- III. Title.
    [DNLM: 1. Patient Care Planning—Handbooks. 2. Nursing Process—Handbooks. WY
49 D651na 1999]
RT49.D64 1999
610.73—dc21

                                                                        99-042875

To our spouses, children, parents, and friends, who much of the time have had to manage without us while we work and dream, as well as cope with our struggles and frustrations.

The Doenges families: the late Dean, Jim, Barbara, and Bob Lanza; David, Monita, Matthew, and Tyler; John, Holly, Nicole, and Kelsey; and the Daigle family, Nancy, Jim, Jennifer, and Jonathan.

The Moorhouse family: Jan, Paul, Jason, Ellaina, Alexa, and Mary Isabella.

To Mary and Marilynn, couldn't have done it without you—Alice.

In loving memory of my mother, Norma Loughmiller and my late husband Bill, my biggest promoters in my early days of writing.

To our FAD family, especially Bob Martone, Ruth De George, Bob Butler, whose support is so vital to the completion of a project of this magnitude.

To the nurses we are writing for, who daily face the challenge of caring for the acutely ill patient and are looking for a practical way to organize and document this care. We believe that nursing diagnosis and these guides will help.

To NANDA and to the International nurses who are developing and using nursing diagnoses—here we come!

Finally, to the late Mary Lisk Jeffries, who initiated the original project. The memory of our early friendship and struggles remains with us. We miss her and wish she were here to see the growth of the profession and how nursing diagnosis has contributed to the process.

INTRODUCTION

We are often asked how we came to write the care plan books. In the late 1970s we were involved with some publishing efforts that did not come to fruition. In this work we had included care plans, so ensuing discussions revolved around the need for a Care Plan book. We spent a year struggling to write care plans before we realized our major difficulty was the lack of standardized labels for patient problems. At that time, we were given a list of nursing diagnoses from the Clearinghouse for Nursing Diagnosis, which became the North American Nursing Diagnosis Association (NANDA). This work answered our need by providing concise titles that could be used in various care plans and followed across the spectrum of patient care. We believed these nursing diagnosis labels would both define and focus nursing care.

Because we had long been involved in direct patient care in our nursing careers, we knew there was a need for guidelines to assist nurses in planning care. As we began to write, our focus was the nurse in a small rural community who at 2 AM needed the answer to a burning question for her patient and had few resources available. We believed the book would give definition and direction to the development and use of individualized nursing care. Thus, in the first edition, the theory of nursing process, diagnosis, and intervention was brought to the clinical setting for implementation by the nurse. We also anticipated that nursing students would appreciate having access to these guidelines as they struggled to learn how to give nursing care. Therefore, we did not consider the book to be an end in itself, but rather a vehicle for the continuing growth and development of the profession. Obviously we struck a cord and met a need, because the first edition was an immediate success.

In becoming involved with NANDA, we acknowledged that maintaining a strict adherence to their wording, while adding our own clearly identified recommendations, would help develop this neophyte standardized language and would promote the growth of nursing as a profession. We have continued our involvement with NANDA, promoting the use of the language by practicing nurses in the United States and around the world and encouraging them to participate in updating and refining the diagnoses. The wide use of our books within the student population has supported and fostered the acceptance of both the activity of diagnosing patient problems/needs and the use of standardized language.

Nursing instructors initially expressed concern that students would simply copy the plans of care and thus limit their learning. However, as students used the plans to individualize care and to develop practice priorities and patient care outcomes, the book met with more acceptance. Instructors began not only to recommend the book, but also to adopt it as an adjunct text. Today, it remains the best selling nursing care plan book recognized as an important adjunct for student learning.

In writing the second edition, we recognized the need for an assessment tool with a nursing focus instead of a medical focus. Not finding one that met our needs, we constructed our own. To facilitate problem identification, we categorized the nursing diagnosis labels and the information obtained in the patient assessment database into a framework entitled "Diagnostic Divisions." Our philosophy is to provide a way in which to gather information and to intervene beneficially, while thinking about the rationale for every action we take and the standardized language that best expresses it. When nurses do this they are defining their practice and are able to identify it with a code and charge for it. By doing this, we promote patient protection (quality of care issue), provide for the definition and protection of nursing practice, and the protection of the individual (legal implications). The latter is important because we live in a litigation-minded society and the nurse's license and livelihood are at stake.

One of the most significant achievements in the healthcare field over the past 20 or more years has been the emergence of the nurse as an active coordinator and initiator of patient care. Although the transition from physician's helpmate to healthcare professional has been painfully slow and is not yet complete, the importance of the nurse within the system can no longer be denied or ignored. Today's nurse designs nursing care interventions that move the total patient toward improved health and maximum independence.

Professional care standards, and healthcare providers and consumers will continue to increase the expectations for nurses' performance. Each day brings new challenges in patient care and the struggle to understand the mysteries of body function and human responses to actual and potential health problems. To meet these challenges competently, the nurse must have up-to-date assessment skills and a working knowledge of pathophysiological concepts concerning the common diseases/conditions presented. We believe that this book is a tool, providing a means of attaining that competency.

In the past, plans of care were viewed principally as learning tools for students and seemed to have little relevance after graduation. However, the need for a written format to communicate and document patient care has been recognized in all care settings. In addition, healthcare policy, governmental regulations, and third-party payor requirements have created the need to validate many things, including appropriateness of care provided, staffing patterns, and monetary charges. Thus, although the student's "case studies" were considered too cumbersome to be practical in the clinical setting, it has long been recognized that the patient plan of care meets certain needs and therefore its appropriate use was validated.

The practicing nurse, as well as the nursing student, can welcome this text as a ready reference in clinical practice. It is designed for use in the acute care, community, and homecare settings. It is organized by systems for easy reference.

Chapter 1 examines current issues and trends and their implications for the nursing profession. An overview of cultural, community, sociological, and ethical concepts affecting the nurse is included. The importance of the nurse's role in collaboration and coordination with other healthcare professionals is integrated throughout the plans of care.

Chapter 2 reviews the historical use of the nursing process in formulating plans of care and the nurse's role in the delivery of that care. Nursing diagnosis, outcomes, and interventions are discussed to assist the nurse in understanding her or his role in the nursing process. In this book, we have also linked NANDA diagnoses with Nursing Intervention Classification (NIC) and Nursing Outcomes Classification (NOC) language.

Chapter 3 discusses care plan construction and describes the use and adaptation of the guides presented in this book. A nursing-based assessment tool is provided to assist the nurse in identifying appropriate nursing diagnoses. Finally, a sample patient situation (with individual database and a corresponding plan of care) is included to demonstrate how critical thinking is used to adapt nursing process theory to practice.

Chapters 4 through 15 present plans of care that include information from multiple disciplines to assist the nurse in providing holistic care. Each plan includes a Patient Assessment Database (presented in a nursing format) and associated Diagnostic Studies. After the database is collected, Nursing Priorities are sifted from the information to help focus and structure the care. Discharge Goals are created to identify what should be generally accomplished by the time of discharge from the care setting. Mean length of stay information provides a general idea of time constraints in achieving the discharge goals. Next, Desired Patient Outcomes are stated in measurable behavioral terms to evaluate both the patient's progress and the effectiveness of care provided.

The nursing diagnoses listed in the plans of care are developed by identifying "may be related to" and "possibly evidenced by" factors that provide an explanation of patient problems/needs.

Corresponding actions/interventions are designed to promote resolution of the identified patient needs. The nurse acting independently or collaboratively within the health team then uses a decision-making model to organize and prioritize nursing interventions. No attempt is made in this book to indicate whether independent or collaborative actions come first because this must be dictated by the individual situation. We do, however, believe that every collaborative action has a component that the nurse must identify and for which nursing has responsibility and accountability.

Rationales for the nursing actions (which are not required in the customary plan of care) are included to assist the nurse in deciding whether the interventions are appropriate for an individual patient. Additional information is provided to further assist the nurse in identifying and planning for rehabilitation as the patient progresses toward discharge and across all care settings. A bibliography is provided as a reference and to allow further research as desired.

This book is designed for students who will find the plans of care helpful as they learn and develop skills in applying the nursing process and using nursing diagnoses. It will complement their classroom work and support the critical thinking process. The book also provides a ready reference for the practicing nurse as a catalyst for thought in planning, evaluating, and documenting care.

As a final note, this book is not intended to be a procedure manual, and efforts have been made to avoid detailed descriptions of techniques or protocols that might be viewed as individual or regional in nature. Instead the reader is referred to a procedure manual or text covering Standards of Care if detailed direction is desired.

As we always say when we sign a book "Use and enjoy." MD, MM, and AG

CONTRIBUTORS

Nancy Lea Carter, RN, MA, ONC
Clinical Nurse, Orthopedics
Presbyterian Medical Center
Albuquerque, New Mexico

Rebecca D. Ellis, RN, MS, NP
Multiple Sclerosis Nurse Practitioner/
  Coordinator
Department of Veterans Affairs
Medical Center, Denver, Colorado

Christie A. Hinds, RN, SNP, MSN, ANP
Director: HIV Patient Care
FHL Health Care, Inc.
Colorado Springs, Colorado

Laura Ruth Johnson, RN, BSN, MNED
Clinical Educator, Surgery
Penrose Community Hospital
Colorado Springs, Colorado

Ginger Pittman, RN, CNN
Education Coordinator
Pikes Peak Dialysis Center, Inc.
Colorado Springs, Colorado

Tracy Steinberg, RN, MSN, CNS
Transplant Coordinator
Division of Transplant Surgery
University of Colorado Health Sciences
  Center
Denver, Colorado

Geri L. Tierney, RN, BSN, ONC
Coordinator, Total Joint Program
The Penrose-St. Francis Healthcare
  System
Colorado Springs, Colorado

Linda White, RN, BSN, CDE
Clinical Director/Nurse Educator
Diabetes Education and Support Center
Colorado Springs, Colorado

Anne Zobec, RN, MS, CS, AOCN
Clinical Nurse Specialist
Medical/Surgical/Oncology
Penrose-St. Francis Health Care System
Colorado Springs, Colorado

CONTENTS IN BRIEF

A table of contents including nursing diagnoses follows.

DETAILED CONTENTS

INDEX OF NURSING DIAGNOSES appears on pages 967–971

Issues and Trends in Medical/Surgical Nursing

THE CHANGING HEALTHCARE ENVIRONMENT

Understanding trends and current issues in medical/surgical nursing care requires looking at the overall trends and the restructuring within the healthcare industry. The impetus to restructure healthcare is due in part to the rapidly rising cost of healthcare delivery, the increasing numbers of uninsured or underinsured consumers, and the need for allocation of resources. In addition, technological advances, the needs of special populations, changing roles for healthcare providers, ethical issues, and liability concerns will all affect the way nursing is provided in the future. Nurses must be aware of these influences and be actively involved in formulating policies and standards of practice so that care continues to be provided at a high level of quality and patient satisfaction.

HEALTHCARE COSTS AND THE ALLOCATION OF RESOURCES

Healthcare expenditures continue to rise. Public Law 98-21 changed the method of payment for federally subsidized inpatient healthcare services from a cost-based retrospective payment system to a prospective payment system based on the 467 diagnoses or diagnosis-related-groups, referred to as DRGs. Now this system is being upgraded to better reflect severity of patient condition/care needs (all patient related or APR-DRGs). Most states are reconsidering (and some have enacted)

options to similarly curb Medicaid reimbursement. Both government and private payors of healthcare are pursuing various methods of cost containment. Solutions include managed care and, in some cases, special incentives for the consumer (such as providing physical fitness/smoking cessation programs) and/or provider (bonus checks when the cost of care is below projected costs). Most insurance plans include preauthorization, early hospital discharge, outpatient services, and some home care; third-party payors are negotiating with healthcare providers, agencies, and facilities to lower reimbursement rates or even to capitate fees (providing services for a preset fee regardless of actual cost) based on both the numbers and specific demographics of the insured population.

MANAGED CARE: RESTRUCTURING HEALTHCARE

With changes in reimbursement, the shift to managed care has forced hospitals to restructure by borrowing methods used in industry, such as re-engineering and work redesign, or by using methods developed specifically for the healthcare arena . . . accelerated clinical improvement aimed at reducing costs without jeopardizing quality and consumer satisfaction. Restructuring the workforce and patient care system was initially accomplished through mergers and consolidations of services, by downsizing professional staff through attrition, early retirement, and layoffs, and by shifting care from registered nurses (RNs) to licensed practical nurses (LPNs) and unlicensed personnel (UAPs). Healthcare professionals have expressed great concern regarding the effect of downsizing on the quality of care provided as well as on the perceived decline in consumer satisfaction. Indeed, studies (Blegen, 1998; Prescott, 1993) have shown that a higher ratio of professional nurses on staff improves patient outcomes and lowers mortality rates.

Responding to these concerns, some hospitals have formed collaborative practice teams whose goal is to revise the patient care system by reducing redundancy of services and eliminating nonproductive activities, relocating ancillary services (such as laboratory and x-ray services), implementing cross-training of staff to enhance care-provider qualifications, implementing computerization, streamlining documentation, and developing structured care methodologies.

The reduction in the number of individuals providing direct patient care has necessitated problem-solving activities that help nurses "work smarter." Computers have advanced beyond billing and order-entry functions. Bedside terminal or hand-held units allow immediate data entry and file and data retrieval. Beepers and cordless phones facilitate communication between patient and nurse, reducing response time. Documentation time has been reduced through streamlining, such as using detailed flow sheets, charting "by exception," generating computerized plans of care, and developing clinical pathways.

Clinical pathways identify specific outcomes (important in the trend of "outcomes-based" patient care) and corresponding activities for a given diagnosis. The use of clinical pathways provides a mechanism for modifying care to reflect clinical innovations and research findings. Clinical pathways may be useful as well for identification of actual/potential outlyers, allowing reallocation of resources to maximize patient outcomes in a timely manner while controlling costs.

Other structured care methodologies promoting standardization of care processes include the use of algorithms, guidelines, protocols, and standing orders. Medicine is developing criteria such as the computer program APACHE (Acute Physiology and Chronic Health Evaluation) to choose appropriate treatment options and help allocate resources. This program provides data on the likely outcomes of various treatments in specific patient populations. Thus, reimbursement could be tied to a scoring system reflecting the likelihood of survival.

The advancement of knowledge continues with the work of the U.S. Department of Health and Human Services' Agency for Health Care Policy and Research (AHCPR), whose purpose is to enhance the quality, appropriateness, and effectiveness of healthcare services and access to these services. Multidisciplinary panels of clinicians (including nurses) are conducting the arduous process of creating clinical practice and patient teaching guidelines addressing specific patient care situations. These guidelines are intended to assist in the prevention, diagnosis, treatment, and management of clinical conditions and to provide a resource by which patient care can be evaluated, the provider held accountable, and reimbursement justified. These processes tend to stabilize care practices and system processes that are designed to improve outcomes. Shifting some routine care activities from the nurse to the patient/family may also permit better use of nursing time and efforts. In addition, promotion of self-care through participation in planning care and setting goals, self-administration of some medications, and self-guided tutorials/education modules provide opportunities for the patient/family to maximize the hospital experience and demonstrate newly learned skills.

The need to provide services at lower costs has forced hospitals to seek alternatives to inpatient care. Currently their emphasis is on outpatient services and affiliations with other provider groups to provide a wider continuum of patient care. Healthcare networks have been created, some of which encompass a major hub or tertiary hospital and smaller affiliating hospitals, freestanding emergency clinics and surgical centers, subacute units, rehabilitation centers, long-term care facilities, and home care agencies. These networks are designed to meet all the patient's healthcare needs while keeping all the revenue within the network. However, this practice has the potential of limiting competition, thereby causing the decline of independent healthcare agencies, especially when doctors, pharmacies, and equipment supply houses join one network.

One innovation is the community nursing organization (CNO), which offers direct access to professional nursing care and nursing coordination of all services with community-based care delivery. The Healthcare Financing Administration (HCFA) developed this nursing model to provide nurses and Medicare beneficiaries a new way to work together to promote health and manage acute or chronic illnesses. At four demonstration sites, all members are seen a minimum of twice a year to evaluate their health and to develop or check on progress of a plan of care.

Significant changes in patient care management are taking place in the areas of case management, disease-state management, and evidence-based care. Case management services are now provided across all settings from traditional case managers for insurers to entrepreneurial "continuum of care" specialty areas and alternate sites, including outpatient, subacute, and home care.

Healthcare delivery systems use managed care to keep patients out of acute care hospitals by providing early intervention and using other less costly services within the network. Whether the "case manager" is a physician, nurse, or insurance adjuster, all individuals involved in care are responsible for evaluating both the therapeutic benefit and cost-effectiveness of the services provided. This need is especially critical for end-of-life care, for which a high percentage of healthcare dollars are spent.

In the acute care setting, the coordination and evaluation of interdisciplinary care may be reflected in clinical or critical pathways. Clinical pathways have been developed for many specific conditions/procedures based on the DRG or the agency expected length of stay (ELOS). If the patient's course varies from the standardized pathway, further evaluation and additional intervention may be needed. Although clinical pathways are useful for patients who fall within an expected course of illness, their lack of flexibility to accommodate preexisting multiple diagnoses (e.g., coronary bypass surgery in a patient with cronic obstructive pulmonary disease [COPD] and chronic renal insufficiency) or the development of complications generally precludes their use when greater individualization of care is required. In addition, because pathways generally address a specific episode of care, they may not focus on care over a continuum.

NURSING CARE COSTS

Nurses have always been mainstays of care for people throughout the life span and especially at the end of their lives and have continued to play a vital role in promoting responsible, appropriate, and ethical care.

Today the nurse's attention is focused on providing nursing care to patients within the guidelines of prospective reimbursement and capitation, scarce dollars, limited time, reduced beds and staff, and restricted numbers of therapy and home care visits. Quantifying the contribution of nursing to patient care requires identification of the level of nursing care necessary for each patient and translating that into direct "billing" of services rendered. In those facilities/agencies already billing for nursing services, the patient plan of care is an integral part of the justification of nursing care costs.

The what and how of the work of nursing have been explained in part in a number of existing publications that help to operationalize the work of nursing. The North American Nursing Diagnosis Association (NANDA) developed a taxonomy (1989) that began a classification schema to categorize and classify nursing diagnostic labels. In 1992, the Iowa Intervention Project: Nursing Intervention Classification (NIC) directed our focus to the content and process of nursing care by identifying and standardizing some of the direct care activities nurses perform. Now a second

group, the Iowa Outcomes Project: Nursing Outcomes Classification (NOC) has addressed patient outcomes responsive to and associated with nursing interventions.

EARLY DISCHARGE

Patients are discharged from acute care as soon as they are out of danger or their condition is stabilized, but they may still require specialized care. Subacute or transitional units can provide routine services (such as monitoring), ongoing therapies and complex care (such as intravenous [IV] therapy, pain and wound management, airway care, and ventilator weaning), as well as rehabilitation services, and postsurgical recovery care.

Shorter hospital stays have also shifted recovery care to the home setting. Families are expected to be more involved in postdischarge care. Although the rate of nosocomial infections may decline, patients could be "abandoned" or recovery delayed or prolonged if the family's personal resources cannot meet the new challenges associated with the recovery process.

AGING POPULATION

The increased mean age of patients requiring hospitalization necessitates some changes in the way their healthcare is provided. A general lack of knowledge among healthcare providers regarding special needs of the elderly, along with limited resources to meet these needs and the high incidence of adverse events (such as confusion, falls, and incontinence), can contribute to instances of suboptimal patient care. At the least, these factors have resulted in prolonged facility stays and increased the number and complexity of treatments, readmissions, and adverse outcomes. To this end, the nursing profession is working to develop models that will improve the care provided to this population (e.g., Nurses Improving Care to the Hospitalized Elderly [NICHE] Project). The provision of primary nurse case managers to follow chronically ill patients across the continuum of care and other projects such as the community nursing organization (CNO) work to assure that the elderly patients are not lost to follow-up and receive ongoing monitoring for timely, cost-effective intervention.

Healthcare decision making has changed dramatically in recent decades, with an explicit acknowledgment of the patient's right to determine the course of care. There has been a long-standing allegiance by the nursing profession to the patient's role in decision making, but nurses in elder care fear that the interpretation and use of advance directives are creating ethical conflicts regarding the withdrawal or withholding of treatment or care, especially when the patient is concerned about being a "burden to others." Living wills and advance directives cannot be expected to anticipate all situations patients may encounter; however, they can provide information to a proxy (named in a medical durable power of attorney) to help in the decision-making process. However, even with advance directives in place, patients have a right to change their minds and redefine their wishes, based on changes in their health status/care options.

TECHNOLOGICAL ADVANCES

Technology continues to evolve at an astounding rate in both treatment and equipment. The purpose of technology is to improve clinical decision making and symptom management, facilitate early detection/prevention of illness, and enhance self-care and patient outcomes. In the near future, expanded use of monoclonal antibodies to carry chemotherapy agents or radionuclides to cancer cells will reduce adverse reactions and possibly the need for acute care. Endotoxin antibodies (immune system molecules that can mediate sepsis) and gene therapy have been developed that could manage or even eliminate hereditary diseases, thus reducing high-cost therapy needs. Equipment developments include user-friendly ventilators, smaller implantable ventricular-assist devices, and artificial hearts that allow patients to leave acute care settings more quickly. The cost of care and the incidence of complications or adverse outcomes have been reduced with the use of such procedures as noninvasive monitoring of pulmonary and cardiac functions, near-infrared spectroscopy for noninvasive intracranial pressure monitoring, tube locators to verify placement of catheters or enteral tubes, and bedside monitoring of many laboratory studies (such as electrolytes, blood urea nitrogen [BUN], hematocrit, glucose, and coagulation times). Additionally, point-of-care computer systems are being refined in an effort to cut documentation time and to track nursing time for the costing of care. Computers providing real-time updating of the patient plan of care enable the nurse to process data from monitoring activities and facilitate evaluation of the effectiveness of nursing actions and other therapies.

We are living in an age of escalating uncertainty and tension. Scientific and technological advances we so covet are the same advances that strip life of its simplicity. In the future, technologies can and will be created to support and, in some cases, replace dependent and interdependent activities of nursing. As a result of the efficiencies afforded by advances in automation and information management, the focus of nursing practice could shift from the "to do's" reflected in the tasks to what nurses know in relation to being with persons. Concrete activities, such as inserting an intravenous line, assessing for respiratory sounds, and providing patient teaching, do not reflect what nurses believe and value as the most important elements of practice. Patients in a technologically driven healthcare system will still feel the need to be comforted, listened to, and treated with dignity and respect.

As technology changes and more people become knowledgeable partners in healthcare, many are choosing alternative therapies and modalities. Billions of dollars are spent yearly for multiple types of therapies not provided by physicians, ranging from guided imagery and meditation to homeopathy and acupuncture. Nurses have long placed emphasis on the psychosocial, spiritual, and physical needs of their patients within the medical regimen. Today, nurses need to be knowledgeable and open-minded regarding alternative therapies—supporting patient choices and learning and evaluating new techniques, as appropriate.

FUTURE OF NURSING

Healthcare reform remains the focus of much writing and debate into the new century. Questions still abound about what constitutes healthcare reform. Whether brought about by statute, insurance payors, or healthcare providers, the changes in healthcare delivery are continuing and far-reaching.

We still believe that a nursing perspective is essential if nurses are to position themselves for a role in the future health care system. As Virginia Henderson said, "The beauty of nursing is the combination of the heart, head, and hands" (Buerhaus, 1998).

In general, the public's image of nursing remains positive; however, expectations may be limited because people are not usually aware of nurses' varied capabilities or their advanced practice potential. Although the public expects nurses to demonstrate technical competence and academic knowledge, it is also now demanding better consumer service, that is, friendliness, attention to the patient's personal or special needs, concern for privacy, information about tests and therapies, and inclusion of the family in the information loop.

As the number of RNs in acute care facilities declines and as they are replaced with less knowledgeable LPNs and UAPs, nurses need to delegate appropriately and use team members effectively and safely. Nurses, who now have less time for nonclinical activities, are nonetheless spending more time collaborating with a variety of healthcare professionals to manage and coordinate care and communicate data regarding effectiveness of therapies. To ensure that patients are getting what they need without wasting healthcare dollars, nurses must be knowledgeable about costs and reimbursement plans, as well as the relative benefits of treatment options. Nurses are interacting more with families, providing them with the information they need to make treatment decisions that reflect the patient's goals and values, and incorporating them into the caregiving process in preparation for the patient's discharge.

Downsizing produced an additional stimulus to nurses to broaden their skill base through cross-training and certification to document their expertise in a given area. Cutting staff requires that those nurses who remain are flexible and perhaps trained to work in more than one clinical area. Healthcare systems can no longer employ RNs in roles that do not directly, critically, and clearly contribute to the outcomes of the organization. Today's nurse must be technically competent, skilled at critical thinking and problem solving, able to work with a variety of people, and fiscally responsible. This is not enough, however, because the outcomes of nursing care are the true measurement of the ability to provide care. Nurses are identifying new practice environments in which to use their skills. They are also working to further define nursing practice and the special contribution that nursing will continue to offer. Nursing's contribution must be defined in the language of outcomes, because that is how services will be evaluated and reimbursed. If nursing cannot define its contribution, then, as far as the reimburser is concerned, the contribution does not exist.

The recent focus of growth in the profession has been the effort to standardize nursing language to better demonstrate what nursing is and what nurses do. As of this edition, several versions of standardized nursing languages have been recognized by the American Nurses Association (ANA) and submitted to the National Library of Medicine for inclusion in the Unified Medical Language System Metathesaurus. These nursing languages (NANDA, NIC/NOC, Omaha System, Home Healthcare Classification, and Ozbolt Patient Care Data Set) enhance the ability of nurses to communicate and document the care they provide, and charge for these services. This facilitates the recognition of nursing's contribution to patient care and promotes the view that nursing is a revenue-generating department.

In the midst of this whirlwind of change, as we experiment with new ways to provide cost-effective care within a specified time frame, it is imperative that we build on the foundation of the profession; that is, nursing is a science as well as an art, and nursing practice is rooted in the scientific process. Whether or not we choose to rename the steps we engage in (assessing patients' needs, choosing actions to meet those needs, and evaluating the effectiveness of those actions), our purpose remains the same—the diagnosis and treatment of human responses to health and illness. If we allow our nursing focus to be replaced by the medical model, our practice will be subsumed, and much more will be lost than the essence of our profession.

CONCLUSION

Rapid and continuous changes in the healthcare environment have greatly increased the responsibilities facing today's nurse. To fulfill these responsibilities, planning and documentation of care are essential to satisfy patient needs and meet legal obligations. Documentation of the necessary impact of nursing on desired patient outcomes provides a basis for evaluating continuing care needs, dealing with legal concerns, and determining payment.

Therefore, as nurses work collaboratively with other disciplines to provide patient care, we need to continue to identify and document the nursing care needs of patients through the use of the nursing process and nursing diagnosis. Although this journey into change is not optional, nursing does have the opportunity and responsibility to take an active role in shaping that change.

What lies ahead for nursing and care planning? Definitely, a tremendously exciting and exacting challenge!

The Nursing Process: Planning Care with Nursing Diagnoses

Nursing care is a key factor in achieving positive patient outcomes and in the maintenance, rehabilitation, and prevention aspects of healthcare. To this end, the nursing profession has identified a problem-solving process that "combines the most desirable elements of the art of nursing with the most relevant elements of systems theory, using the scientific method" (Shore, 1988).

Prospective/capitated payment plans, movement from acute care (hospital) to community settings, freestanding care centers, home health services, the development and revision of specialty standards of care (e.g., AACN [American Association of Critical-Care Nurses]), and other changes in the healthcare system have reaffirmed the need for a common framework of communication and documentation. In addition, hospitals accredited by the Joint Commission on Accreditation of Healthcare Organizations (JCAHO) must meet standards that further specify the parameters of patient assessment and documentation of care.

The what and how of the work of nursing have been explained in part in a number of existing publications that help to operationalize the work of nursing. The publication of the *American Nurses Association (ANA) Social Policy Statement* (1980), which defined nursing as the "diagnosis and treatment of human responses to actual and potential health problems," as well as the *ANA Standards of Clinical Nursing Practice* (1991), describing the patient care process and standards for professional performance, provided impetus and support for the use of nursing diagnosis in the practice setting. This work has been ongoing for more than 25 years, beginning with efforts to identify patient problems/needs for which nurses are accountable.

The work of the North American Nursing Diagnosis Association (NANDA) to develop nursing diagnostic labels is now being complemented by the Iowa Intervention Project: Nursing Interventions Classification (NIC), which has directed our focus to the content and process of nursing care by identifying and standardizing the care activities nurses perform. The Iowa Outcomes Project: Nursing Outcomes Classification (NOC) is now fully involved and is extending its scope by describing outcomes that are responsive to nursing intervention and developing corresponding measurement scales.

The linkage of nursing diagnoses to specific nursing interventions and patient outcomes has involved several standardized nursing languages (e.g., Omaha System, Home Healthcare Classification, Ozbolt Patient Care Data Set) for the purpose of helping to ensure high-quality nursing care and continuity of care for the patient who moves from one area of the healthcare system to another. Evaluating care and documenting it help ensure that the care is appropriate and available as the patient/family receives care in different settings.

The original concept of *nursing process* was introduced in the 1950s as a three-step process of assessment, planning, and evaluation based on the scientific method of observing, measuring, gathering data, and analyzing the findings. Over time, this process became part of the conceptual framework of all nursing curricula and is accepted as part of the legal definition of nursing in the nurse practice acts of most states. Years of study, use, and refinement have led nurses to expand the nursing process to five steps: (1) assessment, including focus assessments (systematic collection of data relating to patients and their problems/needs),

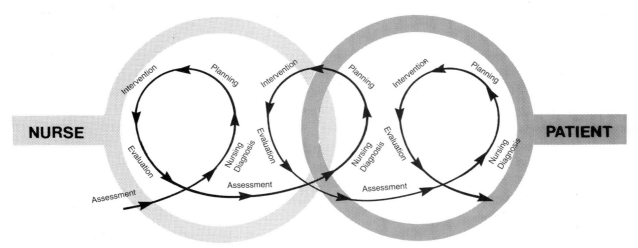

FIGURE 2–1. Diagram of the nursing process. The steps of the nursing process are interrelated, forming a continuous circle of thought and action that is both dynamic and cyclic.

(2) problem identification (analysis and interpretation of data), (3) planning (choice of solutions, prioritizing and goal setting), (4) implementation (putting the plan into action), and (5) evaluation (assessing the effectiveness of the plan and changing the plan as indicated by current needs). These five steps are central to nursing actions and the delivery of high-quality, individualized patient care in any setting.

When a patient enters the healthcare system, the nurse uses these steps of the nursing process to achieve the desired patient outcomes and goals. They evaluate the effectiveness of the plan of care by determining if the desired outcomes and goals have been reached, whether the patient's problems have been resolved, or if problems remain unresolved at the time of discharge. If problems are unresolved, plans must be made for further assessment, additional problem/ need identification, alteration of outcomes and goals, and/or changes of interventions in home care settings.

Although nurses use the nursing process terms as separate, progressive steps, they are, in reality, interrelated elements. Together, they form a continuous circle of thought and action throughout the patient's contact with the healthcare system. The process combines all the skills of critical thinking and creates a method of active problem solving that is both dynamic and cyclic. Figure 2–1 visualizes the way this cyclic process works.

The critical element for providing effective planned nursing care is its relevance as identified in patient assessments. According to *ANA Standards of Clinical Nursing Practice* (ANA, 1991), patient assessment is required in the following areas: physical, psychological, sociocultural, spiritual, cognitive, functional abilities, developmental, economic, and lifestyle. These assessments, combined with the results of medical findings and diagnostic studies, are documented in the patient database and form a strong foundation for developing the patient's plan of care.

PLANNING CARE

Medicine and nursing, as well as other health disciplines, are interrelated and therefore have implications for each other. This interrelationship allows exchange of information, ideas, and thoughts and development of plans of care that include all data pertinent to the individual patient and/or family.

The plan of care contains not only the actions initiated by medical and nursing orders but also the written coordination of care provided by all related healthcare disciplines. The nurse is often the person responsible for coordinating these different activities into a functional plan, which is essential in providing holistic care for the patient. Although independent nursing actions are an integral part of this process, collaborative actions based on the medical regimen or orders from other disciplines are also included in the care of the patient, and it is the responsibility of the practitioner to find the nursing component when functioning within a collaborative team. We believe that nursing is a part of collaborative practice, and, as such, nursing has responsibility and accountability in every collaborative problem in which the nurse interacts with the patient. In this book, collaborative actions are written in conjunction with other disciplines to assist the nurse in choosing appropriate interventions for the individual and the care setting. The educational background and expertise of the nurse, standing protocols, delegation of tasks, the use of care partners, and the area of practice (rural or urban, acute care or community care settings) can influence whether an intervention is actually an independent nursing function or requires collaboration.

The written plan of care communicates the patient's past and present health status and current needs to all members of the healthcare team. It identifies problems solved and those yet to be solved, approaches that have been successful, and patterns of patient responses. The plan of care documents patient care in areas of liability, accountability, and quality improvement. It also provides a mechanism to help ensure continuity of care when the patient leaves a care setting while still needing services.

COMPONENTS OF THE PLAN OF CARE

For each plan of care presented in this book, a patient assessment database is established from information obtained from the history, physical examination, and diagnostic studies. Nursing priorities are then determined and ranked. Priorities represent a general ranking system for the nursing diagnoses in the plan of care and may be reworded and reorganized with timelines, according to the individual patient and situation, to create short- and long-term goals. The nursing diagnosis then follows, with possible related factors (etiology) and corresponding signs and symptoms (cues), when present. Desired patient outcomes for each problem/need are followed by appropriate independent and collaborative interventions with accompanying rationales.

Patient Database

In this book, each selected medical condition has an accompanying patient database that includes subjective ("may report") and objective ("may exhibit") data that would likely be collected through the history-taking interview, physical assessment, diagnostic studies, and review of prior records. The patient database is organized within the 13 categories of the Diagnostic Divisions. A sample medical/surgical assessment tool, definitions of the divisions, and a patient situation are included in Chapter 3.

Interviewing: Interviewing provides data that the nurse obtains from the patient and significant others through conversation and observation. The information includes the individual's perceptions, that is, what the patient wants to share. The data may be collected during one or more contact periods and should include all relevant information. Organizing and updating this data assists in the ongoing identification of patient care needs and nursing diagnoses. All participants in the interview process need to know that collected data are used in planning the patient's care.

Physical Assessment: During this aspect of information gathering, the nurse exercises perceptual and observational skills, through the senses of sight, hearing, touch, and smell. The duration and depth of any physical assessment depends on the current condition of the patient and the urgency of the situation but usually includes inspection, palpation, percussion, and auscultation. In this book, the physical assessment data are presented within the patient database as *objective* data.

Diagnostic Studies: Laboratory and other diagnostic studies are included as part of the data-gathering process. The nurse needs to be aware of significant test results that require reporting to the physician and/or initiation of specific nursing interventions. Some tests are used to diagnose disease, whereas others are useful in following the course of a disease or in adjusting therapies. In many cases, the relationship of the test to the pathological physiology is clear, but in other cases it is not. This is the result of the interrelationship between various organs and body systems. Interpretation of diagnostic test results should be integrated with the history and physical findings.

Nursing Priorities

In this book, nursing priorities are listed in a certain order to facilitate the ranking of selected associated nursing diagnoses that appear in the plan of care guidelines. In any given patient situation, nursing priorities differ on the basis of specific patient need and can vary from minute to minute. A nursing diagnosis that is a priority today may be less of a priority tomorrow, depending on the fluctuating physical and psychosocial condition of the patient or the patient's changing responses to the existing condition.

For example, nursing priorities for a patient diagnosed with severe hypertension would include:

1. Maintain/enhance cardiovascular functioning
2. Prevent complications
3. Provide information about disease process, prognosis, and treatment regimen
4. Support active patient control of condition

Discharge Goals

Once the nursing priorities are determined, the next step is to establish goals of treatment. In this book, each medical condition has established discharge goals, which are broadly stated and reflect the desired general status of the patient on discharge or transfer to another care setting.

Discharge goals for a patient with severe hypertension would include:

1. Blood pressure within acceptable limits for individual
2. Cardiovascular and systemic complications prevented/minimized
3. Disease process/prognosis and therapeutic regimen understood
4. Necessary lifestyle/behavioral changes initiated

Nursing Diagnosis (Problem/Need Identification)

Nursing diagnoses are a uniform way of identifying, focusing on, and dealing with specific patient needs and responses to actual and high-risk problems. Nursing diagnosis labels provide a format for expressing the problem identification portion of the nursing process. In 1989, NANDA developed a taxonomy that began a classification schema to categorize and classify nursing diagnostic labels. The NANDA definition of nursing diagnosis (1990) further clarified the second step of the nursing process (i.e., problem identification/diagnosis). The definition of *nursing diagnosis* developed by NANDA is presented in Box 2–1.

There are several steps involved in the process of problem/need identification. Integrating these steps provides a systematic approach to accurately identifying nursing diagnoses.

1. Collecting a patient database (nursing interview, physical assessment, and diagnostic studies), combined with information collected by other healthcare providers.
2. Reviewing and analyzing the patient data.
3. Synthesizing the gathered patient data as a whole and then labeling your clinical judgment about the patient's response to these actual or high-risk problems/life processes.
4. Comparing and contrasting the relationships among your clinical judgments against related factors and defining characteristics for the selected nursing diagnosis. This step is crucial to choosing the appropriate nursing diagnosis label to be used in creating a specific patient diagnostic statement.
5. Combining the nursing diagnosis with the related factors and defining characteristics to create the patient diagnostic statement. For example, the diagnostic statement for a paraplegic patient with a decubitus ulcer could read: Impaired Skin Integrity related to pressure, circulatory impairment, and decreased sensation evidenced by draining wound, sacral area.

The nursing diagnosis is as correct as the present information allows because it is supported by the immediate data collected. It documents the patient's situation at the present time and should reflect changes as they occur in the patient's condition. Accurate need identification and diagnostic labeling provide the basis for selecting nursing interventions.

The nursing diagnosis may be a physical or a psychosocial response. Physical nursing diagnoses include those that pertain to physical processes, such as circulation (Altered Tissue Perfusion), ventilation (Impaired

BOX 2–1. NANDA Definition of Nursing Diagnosis

Nursing diagnosis is a clinical judgment about individual, family, or community responses to actual and potential health problems/life processes. Nursing diagnoses provide the basis for selection of nursing interventions to achieve outcomes for which the nurse is accountable.

Gas Exchange), and elimination (Constipation). Psychosocial nursing diagnoses include those that pertain to the mind (Acute Confusion), emotions (Fear), or lifestyle/relationships (Altered Role Performance). Unlike medical diagnoses, nursing diagnoses change as the patient progresses through various stages of illness/maladaptation to resolution of the problem or to the conclusion of the condition. Each decision the nurse makes is time-dependent and, with additional information gathered at a later point in time, decisions may change. For example, the initial problems/needs for a patient undergoing cardiac surgery may be Pain; Cardiac Output, decreased; Airway Clearance; and Risk for Infection. As the patient progresses, problems/needs are likely to shift to Activity Intolerance, Knowledge Deficit, and Role Performance.

Diagnostic reasoning is used to ensure the accuracy of the patient diagnostic statement. The defining characteristics and related factors associated with the chosen nursing diagnosis are reviewed and compared with the patient data. If the diagnosis is not consistent with a majority of the cues or is not supported by relevant cues, additional data may be required or another nursing diagnosis needs to be investigated.

Desired Patient Outcomes

A desired patient outcome is defined as the result of achievable nursing interventions and patient responses that is desired by the patient and/or caregiver and attainable within a defined time period, given the present situation and resources. These desired outcomes are the measurable steps toward achieving the previously established discharge goals and are used to evaluate the patient's response to nursing interventions. (The fifth step of the nursing process, evaluation, is addressed in the sample patient situation provided in Chapter 3.) Useful desired patient outcomes must:

1. Be specific.
2. Be realistic.
3. Be measurable.
4. Indicate a definite time frame for achievement.
5. Consider patient's desires and resources.

Desired patient outcomes are written by listing items and/or behaviors that can be observed and monitored to determine whether an acceptable outcome has been achieved within a specified time frame. Action verbs and time frames are used; for example, "patient will ambulate, using cane, within 48 hours of surgery." The action verbs describe the patient's behavior to be evaluated. Time frames are dependent on the patient's projected or anticipated length of stay, often determined by diagnosis-related group (DRG) classification and considering the presence of complications or extenuating circumstances (e.g., age, debilitating disease process). The recent work of NOC in identifying 190 outcomes does not currently address patient groups, but some of the outcomes may be modified to address aggregates. Although the NOC outcomes are listed in general terms (e.g., Ambulation: Walking), 12 indicators are included for this outcome that can be measured by a 5-point Likert-type scale ranging from "dependent, does not participate" to "completely independent." This facilitates tracking patients across care settings and can demonstrate patient progress even when outcomes are not met.

When outcomes are properly written, they provide direction for planning and validating the selected nursing interventions. Consider the two following patient outcomes: "identifies individual nutritional needs within 36 hours" and "formulates a dietary plan based on identified nutritional needs within 72 hours." Based on the clarity of these outcomes, the nurse can select nursing interventions to ensure that the patient's dietary knowledge is assessed, individual needs identified, and nutritional education presented. Often, the patient outcomes identified are not unique to nursing, as we provide care in a team approach with other disciplines. However, the NOC indicators for outcomes are more sensitive to nursing interventions. Other team members can use the majority of NOC labels and identify different indicators relative to their specialty focus to demonstrate their contribution to patient improvement or track deterioration. In this book, the identified outcomes in each plan of care are organized by using NOC labels (which are boxed to call attention to their introduction in this text).

Planning (Goals and Actions/Interventions)

Nursing interventions are prescriptions for specific behaviors expected from the patient and actions to be carried out/facilitated by nurses. These actions/interventions are selected to assist the patient in achieving the stated desired patient outcomes and discharge goals. The expectation is that the prescribed behavior will benefit the patient/family in a predictable way, related to the identified problem and chosen outcomes. These interventions have the intent of individualizing care by meeting a specific patient need and should incorporate identified patient strengths when possible.

Nursing interventions should be specific and clearly stated, beginning with an action verb. Qualifiers of how, when, where, time/frequency, and amount provide the content of the planned activity; for example, "assist as needed with self-care activities each morning," "record respiratory and pulse rates before, during, and after activity," and "instruct family in post-discharge care."

The NIC project has identified 433 interventions (both direct and indirect) that are stated in general terms, such as Respiratory Monitoring. Each label has a varied number of activities that may be chosen to accomplish the intervention. The interventions encompass a broad range of nursing practice, with some requiring specialized training/advanced certification. Others may be appropriate for delegation to other care providers (e.g., LPNs, nursing assistants, unlicensed personnel) but still require planning and evaluation by registered nurses. In this text, these NIC labels are boxed to help the user begin to identify how they are to be used.

This book divides the nursing interventions/actions into independent (nurse initiated) and collaborative (initiated by/performed in conjunction with other care providers) under the appropriate NIC labels. Examples of these two different professionally initiated actions are:

- Independent: Provide calm, restful surroundings, minimize environmental activity/noise, and limit numbers of visitors and length of stay.
- Collaborative: Administer antianxiety medication as indicated.

Rationale

Although rationales do not appear on agency plans of care, they are included in this book to assist the student and practicing nurse in associating the pathophysiological and/or psychological principles with the selected nursing intervention. This will help the nurse determine whether an intervention is appropriate for a specific patient.

CONCLUSION

This book is intended to facilitate the application of the nursing process and the use of nursing diagnosis in medical/surgical patients. Each plan of care guideline was designed to provide generalized information on the associated medical condition. The guidelines can be modified either by using portions of the information provided or by adding more patient care information to the existing guides. The plan of care guidelines were developed according to the NANDA recommendations, except in a few examples where the authors believed more clarification and enhancement were required. The ongoing controversy on the validity of the NANDA-approved nursing diagnosis Knowledge Deficit is one example where further clarification was added. The term "Learning Need" has been added to the nursing diagnosis label. Also, some diagnoses, such as Anxiety/Fear, have been combined for convenience; the combination indicates that two or more factors may be involved, and the nurse can then choose the most appropriate diagnosis for a specific patient. We recognize that not all of the NANDA-approved nursing diagnoses have been used in these plan of care guidelines, but we hope that these guidelines will assist you in determining your patients' needs, outcomes, and nursing interventions.

Next, Chapter 3 will assist you in applying and adapting theory to practice.

Critical Thinking: Adaptation of Theory to Practice

Critical thinking is defined as the "intellectually disciplined process of actively and skillfully conceptualizing, applying, analyzing, synthesizing and evaluating information gathered from or generated by observation, experience, reflection, reasoning, or communication, as a guide to belief and action" (National Council for Excellence in Critical Thinking, 1992). Critical thinking requires cognitive, psychomotor, and affective skills to use the tools of a comprehensive knowledge base, the nursing process, and established standards of care, as well as nursing research, to analyze data and plan a course of action based on new insights and conclusions. Although critical thinking skills are used in all aspects of nursing practice, they are most evident when assessment data are analyzed to identify relevant information, make decisions about patient needs, and develop an individualized plan of care. Therefore, patient assessment is the foundation on which identification of individual needs, responses, and problems is based.

To facilitate the steps of assessing and diagnosing in the nursing process and to aid in the critical thinking process, assessment databases have been developed (Fig. 3–1) that use a nursing focus instead of the traditional medical approach of review of systems. To achieve this nursing focus, we have grouped the North American Nursing Diagnosis Association (NANDA) nursing diagnoses into related categories titled "Diagnostic Divisions" (Table 3–1), which reflect a blending of theories, primarily Maslow's Hierarchy of Needs and a self-care philosophy. These divisions serve as the framework or outline for collection of data and direct the nurse to the corresponding nursing diagnosis labels.

Because these divisions are based on human responses/needs and are not specific "systems," information may be recorded in more than one area. For this reason, the nurse is encouraged to keep an open mind and to collect as much data as possible before choosing the nursing diagnosis label. The results (synthesis) of the collected data are written concisely (patient diagnostic statements) to best reflect the patient's situation.

From the specific data recorded in the database, the related/risk factors (etiology) and signs and symptoms can be identified, and an individualized patient diagnostic statement can be formulated according to the problem, etiology, and signs/symptoms (PES) format to accurately represent the patient's situation. For example, the diagnostic statement may read: Altered peripheral tissue perfusion related to decreased arterial flow, evidenced by decreased pulses, pale/cool feet, thick brittle nails, numbness/tingling of feet when walks $\frac{1}{4}$ mile.

Desired patient outcomes are identified to facilitate choosing appropriate interventions and to serve as evaluators of both nursing care and patient response. These outcomes also form the framework for documentation.

Interventions are designed to specify the action of the nurse, the patient, and/or significant other(s). They are not all-inclusive, because such basic nursing actions as "bathe the patient" or "notify the physician of changes" have been left out. It is expected that these are included in routine patient care. Sometimes controversial issues or treatments are presented for the sake of information and/or because alternate therapies may be used in different care settings or geographic locations.

Interventions need to promote the patient's movement toward health and independence. This requires involvement of the patient in his or her own care, including participation in decisions about the care activities and projected outcomes. This promotes patient responsibility, negating the idea that healthcare providers control patients' lives.

To assist in visualizing this critical thinking process, a prototype patient situation (pp. 20–24) is provided as an example of data collection and construction of a plan of care. As the patient assessment database is reviewed, the nurse can identify the related or risk factors and defining characteristics (signs/symptoms) that were used to formulate the patient diagnostic statements. The addition of timelines to specific patient outcomes and goals reflects the anticipated length of stay and individual patient/nurse expectations. Interventions are based on concerns/needs identified by the patient and nurse during data collection, in addition to physician orders. Although not normally included in a plan of care, rationales are included in this sample for the purpose of explaining or clarifying the choice of interventions. Finally, to complete the learning experience, we present samples of the evaluation step, based on the patient situation.

ADULT MEDICAL/SURGICAL ASSESSMENT TOOL
General Information

Name: _____

Age: _____ DOB: _____ Gender: _____ Race: _____

Admission Date: _____ Time: _____ From: _____

Source of Information: _____ Reliability (1–4 with 4 being very reliable): _____

Activity/Rest

Subjective (Reports)

Occupation: _____ Usual activities: _____

Leisure time activities/hobbies: ____

Limitations imposed by condition: ____

Sleep: Hours: ____ Naps: ____ Aids: ____

   Insomnia: Related to: _____

   Rested on awakening: _____

   Excessive grogginess: _____

Feelings of boredom/dissatisfaction: _____

Objective (Exhibits)

Observed response to activity:

   Cardiovascular: ____ Respiratory: ____

Mental status (e.g., withdrawn/lethargic): ____

Neuromuscular assessment:

   Muscle mass/tone: _____ Posture: _____

   Tremors: _____ ROM: _____ Strength: _____

   Deformity: _____

Circulation

Subjective (Reports)

History of: Hypertension: _____ Heart trouble: _____

   Rheumatic fever: _____ Ankle/leg edema: _____

   Phlebitis: _____

   Slow healing: _____ Claudication: _____

   Dysreflexia: _____

   Bleeding tendencies/episodes: ____

   Palpitations: _____ Syncope: _____

Objective (Exhibits)

BP: R and L: Lying/sit/stand: ____

   Pulse pressure: _____ Ausculatory gap: _____

Pulses (palpation): _____ Carotid: _____

   Temporal: ____ Jugular: ____ Radial: ____

   Femoral: ____ Popliteal: ____

   Posttibial: ____ Dorsalis pedis: ____

Cardiac (palpation): Thrill: ____ Heaves: ____

FIGURE 3–1. Adult medical-surgical assessment tool. This is a suggested guide and tool for creating a database reflecting a nursing focus. Although the diagnostic divisions are alphabetized here for ease of presentation, they can be prioritized or rearranged in any manner to meet individual needs. In addition, this assessment tool can be adapted to meet the needs of specific patient populations.

Extremities: Numbness/Tingling: _____
Cough/hemoptysis: _____
Change in frequency/amount of urine: _____

Heart sounds: Rate: _____ Rhythm: _____
    Quality: _____ Friction rub: _____
    Murmur: _____
Vascular bruit: _____
    Jugular vein distension (JVD): _____
Breath sounds: _____
Extremities: Temperature: _____ Color: _____
    Capillary refill: _____ Homans' sign: _____
    Varicosities: _____ Nail abnormalities: _____
    Edema: _____
    Distribution/quality of hair: _____
    Trophic skin changes: _____
Color: General: _____ Mucous membranes: _____
    Lips: _____ Nail beds: _____ Conjunctiva: _____
    Sclera: _____
Diaphoresis: _____

Ego Integrity

Subjective (Reports)
Stress factors: _____
Ways of handling stress: _____
Financial concerns: _____
Relationship status: _____
Cultural factors/ethnic ties: _____
Religion: _____ Practicing: _____
Lifestyle: _____ Recent changes: _____
Sense of connectedness/harmony with self: _____
    Feelings of: Helplessness: _____
    Hopelessness: _____ Powerlessness: _____

Objective (Exhibits)
Emotional status (check those that apply):
    Calm: _____ Anxious: _____ Angry: _____
    Withdrawn/Fearful: _____ Irritable: _____
    Restive: _____ Euphoric: _____
Observed physiological response(s): _____
Changes in energy field:
    Temperature: _____ Color: _____
    Distribution: _____ Movement: _____
    Sounds: _____

Elimination

Subjective (Reports)
Usual bowel pattern: _____
Laxative use: _____
Character of stool: _____ Last BM: _____
History of bleeding: _____ Hemorrhoids: _____
Constipation: _____ Diarrhea: _____
Usual voiding pattern: _____
    Incontinence/when: _____ Urgency: _____
    Frequency: _____ Retention: _____
Character of urine: _____
Pain/burning/difficulty voiding: _____
History of kidney/bladder disease: _____
    Diuretic use: _____

Objective (Exhibits)
Abdomen: Tender: _____ Soft/firm: _____
    Palpable mass: _____ Size/girth: _____
    Bowel sounds: location/type: _____
Hemorrhoids: _____ Stool guaiac: _____
Bladder palpable: _____
Overflow voiding: _____
CVA tenderness: _____

FIGURE 3–1. (*continued*)

Food/Fluid

Subjective (Reports)

Usual diet (type): ____ Last meal/intake: ____

Dietary pattern/content: B : ____ L: ____ D: ____

Carbohydrate/protein/fat intake: g/d ____

Number of meals daily: ____

Vitamin/food supplement use: ____

Loss of appetite: ____ Nausea/vomiting: ____

Heartburn/indigestion: ____Related to: ____

   Relieved by: ____

Food preferences: ____

Food prohibitions: ____

Allergy/food intolerance: ____

Mastication/swallowing problems: ____

   Dentures: ____

Usual weight: ____ Changes in weight: ____

Diuretic use: ____

Objective (Exhibits)

Current weight: ____ Height: ____ Body build: ____

Skin turgor:____

   Mucous membranes: moist/dry:____

Breath sounds: ____ Crackles: ____ Wheezes: ____

Edema: General: ____ Dependent: ____

   Periorbital: ____ Ascites: ____

Jugular vein distension (JVD): ____

Thyroid enlarged: ____

Condition of teeth/gums: ____

Appearance of tongue: ____

   Mucous membranes: ____ Halitosis: ____

Bowel sounds: ____

Hernia/masses: ____

Urine S/A or Chemstix: ____

Serum glucose (Glucometer): ____

Hygiene

Subjective (Reports)

Activities of daily living: Independent/

   dependent (level): ____

   Mobility: ____ Feeding: ____ Hygiene: ____

   Dressing/grooming: ____ Toileting: ____

Preferred time of personal care/bath: ____

Equipment/prosthetic devices required: ____

Assistance provided by: ____

Objective (Exhibits)

General appearance: ____

Manner of dress: ____ Personal habits: ____

   Body odor: ____ Condition of scalp: ____

   Presence of vermin: ____

Neurosensory

Subjective (Reports)

Fainting spells/dizziness: ____

Headaches: Location: ____ Frequency: ____

Tingling/numbness/weakness (location): ____

Stroke/brain injury (residual effects): ____

Seizures: ____ Type: ____ Aura: ____

   Frequency: ____ Postictal state: ____

   How controlled: ____

Eyes: Vision loss: ____ Last exam: ____

   Glaucoma: ____ Cataract:___

Ears: Hearing loss: ____ Last exam: ____

Sense of smell: ____

Epistaxis:____

Objective (Exhibits)

Mental status (Note duration of change):

   Oriented/disoriented: ____ Person: ____

   Place:____ Time: ____ Situation: ____

   Alert: ____ Drowsy: ____ Lethargic:____

   Stuporous: ____ Comatose: ____

   Cooperative: ____ Combative: ____

   Delusions: ____ Hallucinations: ____

   Affect (describe): ____

   Memory: ____ Recent: ___ Remote: ____

Glasses: ____ Contacts: ____ Hearing aids: ____

Pupil: Shape: ____ Size/reaction: R/L: ____

Facial droop: ____ Swallowing: ____

Handgrasp/release, R/L: ____

Posturing: ____

Deep tendon reflexes: ____

Paralysis: ____

FIGURE 3–1. (*continued*)

Pain/Discomfort

Subjective (Reports)

Primary focus: ____ Location: ____

    Intensity (0–10 with 10 most severe): ____

    Frequency: ____ Quality: ____

    Duration: ____ Radiation: ____

Precipitating/aggravating factors: ____

How relieved: ____

Associated symptoms: ____

Effect on activities: ____ Relationships: ____

Additional: ____

Objective (Exhibits)

Facial grimacing: ____

    Guarding affected area: ____

    Emotional response: ____

    Narrowed focus: ____

    Change in blood pressure: ____ Pulse: ____

Respiration

Subjective (Reports)

Dyspnea/related to: ____

Cough/sputum: ____

History of bronchitis: ____ Asthma: ____

    Emphysema: ____ Tuberculosis: ____

    Recurrent pneumonia: ____

    Exposure to noxious fumes: ____

Smoker: ____ pack/day: ____

    No. of pack years: ____

Use of respiratory aids: ____ Oxygen: ____

Objective (Exhibits)

Respiratory: Rate: ____ Depth: ____

    Symmetry: ____

Use of accessory muscles: ____ Nasal

    flaring: ____

Fremitus: ____

Breath sounds: ____ Egophony: ____

Cyanosis: ____ Clubbing of fingers: ____

Sputum characteristics: ____

Mentation/restlessness: ____

Safety

Subjective (Reports)

Allergies/sensitivity: ____ Reaction: ____

Exposure to infectious diseases: ____

Previous alteration of immune system: ____

    Cause: ____

History of sexually transmitted disease

    (date/type): ____ Testing: ____

    High-risk behaviors: ____

Blood transfusion/number: ____ When: ____

    Reaction: ____ Describe: ____

Geographic areas lived in/visited: ____

Seat belt/helmet use: ____

History of accidental injuries: ____

    Fractures/dislocations: ____

Arthritis/unstable joints: ____

    Back problems: ____

Changes in moles: ____ Enlarged nodes: ____

Delayed healing: ____

Cognitive limitations: ____

    Impaired vision/hearing: ____

Objective (Exhibits)

Temperature: ____ Diaphoresis: ____

Skin integrity: Scars: ____ Rashes: ____

    Lacerations: ____ Ulcerations: ____

    Ecchymosis: ____ Blisters: ____ Burns

    (degree/percent): ____ Drainage: ____

Mark location of the above on diagram:

General strength: ____ Muscle tone: ____

    Gait: ____ ROM:____

    Paresthesia/paralysis:____

FIGURE 3–1. (*continued*)

Prosthesis: Ambulatory devices:____   Results of cultures: ____
                                             Immune system testing: ____
                                             Tuberculosis testing ____

Sexuality (Component of Ego Integrity and Social Interaction)

Subjective (Reports)

Sexually active: ____   Use of condoms: ____

Birth control method: ____

Sexual concerns/difficulties: ____

Objective (Exhibits)

Comfort level with subject matter: ____

Female:

Subjective (Reports)

Age at menarche: ____   Length of cycle: ____

    Duration: ____   Number of pads uses/d: ____

    Last menstrual period: ____   Pregnant

    now: ____

Bleeding between periods: ____

Menopause: ____   Vaginal lubrication: ____

Vaginal discharge: ____

Surgeries: ____

Hormonal therapy/calcium use: ____

Practices breast self-exam: ____

    Mammogram: ____   Last PAP smear: ____

Objective (Exhibits)

Breast exam: ____

Genital warts/lesions: ____

Discharge: ____

Male:

Subjective (Reports)

Penile discharge: ____

Prostate disorder: ____

Circumcised: ____   Vasectomy: ____

Practice self-exam: Breast: ____   Testicles:___

Objective (Exhibits)

Breast: ____   Testicles: ____

Genital warts/lesions: ____

Discharge: ____

Social Interactions

Subjective (Reports)

Marital status: ____   Years in relationship:____

    Living with: ____   Concerns/stresses: ____

Extended family: ____

    Other support person(s): ____

Role within family structure: ____

Perception of relationships with family

    members: ____

Ethnic affiliation: ____

Strength of ethnic identity: ____

Lives in ethnic community (y/n): ____

Objective (Exhibits)

Speech: ____   Clear: ____   Slurred: ____

    Unintelligible: ____   Aphasic: ____

    Usual speech pattern/impairment: ____

    Use of speech aids: ____

    Use of communication aids: ____

    Laryngectomy present: ____

Verbal/nonverbal communication with

    family/SO(s): ____

    Family interaction (behavioral) pattern: ____

FIGURE 3–1. (*continued*)

Feelings of: Mistrust: ____ Rejection: ____
   Unhappiness: ____ Loneliness/isolation: ____
Problems related to illness/condition: ____
Problems with communication: ____

Teaching/Learning

Subjective (Reports)

Dominant language (specify): ____ Second
   language: ____ Literate: ____
   Education level: ____
   Learning disabilities: (specify): ____
   Cognitive limitations: ____
Where born: ____ If immigrant, how long in
   this country: ____
Health and illness beliefs/practices
   (e.g., complimentary therapies)/customs: ____
Special healthcare concerns (e.g., impact of
   religious/cultural practices): ____
   Health goals: ____
Familial risk factors (indicate relationship):
   Diabetes: ____ Thyroid (specify): ____
   Tuberculosis: ____ Heart disease: ____
   Strokes: ____ High BP: ____ Epilepsy: ____
   Kidney disease: ____ Cancer: ____
   Mental illness: ____ Other: ____

Prescribed medications: Drug: ___ Dose:____
   Times (circle last dose): ____
   Take regularly: ____ Purpose: ____
   Side effects/problems: ____
Nonprescription drugs: OTC drugs: ____
   Herbal supplements: ____
   Street drugs: ____ Tobacco: ____
   Smokeless tobacco: ____
Alcohol (amount/frequency): ____
Admitting diagnosis per provider: ____
Reason for admission per patient: ____
History of current complaint: ____
Patient expectations of care: ____
Previous illnesses and/or hospitalizations/
   surgeries: ____
Evidence of failure to improve: ____
Last complete physical exam: ____

Discharge Plan Considerations

DRG projected mean length of stay: ____
Date information obtained: ____
Anticipated date of discharge: ____
Resources available: Persons: ____
   Financial: ____ Community: ____ Support
   groups: ____ Socialization: ____
Areas that may require alteration/assistance:
   Food preparation: ____ Shopping: ____
   Transportation: ____ Ambulation: ____
   Medication/IV therapy: ____
   Treatments: ____ Wound care: ____
   Supplies: ____ Self-care (specify): ____
   Homemaker/maintenance (specify): ____
   Physical layout of home (specify): ____

Anticipated changes in living situation after
   discharge: ____
Living facility other than home (specify): ____
Referrals (date, source, services): ____
   Social Services: ____ Rehabilitation services: ____
   Dietary: ____ Home care: ____
   Resp/O$_2$: ____ Equipment: ____
   Supplies: ____ Other: ____

FIGURE 3–1. (*continued*)

After data are collected, and areas of concern/need identified, the nurse is directed to the Diagnostic Divisions to review the list of nursing diagnoses that fall within the individual categories and to choose the specific diagnostic label that accurately describes the data. Then, with the addition of etiology or related/risk factors (when known) and signs and symptoms or cues (defining characteristics), the client diagnostic statement emerges.

Activity/Rest—Ability to engage in necessary/desired activities of life (work and leisure) and to obtain adequate sleep/rest

Activity intolerance
Activity intolerance, risk for
Disuse Syndrome, risk for
Diversional Activity deficit
Fatigue
*Mobility, impaired bed
*Mobility, impaired wheelchair
*Sleep Deprivation
Sleep Pattern disturbance
*Transfer Ability, impaired wheelchair
*Walking, impaired

Circulation—Ability to transport oxygen and nutrients necessary to meet cellular needs

Adaptive Capacity: Intracranial, decreased
Autonomic Dysreflexia
*Autonomic Dysreflexia, risk for
Cardiac Output, decreased
Tissue Perfusion, altered (specify): renal, cerebral, cardiopulmonary, gastrointestinal, peripheral

Ego Integrity—Ability to develop and use skills and behaviors to integrate and manage life experiences

Adjustment, impaired
Anxiety [specify level]
*Anxiety, death
Body Image disturbance
Coping, defensive
Coping, Individual, ineffective
Decisional Conflict (specify)
Denial, ineffective
Energy Field disturbance
Fear
Grieving, anticipatory
Grieving, dysfunctional
Hopelessness
Personal Identity disturbance
Post-Trauma Syndrome
*Post-Trauma Syndrome, risk for
Powerlessness
Rape-Trauma Syndrome
Rape-Trauma Syndrome: compound reaction
Rape-Trauma Syndrome: silent reaction
Relocation Stress Syndrome
Self-Esteem, chronic low
Self-Esteem disturbance
Self-Esteem, situational low
*Sorrow, chronic
Spiritual Distress (distress of the human spirit)
*Spiritual Distress, risk for
Spiritual Well-Being, potential for enhanced

Elimination—Ability to excrete waste products

Bowel Incontinence
Constipation
Constipation, perceived
*Constipation, risk for
Diarrhea
Urinary Elimination, altered
Urinary Incontinence, functional
Urinary Incontinence, reflex
*Urinary Incontinence, risk for urge
[Urinary] Incontinence, stress
[Urinary] Incontinence, total
[Urinary] Incontinence, urge
Urinary Retention [acute/chronic]

Food/Fluid—Ability to maintain intake of and utilize nutrients and liquids to meet physiologic needs

Breastfeeding, effective
Breastfeeding, ineffective
Breastfeeding, interrupted
*Dentition, altered
*Failure to Thrive, adult
[Fluid Volume deficit hypertonic/hypotonic]
Fluid Volume deficit [isotonic]
Fluid Volume risk for deficit
Fluid Volume excess
*Fluid Volume risk for imbalance
Infant Feeding Pattern, ineffective
*Nausea
Nutrition: altered, less than body requirements
Nutrition: altered, more than body requirements
Nutrition: altered, risk for more than body requirements
Oral Mucous Membrane, altered
Swallowing, impaired

Hygiene—Ability to perform activities of daily living

Self-Care deficit: feeding, bathing/hygiene, dressing/grooming, toileting

Neurosensory—Ability to perceive, integrate, and respond to internal and external cues

Confusion, acute
Confusion, chronic
Infant Behavior: disorganized
Infant Behavior: risk for disorganized
Infant Behavior: organized, potential for enhanced
Memory, impaired
Peripheral Neurovascular risk for dysfunction
Sensory/Perceptual alterations (specify): visual, auditory, kinesthetic, gustatory, tactile, olfactory
Thought Processes, altered
Unilateral Neglect

Pain/Discomfort—Ability to control internal/external environment to maintain comfort

Pain [acute]
Pain, chronic

Respiration—Ability to provide and use oxygen to meet physiologic needs

Airway Clearance, ineffective
Aspiration, risk for
Breathing Pattern, ineffective
Gas Exchange, impaired
Spontaneous Ventilation, inability to sustain
Ventilatory Weaning Response, dysfunctional (DVWR)

Safety—Ability to provide safe, growth-promoting environment

Body Temperature, risk for altered
Environmental Interpretation Syndrome, impaired
Health Maintenance, altered
Home Maintenance Management, impaired
Hyperthermia
Hypothermia
Infection, risk for
Injury, risk for
*Latex Allergy
*Latex Allergy, risk for
Mobility, impaired physical
Perioperative Positioning Injury, risk for
Poisoning, risk for
Protection, altered
Self-Mutilation, risk for
Skin Integrity, impaired
Skin Integrity, risk for impaired
Suffocation, risk for
*Surgical Recovery, delayed
Thermoregulation, ineffective
Tissue Integrity, impaired
Trauma, risk for
Violence, [actual/] risk for directed at others
Violence, [actual/] risk for self-directed

Sexuality [Component of Ego Integrity and Social Interaction] —Ability to meet requirements/characteristics of male/female role

Sexual dysfunction
Sexuality Patterns, altered

Social Interaction—Ability to establish and maintain relationships

Caregiver Role Strain
Caregiver Role Strain, risk for
Communication, impaired verbal
Community Coping, ineffective
Community Coping, potential for enhanced
Family Coping, ineffective: compromised
Family Coping, ineffective: disabling
Family Coping: potential for growth
Family Processes, altered
Family Processes, altered: alcoholism
Loneliness, risk for
Parent/Infant/Child Attachment, risk for altered
Parental Role conflict
Parenting, altered
Parenting, risk for altered
Role Performance, altered
Social Interaction, impaired
Social Isolation

Teaching/Learning—Ability to incorporate and use information to achieve healthy lifestyle/optimal wellness

*Development, risk for altered
Growth and Development, altered
*Growth, risk for altered
Health-Seeking Behaviors (specify)
Knowledge Deficit [Learning Need] (specify)
Noncompliance [Compliance, altered] (specify)
Therapeutic Regimen: Community, ineffective management
Therapeutic Regimen: Families, ineffective management
Therapeutic Regimen: Individual, effective management
Therapeutic Regimen: Individual, ineffective management

*New diagnoses for 1998
[ ]Author recommendations

PATIENT SITUATION: Diabetes Mellitus

Mr. R.S., a type 2 diabetic (formerly a non-insulin-dependent diabetic or NIDDM) for 5 years, presented to his physician's office with a nonhealing ulcer of 3 weeks' duration on his left foot. Screening studies done in the doctor's office revealed blood glucose (BG) of 356/fingerstick and urine Chemstix of 2%. Because of distance from medical provider and lack of local community services, he is admitted to the hospital.

Admitting Physician's Orders

Culture/Sensitivity and Gram's stain of foot ulcer
Random blood glucose on admission and fingerstick BG qid
CBC, electrolytes, serum lipid profile, glycosylated Hb in AM
Chest x-ray and ECG in AM
DiaBeta 10 mg, PO, bid
Glucophage 500 mg, PO, qd to start—will increase gradually
Humulin N 10 U SC q AM and hs, begin insulin instruction for postdischarge self-care, if necessary
Dicloxacillin 500 mg PO, q6h, start after culture obtained
Darvocet-N 100 mg q4h PRN, pain
Diet—2400 calories ADA/three meals with two snacks
Up in chair ad lib with feet elevated
Foot cradle for bed
Irrigate lesion L foot with normal saline tid then apply wet to dry sterile dressing
Vital signs bid

Patient Assessment Database

Name: R.S. Informant: Patient Reliability (scale 1–4): 3
Age: 67 DOB: 5/3/31 Race: White Gender: M
Admission date: 6/28/98 Time: 7 PM From: Home

ACTIVITY/REST

Reports (Subjective):	Occupation: Farmer
	Usual activities/hobbies: Reading, playing cards "Don't have time to do much. Anyway I'm too tired most of the time to do anything after the chores."
	Limitations imposed by illness: "Have to watch what I order if I eat out."
	Sleep: Hours: 6–8 h/night Naps: No Aids: No
	Insomnia: "Not unless I drink coffee after supper." Usually feels rested when awakens at 4:30 AM
Exhibits (Objective):	Observed response to activity: Limps, favors L foot when walking
	Mental status: Alert/active
	Neuromuscular assessment: Muscle mass/tone: bilaterally equal/firm
	Posture: Erect. ROM: normal all extremities
	Strength: Equal 3 extremities/favors L leg currently

CIRCULATION

Reports (Subjective):	Slow healing: lesion L foot, 3 weeks' duration
	Extremities: Numbness/tingling: "My feet feel cold and tingly like sharp pins poking the bottom of my feet when I walk the quarter mile to the mailbox."
	Cough/character of sputum: Occasional/white
	Change in frequency/amount of urine: Yes, voiding more lately
Exhibits (Objective):	Peripheral pulses: Radials 3+, popliteal, dorsalis, posttibial/pedal, all 1+
	BP: R: Lying: 146/90 Sitting: 140/86 Standing: 138/90
	L: Lying: 142/88 Sitting: 138/88 Standing: 138/84
	Pulse: Apical: 86 Radial: 86 Quality: Strong Rhythm: Regular
	Chest auscultation: Few wheezes clear with cough, no murmurs/rubs.
	JVD: -0-

Extremities: Temperature: Feet cool bilat/legs warm
    Color: Skin: Legs pale Capillary refill: Slow both feet (approx 5 sec)
    Homans' sign: -0- Varicosities: Few enlarged superficial veins both calves
    Nails: Toenails thickened, yellow, brittle
    Distribution and quality of hair: Coarse hair to midcalf, none on ankles/toes
Color: General: Ruddy face/arms Mucous membranes/lips: Pink
    Nail beds: Fingers blanch well Conjunctiva and sclera: White

EGO INTEGRITY

Reports (Subjective):

Stress factors: "Normal farmer's problems: weather, pests, bankers, and so on."
Ways of handling stress: "I get busy with the chores and talk things over with my livestock; they listen real good."
Financial concerns: No insurance; needs to hire someone to do chores while in hospital
Relationship status: Married
Cultural factors: Rural/agrarian, Eastern European descent, American, no ethnic ties
Religion: Protestant/practicing
Lifestyle: Middle class/self-sufficient farmer
Recent changes: -0-
Feelings: "I'm in control of most things, except the weather and this diabetes." Concerned regarding possible therapy, "change from pills to shots"

Exhibits (Objective):

Emotional status: Generally calm; appears frustrated at times
Observed physiological response(s): Occasionally sighs deeply/frowns, fidgeting with coin, shoulders tense, shrugs shoulders/throws up hands

ELIMINATION

Reports (Subjective):

Usual bowel pattern: Most every PM
Last bowel movement: Last night Character of stool: Firm/brown
Bleeding: -0- Hemorrhoids: -0- Constipation: Occasional
Laxative used: Hot prune juice
Urinary: No problems Character of urine: Pale yellow

Exhibits (Objective):

Abdomen tender: No Soft/Firm: Soft Palpable mass: None
Bowel sounds: Active all 4 quads

FOOD/FLUID

Reports (Subjective):

Usual diet (type): 2400 ADA (occasionally "cheats" with dessert, "My wife watches it pretty closely"). Number of meals daily: 3/1 snack
Dietary Pattern: Breakfast: Fruit juice, toast, ham, decaf coffee
Lunch: Meat, potatoes, vegetables, fruit, milk
Dinner: Meat sandwich, soup, fruit, decaf coffee
Snack: Milk/crackers at hs. Usual beverage: Skim milk, 2–3 cups decaf coffee. Drinks "a lot of water"—several qt
Last meal/intake: Dinner: Hot roast beef sandwich, vegetable soup, pear with cheese, decaf coffee
Loss of appetite: "Never, but lately I don't feel as hungry as usual."
Nausea/vomiting: -0- Food allergies: None
Heartburn/food intolerance: Cabbage causes gas, coffee after supper causes heartburn
Mastication/swallowing problems: No Dentures: Partial upper plate
Usual weight: 175 lb Recent changes: Has lost about 4 lb this month
Diuretic therapy: No

Exhibits (Objective):

Wt: 171 lb. Ht: 5'10" Build: Stocky
Skin turgor: Good/leathery
Appearance of tongue: Midline, pink Mucous membranes: Pink, intact
Condition of teeth/gums: Good; no irritation/bleeding noted
Breath sounds: Few wheezes cleared with cough
Bowel sounds: Active all 4 quads
Urine Chemstix: 2% Fingerstick: 356 (Dr. office) Random BG drawn on admission

HYGIENE

Reports (Subjective): Activities of daily living: Independent in all areas
Preferred time of bath: PM

Exhibits (Objective): General appearance: Clean, shaven, short-cut hair, hands rough and dry, skin on feet dry, cracked, and scaly, no body odor
Scalp and eyebrows: Scaly white patches

NEUROSENSORY

Reports (Subjective): Headaches: "Occasionally behind my eyes when I worry too much."
Tingling/Numbness: Feet, once or twice a week (as noted)
Eyes: Vision loss, farsighted, "seems a little blurry now." Examination: 2 years ago
Ears: Hearing loss: R: "Some." L: No (has not been tested)
Nose: Epistaxis: -0-. Sense of smell: "No problems"

Exhibits (Objective): Mental status: Alert, oriented to time, place, person, situation Affect: Concerned
Memory: Remote and recent: clear and intact
Speech: Clear, coherent, appropriate
Pupil reaction: PERLA/small Glasses: Reading Hearing aid: No
Handgrip/release: Strong/equal

PAIN/DISCOMFORT

Reports (Subjective): Primary problem focus: L foot Location: Medial aspect, heel of L foot
Intensity (0–10): 4–5/10 Quality: Dull ache with occasional sharp stabbing sensation
Frequency/duration: "Seems like all the time" Radiation: No
Precipitating factors: Shoes, walking How relieved: ASA, not helping
Additional complaints: Sometimes has back pain following chores/heavy lifting relieved by ASA/liniment rubdown

Exhibits (Objective): Facial grimacing: When lesion border palpated
Guarding affected area: Pulls foot away Emotional response: Tense, irritated

RESPIRATORY

Reports (Subjective): Dyspnea: -0- Cough: Occasional morning cough, white sputum
Emphysema: -0- Bronchitis: -0- Asthma: -0- Tuberculosis: -0-
Smoker: Filters Packs/day: ½ Number of pack years: 25+
Use of respiratory aids: -0-

Exhibits (Objective): Respiratory rate: 22 Depth: Good Symmetry: Equal, bilateral
Auscultation: Few wheezes, clear with cough
Cyanosis: -0- Clubbing of fingers: -0-
Sputum characteristics: None to observe
Mentation/restlessness: Alert/oriented/relaxed

SAFETY

Reports (Subjective): Allergies: -0- Blood transfusions: -0-
Sexually transmitted disease: None
Fractures/dislocations: L clavicle, 1966, fell getting off tractor
Arthritis/unstable joints: "Think I've got some arthritis in my knees."
Back problems: Occasional lower back pain
Vision impaired: Requires glasses for reading
Hearing impaired: Slightly (R), compensates by turning "good ear" toward speaker

Exhibits (Objective): Temperature: 99.4°F, tympanic
Skin integrity: Impaired L foot Scars: R Ing, surgical
Rashes: -0- Bruises: -0- Lacerations: -0- Blisters: -0-
Ulcerations: Medial aspect L heel, 2.5 cm diameter, approximately 3 mm deep, draining small amount cream color/pink-tinged matter, no odor noted
Strength (general): Equal all extremities Muscle tone: Firm
ROM: Good. Gait: Favors L foot Paresthesia/Paralysis: -0-

SEXUALITY: MALE

Reports (Subjective):
Sexually active: Yes Use of condoms: No (monogamous)
Recent changes in frequency/interest: "I've been too tired lately."
Penile discharge: -0- Prostate disorder: -0- Vasectomy: -0-
Last proctoscopic examination: 2 years ago Prostate examination: 1 year ago
Practice self-examination: Breast/testicles: No
Problems/complaints: "I don't have any problems, but you'd have to ask my wife if there are any complaints."

Exhibits (Objective):
Examination: Breast: No masses Testicles: Deferred
Prostate: Deferred

SOCIAL INTERACTIONS

Reports (Subjective):
Marital status: Married, 43 years Living with: Wife
Report of problems: None
Extended family: 1 daughter lives in town (30 miles away); 1 daughter married/grandson, living out of state
Other: Several couples; he and wife play cards/socialize 2 or 3 times a month
Role: Works farm alone; husband/father/grandfather
Report of problems related to illness/condition: None until now
Coping behaviors: "My wife and I have always talked things out. You know the eleventh commandment is 'Thou shalt not go to bed angry.'"

Exhibits (Objective):
Speech: Clear, intelligible
Verbal/Nonverbal communication with family/SO(s): Speaks quietly with wife, looking her in the eye; relaxed posture
Family interaction patterns: Wife sitting at bedside, relaxed, both reading paper, making occasional comments to each other

TEACHING/LEARNING

Reports (Subjective):
Dominant language: English Second language: -0- Literate: Yes
Education level: 2 years of college
Health and illness beliefs/practices/customs: "I take care of the minor problems and only see the doctor when something's broken."
Familial risk factors/relationship:
  Diabetes: Maternal uncle Tuberculosis: Brother died age 27
  Heart Disease: Father died age 78, heart attack
  Strokes: Mother died age 81 High BP: Mother
Prescribed medications:

Drug	Dose	Schedule	Last dose	Purpose
DiaBeta	10 mg bid	8 AM/6 PM	6 PM today	Control diabetes

Home urine glucose monitoring: "Stopped several months ago when I ran out of TesTape. It was always negative anyway."
Take medications regularly: Yes
Nonprescription (OTC) drugs: Occasionally ASA
Use of alcohol (amount/frequency): Socially, occasionally beer
Tobacco: Smokes ½ pack/day
Admitting Diagnosis (physician): Hyperglycemia with nonhealing lesion L foot
Reason for hospitalization (patient): "Sore on foot and the doctor is concerned about my blood sugar, and says I'm supposed to learn this fingerstick test now."
History of current complaint: "Three weeks ago, I got a blister on my foot from breaking in my new boots. It got sore so I lanced it, but it isn't getting any better."
Patient's expectations of this hospitalization: "Clear up this infection and control my diabetes."
Other relevant illness and/or previous hospitalizations/surgeries: 1969 R Ing hernia repair
Evidence of failure to improve: Lesion L foot, 3 weeks
Last physical examination: Complete 1 year ago, office follow-up 3 months ago

Discharge Considerations (as of 6/28):

Anticipated discharge: 7/1/98 (3 days).

Resources: Person: Self, wife Financial: "If this doesn't take too long to heal, we got some savings to cover things." Community supports: Diabetic support group (has not participated)

Anticipated lifestyle changes: Become more involved in management of condition

Assistance needed: May require farm help for several days

Teaching: Learn new medication regimen and wound care, review diet; encourage smoking cessation

Referrals: Supplies: Downtown Pharmacy or AARP

Equipment: Glucometer—AARP

Follow-up: Primary care provider 1 wk after discharge to evaluate wound healing and potential need for additional changes in diabetic regimen

PLAN OF CARE: Mr. R.S.

PATIENT DIAGNOSTIC STATEMENT:

Impaired Skin Integrity related to pressure, altered metabolic state, circulatory impairment, and decreased sensation, as evidenced by draining wound L foot.

> **OUTCOME: Nutritional status: biochemical measures (NOC)**
> **Indicators:**

PATIENT WILL:

Demonstrate correction of metabolic state as evidenced by FBS less than 120 mg/dl within 36 hours (6/30 0700).

> **OUTCOME: Wound healing: secondary intention (NOC)**
> **Indicators:**

PATIENT WILL:

Be free of purulent drainage within 48 hours (6/30 1900).
Display signs of healing with wound edges clean/pink within 60 hours (7/1 0700).

ACTIONS/INTERVENTIONS

Wound Care Activities (NIC)

Irrigate wound with room-temperature sterile NS tid.

Assess wound with each dressing change. Obtain wound tracing on admission and at discharge.

Apply wet to dry sterile dressing. Use paper tape.

Infection Control (NIC)

Follow wound precautions.

Obtain sterile specimen of wound drainage on admission for laboratory analysis.

Administer dicloxacillin 500 mg PO q6h, starting 10 PM. Observe for signs of hypersensitivity: pruritus, urticaria, rash.

Administer antidiabetic medications: 10 U Humulin N insulin SC q AM/hs after fingerstick BG; DiaBeta 10 mg PO bid; Glucophage 500 mg PO qd.

RATIONALE

Cleans wound without harming delicate tissues.

Provides information about effectiveness of therapy and identifies additional needs.

Keeps wound clean/minimizes cross-contamination. Adhesive tape may be abrasive to fragile tissues.

Use of gloves and proper handling on contaminated dressings reduces likelihood of spread of infections.

Culture/sensitivity identifies pathogens and therapy of choice.

Treatment of infection/prevention of complications. Food interferes with drug absorption, requiring scheduling around meals. Although no prior history of penicillin reaction, it may occur at any time.

Treats underlying metabolic dysfunction, reducing hyperglycemia and promoting healing. Glucophage lowers serum glucose levels by improving insulin sensitivity, increasing glucose utilization in the muscles. By using in conjunction with DiaBeta, patient may be able to discontinue insulin once target dosage is achieved (e.g., 2000 mg/day). Increase of 1 tablet per week is necessary to limit side effects of diarrhea, abdominal cramping, vomiting, possibly leading to dehydration and prerenal azotemia.

PATIENT DIAGNOSTIC STATEMENT:

Acute Pain related to physical agent (wound L foot) evidenced by verbal report of pain and guarding behavior.

> **OUTCOMES: Pain Control Behavior (NOC)**
> **Indicators:**

PATIENT WILL:

Report pain is minimized/relieved within 1 hour of analgesic administration (ongoing).

Report absence or control of pain by discharge (7/1).

> **OUTCOME: Pain Disruptive Behavior (NOC)**
> **Indicators:**

Ambulate normally, full weight bearing by discharge (7/1).

ACTIONS/INTERVENTIONS	RATIONALE
Pain Management (NIC)	
Determine pain characteristics through patient's description.	Establishes baseline for assessing improvement/changes.
Place foot cradle on bed/encourage use of loose-fitting slipper, when up.	Avoids direct pressure to area of injury, which could result in vasoconstriction/increased pain.
Administer Darvocet-N 100 mg PO q4h as needed. Document effectiveness.	Provides relief of persistent pain unrelieved by other measures.

PATIENT DIAGNOSTIC STATEMENT:

Altered Peripheral Tissue Perfusion related to decreased arterial flow as evidenced by decreased pulses, pale/cool feet, thick brittle nails, numbness/tingling of feet "when walks 1/4 mile."

> **OUTCOMES: Knowledge: disease process (NOC)**
> **Indicators:**

PATIENT WILL:

Verbalize understanding of relationship between chronic disease (diabetes mellitus) and circulatory changes within 48 hours (1900 6/30).

Demonstrate awareness of safety factors/proper foot care within 48 hours (6/30 1900).

Maintain adequate level of hydration to maximize perfusion (ongoing), as evidenced by balanced intake/output, moist skin/mucous membranes, capillary refill less than 4 sec (ongoing).

ACTIONS/INTERVENTIONS	RATIONALE

Circulatory Care (NIC)

Elevate feet when up in chair. Avoid long periods with feet dependent.

Assess for signs of dehydration. Monitor intake/output. Encourage oral fluids.

Recommend cessation of smoking.

Minimizes interruption of blood flow, reduces venous pooling.

Glycosuria may result in dehydration with consequent reduction of circulating volume and further impairment of peripheral circulation.

Vascular construction associated with smoking and diabetes impairs peripheral circulation.

Peripheral Sensation Management (NIC)

Instruct patient to avoid constricting clothing/socks and ill-fitting shoes.

Reinforce safety precautions regarding use of heating pads, hot water bottles/soaks.

Discuss complications of disease that result from vascular changes: ulceration, gangrene, muscle or bony structure changes.

Review proper foot care as outlined in teaching plan.

Compromised circulation and decreased pain sensation may precipitate or aggravate tissue breakdown.

Heat increases metabolic demands on compromised tissues. Vascular insufficiency alters pain sensation increasing risk of injury.

Although proper control of diabetes mellitus may not prevent complications, severity of effects may be minimized. Diabetic foot complications are the leading cause of nontraumatic lower extremity amputations. Note: Skin dry, cracked, scaly; feet cool, pain when walking a distance suggests mild to medium vascular disease (autonomic neuropathy) that can limit response to infection, impair wound healing, and increase risk of bony deformities.

Altered perfusion of lower extremities may lead to serious/persistent complications at the cellular level.

PATIENT DIAGNOSTIC STATEMENT:

Learning Need regarding diabetic condition, related to misinterpretation of information and/or lack of recall as evidenced by inaccurate follow-through of instructions regarding home glucose monitoring and foot care and failure to recognize signs/symptoms of hyperglycemia.

OUTCOMES: Knowledge: treatment regimen (NOC)
Indicators:

PATIENT WILL:

Perform procedure of home glucose monitoring correctly within 36 hours (6/30 0700).

Verbalize basic understanding of disease process and treatment within 38 hours (6/30 0900).

Explain reasons for actions within 38 hours (6/30 0900).

Perform insulin administration correctly within 60 hours (7/1 0700).

ACTIONS/INTERVENTIONS	RATIONALE

Teaching: Disease Process (NIC)

Determine patient's level of knowledge, priorities of learning needs, desire/need for including wife in instruction.

Establishes baseline and direction for teaching/planning. Involvement of wife, if desired, will provide additional resource for recall/understanding and may enhance patient's follow-through.

Provide teaching guide, *Understanding Your Diabetes*, 6/28 PM. Show film *Living with Diabetes*, 6/29, 4 PM when wife is visiting. Include in group teaching session 6/30 AM. Review information and obtain feedback from patient and wife.

Provides different methods for accessing/reinforcing information and enhances opportunity for learning/understanding.

Discuss factors related to/altering diabetic control, such as stress, illness, exercise.

Drug therapy/diet may need to be altered in response to both short- and long-term stressors.

Review signs/symptoms of hyperglycemia (e.g., fatigue, nausea/vomiting, polyuria/polydipsia). Discuss how to prevent and evaluate this situation and when to seek medical care. Have patient identify appropriate interventions.

Recognition/understanding of these signs/symptoms and timely intervention will aid patient in avoiding recurrences and preventing complications.

Review and provide information about necessity for routine examination of feet and proper foot care (e.g., daily inspection for injuries, pressure areas, corns, calluses; proper nail cutting; daily washing, application of good moisturizing lotion such as Eucerin, Keri, or Nivea bid). Recommend loose-fitting socks, shoes that fit (break new shoes in gradually), and not going barefoot. If foot injury/skin break occurs, wash with soap/dermal cleanser and water, cover with sterile dressing, inspect wound, and change dressing daily; report redness, swelling, or presence of drainage.

Reduces risk of tissue injury, promotes understanding and prevention of stasis ulcer formation and wound healing difficulties.

Instruct regarding prescribed insulin therapy:

May be a temporary treatment of hyperglycemia with infection or may be permanent replacement of oral hypoglycemic agent.

Humulin N insulin, sc.

Intermediate-acting insulin generally lasts 18–28 hrs, with peak effect 6–12 hr.

Keep vial in current use at room temperature (if used within 30 days).

Cold insulin is poorly absorbed.

Store extra vials in refrigerator.

Refrigeration prolongs the drug shelf life by preventing wide fluctuations in temperature.

Roll bottle and shake gently.

Vigorous shaking may create foam, which can interfere with accurate dose withdrawal and damage the insulin molecule.

Choice of injection sites (e.g., across lower abdomen in Z pattern).

Provides for steady absorption of medication. Site is easily visualized and accessible by patient; and Z pattern minimizes tissue damage.

Demonstrate, then observe patient in drawing insulin into syringe, reading syringe markings, and administering dose. Assess for accuracy.

May require several instruction sessions and practice before patient and wife feel comfortable drawing up and injecting medication.

Instruct in signs/symptoms of insulin reaction/hypoglycemia: fatigue, nausea, headache, hunger, sweating, irritability, shakiness, anxiety, difficulty concentrating.

Knowing what to watch for and appropriate treatment (such as ½ cup grape juice for immediate response and snack within ½ hr, e.g., 1 slice bread with peanut butter or cheese, fruit and slice of cheese for sustained effect) may prevent or minimize complications.

Review "sick day rules," e.g., call doctor if too sick to eat normally/stay active; take insulin as ordered. Keep record as noted in Sick Day Guide.

Instruct patient/wife in fingerstick glucose monitoring to be done 4×/day until stable, then bid at rotating times, such as FBS, before dinner, before lunch, and hs. Observe return demonstrations of the procedure.

Recommend patient maintain record/log of fingerstick testing, antidiabetic medication and insulin dosage/site, unusual physiological response, dietary intake. Outline desired goals: e.g., FBS 80–120, premeal 80–140.

Schedule consultation with dietician to restructure meal plan and evaluate food choices.

Discuss other healthcare issues, such as smoking habits, self-monitoring for cancer (breasts/testicles), and reporting changes in general well-being.

Understanding of necessary actions in the event of mild/severe illness promotes competent self-care and reduces risk of hyperglycemia or hypoglycemia.

Fingerstick monitoring provides accurate and timely information regarding diabetic status. Return demonstration verifies correct learning.

Provides accurate record for review by caregivers for assessment of therapy effectiveness/needs.

Calories are unchanged on new orders but have been redistributed to three meals and two snacks. Dietary choices (e.g., increased vitamin C) may enhance healing.

Encourages patient involvement, awareness, and responsibility for own health; promotes wellness. Note: Smoking tends to increase patient's resistance to insulin.

EVALUATION

As nursing care is provided, ongoing assessment evaluates the patient's response to therapy and progress toward accomplishing the desired outcomes. This activity serves as the feedback and control part of the nursing process, through which the status of the individual patient diagnostic statement is judged to be resolved, continuing, or requiring revision.

This process is visualized in Figure 3–2. Observation of Mr. R.S.'s wound reveals that edges are clean and pink and drainage is scant. Therefore, he is progressing toward achieving wound healing, and this problem will continue to be addressed, although no revision in the treatment plan is required at this time.

DOCUMENTATION

To date, a number of charting formats are being used for documentation. These include block notes, with a single entry covering an entire shift (e.g., 7–3 PM); narrative timed notes (e.g., 8:30 AM, ate all of breakfast); the problem-oriented medical record system (POMR or PORS) using the SOAP/SOAPIER approach; and the use of flow sheets with charting by exception, to name a few. The POMR can provide thorough documentation, but it was designed by physicians for episodic care and requires that the entries be tied to a problem identified from a problem list.

A charting system format created by nurses for documentation of frequent/repetitive care is Focus Charting®. It was designed to encourage looking at the patient from a positive rather than a negative (or problem-oriented) perspective by using precise documentation to record the nursing process. Recording of assessment, interventions, and evaluation information in *data, action, and response* (DAR) categories facilitates tracking and following what is happening to the patient at any given moment. Charting focuses on patient and nursing concerns, with the focal point being patient status and the associated nursing care. The focus is always stated in a way that reflects the patient's concern/need rather than a nursing task or medical diagnosis. Thus, the focus can be a patient problem/concern or nursing diagnosis, signs/symptoms of potential importance (e.g., fever, dysrhythmia, edema), a significant event or change in status, or a specific standard of care/hospital policy.

A more recent way to evaluate and document the patient's progress (response to care) is through the use of clinical pathways. These were originally developed as tools for providing care in case management systems and are now used in many settings. A clinical pathway is a type of abbreviated plan of care that is event oriented (task oriented) and provides outcome-based guidelines for goal achievement within a designated length of stay. The pathway incorporates agency and professional standards of care and may be interdisciplinary, depending on the care setting. As a rule, however, the standarized clinical pathways address a specific diagnosis/condition or procedure (e.g., myocardial infarction, total hip replacement, chemotherapy) and do not provide for inclusion of secondary diagnoses or complications (e.g., asthmatic patient in alcohol withdrawal). In short, if the patient does not achieve the daily outcomes or goals of care, the variance is identified, and a separate plan of care must be developed to meet the patient's individual needs. Therefore, although clinical pathways are becoming more common in the clinical setting, they have limited value (in place of more individualized plans of care) as learning tools for students who are working to practice the nursing process, critical thinking, and a holistic approach to meeting patient needs. A sample clinical pathway (Fig. 3–3) reflects R.S.'s primary diagnostic problem: nonhealing lesion, diabetic.

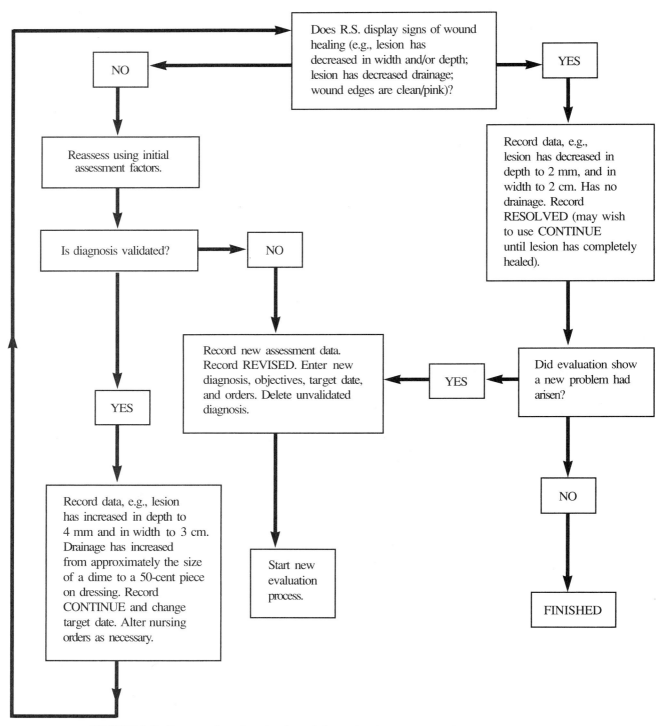

FIGURE 3–2. Outcome-based evaluation of the patient's response to therapy. (Adapted from Cox, HC, et al: *Clinical Applications of Nursing Diagnosis,* ed, 3, FA Davis, Philadelphia, 1996.)

CP: Non-healing Lesion—Diabetic. ELOS: 3 Days—Variations from Designated Pathway Should Be Documented in Progress Notes

ND and Categories of Care	Adm Day 6/28	Day 1 6/29	Day 2 6/30	Day 3 7/1
Impaired skin/ tissue integrity	Actions: Goals:	Actions: Goals: Verbalize understanding of condition; Display blood glucose WNL (ongoing)	Actions: Goals: Be free of signs of dehydration; Wound free of purulent drainage; Verbalize understanding of treatment need; Perform self-care tasks No. 1 & 3 correctly; Explain reasons for actions	Actions: Goals: Wound edges show signs of healing process; Perform self-care tasks: No. 2 correctly; Explain reason for actions; Plan in place to meet discharge needs
Referrals		Dietician & Determine need for: Home care; Physical therapy; Visiting nurse		
Diagnostic studies	Wound culture/sensitivity; Gram stain; Random blood glucose; Fingerstick BG hs	CBC, electrolytes; Glycosylated Hb; Serum lipid profile; ↑ Fingerstick BG qid; Chest X-ray (if indicated); ECG (if indicated)		Fingerstick BG bid if stable
Additional assessments	VS qid; I&O/level of hydration qd; Character of wound tid; Level of knowledge and priorities of learning needs; Observe for signs of antibiotic hypersensitivity reaction	↑ ↑ ↑	↑↑ VS Qshift; ↑; ↑	↑↑ D/C; ↑; ↑
Medications	Antibiotic: *Dicloxacillin* 500 mg PO q6h; Antidiabetic: *Humulin N insulin* 10cc SC tid; Other: NS soaks tid	Anticipated discharge needs; Antibiotic: same; Antidiabetic: same, *Humulin N insulin* 10u SC ᴀᴍ/hs, *DiaBeta* 10 mg PO bid, *Glucophage 500 mg PO qd*; Other: same	Antibiotic: same; Antidiabetic: same; Other: same	Antibiotic: same; Antidiabetic: same; Other: same

FIGURE 3–3. Sample clinical pathway.

CP: Non-healing Lesion—Diabetic. ELOS: 3 Days—Variations from Designated Pathway Should Be Documented in Progress Notes (continued)

ND and Categories of Care	Adm Day 6/28	Day 1 6/29	Day 2 6/30	Day 3 7/1
Patient education	Provide *Understanding Your Diabetes*	Film *Living with Diabetes* Demonstrate and practice self-care activities: 1. Fingerstick BG 2. Insulin admin 3. Wound care 4. Routine foot care	Group sessions: *Diabetic management*	Practice self-care activities 2-*insulin admin* Review discharge instructions
Additional nursing actions	Up ad lib Dressing change tid	→ →	→ →	→ →
Pain	Actions: Goals: State pain relieved or minimized with 1 hr of analgesic administration (ongoing) Verbalize understanding of when to report pain and rating scale used Verbalize understanding of S/C measures No. 1–2 Explain reason for actions	Actions: Goals: Verbalize understanding of S/C measures No. 3 Explain reason for actions	Actions: Goals: Able to participate in usual level: *ambulate full weight bearing*	Actions: Goals: State pain-free/ controlled with medication Verbalize understanding of correct medication use
	→ → →	→ → →	→ → →	→ → →
Additional assessments	Characteristics of pain Level of participation in activities Individual analgesic needs			
Medications Allergies: 0 Patient education	Analgesic: Darvocet-N 100 mg PO q4d PRN Orient to unit/room Guidelines for self-report of pain and rating scale 0–10 Safety/comfort measures: 1 elevation of feet 2 proper footwear	Analgesic: same Safety/comfort measures: *3 prevention of injury*	Analgesic: same	Analgesic: same Review discharge medication instructions: dosage, route, frequency, side effects
Additional nursing actions	Bed cradle as indicated	→	→	→

FIGURE 3–3. *(continued)*

Cardiovascular

HYPERTENSION: SEVERE

Hypertension is defined by the 1992 Joint National Committee on Detection, Evaluation, and Treatment of High Blood Pressure as pressure greater than 140/90 mm Hg and is classified according to the degree of severity. Stage I (mild) is 140/90–159/99. Stage II (moderate) is 160/100–179/108. Stage III (severe) is present when systolic pressure is greater than 180 and diastolic pressure is greater than 110. Stage IV (very severe) occurs when systolic pressure is 210 or greater with diastolic pressure greater than 120. Hypertension is categorized as *primary/essential* (approximately 90% of all cases) or *secondary*, which occurs as a result of an identifiable, sometimes correctable pathological condition, such as renal disease or primary aldosteronism. The goal of treatment is to prevent the long-term sequelae of the disease (i.e., target organ disease [TOD]). African-Americans and the elderly are most prone to this disorder and its sequelae.

CARE SETTING

Although hypertension is usually treated in a community setting, stages III and IV management with symptoms of complications/compromise may require inpatient care, especially when TOD is present. The majority of interventions included here can be used in either setting.

RELATED CONCERNS

Cerebrovascular accident/stroke, page 257
Myocardial infarction (MI), page 75
Psychosocial aspects of care, page 809
Renal failure: acute, page 575
Renal failure: chronic, page 588

Patient Assessment Database
ACTIVITY/REST

May report:	Weakness, fatigue, shortness of breath, sedentary lifestyle
May exhibit:	Elevated heart rate
	Change in heart rhythm
	Tachypnea; shortness of breath with exertion

CIRCULATION

May report:	History of hypertension; presence of atherosclerosis, valvular/coronary artery heart disease (including myocardial infarction [MI], angina, heart failure [HF]) and cerebrovascular disease (reflecting TOD)
	Episodes of palpitations, diaphoresis

May exhibit: Elevated blood pressure (BP) (serial elevated measurements are necessary to confirm diagnosis)

Postural hypotension (may be related to drug regimen)

Pulse: Bounding carotid, jugular, radial pulsations; pulse disparities, e.g., femoral delay as compared with radial or brachial pulsation; absence of/diminished popliteal, posterior tibial, pedal pulses

Apical pulse: Point of maximal impulse (PMI) possibly displaced and/or forceful

Rate/rhythm: Tachycardia, various dysrhythmias

Heart sounds: Accentuated S_2 at base; S_3 (early HF); S_4 (rigid left ventricle/left ventricular hypertrophy)

Murmurs of valvular stenosis

Vascular bruits audible over carotid, femoral, or epigastrium (artery stenosis); jugular venous distension (JVD) (venous congestion)

Extremities: Discoloration of skin, cool temperature (peripheral vasoconstriction); capillary refill possibly slow/delayed (vasoconstriction)

Skin: Pallor, cyanosis, and diaphoresis (congestion, hypoxemia); flushing (pheochromocytoma)

EGO INTEGRITY

May report: History of personality changes, anxiety, depression, euphoria, or chronic anger (may indicate cerebral impairment)

Multiple stress factors (relationship, financial, job related)

May exhibit: Mood swings, restlessness, irritability, narrowed attention span, outbursts of crying

Emphatic hand gestures, tense facial muscles (particularly around the eyes), quick physical movement, expiratory sighs, accelerated speech pattern

ELIMINATION

May report: Past or present renal insult (e.g., infection/obstruction or past history of kidney disease)

FOOD/FLUID

May report: Food preferences, which may include high-salt, high-fat, high-cholesterol foods (e.g., fried foods, cheese, eggs); licorice; high caloric content; low dietary intake of potassium, calcium, and magnesium

Nausea, vomiting

Recent weight changes (gain/loss)

History of diuretic use

May exhibit: Normal weight or obesity

Presence of edema (may be generalized or dependent); venous congestion, JVD

Glycosuria (almost 10% of hypertensive patients are diabetic, reflecting TOD)

NEUROSENSORY

May report: Fainting spells/dizziness

Throbbing, suboccipital headaches (present on awakening and disappearing spontaneously after several hours)

Episodes of numbness and/or weakness on one side of the body, brief periods of confusion or difficulty with speech (transient ischemic attack [TIA]); or history of cerebrovascular accident (CVA)

Visual disturbances (diplopia, blurred vision)

Episodes of epistaxis

May exhibit: Mental status: changes in alertness, orientation, speech pattern/content, affect, thought process, or memory

Motor responses: decreased strength, hand grip, and/or deep tendon reflexes

Optic retinal changes: from mild sclerosis/arterial narrowing to marked retinal and sclerotic changes with edema or papilledema, exudates, hemorrhages, and arterial nicking, dependent on severity/duration of hypertension (TOD)

PAIN/DISCOMFORT

May report: Angina (coronary artery disease/cardiac involvement)

Intermittent pain in legs/claudication (indicative of arteriosclerosis of lower extremity arteries)

Severe occipital headaches as previously noted

Abdominal pain/masses (pheochromocytoma)

RESPIRATION

(Generally associated with advanced cardiopulmonary effects of sustained/severe hypertension)

May report: Dyspnea associated with activity/exertion

Tachypnea, orthopnea, paroxysmal nocturnal dyspnea

Cough with/without sputum production

Smoking history (major risk factor)

May exhibit: Respiratory distress/use of accessory muscles

Adventitious breath sounds (crackles/wheezes)

Pallor or cyanosis

SAFETY

**May report/
exhibit:**   Impaired coordination/gait

Transient episodes of numbness unilateral paresthesias

Light-headedness with position changes

SEXUALITY

May report: Postmenopausal (major risk factor)

TEACHING/LEARNING

May report: Familial risk factors: hypertension, atherosclerosis, heart disease, diabetes mellitus, cerebrovascular/kidney disease

Ethnic/racial risk factors, e.g., more prevalent in African-American and Southeast Asian populations

Use of birth control pills or other hormones; drug/alcohol use

**Discharge plan
considerations:**   **DRG projected mean length of inpatient stay: 3.5 days**

Assistance with self-monitoring of BP

Periodic evaluation of and alterations in medication therapy

Refer to section at end of plan for postdischarge considerations.

DIAGNOSTIC STUDIES

Hemoglobin/hematocrit: Not diagnostic but assesses relationship of cells to fluid volume (viscosity) and may indicate risk factors such as hypercoagulability, anemia.

BUN/creatinine: Provides information about renal perfusion/function.

Glucose: Hyperglycemia (diabetes mellitus is a precipitator of hypertension) may result from elevated catecholamine levels (increases hypertension).

Serum potassium: Hypokalemia may indicate the presence of primary aldosteronism (cause) or be a side effect of diuretic therapy.

Serum calcium: Imbalance may contribute to hypertension.

Lipid panel (total lipids, high-density lipoprotein [HDL], low-density lipoprotein [LDL], cholesterol, triglycerides, phospholipids): Elevated level may indicate predisposition for/presence of atheromatous plaquing.

Thyroid studies: Hyperthyroidism may lead or contribute to vasoconstriction and hypertension.

Serum/urine aldosterone level: May be done to assess for primary aldosteronism (cause).

Urinalysis: Blood, protein, glucose suggest renal dysfunction and/or presence of diabetes.

Creatinine clearance: May be reduced, reflecting renal damage.

Urine vanillylmandelic acid (VMA) (catecholamine metabolite): Elevation may indicate presence of pheochromocytoma (cause); 24-hour urine VMA may be done for assessment of pheochromocytoma if hypertension is intermittent.

Uric acid: Hyperuricemia has been implicated as a risk factor for the development of hypertension.

Renin: Elevated in renovascular and malignant hypertension, salt-wasting disorders.

Urine steroids: Elevation may indicate hyperadrenalism, pheochromocytoma, pituitary dysfunction, Cushing's syndrome.

Intravenous pyelogram (IVP): May identify cause of secondary hypertension, e.g., renal parenchymal disease, renal/ureteral calculi.

Kidney and renography nuclear scan: Evaluates renal status (TOD).

Chest x-ray: May demonstrate obstructing calcification in valve areas; deposits in and/or notching of aorta; cardiac enlargement.

Computer tomography (CT) scan: Assesses for cerebral tumor, cerebrovascular accident (CVA), or encephalopathy or to rule out pheochromocytoma.

Electrocardiogram (ECG): May demonstrate enlarged heart, strain patterns, conduction disturbances. Note: Broad, notched P wave is one of the earliest signs of hypertensive heart disease.

NURSING PRIORITIES

1. Maintain/enhance cardiovascular functioning.
2. Prevent complications.
3. Provide information about disease process/prognosis and treatment regimen.
4. Support active patient control of condition.

DISCHARGE GOALS

1. BP within acceptable limits for individual.
2. Cardiovascular and systemic complications prevented/minimized.
3. Disease process/prognosis and therapeutic regimen understood.
4. Necessary lifestyle/behavioral changes initiated.
5. Plan in place to meet needs after discharge.

NURSING DIAGNOSIS: Cardiac Output, risk for decreased

Risk factors may include
Increased vascular resistance, vasoconstriction
Myocardial ischemia
Ventricular hypertrophy/rigidity

Possibly evidenced by
[Not applicable; presence of signs and symptoms establishes an *actual* diagnosis]

DESIRED OUTCOMES/EVALUATION CRITERIA—PATIENT WILL:

Circulation Status (NOC)

Participate in activities that reduce BP/cardiac workload.
Maintain BP within individually acceptable range.
Demonstrate stable cardiac rhythm and rate within patient's normal range.

ACTIONS/INTERVENTIONS

RATIONALE

Hemodynamic Regulation (NIC)

Independent

Monitor BP. Measure in both arms/thighs three times, 3–5 min apart while patient is at rest, then sitting, then standing for initial evaluation. Use correct cuff size and accurate technique.

Comparison of pressures provides a more complete picture of vascular involvement/scope of problem. Severe hypertension is classified in the adult as a diastolic pressure elevation to 110 mm Hg; progressive diastolic readings above 120 mm Hg are considered first accelerated, then malignant (very severe). Systolic hypertension also is an established risk factor for cerebrovascular disease and ischemic heart disease, when diastolic pressure is elevated.

ACTIONS/INTERVENTIONS	RATIONALE
Independent	
Note presence, quality of central and peripheral pulses.	Bounding carotid, jugular, radial, and femoral pulses may be observed/palpated. Pulses in the legs/feet may be diminished, reflecting effects of vasoconstriction (increased systemic vascular resistance [SVR]) and venous congestion.
Auscultate heart tones and breath sounds.	S_4 heart sound is common in severely hypertensive patients because of the presence of atrial hypertrophy (increased atrial volume/pressure). Development of S_3 indicates ventricular hypertrophy and impaired functioning. Presence of crackles, wheezes may indicate pulmonary congestion secondary to developing or chronic heart failure.
Observe skin color, moisture, temperature, and capillary refill time.	Presence of pallor; cool, moist skin; and delayed capillary refill time may be due to peripheral vasoconstriction or reflect cardiac decompensation/decreased output.
Note dependent/general edema.	May indicate heart failure, renal or vascular impairment.
Provide calm, restful surroundings, minimize environmental activity/noise. Limit the number of visitors and length of stay.	Helps reduce sympathetic stimulation; promotes relaxation.
Maintain activity restrictions, e.g., bedrest/chair rest; schedule periods of uninterrupted rest; assist patient with self-care activities as needed.	Reduces physical stress and tension that affect blood pressure and the course of hypertension.
Provide comfort measures, e.g., back and neck massage, elevation of head.	Decreases discomfort and may reduce sympathetic stimulation.
Instruct in relaxation techniques, guided imagery, distractions.	Can reduce stressful stimuli, produce calming effect, thereby reducing BP.
Monitor response to medications to control blood pressure.	Response to "stepped" drug therapy (consisting of diuretics, angiotensin-converting enzyme [ACE] inhibitors, vascular smooth muscle relaxants, and adrenergic blockers) is dependent on both the individual and the synergistic effects of the drugs. Because of side effects, it is important to use the smallest number and lowest dosage of medications.
Collaborative	
Administer medications as indicated, e.g.:	
Thiazide diuretics, e.g., chlorothiazide (Diuril); hydrochlorothiazide (Esidrix/HydroDIURIL); bendroflumethiazide (Naturetin); indapamide (Lozol); metolazone (Diulo); quinethazone (Hydromox);	Diuretics are considered first-line medications for uncomplicated stage I or II hypertension and may be used alone or in association with other drugs (such as beta blockers) to reduce BP in patients with relatively normal renal function. These diuretics potentiate the effects of other antihypertensive agents as well, by limiting fluid retention, and may reduce the incidence of strokes and heart failure.

Collaborative

Loop diuretics, e.g., furosemide (Lasix); ethacrynic acid (Edecrin); bumetanide (Bumex), torsemide (Demadex);

These drugs produce marked diuresis by inhibiting resorption of sodium and chloride and are effective antihypertensives, especially in patients who are resistant to thiazides or have renal impairment.

Potassium-sparing diuretics, e.g., spironolactone (Aldactone); triamterene (Dyrenium); amiloride (Midamor);

May be given in combination with a thiazide diuretic to minimize potassium loss.

Alpha, beta, or centrally acting adrenergic antagonists, e.g., propranolol (Inderal); acebutolol (Sectral), metoprolol (Lopressor); labetalol (Normodyne); atenolol (Tenormin); nadolol (Corgard); carvedilol (Coreg); methyldopa (Aldomet); clonidine (Catapres); prazosin (Minipress); terazosin (Hytrin); pindolol (Visken);

β-Blockers may be ordered instead of diuretics for patients with ischemic heart disease; obese patients with cardiogenic hypertension; and patients with concurrent supraventricular arrhythmias, angina, or hypertensive cardiomyopathy. Specific actions of these drugs vary, but they generally reduce BP through the combined effect of decreased total peripheral resistance, reduced cardiac output, inhibited sympathetic activity, and suppression of renin release. *Note:* Patients with diabetes should use Cargarol and Visken with caution because they can prolong and mask the hypoglycemic effects of insulin. The elderly may require smaller doses because of the potential for bradycardia and hypotension. African-American patients tend to be less responsive to β-blockers in general and may require increased dosage or use of another drug, e.g., monotherapy with a diuretic.

Calcium channel antagonists, e.g., nifedipine (Procardia); verapamil (Calan); diltiazem (Cardizem); amlodipine (Norvasc); isradipine (DynaCirc); nicardipine (Cardene);

May be necessary to treat severe hypertension when a combination of a diuretic and a sympathetic inhibitor does not sufficiently control BP. Vasodilation of healthy cardiac vasculature and increased coronary blood flow are secondary benefits of vasodilator therapy.

Adrenergic neuron blockers: guanadrel (Hylorel); guanethidine (Ismelin); reserpine (Serpasil);

Reduce arterial and venous constriction activity at the sympathetic nerve endings.

Direct-acting oral vasodilators: hydralazine (Apresoline); minoxidil (Loniten);

Action is to relax vascular smooth muscle, thereby reducing vascular resistance.

Direct-acting parenteral vasodilators: diazoxide (Hyperstat); nitroprusside (Nipride); labetalol (Normodyne);

These are given intravenously for management of hypertensive emergencies.

Ganglion blockers, e.g., guanethidine (Ismelin); trimethaphan (Arfonad); or ACE inhibitors, e.g., captopril (Capoten); enalapril (Vasotec); lisinopril (Zestril); fosinopril (Monopril); ramipril (Altace).

The use of an additional sympathetic inhibitor may be required for its cumulative effect when other measures have failed to control BP or when congestive heart failure (CHF) or diabetes is present.

Implement dietary sodium, fat, and cholesterol restrictions as indicated.

These restrictions can help manage fluid retention and, with associated hypertensive response, decrease myocardial workload.

Prepare for surgery when indicated.

When hypertension is due to pheochromocytoma, removal of the tumor will correct condition.

NURSING DIAGNOSIS: Activity Intolerance

May be related to
Generalized weakness
Imbalance between oxygen supply and demand

Possibly evidenced by
Verbal report of fatigue or weakness
Abnormal heart rate or BP response to activity
Exertional discomfort or dyspnea
ECG changes reflecting ischemia; dysrhythmias

DESIRED OUTCOMES/EVALUATION CRITERIA—PATIENT WILL:

Endurance (NOC)

Participate in necessary/desired activities.
Report a measurable increase in activity tolerance.
Demonstrate a decrease in physiological signs of intolerance.

ACTIONS/INTERVENTIONS	RATIONALE

Energy Management (NIC)

Independent

Assess the patient's response to activity, noting pulse rate over 20 beats per minute (bpm) above resting rate; marked increase in BP during/after activity (systolic pressure increase of 40 mm Hg or diastolic pressure increase of 20 mm Hg); dyspnea or chest pain; excessive fatigue and weakness; diaphoresis; dizziness or syncope.

The stated parameters are helpful in assessing physiological responses to the stress of activity and, if present, are indicators of overexertion.

Instruct patient in energy-conserving techniques, e.g., using chair when showering, sitting to brush teeth or comb hair, carrying out activities at a slower pace.

Energy-saving techniques reduce the energy expenditure, thereby assisting in equalization of oxygen supply and demand.

Encourage progressive activity/self-care when tolerated. Provide assistance as needed.

Gradual activity progression prevents a sudden increase in cardiac workload. Providing assistance only as needed encourages independence in performing activities.

NURSING DIAGNOSIS: Pain [acute], headache

May be related to
Increased cerebral vascular pressure

Possibly evidenced by
Reports of throbbing pain located in suboccipital region, present on awakening, and disappearing spontaneously after being up and about
Reluctance to move head, rubbing head, avoidance of bright lights and noise, wrinkled brow, clenched fists
Reports of stiffness of neck, dizziness, blurred vision, nausea, and vomiting

DESIRED OUTCOMES/EVALUATION CRITERIA—PATIENT WILL:

Pain Control Behavior (NOC)

Report pain/discomfort is relieved/controlled.
Verbalize methods that provide relief.
Follow prescribed pharmacological regimen.

Pain Management (NIC)

Independent

Determine specifics of pain, e.g., location, characteristics, intensity (0–10 scale), onset/duration. Note nonverbal cues.

Facilitates diagnosis of problem and initiation of appropriate therapy. Helpful in evaluating effectiveness of therapy.

Encourage/maintain bedrest during acute phase.

Minimizes stimulation/promotes relaxation.

Provide/recommend nonpharmacological measures for relief of headache, e.g., cool cloth to forehead; back and neck rubs; quiet, dimly lit room; relaxation techniques (guided imagery, distraction); and diversional activities.

Measures that reduce cerebral vascular pressure and that slow/block sympathetic response are effective in relieving headache and associated complications.

Eliminate/minimize vasoconstricting activities that may aggravate headache, e.g., straining at stool, prolonged coughing, bending over.

Activities that increase vasoconstriction accentuate the headache in the presence of increased cerebral vascular pressure.

Assist patient with ambulation as needed.

Dizziness and blurred vision frequently are associated with vascular headache. The patient may also experience episodes of postural hypotension, causing weakness when ambulating.

Provide liquids, soft foods, frequent mouth care if nosebleeds occur or nasal packing has been done to stop bleeding.

Promotes general comfort. Nasal packing may interfere with swallowing or require mouth breathing, leading to stagnation of oral secretions and drying of mucous membranes.

Collaborative

Administer medications as indicated:

Analgesics;

Reduce/control pain and decrease stimulation of the sympathetic nervous system.

Antianxiety agents, e.g., lorazepam (Ativan), diazepam (Valium).

May aid in the reduction of tension and discomfort that is intensified by stress.

NURSING DIAGNOSIS: Nutrition: altered, more than body requirements

May be related to
Excessive intake in relation to metabolic need
Sedentary lifestyle
Cultural preferences

Possibly evidenced by
Weight 10%–20% over ideal for height and frame
Triceps skinfold greater than 15 mm in men and 25 mm in women (maximum for age and sex)
Reported or observed dysfunctional eating patterns

DESIRED OUTCOMES/EVALUATION CRITERIA—PATIENT WILL:

Knowledge: Treatment Regimen (NOC)

Identify correlation between hypertension and obesity.

Nutritional Status: Nutrient Intake (NOC)

Demonstrate change in eating patterns (e.g., food choices, quantity) to attain desirable body weight with optimal maintenance of health.
Initiate/maintain individually appropriate exercise program.

ACTIONS/INTERVENTIONS	RATIONALE

| **Weight Reduction Assistance (NIC)** |

Independent

Assess patient understanding of direct relationship between hypertension and obesity.

Obesity is an added risk with high blood pressure because of the disproportion between fixed aortic capacity and increased cardiac output associated with increased body mass. Reduction in weight may obviate the need for drug therapy or decrease the amount of medication needed for control of BP. *Note:* A recent study indicates that bringing weight within 15% of ideal weight can result in a drop of 10 mm Hg in both systolic and diastolic BP.

Discuss necessity for decreased caloric intake and limited intake of fats, salt, and sugar as indicated.

Faulty eating habits contribute to atherosclerosis and obesity, which predispose to hypertension and subsequent complications, e.g., stroke, kidney disease, heart failure. Excessive salt intake expands the intravascular fluid volume and may damage kidneys, which can further aggravate hypertension. *Note:* A recent study showed that sodium reduction reduced the need for medication by 31%. Weight loss lowered the need for medication by 36% and the combination of the two by 53%.

Determine patient's desire to lose weight.

Motivation for weight reduction is internal. The individual must want to lose weight, or the program most likely will not succeed.

Review usual daily caloric intake and dietary choices.

Identifies current strengths/weaknesses in dietary program. Aids in determining individual need for adjustment/teaching.

Establish a realistic weight reduction plan with the patient, e.g., 1 lb weight loss/wk.

Reducing caloric intake by 500 calories daily theoretically yields a weight loss of 1 lb/wk. Slow reduction in weight is therefore indicative of fat loss with muscle sparing and generally reflects a change in eating habits.

Encourage patient to maintain a diary of food intake, including when and where eating takes place and the circumstances and feelings around which the food was eaten.

Provides a database for both the adequacy of nutrients eaten and the emotional conditions of eating. Helps to focus attention on factors that patient has control over/can change.

Instruct and assist in appropriate food selections, such as a diet rich in fruits, vegetables, and low-fat dairy foods referred to as the DASH (Dietary Approaches to Stop Hypertension) diet and avoiding foods high in saturated fat (butter, cheese, eggs, ice cream, meat) and cholesterol (fatty meat, egg yolks, whole dairy products, shrimp, organ meats).

Avoiding foods high in saturated fat and cholesterol is important in preventing progressing atherogenesis. Moderation and use of low-fat products in place of total abstinence from certain food items may prevent sense of deprivation and enhance cooperation with dietary regimen. The DASH diet, in conjunction with exercise, weight loss, and limits on salt intake, may reduce or even eliminate the need for drug therapy.

Collaborative

Refer to dietitian as indicated.

Can provide additional counseling and assistance with meeting individual dietary needs.

NURSING DIAGNOSIS: Coping, Individual, ineffective

May be related to

Situational/maturational crisis; multiple life changes

Inadequate relaxation; little or no exercise, work overload

Inadequate support systems

Poor nutrition

Unmet expectations; unrealistic perceptions

Inadequate coping methods

Possibly evidenced by

Verbalization of inability to cope or ask for help

Inability to meet role expectations/basic needs or problem-solve

Destructive behavior toward self; overeating, lack of appetite; excessive smoking/drinking, proneness to alcohol abuse

Chronic fatigue/insomnia; muscular tension; frequent head/neck aches; chronic worry, irritability, anxiety, emotional tension, depression

DESIRED OUTCOMES/EVALUATION CRITERIA—PATIENT WILL:

Coping (NOC)

Identify ineffective coping behaviors and consequences.

Verbalize awareness of own coping abilities/strengths.

Identify potential stressful situations and steps to avoid/modify them.

Demonstrate the use of effective coping skills/methods.

ACTIONS/INTERVENTIONS | RATIONALE

Coping Enhancement (NIC)

Independent

Assess effectiveness of coping strategies by observing behaviors, e.g., ability to verbalize feelings and concerns, willingness to participate in the treatment plan.

Adaptive mechanisms are necessary to appropriately alter one's lifestyle, deal with the chronicity of hypertension, and integrate prescribed therapies into daily living.

Note reports of sleep disturbances, increasing fatigue, impaired concentration, irritability, decreased tolerance of headache, inability to cope/problem-solve.

Manifestations of maladaptive coping mechanisms may be indicators of repressed anger and have been found to be major determinants of diastolic BP.

Assist patient to identify specific stressors and possible strategies for coping with them.

Recognition of stressors is the first step in altering one's response to the stressor.

Include patient in planning of care, and encourage maximum participation in treatment plan.

Involvement provides the patient with an ongoing sense of control, improves coping skills, and can enhance cooperation with therapeutic regimen.

Encourage patient to evaluate life priorities/goals. Ask questions such as "Is what you are doing getting you what you want?"

Focuses patient's attention on reality of present situation relative to patient's view of what is wanted. Strong work ethic, need for "control," and outward focus may have led to lack of attention to personal needs.

Assist patient to identify and begin planning for necessary lifestyle changes. Assist to adjust, rather than abandon, personal/family goals.

Necessary changes should be realistically prioritized so patient can avoid being overwhelmed and feeling powerless.

NURSING DIAGNOSIS: Knowledge Deficit [Learning Need] regarding condition, treatment plan, self care and discharge needs

May be related to
Lack of knowledge/recall
Information misinterpretation
Cognitive limitation
Denial of diagnosis

Possibly evidenced by
Verbalization of the problem
Request for information
Statement of misconception
Inaccurate follow-through of instructions; inadequate performance of procedures
Inappropriate or exaggerated behaviors, e.g., hostile, agitated, apathetic

DESIRED OUTCOMES/EVALUATION CRITERIA—PATIENT WILL:

Knowledge: Disease Process (NOC)

Verbalize understanding of disease process and treatment regimen.
Identify drug side effects and possible complications that necessitate medical attention.
Maintain BP within individually acceptable parameters.

Knowledge: Treatment Regimen (NOC)

Describe reasons for therapeutic actions/treatment regimen.

ACTIONS/INTERVENTIONS	RATIONALE
Teaching: Disease Process (NIC)	
Independent	
Assess readiness and blocks to learning. Include significant other (SO).	Misconceptions and denial of the diagnosis because of long-standing feelings of well-being may interfere with patient/SO willingness to learn about disease, progression, and prognosis. If the patient does not accept the reality of a life-threatening condition requiring continuing treatment, lifestyle/behavioral changes will not be initiated/sustained.
Define and state the limits of desired BP. Explain hypertension and its effects on the heart, blood vessels, kidneys, and brain.	Provides basis for understanding elevations of BP and clarifies frequently used medical terminology. Understanding that high BP can exist without symptoms is central to enabling patient to continue treatment, even when feeling well.
Avoid saying "normal" BP, and use the term "well-controlled" to describe patient's BP within desired limits.	Because treatment for hypertension is lifelong, conveying the idea of "control" helps the patient understand the need for continued treatment/medication.
Assist the patient in identifying modifiable risk factors, e.g., obesity; diet high in sodium, saturated fats, and cholesterol; sedentary lifestyle; smoking; alcohol intake (more than 2 oz/day on a regular basis); stressful lifestyle.	These risk factors have been shown to contribute to hypertension and cardiovascular and renal disease.

ACTIONS/INTERVENTIONS	RATIONALE

Independent

Problem-solve with patient to identify ways in which appropriate lifestyle changes can be made to reduce modifiable risk factors.

Changing "comfortable/usual" behavior patterns can be very stressful. Support, guidance, and empathy can enhance the patient's success in accomplishing these tasks.

Discuss importance of eliminating smoking, and assist patient in formulating a plan to quit smoking.

Nicotine increases catecholamine discharge, resulting in increased heart rate, BP, vasoconstriction, and myocardial workload, and reduces tissue oxygenation.

Reinforce the importance of cooperation with treatment regimen and keeping follow-up appointments.

Lack of cooperation is a common reason for failure of antihypertensive therapy. Therefore, ongoing evaluation for patient cooperation is critical to successful treatment. Compliance usually improves when the patient understands causative factors and consequences of inadequate intervention and health maintenance.

Instruct and demonstrate technique of BP self-monitoring. Evaluate patient's hearing, visual acuity, manual dexterity, and coordination.

Monitoring BP at home is reassuring to the patient because it provides visual/positive reinforcement for efforts in following the medical regimen and promotes early detection of deleterious changes.

Help patient develop a simple, convenient schedule for taking medications.

Individualizing medication schedule to fit the patient's personal habits/needs may facilitate cooperation with long-term regimen.

Explain prescribed medications along with their rationale, dosage, expected and adverse side effects, and idiosyncrasies, e.g.:

Adequate information and understanding that side effects (e.g., mood changes, initial weight gain, dry mouth) are common and often subside with time can enhance cooperation with treatment plan.

Diuretics: Take daily doses (or larger dose) in the early morning;

Scheduling minimizes nighttime urination.

Weigh self on a regular schedule and record;

Primary indicator of effectiveness of diuretic therapy.

Avoid/limit alcohol intake;

The combined vasodilating effect of alcohol and the volume-depleting effect of a diuretic greatly increases the risk of orthostatic hypotension.

Notify physician if unable to tolerate food or fluid;

Dehydration can develop rapidly if intake is poor and patient continues to take a diuretic.

Antihypertensives: Take prescribed dose on a regular schedule; avoid skipping, altering, or making up doses; and do not discontinue without notifying the healthcare provider;

Abruptly discontinuing drug causes rebound hypertension that may lead to severe complications.

Rise slowly from a lying to standing position, sitting for a few minutes before standing. Sleep with the head slightly elevated.

Measures reduce severity of orthostatic hypotension associated with the use of vasodilators and diuretics.

Suggest frequent position changes, leg exercises when lying down.

Decreases peripheral venous pooling that may be potentiated by vasodilators and prolonged sitting/standing.

Recommend avoiding hot baths, steam rooms, and saunas, especially with concomitant use of alcoholic beverages.

Prevents vasodilation with potential for dangerous side effects of syncope and hypotension.

Instruct the patient to consult healthcare provider before taking other prescription or over-the-counter (OTC) medications.

Precaution is important in preventing potentially dangerous drug interactions. Any drug that contains a sympathetic nervous stimulant may increase BP or counteract antihypertensive effects.

ACTIONS/INTERVENTIONS

Independent

Instruct patient about increasing intake of foods/fluids high in potassium, e.g., oranges, bananas, figs, dates, tomatoes, potatoes, raisins, apricots, Gatorade, and fruit juices and foods/fluids high in calcium, e.g., low-fat milk, yogurt, or calcium supplements, as indicated.

Review signs/symptoms requiring notification of healthcare provider, e.g., headache present on awakening that does not abate; sudden and continued increase of BP; chest pain/shortness of breath; irregular/increased pulse rate; significant weight gain (2 lb/day or 5 lb/wk) or peripheral/abdominal swelling; visual disturbances; frequent, uncontrollable nose bleeds; depression/emotional lability; severe dizziness or episodes of fainting; muscle weakness/cramping; nausea/vomiting; excessive thirst.

Explain rationale for prescribed dietary regimen (usually a diet low in sodium, saturated fat, and cholesterol).

Help patient identify sources of sodium intake (e.g., table salt, salty snacks, processed meats and cheeses, sauerkraut, sauces, canned soups and vegetables, baking soda, baking powder, monosodium glutamate). Stress the importance of reading ingredient labels of foods and OTC drugs.

Encourage patient to decrease or eliminate caffeine, e.g., coffee, tea, cola, chocolate.

Stress importance of planning/accomplishing daily rest periods.

Recommend that patient monitor own physiological response to activity (e.g., pulse rate, shortness of breath), report a decreased tolerance to activity, and stop activity that causes chest pain, shortness of breath, dizziness, extreme fatigue, or weakness.

Encourage patient to establish an individual exercise program incorporating aerobic exercise (walking, swimming) within the patient's capabilities. Stress the importance of avoiding isometric activity.

Demonstrate application of ice pack to the back of the neck and pressure over the distal third of nose, and recommend that patient lean the head forward, if nose bleed occurs.

Provide information regarding community resources, and support the patient in making lifestyle changes. Initiate referrals as indicated.

RATIONALE

Diuretics can deplete potassium levels. Dietary replacement is more palatable than drug supplements and may be all that is needed to correct deficit. Some studies show that 400 mg of calcium/day can lower systolic and diastolic BP. Correcting mineral deficiencies can also affect BP.

Early detection of developing complications/decreased effectiveness of drug regimen or adverse reactions to it allows for timely intervention.

Excess saturated fats, cholesterol, sodium, alcohol, and calories have been defined as nutritional risks in hypertension. A diet low in fat and high in polyunsaturated fat reduces BP, possibly through prostaglandin balance in both normotensive and hypertensive people.

Two years on a moderate low-salt diet may be sufficient to control mild hypertension or reduce the amount of medication required.

Caffeine is a cardiac stimulant and may adversely affect cardiac function/reserves.

Alternating rest and activity increases tolerance to activity progression.

The patient's involvement in monitoring own activity tolerance is vital to safely resuming and/or modifying activities of daily living.

Besides helping to lower BP, aerobic activity aids in toning the cardiovascular system. Isometric exercise can increase serum catecholamine levels, further elevating BP.

Nasal capillaries may rupture as a result of excessive vascular pressure. Cold and pressure constrict capillaries to slow or halt bleeding. Leaning forward reduces the amount of blood that is swallowed.

Community resources such as the American Heart Association, "coronary clubs," stop smoking clinics, alcohol (drug) rehabilitation, weight loss programs, stress management classes, and counseling services may be helpful in the patient's efforts to initiate and maintain lifestyle changes.

POTENTIAL CONSIDERATIONS following acute hospitalization (dependent on patient's age, physical condition/presence of complications, personal resources, and life responsibilities)

Activity intolerance—frequently occurs as a result of alterations in cardiac output and side effects of medication.

Nutrition: altered, more than body requirements—obesity is often present and a factor in blood pressure control.

Therapeutic Regimen: Individual, ineffective management—result of the complexity of the therapeutic regimen, required lifestyle changes, side effects of medication, and frequent feelings of general well-being ("I'm not really sick").

Sexuality Patterns, altered—interference in sexual functioning may occur because of activity intolerance and side effects of medication.

Family Coping: potential for growth—opportunity exists for family members to support patient while reducing risk factors for themselves and improving quality of life for family as a whole.

HEART FAILURE: CHRONIC

Failure of the left and/or right chambers of the heart results in insufficient output to meet tissue needs and causes pulmonary and systemic vascular congestion. This disease condition is termed *heart failure* (HF). Despite diagnostic and therapeutic advances, HF continues to be associated with high morbidity and mortality. (Agency for Health Care Policy and Research [AHCPR] guidelines [6/94] promote the term *heart failure* [HF] in place of *congestive heart failure* [CHF] because many patients with heart failure do not manifest pulmonary or systemic congestion.) The New York Heart Association functional classification system for HF includes classes I to IV. Common causes of HF include ventricular dysfunction, cardiomyopathies, hypertension, coronary artery disease, valvular disease, and dysrhythmias.

CARE SETTING

Although generally managed at the community level, inpatient stay may be required for periodic exacerbation of failure/development of complications.

RELATED CONCERNS

Myocardial infarction, page 75
Hypertension, page 33
Cardiac surgery, page 102
Digitalis toxicity, page 90
Dysrhythmias, page 90
Psychosocial aspects of care, page 809

Patient Assessment Database

ACTIVITY/REST

May report:	Fatigue/exhaustion progressing throughout the day; exercise intolerance
	Insomnia
	Chest pain/pressure with activity
	Dyspnea at rest or with exertion
May exhibit:	Restlessness, mental status changes, e.g., anxiety and lethargy
	Vital sign changes with activity

CIRCULATION

May report:	History of hypertension, recent/acute multiple MIs, previous episodes of HF, valvular heart disease, cardiac surgery, endocarditis, systemic lupus erythematosus (SLE), anemia, septic shock
	Swelling of feet, legs, abdomen, "belt too tight" (right-sided failure)
May exhibit:	BP may be low (pump failure), normal (mild or chronic HF), or high (fluid overload/increased SVR)
	Pulse pressure may be narrow, reflecting reduced stroke volume
	Tachycardia (may be left- or right-sided failure)
	Dysrhythmias, e.g., atrial fibrillation, premature ventricular contractions/tachycardia, heart blocks
	Apical pulse: PMI may be diffuse and displaced inferiorly to the left
	Heart sounds: S_3 (gallop) is diagnostic of congestive failure; S_4 may occur; S_1 and S_2 may be softened
	Systolic and diastolic murmurs may indicate the presence of valvular stenosis or insufficiency, both atrial and ventricular
	Pulses: Peripheral pulses diminished; central pulses may be bounding, e.g., visible jugular, carotid, abdominal pulsations; alteration in strength of beat may be noted
	Color ashen, pale, dusky, or even cyanotic
	Nailbeds pale or cyanotic, with slow capillary refill
	Liver may be enlarged/palpable, positive hepatojugular reflex
	Breath sounds: Crackles, rhonchi

Edema may be dependent, generalized, or pitting, especially in extremities; JVD may be present.

EGO INTEGRITY

May report: Anxiety, apprehension, fear
Stress related to illness/financial concerns (job/cost of medical care)

May exhibit: Various behavioral manifestations, e.g., anxiety, anger, fear, irritability

ELIMINATION

May report: Decreased voiding, dark urine
Night voiding (nocturia)
Diarrhea/constipation

FOOD/FLUID

May report: Loss of appetite/anorexia
Nausea/vomiting
Significant weight gain (may not respond to diuretic use)
Lower extremity swelling
Tight clothing/shoes
Diet high in salt/processed foods, fat, sugar, and caffeine
Use of diuretics

May exhibit: Rapid/continuous weight gain
Abdominal distension (ascites); edema (general, dependent, pitting, brawny)
Abdominal tenderness (ascites, hepatic engorgement)

HYGIENE

May report: Fatigue/weakness, exhaustion during self-care activities

May exhibit: Appearance indicative of neglect of personal care

NEUROSENSORY

May report: Weakness, dizziness, fainting episodes

May exhibit: Lethargy, confusion, disorientation
Behavior changes, irritability

PAIN/DISCOMFORT

May report: Chest pain, chronic or acute angina
Right upper abdominal pain (right-sided heart failure [RHF])
Generalized muscle aches/pains

May exhibit: Nervousness, restlessness
Narrowed focus (withdrawal)
Guarding behavior

RESPIRATION

May report: Dyspnea on exertion, sleeping sitting up or with several pillows
Cough with/without sputum production, dry/hacking—especially when recumbent
History of chronic lung disease
Use of respiratory aids, e.g., oxygen and/or medications

May exhibit: Tachypnea; shallow, labored breathing; use of accessory muscles, nasal flaring
Cough: Dry/hacking/nonproductive or may be gurgling with/without sputum production
Sputum may be blood-tinged, pink/frothy (pulmonary edema)
Breath sounds may be diminished, with bibasilar crackles and wheezes
Mentation may be diminished; lethargy, restlessness present
Color: pallor or cyanosis

SAFETY

May exhibit: Changes in mentation/confusion
Loss of strength/muscle tone
Skin excoriations, rashes

SOCIAL INTERACTION

May report: Decreased participation in usual social activities

TEACHING/LEARNING

May report: Use/misuse of cardiac medications, e.g., β-blockers, calcium channel blockers
Recent/recurrent hospitalizations
Evidence of failure to improve

Discharge plan considerations **DRG projected mean length of inpatient stay: 5.5 days**
Assistance with shopping, transportation, self-care needs, homemaker/maintenance tasks
Alteration in medication use/therapy
Changes in physical layout of home

Refer to section at end of plan for postdischarge considerations.

DIAGNOSTIC STUDIES

ECG: Ventricular or atrial hypertrophy, axis deviation, ischemia, and damage patterns may be present. Dysrhythmias, e.g., tachycardia, atrial fibrillation, conduction delays, frequent premature ventricular contractions (PVCs) may be present. Persistent ST-T segment elevation 6 weeks or more after myocardial infarction suggests presence of ventricular aneurysm (may cause cardiac dysfunction/failure).

Sonograms (echocardiogram, Doppler and transesophageal echocardiogram): May reveal enlarged chamber dimensions, alterations in valvular function/structure, decreased ventricular contractility.

Heart scan (multigated acquisition [MUGA]): Measures cardiac volume during both systole and diastole, ejection fraction, and estimates wall motion.

Exercise or pharmacological stress myocardial perfusion (e.g., persantine thallium scan): Determines presence of myocardial ischemia and wall motion abnormalities.

Positron-emission tomography (PET) scan: More sensitive test than scintigraphy for evaluation of myocardial ischemia/detecting viable myocardium.

Cardiac catheterization: Abnormal pressures are indicative and help differentiate right- versus left-sided heart failure, as well as valve stenosis or insufficiency. Also assesses patency of coronary arteries. Contrast injected into the ventricles reveals abnormal size and ejection fraction/altered contractility.

Chest x-ray: May show enlarged cardiac shadow reflecting chamber dilation/hypertrophy or changes in blood vessels reflecting increased pulmonary pressure. Abnormal contour, e.g., bulging of left cardiac border, may suggest ventricular aneurysm.

Liver enzymes: Elevated in liver congestion/failure.

Digoxin and other cardiac drug levels: Determine therapeutic range and correlate with patient response.

Bleeding and clotting times: Determine therapeutic range; identify those at risk for excessive clot formation.

Electrolytes: May be altered because of fluid shifts/decreased renal function, diuretic therapy.

Pulse oximetry: Oxygen saturation may be low, especially when acute HF is imposed on chronic obstructive pulmonary disease (COPD) or chronic HF.

Arterial blood gases (ABGs): Left ventricular failure is characterized by mild respiratory alkalosis (early) or hypoxemia with an increased PCO_2 (late).

BUN, creatinine: Elevated BUN suggests decreased renal perfusion. Elevation of both BUN and creatinine is indicative of renal failure.

Serum albumin/transferrin: May be decreased as a result of reduced protein intake or reduced protein synthesis in congested liver.

Complete blood count (CBC): May reveal anemia, polycythemia, or dilutional changes indicating water retention. WBCs may be elevated, reflecting recent/acute MI, pericarditis, or other inflammatory or infectious states.

Erythrocyte sedimentation rate (ESR): May be elevated, indicating acute inflammatory reaction.

Thyroid studies: Increased thyroid activity suggests thyroid hyperactivity as precipitator of HF.

NURSING PRIORITIES

1. Improve myocardial contractility/systemic perfusion.
2. Reduce fluid volume overload.
3. Prevent complications.
4. Provide information about disease/prognosis, therapy needs, and prevention of recurrences.

DISCHARGE GOALS

1. Cardiac output adequate for individual needs.
2. Complications prevented/resolved.
3. Optimum level of activity/functioning attained.
4. Disease process/prognosis and therapeutic regimen understood.
5. Plan in place to meet needs after discharge.

NURSING DIAGNOSIS: Cardiac Output, decreased

May be related to
Altered myocardial contractility/inotropic changes
Alterations in rate, rhythm, electrical conduction
Structural changes (e.g., valvular defects, ventricular aneurysm)

Possibly evidenced by
Increased heart rate (tachycardia), dysrhythmias, ECG changes
Changes in BP (hypotension/hypertension)
Extra heart sounds (S_3, S_4)
Decreased urine output
Diminished peripheral pulses
Cool, ashen skin; diaphoresis
Orthopnea, crackles, JVD, liver engorgement, edema
Chest pain

DESIRED OUTCOMES/EVALUATION CRITERIA—PATIENT WILL:

> **Cardiac Pump Effectiveness (NOC)**

Display vital signs within acceptable limits, dysrhythmias absent/controlled, and no symptoms of failure (e.g., hemodynamic parameters within acceptable limits, urinary output adequate).
Report decreased episodes of dyspnea, angina.
Participate in activities that reduce cardiac workload.

ACTIONS/INTERVENTIONS	RATIONALE

> **Hemodynamic Regulation (NIC)**

Independent

Auscultate apical pulse; assess heart rate, rhythm (document dysrhythmia if telemetry available).

Tachycardia is usually present (even at rest) to compensate for decreased ventricular contractility. Premature atrial contractions (PACs), paroxysmal atrial tachycardia (PAT), PVCs, multifocal atrial tachycardia (MAT), and atrial fibrillation (AF) are common dysrhythmias associated with HF, although others may also occur. *Note:* Intractable ventricular dysrhythmias unresponsive to medication suggest ventricular aneurysm.

ACTIONS/INTERVENTIONS	RATIONALE
Independent	
Note heart sounds.	S_1 and S_2 may be weak because of diminished pumping action. Gallop rhythms are common (S_3 and S_4), produced as blood flows into noncompliant/distended chambers. Murmurs may reflect valvular incompetence/stenosis.
Palpate peripheral pulses.	Decreased cardiac output may be reflected in diminished radial, popliteal, dorsalis pedis, and posttibial pulses. Pulses may be fleeting or irregular to palpation, and pulsus alternans (strong beat alternating with weak beat) may be present.
Monitor BP.	In early, moderate, or chronic HF, BP may be elevated because of increased SVR. In advanced HF, the body may no longer be able to compensate, and profound/irreversible hypotension may occur.
Inspect skin for pallor, cyanosis.	Pallor is indicative of diminished peripheral perfusion secondary to inadequate cardiac output, vasoconstriction, and anemia. Cyanosis may develop in refractory HF. Dependent areas are often blue or mottled as venous congestion increases.
Monitor urine output, noting decreasing output and dark/concentrated urine.	Kidneys respond to reduced cardiac output by retaining water and sodium. Urine output is usually decreased during the day because of fluid shifts into tissues but may be increased at night because fluid returns to circulation when patient is recumbent.
Note changes in sensorium, e.g., lethargy, confusion, disorientation, anxiety, and depression.	May indicate inadequate cerebral perfusion secondary to decreased cardiac output.
Encourage rest, semirecumbent in bed or chair. Assist with physical care as indicated.	Physical rest should be maintained during acute or refractory HF to improve efficiency of cardiac contraction and to decrease myocardial oxygen demand/consumption and workload.
Provide quiet environment; explain medical/nursing management; help patient avoid stressful situations; listen/respond to expressions of feelings/fears.	Psychological rest helps reduce emotional stress, which can produce vasoconstriction, elevating BP and increasing heart rate/work.
Provide bedside commode. Have patient avoid activities eliciting a vasovagal response, e.g., straining during defecation, holding breath during position changes.	Commode use decreases work of getting to bathroom or struggling to use bedpan. Vasovagal maneuver causes vagal stimulation followed by rebound tachycardia, which further compromises cardiac function/output.
Elevate legs, avoiding pressure under knee. Encourage active/passive exercises. Increase ambulation/activity as tolerated.	Decreases venous stasis and may reduce incidence of thrombus/embolus formation.
Check for calf tenderness, diminished pedal pulse, swelling, local redness, or pallor of extremity.	Reduced cardiac output, venous pooling/stasis, and enforced bedrest increases risk of thrombophlebitis.
Withhold digitalis preparation as indicated, and notify physician if marked changes occur in cardiac rate or rhythm or signs of digitalis toxicity occur.	Incidence of toxicity is high (20%) because of narrow margin between therapeutic and toxic ranges. Digoxin may have to be discontinued in the presence of toxic drug levels, a slow heart rate, or low potassium level. (Refer to CP: Dysrhythmias, ND: Poisoning, risk for digitalis toxicity, p. 97.)

ACTIONS/INTERVENTIONS	RATIONALE
Collaborative	
Administer supplemental oxygen as indicated.	Increases available oxygen for myocardial uptake to combat effects of hypoxia/ischemia.
Administer medications as indicated:	A variety of medications may be used to increase stroke volume, improve contractility, and reduce congestion.
Diuretics, e.g., furosemide (Lasix), ethacrynic acid (Edecrin), bumetanide (Bumex), spironolactone (Aldactone);	Diuretics, in conjunction with restriction of dietary sodium and fluids, often lead to clinical improvement in patients with stages I and II HF. In general, type and dosage of diuretic depends on cause and degree of HF and state of renal function. Preload reduction is most useful in treating patients with a relatively normal cardiac output accompanied by congestive symptoms. Loop diuretics block chloride reabsorption, thus interfering with the reabsorption of sodium and water.
Vasodilators, e.g., nitrates (Nitro-Dur, Isordil), arteriodilators, e.g., hydralazine (Apresoline), combination drugs, e.g., prazosin (Minipress);	Vasodilators are the mainstay of treatment in HF and are used to increase cardiac output, reducing circulating volume (venodilators) and decreasing SVR, thereby reducing ventricular workload. *Note:* Parenteral vasodilators (e.g., Nipride) are reserved for patients with severe HF or those unable to take oral medications.
ACE inhibitors: e.g., captopril (Capoten), lisinopril (Prinivil), enalapril (Vasotec), quinapril (Accupril), ramipril (Altace), fosinopril (Monopril);	ACE inhibitors represent first-line therapy to control heart failure by decreasing venticular filling pressures and SVR while increasing cardiac output with little or no change in BP and HR.
Digoxin (Lanoxin);	Increases force of myocardial contraction when diminished contractility is the cause of HF and slows heart rate by decreasing conduction velocity and prolonging refractory period of the atrioventricular (AV) junction to increase cardiac efficiency/output.
Inotropic agents, e.g., amrinone (Inocor), milrinone (Primacor), vesnarinone (Arkin-Z);	These medications are useful for short-term treatment of HF unresponsive to cardiac glycosides, vasodilators, and diuretics in order to increase myocardial contractility and produce vasodilation. Positive inotropic properties have reduced mortality rates 50% and improved quality of life.
Beta-adrenergic receptor antagonists, e.g., carvedilol (Careg), bisoprolol (Zebeta), metoprolol (Lopressor);	Useful in the treatment of HF by blocking the cardiac effects of chronic adrenergic stimulation. Many patients experience improved activity tolerance and ejection fraction.
Morphine sulfate;	Decreases vascular resistance and venous return, reducing myocardial workload, especially when pulmonary congestion is present. Allays anxiety and breaks the feedback cycle of anxiety to catecholamine release to anxiety.
Antianxiety agents/sedatives;	Promote rest/relaxation, reducing oxygen demand and myocardial workload.

ACTIONS/INTERVENTIONS	RATIONALE
Collaborative	
Anticoagulants, e.g., low-dose heparin, warfarin (Coumadin).	May be used prophylactically to prevent thrombus/embolus formation in presence of risk factors such as venous stasis, enforced bedrest, cardiac dysrhythmias, and history of previous thrombolic episodes.
Administer IV solutions, restricting total amount as indicated. Avoid saline solutions.	Because of existing elevated left ventricular pressure, patient may not tolerate increased fluid volume (preload). Patients with HF also excrete less sodium, which causes fluid retention and increases myocardial workload.
Monitor/replace electrolytes.	Fluid shifts and use of diuretics can alter electrolytes (especially potassium and chloride), which affect cardiac rhythm and contractility.
Monitor serial ECG and chest x-ray changes.	ST segment depression and T wave flattening can develop because of increased myocardial oxygen demand, even if no coronary artery disease is present. Chest x-ray may show enlarged heart and changes of pulmonary congestion.
Measure cardiac output and other functional parameters as indicated.	Cardiac index, preload/afterload, contractility, and cardiac work can be measured noninvasively by using thoracic electrical bioimpedance (TEB) technique. Useful in determining effectiveness of therapeutic interventions and response to activity.
Monitor laboratory studies, e.g., BUN, creatinine;	Elevation of BUN/creatinine reflects kidney hypoperfusion/failure.
Liver function studies (AST, LDH);	May be elevated because of liver congestion and indicate need for smaller dosages of medications that are detoxified by the liver.
Prothrombin time (PT)/activated partial thromboplastin time (aPTT) coagulation studies.	Measures changes in coagulation processes or effectiveness of anticoagulant therapy.
Prepare for insertion/maintain pacemaker, if indicated.	May be necessary to correct bradydysrhythmias unresponsive to drug intervention, which can aggravate congestive failure/produce pulmonary edema.
Prepare for surgery as indicated, e.g., valve replacement, angioplasty, coronary artery bypass grafting (CABG);	Heart failure due to ventricular aneurysm or valvular dysfunction may require aneurysmectomy or valve replacement to improve myocardial contractility/function. Revascularization of cardiac muscle by CABG may be done to improve cardiac function.
Cardiomyoplasty;	Cardiomyoplasty, an experimental procedure in which the latissimus dorsi muscle is wrapped around the heart and electrically stimulated to contract with each heartbeat, may be done to augment ventricular function while the patient is awaiting cardiac transplantation or when transplantation is not an option.

ACTIONS/INTERVENTIONS

Collaborative

Transmyocardial revascularization;

Assist with/maintain mechanical circulatory support system, such as IABP or VAD, when indicated.

RATIONALE

Other new surgical techniques include transmyocardial revascularization using CO_2 laser technology, in which a laser is used to create multiple 1-mm diameter channels in viable but underperfused cardiac muscle.

An intra-aortic balloon pump (IABP) may be inserted as a temporary support to the failing heart in the critically ill patient with potentially reversible HF. A battery-powered ventricular assist device (VAD) may also be used, positioned between the cardiac apex and the descending thoracic or abdominal aorta. This device receives blood from the left ventricle (LV) and ejects it into the systemic circulation, often allowing the patient to resume a nearly normal lifestyle while awaiting heart transplantation. With end-stage HF, cardiac transplantation may be indicated.

NURSING DIAGNOSIS: Activity Intolerance

May be related to:
Imbalance between oxygen supply/demand
Generalized weakness
Prolonged bedrest/immobility

Possibly evidenced by
Weakness, fatigue
Changes in vital signs, presence of dysrhythmias
Dyspnea
Pallor, diaphoresis

DESIRED OUTCOMES/EVALUATION CRITERIA—PATIENT WILL:

Endurance (NOC)

Participate in desired activities; meet own self-care needs.
Achieve measurable increase in activity tolerance, evidenced by reduced fatigue and weakness and vital signs within acceptable limits during activity.

ACTIONS/INTERVENTIONS

Energy Management (NIC)

Independent

Check vital signs before and immediately after activity, especially if patient is on vasodilators, diuretics, or β-blockers.

RATIONALE

Orthostatic hypotension can occur with activity because of medication effect (vasodilation), fluid shifts (diuresis), or compromised cardiac pumping function.

ACTIONS/INTERVENTIONS

Independent

Document cardiopulmonary response to activity. Note tachycardia, dysrhythmias, dyspnea, diaphoresis, pallor.

Assess for other precipitators/causes of fatigue, e.g., treatments, pain, medications.

Evaluate accelerating activity intolerance.

Provide assistance with self-care activities as indicated. Intersperse activity periods with rest periods.

Collaborative

Implement graded cardiac rehabilitation/activity program.

RATIONALE

Compromised myocardium/inability to increase stroke volume during activity may cause an immediate increase in heart rate and oxygen demands, thereby aggravating weakness and fatigue.

Fatigue is a side effect of some medications (e.g., β-blockers, tranquilizers, and sedatives). Pain and stressful regimens also extract energy and produce fatigue.

May denote increasing cardiac decompensation rather than overactivity.

Meets patient's personal care needs without undue myocardial stress/excessive oxygen demand.

Strengthens and improves cardiac function under stress, if cardiac dysfunction is not irreversible. Gradual increase in activity avoids excessive myocardial workload and oxygen consumption.

NURSING DIAGNOSIS: Fluid Volume excess

May be related to
Reduced glomerular filtration rate (decreased cardiac output)/increased antidiuretic hormone (ADH) production, and sodium/water retention

Possibly evidenced by
Orthopnea, S_3 heart sound
Oliguria, edema, JVD, positive hepatojugular reflex
Weight gain
Hypertension
Respiratory distress, abnormal breath sounds

DESIRED OUTCOMES/EVALUATION CRITERIA—PATIENT WILL:

Fluid Balance (NOC)

Demonstrate stabilized fluid volume with balanced intake and output, breath sounds clear/clearing, vital signs within acceptable range, stable weight, and absence of edema.
Verbalize understanding of individual dietary/fluid restrictions.

ACTIONS/INTERVENTIONS

Fluid Management (NIC)

Independent

Monitor urine output, noting amount and color, as well as time of day when diuresis occurs.

RATIONALE

Urine output may be scanty and concentrated (especially during the day) because of reduced renal perfusion. Recumbency favors diuresis; therefore urine output may be increased at night/during bedrest.

ACTIONS/INTERVENTIONS	RATIONALE

Independent

Monitor/calculate 24-hour intake and output (I&O) balance.	Diuretic therapy may result in sudden/excessive fluid loss (circulating hypovolemia), even though edema/ascites remains.
Maintain chair or bedrest in semi-Fowler's position during acute phase.	Recumbency increases glomerular filtration and decreases production of ADH, thereby enhancing diuresis.
Establish fluid intake schedule if fluids are medically restricted, incorporating beverage preferences when possible. Give frequent mouth care/ice chips as part of fluid allotment.	Involving patient in therapy regimen may enhance sense of control and cooperation with restrictions.
Weigh daily.	Documents changes in/resolution of edema in response to therapy. A gain of 5 lb represents approximately 2 L of fluid. Conversely, diuretics can result in rapid/excessive fluid shifts and weight loss.
Assess for distended neck and peripheral vessels. Inspect dependent body areas for edema with/without pitting; note presence of generalized body edema (anasarca).	Excessive fluid retention may be manifested by venous engorgement and edema formation. Peripheral edema begins in feet/ankles (or dependent areas) and ascends as failure worsens. Pitting edema is generally obvious only after retention of at least 10 lb of fluid. Increased vascular congestion (associated with RHF) eventually results in systemic tissue edema.
Change position frequently. Elevate feet when sitting. Inspect skin surface, keep dry, and provide padding as indicated. (Refer to ND: Skin Integrity, risk for impaired, p. 58.)	Edema formation, slowed circulation, altered nutritional intake, and prolonged immobility/bedrest are cumulative stressors that affect skin integrity and require close supervision/preventive interventions.
Auscultate breath sounds, noting decreased and/or adventitious sounds, e.g., crackles, wheezes. Note presence of increased dyspnea, tachypnea, orthopnea, paroxysmal nocturnal dyspnea, persistent cough.	Excess fluid volume often leads to pulmonary congestion. Symptoms of pulmonary edema may reflect acute left-sided HF. RHF's respiratory symptoms (dyspnea, cough, orthopnea) may have slower onset but are more difficult to reverse.
Investigate reports of sudden extreme dyspnea/air hunger, need to sit straight up, sensation of suffocation, feelings of panic or impending doom.	May indicate development of complications (pulmonary edema/embolus) and differs from orthopnea and paroxysmal nocturnal dyspnea in that it develops much more rapidly and requires immediate intervention.
Monitor BP and central venous pressure (CVP) (if available).	Hypertension and elevated CVP suggest fluid volume excess and may reflect developing/increasing pulmonary congestion, HF.
Assess bowel sounds. Note complaints of anorexia, nausea, abdominal distension, constipation.	Visceral congestion (occurring in progressive HF) can alter gastric/intestinal function.
Provide small, frequent, easily digestible meals.	Reduced gastric motility can adversely affect digestion and absorption. Small, frequent meals may enhance digestion/prevent abdominal discomfort.
Measure abdominal girth, as indicated.	In progressive RHF, fluid may shift into the peritoneal space, causing increasing abdominal girth (ascites).
Encourage verbalization of feelings regarding limitations.	Expression of feelings/concerns may decrease stress/anxiety, which is an energy drain that can contribute to feelings of fatigue.

ACTIONS/INTERVENTIONS	RATIONALE
Independent	
Palpate abdomen. Note reports of right upper quadrant pain/tenderness.	Advancing HF leads to venous congestion, resulting in abdominal distension, liver engorgement (hepatomegaly), and pain. This can alter liver function and impair/prolong drug metabolism.
Note increased lethargy, hypotension, muscle cramping.	Signs of potassium and sodium deficits that may occur because of fluid shifts and diuretic therapy.
Collaborative	
Administer medications as indicated:	
Diuretics, e.g., furosemide (Lasix), bumetanide (Bumex);	Increases rate of urine flow and may inhibit reabsorption of sodium/chloride in the renal tubules.
Thiazides with potassium-sparing agents, e.g., spironolactone (Aldactone);	Promotes diuresis without excessive potassium losses.
Potassium supplements, e.g., K-Dur.	Replaces potassium that is lost as a common side effect of diuretic therapy, which can adversely affect cardiac function.
Maintain fluid/sodium restrictions as indicated.	Reduces total body water/prevents fluid reaccumulation.
Consult with dietitian.	May be necessary to provide diet acceptable to patient that meets caloric needs within sodium restriction.
Monitor chest x-ray.	Reveals changes indicative of increase/resolution of pulmonary congestion.
Assist with rotating tourniquets/phlebotomy, dialysis, or ultrafiltration as indicated.	Although not frequently used, mechanical fluid removal rapidly reduces circulating volume, especially in pulmonary edema refractory to other therapies.

NURSING DIAGNOSIS: Gas Exchange, risk for impaired

Risk factors may include
Alveolar-capillary membrane changes, e.g., fluid collection/shifts into interstitial space/alveoli

Possibly evidenced by
[Not applicable; presence of signs and symptoms establishes an *actual* diagnosis]

DESIRED OUTCOMES/EVALUATION CRITERIA—PATIENT WILL:

Respiratory Status: Gas Exchange (NOC)

Demonstrate adequate ventilation and oxygenation of tissues by ABGs/oximetry within patient's normal ranges and free of symptoms of respiratory distress.
Participate in treatment regimen within level of ability/situation.

ACTIONS/INTERVENTIONS	RATIONALE

Airway Management (NIC)

Independent

Auscultate breath sounds, noting crackles, wheezes.	Reveals presence of pulmonary congestion/collection of secretions, indicating need for further intervention.
Instruct patient in effective coughing, deep breathing.	Clears airways and facilitates oxygen delivery.
Encourage frequent position changes.	Helps prevent atelectasis and pneumonia.
Maintain chair/bedrest, with head of bed elevated 20–30 degrees, semi-Fowler's position. Support arms with pillows.	Reduces oxygen consumption/demands and promotes maximal lung inflation.

Collaborative

Monitor/graph serial ABGs, pulse oximetry.	Hypoxemia can be severe during pulmonary edema. Compensatory changes are usually present in chronic HF. Note: In patients with abnormal cardiac index, research suggests pulse oximeter measurements may exceed actual oxygen saturation by up to 7%.
Administer supplemental oxygen as indicated.	Increases alveolar oxygen concentration, which may correct/reduce tissue hypoxemia.
Administer medications as indicated:	
Diuretics, e.g., furosemide (Lasix);	Reduces alveolar congestion, enhancing gas exchange.
Bronchodilators, e.g., aminophylline.	Increases oxygen delivery by dilating small airways and exert mild diuretic effect to aid in reducing pulmonary congestion.

NURSING DIAGNOSIS: Skin Integrity, risk for impaired

Risk factors may include
Prolonged bedrest
Edema, decreased tissue perfusion

Possibly evidenced by
[Not applicable; presence of signs and symptoms establishes an *actual* diagnosis]

DESIRED OUTCOMES/EVALUATION CRITERIA—PATIENT WILL:

Tissue Perfusion: Peripheral (NOC)

Maintain skin integrity.
Demonstrate behaviors/techniques to prevent skin breakdown.

ACTIONS/INTERVENTIONS	RATIONALE

Pressure Management (NIC)

Independent

Inspect skin, noting skeletal prominences, presence of edema, areas of altered circulation/pigmentation, or obesity/emaciation.

Skin is at risk because of impaired peripheral circulation, physical immobility, and alterations in nutritional status.

Provide gentle massage around reddened or blanched areas.

Improves blood flow, minimizing tissue hypoxia. *Note:* Direct massage of compromised area may cause tissue injury.

Encourage frequent position changes in bed/chair, assist with active/passive range of motion (ROM) exercises.

Reduces pressure on tissues, improving circulation and reducing time any one area is deprived of full blood flow.

Provide frequent skin care; minimize contact with moisture/excretions.

Excessive dryness or moisture damages skin and hastens breakdown.

Check fit of shoes/slippers and change as needed.

Dependent edema may cause shoes to fit poorly, increasing risk of pressure and skin breakdown on feet.

Avoid intramuscular route for medication.

Interstitial edema and impaired circulation impede drug absorption and predispose to tissue breakdown/development of infection.

Collaborative

Provide alternating pressure/egg-crate mattress, sheepskin elbow/heel protectors.

Reduces pressure to skin, may improve circulation.

NURSING DIAGNOSIS: Knowledge Deficit [Learning Need] regarding condition, treatment regimen, self care, and discharge needs

May be related to
Lack of understanding/misconceptions about interrelatedness of cardiac function/disease/failure

Possibly evidenced by
Questions
Statements of concern/misconceptions
Recurrent, preventable episodes of HF

DESIRED OUTCOMES/EVALUATION CRITERIA—PATIENT WILL:

Knowledge: Disease Process (NOC)

Identify relationship of ongoing therapies (treatment program) to reduction of recurrent episodes and prevention of complications.
List signs/symptoms that require immediate intervention.
Identify own stress/risk factors and some techniques for handling.
Initiate necessary lifestyle/behavioral changes.

ACTIONS/INTERVENTIONS	RATIONALE

Teaching: Disease Process (NIC)

Independent

Discuss normal heart function. Include information regarding patient's variance from normal function. Explain difference between heart attack and HF.

Knowledge of disease process and expectations can facilitate adherence to prescribed treatment regimen.

Reinforce treatment rationale. Include SO/family members in teaching as appropriate, especially for complicated regimens such as dobutamine infusion home therapy when patient does not respond to customary combination therapy or cannot be weaned from dobutamine, or those awaiting heart transplant.

Patient may believe it is acceptable to alter postdischarge regimen when feeling well and symptom-free or when feeling below par, which can increase the risk of exacerbation of symptoms. Understanding of regimen, medications, and restrictions may augment cooperation with control of symptoms. Home IV therapy requires a significant commitment by caregivers to operate/troubleshoot infusion pump, change dressing for peripherally inserted central catheter (PICC) line, monitor I&O and signs/symptoms of HF.

Encourage developing a regular home exercise program, and provide guidelines for sexual activity.

Promotes maintenance of muscle tone and organ function for overall sense of well-being. Changing sexual habits may be difficult (e.g., sex in morning when well rested, patient on top, inclusion of other physical expressions of affection) but provides opportunity for continuing satisfying sexual relationship.

Discuss importance of being as active as possible without becoming exhausted and of rest between activities.

Excessive physical activity or overexertion can further weaken the heart, exacerbating failure, and necessitates adjustment of exercise program.

Discuss importance of sodium limitation. Provide list of sodium content of common foods that are to be avoided/limited. Encourage reading of labels on food and drug packages.

Dietary intake of sodium above 3 g/day can offset effect of diuretic. Most common source of sodium is table salt and obviously salty foods, although canned soups/vegetables, luncheon meats, and dairy products also may contain high levels of sodium.

Refer to dietitian for counseling specific to individual needs/dietary customs.

Identifies dietary needs, especially in presence of nausea/vomiting and resulting wasting syndrome (cardiac cachexia). Eating six small meals and using liquid dietary supplements and vitamin supplements can limit inappropriate weight loss.

Review medications, purpose, and side effects. Provide both oral and written instructions.

Understanding therapeutic needs and importance of prompt reporting of side effects can prevent occurrence of drug-related complications. Anxiety may block comprehension of input or details, and patient/SO may refer to written material at later date to refresh memory.

Recommend taking diuretic early in morning.

Provides adequate time for drug effect before bedtime to prevent/limit interruption of sleep.

Instruct and receive return demonstration of ability to take and record daily pulse and blood pressure and when to notify healthcare provider, e.g., parameters above/below preset rate, changes in rhythm/regularity.

Promotes self-monitoring of condition/drug effect. Early detection of changes allows for timely intervention and may prevent complications, such as digitalis toxicity.

ACTIONS/INTERVENTIONS	RATIONALE

Independent

Explain and discuss patient's role in control of risk factors (e.g., smoking) and precipitating or aggravating factors (e.g., high-salt diet, inactivity/overexertion, exposure to extremes in temperature).

Adds to body of knowledge and permits patient to make informed decisions regarding control of condition and prevention of recurrence/complications. Smoking potentiates vasoconstriction; sodium intake promotes water retention/edema formation; improper balance between activity and rest and exposure to temperature extremes may result in exhaustion/increased myocardial workload and increased risk of respiratory infections. Alcohol can depress cardiac contractility. Limitation of alcohol use to social occasions or maximum of 1 drink/day may be tolerated unless cardiomyopathy is alcohol-induced (requiring complete abstinence).

Review signs/symptoms that require immediate medical attention, e.g., rapid/significant weight gain, edema, shortness of breath, increased fatigue, cough, hemoptysis, fever.

Self-monitoring increases patient responsibility in health maintenance and aids in prevention of complications, e.g., pulmonary edema, pneumonia. Weight gain of more than 3 lb in a week requires medical evaluation/adjustment of diuretic therapy. *Note:* Patient should weigh self daily in morning without clothing, after voiding and before eating.

Provide opportunities for patient/SO to ask questions, discuss concerns, and make necessary lifestyle changes.

Chronicity and recurrent/debilitating nature of HF often exhausts coping abilities and supportive capacity of both patient and SO, leading to depression.

Discuss general health risks (such as infection), recommending avoidance of crowds and individuals with respiratory infections, obtaining yearly influenza immunization and one-time pneumonia immunization.

This population is at increased risk for infection because of circulatory compromise.

Stress importance of reporting signs/symptoms of digitalis toxicity, e.g., development of gastrointestinal (GI) and visual disturbances, changes in pulse rate/rhythm, worsening of heart failure.

Early recognition of developing complications and involvement of healthcare provider may prevent toxicity/hospitalization.

Identify community resources/support groups and visiting home health nurse as indicated.

May need additional assistance with self-monitoring/home management, especially when HF is progressive.

Discuss importance of advance directives and of communicating plan/wishes to family and primary care providers.

Up to 50% of all deaths from heart failure are sudden, with many occurring at home, possibly without significant worsening of symptoms. If patient chooses to refuse life-support measures, an alternative contact person (rather than 911) needs to be designated, should cardiac arrest occur.

POTENTIAL CONSIDERATIONS following discharge from care setting (dependent on patient's age, physical condition/presence of complications, personal resources, and life responsibilities)

Activity intolerance—poor cardiac reserve, side effects of medication, generalized weakness.
Fluid Volume excess or deficit—changes in glomerular filtration rate, diuretic use, individual fluid/salt intake.
Skin Integrity, impaired—decreased activity level, prolonged sitting, presence of edema, altered circulation.
Therapeutic Regimen: Individual, ineffective management—complexity of regimen, economic limitations.
Home Maintenance Management, impaired—chronic/debilitating condition, insufficient finances, inadequate support systems.
Self-Care deficit—decreased strength/endurance, depression.

Sample CP: Heart Failure, Hospital. ELOS 4 Days Cardiology or Medical Unit

ND and Categories of Care	Day 1 _____	Day 2 _____	Day 3 _____	Day 4 _____
Decreased cardiac output R/T decreased myocardial contractility, altered electrical conduction, structural changes	**Goals** Participate in actions to reduce cardiac workload	Display VS within acceptable limits; dysrhythmias controlled; pulse oximetry within acceptable range Meet own self-care needs with assistance as necessary	→ Dysrhythmias controlled or absent → Free of signs of respiratory distress → Demonstrate measurable increase in activity tolerance	→
Fluid Volume Excess R/T compromised regulatory mechanism	Verbalize understanding of fluid/food restrictions	Verbalize understanding of general condition and healthcare needs Breath sounds clearing Urinary output adequate Weight loss (reflecting fluid loss)	Plan for lifestyle/ behavior changes Breath sounds clear Balanced I&O Edema resolving	Plan in place to meet postdischarge needs Weight stable (continued loss if edema present)
Referrals	Cardiology Dietitian	Cardiac Rehab Occupational therapist (for ADLs) Social Services Home care	Community Resources	
Diagnostic studies	ECG Echo-Doppler CXR ABGs/Pulse oximetry Cardiac enzymes BUN/CR CBC/electrolytes, MG++ PT/aPTT Liver function studies Serum glucose Albumin Uric acid Digoxin level (as indicated) UA	Echo-Doppler (if not done day 1) or MUGA Cardiac enzymes (if ↑) BUN/Cr Electrolytes PT/aPTT (if on anticoagulants)	CXR BUN/Cr Electrolytes PT/aPTT (as indicated) Repeat digoxin level (if indicated)	
Additional assessments	Apical pulse, heart/breath sounds q8h Cardiac rhythm (Telemetry)q4h BP, P, R *q2h until stable, q4h* Temp *q8h* I&O *q8h* Weight *qAM* Peripheral edema *q8h* → Peripheral pulses *q8h* → Sensorium q8h → DVT check *qd* → Response to activity → Response to therapeutic interventions →	→ → → q8h → → →	→ bid → D/C → → → → bid → bid → bid → → →	→ → → → → D/C → → qd → D/C → D/C → → →

ND and Categories of Care	Day 1 _____	Day 2 _____	Day 3 _____	Day 4 _____
Medications Allergies:	IV diuretic	→ PO	→	→
	ACE inhibitor	→	→	→
	Digoxin	→	→	→
	PO/Cutaneous nitrates	→	→	→
	Morphine sulfate	→	→ D/C	
	Daytime/hs sedation	→	→	→ D/C
	PO/low-dose anticoagulant	→	→ PO or D/C	→
	IV/PO potassium	→	→ D/C	
	Stool softener/laxative	→	→	→

Patient education	Orient to unit/room
	Review advanced
	  directives
	Discuss expected
	  outcomes, diagnostic
	  tests/results
	Fluid/nutritional
	  restrictions/needs
		Cardiac education per
		  protocol
		Review medications:
		  Dose, time, route,
		  purpose, side effects
		Progressive activity
		  program
		Skin care
			Signs/symptoms to
			  report to healthcare
			  provider
			Plan for homecare
			  needs
				Provide written
				  instructions for
				  homecare
				Schedule for follow-
				  up appointments

Additional nursing
  actions
	Bed/chair rest	→ BPR/Ambulate as
		  tolerated, cardiac
		  program
			→ Up ad lib/graded
			  program
				→

	Assist with physical care	→	→	→
	Egg-crate mattress	→	→	→ (send home)
	Dysrhythmia/angina care per protocol	→	→	→
	Supplemental O$_2$	→	→ D/C	
	Cardiac diet	→	→	→

ANGINA PECTORIS

The classic symptom of coronary artery disease (CAD) is angina—pain caused by inadequate flow of oxygen to the myocardium. Angina has three major forms: (1) stable (precipitated by effort, of short duration, and easily relieved), (2) unstable (longer lasting, more severe, may not be relieved by rest/nitroglycerin; may also be new onset of pain with exertion or recent acceleration in severity of pain), and (3) variant (chest pain at rest with ECG changes). The AHCPR guidelines of May 1994 state that unstable angina is a transitory syndrome that causes significant disability and death in the United States. In most but not all patients presenting with angina, symptoms are caused by significant CAD.

CARE SETTING

Patients judged to be at intermediate or high likelihood of significant CAD are often hospitalized for further evaluation and therapeutic intervention. Classification of angina (provided by Canadian Cardiovascular Society Classification [CCSC]) aids in determining the risk of adverse outcomes for patients with unstable angina and, therefore, level of treatment needs. Class III angina is identified as occurring if the patient walks less than two blocks and normal activity is markedly limited, and class IV angina occurs at rest or with minimal activity and level of activity is severely limited. These two classes may require inpatient evaluation/therapeutic adjustments.

RELATED CONCERNS

Cardiac surgery, page 102
Dysrhythmias, page 90
Heart failure: chronic, page 47
Myocardial infarction, page 75
Psychosocial aspects of care, page 809

Patient Assessment Database

ACTIVITY/REST

May report:	Sedentary lifestyle, weakness
	Fatigue, feeling incapacitated after exercise
	Chest pain with exertion or at rest
	Awakened by chest pain
May exhibit:	Exertional dyspnea

CIRCULATION

May report:	History of heart disease, hypertension, obesity in self/family
May exhibit:	Tachycardia, dysrhythmias
	Blood pressure normal, elevated, or decreased
	Heart sounds: May be normal; late S_4 or transient late systolic murmur (papillary muscle dysfunction) may be evident during pain
	Moist, cool, pale skin/mucous membranes in presence of vasoconstriction

FOOD/FLUID

May report:	Nausea, "heartburn"/epigastric distress with eating
	Diet high in cholesterol/fats, salt, caffeine, liquor
May exhibit:	Belching, gastric distension

EGO INTEGRITY

May report:	Stressors of work, family, others
May exhibit:	Apprehension, uneasiness

PAIN/DISCOMFORT

May report:	Substernal or anterior chest pain that may radiate to jaw, neck, shoulders, and upper extremities (to left side more than right)

Quality: Varies from transient/mild to moderate, heavy pressure, tightness, squeezing, burning

Duration: Usually less than 15 min, rarely more than 30 min (average 3 min)

Precipitating factors: Physical exertion or great emotion, such as anger or sexual arousal; exercise in weather extremes; or may be unpredictable and/or occur during rest

Relieving factors: Pain may be responsive to particular relief mechanisms (e.g., rest, antianginal medications)

New or ongoing chest pain that has changed in frequency, duration, character, or predictability (i.e., unstable, variant, Prinzmetal's)

May exhibit: Facial grimacing, placing fist over midsternum, rubbing left arm, muscle tension, restlessness

Autonomic responses, e.g., tachycardia, blood pressure changes

RESPIRATION

May report: Dyspnea worse with exertion

History of smoking

May exhibit: Respirations: Increased rate/rhythm and alteration in depth

TEACHING/LEARNING

May report: Family history or risk factors of CAD, hypertension, stroke, diabetes, cigarette smoking, hyperlipidemia

Use/misuse of cardiac, hypertensive, or OTC drugs

Regular alcohol use, illicit drug use, e.g., cocaine, amphetamines

Discharge plan considerations: **DRG projected mean length of inpatient stay: 3.2–4.2 days**

Alteration in medication use/therapy

Assistance with homemaker/maintenance tasks

Changes in physical layout of home

Refer to section at end of plan for postdischarge considerations.

DIAGNOSTIC STUDIES

ECG: Usually normal when patient at rest; depression of the ST segment or T wave inversion signifies ischemia. Dysrhythmias and heart block may also be present. Significant Q waves are consistent with a prior MI.

24-hour ECG monitoring (Holter): Done to see whether pain episodes correlate with or change during exercise or activity. ST depression without pain is highly indicative of ischemia.

Exercise or pharmacological stress electrocardiography: Provides more diagnostic information, such as duration and level of activity attained before onset of angina. A markedly positive test is indicative of severe CAD.

Cardiac enzymes (AST, CPK, CK and CK-MB; LDH and isoenzymes LD_1, LD_2): Usually within normal limits (WNL), elevation indicates myocardial damage.

Chest x-ray: Usually normal; however, infiltrates may be present, reflecting cardiac decompensation or pulmonary complications.

PCO_2, potassium and myocardial lactate: May be elevated during anginal attack (all play a role in myocardial ischemia and may perpetuate it).

Serum lipids (total lipids, lipoprotein electrophoresis, and isoenzymes [HDL, LDL, VLDL]; cholesterol, triglycerides; phospholipids): May be elevated (CAD risk factor).

Echocardiogram: May reveal abnormal valvular action as cause of chest pain.

Nuclear imaging studies (rest or stress scan):

   Thallium 201: Ischemic regions appear as areas of decreased thallium uptake.

   MUGA: Evaluates specific and general ventricle performance, regional wall motion, and ejection fraction.

Cardiac catheterization with angiography: Definitive test for CAD in patients with known ischemic disease with angina or incapacitating chest pain, in patients with cholesterolemia and familial heart disease who are experiencing chest pain, and in patients with abnormal resting ECGs. Abnormal results are present in valvular disease, altered contractility, ventricular failure, and circulatory abnormalities. *Note:* Ten percent of patients with unstable angina have normal-appearing coronary arteries.

Ergonovine (Ergotrate) injection: On occasion, may be used for patients who have angina at rest to demonstrate hyperspastic coronary vessels. (Patients with resting angina usually experience chest pain, ST elevation, or depression and/or pronounced rise in left ventricular end-diastolic pressure [LVEDP], fall in systemic systolic pressure, and/or high-grade coronary artery narrowing. Some patients may also have severe ventricular dysrhythmias.)

NURSING PRIORITIES

1. Relieve/control pain.
2. Prevent/minimize development of myocardial complications.
3. Provide information about disease process/prognosis and treatment.
4. Support patient/SO in initiating necessary lifestyle/behavioral changes.

DISCHARGE GOALS

1. Achieves desired activity level; meets self-care needs with minimal or no pain.
2. Free of complications.
3. Disease process/prognosis and therapeutic regimen understood.
4. Participating in treatment program, behavioral changes.
5. Plan in place to meet needs after discharge.

NURSING DIAGNOSIS: Pain [acute]

May be related to
Decreased myocardial blood flow
Increased cardiac workload/oxygen consumption

Possibly evidenced by
Reports of pain varying in frequency, duration, and intensity (especially as condition worsens)
Narrowed focus
Distraction behaviors (moaning, crying, pacing, restlessness)
Autonomic responses, e.g., diaphoresis, blood pressure and pulse rate changes, pupillary dilation, increased/decreased respiratory rate

DESIRED OUTCOMES/EVALUATION CRITERIA—PATIENT WILL:

Pain Level (NOC)

Report anginal episodes decreased in frequency, duration, and severity.
Demonstrate relief of pain as evidenced by stable vital signs, absence of muscle tension, restlessness.

ACTIONS/INTERVENTIONS	RATIONALE

Pain Management (NIC)

Independent

Instruct patient to notify nurse immediately when chest pain occurs.

Pain and decreased cardiac output may stimulate the sympathetic nervous system to release excessive amounts of norepinephrine, which increases platelet aggregation and release of thromboxane A_2. This potent vasoconstrictor causes coronary artery spasm, which can precipitate, complicate, and/or prolong an anginal attack. Unbearable pain may cause vasovagal response, decreasing BP and heart rate.

ACTIONS/INTERVENTIONS	RATIONALE
Independent	
Assess and document patient response/effects of medication.	Provides information about disease progression. Aids in evaluating effectiveness of interventions and may indicate need for change in therapeutic regimen.
Identify precipitating event, if any; frequency, duration, intensity, and location of pain.	Helps differentiate this chest pain and aids in evaluating possible progression to unstable angina. (Stable angina usually lasts 3–15 min and is often relieved by rest and sublingual nitroglycerin (NTG); unstable angina is more intense, may last up to 30–45 min, and may not be relieved by NTG/rest.)
Observe for associated symptoms, e.g., dyspnea, nausea/vomiting, dizziness, palpitations, desire to micturate.	Decreased cardiac output (which may occur during ischemic myocardial episode) stimulates sympathetic/parasympathetic nervous system, causing a variety of vague sensations that patient may not identify as related to anginal episode.
Evaluate reports of pain in jaw, neck, shoulder, arm, or hand (typically on left side).	Cardiac pain may radiate, e.g., pain is often referred to more superficial sites served by the same spinal cord nerve level.
Place patient at complete rest during anginal episodes.	Reduces myocardial oxygen demand to minimize risk of tissue injury/necrosis.
Elevate head of bed if patient is short of breath.	Facilitates gas exchange to decrease hypoxia and resultant shortness of breath.
Monitor heart rate/rhythm.	Patients with unstable angina have an increased risk of acute life-threatening dysrhythmias, which occur in response to ischemic changes and/or stress.
Monitor vital signs every 5 min during anginal attack.	Blood pressure may initially rise because of sympathetic stimulation, then fall if cardiac output is compromised. Tachycardia also develops in response to sympathetic stimulation and may be sustained as a compensatory response if cardiac output falls.
Stay with patient who is experiencing pain or appears anxious.	Anxiety releases catecholamines, which increase myocardial workload and can escalate/prolong ischemic pain. Presence of nurse can reduce feelings of fear and helplessness.
Maintain quiet, comfortable environment; restrict visitors as necessary.	Mental/emotional stress increases myocardial workload.
Provide light meals. Have patient rest for 1 hr after meals.	Decreases myocardial workload associated with work of digestion, reducing risk of anginal attack.
Collaborative	
Provide supplemental oxygen as indicated.	Increases oxygen available for myocardial uptake/reversal of ischemia.

Collaborative

Administer antianginal medication(s) promptly as indicated:

Nitroglycerin: Sublingual (Nitrostat), buccal or oral tablets, metered-dose spray;

Sustained-release tablets, caplets (Nitrong, Nitrocap T.D.), chewable tablets (Isordil, Sorbitrate), patches, transmucosal ointment (Nitro-Dur, Transderm-Nitro);

β-blockers, e.g., atenolol (Tenormin), nadolol (Corgard), metroprolol (Lopressor), propranolol (Inderal);

Analgesics, e.g., acetaminophen (Tylenol);

Morphine sulphate (MS).

Calcium channel antagonists, e.g., nifedipine (Procardia); felodipine (Plendil); isradipine (DynaCirc); diltiazem (Cardizem).

Monitor serial ECG changes.

Nitroglycerin has been the standard for treating and preventing anginal pain for more than 100 yr. Today it is available in many forms and is still the cornerstone of antianginal therapy. Rapid vasodilator effect lasts 10–30 min and can be used prophylactically to prevent, as well as abort, anginal attacks. Long-acting preparations are used to prevent recurrences. May cause headache, dizziness, lightheadedness—symptoms that usually pass quickly. If headache is intolerable, alteration of dose or discontinuation of drug may be necessary.

Reduces frequency and severity of attack by producing prolonged/continuous vasodilation.

Reduces angina by reducing the heart's workload. (Refer to ND: Cardiac Output, decreased, following.) *Note:* Often these drugs alone are sufficient to relieve angina in less severe conditions.

Usually sufficient analgesia for relief of headache caused by dilation of cerebral vessels in response to nitrates.

Potent narcotic analgesic may be used in acute onset because of its several beneficial effects, e.g., causes peripheral vasodilation and reduces myocardial workload; has a sedative effect to produce relaxation; interrupts the flow of vasoconstricting catecholamines and thereby effectively relieves severe chest pain. MS is given IV for rapid action and because decreased cardiac output compromises peripheral tissue absorption.

Have an antianginal effect because of direct coronary vasodilation.

Ischemia during anginal attack may cause transient ST segment depression or elevation and T wave inversion. Serial tracings verify ischemic changes, which may disappear when patient is pain-free. They also provide a baseline against which to compare later pattern changes.

NURSING DIAGNOSIS: Cardiac Output, risk for decreased

Risk factors may include
Inotropic changes (transient/prolonged myocardial ischemia, effects of medications)
Alterations in rate/rhythm and electrical conduction

Possibly evidenced by
[Not applicable; presence of signs and symptoms establishes an *actual* diagnosis]

DESIRED OUTCOMES/EVALUATION CRITERIA—PATIENT WILL:

Cardiac Pump Effectiveness (NOC)

Report/display decreased episodes of dyspnea, angina, and dysrhythmias.
Demonstrate increased activity tolerance.
Participate in behaviors/activities that reduce the workload of the heart.

ACTIONS/INTERVENTIONS	RATIONALE
Hemodynamic Regulation (NIC)	
Independent	**Independent**
Maintain bedrest in position of comfort during acute episodes.	Decreases oxygen consumption/demand reducing myocardial workload and risk of decompensation.
Monitor vital signs (e.g., heart rate, BP) and cardiac rhythm.	Tachycardia may be present because of pain, anxiety, hypoxemia, and reduced cardiac output. Changes may also occur in BP (hypertension or hypotension) because of cardiac response. ECG changes reflecting ischemia/dysrhythmias indicate need for additional evaluation and therapeutic intervention.
Auscultate breath sounds and heart sounds. Listen for murmurs.	S_3, S_4, or crackles can occur with cardiac decompensation or some medications (especially β-blockers). Development of murmurs may reveal a valvular cause for chest pain (e.g., aortic stenosis, mitral stenosis) or papillary muscle rupture.
Provide for adequate rest periods. Assist with/perform self-care activities, as indicated.	Conserves energy, reduces cardiac workload.
Stress importance of avoiding straining/bearing down, especially during defecation.	Valsalva maneuver causes vagal stimulation, reducing heart rate (bradycardia), which may be followed by rebound tachycardia, both of which may impair cardiac output.
Encourage immediate reporting of pain for prompt administration of medications as indicated.	Timely interventions can reduce oxygen consumption and myocardial workload and may prevent/minimize cardiac complications.
Monitor for and document effects of/adverse response to medications, noting BP, heart rate, and rhythm (especially when giving combination of calcium antagonists, β-blockers, and nitrates).	Desired effect is to decrease myocardial oxygen demand by decreasing ventricular stress. Drugs with negative inotropic properties can decrease perfusion to an already ischemic myocardium. Combination of nitrates and β-blockers may have cumulative effect on cardiac output.
Assess for signs and symptoms of heart failure.	Angina is only a symptom of underlying pathology causing myocardial ischemia. Disease may compromise cardiac function to point of decompensation.

ACTIONS/INTERVENTIONS	RATIONALE
Independent	
Evaluate mental status, noting development of confusion, disorientation.	Reduced perfusion of the brain can produce observable changes in sensorium.
Note skin color and presence/quality of pulses.	Peripheral circulation is reduced when cardiac output falls, giving the skin a pale or gray color (depending on level of hypoxia) and diminishing the strength of peripheral pulses.
Collaborative	
Administer supplemental oxygen as needed.	Increases oxygen available for myocardial uptake to improve contractility, reduce ischemia, and reduce lactic acid levels.
Monitor pulse oximetry or ABGs as indicated.	Determines adequacy of respiratory function and/or O₂ therapy.
Measure cardiac output and other functional parameters as indicated.	Cardiac index, preload/afterload, contractility, and cardiac work can be measured noninvasively thorough various means, including thoracic electrical bioimpedance (TEB) technique. Useful in evaluating response to therapeutic interventions and identifying need for more aggressive/emergency care.
Administer medications as indicated:	
Calcium channel blockers, e.g., diltiazem (Cardizem), nifedipine (Procardia), verapamil (Calan);	Although differing in mode of action, calcium channel blockers play a major role in preventing and terminating ischemia induced by coronary artery spasm and in reducing vascular resistance, thereby decreasing BP and cardiac workload. *Note:* Procardia should be used in conjunction with β-blockers.
β-Blockers, e.g., atenolol (Tenormin), nadolol (Corgard), propranolol (Inderal), esmolol (Brevibloc);	These medications decrease cardiac workload by reducing heart rate and systolic BP. *Note:* Overdosage produces cardiac decompensation.
Acetylsalicylic acid (ASA), other antiplatelet agents, e.g., ticlopidine (Ticlid);	Useful in unstable angina, ASA diminishes platelet aggregation/clot formation. For patients with major GI intolerance, alternate drugs may be indicated.
IV heparin.	Bolus, followed by continuous infusion, is recommended to help reduce risk of subsequent MI and recurrent unstable angina for patients diagnosed with intermediate or high-risk unstable angina.
Monitor laboratory studies e.g., partial thromboplastin time (PTT), aPTT.	Evaluates therapy needs/effectiveness.
Discuss purpose and prepare for stress testing and cardiac catheterization, when indicated.	Stress testing provides information about the health/strength of the ventricles.

ACTIONS/INTERVENTIONS

Collaborative

Prepare for surgical intervention, angioplasty with/ without intracoronary stent placement, valve replacement, CABG, if indicated.

RATIONALE

Angioplasty (also called percutaneous transluminal coronary angioplasty [PTCA]) increases coronary blood flow by compression of atheromatous lesions and dilation of the vessel lumen in an occluded coronary artery. Intracoronary stents may be placed at the time of PTCA to provide structural support within the coronary artery and improve the odds of long-term patency. This procedure is preferred over the more invasive CABG surgery. CABG is the recommended treatment when testing confirms myocardial ischemia as a result of left main coronary artery disease or symptomatic three-vessel disease, especially those with left ventricular dysfunction.

Prepare for transfer to critical care unit if condition warrants.

Profound/prolonged chest pain with decreased cardiac output reflects development of complications requiring more intense/emergency interventions.

NURSING DIAGNOSIS: Anxiety [specify level]

May be related to
Situational crises
Threat to self-concept (altered image/abilities)
Underlying pathophysiological response
Threat to or change in health status (disease course that can lead to further compromise, debility, even death)
Negative self-talk

Possibly evidenced by
Expressed concern regarding changes in life events
Increased tension/helplessness
Apprehension, uncertainty, restlessness
Association of diagnosis with loss of healthy body image, loss of place/influence
View of self as noncontributing member of family/society
Fear of death as an imminent reality

DESIRED OUTCOMES/EVALUATION CRITERIA—PATIENT WILL:

Anxiety Control (NOC)

Verbalize awareness of feelings of anxiety and healthy ways to deal with them.
Report anxiety is reduced to a manageable level.
Express concerns about effect of disease on lifestyle, position within family and society.
Demonstrate effective coping strategies/problem-solving skills.

ACTIONS/INTERVENTIONS

Anxiety Reduction (NIC)

Independent

Explain purpose of tests and procedures, e.g., stress testing.

RATIONALE

Reduces anxiety attributable to fear of unknown diagnosis and prognosis.

ACTIONS/INTERVENTIONS	RATIONALE
Independent	
Promote expression of feelings and fears, e.g., denial, depression, and anger. Let patient/SO know these are normal reactions. Note statements of concern, such as "Heart attack is inevitable."	Unexpressed feelings may create internal turmoil and affect self-image. Verbalization of concerns reduces tension, verifies level of coping, and facilitates dealing with feelings. Presence of negative self-talk can increase level of anxiety and may contribute to exacerbation of angina attacks.
Encourage family and friends to treat patient as before.	Reassures patient that role in the family and business has not been altered.
Tell patient the medical regimen has been designed to reduce/limit future attacks and increase cardiac stability.	Encourages patient to test symptom control (e.g., no angina with certain levels of activity), to increase confidence in medical program, and integrate abilities into perceptions of self. (Refer to CP: Psychosocial Aspects of Care, ND: Anxiety [specify level]/Fear for additional considerations, p. 811).
Collaborative	
Administer sedatives, tranquilizers, as indicated.	May be desired to help patient to relax until physically able to re-establish adequate coping strategies.

NURSING DIAGNOSIS: Knowledge Deficit [Learning Need] regarding condition, treatment needs, self care and discharge needs

May be related to
Lack of exposure
Inaccurate/misinterpretation of information
Unfamiliarity with information resources

Possibly evidenced by
Questions; statement of concerns
Request for information
Inaccurate follow-through of instructions

DESIRED OUTCOMES/EVALUATION CRITERIA—PATIENT WILL:
Participate in learning process.
Assume responsibility for own learning, looking for information and asking questions.

Knowledge: Disease Process (NOC)

Verbalize understanding of condition/disease process and potential complications.

Knowledge: Treatment Regimen (NOC)

Verbalize understanding of /participate in therapeutic regimen.
Initiate necessary lifestyle changes.

ACTIONS/INTERVENTIONS	RATIONALE

Teaching: Disease Process (NIC)

Independent

Discuss pathophysiology of condition. Stress need for preventing and managing anginal attacks.

Patients with angina need to learn why it occurs and what they can do to control it. This is the focus of therapeutic management to reduce likelihood of myocardial infarction and promote healthy heart lifestyle.

Review significance of cholesterol levels and differentiate between LDL and HDL factors. Emphasize importance of periodic laboratory measurements.

Although recommended LDL is ±160 mg/dL, patients with two or more risk factors (e.g., smoking, hypertension, diabetes mellitus, positive family history) should keep LDL ±130 mg/dL and those with diagnosis of CAD need to keep LDL below 100 mg/dL. HDL below 35–45 is considered a risk factor; a level above 60 mg/dL is considered an advantage.

Encourage avoidance of factors/situations that may precipitate anginal episode, e.g., emotional stress, extensive or intense physical exertion, ingestion of large/heavy meal, especially at bedtime, exposure to extremes in environmental temperature.

May reduce incidence/severity of ischemic episodes. Helps patient manage symptoms.

Assist patient/SO to identify sources of physical and emotional stress and discuss ways that they can be avoided.

This is a crucial step in limiting/preventing anginal attacks.

Review importance of weight control, cessation of smoking, dietary changes, and exercise.

Knowledge of the significance of risk factors provides patient with opportunity to make needed changes. Patients with high cholesterol who do not respond to 6-month program of low-fat diet and regular exercise will require medication.

Encourage patient to follow prescribed reconditioning program; caution to avoid exhaustion.

Fear of triggering attacks may cause patient to avoid participation in activity that has been prescribed to enhance recovery (increase myocardial strength and form collateral circulation).

Discuss impact of illness on desired lifestyle and activities, including work, driving, sexual activity, and hobbies. Provide information, privacy, or consultation, as indicated.

Patient may be reluctant to resume/continue usual activities because of fear of anginal attack or death. Patient should take nitroglycerin prophylactically before any activity that is known to precipitate angina.

Demonstrate how/encourage patient to monitor own pulse and BP during/after activities, when appropriate, and to schedule/simplify activities, avoid strain, and take rest periods.

Allows patient to identify those activities that can be modified to avoid cardiac stress and stay below the anginal threshold.

Discuss steps to take when anginal attacks occur, e.g., cessation of activity, keeping "rescue" NTG on hand, administration of prn medication, use of relaxation techniques.

Being prepared for an event takes away the fear that patient will not know what to do if attack occurs.

ACTIONS/INTERVENTIONS	RATIONALE

Independent

Review prescribed medications for control/prevention of anginal attacks;

Angina is a complicated condition that often requires the use of many drugs given to decrease myocardial workload, improve coronary circulation, and control the occurrence of attacks.

Lipid-lowering agents, e.g., bile acid sequestrants, e.g., cholestyramine (Questran), colestipal (Colestid), nicotinic acid, and HMG-CoA reductase inhibitors, e.g., pravastatin (Pravachol), lovastatin (Mevacor), simvastatin (Zocor).

These drugs are considered first-line agents for lowering serum cholesterol levels. *Note:* Questran/ Colestid may inhibit absorption of fat-soluble vitamins and some drugs such as Coumadin, Lanoxin, and Inderal. The HMG-CoA reductase inhibitors may cause photosensitivity.

Stress importance of checking with physician before taking OTC drugs.

OTC drugs may potentiate or negate prescribed medications.

Discuss ASA and other antiplatelet agents as indicated.

May be given prophylactically on a daily basis to decrease platelet aggregation and improve coronary circulation. May prolong survival rate of patients with unstable angina.

Review symptoms to be reported to physician, e.g., increase in frequency/duration of attacks, changes in response to medications.

Knowledge of expectations can avoid undue concern for insignificant reasons or delay in treatment of important symptoms.

Discuss importance of follow-up appointments.

Angina is a symptom of progressive coronary artery disease that should be monitored and may require occasional adjustment of treatment regimen.

POTENTIAL CONSIDERATIONS following discharge from care setting (dependent on patient's age, physical condition/presence of complications, personal resources, and life responsibilities)

Pain [acute]—episodes of decreased myocardial blood flow/ischemia

Activity intolerance—imbalance between oxygen supply/demand, sedentary/stressful lifestyle

Denial, ineffective—learned response patterns (e.g., avoidance), cultural factors, personal and family value systems

Family Processes, altered—situational transition and crisis

Home Maintenance Management, impaired—altered ability to perform tasks, inadequate support systems, reluctance to request assistance

MYOCARDIAL INFARCTION

Myocardial infarction (MI) is caused by marked reduction/loss of blood flow through one or more of the coronary arteries, resulting in cardiac muscle ischemia and necrosis.

CARE SETTING

Inpatient acute hospital, step-down, or medical unit.

RELATED CONCERNS

Angina pectoris, page 64
Dysrhythmias, page 90
Heart failure: chronic, page 47
Psychosocial aspects of care, page 809
Thrombophlebitis: deep vein thrombosis, page 115

Patient Assessment Database

ACTIVITY/REST

May report:	Weakness, fatigue, loss of sleep
	Sedentary lifestyle, sporadic exercise schedule
May exhibit:	Tachycardia, dyspnea with rest/activity

CIRCULATION

May report:	History of previous MI, CAD, HF, hypertension, diabetes mellitus
May exhibit:	Blood pressure (BP) may be normal, increased, or decreased; postural changes may be noted from lying to sitting/standing
	Pulse may be normal; full/bounding, or have a weak/thready quality with delayed capillary refill; irregularities (dysrhythmias) may be present
	Heart sounds S_3/S_4 may reflect a pathological condition (e.g., cardiac failure, decreased ventricular contractility, or compliance)
	Murmurs may reflect valvular insufficiency or papillary muscle dysfunction
	Friction rub (suggests pericarditis)
	Heart rate regular or irregular; tachycardia/bradycardia may be present
	Edema: Jugular vein distention, peripheral/dependent edema, generalized edema
	Color: Pallor or cyanosis/mottling of skin, nailbeds, mucous membranes, and lips may be noted

EGO INTEGRITY

May report:	Denial of significance of symptoms/presence of condition
	Fear of dying, feelings of impending doom
	Anger at inconvenience of illness/"unnecessary" hospitalization
	Worry about family, job, finances
May exhibit:	Denial, withdrawal, anxiety, lack of eye contact
	Irritability, anger, combative behavior
	Focus on self/pain

ELIMINATION

May exhibit:	Normal or decreased bowel sounds

FOOD/FLUID

May report:	Nausea, loss of appetite, belching, indigestion/heartburn
May exhibit:	Poor skin turgor; dry or diaphoretic skin
	Vomiting

HYGIENE

May report/ exhibit: Difficulty in performing care tasks

NEUROSENSORY

May report: Dizziness, fainting spells in or out of bed (upright or at rest)

May exhibit: Changes in mentation
Weakness

PAIN/DISCOMFORT

May report: Sudden onset of chest pain unrelieved by rest or nitroglycerin (although most pain is deep and visceral, 20% of MIs are painless)

Location: Typically anterior chest (substernal, precordium); may radiate to arms, jaws, face; may have atypical location such as epigastrium/abdomen; elbow, jaw, back, neck

Quality: Crushing, constricting, viselike, squeezing, heavy, steady

Intensity: Usually 10 on a scale of 0–10 or "worst pain ever experienced." *Note:* Pain is sometimes absent in postoperative patients, those with diabetes mellitus or hypertension, or the elderly

Precipitating factor: May/may not be associated with activity

May exhibit: Facial grimacing, changes in body posture, may place clenched fist on midsternum when describing pain

Crying, groaning, squirming, stretching

Withdrawal, lack of eye contact

Autonomic responses: Changes in heart rate/rhythm, BP, respirations, skin color/moisture, level of consciousness

RESPIRATION

May report: Dyspnea with/without exertion, nocturnal dyspnea
Cough with/without sputum production
History of smoking, chronic respiratory disease

May exhibit: Increased respiratory rate, shallow/labored breathing
Pallor or cyanosis
Breath sounds clear or crackles/wheezes
Sputum clear, pink-tinged

SOCIAL INTERACTION

May report: Recent stress, e.g., work, family
Difficulty coping with recent/current stressors, e.g., money, work, family problems made worse by this illness/hospitalization

May exhibit: Difficulty resting quietly, overemotional responses (intense anger, fear)
Withdrawal from family

TEACHING/LEARNING

May report: Family history of heart disease/MI, diabetes, stroke, hypertension, peripheral vascular disease
Use of tobacco

Discharge plan considerations: **DRG projected length of inpatient stay: 4.9–7.0 days; (2–4 days/critical care unit [CCU])**
May require assistance with food preparation, shopping, transportation, homemaking/maintenance tasks; physical layout of home

DIAGNOSTIC STUDIES

ECG: ST elevation signifying ischemia, peaked upright or inverted T wave indicating injury; development of Q waves signifying prolonged ischemia or necrosis.

Cardiac enzymes and isoenzymes:

CPK-MB (isoenzyme in cardiac muscle): Elevate within 4–8 hr, peak in 12–20 hr, return to normal in 48–72 hr.

LDH: Elevates within 8–24 hr, peaks within 72–144 hr, and may take as long as 14 days to return to normal. An LDH_1 greater than LDH_2 (flipped ratio) helps confirm/diagnose MI if not detected in acute phase.

Troponins: Troponin I (cTnI) and troponin T (cTnT): Levels are elevated at 3–12 hr, peak at 24–48 hr, and return to baseline over 5–14 days. These enzymes have increased specificity for necrosis and are therefore useful in diagnosing postoperative MI when MB-CPK may be elevated related to skeletal trauma.

Electrolytes: Imbalances of sodium and potassium can alter conduction and compromise contractility.

WBC: Leukocytosis (10,000–20,000) usually appears on the second day after MI because of the inflammatory process.

Sedimentation rate (ESR): Rises on second or third day after MI, indicating inflammatory response.

Chemistry profiles: May be abnormal, depending on acute/chronic abnormal organ function/perfusion.

ABGs/pulse oximetry: May indicate hypoxia or acute/chronic lung disease processes.

Lipids (total lipids, HDL, LDL, VLDL, total cholesterol, triglycerides, phospholipids): Elevations may reflect arteriosclerosis as a cause for coronary narrowing or spasm.

Chest x-ray: May be normal or show an enlarged cardiac shadow suggestive of HF or ventricular aneurysm.

Two-dimensional echocardiogram: May be done to determine dimensions of chambers, septal/ventricular wall motion, ejection fraction (blood flow), and valve configuration/function.

Nuclear imaging studies:

> *Persantine Thallium:* Evaluate myocardial blood flow and status of myocardial cells, e.g., location/extent of acute/previous MI.
>
> *Cardiac blood imaging/MUGA:* Evaluates specific and general ventricular performance, regional wall motion, and ejection fraction.
>
> *Technetium:* Accumulates in ischemic cells, outlining necrotic area(s).

Coronary angiography: Visualizes narrowing/occlusion of coronary arteries and is usually done in conjunction with measurements of chamber pressures and assessment of left ventricular function (ejection fraction). Procedure is not usually done in acute phase of MI unless angioplasty or emergency heart surgery is imminent.

Digital subtraction angiography (DSA): Technique used to visualize status of arterial bypass grafts and to detect peripheral artery disease.

MRI: Allows visualization of blood flow, cardiac chambers/intraventricular septum, valves, vascular lesions, plaque formations, areas of necrosis/infarction, and blood clots.

Exercise stress test: Determines cardiovascular response to activity (often done in conjunction with thallium imaging in the recovery phase).

NURSING PRIORITIES

1. Relieve pain, anxiety.
2. Reduce myocardial workload.
3. Prevent/detect and assist in treatment of life-threatening dysrhythmias or complications.
4. Promote cardiac health, self-care.

DISCHARGE GOALS

1. Chest pain absent/controlled.
2. Heart rate/rhythm sufficient to sustain adequate cardiac output/tissue perfusion.
3. Achievement of activity level sufficient for basic self-care.
4. Anxiety reduced/managed.
5. Disease process, treatment plan, and prognosis understood.
6. Plan in place to meet needs after discharge.

ACTIONS/INTERVENTIONS	RATIONALE
Pain Management (NIC)	
Independent	
Monitor/document characteristics of pain, noting verbal reports, nonverbal cues (e.g., moaning, crying, restlessness, diaphoresis, clutching chest, rapid breathing), and hemodynamic response (BP/heart rate changes).	Variation of appearance and behavior of patients in pain may present a challenge in assessment. Most patients with an acute MI appear ill, distracted, and focused on pain. Verbal history and deeper investigation of precipitating factors should be postponed until pain is relieved. Respirations may be increased as a result of pain and associated anxiety; release of stress-induced catecholamines increases heart rate and BP.
Obtain full description of pain from patient including location, intensity (0–10), duration, characteristics (dull/crushing), and radiation. Assist patient to quantify pain by comparing it to other experiences.	Pain is a subjective experience and must be described by the patient. Provides baseline for comparison to aid in determining effectiveness of therapy, resolution/progression of problem.
Review history of previous angina, anginal equivalent, or MI pain. Discuss family history if pertinent.	May differentiate current pain from preexisting patterns, as well as identify complications such as extension of infarction, pulmonary embolus, or pericarditis.
Instruct patient to report pain immediately.	Delay in reporting pain hinders pain relief/may require increased dosage of medication to achieve relief. In addition, severe pain may induce shock by stimulating the sympathetic nervous system, thereby creating further damage and interfering with diagnostics and relief of pain.
Provide quiet environment, calm activities, and comfort measures (e.g., dry/wrinkle-free linens, backrub). Approach the patient calmly and confidently.	Decreases external stimuli, which may aggravate anxiety and cardiac strain, limit coping abilities and adjustment to current situation.
Assist/instruct in relaxation techniques, e.g., deep/slow breathing, distraction behaviors, visualization, guided imagery.	Helpful in decreasing perception of/response to pain. Provides a sense of having some control over the situation, increase in positive attitude.

ACTIONS/INTERVENTIONS	RATIONALE

Independent

Check vital signs before and after narcotic medication.

Hypotension/respiratory depression can occur as a result of narcotic administration. These problems may increase myocardial damage in presence of ventricular insufficiency.

Collaborative

Administer supplemental oxygen by means of nasal cannula or face mask, as indicated.

Increases amount of oxygen available for myocardial uptake and thereby may relieve discomfort associated with tissue ischemia.

Administer medications as indicated, e.g.:

Antianginals, e.g., nitroglycerin (Nitro-Bid, Nitrostat, Nitro-Dur);

Nitrates are useful for pain control by coronary vasodilating effects, which increase coronary blood flow and myocardial perfusion. Peripheral vasodilation effects reduce the volume of blood returning to the heart (preload), thereby decreasing myocardial workload and oxygen demand.

β-Blockers, e.g., atenolol (Tenormin), pindolol (Visken), propranolol (Inderal);

Important second-line agents for pain control through effect of blocking sympathetic stimulation, thereby reducing heart rate, systolic BP, and myocardial oxygen demand. May be given alone or with nitrates. *Note:* β-Blockers may be contraindicated if myocardial contractility is severely impaired because negative inotropic properties can further reduce contractility.

Analgesics, e.g., morphine, meperidine (Demerol).

Although intravenous (IV) morphine is the usual drug of choice, other injectable narcotics may be used in acute-phase/recurrent chest pain unrelieved by nitroglycerin to reduce severe pain, provide sedation, and decrease myocardial workload. IM injections should be avoided, if possible, because they can alter the CPK diagnostic indicator and are not well absorbed in underperfused tissue.

NURSING DIAGNOSIS: Activity Intolerance

May be related to
Imbalance between myocardial oxygen supply and demand
Presence of ischemia/necrotic myocardial tissues
Cardiac depressant effects of certain drugs (β-blockers, antidysrhythmics)

Possibly evidenced by
Alterations in heart rate and BP with activity
Development of dysrhythmias
Changes in skin color/moisture
Exertional angina
Generalized weakness

DESIRED OUTCOMES/EVALUATION CRITERIA—PATIENT WILL:

Endurance (NOC)

Demonstrate measurable/progressive increase in tolerance for activity with heart rate/rhythm and BP within patient's normal limits and skin warm, pink, dry.
Report absence of angina with activity.

Energy Management (NIC)

Independent

Record/document heart rate, rhythm, and BP changes before, during, and after activity, as indicated. Correlate with reports of chest pain/shortness of breath. (Refer to ND: Cardiac Output, decreased risk for, p. 82.)

Trends determine patient's response to activity and may indicate myocardial oxygen deprivation that may require decrease in activity level/return to bedrest, changes in medication regimen, or use of supplemental oxygen.

Encourage rest (bed/chair) initially. Thereafter, limit activity on basis of pain/or adverse cardiac response. Provide nonstress diversional activities.

Reduces myocardial workload/oxygen consumption, reducing risk of complications (e.g., extension of MI). *Note:* American Heart Association/American College of Cardiology guidelines (1996) suggest that patients with cardiac conditions should not be kept in bed longer than 24 hr. Patients with uncomplicated MI are encouraged to engage in mild activity out of bed, including short walks when 12 hr postincident.

Instruct patient to avoid increasing abdominal pressure, e.g., straining during defecation.

Activities that require holding the breath and bearing down (Valsalva maneuver) can result in bradycardia (temporarily reduced cardiac output) and rebound tachycardia with elevated BP.

Explain pattern of graded increase of activity level, e.g., getting up to commode or sitting in chair, progressive ambulation, and resting after meals.

Progressive activity provides a controlled demand on the heart, increasing strength and preventing overexertion.

Review signs/symptoms reflecting intolerance of present activity level or requiring notification of nurse/physician.

Palpitations, pulse irregularities, development of chest pain, or dyspnea may indicate need for changes in exercise regimen or medication.

Collaborative

Refer to cardiac rehabilitation program.

Provides continued support/additional supervision and participation in recovery and wellness process.

NURSING DIAGNOSIS: Anxiety [specify level]/Fear

May be related to
Threat to or change in health and socioeconomic status
Threat of loss/death
Unconscious conflict about essential values, beliefs, and goals of life
Interpersonal transmission/contagion

Possibly evidenced by
Fearful attitude
Apprehension, increased tension, restlessness, facial tension
Uncertainty, feelings of inadequacy
Somatic complaints/sympathetic stimulation
Focus on self, expressions of concern about current and future events
Fight (e.g., belligerent attitude) or flight behavior

DESIRED OUTCOMES/EVALUATION CRITERIA—PATIENT WILL:

Anxiety/Fear Control (NOC)

Recognize feelings.
Identify causes, contributing factors.
Verbalize reduction of anxiety/fear.
Demonstrate positive problem-solving skills.
Identify/use resources appropriately.

ACTIONS/INTERVENTIONS	RATIONALE

Anxiety Reduction (NIC)

Independent

Identify and acknowledge patient's perception of threat/situation. Encourage expressions of—and do not deny—feelings of anger, grief, sadness, fear.	Coping with the pain and emotional trauma of an MI is difficult. Patient may fear death and/or be anxious about immediate environment. Ongoing anxiety (related to concerns about impact of heart attack on future lifestyle, matters left unattended/unresolved, and effects of illness on family) may be present in varying degrees for some time and may be manifested by symptoms of depression.
Note presence of hostility, withdrawal, and/or denial (inappropriate affect or refusal to comply with medical regimen).	Research into survival rates between type A and type B individuals and the impact of denial has been ambiguous; however, studies show some correlation between degree/expression of anger or hostility and an increased risk for MI.
Maintain confident manner (without false reassurance).	Patient and SO can be affected by the anxiety/uneasiness displayed by health team members. Honest explanations can alleviate anxiety.
Observe for verbal/nonverbal signs of anxiety and stay with patient. Intervene if patient displays destructive behavior.	Patient may not express concern directly, but words/actions may convey sense of agitation, aggression, and hostility. Intervention can help patient to regain control of own behavior.
Accept but do not reinforce use of denial. Avoid confrontations.	Denial can be beneficial in decreasing anxiety but can postpone dealing with the reality of the current situation. Confrontation can promote anger and increase use of denial reducing cooperation, and possibly impeding recovery.
Orient patient/SO to routine procedures and expected activities. Promote participation when possible.	Predictability and information can decrease anxiety for patient.
Answer all questions factually. Provide consistent information; repeat as indicated.	Accurate information about the situation reduces fear, strengthens nurse-patient relationship, and assists patient/SO to deal realistically with situation. Attention span may be short, and repetition of information helps with retention.
Encourage patient/SO to communicate with one another, sharing questions and concerns.	Sharing information elicits support/comfort and can relieve tension of unexpressed worries.
Provide privacy for patient and SO.	Allows needed time for personal expression of feelings; may enhance mutual support and promote more adaptive behaviors.
Provide rest periods/uninterrupted sleep time, quiet surroundings, with patient controlling type, amount of external stimuli.	Conserves energy and enhances coping abilities.
Support normality of grieving process, including time necessary for resolution.	Can provide reassurance that feelings are normal response to situation/perceived changes.
Encourage independence, self-care, and decision making within accepted treatment plan.	Increased independence from staff promotes self-confidence and reduces feelings of abandonment that can accompany transfer from coronary unit/discharge from hospital.

ACTIONS/INTERVENTIONS	RATIONALE

Independent

Encourage discussion about postdischarge expectations.	Helps patient/SO identify realistic goals, thereby reducing risk of discouragement in face of the reality of limitations of condition/pace of recuperation.

Collaborative

Administer antianxiety/hypnotics as indicated, e.g., diazepam (Valium), lorazepam (Ativan), flurazepam (Dalmane).	Promotes relaxation/rest and reduces feelings of anxiety.

NURSING DIAGNOSIS: Cardiac Output, risk for decreased

Risk factors may include
Changes in rate, rhythm, electrical conduction
Reduced preload/increased SVR
Infarcted/dyskinetic muscle, structural defects, e.g., ventricular aneurysm, septal defects

Possibly evidenced by
[Not applicable; presence of signs and symptoms establishes *actual* diagnosis]

DESIRED OUTCOMES/EVALUATION CRITERIA—PATIENT WILL:

Cardiac Pump Effectiveness (NOC)

Maintain hemodynamic stability, e.g., BP, cardiac output within normal range, adequate urinary output, decreased frequency/absence of dysrhythmias.
Report decreased episodes of dyspnea, angina.
Demonstrate an increase in activity tolerance.

ACTIONS/INTERVENTIONS	RATIONALE

Cardiac Care: Acute (NIC)

Independent

Auscultate BP. Compare both arms and obtain lying, sitting, and standing pressures when able.	Hypotension may occur related to ventricular dysfunction, hypoperfusion of the myocardium, and vagal stimulation. However, hypertension is also a common phenomenon, possibly related to pain, anxiety, catecholamine release, and/or preexisting vascular problems. Orthostatic (postural) hypotension may be associated with complications of infarct, e.g., HF.
Evaluate quality and equality of pulses, as indicated.	Decreased cardiac output results in diminished weak/thready pulses. Irregularities suggest dysrhythmias, which may require further evaluation/monitoring.

ACTIONS/INTERVENTIONS	RATIONALE
Independent	
Auscultate heart sound:	
Note development of S_3, S_4;	S_3 is usually associated with HF, but it may also be noted with the mitral insufficiency (regurgitation) and left ventricular overload that can accompany severe infarction. S_4 may be associated with myocardial ischemia, ventricular stiffening, and pulmonary or systemic hypertension.
Presence of murmurs/rubs.	Indicates disturbances of normal blood flow within the heart, e.g., incompetent valve, septal defect, or vibration of papillary muscle/chordae tendinea (complication of MI). Presence of rub with an infarction is also associated with inflammation, e.g., pericardial effusion and pericarditis.
Auscultate breath sounds.	Crackles reflecting pulmonary congestion may develop because of depressed myocardial function.
Monitor heart rate and rhythm. Document dysrhythmias via telemetry.	Heart rate and rhythm respond to medication, activity and developing complications. Dysrhythmias (especially premature ventricular contractions or progressive heart blocks) can compromise cardiac function or increase ischemic damage. Acute or chronic atrial flutter/fibrillation may be seen with coronary artery or valvular involvement and may or may not be pathological.
Note response to activity and promote rest appropriately. (Refer to ND: Activity intolerance, p. 79.)	Overexertion increases oxygen consumption/demand and can compromise myocardial function.
Provide small/easily digested meals. Limit caffeine intake, e.g., coffee, chocolate, cola.	Large meals may increase myocardial workload and cause vagal stimulation, resulting in bradycardia/ectopic beats. Caffeine is a direct cardiac stimulant that can increase heart rate. *Note:* New guidelines suggest no need to restrict caffeine in regular coffee drinkers.
Have emergency equipment/medications available.	Sudden coronary occlusion, lethal dysrhythmias, extension of infarct, and unrelenting pain are situations that may precipitate cardiac arrest, requiring immediate life-saving therapies/transfer to CCU.
Collaborative	
Administer supplemental oxygen, as indicated.	Increases amount of oxygen available for myocardial uptake, reducing ischemia and resultant cellular irritation/dysrhythmias.
Measure cardiac output and other functional parameters as appropriate.	Cardiac index, preload/afterload, contractility, and cardiac work can be measured noninvasively with thoracic electrical bioimpedance (TEB) technique. Useful in evaluating response to therapeutic interventions and identifying need for more aggressive/emergency care.
Maintain IV/hep-lock access as indicated.	Patent line is important for administration of emergency drugs in presence of persistent lethal dysrhythmias or chest pain.

ACTIONS/INTERVENTIONS	RATIONALE
Collaborative	
Review serial ECGs.	Provides information regarding progression/resolution of infarction, status of ventricular function, electrolyte balance, and effects of drug therapies.
Review chest x-ray.	May reflect pulmonary edema related to ventricular dysfunction.
Monitor laboratory data: e.g., cardiac enzymes, ABGs, electrolytes.	Enzymes monitor resolution/extension of infarction. Presence of hypoxia indicates need for supplemental oxygen. Electrolyte imbalance, e.g., hypokalemia/hyperkalemia, adversely affects cardiac rhythm/contractility.
Administer antidysrhythmic drugs as indicated. (Refer to CP: Dysrhythmias, p. 90.)	Dysrhythmias are usually treated symptomatically, except for PVCs, which are often treated prophylactically. Early inclusion of ACE inhibitor therapy (especially in presence of large anterior MI, ventricular aneurysm, or HF) enhances ventricular output, increases survival, and may slow progression of HF. *Note:* Use of routine lidocaine is no longer recommended.
Assist with insertion/maintain pacemaker, when used.	Pacing may be a temporary support measure during acute phase or may be needed permanently if infarction severely damages conduction system, impairing systolic function. Evaluation is based on echocardiography or radionuclide ventriculography.

NURSING DIAGNOSIS: Tissue Perfusion, risk for altered

Risk factors may include
Reduction/interruption of blood flow, e.g., vasoconstriction, hypovolemia/shunting, and thromboembolic formation

Possibly evidenced by
[Not applicable; presence of signs and symptoms establishes an *actual* diagnosis]

DESIRED OUTCOMES/EVALUATION CRITERIA—PATIENT WILL:

Cardiac Pump Effectiveness (NOC)

Demonstrate adequate perfusion as individually appropriate, e.g., skin warm and dry, peripheral pulses present/strong, vital signs within patient's normal range, patient alert/oriented, balanced I&O, absence of edema, free of pain/discomfort.

ACTIONS/INTERVENTIONS	RATIONALE
Circulatory Care (NIC)	
Independent	
Investigate sudden changes or continued alterations in mentation, e.g., anxiety, confusion, lethargy, stupor.	Cerebral perfusion is directly related to cardiac output and is also influenced by electrolyte/acid-base variations, hypoxia, and systemic emboli.

ACTIONS/INTERVENTIONS	RATIONALE
Independent	
Inspect for pallor, cyanosis, mottling, cool/clammy skin. Note strength of peripheral pulse.	Systemic vasoconstriction resulting from diminished cardiac output may be evidenced by decreased skin perfusion and diminished pulses. (Refer to ND: Cardiac Output, risk for decreased, p. 82.)
Assess for Homans' sign (pain in calf on dorsiflexion), erythema, edema.	Indicators of deep vein thrombosis (DVT), although DVT can be present without a positive Homans' sign.
Encourage active/passive leg exercises, avoidance of isometric exercises.	Enhances venous return, reduces venous stasis, and decreases risk of thrombophlebitis; however, isometric exercises can adversely affect cardiac output by increasing myocardial work and oxygen consumption.
Instruct patient in application/periodic removal of antiembolic hose, when used.	Limits venous stasis, improves venous return, and reduces risk of thrombophlebitis in patient who is limited in activity.
Monitor respirations, note work of breathing.	Cardiac pump failure and/or ischemic pain may precipitate respiratory distress; however, sudden/continued dyspnea may indicate thromboembolic pulmonary complications.
Assess GI function, noting anorexia, decreased/absent bowel sounds, nausea/vomiting, abdominal distention, constipation.	Reduced blood flow to mesentery can produce GI dysfunction, e.g., loss of peristalsis. Problems may be potentiated/aggravated by use of analgesics, decreased activity, and dietary changes.
Monitor intake, note changes in urine output. Record urine specific gravity as indicated.	Decreased intake/persistent nausea may result in reduced circulating volume, which negatively affects perfusion and organ function. Specific gravity measurements reflect hydration status and renal function.
Collaborative	
Monitor laboratory data, e.g., ABGs, BUN, creatinine, electrolytes, coagulation studies (PT, aPTT, clotting times).	Indicators of organ perfusion/function. Abnormalities in coagulation may occur as a result of therapeutic measures (e.g., heparin/Coumadin use and some cardiac drugs).
Administer medications as indicated, e.g.:	
Aspirin;	Aspirin is used as antiplatelet therapy, which reduces mortality in MI patients, and is taken daily. Aspirin also reduces coronary reocclusion after percutaneous transluminal coronary angioplasty (PTCA).
Heparin/warfarin sodium (Coumadin);	Low-dose heparin is given during PTCA and may be given prophylactically in high-risk patients (e.g., atrial fibrillation, obesity, ventricular aneurysm, or history of thrombophlebitis) to reduce risk of thrombophlebitis or mural thrombus formation. Coumadin is the drug of choice for long-term/postdischarge anticoagulant therapy.
Cimetidine (Tagamet), ranitidine (Zantac), antacids.	Reduces or neutralizes gastric acid, preventing discomfort and gastric irritation, especially in presence of reduced mucosal circulation.

ACTIONS/INTERVENTIONS

Collaborative

Assist with perfusion therapy:

Administer thrombolytic agents, e.g., alteplase (Activase, rt-PA), reteplase (Retavase), streptokinase (Streptase), anistraplase (APSAC), urokinase (Abbokinase);

Prepare for PTCA, also called balloon angioplasty, possibly with intracoronary stents;

Transfer to critical care.

RATIONALE

Thrombolytic therapy is the treatment of choice (when initiated within 6 hr) to dissolve the clot (if that is the cause of the MI) and restore perfusion of the myocardium.

This procedure is employed to open partially blocked coronary arteries before they become totally blocked. The mechanism includes a combination of vessel stretching and plaque compression. Intracoronary stents may be placed at the time of PTCA to provide structural support within the coronary artery and improve the odds of long-term patency.

More intensive monitoring and aggressive interventions are necessary to promote optimum outcome.

NURSING DIAGNOSIS: Fluid Volume risk for excess

Risk factors may include
Decreased organ perfusion (renal)
Increased sodium/water retention
Increased hydrostatic pressure or decreased plasma proteins (sequestering of fluid in interstitial space/tissues)

Possibly evidenced by
[Not applicable; presence of signs and symptoms establishes an *actual* diagnosis]

DESIRED OUTCOMES/EVALUATION CRITERIA—PATIENT WILL:

Fluid Balance (NOC)

Maintain fluid balance as evidenced by BP within patient's normal limits.
Be free of peripheral/venous distension and dependent edema, with lungs clear and weight stable.

ACTIONS/INTERVENTIONS

Fluid Management (NIC)

Independent

Auscultate breath sounds for presence of crackles.

Note JVD, development of dependent edema.

Measure I&O, noting decrease in output, concentrated appearance. Calculate fluid balance.

Weigh daily.

RATIONALE

May indicate pulmonary edema secondary to cardiac decompensation.

Suggests developing congestive failure/fluid volume excess.

Decreased cardiac output results in impaired kidney perfusion, sodium/water retention, and reduced urine output.

Sudden changes in weight reflect alterations in fluid balance.

ACTIONS/INTERVENTIONS

Independent

Maintain total fluid intake at 2000 ml/24 hr within cardiovascular tolerance.

Collaborative

Provide low-sodium diet/beverages.

Administer diuretics, e.g., furosemide (Lasix), spironolactone with hydrochlorothiazide (Aldactazide), hydralazine (Apresoline).

Monitor potassium as indicated.

RATIONALE

Meets normal adult body fluid requirements but may require alteration/restriction in presence of cardiac decompensation.

Sodium enhances fluid retention and should therefore be restricted during active MI phase and/or if heart failure is present.

May be necessary to correct fluid overload. Drug choice is usually dependent on acute/chronic nature of symptoms.

Hypokalemia can limit effectiveness of therapy and can occur with use of potassium-depleting diuretics.

NURSING DIAGNOSIS: Knowledge Deficit [Learning Need] regarding cause/treatment of condition, self care, and discharge needs

May be related to
Lack of information/misunderstanding of medical condition/therapy needs
Unfamiliarity with information resources
Lack of recall

Possibly evidenced by
Questions; statement of misconception
Failure to improve on previous regimen
Development of preventable complications

DESIRED OUTCOMES/EVALUATION CRITERIA—PATIENT WILL:

> **Knowledge: Disease Process (NOC)**

Verbalize understanding of condition, potential complications, individual risk factors, and function of pacemaker (if used).
Relate signs of pacemaker failure.

> **Knowledge: Treatment Regimen (NOC)**

Verbalize understanding of therapeutic regimen.
List desired action and possible adverse side effects of medications.
Correctly perform necessary procedures and explain reasons for actions.

ACTIONS/INTERVENTIONS

> **Teaching: Individual (NIC)**

Independent

Assess patient/SO level of knowledge and ability/desire to learn.

RATIONALE

Necessary for creation of individual instruction plan. Reinforces expectation that this will be a "learning experience." Verbalization identifies misunderstandings and allows for clarification.

ACTIONS/INTERVENTIONS	RATIONALE

Independent

Be alert to signs of avoidance, e.g., changing subject away from information being presented or extremes of behavior (withdrawal/euphoria).

Natural defense mechanisms, such as anger or denial of significance of situation, can block learning, affecting patient's response and ability to assimilate information. Changing to a less formal/structured style may be more effective until patient/SO is ready to accept/deal with current situation.

Present information in varied learning formats, e.g., programmed books, audiovisual tapes, question-and-answer sessions, group activities.

Using multiple learning methods enhances retention of material.

Cardiac Care: Rehabilitation (NIC)

Reinforce explanations of risk factors, dietary/activity restrictions, medications, and symptoms requiring immediate medical attention.

Provides opportunity for patient to retain information and to assume control/participate in rehabilitation program. *Note:* Routine use of supplements/herbal remedies (e.g., ginkgo biloba, garlic, vitamin E) can result in alterations in blood clotting, especially when anticoagulant/ASA therapy is prescribed.

Encourage identification/reduction of individual risk factors, e.g., smoking/alcohol consumption, obesity.

These behaviors/chemicals have direct adverse effects on cardiovascular function and may impede recovery, increase risk for complications.

Warn against isometric activity, Valsalva maneuver, and activities requiring arms positioned above head.

These activities greatly increase cardiac workload and myocardial oxygen consumption and may adversely affect myocardial contractility/output.

Review programmed increases in levels of activity. Educate patient regarding gradual resumption of activities, e.g., walking, work, recreational and sexual activity. Provide guidelines for gradually increasing activity and instruction regarding target heart rate and pulse taking, as appropriate.

Gradual increase in activity increases strength and prevents overexertion, may enhance collateral circulation, and allows return to normal lifestyle. *Note:* Sexual activity can be safely resumed once patient can accomplish activity equivalent to climbing two flights of stairs without adverse cardiac effects.

Identify alternate activities for "bad weather" days, such as measured walking in house or shopping mall.

Provides for continuing daily activity program.

Review signs/symptoms requiring reduction in activity and notification of healthcare provider. Differentiate between increased heart rate that normally occurs during various activities and worsening signs of cardiac stress (e.g., chest pain, dyspnea, palpitations, increased heart rate lasting more than 15 min after cessation of activity, excessive fatigue the following day).

Pulse elevations beyond established limits, development of chest pain, or dyspnea may require changes in exercise and medication regimen.

Stress importance of follow-up care and identify community resources/support groups, e.g., cardiac rehabilitation programs, "coronary clubs," smoking cessation clinics.

Reinforces that this is an ongoing/continuing health problem for which support/assistance is available postdischarge.

Emphasize importance of contacting physician if chest pain, change in anginal pattern, or other symptoms recur.

Timely evaluation/intervention may prevent complications.

Stress importance of reporting development of fever in association with diffuse/atypical chest pain (pleural, pericardial) and joint pain.

Post-MI complication of pericardial inflammation (Dressler's syndrome) requires further medical evaluation/intervention.

ACTIONS/INTERVENTIONS	RATIONALE
Independent	
Encourage patient/SO to share concerns/feelings. Discuss signs of pathological depression versus transient feelings frequently associated with major life events. Recommend seeking professional help if depressed feelings persist.	Depressed patients have a greater risk of dying 6–18 mo following a heart attack. Timely intervention may be beneficial. *Note:* Serotonin reuptake inhibitors (SSRIs), e.g., paroxetine (Paxil), have been found to be as effective as tricyclic antidepressants but with significantly fewer adverse cardiac complications.

POTENTIAL CONSIDERATIONS following discharge from care setting (dependent on patient's age, physical condition/presence of complications, personal resources, and life responsibilities)

Activity intolerance—imbalance between myocardial oxygen supply/demand.

Grieving, anticipatory—perceived loss of general well-being, required changes in lifestyle, confronting mortality.

Decisional Conflict (treatment)—multiple/divergent sources of information, perceived threat to value system, support system deficit.

Family Processes, altered—situational transition and crisis.

Home Maintenance Management, impaired—altered ability to perform tasks, inadequate support systems, reluctance to request assistance.

DYSRHYTHMIAS (INCLUDING DIGITALIS TOXICITY)

A cardiac dysrhythmia is any disturbance in the normal rhythm of the electrical excitation of the heart. It can be the result of a primary cardiac disorder, a response to a systemic condition, the result of electrolyte imbalance or drug toxicity. Dysrhythmias vary in severity and in their effects on cardiac function, which are partially influenced by the site of origin (ventricular or supraventricular).

CARE SETTING

Generally, minor dysrhythmias are monitored and treated in the community setting; however, potential life-threatening situations usually require a short inpatient stay.

RELATED CONCERNS

Angina pectoris, page 64
Heart failure: chronic, page 47
Myocardial infarction, page 75
Psychosocial aspects of care, page 809

Patient Assessment Database

ACTIVITY/REST

May report: Generalized weakness and exertional fatigue

May exhibit: Changes in heart rate/BP with activity/exercise

CIRCULATION

May report: History of previous/acute MI (90%–95% experience dysrhythmias), cardiomyopathy, HF, valvular heart disease, hypertension, use of pacemaker
                      Pulse: Fast, slow, or irregular; palpitations, skipped beats

May exhibit: BP changes (hypertension or hypotension) during episodes of dysrhythmia
                      Pulses may be irregular, e.g., skipped beats; pulsus alternans (regular strong beat/weak beat); bigeminal pulse (irregular strong beat/weak beat)
                      Pulse deficit (difference between apical pulse and radial pulse)
                      Heart sounds: irregular rhythm, extra sounds, dropped beats
                      Skin color and moisture changes, e.g., pallor, cyanosis, diaphoresis (heart failure, shock)
                      Edema dependent, generalized, JVD (in presence of heart failure)
                      Urine output decreased if cardiac output is severely diminished

EGO INTEGRITY

May report: Feeling nervous (certain tachydysrhythmias), sense of impending doom
                      Stressors related to current medical problems

May exhibit: Anxiety, fear, withdrawal, anger, irritability, crying

FOOD/FLUID

May report: Loss of appetite, anorexia
                      Food intolerance (with certain medications)
                      Nausea/vomiting
                      Changes in weight

May exhibit: Weight gain or loss
                      Edema
                      Changes in skin moisture/turgor
                      Respiratory crackles

NEUROSENSORY

May report: Dizzy spells, fainting, headaches

May exhibit:	Mental status/sensorium changes, e.g., disorientation, confusion, loss of memory; changes in usual speech pattern/consciousness, stupor, coma
	Behavioral changes, e.g., combativeness, lethargy, hallucinations
	Pupil changes (equal and react to light)
	Loss of deep tendon reflexes with life-threatening dysrhythmias (ventricular tachycardia, severe bradycardia)

PAIN/DISCOMFORT

May report:	Chest pain, mild to severe, which may or may not be relieved by antianginal medication
May exhibit:	Distraction behaviors, e.g., restlessness

RESPIRATION

May report:	Chronic lung disease
	History of or current tobacco use
	Shortness of breath
	Coughing (with/without sputum production)
May exhibit:	Changes in respiratory rate/depth during dysrhythmia episode
	Breath sounds: Adventitious sounds (crackles, rhonchi, wheezing) may be present, indicating respiratory complications, such as left-sided heart failure (pulmonary edema) or pulmonary thromboembolic phenomena
	Hemoptysis

SAFETY

May exhibit:	Fever
	Skin: Rashes (medication reaction)
	Loss of muscle tone/strength

TEACHING/LEARNING

May report:	Familial risk factors, e.g., heart disease, stroke
	Use/misuse of prescribed medications, such as heart medications (e.g., digitalis), anticoagulants (e.g., warfarin [Coumadin]), phenothiazines (e.g., diazepam [Valium]), tricyclic antidepressants (e.g., amitriptyline [Elavil]), or antipsychotic agents (e.g., fluphenazine [Prolixin], chlorpromazine [Thorazine]), or OTC medications (e.g., cough syrup and analgesics containing ASA)
	Stimulant abuse, including caffeine/nicotine
	Lack of understanding about disease process/therapeutic regimen
	Evidence of failure to improve, e.g., recurrent/intractable dysrhythmias that are life threatening
Discharge plan considerations:	**DRG projected mean length of inpatient stay: 3.9 days**
	Alteration of medication use/therapy
	Refer to section at end of plan for postdischarge considerations.

DIAGNOSTIC STUDIES

ECG: Reveals type/source of dysrhythmia and effects of electrolyte imbalances and cardiac medications. Demonstrates patterns of ischemic injury and conduction aberrance. *Note:* Exercise ECG can reveal dysrhythmias occurring only when patient is not at rest (can be diagnostic for cardiac cause of syncope).

Extended or event monitoring (e.g., Holter monitor): Extended ECG tracing (24 hr to weeks) may be desired to determine which dysrhythmias may be causing specific symptoms when patient is active (home/work) or at rest. May also be used to evaluate pacemaker function, antidysrhythmia drug effect, or effectiveness of cardiac rehabilitation.

Signal-averaged ECG (SAE): May be used to screen high-risk patients (especially post-MI or unexplained syncope) for ventricular dysrhythmias, presence of delayed conduction, and late potentials (as occurs with sustained ventricular tachycardia).

Chest x-ray: May show enlarged cardiac shadow due to ventricular or valvular dysfunction.

Myocardial imaging scans: May demonstrate ischemic/damaged myocardial areas that could impede normal conduction or impair wall motion and pumping capabilities.

Electrophysiologic (EP) studies: Provides cardiac mapping of entire conduction system to evaluate normal and abnormal pathways of electrical conduction. Used to diagnose dysrhythmias and evaluate effectiveness of medication or pacemaker therapies.

Electrolytes: Elevated or decreased levels of potassium, calcium, and magnesium can cause dysrhythmias.

Drug screen: May reveal toxicity of cardiac drugs, presence of street drugs, or suggest interaction of drugs, e.g., digitalis and quinidine.

Thyroid studies: Elevated or depressed serum thyroid levels can cause/aggravate dysrhythmias.

Sedimentation rate (ESR): Elevation may indicate acute/active inflammatory process, e.g., endocarditis, as a precipitating factor for dysrhythmias.

ABGs/pulse oximetry: Hypoxemia can cause/exacerbate dysrhythmias.

NURSING PRIORITIES

1. Prevent/treat life-threatening dysrhythmias.
2. Support patient/SO in dealing with anxiety/fear of potentially life-threatening situation.
3. Assist in identification of cause/precipitating factors.
4. Review information regarding condition/prognosis/treatment regimen.

DISCHARGE GOALS

1. Free of life-threatening dysrhythmias and complications of impaired cardiac output/tissue perfusion.
2. Anxiety reduced/managed.
3. Disease process, therapy needs, and prevention of complications understood.
4. Plan in place to meet needs after discharge.

NURSING DIAGNOSIS: Cardiac Output, risk for decreased

Risk factors may include
Altered electrical conduction
Reduced myocardial contractility

Possibly evidenced by:
[Not applicable; presence of signs and symptoms establishes an *actual* diagnosis.]

DESIRED OUTCOMES/EVALUATION CRITERIA—PATIENT WILL:

Cardiac Pump Effectiveness (NOC)

Maintain/achieve adequate cardiac output as evidenced by BP/pulse within normal range, adequate urinary output, palpable pulses of equal quality, usual level of mentation.
Display reduced frequency/absence of dysrhythmia(s).
Participate in activities that reduce myocardial workload.

ACTIONS/INTERVENTIONS	RATIONALE
Hemodynamic Regulation (NIC)	
Independent	
Palpate pulses (radial, carotid, femoral, dorsalis pedis), noting rate, regularity, amplitude (full/thready), and symmetry. Document presence of pulsus alternans, bigeminal pulse, or pulse deficit.	Differences in equality, rate, and regularity of pulses are indicative of the effect of altered cardiac output on systemic/peripheral circulation.
Auscultate heart sounds, noting rate, rhythm, presence of extra heartbeats, dropped beats.	Specific dysrhythmias are more clearly detected audibly than by palpation. Hearing extra heartbeats or dropped beats helps identify dysrhythmias in the unmonitored patient.

ACTIONS/INTERVENTIONS

Independent

Monitor vital signs. Assess adequacy of cardiac output/tissue perfusion, noting significant variations in BP/pulse rate equality, respirations, changes in skin color/temperature, level of consciousness/sensorium, and urine output during episodes of dysrhythmias.

Determine type of dysrhythmia and document with rhythm strip (if cardiac/telemetry monitoring is available):

  Sinus tachycardia;

  Sinus bradycardia;

Atrial dysrhythmias, e.g., PACs, atrial flutter, atrial fibrillation (AF), atrial supraventricular tachycardias (i.e., PAT, MAT, SVT);

Ventricular dysrhythmias; e.g., premature ventricular contractions/ventricular premature beats (PVCs/VPBs), ventricular tachycardia (VT), ventricular flutter/fibrillation (VF);

RATIONALE

Although not all dysrhythmias are life-threatening, immediate treatment may be required to terminate dysrhythmia in the presence of alterations in cardiac output and tissue perfusion.

Useful in determining need for/type of intervention required.

Tachycardia can occur in response to stress, pain, fever, infection, coronary artery blockage, valvular dysfunction, hypovolemia, hypoxia, or as a result of decreased vagal tone or of increased sympathetic nervous system activity associated with the release of catecholamines. Although it generally does not require treatment, persistent tachycardia may worsen underlying pathology in patients with ischemic heart disease because of shortened diastolic filling time and increased oxygen demands. These patients may require medications.

Bradycardia is common in patients with acute MI (especially anterior and inferior) and is the result of excessive parasympathetic activity, blocks in conduction to the SA or AV nodes, or loss of automaticity of the heart muscle. Patients with severe heart disease may not be able to compensate for a slow rate by increasing stroke volume. Therefore, decreased cardiac output, HF, and potentially lethal ventricular dysrhythmias may occur.

PACs can occur as a response to ischemia and are normally harmless but can precede or precipitate atrial fibrillation. Acute and chronic atrial flutter and/or fibrillation can occur with coronary artery or valvular disease and may or may not be pathological. Rapid atrial flutter/fibrillation reduces cardiac output as a result of incomplete ventricular filling (shortened cardiac cycle) and increased oxygen demand.

PVCs or VPBs reflect cardiac irritability and are commonly associated with MI, digitalis toxicity, coronary vasospasm, and misplaced temporary pacemaker leads. Frequent, multiple, or multifocal PVCs result in diminished cardiac output and may lead to potentially lethal dysrhythmias, e.g., VT or sudden death/cardiac arrest from ventricular flutter/fibrillation. *Note:* Intractable ventricular dysrhythmias unresponsive to medication may reflect ventricular aneurysm. *Note:* Polymorphic VT (torsades de pointes) is recognized by inconsistent shape of QRS complexes and is often drug related, e.g., procainamide (Pronestyl), quinidine (Quinaglute), disopyramide (Norpace), and sotalol (Betapace).

ACTIONS/INTERVENTIONS	RATIONALE

Independent

Heart blocks.

Reflect altered transmission of impulses through normal conduction channels (slowed, altered) and may be the result of MI, coronary artery disease with reduced blood supply to sinoatrial (SA) or atrioventricular (AV) nodes, drug toxicity, and sometimes cardiac surgery. Progressing heart block is associated with slowed ventricular rates, decreased cardiac output, and potentially lethal ventricular dysrhythmias or cardiac standstill.

Provide calm/quiet environment. Review reasons for limitation of activities during acute phase.

Reduces stimulation and release of stress-related catecholamines, which can cause/aggravate dysrhythmias and vasoconstriction, increasing myocardial workload.

Demonstrate/encourage use of stress management behaviors, e.g., relaxation techniques, guided imagery, slow/deep breathing.

Promotes patient participation in exerting some sense of control in a stressful situation.

Investigate reports of chest pain, documenting location, duration, intensity (0–10 scale), and relieving/aggravating factors. Note nonverbal pain cues, e.g., facial grimacing, crying, changes in BP/heart rate.

Reasons for chest pain are variable and depend on underlying cause. However, chest pain may indicate ischemia due to altered electrical conduction, decreased myocardial perfusion, or increased oxygen need (e.g., impending/evolving MI).

Be prepared to initiate cardiopulmonary resuscitation (CPR) as indicated.

Development of life-threatening dysrhythmias requires prompt intervention to prevent ischemic damage/death.

Collaborative

Monitor laboratory studies, e.g.

Electrolytes;

Imbalance of electrolytes, such as potassium, magnesium, and calcium, adversely affects cardiac rhythm and contractility.

Drug levels.

Reveal therapeutic/toxic level of prescription medications or street drugs that may affect/contribute to presence of dysrhythmias.

Administer supplemental oxygen as indicated.

Increases amount of oxygen available for myocardial uptake, which decreases irritability caused by hypoxia.

Administer medications as indicated:

Dysrhythmias are generally treated symptomatically.

Potassium;

Correction of hypokalemia may be sufficient to terminate some ventricular dysrhythmias.

Antidysrhythmics, such as:

Class I drugs:

Class I drugs depress depolarization and alter repolarization, stabilizing the cell. These drugs are divided into groups a, b, and c, based on their unique effects.

ACTIONS/INTERVENTIONS	RATIONALE
Collaborative	

Class Ia, e.g., disopyramide (Norpace), procainamide (Pronestyl, Procan SR), quinidine (Quinaglute, Cardioquin);

These drugs increase action potential, duration, and effective refractory period and decrease membrane responsiveness, prolonging both QRS complex and QT interval. Useful for treatment of atrial and ventricular premature beats, repetitive dysrhythmias (e.g., atrial tachycardias and atrial flutter/fibrillation). *Note:* Myocardial depressant effects may be potentiated when class Ia drugs are used in conjunction with any drugs possessing similar properties.

Class Ib, e.g., lidocaine (Xylocaine), phenytoin (Dilantin), tocainide (Tonocard), mexiletine (Mexitil);

These drugs shorten the duration of the refractory period (QT interval), and their action depends on the tissue affected and the level of extracellular potassium. Drugs of choice for ventricular dysrhythmias, they are also effective for automatic and re-entrant dysrhythmias and digitalis-induced dysrhythmias. *Note:* These drugs may aggravate myocardial depression.

Class Ic, e.g., flecainide (Tambocor), propafenone (Rhythmol), encainide (Enkaid);

These drugs slow conduction by depressing SA node automaticity and decreasing conduction velocity through the atria, ventricles, and Purkinje fibers. The result is prolongation of the PR interval and lengthening of the QRS complex. They suppress and prevent all types of ventricular dysrhythmias. *Note:* Flecainide increases risk of drug-induced dysrhythmias post-MI. Propafenone can worsen or cause new dysrhythmias, a tendency called the "proarrhythmic effect." Encainide is available only for patients who demonstrated a good result before the drug was removed from the market.

Class II drugs: e.g., propranolol (Inderal), nadolol (Corgard), acebutolol (Sectral), esmolol (Brevibloc), sotalol (Betapace);

Beta-adrenergic blockers have antiadrenergic properties and decrease automaticity. Therefore, they are useful in the treatment of dysrhythmias caused by SA and AV node dysfunction (e.g., SVTs, atrial flutter or fibrillation). *Note:* These drugs may exacerbate bradycardia and cause myocardial depression, especially when combined with drugs that have similar properties.

Class III drugs: e.g., bretylium tosylate (Bretylol), amiodarone (Cordarone), sotalol (Betapace);

These drugs prolong the refractory period and action potential duration, consequently prolonging the QT interval. They are used to terminate ventricular fibrillation and other life-threatening ventricular dysrhythmias/sustained ventricular tachyarrhythmias, especially when lidocaine/procainamide are not effective. *Note:* Sotalol is a nonselective β-blocker with characteristics of both class II and class III.

ACTIONS/INTERVENTIONS	RATIONALE
Collaborative	
Class IV drugs: e.g., verapamil (Calan), nifedipine (Procardia), diltiazem (Cardizem);	Calcium antagonists (also called calcium channel blockers) slow conduction time through the AV node (prolonging PR interval) to decrease ventricular response in SVTs, atrial flutter/fibrillation.
Miscellaneous e.g., atropine sulfate, isoproterenol (Isuprel), cardiac glycosides: digoxin (Lanoxin);	Useful in treating bradycardia by increasing SA and AV conduction and enhancing automaticity. Cardiac glycosides may be used alone or in combination with other antidysrhythmic drugs to reduce ventricular rate in presence of uncontrolled/poorly tolerated atrial tachycardias or flutter/fibrillation.
Adenosine (Adenocard).	Unclassified first-line treatment for paroxysmal supraventricular tachycardia (PAT). Slows conduction and interrupts reentry pathways in AV node. *Note:* Contraindicated in patients with second- or third-degree heart block or those with sick sinus syndrome who do not have a functioning pacemaker.
Prepare for/assist with elective cardioversion.	May be used in atrial fibrillation or certain unstable dysrhythmias to restore normal heart rate/relieve symptoms of heart failure.
Assist with insertion/maintain pacemaker function.	Temporary pacing may be necessary to accelerate impulse formation or override tachydysrhythmias and ectopic activity, to maintain cardiovascular function until spontaneous pacing is restored or permanent pacing is initiated.
Insert/maintain IV access.	Patent access line may be required for administration of emergency drugs.
Prepare for invasive diagnostic procedures/surgery as indicated.	Differential diagnosis of underlying cause may be required to formulate appropriate treatment plan. Resection of ventricular aneurysm may be required to correct intractable ventricular dysrhythmias unresponsive to medical therapy. Surgery, e.g., CABG, may be indicated to enhance circulation to myocardium and conduction system.
Prepare for implantation of cardioverter/defibrillator (ICD) when indicated.	This device may be surgically implanted in those patients with recurrent, life-threatening ventricular dysrhythmias unresponsive to tailored drug therapy. The latest generation of devices can provide multilevel ("tiered") therapy, that is, antitachycardia and antibradycardia pacing, cardioversion, or defibrillation, depending on how each device is programmed.

> **NURSING DIAGNOSIS: Poisoning, risk for digitalis toxicity**
>
> **Risk factors may include**
> Limited range of therapeutic effectiveness, lack of education/proper precautions, reduced vision/cognitive limitations
>
> **Possibly evidenced by**
> [Not applicable; presence of signs and symptoms establishes an *actual* diagnosis]
>
> **DESIRED OUTCOMES/EVALUATION CRITERIA—PATIENT WILL:**
>
> **Knowledge: Medication (NOC)**
>
> Verbalize understanding of individual prescription, how it interacts with other drugs/substances, and importance of maintaining prescribed regimen.
> Recognize signs of digitalis overdose and developing heart failure, and what to report to physician.
>
> **Cardiac Pump Effectiveness (NOC)**
>
> Be free of signs of toxicity; display serum drug level within individually acceptable range.

ACTIONS/INTERVENTIONS	RATIONALE
Medication Management (NIC)	
Independent	
Explain patient's specific type of digitalis preparation and its specific therapeutic use.	Reduces confusion due to digitalis preparations varying in name (although they may be similar), dosage strength, and onset and duration of action. Up to 15% of all patients receiving digitalis develop toxicity at some time during the course of therapy because of its narrow therapeutic range.
Instruct patient not to change dose for any reason, not to omit dose (unless instructed to, depending on pulse rate), not to increase dose or take extra doses, and to contact doctor if more than one dose is omitted.	Alterations in drug regimen can reduce therapeutic effects, result in toxicity, and cause complications.
Advise patient that digitalis may interact with many other drugs (e.g., barbiturates, neomycin, cholestyramine, quinidine, and antacids) and that physician should be informed that digitalis is taken whenever new medications are prescribed. Advise patient not to use OTC drugs (e.g., laxatives, antidiarrheals, antacids, cold remedies, diuretics, herbals) without first checking with the pharmacist or healthcare provider.	Knowledge may help prevent dangerous drug interactions.
Review importance of dietary and supplemental intake of potassium, calcium, and magnesium.	Maintaining electrolytes at normal ranges may prevent or limit development of toxicity and correct many associated dysrhythmias.

ACTIONS/INTERVENTIONS	RATIONALE

Anxiety Reduction (NIC)

Independent

Provide information and have the patient/SO verbalize understanding of toxic signs/symptoms to report to the healthcare provider.

Nausea, vomiting, diarrhea, unusual drowsiness, confusion, very slow or very fast irregular pulse, thumping in chest, double/blurred vision, yellow/green tint or halos around objects, flickering color forms or dots, altered color perception, and worsening heart failure (e.g., dependent/generalized edema, dyspnea, decreased amount/frequency of voiding) indicate need for prompt evaluation/intervention. Mild symptoms of toxicity may be managed with a brief drug holiday. *Note:* In severe/refractory heart failure, altered cardiac binding of digitalis may result in toxicity, even with previously appropriate drug doses.

Discuss necessity of periodic laboratory evaluation:

    Serum digoxin (Lanoxin) or digitoxin (Crystodigin) level;

Digitalis has a narrow therapeutic serum range, with toxicity occurring at levels that are dependent on individual response. Laboratory levels are evaluated in conjunction with clinical manifestations and ECG to determine individual therapeutic levels/resolution of toxicity.

    Electrolytes, BUN, creatinine, liver function studies.

Abnormal levels of potassium, calcium, or magnesium increase the heart's sensitivity to digitalis. Impaired kidney function can cause digoxin (mainly excreted by the kidney) to accumulate to toxic levels. Digitoxin levels (mainly excreted by the bowel) are affected by impaired liver function.

Collaborative

Administer other appropriate antidysrhythmia medications, e.g., lidocaine (Xylocaine), propranolol (Inderal), and procainamide (Pronestyl).

May be necessary to maintain/improve cardiac output in presence of excess effect of digitalis.

Prepare patient for transfer to CCU as indicated (e.g., dangerous dysrhythmias/exacerbation of heart failure).

In the presence of digitalis toxicity, patients frequently require intensive monitoring until therapeutic levels have been restored. Because all digitalis preparations have long serum half-lives, stabilization can take several days.

NURSING DIAGNOSIS: Knowledge Deficit [Learning Need] regarding cause, treatment, self care, and discharge needs

May be related to

Lack of information/misunderstanding of medical condition/therapy needs

Unfamiliarity with information resources

Lack of recall

Possibly evidenced by

Questions, statement of misconception

Failure to improve on previous regimen

Development of preventable complications

DESIRED OUTCOMES/EVALUATION CRITERIA—PATIENT WILL:

Knowledge: Disease Process (NOC)

Verbalize understanding of condition, prognosis, and function of pacemaker (if used).

Relate signs of pacemaker failure.

Knowledge: Treatment Regimen (NOC)

Verbalize understanding of therapeutic regimen.

List desired action and possible adverse side effects of medications.

Correctly perform necessary procedures and explain reasons for actions.

ACTIONS/INTERVENTIONS

RATIONALE

Teaching: Disease Process (NIC)

Independent

Assess patient/SO level of knowledge and ability/desire to learn.

Necessary for creation of individual instruction plan. Reinforces expectation that this will be a "learning experience." Verbalization identifies misunderstandings and allows for clarification.

Be alert to signs of avoidance, e.g., changing subject away from information being presented or extremes of behavior (withdrawal/euphoria).

Natural defense mechanisms, such as anger or denial of significance of situation, can block learning, affecting patient's response and ability to assimilate information. Changing to a less formal/structured style may be more effective until patient/SO is ready to accept/deal with current situation.

Present information in varied learning formats, e.g., programmed books, audiovisual tapes, question-and-answer sessions, group activities.

Multiple learning methods may enhance retention of material.

Provide information in written form for patient/SO to take home.

Follow-up reminders may enhance patient's understanding and cooperation with the desired regimen. Written instructions are a helpful resource when patient is not in direct contact with healthcare team.

Reinforce explanations of risk factors, dietary/activity restrictions, medications, and symptoms requiring immediate medical attention.

Provides opportunity for patient to retain information and to assume control/participate in rehabilitation program.

Encourage identification/reduction of individual risk factors, e.g., smoking and alcohol consumption, obesity.

These behaviors/chemicals have direct adverse effect on cardiovascular function and may impede recovery and increase risk for complications.

ACTIONS/INTERVENTIONS	RATIONALE

Independent

Review normal cardiac function/electrical conduction.	Provides a knowledge base to understand individual variations and to understand reasons for therapeutic interventions.
Explain/reinforce specific dysrhythmia problem and therapeutic measures to patient/SO.	Ongoing/updated information (e.g., whether the problem is resolving or may require long-term control measures) can decrease anxiety associated with the unknown and prepare patient/SO to make necessary lifestyle adaptations. Educating the SO may be especially important if the patient is elderly, visually or hearing impaired, or unable or even unwilling to learn/follow instructions. Repeated explanations may be needed because anxiety and/or bulk of new information can block/limit learning.
Identify adverse effects/complications of specific dysrhythmias, e.g., fatigue, dependent edema, progressive changes in mentation, vertigo.	Dysrhythmias may decrease cardiac output, manifested by symptoms of developing cardiac failure/altered cerebral perfusion. Tachydysrhythmias may also be accompanied by debilitating anxiety/feelings of impending doom.
Instruct and document teaching regarding medications. Include why the drug is needed (desired action), how and when to take the drug, what to do if a dose is forgotten (dosage and usage information), and expected side effects or possible adverse reactions/interactions with other prescribed/OTC drugs or substances (alcohol, tobacco, herbal remedies), as well as what and when to report to the physician.	Information necessary for patient to make informed choices and to manage medication regimen. *Note:* Use of herbal remedies in conjunction with drug regimen may result in adverse effects (e.g., cardiac stimulation, impaired clotting), necessitating evaluation of product for safe use.
Encourage development of regular exercise routine, avoiding overexertion. Identify signs/symptoms requiring immediate cessation of activities, e.g., dizziness, light-headedness, dyspnea, chest pain.	When dysrhythmias are properly managed, normal activity should not be affected. Exercise program is useful in improving overall cardiovascular well-being.
Review individual dietary needs/restrictions, e.g., potassium, caffeine.	Depending on specific problem, patient may need to increase dietary potassium, such as when potassium-depleting diuretics are used. Caffeine may be limited to prevent cardiac excitation.
Demonstrate proper pulse-taking technique. Recommend weekly checking of pulse for 1 full minute or daily recording of pulse before medication and during exercise as appropriate. Identify situations requiring immediate medical intervention, e.g., dizziness or irregular heartbeat, fainting, chest pain.	Continued self-observation/monitoring provides for timely intervention to avoid complications. Medication regimen may be altered or further evaluation may be required when heart rate varies from desired rate or pacemaker's preset rate.
Review safety precautions, techniques to evaluate/maintain pacemaker or ICD function, and symptoms requiring medical intervention, e.g., report pulse rate below set limit for demand pacing or less than low-limit rate for rate-adaptive pacers, prolonged hiccups.	Promotes self-care, provides for timely interventions to prevent serious complications. Instructions/concerns depend on function and type of device, as well as the patient's condition and presence/absence of family or caregivers.
Recommend wearing medical alert bracelet or necklace and carrying pacemaker ID card.	Allows for appropriate evaluation and timely intervention, especially if patient is unable to respond in an emergency situation.

ACTIONS/INTERVENTIONS

Independent

Discuss environmental safety concerns, e.g., microwave ovens and other electrical appliances (including electrical blankets, razors, radio/TV), can be safely operated if they are properly grounded and in good repair. There is no problem with metal detectors, although pacemaker may trigger sensitive detectors. Although cordless phones are safe, cellular phones held directly over pacemaker may cause interference, so it is recommended that patient not carry phone in shirt pocket when phone is on. Additionally, high-voltage areas, magnetic fields, and radiation can interfere with optimal pacemaker function, so patient should avoid high-tension electric wires, arc welding, and large industrial magnets, e.g., demolition sites and MRI.

RATIONALE

Aids in clarifying misconceptions and fears and encourages patient to be proactive in avoiding potentially harmful situations.

POTENTIAL CONSIDERATIONS following discharge from care setting (dependent on patient's age, physical condition/presence of complications, personal resources, and life responsibilities)

Activity intolerance—imbalance between oxygen supply/demand.
Therapeutic Regimen: Individual, ineffective management—complexity of therapeutic regimen, decisional conflicts, economic difficulties, inadequate number/types of cues to action.

CARDIAC SURGERY: POSTOPERATIVE CARE—CORONARY ARTERY BYPASS GRAFT, CARDIOMYOPLASTY, VALVE REPLACEMENT

The goal of treatment for heart disease is to maximize cardiac output. Surgically, this may be done by improving myocardial muscle function and blood flow through procedures such as CABG, wrapping the latissimus dorsi muscle around the heart, and/or repair or replacement of defective valves. Of the three types of cardiac surgery: (1) reparative (e.g., closure of atrial or ventricular septal defect, repair of mitral stenosis), (2) reconstructive (e.g., CABG, reconstruction of an incompetent valve), and (3) substitutional (e.g., valve replacement, cardiac transplant), reparative surgeries are more likely to produce cure or prolonged improvement.

CARE SETTING

Inpatient acute hospital on a surgical or post-ICU step-down unit.

RELATED CONCERNS

Angina pectoris, page 64
Heart failure: chronic, page 47
Dysrhythmias, page 90
Myocardial infarction, page 75
Hemothorax/pneumothorax, page 165
Psychosocial aspects of care, page 809
Surgical intervention, page 828

Patient Assessment Database

The preoperative data presented here depend on the specific disease process and underlying cardiac condition/reserve.

ACTIVITY/REST

May report:	History of exercise intolerance
	Generalized weakness, fatigue
	Inability to perform expected/usual life activities
	Insomnia/sleep disturbance
May exhibit:	Abnormal heart rate, BP changes with activity
	Exertional discomfort or dyspnea
	ECG changes/dysrhythmias

CIRCULATION

May report:	History of recent/acute MI, three (or more) vessel coronary artery disease, valvular heart disease, hypertension
May exhibit:	Variations in BP, heart rate/rhythm
	Abnormal heart sounds: S_3/S_4, murmurs
	Pallor/cyanosis of skin or mucous membranes
	Cool/cold, clammy skin
	Edema, JVD
	Diminished peripheral pulses
	Abnormal breath sounds: crackles
	Restlessness/other changes in mentation or sensorium (severe cardiac decompensation)

EGO INTEGRITY

May report:	Feeling frightened/apprehensive, helpless
	Distress over current events (anger/fear)
	Fear of death/eventual outcome of surgery, possible complications
	Fear about changes in lifestyle/role functioning
May exhibit:	Apprehension, restlessness
	Facial/general tension; withdrawal/lack of eye contact

Focus on self; hostility, anger; crying
Changes in heart rate, BP, breathing patterns

FOOD/FLUID

May report: Change in weight
Loss of appetite
Abdominal pain, nausea/vomiting
Change in urine frequency/amount

May exhibit: Weight gain/loss
Dry skin, poor skin turgor
Postural hypotension
Diminished/absent bowel sounds
Edema (generalized, dependent, pitting)

NEUROSENSORY

May report: Fainting spells, vertigo
May exhibit: Changes in orientation or usual response to stimuli
Restlessness; irritability, exaggerated emotional responses; apathy

PAIN/DISCOMFORT

May report: Chest pain, angina

RESPIRATION

May report: Shortness of breath
May exhibit: Crackles
Productive cough

SAFETY

May report: Infectious episode with valvular involvement or myopathy

TEACHING/LEARNING

May report: Familial risk factors of diabetes, heart disease, hypertension, strokes
Use of various cardiovascular drugs
Failure to improve

Postoperative

PAIN/DISCOMFORT

May report: Incisional discomfort
Pain/paresthesia of shoulders, arms, hands, legs
May exhibit: Guarding
Facial mask of pain; grimacing
Distraction behaviors; moaning; restlessness
Changes in BP/pulse/respiratory rate

RESPIRATION

May report: Inability to cough or take a deep breath
May exhibit: Decreased chest expansion
Splinting/muscle guarding
Dyspnea (normal response to thoracotomy)
Areas of diminished or absent breath sounds (atelectasis)
Anxiety
Changes in ABGs/pulse oximetry

May exhibit: Oozing/bleeding from chest or donor site incisions

TEACHING/LEARNING

Discharge plan considerations: **DRG projected mean length of inpatient stay: 4.7 days, acute care (additional days may be divided among multiple levels of care)**

Short-term assistance with food preparation, shopping, transportation, self-care needs, and homemaker/home maintenance tasks

Refer to section at end of plan for postdischarge considerations.

DIAGNOSTIC STUDIES (POSTOPERATIVE)

Hemoglobin/Hematocrit: A low Hb reduces oxygen-carrying capacity and indicates need for red blood cell replacement. Elevation of Hct suggests dehydration/need for fluid replacement.

Coagulation studies: Various studies may be done (e.g., platelet count, bleeding and clotting time) to determine therapeutic level of anticoagulant therapy when used.

Electrolytes: Imbalances (hyperkalemia/hypokalemia, hypernatremia/hyponatremia, and hypocalcemia) can affect cardiac function and fluid balance.

ABGs: Verifies oxygenation status, effectiveness of respiratory function, and acid-base balance.

Pulse oximetry: Provides noninvasive measure of oxygenation at tissue level.

BUN/Creatinine: Reflects adequacy of renal and liver perfusion/function.

Amylase: Elevation is occasionally seen in high-risk patients, e.g., those with heart failure undergoing valve replacement.

Glucose: Fluctuations may occur because of preoperative nutritional status, presence of diabetes/organ dysfunction, rate of dextrose infusions.

Cardiac enzymes/Isoenzymes: Elevated in the presence of acute, recent, or perioperative MI.

Chest x-ray: Reveals heart size and position, pulmonary vasculature, and changes indicative of pulmonary complications (e.g., atelectasis). Verifies condition of valve prosthesis and sternal wires, position of pacing leads, intravascular/cardiac lines.

ECG: Identifies changes in electrical, mechanical function such as might occur in immediate postoperative phase, acute/perioperative MI, valve dysfunction, and/or pericarditis.

Cardiac echocardiogram/Catheterization: Measures chamber pressures and pressure gradients across valves, identifies occlusions of arteries, impaired coronary perfusion, and possible wall motion abnormalities.

Transesophageal echocardiography: Useful in diagnosing cardiac valve and chamber abnormalities, such as regurgitation, shunting, or stenosis in patients in whom transthoracic approach is not feasible.

Nuclear studies (e.g., thallium-201, DPY-thallium/Persantine): Heart scans demonstrate coronary artery disease, heart chamber dimensions, and presurgical/postsurgical functional capabilities.

NURSING PRIORITIES

1. Support hemodynamic stability/ventilatory function.
2. Promote relief of pain/discomfort.
3. Promote healing.
4. Provide information about postoperative expectations and treatment regimen.

DISCHARGE GOALS

1. Activity tolerance adequate to meet self-care needs.
2. Pain alleviated/managed.
3. Complications prevented/minimized.
4. Incisions healing.
5. Postdischarge medications, exercise, diet, therapy understood.
6. Plan in place to meet needs after discharge.

> **NURSING DIAGNOSIS: Cardiac Output, risk for decreased**
>
> **Risk factors may include**
>
> Decreased myocardial contractility secondary to temporary factors (e.g., ventricular wall surgery, recent MI, response to certain medications/drug interactions)
>
> Decreased preload (hypovolemia)
>
> Alterations in electrical conduction (dysrhythmias)
>
> **Possibly evidenced by**
>
> [Not applicable; presence of signs and symptoms establishes an *actual* diagnosis]
>
> **DESIRED OUTCOMES/EVALUATION CRITERIA—PATIENT WILL:**
>
> **Tissue Perfusion: Cardiac (NOC)**
>
> Report/display decreased episodes of angina and dysrhythmias.
>
> Demonstrate an increase in activity tolerance.
>
> Participate in activities that maximize/enhance cardiac function.

ACTIONS/INTERVENTIONS	RATIONALE
Hemodynamic Regulation (NIC)	
Independent	
Monitor/document trends in heart rate and BP, especially noting hypertension. Be aware of specific systolic/diastolic limits defined for patient.	Tachycardia is a common response to discomfort and anxiety, inadequate blood/fluid replacement, and the stress of surgery. However, sustained tachycardia increases cardiac workload and can decrease effective cardiac output. Hypertension can occur (fluid excess or preexisting condition), placing stress on suture lines of new grafts and changing blood flow/pressure within heart chambers and across valves, with increased risk for various complications. Hypotension may result from fluid deficit, dysrhythmias, heart failure/shock.
Monitor/document cardiac dysrhythmias. Observe patient response to dysrhythmias, e.g., drop in BP.	Life-threatening dysrhythmias can occur because of electrolyte imbalance, myocardial ischemia, or alterations in the heart's electrical conduction. Decreased cardiac output and hemodynamic compromise that occur with dysrhythmias require prompt intervention.
Observe for changes in usual mental status/orientation/body movement or reflexes, e.g., onset of confusion, disorientation, restlessness, reduced response to stimuli, stupor.	May indicate decreased cerebral blood flow or oxygenation as a result of diminished cardiac output (sustained or severe dysrhythmias, low BP, heart failure, or thromboembolic phenomena).
Record skin temperature/color and quality/equality of peripheral pulses.	Warm, pink skin and strong, equal pulses are general indicators of adequate cardiac output.
Measure/document I&O and fluid balance.	Useful in determining fluid needs or identifying fluid excesses, which can compromise cardiac output/oxygen consumption.
Schedule uninterrupted rest/sleep periods. Assist with self-care activities as needed.	Prevents fatigue/overexhaustion and excessive cardiovascular stress.
Monitor graded activity program. Note patient response, vital signs before/during/after activity, development of dysrhythmias.	Regular exercise stimulates circulation/cardiovascular tone and promotes feeling of well-being. Progression of activity depends on cardiac tolerance.

ACTIONS/INTERVENTIONS

Independent

Evaluate presence/degree of anxiety/emotional duress. Encourage the use of relaxation techniques, e.g., deep breathing, diversional activities.

Inspect for JVD, peripheral or dependent edema, congestion in lungs, shortness of breath, change in mental status.

Investigate reports of angina/severe chest pain accompanied by restlessness, diaphoresis, ECG changes.

Investigate/report profound hypotension (unresponsive to fluid challenge), tachycardia, distant heart sounds, stupor/coma.

Collaborative

Review serial ECGs.

Measure cardiac output and other functional parameters as indicated.

Administer IV fluids/blood transfusions as needed.

Administer supplemental oxygen as appropriate.

Administer electrolytes and medications as indicated, e.g., electrolyte solutions/potassium, antidysrhythmics, β-blockers, digitalis, diuretics, anticoagulants.

Maintain surgically placed pacing wires (atrial/ventricular) and initiate pacing if indicated.

RATIONALE

Excessive/escalating emotional reactions can affect vital signs and SVR, eventually affecting cardiac function.

May be indicative of heart failure (acute or chronic).

Although not a common complication of CABG, perioperative or postoperative MI can occur.

Development of cardiac tamponade can rapidly progress to cardiac arrest because of the heart's inability to fill adequately for effective cardiac output. *Note:* This is a relatively rare, life-threatening complication that usually occurs in the immediate postoperative period but can occur later in the recovery phase.

Most frequently done to follow the progress in normalization of electrical conduction patterns/ventricular function after surgery or to identify complications, e.g., perioperative MI.

Useful in evaluating response to therapeutic interventions and identifying need for more aggressive/emergency care. *Note:* Cardiac index, preload/afterload, contractility, and cardiac work can be measured noninvasively by using thoracic electrical bioimpedance (TEB) technique.

IV fluids may be discontinued before discharge from the intensive care unit (ICU), or one line (central/peripheral) may remain in place for fluid replacement and/or emergency cardiac medications. Red blood cell (RBC) replacement may be indicated on occasion to restore/maintain adequate circulating volume and enhance oxygen-carrying capacity.

Promotes maximal oxygenation, which can reduce cardiac workload and aid in resolving myocardial ischemia and dysrhythmias.

Patient needs are variable, depending on type of surgery (CABG or valve replacement), response to surgical intervention, and preexisting conditions (e.g., general health, age, type of heart disease). Electrolytes, antidysrhythmics, and other heart medications may be required on a short-term or long-term basis to maximize cardiac contractility/output.

May be required to support cardiac output in presence of conduction disturbances (severe dysrhythmias) that compromise cardiac function.

NURSING DIAGNOSIS: Pain [acute]/[Discomfort]

May be related to
Sternotomy (mediastinal incision) and/or donor site (leg/arm incision)
Myocardial ischemia (acute MI, angina)
Tissue inflammation/edema formation
Intraoperative nerve trauma

Possibly evidenced by
Reports of incisional discomfort/pain; paresthesia; pain in hand, arm, shoulder
Anxiety, restlessness, irritability
Distraction behaviors
Increased heart rate

DESIRED OUTCOMES/EVALUATION CRITERIA—PATIENT WILL:

Pain Level (NOC)

Verbalize relief/absence of pain.
Demonstrate relaxed body posture, ability to rest/sleep appropriately.

Pain Control Behavior (NOC)

Differentiate surgical discomfort from angina/preoperative heart pain.

ACTIONS/INTERVENTIONS	RATIONALE
Pain Management (NIC)	
Independent	
Note type/location of incision(s).	Newer (MIDCABG) procedures may require only a "mini" chest incision, with minimal pain.
Encourage patient to report type, location, and intensity of pain, rating on a scale of 0–10. Note associated symptoms. Ask the patient how this compares with preoperative chest pain.	Pain is perceived, manifested, and tolerated individually. It is important for the patient to differentiate incisional pain from other types of chest pain, such as angina or discomfort from chest tubes. Many CABG patients do not experience severe discomfort in chest incision and may complain more often of donor site incision discomfort. Severe pain in either area should be investigated further for possible complications.
Observe for anxiety, irritability, crying, restlessness, sleep disturbances.	These nonverbal cues may indicate the presence/degree of pain being experienced.
Monitor vital signs.	Heart rate usually increases with pain, although a bradycardiac response can occur in a severely diseased heart. BP may be elevated slightly with incisional discomfort but may be decreased or unstable if chest pain is severe and/or myocardial damage is occurring.
Identify/promote position of comfort, using adjuncts as necessary.	Pillows/blanket rolls are useful in supporting extremities, maintaining body alignment, and splinting incisions to reduce muscle tension/promote comfort.
Suggest use of saltwater gargle, throat lozenges, or spray.	Helps relieve discomfort in throat associated with endotracheal tube.

107

ACTIONS/INTERVENTIONS	RATIONALE
Independent	
Provide comfort measures (e.g., back rubs, position changes), assist with self-care activities, and encourage diversional activities as indicated.	May promote relaxation/redirect attention and reduce analgesic dosage needs/frequency.
Schedule care activities to balance with adequate periods of sleep/rest.	Rest and sleep are vital for cardiac healing (balance between oxygen demand and consumption) and can enhance coping with stress and discomfort.
Identify/encourage use of behaviors such as guided imagery, distractions, visualizations, deep breathing.	Relaxation techniques aid in management of stress, promote sense of well-being, may reduce analgesic needs, and promote healing.
Tell patient that it is acceptable, even preferable, to request analgesics as soon as discomfort becomes noticeable.	Presence of pain causes muscle tension, which can impair circulation, slow healing process, and intensify pain.
Medicate before procedures/activities as indicated.	Patient comfort and cooperation in respiratory treatments, ambulation, and procedures (e.g., removal of chest tubes, pacemaker wires, and suture removal) are facilitated by maximum analgesic blood level.
Investigate reports of pain in unusual areas (e.g., calves of legs, abdomen) or vague complaints of discomfort, especially when accompanied by changes in mentation, vital signs, respiratory rate.	May be an early manifestation of developing complication, e.g., thrombophlebitis, infection, gastrointestinal dysfunction.
Note reports of pain and/or numbness in ulnar area (fourth and fifth digits) of the hand, often accompanied by pain/discomfort of the arms and shoulders. Tell the patient that the problem usually resolves with time.	Indicative of a stretch injury of the brachial plexus as a result of the position of the arms during surgery. No specific treatment is currently useful.
Collaborative	
Administer medications as indicated, e.g., propoxyphene and acetaminophen (Darvocet-N), acetaminophen and oxycodone (Tylox).	Usually provides for adequate control of pain and reduces muscle tension, which improves patient comfort and promotes healing.

NURSING DIAGNOSIS: Role Performance, altered

May be related to
Situational crisis (dependent role)/recuperative process
Uncertainty about future

Possibly evidenced by
Delay/alteration in physical capacity to resume role
Change in usual role or responsibility
Change in self/others' perception of role

DESIRED OUTCOMES/EVALUATION CRITERIA—PATIENT WILL:

Psychosocial Adjustment: Life Change (NOC)

Verbalize realistic perception and acceptance of self in changed role.
Talk with SO about situation and changes that have occurred.
Develop realistic plans for adapting to perceived role changes.

ACTIONS/INTERVENTIONS	RATIONALE
Collaborative	
Assess patient role in family constellation. Identify concerns about role dysfunction/interruption, e.g., recuperation, health-illness transitions.	Helps to know patient responsibilities and how illness affects this role. Dependent role of the patient provokes anxiety and concern about how the patient will be able to manage usual role responsibilities.
Assess level of anxiety, patient's perception of degree of threat to self/life.	Information provides baseline for identifying/individualizing plan of care.
Note cultural factors affecting role changes.	Cultural expectations regarding male/female illness role can determine how patient/SO reacts to and deals with current situation and may affect future adaptation to perceived changes.
Maintain positive attitude toward the patient, providing opportunities for the patient to exercise control as much as possible.	Helps patient to accept changes that are occurring and to begin to realize that control over self/situation is possible.
Assist patient/SO to develop strategies for dealing with changes, e.g., shift responsibilities to other family members/friends or neighbors, acquire temporary assistance (homemaker/yardwork), investigate avenues for financial assistance.	Planning for changes that may occur/be required promotes sense of control and accomplishment without loss of self-esteem.
Acknowledge reality of grieving process related to change in usual role (even if only temporary) and help patient to deal realistically with feelings of anger and sadness.	Cardiac surgery constitutes a dramatic point in the patient's life, which will never be the same again. These feelings need to be recognized and dealt with by the patient/family to move forward.

NURSING DIAGNOSIS: Breathing Pattern, risk for ineffective

Risk factors may include

Inadequate ventilation (pain/muscular weakness)

Diminished oxygen-carrying capacity (blood loss)

Decreased lung expansion (atelectasis or pneumothorax/hemothorax)

Possibly evidenced by

[Not applicable; presence of signs and symptoms establishes an *actual* diagnosis]

DESIRED OUTCOMES/EVALUATION CRITERIA—PATIENT WILL:

Respiratory Status: Ventilation (NOC)

Maintain a normal/effective respiratory pattern free of cyanosis and other signs/symptoms of hypoxia with breath sounds equal bilaterally, lung fields clearing.

Display complete reexpansion of lungs with absence of pneumothorax/hemothorax.

Respiratory Monitoring (NIC)

Independent

Evaluate respiratory rate and depth. Note respiratory effort, e.g., presence of dyspnea, use of accessory muscles, nasal flaring.	Patient responses are variable. Rate and effort may be increased by pain, fear, fever, diminished circulating volume (blood or fluid loss), accumulation of secretions, hypoxia, or gastric distention. Respiratory suppression (decreased rate) can occur from excessive use of narcotic analgesics. Early recognition and treatment of abnormal ventilation may prevent complications.
Auscultate breath sounds. Note areas of diminished/absent breath sounds and presence of adventitious sounds, e.g., crackles or rhonchi.	Breath sounds are often diminished in lung bases for a period of time following surgery because of normally occurring atelectasis. Loss of active breath sounds in an area of previous ventilation may reflect collapse of the lung segment, especially if chest tubes have recently been removed. Crackles or rhonchi may be indicative of fluid accumulation (interstitial edema, pulmonary edema, or infection) or partial airway obstruction (pooling of secretions).
Observe chest excursion. Investigate decreased expansion or lack of symmetry in chest movement.	Air or fluid in the pleural space prevents complete expansion (usually on one side) and requires further assessment of ventilation status.
Observe character of cough and sputum production.	Frequent coughing may simply be throat irritation from operative endotracheal tube (ET) placement or can reflect pulmonary congestion. Purulent sputum suggests onset of pulmonary infection.
Inspect skin and mucous membranes for cyanosis.	Cyanosis of lips, nailbeds, or earlobes or general duskiness may indicate a hypoxic condition due to heart failure or pulmonary complications. General pallor (commonly present in immediate postoperative period) may indicate anemia from blood loss/insufficient blood replacement or RBC destruction from cardiopulmonary bypass pump.
Elevate head of bed, place in upright or semi-Fowler's position. Assist with early ambulation/increased time out of bed.	Stimulates respiratory function/lung expansion. Effective in preventing and resolving pulmonary congestion.
Encourage patient participation/responsibility for deep-breathing exercises, use of adjuncts, and coughing, as indicated.	Aids in reexpansion/maintaining patency of small airways, especially after removal of chest tubes. Coughing is not necessary unless wheezes/rhonchi are present, indicating retention of secretions.
Reinforce splinting of chest with pillows during deep breathing/coughing.	Reduces incisional tension, promotes maximal lung expansion, and may enhance effectiveness of cough effort.
Explain that coughing/respiratory treatments will not loosen/damage grafts or reopen chest incision.	Provides reassurance that injury will not occur and may enhance cooperation with therapeutic regimen.

ACTIONS/INTERVENTIONS	RATIONALE

Independent

Encourage maximal fluid intake within cardiac reserves.	Adequate hydration helps liquefy secretions, facilitating expectoration.
Medicate with analgesic before respiratory treatments, as indicated.	Allows for easier chest movement and reduces discomfort related to incisional pain, facilitating patient cooperation with/effectiveness of respiratory treatments.
Record response to deep-breathing exercises or other respiratory treatment, noting breath sounds (before/after treatment), cough/sputum production.	Documents effectiveness of therapy or need for more aggressive interventions.
Investigate/report respiratory distress, diminished or absent breath sounds, tachycardia, severe agitation, drop in BP.	Although not a common complication, hemothorax/pneumothorax may occur following removal of the chest tubes and requires prompt intervention to maintain respiratory function.

Collaborative

Review chest x-ray reports and laboratory studies (ABGs, Hb) as indicated.	Monitors effectiveness of respiratory therapy and/or documents developing complications. A blood transfusion may be needed if blood loss is the reason for respiratory hypoxemia.
Assist with use of incentive spirometer.	Used to maximize lung inflation, reduce atelectasis, and prevent pulmonary complications.
Administer supplemental oxygen by cannula or mask, as indicated.	Enhances oxygen delivery to the lungs for circulatory uptake, especially in presence of reduced/altered ventilation.
Assist with reinsertion of chest tubes or thoracentesis if indicated.	Re-expands lung by removal of accumulated blood/air and restoration of negative pleural pressure.

NURSING DIAGNOSIS: Skin Integrity, impaired

May be related to
Surgical incisions, puncture wounds

Possibly evidenced by
Disruption of skin surface

DESIRED OUTCOMES/EVALUATION CRITERIA—PATIENT WILL:

Wound Healing: Primary Intention (NOC)

Demonstrate behaviors/techniques to promote healing, prevent complications.
Display timely wound healing.

ACTIONS/INTERVENTIONS	RATIONALE

Incision Site Care (NIC)

Independent

Inspect all incisions. Evaluate healing progress. Review expectations for healing with patient.

Healing begins immediately, but complete healing takes time. Chest incision heals first (minimal muscle tissue), but donor site incision (when saphenous vein is used) requires more time (more muscle tissue, longer incision, slower circulation). As healing progresses, the incision lines may appear dry, with crusty scabs. Underlying tissue may look bruised and feel tense, warm, and lumpy (resolving hematoma).

Suggest wearing soft cotton shirts and loose-fitting clothing, leaving incisions open to air as much as possible, covering/padding portion of incisions as necessary.

Reduces suture line irritation and pressure from clothing. Leaving incisions open to air promotes healing process and may reduce risk of infection.

Have patient shower in warm water, washing incisions gently. Tell patient to avoid tub baths until approved by physician.

Keeps incision clean, promotes circulation/healing. *Note:* "Climbing" out of tub requires use of arms and pectoral muscles, which can put undue stress on sternotomy.

Encourage elevation of legs when sitting up in chair.

Promotes circulation, reduces edema to improve tissue healing.

Review normal signs of healing, e.g., itching along wound line, bruising, slight redness, scabbing. Instruct to watch for/report to physician: places in incision that do not heal; reopening of healed incision; any drainage (bloody or purulent); localized area that is swollen with redness, feels increasingly painful, and is hot to touch; temperature greater than 101.5°F (38.6°C) for longer than 24 hr.

Helps patient understand expected progression of healing and recognize signs of complications/nonhealing requiring further evaluation/intervention.

Promote adequate nutritional and fluid intake.

Helps to maintain good circulating volume for tissue perfusion and meets cellular energy requirements to facilitate tissue regeneration/healing process.

Collaborative

Obtain specimen of wound drainage as indicated.

If infection occurs, local and systemic treatments may be required, e.g., peroxide/saline/Betadine soaks, antibiotic therapy.

NURSING DIAGNOSIS: Knowledge Deficit [Learning Need] regarding condition, postoperative care, self care, and discharge needs

May be related to

Lack of exposure/recall

Information misinterpretation

Possibly evidenced by

Questions/requests for information

Verbalization of problem, statement of misconception

Inaccurate follow-through of instructions

DESIRED OUTCOMES/EVALUATION CRITERIA—PATIENT WILL:

Knowledge: Disease Process (NOC)

Participate in learning process.

Assume responsibility for own learning.

Begin to look for information/ask questions.

Verbalize understanding of condition, prognosis, and potential complications.

Knowledge: Treatment Regimen (NOC)

Describe reasons for therapeutic actions.

ACTIONS/INTERVENTIONS	RATIONALE
Teaching: Disease Process (NIC)	
Independent	
Reinforce surgeon's explanation of particular surgical procedure, providing diagram as appropriate.	Provides individually specific information, creating knowledge base for subsequent learning regarding home management.
Incorporate this information into discussion about short- and long-term recovery expectations.	Length of rehabilitation and prognosis are dependent on type of surgical procedure, preoperative physical condition, and duration/severity of complications.
Cardiac Care: Rehabilitation (NIC)	
Reinforce continuation of breathing exercises, incentive spirometry, and coughing with splinting incision.	Promotes alveolar ventilation, reducing risk of lung congestion.
Discuss routine/prophylactic medications and OTC drug use. Stress importance of checking with physician before taking any drugs.	Dependent on type of valve replacement (i.e., synthetic) and presence of atrial fibrillation, anticoagulant therapy may be indicated. Also, antibiotic agent may be required when dental care is provided. Potential for drug interactions must be considered before adding therapeutic agents to regimen. *Note:* Using herbal products (e.g., ginkgo biloba, garlic, vitamins) can alter coagulation and have an adverse effect when taken with anticoagulants.
Review prescribed cardiac rehabilitation/exercise program and progress to date. Assist patient/SO to set realistic goals.	Individual capabilities and expectations depend on type of surgery, underlying cardiac function, and prior physical conditioning.
Encourage participation in home routines, e.g., self-care, cooking. Suggest alternating rest periods with activity and light tasks with heavy tasks. Avoid heavy lifting, isometric/strenuous upper-body exercise.	Prevents excessive fatigue/overexhaustion. *Note:* Strenuous use of arms can place undue stress on sternotomy.

ACTIONS/INTERVENTIONS	RATIONALE

Independent

Problem-solve with patient/SO ways to continue progressive activity program during temperature extremes and high wind/pollution days, e.g., walking predetermined distance within own house or local indoor shopping mall/exercise track.	Having a plan forestalls giving up exercise because of interferences such as weather.
Schedule rest periods and short naps several times a day.	Rest and sleep enhance coping abilities, reduce nervousness (common in this phase), and promote healing.
Reinforce physician's time limitations about lifting, driving, returning to work, resuming sexual activity, and exercising that involves upper extremities.	These restrictions are present until after the first postoperative office visit for assessment of sternum healing.
Discuss issues concerning resumption of sexual activity, e.g., comparison of stress sexual intercourse with other activities;	Concerns about sexual activity often go unexpressed, but patients usually desire information about what to expect. In general, patient can safely engage in sex when activity level has advanced to point at which patient can climb two flights of stairs (which is about the same amount of energy expenditure).
Position recommendations;	Patient should avoid positions that restrict breathing (sexual activity increases oxygen demand and consumption). Patient with sternotomy should not support self or partner with arms (breastbone healing, support muscles stretched).
Expectations of sexual performance;	Impotence appears to occur with some regularity in postoperative cardiac surgery patients. Although etiology is unknown, condition usually resolves in time without specific intervention. If situation persists, may require further evaluation.
Appropriate timing, e.g., avoid sexual intercourse following heavy meal, during periods of emotional distress, when patient is fatigued/exhausted;	Timing of activity may reduce occurrence of complications/angina.
Pharmacological considerations.	Some patients may require antianginal medications (prophylactically) before sexual activity.
Identify services/resources available after discharge. Provide telephone contact number/schedule follow-up calls as appropriate. Include referral names for home care services, as indicated.	Facilitates transition to home; provides for ongoing monitoring, continuation of prescribed therapies, opportunity to discuss concerns.

POTENTIAL CONSIDERATIONS following discharge from care setting (dependent on patient's age, physical condition/presence of complications, personal resources, and life responsibilities)

Activity intolerance—generalized weakness, sedentary lifestyle.
Skin/Tissue Integrity, impaired—surgical incisions, puncture wounds.
Home Maintenance Management, impaired—altered ability to perform tasks, inadequate support systems, reluctance to request assistance.
Infection, risk for—broken skin, traumatized tissue, invasive procedures, decreased hemoglobin.
Self-Care deficit—decreased strength and endurance, discomfort.
Role Performance, altered—situational crisis/recuperative process, uncertainty about future.

THROMBOPHLEBITIS: DEEP VEIN THROMBOSIS (INCLUDING PULMONARY EMBOLI CONSIDERATIONS)

Thrombophlebitis is a condition in which a clot forms in a vein, associated with inflammation/trauma of the vein wall or a partial obstruction of the vein. Clot formation is related to (1) stasis of blood flow, (2) abnormalities in the vessel walls, and (3) alterations in the clotting mechanism (Virchow's triad). Young women and the elderly are at greatest risk.

Thrombophlebitis can affect superficial or deep veins. Although both conditions can cause symptoms, DVT is more serious in terms of potential complications, including pulmonary embolism, postphlebotic syndrome, chronic venous insufficiency, and vein valve destruction. *Note:* Approximately 50% of patients with DVT are asymptomatic.

CARE SETTING

Primarily treated at the community level, with short inpatient stay generally indicated in the presence of embolization.

RELATED CONCERNS

Surgical intervention, page 828
Mechanical ventilation, page 188
Fractures, page 680
Psychosocial aspects of care, page 809

Patient Assessment Database

ACTIVITY/REST

May report:	Occupation that requires sitting or standing for long periods of time Lengthy immobility (e.g., orthopedic trauma, long hospitalization/bedrest, prolonged sitting/travel, complicated pregnancy); paralysis/progressive debilitating condition Pain with activity/prolonged standing Fatigue/weakness of affected extremity, general malaise
May exhibit:	Generalized or extremity weakness

CIRCULATION

May report:	History of previous peripheral vascular disease, venous thrombosis, preexisting varices Presence of other predisposing factors, e.g., hypertension (pregnancy-induced), diabetes mellitus, MI/valvular heart disease, thrombotic cerebrovascular accident
May exhibit:	Tachycardia Peripheral pulse may be diminished in the affected extremity (DVT) Varicosities and/or hardened, bumpy/knotty vein (thrombus) Skin color/temperature in affected extremity (calf/thigh): pale, cool, edematous (DVT); pinkish red, warm along the course of the vein (superficial) Positive Homans' sign (absence does not rule out DVT because only about 33% of patients have a positive sign)

FOOD/FLUID

May exhibit:	Poor skin turgor, dry mucous membranes (dehydration predisposes to hypercoagulability) Obesity (predisposes to stasis and pelvic vein pressure) Edema of affected extremity (dependent on location of thrombus)

PAIN/DISCOMFORT

May report:	Throbbing, tenderness, aching pain aggravated by standing or movement of affected extremity, groin tenderness
May exhibit:	Guarding of affected extremity

SAFETY

May report: History of direct or indirect injury to extremity or vein (e.g., major trauma/fractures, orthopedic/pelvic surgery, prolonged labor with fetal head pressure on pelvic veins, intravenous therapy)

Presence of malignancy (particularly of the pancreas, lung, GI system, prostate)

May exhibit: Fever, chills

TEACHING/LEARNING

May report: Use of oral contraceptives/estrogens; recent anticoagulant therapy (predisposes to hypercoagulability)

Recurrence/lack of resolution of previous thrombophlebotic episode

Discharge plan considerations: **DRG projected mean length of inpatient stay: 5.8 days**

Temporary assistance with shopping, transportation, and homemaker/maintenance tasks

Properly fitted antiembolic hose

DIAGNOSTIC STUDIES

Hematocrit: Hemoconcentration (elevated Hct) potentiates risk of thrombus formation.

Coagulation profile: PT, PTT, and platelets may reveal hypercoagulability.

Antithrombin: Useful in determining cause of impaired coagulation/hypercoagulation and in the management of venous thrombotic disease. Elevated in DVT.

Noninvasive vascular studies (Doppler ultrasound, compression ultrasonography, impedance plethysmography, and duplex venous scanning): Changes in blood flow and volume identify venous occlusion, vascular damage, and vascular insufficiency. Ultrasonography appears to be most accurate noninvasive method for diagnosing multiple proximal DVT (iliac, femoral, popliteal) but is less reliable in detecting isolated calf vein thrombi.

Trendelenburg test: May demonstrate vessel valve incompetence.

Venography: Radiographically confirms diagnosis through changes in blood flow and/or size of channels. *Note:* This study carries a risk of inducing DVT and therefore is reserved for patients with negative or difficult-to-interpret noninvasive studies in the presence of high clinical suspicion.

MRI: May be useful in assessing blood flow turbulence and movement, venous valvular competence.

NURSING PRIORITIES

1. Maintain/enhance tissue perfusion, facilitate resolution of thrombus.
2. Promote optimal comfort.
3. Prevent complications.
4. Provide information about disease process/prognosis and treatment regimen.

DISCHARGE GOALS

1. Tissue perfusion improved in affected limb.
2. Pain/discomfort relieved.
3. Complications prevented/resolved.
4. Disease process/prognosis and therapeutic needs understood.
5. Plan in place to meet needs after discharge.

NURSING DIAGNOSIS: Tissue Perfusion, altered peripheral

May be related to

Decreased blood flow/venous stasis (partial or complete venous obstruction)

Possibly evidenced by

Tissue edema, pain

Diminished peripheral pulses, slow/diminished capillary refill

Skin color changes (pallor, erythema)

DESIRED OUTCOMES/EVALUATION CRITERIA—PATIENT WILL:

Tissue Perfusion: Peripheral (NOC)

Demonstrate improved perfusion as evidenced by peripheral pulses present/equal, skin color and temperature normal, absence of edema.

Engage in behaviors/actions to enhance tissue perfusion.

Display increasing tolerance to activity.

ACTIONS/INTERVENTIONS	RATIONALE

Embolus Care: Peripheral (NIC)

Independent

Evaluate circulatory and neurological studies of involved extremity—both sensory and motor. Inspect for skin color and temperature changes, as well as edema (from groin to foot). Note symmetry of calves; measure and record calf circumference. Report proximal progression of inflammatory process, traveling pain.	Symptoms help distinguish between superficial thrombophlebitis and DVT. Redness, heat, tenderness, and localized edema are characteristic of superficial involvement. Pallor and coolness of extremity are characteristic of DVT. Calf vein involvement is associated with absence of edema; femoral vein involvement is associated with mild to moderate edema; iliofemoral vein thrombosis is characterized by severe edema.
Examine extremity for obviously prominent veins. Palpate gently for local tissue tension, stretched skin, knots/bumps along course of vein.	Distention of superficial veins can occur in DVT because of backflow through communicating veins. Thrombophlebitis in superficial veins may be visible or palpable.
Assess capillary refill and check for Homans' sign.	Diminished capillary refill usually present in DVT. Positive Homans' sign (deep calf pain in affected leg upon dorsiflexion of foot) is not as consistent a clinical manifestation as once thought and may or may not be present.
Promote bedrest initially, with legs elevated above heart level during acute phase.	Until treatment is instituted, limitation of activity minimizes the possibility of dislodging thrombus/creating emboli.
Elevate legs when in bed or chair, as indicated.	Reduces tissue swelling and rapidly empties superficial and tibial veins, preventing overdistension and thereby increasing venous return. *Note:* Some physicians believe that elevation may potentiate release of thrombus, thus increasing risk of embolization and decreasing circulation to the most distal portion of the extremity.

ACTIONS/INTERVENTIONS

Independent

Initiate active or passive exercises while in bed (e.g., flex/extend/rotate foot periodically). Assist with gradual resumption of ambulation (e.g., walking 10 min/hr) as soon as patient is permitted out of bed.

Caution patient to avoid crossing legs or hyperflexion at knee (seated position with legs dangling, or lying in jackknife position).

Instruct patient to avoid rubbing/massaging the affected extremity.

Encourage deep-breathing exercises.

Increase fluid intake to at least 2000 ml/day, within cardiac tolerance.

Collaborative

Apply warm, moist compresses or heat cradle to affected extremity if indicated.

Administer anticoagulants, e.g.:

Heparin via continuous or intermittent IV, intermittent subcutaneous (SC) injections, and/or PO coumarin derivatives (Coumadin);

Thrombolytic agents, e.g., streptokinase, urokinase.

RATIONALE

These measures are designed to increase venous return from lower extremities and reduce venous stasis, as well as improve general muscle tone/strength. They also promote normal organ function and enhance general well-being.

Physical restriction of circulation impairs blood flow and increases venous stasis in pelvic, popliteal, and leg vessels, thus increasing swelling and discomfort.

This activity potentiates risk of fragmenting/dislodging thrombus, causing embolization, and increasing risk of complications.

Increases negative pressure in thorax, which assists in emptying large veins.

Dehydration increases blood viscosity and venous stasis, predisposing to thrombus formation.

May be prescribed to promote vasodilation and venous return and resolution of local edema. *Note:* May be contraindicated in presence of arterial insufficiency, in which heat can increase cellular oxygen consumption/nutritional needs, furthering imbalance between supply and demand.

Heparin is preferred initially because of its prompt, predictable, antagonistic action on thrombin as it is formed and also because it removes activated coagulation factors XII, XI, IX, and X (intrinsic pathway), preventing further clot formation. Coumadin has a potent depressant effect on liver formation of prothrombin from vitamin K and impairs formation of factors VII, IX, and X (extrinsic pathway). Coumadin is generally used for long-term/postdischarge therapy to keep international normalized ratio (INR) at 2–3. *Note:* A new low molecular weight heparin derivative, enoxaparin (Lovenox) is a fast-acting substance (given SC for 7–10 days) that prevents the conversion of factor Xa to thrombin, allowing earlier discharge in some patients.

May be used for treatment of acute (less than 5 days old) or massive DVT to prevent valvular damage and development of chronic venous insufficiency. Heparin is usually begun several hours after the completion of thrombolytic therapy.

ACTIONS/INTERVENTIONS	RATIONALE
Collaborative	
Monitor laboratory studies as indicated: PT, PTT, aPTT, CBC;	Monitors anticoagulant therapy and presence of risk factors, e.g., hemoconcentration and dehydration, which potentiate clot formation. *Note:* Lovenox does not require serial monitoring because PT and aPTT are not affected.
Platelet count, platelet/aggregation test, antiheparin antibody assay.	On occasion, platelet count may decrease as a result of an immune reaction leading to platelet aggregation or the formation of "white clots." If bacteremia/DIC have been ruled out, condition may be the result of heparin-induced thrombocytopenia and thrombosis (HITT), requiring a change to Coumadin or other agents, e.g., dipyridamole (Persantine) and ASA.
Apply/regulate graduated compression stockings, intermittent pneumatic compression, if indicated.	Sequential compression devices may be used to improve blood flow velocity and empty vessels by providing artificial muscle-pumping action.
Apply elastic support hose following acute phase. Take care to avoid tourniquet effect.	Properly fitted support hose are useful (once ambulation has begun) to minimize or delay development of postphlebotic syndrome. They must exert a sustained, evenly distributed pressure over entire surface of calves and thighs to reduce the caliber of superficial veins and increase blood flow to deep veins.
Prepare for surgical intervention when indicated.	Thrombectomy (excision of thrombus) is occasionally necessary if inflammation extends proximally or circulation is severely restricted. Multiple/recurrent thrombotic episodes unresponsive to medical treatment (or when anticoagulant therapy is contraindicated) may require insertion of a vena caval screen/umbrella.

NURSING DIAGNOSIS: Pain [acute]/[Discomfort]

May be related to

Diminished arterial circulation and oxygenation of tissues with production/accumulation of lactic acid in tissues

Inflammatory process

Possibly evidenced by

Reports of pain, tenderness, aching/burning

Guarding of affected limb

Restlessness, distraction behaviors

DESIRED OUTCOMES/EVALUATION CRITERIA—PATIENT WILL:

Pain Control Behavior (NOC)

Report pain/discomfort is alleviated or controlled.

Verbalize methods that provide relief.

Display relaxed manner; be able to sleep/rest and engage in desired activity.

ACTIONS/INTERVENTIONS	RATIONALE

Pain Management (NIC)

Independent

Assess degree and characteristics of discomfort/pain. Note guarding of extremity. Palpate leg with caution.	Degree of pain is directly related to extent of circulatory deficit, inflammatory process, degree of tissue ischemia, and extent of edema associated with thrombus development. Changes in characteristics of pain may indicate progression of problem/development of complications.
Maintain bedrest during acute phase.	Reduces discomfort associated with muscle contraction and movement.
Elevate affected extremity.	Encourages venous return to facilitate circulation, reducing stasis/edema formation.
Provide foot cradle.	Cradle keeps pressure of bedclothes off the affected leg, thereby reducing pressure discomfort.
Encourage patient to change position frequently.	Decreases/prevents muscle fatigue, helps minimize muscle spasm, maximizes circulation to tissues.
Monitor vital signs, noting elevated temperature.	Elevations in heart rate may indicate increased pain/discomfort or occur in response to fever and inflammatory process. Fever can also increase patient's discomfort.
Investigate reports of sudden and/or sharp chest pain, accompanied by dyspnea, tachycardia, and apprehension, or development of a new pain with signs of another site of vascular involvement.	These signs/symptoms suggest presence of pulmonary emboli as a complication of DVT, or peripheral arterial occlusion associated with heparin-induced thrombocytopenia and thrombosis (HITT). Both conditions require prompt medical evaluation and treatment.

Collaborative

Administer medications, as indicated:	
Analgesics (narcotic/nonnarcotic);	Relieves pain and decreases muscle tension.
Antipyretics, e.g., acetaminophen (Tylenol).	Reduces fever and inflammation. *Note:* Risk of bleeding may be increased by concurrent use of drugs that affect platelet function, e.g., ASA and nonsteroidal anti-inflammatory drugs (NSAIDs).
Apply moist heat to extremity, if indicated.	Causes vasodilation, which increases circulation, relaxes muscles, and may stimulate release of natural endorphins.

NURSING DIAGNOSIS: Gas Exchange, impaired (in presence of pulmonary embolus)

May be related to
Altered blood flow to alveoli or to major portions of the lung
Alveolar-capillary membrane changes (atelectasis, airway/alveolar collapse, pulmonary edema/effusion, excessive secretions/active bleeding)

Possibly evidenced by
Profound dyspnea, restlessness, apprehension, somnolence, cyanosis
Changes in ABGs/pulse oximetry, e.g., hypoxemia and hypercapnia

DESIRED OUTCOMES/EVALUATION CRITERIA—PATIENT WILL:

Respiratory Status: Gas Exchange (NOC)

Demonstrate adequate ventilation/oxygenation by ABGs within patient's normal range.
Report/display resolution or absence of symptoms of respiratory distress.

ACTIONS/INTERVENTIONS	RATIONALE
Embolus Care: Pulmonary (NIC)	
Independent	
Note respiratory rate and depth, work of breathing (use of accessory muscles/nasal flaring, pursed-lip breathing).	Tachypnea and dyspnea accompany pulmonary obstruction. Dyspnea ("air hunger") and increased work of breathing may be first or only sign of subacute pulmonary embolus (PE). Severe respiratory distress/failure accompanies moderate to severe loss of functional lung units.
Auscultate lungs for areas of decreased/absent breath sounds and the presence of adventitious sounds, e.g., crackles.	Nonventilated areas may be identified by absence of breath sounds. Crackles occur in fluid-filled tissues/airways or may reflect cardiac decompensation.
Observe for generalized duskiness and cyanosis in "warm tissues" such as earlobes, lips, tongue, and buccal membranes.	Indicative of systemic hypoxemia.
Monitor vital signs. Note changes in cardiac rhythm.	Tachycardia, tachypnea, and changes in BP are associated with advancing hypoxemia and acidosis. Rhythm alterations and extra heart sounds may reflect increased cardiac workload related to worsening ventilation imbalance.
Assess level of consciousness/mentation changes.	Systemic hypoxemia may be demonstrated initially by restlessness and irritability, then by progressively decreased mentation.
Assess activity tolerance, e.g., reports of weakness/fatigue, vital sign changes, increased dyspnea during exertion. Encourage rest periods, and limit activities to patient tolerance.	These parameters assist in determining patient response to resumed activities and ability to participate in self-care.
Airway Management (NIC)	
Institute measures to restore/maintain patent airways, e.g., coughing, suctioning.	Plugged/collapsed airways reduce number of functional alveoli, negatively affecting gas exchange.

ACTIONS/INTERVENTIONS	RATIONALE

Independent

Elevate head of bed as patient requires/tolerates.	Promotes maximal chest expansion, making it easier to breathe and enhancing physiological/psychological comfort.
Assist with frequent changes of position, and get patient out of bed/ambulate as tolerated.	Turning and ambulation enhance aeration of different lung segments, thereby improving oxygen diffusion.
Assist patient to deal with fear/anxiety that may be present:	Feelings of fear and severe anxiety are associated with inability to breathe and may actually increase oxygen consumption/demand.
Encourage expression of feelings, inform patient/SOs of normalcy of anxious feelings, sense of impending doom;	Understanding basis of feelings may help patient regain some sense of control over emotions.
Provide brief explanations of what is happening and expected effects of interventions;	Allays anxiety related to unknown and may help reduce fears concerning personal safety.
Monitor frequently, arrange for individual (volunteer, family, others) to stay with patient as indicated.	Provides assurance that changes in condition will be noted and that assistance is readily available.

Collaborative

Embolus Care: Pulmonary (NIC)	
Prepare for lung scan.	May reveal pattern of abnormal perfusion in areas of ventilation (ventilation/perfusion mismatch), confirming diagnosis of pulmonary embolus (PE) and degree of obstruction. Absence of both ventilation and perfusion reflects alveolar congestion/airway obstruction.
Monitor serial ABGs/pulse oximetry.	Hypoxemia is present in varying degrees, depending on the amount of airway obstruction, usual cardiopulmonary function, and presence/degree of shock. Respiratory alkalosis and metabolic acidosis may also be present.

Airway Management (NIC)	
Administer supplemental oxygen by appropriate method.	Maximizes available oxygen for gas exchange, reducing work of breathing. *Note:* If obstruction is large or hypoxemia does not respond to supplemental oxygenation, it may be necessary to move patient to critical care area for intubation and mechanical ventilation.
Administer fluids (IV/PO) as indicated.	Increased fluids may be given to reduce hyperviscosity of blood (potentiates thrombus formation) or to support circulating volume/tissue perfusion.
Administer medications as indicated:	
Thrombolytic agents, e.g., streptokinase (Kabikinase, Streptase), urokinase (Abbokinase), alteplase (t-PA, Activase);	Indicated in massive pulmonary obstruction when the patient is seriously hemodynamically threatened. *Note:* These patients will probably be initially cared for in/transferred to the critical care setting.

ACTIONS/INTERVENTIONS	RATIONALE
Collaborative	
Morphine sulfate, antianxiety agents.	May be necessary initially to control pain/anxiety and improve work of breathing, maximizing gas exchange.
Provide supplemental humidification, e.g., ultrasonic nebulizers.	Delivers moisture to mucous membranes and helps liquefy secretions to facilitate airway clearance.
Assist with chest physiotherapy (e.g., postural drainage and percussion of nonaffected area, blow bottles/incentive spirometer).	Facilitates deeper respiratory effort and promotes drainage of secretions from lung segments into bronchi, where they may more readily be removed by coughing/suctioning.
Prepare for/assist with bronchoscopy.	May be done to remove blood clots and clear airways.
Prepare for surgical intervention if indicated.	Vena caval ligation or insertion of an intracaval umbrella may be useful for patients who experience recurrent emboli despite adequate anticoagulation, when anticoagulation is contraindicated, or when septic emboli arising from below the renal veins do not respond to treatment. Additionally, pulmonary embolectomy may be considered in life-threatening situations.

NURSING DIAGNOSIS: Knowledge Deficit [Learning Need] regarding condition, treatment program, self care, and discharge needs

May be related to
Lack of exposure or recall
Misinterpretation of information
Unfamiliarity with information resources

Possibly evidenced by
Request for information, statement of misconception
Inaccurate follow-through of instructions
Development of preventable complications

DESIRED OUTCOMES/EVALUATION CRITERIA—PATIENT WILL:

Knowledge: Disease Process (NOC)

Verbalize understanding of disease process, treatment regimen, and limitations.
Participate in learning process.
Identify signs/symptoms requiring medical evaluation.

Knowledge: Treatment Regimen (NOC)

Correctly perform therapeutic actions and explain reasons for actions.

ACTIONS/INTERVENTIONS	RATIONALE

Teaching: Disease Process (NIC)

Independent

Review pathophysiology of condition and signs/symptoms of possible complications, e.g., pulmonary emboli, chronic venous insufficiency, venous stasis ulcers (postphlebotic syndrome).

Provides a knowledge base from which patient can make informed choices and understand/identify healthcare needs. Up to 33% experience a recurrence of DVT.

Explain purpose of activity restrictions and need for balance between activity/rest.

Rest reduces oxygen and nutrient needs of compromised tissues and decreases risk of fragmentation of thrombosis. Balancing rest with activity prevents exhaustion and further impairment of cellular perfusion.

Establish appropriate exercise/activity program.

Aids in developing collateral circulation, enhances venous return, and prevents recurrence.

Problem-solve solutions to predisposing factors that may be present, e.g., employment that requires prolonged standing/sitting, wearing restrictive clothing (girdles/garters), use of oral contraceptives, obesity, prolonged bedrest/immobility, dehydration.

Actively involves patient in identifying and initiating lifestyle/behavior changes to promote health and prevent recurrence of condition/development of complications.

Recommend sitting with feet touching the floor, avoiding crossing of legs.

Prevents excess pressure on the popliteal space.

Discuss purpose, dosage of anticoagulant. Emphasize importance of taking drug as prescribed.

Promotes patient safety by reducing risk of inadequate therapeutic response/deleterious side effects.

Identify safety precautions, e.g., use of soft toothbrush, electric razor for shaving, gloves for gardening, avoiding sharp objects (including toothpicks), walking barefoot, engaging in rough sports/activities, or forceful blowing of nose.

Reduces the risk of traumatic injury, which potentiates bleeding/clot formation.

Review possible drug interactions, and stress need to read ingredient labels of OTC drugs.

Salicylates and excess alcohol decrease prothrombin activity, whereas vitamin K (multivitamins, bananas, leafy green vegetables) increases prothrombin activity. Barbiturates increase metabolism of coumarin drugs; antibiotics alter intestinal flora and may interfere with vitamin K synthesis.

Identify untoward anticoagulant effects requiring medical attention, e.g., bleeding from mucous membranes (nose, gums), continued oozing from cuts/punctures, severe bruising after minimal trauma, development of petechiae.

Early detection of deleterious effects of therapy (prolongation of clotting time) allows for timely intervention and may prevent serious complications. *Note:* Even regular use of acetaminophen may prolong clotting times. In addition, use of herbal products, such as ginkgo biloba, garlic, vitamin E, also impair clotting and should be avoided during anticoagulant therapy.

Stress importance of medical follow-up/laboratory testing.

Understanding that close supervision of anticoagulant therapy is necessary (therapeutic dosage range is narrow and complications may be deadly) promotes patient participation.

Encourage wearing of medical-alert identification bracelet/tag, as indicated.

Alerts emergency healthcare providers to use of anticoagulants.

Review purpose and demonstrate correct application/removal of antiembolic hose.

Understanding may enhance cooperation with prescribed therapy and prevent improper/ineffective use.

ACTIONS/INTERVENTIONS	RATIONALE
Independent	
Instruct in meticulous skin care of lower extremities, e.g., prevent/promptly treat breaks in skin and report development of lesions/ulcers or changes in skin color.	Chronic venous congestion/postphlebotic syndrome may develop (especially in presence of severe vascular involvement and/or recurrent episodes), potentiating risk of stasis ulcers/infection.

POTENTIAL CONSIDERATIONS following discharge from care setting (dependent on patient's age, physical condition/presence of complications, personal resources, and life responsibilities)

Therapeutic Regimen: Individual, ineffective management—perceived seriousness of condition, susceptibility to recurrence, benefit of therapy.

Respiratory

CHRONIC OBSTRUCTIVE PULMONARY DISEASE (COPD) AND ASTHMA

All respiratory diseases characterized by chronic obstruction to airflow fall under the broad classification of COPD, also known as chronic airflow limitations (CAL). *COPD* is a condition of chronic dyspnea with expiratory airflow limitation that does not significantly fluctuate. Within that broad category, the primary cause of the obstruction may vary; examples include airway inflammation, mucus plugging, narrowed airway lumina, or airway destruction. The term COPD includes chronic bronchitis and emphysema. Although asthma also involves airway inflammation and periodic narrowing of the airway lumina (hyperreactivity), the condition is the result of individual response to a wide variety of stimuli/triggers and is therefore episodic in nature with fluctuations/exacerbations of symptoms. Because patient response and therapy needs can be similar, asthma has been included in this plan of care.

Asthma: Characterized by reversible inflammation and constriction of bronchial smooth muscle, hypersecretion of mucus, and edema. Precipitating factors include allergens, emotional upheaval, cold weather, exercise, chemicals, medications, and viral infections.

Chronic bronchitis: Widespread inflammation of airways with narrowing or blocking of airways, increased production of mucoid sputum, and marked cyanosis.

Emphysema: Most severe form of COPD, characterized by recurrent inflammation that damages and eventually destroys alveolar walls to create large blebs or bullae (air spaces) and collapsed bronchioles on expiration (airtrapping).

Note: Chronic bronchitis and emphysema coexist in many patients and are most commonly seen in hospitalized COPD patients when acute exacerbations occur. Chronic bronchitis and emphysema are usually irreversible, although some effects can be mediated.

CARE SETTING

Primarily community level; however, severe exacerbations may necessitate emergency and/or inpatient stay.

RELATED CONCERNS

Heart failure: chronic, page 47
Pneumonia: microbial, page 140
Psychosocial aspects of care, page 809
Ventilatory assistance (mechanical), page 188
Surgical intervention, page 828

Patient Assessment Database

ACTIVITY/REST

May report: Fatigue, exhaustion, malaise
Inability to perform basic activities of daily living (ADLs) because of breathlessness
Inability to sleep, need to sleep sitting up
Dyspnea at rest or in response to activity or exercise

May exhibit: Fatigue
Restlessness, insomnia
General debilitation/loss of muscle mass

CIRCULATION

May report: Swelling of lower extremities

May exhibit: Elevated blood pressure (BP)
Elevated heart rate/severe tachycardia, dysrhythmias
Distended neck veins (advanced disease)
Dependent edema, may not be related to heart disease
Faint heart sounds (due to increased anteroposterior [AP] chest diameter)
Skin color/mucous membranes may be pale or bluish/cyanotic; clubbing of nails and peripheral cyanosis; pallor (can indicate anemia)

EGO INTEGRITY

May report: Increased stress factors
Changes in lifestyle
Feelings of hopelessness, loss of interest in life

May exhibit: Anxious, fearful, irritable behavior, emotional distress
Apathy, dull affect, withdrawal

FOOD/FLUID

May report: Nausea (side effect of medication/mucus production)
Poor appetite/anorexia (emphysema)
Inability to eat because of respiratory distress
Persistent weight loss, decreased muscle mass/subcutaneous fat (emphysema) or weight gain may reflect edema (bronchitis, prednisone use)

May exhibit: Poor skin turgor
Dependent edema
Diaphoresis
Abdominal palpation may reveal hepatomegaly (bronchitis)

HYGIENE

May report: Decreased ability/increased need for assistance with ADLs

May exhibit: Poor hygiene, body odor

RESPIRATION

May report: Variable levels of dyspnea, such as insidious and progressive onset (predominant symptom in emphysema), especially on exertion; seasonal or episodic occurrence of breathlessness (asthma); sensation of chest tightness, inability to breathe (asthma); chronic "air hunger"
Persistent cough with sputum production (gray, white, or yellow), which may be copious (chronic bronchitis); intermittent cough episodes, usually nonproductive in early stages, although they may become productive (emphysema); paroxysms of cough (asthma)
History of recurrent pneumonia, long-term exposure to chemical pollution/respiratory irritants (e.g., cigarette smoke), or occupational dust/fumes (e.g., cotton, hemp, asbestos, coal dust, sawdust)
Familial and hereditary factors, i.e., deficiency of α_1-antitrypsin (emphysema)
Use of oxygen at night or continuously

May exhibit: Respirations: Usually rapid, may be shallow; prolonged expiratory phase with grunting, pursed-lip breathing (emphysema)

Assumption of three-point ("tripod") position for breathing (especially with acute exacerbation of chronic bronchitis)

Use of accessory muscles for respiration, e.g., elevated shoulder girdle, retraction of supraclavicular fossae, flaring of nares

Chest may appear hyperinflated with increased AP diameter (barrel-shaped); minimal diaphragmatic movement

Breath sounds may be faint with expiratory wheezes (emphysema); scattered, fine, or coarse moist crackles (bronchitis); rhonchi, wheezing throughout lung fields on expiration, and possibly during inspiration, progressing to diminished or absent breath sounds (asthma)

Percussion may reveal hyperresonance over lung fields (e.g., air-trapping with emphysema) or dullness over lung fields (e.g., consolidation, fluid, mucus)

Difficulty speaking sentences of more than four or five words at one time; loss of voice

Color: Pallor with cyanosis of lips, nailbeds; overall duskiness; ruddy color (chronic bronchitis, "blue bloaters"); normal skin color despite abnormal gas exchange and rapid respiratory rate (moderate emphysema, known as "pink puffers")

Clubbing of the fingernails (emphysema)

SAFETY

May report: History of allergic reactions or sensitivity to substances/environmental factors

Recent/recurrent infections

Flushing/perspiration (asthma)

SEXUALITY

May report: Decreased libido

SOCIAL INTERACTION

May report: Dependent relationship(s)

Insufficient support from/to partner/significant other (SO); lack of support systems

Prolonged disease or disability progression

May exhibit: Inability to converse/maintain voice because of respiratory distress

Limited physical mobility

Neglectful relationships with other family members

Inability to perform/inattention to employment responsibilities, absenteeism/confirmed disability

TEACHING/LEARNING

May report: Use/misuse of respiratory drugs

Smoking/difficulty stopping smoking; chronic exposure to second-hand smoke, smoking substances other than tobacco

Regular use of alcohol

Failure to improve

Discharge plan considerations: **DRG projected mean length of inpatient stay: 5.2 days**

Episodic or long-term assistance with shopping, transportation, self-care needs, homemaker/home maintenance tasks

Changes in medication/therapeutic treatments, use of supplemental oxygen, ventilator support

Refer to section at end of plan for postdischarge considerations.

DIAGNOSTIC STUDIES

Chest x-ray: May reveal hyperinflation of lungs, flattened diaphragm, increased retrosternal air space, decreased vascular markings/bullae (emphysema), increased bronchovascular markings (bronchitis), normal findings during periods of remission (asthma).

Pulmonary function tests: Done to determine cause of dyspnea, whether functional abnormality is obstructive or restrictive, to estimate degree of dysfunction, and to evaluate effects of therapy, e.g., bronchodilators. Exercise pulmonary function studies may also be done to evaluate activity tolerance in those with known pulmonary impairment/progression of disease.

The forced expiratory volume over 1 second (FEV_1) and all other measurements of expiratory airflow: Reduced FEV_1 is not only the standard way of assessing the clinical course and response to therapy, but also an important predictor of prognosis.

Total lung capacity (TLC), functional residual capacity (FRC), and residual volume (RV): May be increased, indicating air-trapping.

Arterial blood gases (ABGs): Estimate progression of chronic disease process, e.g., most often PaO_2 is decreased, and $PaCO_2$ is normal or increased in chronic bronchitis and emphysema, but is often decreased in asthma; pH normal or acidotic, mild respiratory alkalosis secondary to hyperventilation (moderate emphysema or asthma).

Bronchogram: Can show cylindrical dilation of bronchi on inspiration; bronchial collapse on forced expiration (emphysema); enlarged mucous ducts (bronchitis).

Lung scan: Perfusion/ventilation studies may be done to differentiate between the various pulmonary diseases. COPD is characterized by a mismatch of perfusion and ventilation (i.e., areas of abnormal ventilation in area of perfusion defect).

Complete blood count (CBC) and differential: Increased hemoglobin (advanced emphysema), increased eosinophils (asthma).

Blood chemistry: α_1-Antitrypsin done to verify deficiency and diagnosis of primary emphysema.

Sputum culture: Determines presence of infection, identifies pathogen.

Cytologic examination: Rules out underlying malignancy or allergic disorder.

Electrocardiogram (ECG): Right axis deviation, peaked P waves (severe asthma); atrial dysrhythmias (bronchitis), tall, peaked P waves in leads II, III, AVF (bronchitis, emphysema); vertical QRS axis (emphysema).

Exercise ECG, stress test: Helps in assessing degree of pulmonary dysfunction, evaluating effectiveness of bronchodilator therapy, planning/evaluating exercise program.

NURSING PRIORITIES

1. Maintain airway patency.
2. Assist with measures to facilitate gas exchange.
3. Enhance nutritional intake.
4. Prevent complications, slow progression of condition.
5. Provide information about disease process/prognosis and treatment regimen.

DISCHARGE GOALS

1. Ventilation/oxygenation adequate to meet self-care needs.
2. Nutritional intake meeting caloric needs.
3. Infection treated/prevented.
4. Disease process/prognosis and therapeutic regimen understood.
5. Plan in place to meet needs after discharge.

NURSING DIAGNOSIS: Airway Clearance, ineffective

May be related to
Bronchospasm
Increased production of secretions, retained secretions, thick, viscous secretions
Decreased energy/fatigue

Possibly evidenced by
Statement of difficulty breathing
Changes in depth/rate of respirations, use of accessory muscles
Abnormal breath sounds, e.g., wheezes, rhonchi, crackles
Cough (persistent), with/without sputum production

DESIRED OUTCOMES/EVALUATION CRITERIA—PATIENT WILL:

Respiratory Status: Ventilation (NOC)

Maintain patent airway with breath sounds clear/clearing.
Demonstrate behaviors to improve airway clearance, e.g., cough effectively and expectorate secretions.

ACTIONS/INTERVENTIONS	RATIONALE

Airway Management (NIC)

Independent

Auscultate breath sounds. Note adventitious breath sounds, e.g., wheezes, crackles, rhonchi.

Some degree of bronchospasm is present with obstructions in airway and may/may not be manifested in adventitious breath sounds, e.g., scattered, moist crackles (bronchitis); faint sounds, with expiratory wheezes (emphysema); or absent breath sounds (severe asthma).

Assess/monitor respiratory rate. Note inspiratory/expiratory ratio.

Tachypnea is usually present to some degree and may be pronounced on admission or during stress/concurrent acute infectious process. Respirations may be shallow and rapid with prolonged expiration in comparison to inspiration.

Note presence/degree of dyspnea, e.g., reports of "air hunger," restlessness, anxiety, respiratory distress, use of accessory muscles. Use 0–10 scale or American Thoracic Society's "Grade of Breathlessness Scale" to rate breathing difficulty. Ascertain precipitating factors when possible. Differentiate acute episode from exacerbation of chronic dyspnea.

Respiratory dysfunction is variable depending on the underlying process, e.g., infection, allergic reaction, and the stage of chronicity in a patient with established COPD. *Note:* Rapid onset of acute dyspnea may reflect pulmonary embolus.

Assist the patient to assume position of comfort, e.g., elevate head of bed, have patient lean on overbed table or sit on edge of bed.

Elevation of the head of the bed facilitates respiratory function by use of gravity; however, the patient in severe distress will seek the position that most eases breathing. Supporting arms/legs with table, pillows, and so on helps reduce muscle fatigue and can aid chest expansion.

Keep environmental pollution to a minimum, e.g., dust, smoke, and feather pillows according to individual situation.

Precipitators of allergic type of respiratory reactions that can trigger/exacerbate onset of acute episode.

Encourage/assist with abdominal or pursed-lip breathing exercises.

Provides the patient with some means to cope with/control dyspnea and reduce air-trapping.

Observe characteristics of cough, e.g., persistent, hacking, moist. Assist with measures to improve effectiveness of cough effort.

Cough can be persistent but ineffective, especially if the patient is elderly, acutely ill, or debilitated. Coughing is most effective in an upright or in a head-down position after chest percussion.

Increase fluid intake to 3000 mL/day within cardiac tolerance. Provide warm/tepid liquids. Recommend intake of fluids between, instead of during, meals.

Hydration helps decrease the viscosity of secretions, facilitating expectoration. Using warm liquids may decrease bronchospasm. Fluids during meals can increase gastric distension and pressure on the diaphragm.

Collaborative

Administer medications as indicated:

β-agonists: epinephrine (Adrenalin, Vaponefrin), albuterol (Proventil, Ventolin), terbutaline (Brethine, Brethaire), isoetharine (Bronkosol, Bronkometer), salmeterol (Serevent);

Inhaled β_2-adrenergic agonists are first-line therapies for rapid symptomatic improvement in severe bronchoconstriction. These medications relax smooth muscles and reduce local congestion, reducing airway spasm, wheezing, and mucous production. Medications may be oral, injected, or inhaled. Serevent is longer acting and can be used in combination with short-acting agents as needed.

ACTIONS/INTERVENTIONS

Collaborative

Bronchodilators: e.g., anticholinergic agents: ipratropium (Atrovent);

Xanthines, e.g., aminophylline, oxtriphylline (Choledyl), theophylline (Bronkodyl, Theo-Dur);

Leukotriene antagonists: zafirlukast (Accolate); zileuton (Zyflo);

Cromolyn (Intal), flunisolide (AeroBid);

Oral, IV, and inhaled steroids: methylprednisolone (Medrol), dexamethasone (Decadron); antihistamines, e.g., beclomethasone (Vanceril, Beclovent), triamcinolone (Azmacort); fluticasone (Flovent);

Antimicrobials;

Analgesics, cough suppressants/antitussives, e.g., codeine, dextromethorphan products (Benylin DM, Comtrex, Novahistine);

Artificial surfactant, e.g., colfosceril palmitate (Exosurf).

Provide supplemental humidification, e.g., ultrasonic nebulizer, aerosol room humidifier.

Assist with respiratory treatments, e.g., intermittent positive pressure breathing (IPPB), spirometry, chest physiotherapy.

RATIONALE

Inhaled anticholinergic agents are now considered the first-line drugs for patients with stable COPD because studies indicate they have a longer duration of action with less toxicity potential while still providing the effective relief of the β-agonists.

Decreases mucosal edema and smooth muscle spasm (bronchospasm) by indirectly increasing cyclic adenosine monophosphate (AMP). May also reduce muscle fatigue/respiratory failure by increasing diaphragmatic contractility. Use of theophylline may be of little or no benefit in presence of adequate β-agonist regimen; however, it may sustain bronchodilation because effect of β-agonist diminishes between doses.

Reduces leukotriene activity to limit inflammatory response. In mild to moderate asthma, reduces need for inhaled β_2-agonists and systemic corticosteroids. Not effective in acute exacerbations because there is no bronchodilator effect.

Decreases local airway inflammation and edema by inhibiting effects of histamine and other mediators.

May be used to prevent allergic reactions/inhibit release of histamine, reducing severity and frequency of airway spasm, respiratory inflammation, and dyspnea. *Note:* Inhaled corticosteroids may cause local immunosuppression resulting in oral candidiasis infection.

Various antimicrobials may be indicated for control of respiratory infection/pneumonia. *Note:* Even in the absence of pneumonia, therapy may enhance airflow and improve outcome.

Persistent, exhausting cough may need to be suppressed to conserve energy and permit the patient to rest.

Research suggests aerosol administration may enhance expectoration of sputum, improve pulmonary function, and reduce lung volumes (air-trapping).

Humidity helps reduce viscosity of secretions, facilitating expectoration, and may reduce/prevent formation of thick mucous plugs in bronchioles.

Breathing exercises help enhance diffusion; aerosol/nebulizer medications can reduce bronchospasm and stimulate expectoration. Postural drainage and percussion enhance removal of excessive/sticky secretions and improve ventilation of bottom lung segments. *Note:* Chest physiotherapy may aggravate bronchospasms in asthmatics.

ACTIONS/INTERVENTIONS

Collaborative

Monitor/graph serial ABGs, pulse oximetry, chest x-ray.

RATIONALE

Establishes baseline for monitoring progression/regression of disease process and complications. *Note:* Pulse oximetry readings detects changes in saturation as they are happening, helping to identify trends before patient is symptomatic. However, studies have shown that the accuracy of pulse oximetry may be questioned if the patient has severe peripheral vasoconstriction.

NURSING DIAGNOSIS: Gas Exchange, impaired

May be related to
Altered oxygen supply (obstruction of airways by secretions, bronchospasm; air-trapping)
Alveoli destruction

Possibly evidenced by
Dyspnea
Confusion, restlessness
Inability to move secretions
Abnormal ABG values (hypoxia and hypercapnia)
Changes in vital signs
Reduced tolerance for activity

DESIRED OUTCOMES/EVALUATION CRITERIA—PATIENT WILL:

Respiratory Status: Gas Exchange (NOC)

Demonstrate improved ventilation and adequate oxygenation of tissues by ABGs within patient's normal range and be free of symptoms of respiratory distress.
Participate in treatment regimen within level of ability/situation.

ACTIONS/INTERVENTIONS

Acid/Base Management (NIC)

Independent

Assess respiratory rate, depth. Note use of accessory muscles, pursed-lip breathing, inability to speak/converse.

Elevate head of bed, assist patient to assume position to ease work of breathing. Include periods of time in prone position as tolerated. Encourage deep-slow or pursed-lip breathing as individually needed/tolerated.

Assess/routinely monitor skin and mucous membrane color.

RATIONALE

Useful in evaluating the degree of respiratory distress and/or chronicity of the disease process.

Oxygen delivery may be improved by upright position and breathing exercises to decrease airway collapse, dyspnea, and work of breathing. *Note:* Recent research supports use of prone position to increase PaO_2.

Cyanosis may be peripheral (noted in nailbeds) or central (noted around lips/or earlobes). Duskiness and central cyanosis indicate advanced hypoxemia.

ACTIONS/INTERVENTIONS	RATIONALE

Independent

Encourage expectoration of sputum; suction when indicated.	Thick, tenacious, copious secretions are a major source of impaired gas exchange in small airways. Deep suctioning may be required when cough is ineffective for expectoration of secretions.
Auscultate breath sounds, noting areas of decreased airflow and/or adventitious sounds.	Breath sounds may be faint because of decreased airflow or areas of consolidation. Presence of wheezes may indicate bronchospasm/retained secretions. Scattered moist crackles may indicate interstitial fluid/cardiac decompensation.
Palpate for fremitus.	Decrease of vibratory tremors suggests fluid collection or air-trapping.
Monitor level of consciousness/mental status. Investigate changes.	Restlessness and anxiety are common manifestations of hypoxia. Worsening ABGs accompanied by confusion/somnolence are indicative of cerebral dysfunction due to hypoxemia.
Evaluate level of activity tolerance. Provide calm, quiet environment. Limit patient's activity or encourage bed/chair rest during acute phase. Have patient resume activity gradually and increase as individually tolerated.	During severe/acute/refractory respiratory distress the patient may be totally unable to perform basic self-care activities because of hypoxemia and dyspnea. Rest interspersed with care activities remains an important part of treatment regimen. An exercise program is aimed at increasing endurance and strength without causing severe dyspnea and can enhance sense of well-being.
Evaluate sleep patterns, note reports of difficulties and whether patient feels well rested. Provide quiet environment, group care/monitoring activities to allow periods of uninterrupted sleep; limit stimulants, e.g., caffeine; encourage position of comfort.	Multiple external stimuli and presence of dyspnea may prevent relaxation and inhibit sleep.
Monitor vital signs and cardiac rhythm.	Tachycardia, dysrhythmias, and changes in BP can reflect effect of systemic hypoxemia on cardiac function.

Collaborative

Monitor/graph serial ABGs and pulse oximetry.	$PaCO_2$ usually elevated (bronchitis, emphysema) and PaO_2 is generally decreased, so that hypoxia is present in a greater or lesser degree. *Note:* A "normal" or increased $PaCO_2$ signals impending respiratory failure for asthmatics.
Administer supplemental oxygen judiciously as indicated by ABG results and patient tolerance.	May correct/prevent worsening of hypoxia. *Note:* In chronic emphysema, patient's respiratory drive is determined by the CO_2 level and may be eliminated by excess elevation of PaO_2.
Administer antianxiety, sedative, or narcotic agents with caution.	May be used to control anxiety/restlessness, which increases oxygen consumption/demand, exacerbating dyspnea. Must be monitored closely because depressive effect may lead to respiratory failure.

RESPIRATORY: Chronic Obstructive Pulmonary Disease (COPD) and Asthma

133

ACTIONS/INTERVENTIONS

Collaborative

Assist with noninvasive positive pressure ventilation (NIPPV) or intubation, institution/maintenance of mechanical ventilation; transfer to critical care area depending on patient directives.

Prepare for surgical intervention as appropriate.

RATIONALE

Development of/impending respiratory failure requires prompt life-saving measures. *Note:* NIPPV provides periodic ventilatory support without intubation and may be useful in the home setting as well to treat chronic respiratory failure or limit acute exacerbations in patients who are able to maintain spontaneous respiratory effort.

Screened candidates may benefit from lung volume reduction surgery (LVRS) in which hyperinflated giant bullae/cysts are removed, e.g., those occupying at least one-third of the involved lobe, or areas of lung tissue with small cystic disease. In the absence of fibrosis, this procedure removes ineffective lung tissue, allowing for better expansion and maximal blood flow to healthy tissues, thus increasing alveolar gas exchange.

NURSING DIAGNOSIS: Nutrition: altered, less than body requirements

May be related to
Dyspnea; sputum production
Medication side effects; anorexia, nausea/vomiting
Fatigue

Possibly evidenced by
Weight loss; loss of muscle mass, poor muscle tone
Reported altered taste sensation; aversion to eating, lack of interest in food

DESIRED OUTCOMES/EVALUATION CRITERIA—PATIENT WILL:

Nutritional Status (NOC)

Display progressive weight gain toward goal as appropriate.
Demonstrate behaviors/lifestyle changes to regain and/or maintain appropriate weight.

ACTIONS/INTERVENTIONS

Nutrition Therapy (NIC)

Independent

Assess dietary habits, recent food intake. Note degree of difficulty with eating. Evaluate weight and body size (mass).

RATIONALE

The patient in acute respiratory distress is often anorectic because of dyspnea, sputum production, medications. In addition, many COPD patients habitually eat poorly, even though respiratory insufficiency creates a hypermetabolic state with increased caloric needs. As a result, patient often is admitted with some degree of malnutrition. People who have emphysema are often thin with wasted musculature.

ACTIONS/INTERVENTIONS

Independent

Auscultate bowel sounds.

Give frequent oral care, remove expectorated secretions promptly, provide specific container for disposal of secretions and tissues.

Encourage a rest period of 1 hr before and after meals. Provide frequent small feedings.

Avoid gas-producing foods and carbonated beverages.

Avoid very hot or very cold foods.

Weigh as indicated.

Collaborative

Consult dietitian/nutritional support team to provide easily digested, nutritionally balanced meals by appropriate means, e.g., oral, supplemental/tube feedings, parenteral nutrition. (Refer to CP: Total Nutritional Support: Parenteral/Enteral Feeding, p. 508.)

Review laboratory studies, e.g., serum albumin/prealbumin, transferrin, amino acid profile, iron, nitrogen balance studies, glucose, liver function studies, electrolytes.

Administer supplemental oxygen during meals as indicated.

RATIONALE

Diminished/hypoactive bowel sounds may reflect decreased gastric motility and constipation (common complication) related to limited fluid intake, poor food choices, decreased activity, and hypoxemia.

Noxious tastes, smells, and sights are prime deterrents to appetite and can produce nausea and vomiting with increased respiratory difficulty.

Helps reduce fatigue during mealtime and provides opportunity to increase total caloric intake.

Can produce abdominal distension, which hampers abdominal breathing and diaphragmatic movement and can increase dyspnea.

Extremes in temperature can precipitate/aggravate coughing spasms.

Useful in determining caloric needs, setting weight goal, and evaluating adequacy of nutritional plan. *Note:* Weight loss may continue initially, despite adequate intake, as edema is resolving.

Method of feeding and caloric requirements are based on individual situation/needs to provide maximal nutrients with minimal patient effort/energy expenditure.

Evaluates/treats deficits and monitors effectiveness of nutritional therapy.

Decreases dyspnea and increases energy for eating, enhancing intake.

NURSING DIAGNOSIS: Infection, risk for

Risk factors may include
Inadequate primary defenses (decreased ciliary action, stasis of secretions)
Inadequate acquired immunity (tissue destruction, increased environmental exposure)
Chronic disease process
Malnutrition

Possibly evidenced by
[Not applicable; presence of signs and symptoms establishes an *actual* diagnosis]

DESIRED OUTCOMES/EVALUATION CRITERIA—PATIENT WILL:

Knowledge: Infection Control (NOC)

Verbalize understanding of individual causative/risk factors.
Identify interventions to prevent/reduce risk of infection.
Demonstrate techniques, lifestyle changes to promote safe environment.

ACTIONS/INTERVENTIONS	RATIONALE

Infection Protection (NIC)

Independent

Monitor temperature.

Fever may be present because of infection and/or dehydration.

Review importance of breathing exercises, effective cough, frequent position changes, and adequate fluid intake.

These activities promote mobilization and expectoration of secretions to reduce risk of developing pulmonary infection.

Observe color, character, odor of sputum.

Odorous, yellow, or greenish secretions suggest the presence of pulmonary infection.

Demonstrate and assist the patient in disposal of tissues and sputum. Stress proper handwashing (nurse and patient) and use gloves when handling/disposing of tissues, sputum containers.

Prevents spread of fluid-borne pathogens.

Monitor visitors; provide masks as indicated.

Reduces potential for exposure to infectious illnesses, e.g., upper respiratory infection (URI).

Encourage balance between activity and rest.

Reduces oxygen consumption/demand imbalance and improves patient's resistance to infection, promoting healing.

Discuss need for adequate nutritional intake.

Malnutrition can affect general well-being and lower resistance to infection.

Recommend rinsing mouth with water and spitting, not swallowing, or use of spacer on mouthpiece of inhaled corticosteroids.

Reduces localized immunosuppressive effect of drug and risk of oral candidiasis.

Collaborative

Obtain sputum specimen by deep coughing or suctioning for Gram stain, culture/sensitivity.

Done to identify causative organism and susceptibility to various antimicrobials.

Administer antimicrobials as indicated.

May be given for specific organisms identified by culture and sensitivity, or be given prophylactically because of high risk.

NURSING DIAGNOSIS: Knowledge Deficit [Learning Need] regarding condition, treatment, self care, and discharge needs

May be related to
Lack of information/unfamiliarity with information resources
Information misinterpretation
Lack of recall/cognitive limitation

Possibly evidenced by
Request for information
Statement of concerns/misconception
Inaccurate follow-through of instructions
Development of preventable complications

DESIRED OUTCOMES/EVALUATION CRITERIA—PATIENT WILL:

Knowledge: Disease Process (NOC)

Verbalize understanding of condition/disease process and treatment.
Identify relationship of current signs/symptoms to the disease process and correlate these with causative factors.

Knowledge: Treatment Regimen (NOC)

Initiate necessary lifestyle changes and participate in treatment regimen.

ACTIONS/INTERVENTIONS	RATIONALE
Teaching: Disease Process (NIC)	
Independent	
Explain/reinforce explanations of individual disease process. Encourage patient/SO to ask questions.	Decreases anxiety and can lead to improved participation in treatment plan.
Instruct/reinforce rationale for breathing exercises, coughing effectively, and general conditioning exercises.	Pursed-lip and abdominal/diaphragmatic breathing exercises strengthen muscles of respiration, help minimize collapse of small airways, and provide the individual with means to control dyspnea. General conditioning exercises increase activity tolerance, muscle strength, and sense of well-being.
Stress importance of oral care/dental hygiene.	Decreases bacterial growth in the mouth, which can lead to pulmonary infections.
Discuss importance of avoiding people with active respiratory infections. Stress need for routine influenza/pneumococcal vaccinations.	Decreases exposure to and incidence of acquired acute URIs.
Discuss individual factors that may trigger or aggravate condition, e.g., excessively dry air, wind, environmental temperature extremes, pollen, tobacco smoke, aerosol sprays, air pollution. Encourage patient/SO to explore ways to control these factors in and around the home and work setting.	These environmental factors can induce/aggravate bronchial irritation, leading to increased secretion production and airway blockage.
Review the harmful effects of smoking and advise cessation of smoking by patient and/or SO.	Cessation of smoking may slow/halt progression of COPD. Even when patient wants to stop smoking, support groups and medical monitoring may be needed. *Note:* Research studies suggest that "side-stream" or "second-hand" smoke can be as detrimental as actually smoking.
Provide information about activity limitations and alternating activities with rest periods to prevent fatigue; ways to conserve energy during activities (e.g., pulling instead of pushing, sitting instead of standing while performing tasks); use of pursed-lip breathing, side-lying position, and possible need for supplemental oxygen during sexual activity.	Having this knowledge can enable patient to make informed choices/decisions to reduce dyspnea, maximize activity level, perform most desired activities, and prevent complications.

137

ACTIONS/INTERVENTIONS	RATIONALE

Independent

Discuss importance of medical follow-up care, periodic chest x-rays, sputum cultures.

Monitoring disease process allows for alterations in therapeutic regimen to meet changing needs and may help prevent complications.

Review oxygen requirements/dosage for patient who is discharged on supplemental oxygen. Discuss safe use of oxygen and refer to supplier as indicated.

Reduces risk of misuse (too little/too much) and resultant complications. Promotes environmental/physical safety.

Instruct patient/SO in use of NIPPV as appropriate. Problem-solve possible side effects and identify adverse signs/symptoms, e.g., increased dyspnea, fatigue, daytime drowsiness, or headaches on awakening.

NIPPV may be used at night/periodically during day to decrease CO_2 level, improve quality of sleep, and enhance functional level during the day. Signs of increasing CO_2 level indicate need for more aggressive therapy.

Instruct asthmatic patient in use of peak flow meter, as appropriate.

Peak flow level can drop before patient exhibits any signs/symptoms of asthma during the "first time" after exposure to a trigger. Regular use of the peak flow meter may reduce the severity of the attack because of earlier intervention.

Provide information/encourage participation in support groups, e.g., American Lung Association, public health department.

These patients and their SOs may experience anxiety, depression, and other reactions as they deal with a chronic disease that has an impact on their desired lifestyle. Support groups and/or home visits may be desired or needed to provide assistance, emotional support, and respite care.

Refer for evaluation of home care if indicated. Provide a detailed plan of care and baseline physical assessment to home care nurse as needed on discharge from acute care.

Provides for continuity of care. May help reduce frequency of rehospitalization.

Teaching: Prescribed Medications (NIC)

Discuss respiratory medications, side effects, adverse reactions.

Frequently these patients are simultaneously on several respiratory drugs that have similar side effects and potential drug interactions. It is important that the patient understand the difference between nuisance side effects (medication continued), and untoward or adverse side effects (medication possibly discontinued/dosage changed).

Demonstrate technique for using a metered-dose inhaler (MDI), such as how to hold it, taking 2–5 min between puffs, cleaning the inhaler.

Proper administration of drug enhances delivery and effectiveness.

Devise system for recording prescribed intermittent drug/inhaler usage.

Reduces risk of improper use/overdosage of prn medications, especially during acute exacerbations, when cognition may be impaired.

Recommend avoidance of sedative antianxiety agents unless specifically prescribed/approved by physician treating respiratory condition.

Although the patient may be nervous and feel the need for sedatives, these can depress respiratory drive and protective cough mechanisms. *Note:* These drugs may be used prophylactically when patient is unable to avoid situations known to increase stress/trigger respiratory response.

POTENTIAL CONSIDERATIONS following acute hospitalization (dependent on patient's age, physical condition/presence of complications, personal resources, and life responsibilities)

Self-Care deficit, specify—intolerance to activity, decreased strength/endurance, depression, severe anxiety.

Home Maintenance Management, impaired—intolerance to activity, inadequate support system, insufficient finances, unfamiliarity with neighborhood resources.

Infection, risk for—decreased ciliary action, stasis of secretions, tissue destruction, increased environmental exposure, chronic disease process, malnutrition.

PNEUMONIA: MICROBIAL

Pneumonia is an inflammation of the lung parenchyma, usually associated with the filling of the alveoli with fluid. Primary pneumonia is caused by the patient's inhaling or aspirating a pathogen. Secondary pneumonia ensues from lung damage caused by the spread of bacteria from an infection elsewhere in the body. Likely causes include various infectious agents, chemical irritants, and radiation therapy. This plan of care deals with bacterial and viral pneumonias, e.g., pneumococcal pneumonia, pneumocystis carinii, *Haemophilus influenzae,* mycoplasma, and Gram-negative microbes.

CARE SETTING

Most patients are treated as outpatients; however, persons at higher risk (e.g., with ongoing/chronic health problems) are treated in the hospital, as are those already hospitalized for other reasons.

RELATED CONCERNS

AIDS, page 765
Chronic obstructive pulmonary disease (COPD), page 126
Psychosocial aspects of care, page 809
Sepsis/Septicemia, page 741
Surgical intervention, page 828

Patient Assessment Database

ACTIVITY/REST

May report:	Fatigue, weakness
	Insomnia
May exhibit:	Lethargy
	Decreased tolerance to activity

CIRCULATION

May report:	History of recent/chronic heart failure (HF)
May exhibit:	Tachycardia
	Flushed appearance or pallor

EGO INTEGRITY

May report:	Multiple stressors, financial concerns

FOOD/FLUID

May report:	Loss of appetite, nausea/vomiting
May exhibit:	Distended abdomen
	Hyperactive bowel sounds
	Dry skin with poor turgor
	Cachectic appearance (malnutrition)

NEUROSENSORY

May report:	Frontal headache (influenza)
May exhibit:	Changes in mentation (confusion, somnolence)

PAIN/DISCOMFORT

May report:	Headache
	Chest pain (pleuritic), aggravated by cough; substernal chest pain (influenza)
	Myalgia, arthralgia
May exhibit:	Splinting/guarding over affected area (patient commonly lies on affected side to restrict movement)

RESPIRATION

May report:	History of recurrent/chronic URIs, tuberculosis or COPD, cigarette smoking
	Progressive dyspnea
	Cough: Dry hacking (initially) progressing to productive cough
May exhibit:	Tachypnea; shallow grunting respirations, use of accessory muscles, nasal flaring
	Sputum: Pink, rusty, or purulent
	Percussion: Dull over consolidated areas
	Fremitus: Tactile and vocal, gradually increases with consolidation
	Pleural friction rub
	Breath sounds: Diminished or absent over involved area, or bronchial breath sounds over area(s) of consolidation; coarse inspiratory crackles
	Color: Pallor or cyanosis of lips/nailbeds

SAFETY

May report:	Recurrent chills
	History of altered immune system: i.e., systemic lupus erythematosus (SLE), AIDS, steroid or chemotherapy use, institutionalization, general debilitation
	Fever (e.g., 102°F–104°F/39°C–40°C)
May exhibit:	Diaphoresis
	Shaking
	Rash may be noted in cases of rubeola or varicella

TEACHING/LEARNING

May report:	History of recent surgery; chronic alcohol use; intravenous (IV) drug therapy or abuse; immunosuppressive therapy
Discharge plan considerations:	**DRG projected mean length of inpatient stay: 4.3 to 8.3 days**
	Assistance with self-care, homemaker tasks.
	Oxygen may be needed, especially if recovery is prolonged or other predisposing condition exists.

Refer to section at end of plan for postdischarge considerations.

DIAGNOSTIC STUDIES

Chest x-ray: Identifies structural distribution (e.g., lobar, bronchial); may also reveal multiple abscesses/infiltrates, empyema (staphylococcus); scattered or localized infiltration (bacterial); or diffuse/extensive nodular infiltrates (more often viral). In mycoplasmal pneumonia, chest x-ray may be clear.

Fiberoptic bronchoscopy: May be both diagnostic (qualitative cultures) and therapeutic (re-expansion of lung segment).

ABGs/Pulse oximetry: Abnormalities may be present, depending on extent of lung involvement and underlying lung disease.

Gram stain/Cultures: Sputum collection; needle aspiration of empyema, pleural, and transtracheal or transthoracic fluids; lung biopsies and blood cultures may be done to recover causative organism. More than one type of organism may be present; common bacteria include *Diplococcus pneumonia, Staphylococcus aureus,* α-hemolytic *Streptococcus, Haemophilus influenzae;* cytomegalovirus (CMV). *Note:* Sputum cultures may not identify all offending organisms. Blood cultures may show transient bacteremia.

CBC: Leukocytosis usually present, although a low white blood cell (WBC) count may be present in viral infection, immunosuppressed conditions such as AIDS, and overwhelming bacterial pneumonia. Erythrocyte sedimentation rate (ESR) is elevated.

Serologic studies, e.g., viral or Legionella titers, cold agglutinins: Assist in differential diagnosis of specific organism.

Lung function studies: Volumes may be decreased (congestion and alveolar collapse); airway pressure may be increased and compliance decreased. Shunting is present (hypoxemia).

Electrolytes: Sodium and chloride may be low.

Bilirubin: May be increased.

Percutaneous aspiration/Open biopsy of lung tissues: May reveal typical intranuclear and cytoplasmic inclusions (CMV), characteristic giant cells (rubeola).

NURSING PRIORITIES

1. Maintain/improve respiratory function.
2. Prevent complications.
3. Support recuperative process.
4. Provide information about disease process/prognosis and treatment.

DISCHARGE GOALS

1. Ventilation and oxygenation adequate for individual needs.
2. Complications prevented/minimized.
3. Disease process/prognosis and therapeutic regimen understood.
4. Lifestyle changes identified/initiated to prevent recurrence.
5. Plan in place to meet needs after discharge.

NURSING DIAGNOSIS: Airway Clearance, ineffective

May be related to
Tracheal bronchial inflammation, edema formation, increased sputum production
Pleuritic pain
Decreased energy, fatigue

Possibly evidenced by
Changes in rate, depth of respirations
Abnormal breath sounds, use of accessory muscles
Dyspnea, cyanosis
Cough, effective or ineffective; with/without sputum production

DESIRED OUTCOMES/EVALUATION CRITERIA—PATIENT WILL:

Respiratory Status: Ventilation (NOC)

Identify/demonstrate behaviors to achieve airway clearance.
Display patent airway with breath sounds clearing, absence of dyspnea, cyanosis.

ACTIONS/INTERVENTIONS	RATIONALE
Airway Management (NIC)	
Independent	
Assess rate/depth of respirations and chest movement.	Tachypnea, shallow respirations, and asymmetric chest movement are frequently present because of discomfort of moving chest wall and/or fluid in lung.
Auscultate lung fields, noting areas of decreased/absent airflow and adventitious breath sounds, e.g., crackles, wheezes.	Decreased airflow occurs in areas consolidated with fluid. Bronchial breath sounds (normal over bronchus) can also occur in consolidated areas. Crackles, rhonchi, and wheezes are heard on inspiration and/or expiration in response to fluid accumulation, thick secretions, and airway spasm/obstruction.
Elevate head of bed, change position frequently.	Lowers diaphragm, promoting chest expansion, aeration of lung segments, mobilization and expectoration of secretions.
Assist patient with frequent deep-breathing exercises. Demonstrate/help patient learn to perform activity, e.g., splinting chest and effective coughing while in upright position.	Deep breathing facilitates maximum expansion of the lungs/smaller airways. Coughing is a natural self-cleaning mechanism, assisting the cilia to maintain patent airways. Splinting reduces chest discomfort, and an upright position favors deeper, more forceful cough effort.

ACTIONS/INTERVENTIONS

Independent

Suction as indicated.

Force fluids to at least 2500 mL/day (unless contraindicated). Offer warm, rather than cold, fluids.

Collaborative

Assist with/monitor effects of nebulizer treatments and other respiratory physiotherapy, e.g., incentive spirometer, IPPB, percussion, postural drainage. Perform treatments between meals and limit fluids when appropriate.

Administer medications as indicated: mucolytics, expectorants, bronchodilators, analgesics.

Provide supplemental fluids, e.g., IV, humidified oxygen, and room humidification.

Monitor serial chest x-rays, ABGs, pulse oximetry readings. (Refer to ND: Gas Exchange, impaired, following.)

Assist with bronchoscopy/thoracentesis, if indicated.

RATIONALE

Stimulates cough or mechanically clears airway in patient who is unable to do so because of ineffective cough or decreased level of consciousness.

Fluids (especially warm liquids) aid in mobilization and expectoration of secretions.

Facilitates liquification and removal of secretions. Postural drainage may not be effective in interstitial pneumonias or those causing alveolar exudate/destruction. Coordination of treatments/schedules and oral intake reduces likelihood of vomiting with coughing, expectorations.

Aids in reduction of bronchospasm and mobilization of secretions. Analgesics are given to improve cough effort by reducing discomfort, but should be used cautiously because they can decrease cough effort/depress respirations.

Fluids are required to replace losses (including insensible) and aid in mobilization of secretions. *Note:* Some recent studies indicate that room humidification has been found to provide minimal benefit and is thought to increase the risk of transmitting infection.

Follows progress and effects of disease process/therapeutic regimen and facilitates necessary alterations in therapy.

Occasionally needed to remove mucous plugs, drain purulent secretions, and/or prevent atelectasis.

NURSING DIAGNOSIS: Gas Exchange, impaired

May be related to

Alveolar-capillary membrane changes (inflammatory effects)

Altered oxygen-carrying capacity of blood/release at cellular level (fever, shifting oxyhemoglobin curve)

Altered delivery of oxygen (hypoventilation)

Possibly evidenced by

Dyspnea, cyanosis

Tachycardia

Restlessness/changes in mentation

Hypoxia

DESIRED OUTCOMES/EVALUATION CRITERIA—PATIENT WILL:

Respiratory Status: Gas Exchange (NOC)

Demonstrate improved ventilation and oxygenation of tissues by ABGs within patient's acceptable range and absence of symptoms of respiratory distress.

Participate in actions to maximize oxygenation.

ACTIONS/INTERVENTIONS	RATIONALE

Acid-Base Management (NIC)

Independent

Assess respiratory rate, depth, and ease.

Manifestations of respiratory distress are dependent on/and indicative of the degree of lung involvement and underlying general health status.

Observe color of skin, mucous membranes, and nail-beds, noting presence of peripheral cyanosis (nail-beds) or central cyanosis (circumoral).

Cyanosis of nailbeds may represent vasoconstriction or the body's response to fever/chills; however, cyanosis of earlobes, mucous membranes, and skin around the mouth ("warm membranes") is indicative of systemic hypoxemia.

Assess mental status.

Restlessness, irritation, confusion, and somnolence may reflect hypoxemia/decreased cerebral oxygenation.

Monitor heart rate/rhythm.

Tachycardia is usually present as a result of fever/dehydration but may represent a response to hypoxemia.

Monitor body temperature, as indicated. Assist with comfort measures to reduce fever and chills, e.g., addition/removal of bedcovers, comfortable room temperature, tepid or cool water sponge bath.

High fever (common in bacterial pneumonia and influenza) greatly increases metabolic demands and oxygen consumption and alters cellular oxygenation.

Maintain bedrest. Encourage use of relaxation techniques and diversional activities.

Prevents overexhaustion and reduces oxygen consumption/demands to facilitate resolution of infection.

Elevate head and encourage frequent position changes, deep breathing, and effective coughing.

These measures promote maximal inspiration, enhance expectoration of secretions to improve ventilation. (Refer to ND: Airway Clearance, ineffective, p. 158.)

Assess level of anxiety. Encourage verbalization of concerns/feelings. Answer questions honestly. Visit frequently, arrange for SO/visitors to stay with patient as indicated.

Anxiety is a manifestation of psychological concerns and physiological responses to hypoxia. Providing reassurance and enhancing sense of security can reduce the psychological component, thereby decreasing oxygen demand and adverse physiological response.

Observe for deterioration in condition, noting hypotension, copious amounts of pink/bloody sputum, pallor, cyanosis, change in level of consciousness, severe dyspnea, restlessness.

Shock and pulmonary edema are the most common causes of death in pneumonia and require immediate medical intervention.

Collaborative

Administer oxygen therapy by appropriate means, e.g., nasal prongs, mask, Venturi mask.

The purpose of oxygen therapy is to maintain PaO_2 above 60 mm Hg. Oxygen is administered by the method that provides appropriate delivery within the patient's tolerance.

Monitor ABGs, pulse oximetry.

Follows progress of disease process and facilitates alterations in pulmonary therapy.

Prepare for/transfer to critical care setting if indicated.

Intubation and mechanical ventilation may be required in the event of severe respiratory insufficiency. (Refer to CP: Mechanical Ventilation, p. 188.)

NURSING DIAGNOSIS: Infection, risk for [spread]

Risk factors may include:

Inadequate primary defenses (decreased ciliary action, stasis of respiratory secretions)

Inadequate secondary defenses (presence of existing infection, immunosuppression), chronic disease, malnutrition

Possibly evidenced by:

[Not applicable; presence of signs and symptoms establishes an *actual* diagnosis]

DESIRED OUTCOMES/EVALUATION CRITERIA—PATIENT WILL:

Infection Status (NOC)

Achieve timely resolution of current infection without complications.

Knowledge: Infection Control (NOC)

Identify interventions to prevent/reduce risk/spread of/secondary infection.

ACTIONS/INTERVENTIONS	RATIONALE

Infection Control (NIC)

Independent

Monitor vital signs closely, especially during initiation of therapy.	During this period of time, potentially fatal complications (hypotension/shock) may develop.
Instruct patient concerning the disposition of secretions (e.g., raising and expectorating versus swallowing) and reporting changes in color, amount, odor of secretions.	Although patient may find expectoration offensive and attempt to limit or avoid it, it is essential that sputum be disposed of in a safe manner. Changes in characteristics of sputum reflect resolution of pneumonia or development of secondary infection.
Demonstrate/encourage good handwashing technique.	Effective means of reducing spread/acquisition of infection.
Change position frequently and provide good pulmonary toilet.	Promotes expectoration, clearing of infection.
Limit visitors as indicated.	Reduces likelihood of exposure to other infectious pathogens.
Institute isolation precautions as individually appropriate.	Dependent on type of infection, response to antibiotics, patient's general health, and development of complications, isolation techniques may be desired to prevent spread/protect patient from other infectious processes.
Encourage adequate rest balanced with moderate activity. Promote adequate nutritional intake.	Facilitates healing process and enhances natural resistance.
Monitor effectiveness of antimicrobial therapy.	Signs of improvement in condition should occur within 24–48 hr.
Investigate sudden changes/deterioration in condition, such as increasing chest pain, extra heart sounds, altered sensorium, recurring fever, changes in sputum characteristics.	Delayed recovery or increase in severity of symptoms suggests resistance to antibiotics or secondary infection. Complications affecting any/all organ systems include lung abscess/empyema, bacteremia, pericarditis/endocarditis, meningitis/encephalitis, and superinfections.

145

ACTIONS/INTERVENTIONS	RATIONALE
Collaborative	
Administer antimicrobials as indicated by results of sputum/blood cultures: e.g., penicillins, erythromycin (E-mycin), tetracycline (Achromycin), doxycycline hyclate (Vibramycin), amikacin (Amikin); cephalosporins: amantadine (Symmetrel); sparfloxacin (Zagam).	These drugs are used to combat most of the microbial pneumonias. Combinations of antiviral and antifungal agents may be used when the pneumonia is a result of mixed organisms. *Note:* Vancomycin and third-generation cephalosporins are the treatment of choice for penicillin-resistant streptococcal pneumonia.
Prepare for/assist with diagnostic studies as indicated.	Fiberoptic bronchoscopy (FOB) may be done in patients who do not respond rapidly (within 1–3 days) to antimicrobial therapy to clarify diagnosis and therapy needs.

NURSING DIAGNOSIS: Activity Intolerance

May be related to
Imbalance between oxygen supply and demand
General weakness
Exhaustion associated with interruption in usual sleep pattern because of discomfort, excessive coughing, and dyspnea

Possibly evidenced by
Verbal reports of weakness, fatigue, exhaustion
Exertional dyspnea, tachypnea
Tachycardia in response to activity
Development/worsening of pallor/cyanosis

DESIRED OUTCOMES/EVALUATION CRITERIA—PATIENT WILL:

Endurance (NOC)

Report/demonstrate a measurable increase in tolerance to activity with absence of dyspnea and excessive fatigue, and vital signs within patient's acceptable range.

ACTIONS/INTERVENTIONS	RATIONALE
Energy Management (NIC)	
Independent	
Evaluate patient's response to activity. Note reports of dyspnea, increased weakness/fatigue, and changes in vital signs during and after activities.	Establishes patient's capabilities/needs and facilitates choice of interventions.
Provide a quiet environment and limit visitors during acute phase as indicated. Encourage use of stress management and diversional activities as appropriate.	Reduces stress and excess stimulation, promoting rest.
Explain importance of rest in treatment plan and necessity for balancing activities with rest.	Bedrest is maintained during acute phase to decrease metabolic demands, thus conserving energy for healing. Activity restrictions thereafter are determined by individual patient response to activity and resolution of respiratory insufficiency.

ACTIONS/INTERVENTIONS

Independent

Assist the patient to assume comfortable position for rest/sleep.

Assist with self-care activities as necessary. Provide for progressive increase in activities during recovery phase.

RATIONALE

Patient may be comfortable with head of bed elevated, sleeping in a chair, or leaning forward on overbed table with pillow support.

Minimizes exhaustion and helps to balance oxygen supply and demand.

NURSING DIAGNOSIS: Pain [acute]

May be related to
Inflammation of lung parenchyma
Cellular reactions to circulating toxins
Persistent coughing

Possibly evidenced by
Reports of pleuritic chest pain; headache, muscle/joint pain
Guarding of affected area
Distraction behaviors, restlessness

DESIRED OUTCOMES/EVALUATION CRITERIA—PATIENT WILL:

Pain: Disruptive Effects (NOC)

Verbalize relief/control of pain.
Demonstrate relaxed manner, resting/sleeping and engaging in activity appropriately.

ACTIONS/INTERVENTIONS

Pain Management (NIC)

Independent

Determine pain characteristics, e.g., sharp, constant, stabbing. Investigate changes in character/location/intensity of pain.

Monitor vital signs.

Provide comfort measures, e.g., back rubs, change of position, quiet music/conversation. Encourage use of relaxation/breathing exercises.

Offer frequent oral hygiene.

Instruct and assist patient in chest splinting techniques during coughing episodes. (Refer to ND: Airway Clearance, ineffective, p. 158.)

RATIONALE

Chest pain, usually present to some degree with pneumonia, may also herald the onset of complications of pneumonia, such as pericarditis and endocarditis.

Changes in heart rate or BP may indicate that the patient is experiencing pain, especially when other reasons for changes in vital signs have been ruled out.

Nonanalgesic measures administered with a gentle touch can lessen discomfort and augment therapeutic effects of analgesics. Patient involvement in pain control measures promotes independence and enhances sense of well-being.

Mouth breathing and oxygen therapy can irritate and dry out mucous membranes, potentiating general discomfort.

Aids in control of chest discomfort while enhancing effectiveness of cough effort.

ACTIONS/INTERVENTIONS

Collaborative

Administer analgesics and antitussives as indicated.

RATIONALE

These medications may be used to suppress nonproductive/paroxysmal cough or reduce excess mucus, thereby enhancing general comfort/rest.

NURSING DIAGNOSIS: Nutrition: altered, risk for less than body requirements

Risk factors may include
Increased metabolic needs secondary to fever and infectious process
Anorexia associated with bacterial toxins, the odor and taste of sputum, and certain aerosol treatments
Abdominal distension/gas associated with swallowing air during dyspneic episodes

Possibly evidenced by
[Not applicable; presence of signs and symptoms establishes an *actual* diagnosis]

DESIRED OUTCOMES/EVALUATION CRITERIA—PATIENT WILL:

Nutritional Status (NOC)

Demonstrate increased appetite.
Maintain/regain desired body weight.

ACTIONS/INTERVENTIONS

Nutrition Therapy (NIC)

Independent

Identify factors that are contributing to nausea/vomiting, e.g., copious sputum, aerosol treatments, severe dyspnea, pain.

Provide covered container for sputum and remove at frequent intervals. Assist with/encourage oral hygiene after emesis, after aerosol and postural drainage treatments, and before meals.

Schedule respiratory treatments at least 1 hr before meals.

Auscultate for bowel sounds. Observe/palpate for abdominal distension.

Provide small, frequent meals, including dry foods (toast, crackers) and/or foods that are appealing to patient.

Evaluate general nutritional state, obtain baseline weight.

RATIONALE

Choice of interventions depends on the underlying cause of the problem.

Eliminates noxious sights, tastes, smells from the patient environment and can reduce nausea.

Reduces effects of nausea associated with these treatments.

Bowel sounds may be diminished/absent if the infectious process is severe/prolonged. Abdominal distension may occur as a result of air swallowing or reflect the influence of bacterial toxins on the gastrointestinal (GI) tract.

These measures may enhance intake even though appetite may be slow to return.

Presence of chronic conditions (e.g., COPD or alcoholism) or financial limitations can contribute to malnutrition, lowered resistance to infection, and/or delayed response to therapy.

NURSING DIAGNOSIS: Fluid Volume risk for deficit

Risk factors may include
Excessive fluid loss (fever, profuse diaphoresis, mouth breathing/hyperventilation, vomiting)
Decreased oral intake

Possibly evidenced by
[Not applicable; presence of signs and symptoms establishes an *actual* diagnosis]

DESIRED OUTCOMES/EVALUATION CRITERIA—PATIENT WILL:

Fluid Balance (NOC)

Demonstrate fluid balance evidenced by individually appropriate parameters, e.g., moist mucous membranes, good skin turgor, prompt capillary refill, stable vital signs.

ACTIONS/INTERVENTIONS	RATIONALE
Fluid Management (NIC)	
Independent	
Assess vital sign changes, e.g., increased temperature/prolonged fever, tachycardia, orthostatic hypotension.	Elevated temperature/prolonged fever increases metabolic rate and fluid loss through evaporation. Orthostatic BP changes and increasing tachycardia may indicate systemic fluid deficit.
Assess skin turgor, moisture of mucous membranes (lips, tongue).	Indirect indicators of adequacy of fluid volume, although oral mucous membranes may be dry because of mouth breathing and supplemental oxygen.
Note reports of nausea/vomiting.	Presence of these symptoms reduces oral intake.
Monitor intake and output (I&O), noting color, character of urine. Calculate fluid balance. Be aware of insensible losses. Weigh as indicated.	Provides information about adequacy of fluid volume and replacement needs.
Force fluids to at least 2500 mL/day or as individually appropriate.	Meets basic fluid needs, reducing risk of dehydration.
Collaborative	
Administer medications as indicated, e.g., antipyretics, antiemetics.	Useful in reducing fluid losses.
Provide supplemental IV fluids as necessary.	In presence of reduced intake/excessive loss, use of parenteral route may correct/prevent deficiency.

NURSING DIAGNOSIS: Knowledge Deficit [Learning Need] regarding condition treatment, self care, and discharge needs

May be related to
Lack of exposure
Misinterpretation of information
Altered recall

Possibly evidenced by
Requests for information; statement of misconception
Failure to improve/recurrence

ACTIONS/INTERVENTIONS	RATIONALE
Teaching: Disease Process (NIC)	
Independent	
Review normal lung function, pathology of condition.	Promotes understanding of current situation and importance of cooperating with treatment regimen.
Discuss debilitating aspects of disease, length of convalescence, and recovery expectations. Identify self-care and homemaker needs/resources.	Information can enhance coping and help reduce anxiety and excessive concern. Respiratory symptoms may be slow to resolve, and fatigue and weakness can persist for an extended period. These factors may be associated with depression and the need for various forms of support and assistance.
Provide information in written and verbal form.	Fatigue and depression can affect ability to assimilate information/follow medical regimen.
Stress importance of continuing effective coughing/deep-breathing exercises.	During initial 6–8 wk after discharge, patient is at greatest risk for recurrence of pneumonia.
Emphasize necessity for continuing antibiotic therapy for prescribed period.	Early discontinuation of antibiotics may result in failure to completely resolve infectious process.
Review importance of cessation of smoking.	Smoking destroys tracheobronchial ciliary action, irritates bronchial mucosa, and inhibits alveolar macrophages, compromising body's natural defense against infection.
Outline steps to enhance general health and well-being, e.g., balanced rest and activity, well-rounded diet, avoidance of crowds during cold/flu season and persons with URIs.	Increases natural defenses/immunity, limits exposure to pathogens.
Stress importance of continuing medical follow-up and obtaining vaccinations/immunizations as appropriate.	May prevent recurrence of pneumonia and/or related complications.
Identify signs/symptoms requiring notification of healthcare provider, e.g., increasing dyspnea, chest pain, prolonged fatigue, weight loss, fever/chills, persistence of productive cough, changes in mentation.	Prompt evaluation and timely intervention may prevent/minimize complications.

POTENTIAL CONSIDERATIONS following acute hospitalization (dependent on patient's age, physical condition/presence of complications, personal resources, and life responsibilities)

Fatigue—increased energy requirements to perform ADLs, discomfort, effects of antimicrobial therapy.

Infection, risk for—inadequate secondary response (e.g., leukopenia, suppressed inflammatory response), chronic disease, malnutrition, current use of antibiotics.

Therapeutic Regimen: Individual, ineffective management—complexity of therapeutic regimen, economic difficulties, perceived seriousness/susceptibility.

Sample CP: Bacterial Pneumonia, Hospital. ELOS: 5 Days Medical Unit

ND and Categories of Care	Day 1 ____	Day 2 ____	Day 3 ____	Day 4 ____	Day 5 ____
Impaired gas exchange R/T alveolar congestion, inflammation, hypoventilation	Goals Participate in activities to maximize oxygenation and airway clearance	Demonstrate improving ventilation and oxygenation by lessening symptoms of respiratory distress, ABGs, approaching acceptable levels	Verbalize understanding of general healthcare needs	Initiate activities accepting responsibility for therapeutic regimen within level of ability Plan in place to meet postdischarge needs	Demonstrate ABGs within patient's acceptable range and absence of respiratory distress
Referrals	Pulmonary specialist		Home care Home O$_2$/Resp. Therapist		
Diagnostic studies	CXR ABGs CBC, electrolytes	→ Repeat if pulse ox <87%	Repeat if WBC count elevated, febrile, or ABGs not WNL Hb/Hct		
Additional assessments	Sputum C&S/Gram stain Blood culture Pulse oximetry q4h	↑ DC if 92%			
	Respiratory rate, rhythm, depth, use of accessory muscles, color of skin/mucous membranes q4h	↑	↑ q8h	↑	↑
	Breath sounds q4h	↑	↑ q8h	↑	↑
	Cough/sputum characteristics	↑	↑	↑	↑
	Vital signs q4h	↑	↑ q8h	↑	↑
	I&O q8h	↑	↑	↑	↑
	Weight qd	↑	↑		
Medications Allergies: ____ ____	IV antibiotics	↑	↑ PO	↑	↑
	Bronchodilator via MDI or nebulizer	→ MDI	↑	↑	↑
	Mucolytic	↑	↑	↑	↑
	Antitussives—prn	↑	↑		
	Acetaminophen if temperature above 101°F	↑	D/C		
	Analgesics—prn	→ D/C			

152

Sample CP: Bacterial Pneumonia, Hospital. ELOS: 5 Days Medical Unit (Continued)

ND and Categories of Care	Day 1 _____	Day 2 _____	Day 3 _____	Day 4 _____	Day 5 _____
Patient education	Orient to unit/room Review advance directives Diagnostic tests/results Pulmonary hygiene: T,C,DB, splinting techniques Use of incentive spirometer, MDI Proper handling of secretions, handwashing techniques Relaxation techniques	Adaptive breathing techniques as indicated Pacing of activities Smoking cessation Fluid/nutritional needs, balancing activity/rest	Individual risk factors, prevention of recurrence, vaccinations/immunizations Signs/symptoms to report to healthcare provider	Medications postdischarge: dose, time, route, purpose, side effects Proper use and care of home care equipment (e.g., O_2 concentrator, nebulizer)	Provide written instructions Schedule for follow-up appointments
Additional nursing actions	Position for maximal respiratory effort	→ per self	→	→	
	Assist with physical care		→ as necessary	→ per self	
	Incentive spirometry q4h		→ per self WA	→ per self	
	Supplemental O_2		→	→ D/C	
	Oral care—prn	→ per self	→	→ D/C	
	Suction as indicated		→	→ D/C	
	Screen visitors/staff for URI		→	→ D/C	
	Encourage fluid to 2500 mL/day as tolerated		→	→ per self	

LUNG CANCER: POSTOPERATIVE CARE

Lung cancer is the most common cause of cancer death in the United States and usually develops within the wall or epithelium of the bronchial tree. The two major categories are small cell lung cancers (SCLC), such as oat cell; and non–small cell lung cancers (NSCLC) such as squamous cell, adenocarcinoma, and large cell. Prognosis is generally poor, varying with the type of cancer and extent of involvement at the time of diagnosis. Survival rates are better with NSCLC, especially if treated in early stages. Although NSCLC tumors are frequently associated with metastases, they are generally slow growing.

Treatment options can include combinations of surgery, radiation, and chemotherapy. Surgery is the primary treatment for stage I and stage II tumors. Selected stage III carcinomas may be operable if the tumor is resectable. Surgical procedures for operable tumors of the lung include:

1. Pneumonectomy (removal of an entire lung), performed for lesions originating in the mainstem bronchus or lobar bronchus.
2. Lobectomy (removal of one lobe), preferred for peripheral carcinoma localized in a lobe.
3. Wedge or segmental resection, performed for lesions that are small and well-contained within one segment.
4. Endoscopic laser resection may be done on peripheral tumors to reduce the necessity of cutting through ribs.

CARE SETTING

Inpatient surgical and possibly subacute units.

RELATED CONCERNS

Cancer, page 900
Hemothorax/Pneumothorax, page 165
Psychosocial aspects of care, page 809
Radical neck surgery: laryngectomy (postoperative care), page 173
Surgical intervention, page 828

Patient Assessment Database (Preoperative)

Findings depend on type, duration of cancer, and extent of metastasis.

ACTIVITY/REST

May report:	Fatigue, inability to maintain usual routine, dyspnea with activity
May exhibit:	Lassitude (usually in advanced stage)

CIRCULATION

May exhibit:	Jugular venous distention (JVD) (with vena caval obstruction)
	Heart sounds: Pericardial rub (indicating effusion)
	Tachycardia/dysrhythmias
	Clubbing of fingers

EGO INTEGRITY

May report:	Frightened feelings, fear of outcome of surgery
	Denial of severity of condition/potential for malignancy
May exhibit:	Restlessness, insomnia, repetitive questioning

ELIMINATION

May report:	Intermittent diarrhea (hormonal imbalance, SCLC)
	Increased frequency/amount of urine (hormonal imbalance, epidermoid tumor)

FOOD/FLUID

May report:	Weight loss, poor appetite, decreased food intake
	Difficulty swallowing
	Thirst/increased fluid intake
May exhibit:	Thin, emaciated, or wasted appearance (late stages)

Edema of face/neck, chest, back (vena caval obstruction); facial/periorbital edema (hormonal imbalance, SCLC)

Glucose in urine (hormonal imbalance, epidermoid tumor)

PAIN/DISCOMFORT

May report:
Chest pain (not usually present in early stages and not always in advanced stages), which may/may not be affected by position change

Shoulder/arm pain (particularly with large cell or adenocarcinoma)

Bone/joint pain: Cartilage erosion secondary to increased growth hormones (large cell or adenocarcinoma)

Intermittent abdominal pain

May exhibit:
Distraction behaviors (restlessness, withdrawal)

Guarding/protective actions

RESPIRATION

May report:
Mild cough or change in usual cough pattern and/or sputum production

Shortness of breath

Occupational exposure to pollutants, industrial dusts (e.g., asbestos, iron oxides, coal dust), radioactive material

Hoarseness/change in voice (vocal cord paralysis)

History of smoking

May exhibit:
Dyspnea, aggravated by exertion

Increased tactile fremitus (indicating consolidation)

Brief crackles/wheezes on inspiration or expiration (impaired airflow)

Persistent crackles/wheezes; tracheal shift (space-occupying lesion)

Hemoptysis

SAFETY

May exhibit:
Fever may be present (large cell or adenocarcinoma)

Bruising, discoloration of skin (hormonal imbalance, SCLC)

SEXUALITY

May exhibit:
Gynecomastia (neoplastic hormonal changes, large cell carcinoma)

Amenorrhea/impotence (hormonal imbalance, SCLC)

TEACHING/LEARNING

May report:
Familial risk factors: Cancer (especially lung), tuberculosis

Failure to improve

Discharge plan considerations:
DRG projected mean length of inpatient stay: 9.9 days

Assistance with transportation, medications, treatments, self-care, homemaker/maintenance tasks

Refer to section at end of plan for postdischarge considerations.

DIAGNOSTIC STUDIES

Fiberoptic bronchoscopy: Allows for visualization, regional washings, and cytologic brushing of lesions (large percent of bronchogenic carcinomas may be visualized).

Chest x-ray (PA and lateral), chest computed tomography (CT): Outlines shape, size, and location of lesion. May reveal mass of air in hilar region, pleural effusion, atelectasis, or erosion of ribs or vertebrae.

Cytologic examinations (sputum, pleural, or lymph node): Performed to assess presence/stage of carcinoma.

Biopsy: May be performed on scalene nodes, hilar lymph nodes, or pleura to establish diagnosis.

Mediastinoscopy: Used for staging of carcinoma.

Lung scan: Helpful in determining tumor size/location and for staging.

Pulmonary function studies and ABGs: Assess lung capacity to meet postoperative ventilatory needs.

Skin tests, absolute lymphocyte counts: May be done to evaluate for immunocompetence (common in lung cancers).

Bone scan; CT scan of brain, liver; gallium scan of liver, spleen, bone: Used to detect metastasis.

NURSING PRIORITIES

1. Maintain/improve respiratory function.
2. Control/alleviate pain.
3. Support efforts to cope with diagnosis/situation.
4. Provide information about disease process/prognosis and therapeutic regimen.

DISCHARGE GOALS

1. Oxygenation/ventilation adequate to meet individual activity needs.
2. Pain controlled.
3. Anxiety/fear decreased to manageable level.
4. Free of preventable complications.
5. Disease process/prognosis and planned therapies understood.
6. Plan in place to meet needs after discharge.

NURSING DIAGNOSIS: Gas Exchange, impaired

May be related to
Removal of lung tissue
Altered oxygen supply (hypoventilation)
Decreased oxygen-carrying capacity of blood (blood loss)

Possibly evidenced by
Dyspnea
Restlessness/changes in mentation
Hypoxemia and hypercapnea
Cyanosis

DESIRED OUTCOMES/EVALUATION CRITERIA—PATIENT WILL:

Respiratory Status: Gas Exchange (NOC)

Demonstrate improved ventilation and adequate oxygenation of tissues by ABGs within patient's normal range.
Be free of symptoms of respiratory distress.

ACTIONS/INTERVENTIONS	RATIONALE
Respiratory Management (NIC)	
Independent	
Note respiratory rate, depth, and ease of respirations. Observe for use of accessory muscles, pursed-lip breathing, changes in skin/mucous membrane color, e.g., pallor, cyanosis.	Respirations may be increased as a result of pain or as an initial compensatory mechanism to accommodate for loss of lung tissue; however, increased work of breathing and cyanosis may indicate increasing oxygen consumption and energy expenditures and/or reduced respiratory reserve, e.g., elderly patient or extensive COPD.
Auscultate lungs for air movement and abnormal breath sounds.	Consolidation and lack of air movement on operative side is normal in the pneumonectomy patient; however, the lobectomy patient should demonstrate normal airflow in remaining lobes.

ACTIONS/INTERVENTIONS	RATIONALE
Independent	
Investigate restlessness and changes in mentation/level of consciousness.	May indicate increased hypoxia or complications such as mediastinal shift in pneumonectomy patient when accompanied by tachypnea, tachycardia, and tracheal deviation.
Assess patient response to activity. Encourage rest periods/limit activities to patient tolerance.	Increased oxygen consumption/demand and stress of surgery can result in increased dyspnea and changes in vital signs with activity; however, early mobilization is desired to help prevent pulmonary complications and to obtain and maintain respiratory and circulatory efficiency. Adequate rest balanced with activity can prevent respiratory compromise.
Note development of fever.	Fever within the first 24 hr after surgery is frequently due to atelectasis. Temperature elevation within the fifth to tenth postoperative day usually indicates an infection, e.g., wound or systemic.

Airway Management (NIC)

Maintain patent airway by positioning, suctioning, use of airway adjuncts.	Airway obstruction impedes ventilation, impairing gas exchange. (Refer to ND: Airway Clearance, ineffective, p. 158.)
Reposition frequently, placing patient in sitting positions and supine to side positions.	Maximizes lung expansion and drainage of secretions.
Avoid positioning the patient with a pneumonectomy on the operative side; instead, favor the "good lung down" position.	Recent research shows that positioning patients following lung surgery with their "good lung down" maximizes oxygenation by using gravity to enhance blood flow to the healthy lung, thus creating the best possible match between ventilation and perfusion.
Encourage/assist with deep-breathing exercises and pursed-lip breathing as appropriate.	Promotes maximal ventilation and oxygenation and reduces/prevents atelectasis.

Tube Care: Chest (NIC)

Maintain patency of chest drainage system for lobectomy, segmental/wedge resection patient.	Drains fluid from pleural cavity to promote re-expansion of remaining lung segments.
Note changes in amount/type of chest tube drainage.	Bloody drainage should decrease in amount and change to a more serous composition as recovery progresses. A sudden increase in amount of bloody drainage or return to frank bleeding suggests thoracic bleeding/hemothorax; sudden cessation suggests blockage of tube, requiring further evaluation and intervention.
Observe presence/degree of bubbling in water-seal chamber.	Air leaks immediately postoperative are not uncommon, especially following lobectomy or segmental resection; however, this should diminish as healing progresses. Prolonged or new leaks require evaluation to identify problems in the patient versus the drainage system.

ACTIONS/INTERVENTIONS	RATIONALE

Collaborative

Administer supplemental oxygen via nasal cannula, partial rebreathing mask, or high-humidity face mask, as indicated.

Maximizes available oxygen, especially while ventilation is reduced from anesthetic, depression, or pain, and during period of compensatory physiological shift of circulation to remaining functional alveolar units.

Assist with/encourage use of incentive spirometer or blow bottles.

Prevents/reduces atelectasis and promotes re-expansion of small airways.

Monitor/graph ABGs, pulse oximetry readings. Note hemoglobin (Hb) levels.

Decreasing PaO_2 or increasing $PaCO_2$ may indicate need for ventilatory support. Significant blood loss can result in decreased oxygen-carrying capacity, reducing PaO_2.

NURSING DIAGNOSIS: Airway Clearance, ineffective

May be related to
Increased amount/viscosity of secretions
Restricted chest movement/pain
Fatigue/weakness

Possibly evidenced by
Changes in rate/depth of respiration
Abnormal breath sounds
Ineffective cough
Dyspnea

DESIRED OUTCOMES/EVALUATION CRITERIA—PATIENT WILL:

Respiratory Status: Ventilation (NOC)

Demonstrate patent airway, with fluid secretions easily expectorated, clear breath sounds, and noiseless respirations.

ACTIONS/INTERVENTIONS	RATIONALE

Airway Management (NIC)

Independent

Auscultate chest for character of breath sounds and presence of secretions.

Noisy respirations, rhonchi, and wheezes are indicative of retained secretions and/or airway obstruction.

Assist patient with/instruct in effective deep breathing and coughing with upright position (sitting) and splinting of incision.

Upright position favors maximal lung expansion, and splinting improves force of cough effort to mobilize and remove secretions. Splinting may be done by nurse (placing hands anteriorly and posteriorly over chest wall) and by patient (with pillows) as strength improves.

Observe amount and character of sputum/aspirated secretions. Investigate changes as indicated.

Increased amounts of colorless (or blood-streaked)/watery secretions are normal initially and should decrease as recovery progresses. Presence of thick/tenacious, bloody, or purulent sputum suggests development of secondary problems (e.g., dehydration, pulmonary edema, local hemorrhage, or infection) that require correction/treatment.

ACTIONS/INTERVENTIONS	RATIONALE
Independent	
Suction if cough is weak or rhonchi not cleared by cough effort. Avoid deep endotracheal/nasotracheal suctioning in pneumonectomy patient if possible.	"Routine" suctioning increases risk of hypoxemia and mucosal damage. Deep tracheal suctioning is generally contraindicated following pneumonectomy to reduce the risk of rupture of the bronchial stump suture line. If suctioning is unavoidable, it should be done gently and only to induce effective coughing.
Encourage oral fluid intake (at least 2500 mL/day) within cardiac tolerance.	Adequate hydration aids in keeping secretions loose/enhances expectoration.
Assess for pain/discomfort and medicate on a routine basis and before breathing exercises.	Encourages the patient to move, cough more effectively, and breathe more deeply to prevent respiratory insufficiency.
Collaborative	
Provide/assist with IPPB, incentive spirometer, postural drainage/percussion as indicated.	Improves lung expansion/ventilation and facilitates removal of secretions. *Note:* Postural drainage may be contraindicated in some patients and in any event must be performed cautiously to prevent respiratory embarrassment and incisional discomfort.
Use humidified oxygen/ultrasonic nebulizer. Provide additional fluids via IV as indicated.	Providing maximal hydration helps loosen/liquefy secretions to promote expectoration. Impaired oral intake necessitates IV supplementation to maintain hydration.
Administer bronchodilators, expectorants, and/or analgesics as indicated.	Relieves bronchospasm to improve airflow. Expectorants increase mucous production and liquefy and reduce viscosity of secretions, facilitating removal. Alleviation of chest discomfort promotes cooperation with breathing exercises and enhances effectiveness of respiratory therapies.

NURSING DIAGNOSIS: Pain [acute]

May be related to
Surgical incision, tissue trauma, and disruption of intercostal nerves
Presence of chest tube(s)
Cancer invasion of pleura, chest wall

Possibly evidenced by
Verbal reports of discomfort
Guarding of affected area
Distraction behaviors, e.g., restlessness
Narrowed focus (withdrawal)
Changes in BP, heart/respiratory rate

DESIRED OUTCOMES/EVALUATION CRITERIA—PATIENT WILL:

Pain Level (NOC)

Report pain relieved/controlled.
Appear relaxed and sleep/rest appropriately.
Participate in desired/needed activities.

ACTIONS/INTERVENTIONS	RATIONALE

Pain Management (NIC)

Independent

Ask patient about pain. Determine pain characteristics, e.g., continuous, aching, stabbing, burning. Have patient rate intensity on a 0–10 scale.

Helpful in evaluating cancer-related pain symptoms, which may involve viscera, nerve, or bone tissue. Use of rating scale aids patient in assessing level of pain and provides tool for evaluating effectiveness of analgesics, enhancing patient control of pain.

Assess patient's verbal and nonverbal pain cues.

Discrepancy between verbal/nonverbal cues may provide clues to degree of pain, need for/effectiveness of interventions.

Note possible pathophysiological and psychological causes of pain.

A posterolateral incision is more uncomfortable for the patient than an anterolateral incision. The presence of chest tubes can greatly increase discomfort. In addition, fear, distress, anxiety, and grief over confirmed diagnosis of cancer can impair ability to cope.

Evaluate effectiveness of drug regimen. Encourage sufficient medication to control pain; change medication or time span as appropriate.

Pain perception and pain relief are subjective; thus pain management is best left to the patient's discretion. If the patient is unable to provide input, the nurse should observe physiological and nonverbal signs of pain and administer medications on a regular basis.

Encourage verbalization of feelings about the pain.

Fears/concerns can increase muscle tension and lower threshold of pain perception. (Refer to ND: Fear/Anxiety [specify level], following.)

Provide comfort measures, e.g., frequent changes of position, back rubs, support with pillows. Encourage use of relaxation techniques, e.g., visualization, guided imagery, and appropriate diversional activities.

Promotes relaxation and redirects attention. Relieves discomfort and augments therapeutic effects of analgesia.

Schedule rest periods, provide quiet environment.

Decreases fatigue and conserves energy, enhancing coping abilities.

Assist with self-care activities, breathing/arm exercises, and ambulation.

Prevents undue fatigue and incisional strain. Encouragement and physical assistance/support may be needed for some time before the patient is able or confident enough to perform these activities because of pain or fear of pain.

Collaborative

Administer analgesics routinely as indicated, especially 45–60 min before respiratory treatments, deep-breathing/coughing exercises. Assist with patient-controlled analgesia (PCA) or analgesia through epidural catheter.

Maintaining a more constant drug level avoids cyclic periods of pain, aids in muscle healing, and improves respiratory function and emotional comfort/coping.

NURSING DIAGNOSIS: Fear/Anxiety [specify level]

May be related to
Situational crises
Threat to/change in health status
Perceived threat of death

Possibly evidenced by
Withdrawal
Apprehension
Anger
Increased pain, sympathetic stimulation
Expressions of denial, shock, guilt, insomnia

DESIRED OUTCOMES/EVALUATION CRITERIA—PATIENT WILL:

Fear Control/Anxiety Control (NOC)

Acknowledge and discuss fears/concerns.
Demonstrate appropriate range of feelings and appear relaxed/resting appropriately.
Verbalize accurate knowledge of situation.
Report beginning use of individually appropriate coping strategies.

ACTIONS/INTERVENTIONS	RATIONALE
Anxiety Reduction (NIC)	
Independent	
Evaluate patient/SO level of understanding of diagnosis.	Patient and SO are hearing and assimilating new information that includes changes in self-image and lifestyle. Understanding perceptions of those involved sets the tone for individualizing care and provides information necessary for choosing appropriate interventions.
Acknowledge reality of patient's fears/concerns and encourage expression of feelings.	Support may enable the patient to begin exploring/ dealing with the reality of cancer and its treatment. Patient may need time to identify feelings and even more time to begin to express them.
Provide opportunity for questions and answer them honestly. Be sure that patient and care providers have the same understanding of terms used.	Establishes trust and reduces misperceptions/misinterpretation of information.
Accept, but do not reinforce, patient's denial of the situation.	When extreme denial or anxiety is interfering with progress of recovery, the issues facing the patient need to be explained and resolutions explored.
Note comments/behaviors indicative of beginning acceptance and/or use of effective strategies to deal with situation.	Fear/anxiety will diminish as patient begins to accept/deal positively with reality. Indicator of patient's readiness to accept responsibility for participation in recovery and to "resume life."
Involve patient/SO in care planning. Provide time to prepare for events/treatments.	May help restore some feeling of control/independence to patient who feels powerless in dealing with diagnosis and treatment.
Provide for patient's physical comfort.	It is difficult to deal with emotional issues when experiencing extreme/persistent physical discomfort.

> **NURSING DIAGNOSIS: Knowledge Deficit [Learning Need] regarding condition, treatment, prognosis, self care, and discharge needs**
>
> **May be related to**
> Lack of exposure, unfamiliarity with information/resources
> Information misinterpretation
> Lack of recall
> **Possibly evidenced by**
> Statements of concern; request for information
> Inadequate follow-through of instruction
> Inappropriate or exaggerated behaviors, e.g., hysterical, hostile, agitated, apathetic
> **DESIRED OUTCOMES/EVALUATION CRITERIA—PATIENT WILL:**
>
> | **Knowledge: Disease Process (NOC)** |
>
> Verbalize understanding of ramifications of diagnosis, prognosis, possible complications.
> Participate in learning process.
>
> | **Knowledge: Treatment Regimen (NOC)** |
>
> Verbalize understanding of therapeutic regimen.
> Correctly perform necessary procedures and explain reasons for the actions.
> Initiate necessary lifestyle changes.

ACTIONS/INTERVENTIONS	RATIONALE
Teaching: Disease Process (NIC)	
Independent	
Discuss diagnosis, current/planned therapies and expected outcomes.	Provides individually specific information, creating knowledge base for subsequent learning regarding home management. Radiation or chemotherapy may follow surgical intervention and information is essential to enable the patient/SO to make informed decisions.
Reinforce surgeon's explanation of particular surgical procedure, providing diagram as appropriate. Incorporate this information into discussion about short-/long-term recovery expectations.	Length of rehabilitation and prognosis depend on type of surgical procedure, preoperative physical condition, and duration/degree of complications.
Discuss necessity of planning for follow-up care before discharge.	Follow-up assessment of respiratory status and general health is imperative to assure optimal recovery. Also provides opportunity to readdress concerns/questions at a less stressful time.
Identify signs/symptoms requiring medical evaluations, e.g., changes in appearance of incision, development of respiratory difficulty, fever, increased chest pain, changes in appearance of sputum.	Early detection and timely intervention may prevent/minimize complications.
Help patient determine activity tolerance and set goals.	Weakness and fatigue should lessen as lung(s) heals and respiratory function improves during recovery period, especially if cancer was completely removed. If cancer is advanced, it is emotionally helpful for the patient to be able to set realistic activity goals to achieve optimal independence.

ACTIONS/INTERVENTIONS	RATIONALE
Independent	
Evaluate availability/adequacy of support system(s) and necessity for assistance in self-care/home management.	General weakness and activity limitations may reduce individual's ability to meet own needs.
Recommend alternating rest periods with activity and light tasks with heavy tasks. Stress avoidance of heavy lifting, isometric/strenuous upper body exercise. Reinforce physician's time limitations about lifting.	Generalized weakness and fatigue are usual in the early recovery period but should diminish as respiratory function improves and healing progresses. Rest and sleep enhance coping abilities, reduce nervousness (common in this phase), and promote healing. *Note:* Strenuous use of arms can place undue stress on incision because chest muscles may be weaker than normal for 3–6 months following surgery.
Recommend stopping any activity that causes undue fatigue or increased shortness of breath.	Exhaustion aggravates respiratory insufficiency.
Encourage inspection of incisions. Review expectations for healing with patient.	Healing begins immediately, but complete healing takes time. As healing progresses, incision lines may appear dry, with crusty scabs. Underlying tissue may look bruised and feel tense, warm, and lumpy (resolving hematoma).
Instruct patient/SO to watch for/report places in incision that do not heal or reopening of healed incision, any drainage (bloody or purulent), localized area of swelling with redness or increased pain that is hot to touch.	Signs/symptoms indicating failure to heal, development of complications requiring further medical evaluation/intervention.
Suggest wearing soft cotton shirts and loose-fitting clothing, cover/pad portion of incision as indicated, leave incision open to air as much as possible.	Reduces suture line irritation and pressure from clothing. Leaving incisions open to air promotes healing process and may reduce risk of infection.
Shower in warm water, washing incision gently. Avoid tub baths until approved by physician.	Keeps incision clean, promotes circulation/healing. *Note:* "Climbing" out of tub requires use of arms and pectoral muscles, which can put undue stress on incision.
Support incision with Steri-strips as needed when sutures/staples are removed.	Aids in maintaining approximation of wound edges to promote healing.
Instruct in/provide rationale for arm/shoulder exercises. Have patient/SO demonstrate exercises. Encourage following graded increase in number/intensity of routine repetitions.	Simple arm circles and lifting arms over the head or out to the affected side are initiated on the first or second postoperative day to restore normal range of motion (ROM) of shoulder and to prevent ankylosis of the affected shoulder.
Stress importance of avoiding exposure to smoke, air pollution, and contact with individuals with URIs.	Protects lung(s) from irritation and reduces risk of infection.
Review nutritional/fluid needs. Suggest increasing protein and use of high-calorie snacks as appropriate.	Meeting cellular energy requirements and maintaining good circulating volume for tissue perfusion facilitates tissue regeneration/healing process.
Identify individually appropriate community resources, e.g., American Cancer Society, visiting nurse, social services, home care.	Agencies such as these offer a broad range of services that can be tailored to provide support and meet individual needs.

POTENTIAL CONSIDERATIONS following hospitalization (dependent on patient's age, physical condition/presence of complications, personal resources, and life responsibilities)

Airway Clearance, ineffective—increased amount/viscosity of secretions, restricted chest movement/pain, fatigue/weakness.

Pain [acute]—surgical incision, tissue trauma, disruption of intercostal nerves, presence of distress/anxiety.

Self-Care deficit—decreased strength/endurance, presence of pain, intolerance to activity, depression, presence of therapeutic devices, e.g., IV lines.

Refer to CP, Cancer for other considerations, page 900.

HEMOTHORAX/PNEUMOTHORAX

The lung may collapse partially or completely because of air (pneumothorax), blood (hemothorax), or other fluid (pleural effusion) collecting in the pleural/potential space. The intrathoracic pressure changes induced by increased pleural space volumes reduce lung capacity, causing respiratory distress and gas exchange problems and producing tension on mediastinal structures that can impede cardiac and systemic circulation. Pneumothorax may be traumatic (open or closed) or spontaneous.

CARE SETTING

Inpatient medical or surgical unit.

RELATED CONCERNS

Cardiac surgery: postoperative care, coronary artery bypass graft; cardiomyoplasty; valve replacement, page 102.
Chronic obstructive pulmonary disease (COPD), page 126
Psychosocial aspects of care, page 809
Pulmonary tuberculosis (TB), page 204
Ventilatory assistance (mechanical), page 188

Patient Assessment Database

Findings vary, depending on the amount of air and/or fluid accumulation, rate of accumulation, and underlying lung function.

ACTIVITY/REST

May report: Dyspnea with activity or even at rest

CIRCULATION

May exhibit: Tachycardia; irregular rate/dysrhythmias
S_3 or S_4/gallop heart rhythm (heart failure secondary to effusion)
Apical pulse reveals point of maximal impulse (PMI) displaced in presence of mediastinal shift (with tension pneumothorax)
Hamman's sign (crunching sound correlating with heartbeat, reflecting air in mediastinum)
BP: hypertension/hypotension
JVD

EGO INTEGRITY

May exhibit: Apprehension, irritability

FOOD/FLUID

May exhibit: Recent placement of central venous IV/pressure line (causative factor)

PAIN/DISCOMFORT

May report (depending on the size/area involved): Unilateral chest pain, aggravated by breathing, coughing
Sudden onset of symptoms while coughing or straining (spontaneous pneumothorax)
Sharp, stabbing pain aggravated by deep breathing, possibly radiating to neck, shoulders, abdomen (pleural effusion)

May exhibit: Guarding affected area
Distraction behaviors
Facial grimacing

RESPIRATION

May report: Difficulty breathing, "air hunger"
Coughing (may be presenting symptom)

165

History of recent chest surgery/trauma; chronic lung disease, lung inflammation/infection (empyema/effusion); diffuse interstitial disease (sarcoidosis), malignancies (e.g., obstructive tumor)

Previous spontaneous pneumothorax; spontaneous rupture of emphysematous bulla, subpleural bleb (COPD)

May exhibit: Respiratory: Rate increased/tachypnea

Increased work of breathing, use of accessory muscles in chest, neck; intercostal retractions, forced abdominal expiration

Breath sounds decreased or absent (involved site)

Fremitus decreased (involved site)

Chest percussion: Hyperresonance over air-filled area (pneumothorax); dullness over fluid-filled area (hemothorax)

Chest observation and palpation: Unequal (paradoxic) chest movement (if trauma, flail); reduced thoracic excursion (affected side)

Skin: Pallor, cyanosis, diaphoresis, subcutaneous crepitation (air in tissues on palpation)

Mentation: Anxiety, restlessness, confusion, stupor

Use of positive pressure mechanical ventilation/positive end-expiratory pressure (PEEP) therapy

SAFETY

May report: Recent chest trauma

Radiation/chemotherapy for malignancy

TEACHING/LEARNING

May report: History of familial risk factors: Tuberculosis, cancer

Recent intrathoracic surgery/lung biopsy

Evidence of failure to improve

Discharge plan considerations **DRG projected length of inpatient stay: 6.5 days**

Temporary assistance with self-care, homemaker/maintenance tasks

Refer to section at end of plan for postdischarge considerations.

DIAGNOSTIC STUDIES

Thoracic CT: Recent studies show that CT is more sensitive than x-ray in detecting thoracic injuries, lung contusion, hemothorax and pneumothorax. Early CT may influence therapeutic management.

Chest x-ray: Reveals air and/or fluid accumulation in the pleural space; may show shift of mediastinal structures (heart).

ABGs: Variable depending on degree of compromised lung function, altered breathing mechanics, and ability to compensate. $PaCO_2$ occasionally elevated. PaO_2 may be normal or decreased; oxygen saturation usually decreased.

Thoracentesis: Presence of blood/serosanguinous fluid indicates hemothorax.

Hb: May be decreased, indicating blood loss.

NURSING PRIORITIES

1. Promote/maintain lung re-expansion for adequate oxygenation/ventilation.
2. Minimize/prevent complications.
3. Reduce discomfort/pain.
4. Provide information about disease process, treatment regimen, and prognosis.

DISCHARGE GOALS

1. Adequate ventilation/oxygenation maintained.
2. Complications prevented/resolved.
3. Pain absent/controlled.
4. Disease process/prognosis and therapy needs understood.
5. Plan in place to meet needs after discharge.

NURSING DIAGNOSIS: Breathing Pattern, ineffective

May be related to

Decreased lung expansion (air/fluid accumulation)

Musculoskeletal impairment

Pain/anxiety

Inflammatory process

Possibly evidenced by

Dyspnea, tachypnea

Changes in depth/equality of respirations; altered chest excursion

Use of accessory muscles, nasal flaring

Cyanosis, abnormal ABGs

DESIRED OUTCOMES/EVALUATION CRITERIA—PATIENT WILL:

Respiratory Status: Gas Exchange (NOC)

Establish a normal/effective respiratory pattern with ABGs within patient's normal range.

Be free of cyanosis and other signs/symptoms of hypoxia.

ACTIONS/INTERVENTIONS

Respiratory Monitoring (NIC)

Independent

Identify etiology/precipitating factors, e.g., spontaneous collapse, trauma, malignancy, infection, complication of mechanical ventilation.

Evaluate respiratory function, noting rapid/shallow respirations, dyspnea, reports of "air hunger," development of cyanosis, changes in vital signs.

Monitor for synchronous respiratory pattern when using mechanical ventilator. Note changes in airway pressures.

Auscultate breath sounds.

Note chest excursion and position of trachea.

Assess fremitus.

Assist patient with splinting painful area when coughing, deep breathing.

RATIONALE

Understanding the cause of lung collapse is necessary for proper chest tube placement and choice of other therapeutic measures.

Respiratory distress and changes in vital signs may occur as a result of physiological stress and pain or may indicate development of shock due to hypoxia/hemorrhage.

Difficulty breathing "with" ventilator and/or increasing airway pressures suggests worsening of condition/development of complications (e.g., spontaneous rupture of a bleb creating a new pneumothorax).

Breath sounds may be diminished or absent in a lobe, lung segment, or entire lung field (unilateral). Atelectatic area will have no breath sounds, and partially collapsed areas have decreased sounds. Evaluation also establishes areas of good air exchange and provides a baseline to evaluate resolution of pneumothorax.

Chest excursion is unequal until lung re-expands. Trachea deviates away from affected side with tension pneumothorax.

Voice and tactile fremitus (vibration) is reduced in fluid-filled/consolidated tissue.

Supporting chest and abdominal muscles makes coughing more effective/less traumatic.

ACTIONS/INTERVENTIONS	RATIONALE

Independent

Maintain position of comfort, usually with head of bed elevated. Turn to affected side. Encourage patient to sit up as much as possible.

Promotes maximal inspiration; enhances lung expansion and ventilation in unaffected side.

Maintain a calm attitude, assisting patient to "take control" by using slower/deeper respirations.

Assists the patient to deal with the physiological effects of hypoxia, which may be manifested as anxiety and/or fear.

Tube Care: Chest (NIC)

Once chest tube is inserted:

Check suction control chamber for correct amount of suction (determined by water level, wall/table regulator at correct setting);

Maintains prescribed intrapleural negativity, which promotes optimum lung expansion and/or fluid drainage. *Note:* Dry-seal setups are also used with an automatic control valve (AVC), which provides a one-way valve seal similar to that achieved with the water-seal system.

Check fluid level in water-seal chamber; maintain at prescribed level;

Water in a sealed chamber serves as a barrier that prevents atmospheric air from entering the pleural space should the suction source be disconnected and aids in evaluating whether the chest drainage system is functioning appropriately. *Note:* Underfilling the water-seal chamber leaves it exposed to air, putting the patient at risk for pneumothorax or tension pneumothorax. Overfilling (a more common mistake) prevents air from easily exiting the pleural space, thus preventing resolution of pneumothorax or tension pneumothorax.

Observe water-seal chamber bubbling;

Bubbling during expiration reflects venting of pneumothorax (desired action). Bubbling usually decreases as the lung expands or may occur only during expiration or coughing as the pleural space diminishes. Absence of bubbling may indicate complete lung re-expansion (normal) or represent complications, e.g., obstruction in the tube.

Evaluate for abnormal/continuous water-seal chamber bubbling;

With suction applied, this indicates a persistent air leak that may be from a large pneumothorax at the chest insertion site (patient-centered) or chest drainage unit (system-centered).

Determine location of air leak (patient- or system-centered) by clamping thoracic catheter just distal to exit from chest;

If bubbling stops when catheter is clamped at insertion site, leak is patient-centered (at insertion site or within the patient).

Place petrolatum gauze and/or other appropriate material around the insertion as indicated;

Usually corrects insertion site air leak.

Clamp tubing in stepwise fashion downward toward drainage unit if air leak continues;

Isolates location of a system-centered air leak. *Note:* Recent information indicates that clamping for a suspected leak may be the only time that chest tube should be clamped.

Seal drainage tubing connection sites securely with lengthwise tape or bands according to established policy;

Prevents/corrects air leaks at connector sites.

ACTIONS/INTERVENTIONS

Independent

Monitor water-seal chamber "tidaling." Note whether change is transient or permanent;

Position drainage system tubing for optimal function, e.g., shorten tubing/coil extra tubing on bed, making sure tubing is not kinked or hanging below entrance to drainage container. Drain accumulated fluid as necessary;

Note character/amount of chest tube drainage;

Evaluate need for tube stripping ("milking");

Strip tubes carefully per protocol, in a manner that minimizes excess negative pressure.

If thoracic catheter is disconnected/dislodged:

Observe for signs of respiratory distress. If possible, reconnect thoracic catheter to tubing/suction, using clean technique. If the catheter is dislodged from the chest, cover insertion site immediately with petrolatum dressing and apply firm pressure. Notify physician at once.

After thoracic catheter is removed:

Cover insertion site with sterile occlusive dressing. Observe for signs/symptoms that may indicate recurrence of pneumothorax, e.g., shortness of breath, reports of pain. Inspect insertion site, note character of drainage.

Collaborative

Review serial chest x-rays.

RATIONALE

The water-seal chamber serves as an intrapleural manometer (gauges intrapleural pressure); therefore, fluctuation (tidaling) reflects pressure differences between inspiration and expiration. Tidaling of 2–6 cm during inspiration is normal and may increase briefly during coughing episodes. Continuation of excessive tidal fluctuations may indicate existence of airway obstruction or presence of a large pneumothorax.

Improper position, kinking, or accumulation of clots/fluid in the tubing changes the desired negative pressure and impedes air/fluid evacuation.

Useful in evaluating resolution of condition/development of complication or hemorrhage requiring prompt intervention. *Note:* Some drainage systems are equipped with an autotransfusion device, which allows for salvage of shed blood.

Although routine stripping is not recommended, it may be necessary occasionally to maintain drainage in the presence of fresh bleeding/large blood clots or purulent exudate (empyema).

Stripping is usually uncomfortable for the patient because of the change in intrathoracic pressure, which may induce coughing or chest discomfort. Vigorous stripping can create very high intrathoracic suction pressure, which can be injurious (e.g., invagination of tissue into catheter eyelets, collapse of tissues around the catheter, and/or bleeding from rupture of small blood vessels).

Pneumothorax may recur, requiring prompt intervention to prevent fatal pulmonary and circulatory impairment.

Early detection of a developing complication is essential, e.g., recurrence of pneumothorax, presence of infection.

Monitors progress of resolving hemothorax/pneumothorax and re-expansion of lung. Can identify malposition of endotracheal tube (ET) affecting lung re-expansion.

ACTIONS/INTERVENTIONS

Collaborative

Monitor/graph serial ABGs and pulse oximetry. Review vital capacity/tidal volume measurements.

Administer supplemental oxygen via cannula/mask/mechanical ventilation as indicated.

RATIONALE

Assesses status of gas exchange and ventilation, need for continuation or alterations in therapy.

Aids in reducing work of breathing; promotes relief of respiratory distress and cyanosis associated with hypoxemia.

NURSING DIAGNOSIS: Trauma/Suffocation, risk for

Risk factors may include
Concurrent disease/injury process
Dependence on external device (chest drainage system)
Lack of safety education/precautions

Possibly evidenced by
[Not applicable; presence of signs and symptoms establishes an *actual* diagnosis]

DESIRED OUTCOMES/EVALUATION CRITERIA—PATIENT WILL:

Risk Control (NOC)

Recognize need for/seek assistance to prevent complications.

CAREGIVER WILL:
Correct/avoid environmental and physical hazards.

ACTIONS/INTERVENTIONS

RATIONALE

Teaching: Procedure/Treatment (NIC)

Independent

Review with patient purpose/function of chest drainage unit, taking note of safety features.

Instruct patient to refrain from lying/pulling on tubing.

Identify changes/situations that should be reported to caregivers, e.g., change in sound of bubbling, sudden "air hunger" and chest pain, disconnection of equipment.

Information on how system works provides reassurance, reducing patient anxiety.

Reduces risk of obstructing drainage/inadvertently disconnecting tubing

Timely intervention may prevent serious complications.

Environmental Management: Safety (NIC)

Anchor thoracic catheter to chest wall and provide extra length of tubing before turning or moving patient:

Secure tubing connection sites;

Pad banding sites with gauze/tape.

Secure drainage unit to patient's bed or on stand/cart placed in low-traffic area.

Prevents thoracic catheter dislodgment or tubing disconnection and reduces pain/discomfort associated with pulling or jarring of tubing.

Prevents tubing disconnection.

Protects skin from irritation/pressure.

Maintains upright position and reduces risk of accidental tipping/breaking of unit.

ACTIONS/INTERVENTIONS

Independent

Provide safe transportation if patient is sent off unit for diagnostic purposes. Before transporting: check water-seal chamber for correct fluid level, presence/absence of bubbling; presence/degree/timing of tidaling. Ascertain whether or not chest tube can be clamped or disconnected from suction source.

Monitor thoracic insertion site, noting condition of skin, presence/characteristics of drainage from around the catheter. Change/reapply sterile occlusive dressing as needed.

Observe for signs of respiratory distress if thoracic catheter is disconnected/dislodged. (Refer to ND: Breathing Pattern, ineffective, p. 167.)

RATIONALE

Promotes continuation of optimal evacuation of fluid/air during transport. If patient is draining large amounts of chest fluid or air, tube should not be clamped or suction interrupted because of risk of reaccumulation of fluid/air, compromising respiratory status.

Provides for early recognition and treatment of developing skin/tissue erosion or infection.

Pneumothorax may recur/worsen, compromising respiratory function and requiring emergency intervention.

NURSING DIAGNOSIS: Knowledge Deficit [Learning Need] regarding condition, treatment regimen, self care, and discharge needs

May be related to
Lack of exposure to information

Possibly evidenced by
Expressions of concern, request for information
Recurrence of problem

DESIRED OUTCOMES/EVALUATION CRITERIA—PATIENT WILL:

Knowledge: Disease Process (NOC)

Verbalize understanding of cause of problem (when known).
Identify signs/symptoms requiring medical follow-up.

Knowledge: Treatment Regimen (NOC)

Follow therapeutic regimen and demonstrate lifestyle changes if necessary to prevent recurrence.

ACTIONS/INTERVENTIONS

Teaching: Disease Process (NIC)

Independent

Review pathology of individual problem.

Identify likelihood for recurrence/long-term complications.

RATIONALE

Information reduces fear of unknown. Provides knowledge base for understanding underlying dynamics of condition and significance of therapeutic interventions.

Certain underlying lung diseases such as severe COPD and malignancies may increase incidence of recurrence. In otherwise healthy patients who suffered a spontaneous pneumothorax, incidence of recurrence is 10%–50%. Those who have a second spontaneous episode are at high risk for a third incident (60%).

ACTIONS/INTERVENTIONS	RATIONALE
Independent	
Review signs/symptoms requiring immediate medical evaluation, e.g., sudden chest pain, dyspnea/air hunger, progressive respiratory distress.	Recurrence of pneumothorax/hemothorax requires medical intervention to prevent/reduce potential complications.
Review significance of good health practices, e.g., adequate nutrition, rest, exercise.	Maintenance of general well-being promotes healing and may prevent/limit recurrences.

POTENTIAL CONSIDERATIONS following acute hospitalization (dependent on patient's age, physical condition/presence of complications, personal resources, and life responsibilities)

Infection, risk for—invasive procedure, traumatized tissue/broken skin, decreased ciliary action.
Breathing Pattern, ineffective—recurrence of condition, inflammatory process.

RADICAL NECK SURGERY: LARYNGECTOMY (POSTOPERATIVE CARE)

Head and neck cancer refers to a malignancy that lies above the clavicle but excludes the brain, spinal cord, axial skeleton, and vertebrae. Head and neck cancer accounts for 5.5% of all malignant disease. The majority of the laryngeal neoplasms (95%) are squamous cell carcinomas that arise from the oral cavity. When cancer is limited to the vocal cords (intrinsic), spread may be slow. When the cancer involves the epiglottis (extrinsic), metastasis is more common. Current treatment choices include surgery, radiation, and chemotherapy. Carbon dioxide laser may be used for early stage disease. This plan of care focuses on nursing care of the patient undergoing radical surgery of the neck, including laryngectomy.

Partial laryngectomy: Tumors that are limited to one vocal cord are removed and a temporary tracheotomy is performed to maintain the airway. After recovery from surgery, the patient will have a voice but it will be hoarse.

Hemilaryngectomy: When there is a possibility the cancer includes one true and one false vocal cord, they are removed along with an arytenoid cartilage and half of the thyroid cartilage. Temporary tracheotomy is performed, and the patient's voice will be hoarse after surgery.

Supraglottic laryngectomy: When the tumor is located in the epiglottis or false vocal cords, radical neck dissection is done and tracheotomy performed. The patient's voice remains intact; however, swallowing is more difficult because the epiglottis has been removed.

Total laryngectomy: Advanced cancers that involve a large portion of the larynx require removal of the entire larynx, the hyoid bone, the cricoid cartilage, two or three tracheal rings, and the strap muscles connected to the larynx. A permanent opening is created in the neck into the trachea, and a laryngectomy tube is inserted to keep the stoma open. The lower portion of the posterior pharynx is removed when the tumor extends beyond the epiglottis, with the remaining portion sutured to the esophagus after a nasogastric tube is inserted. The patient must breathe through a permanent tracheostomy, with normal speech no longer possible. Swallowing is not a long-term problem because there is no connection between the esophagus and trachea.

CARE SETTING

Inpatient surgical and possibly subacute units.

RELATED CONCERNS

Cancer, page 900
Psychosocial aspects of care, page 809
Surgical intervention, page 828
Total nutritional support: parenteral/enteral feeding, page 508

Patient Assessment Database

Preoperative data presented here depend on the specific type/location of cancer process and underlying complications.

EGO INTEGRITY

May report:	Feelings of fear about loss of voice, dying, occurrence/recurrence of cancer
	Concern about how surgery will affect family relationships, ability to work, and finances
May exhibit:	Anxiety, depression, anger, and withdrawal
	Denial

FOOD/FLUID

May report:	Difficulty swallowing (dysphagia)
May exhibit:	Difficulty handling oral secretions, chokes easily
	Swelling, ulcerations, masses may be noted depending on location of cancer
	Oral inflammation/drainage, poor dental hygiene
	Leukoplakia, erythroplasia of oral cavity
	Halitosis
	Swelling of tongue
	Altered gag reflex and facial paralysis

HYGIENE

May exhibit: Neglect of dental hygiene
Need for assistance in basic care

NEUROSENSORY

May report: Diplopia (double vision)
Deafness
Tingling, paresthesia of facial muscles

May exhibit: Hemiparalysis of face (parotid and submandibular involvement), persistent hoarseness or loss of voice (dominant and earliest symptom of intrinsic laryngeal cancer)
Difficulty swallowing
Conduction deafness
Disruption of mucous membranes

PAIN/DISCOMFORT

May report: Chronic sore throat, "lump in throat"
Referred pain to ear, facial pain (late stage, probably metastatic)
Pain/burning sensation with swallowing (especially with hot liquids or citrus juices), local pain in oropharynx

(Postoperative)   Sore throat or mouth (pain is not usually reported as severe following head and neck surgery, as compared with pain noted before surgery)

May exhibit: Guarding behaviors
Restlessness
Facial mask of pain
Alteration in muscle tone

RESPIRATION

May report: History of smoking (including cigars)/chewing tobacco
Occupation working with hardwood sawdust, toxic chemicals/fumes, heavy metals
History of voice overuse, e.g., professional singer or auctioneer
History of chronic lung disease
Cough with/without sputum
Bloody nasal drainage

May exhibit: Blood-tinged sputum, hemoptysis
Dyspnea (late)

SAFETY

May report: Excessive sun exposure over a period of years or radiation therapy
Visual/hearing changes

May exhibit: Masses/enlarged nodes

SOCIAL INTERACTION

May report: Lack of family/support system (may be result of age group or behaviors, e.g., alcoholism)
Concerns about ability to communicate, engage in social interactions

May exhibit: Persistent hoarseness, change in voice pitch
Muffled/garbled speech, reluctance to speak
Hesitancy/reluctance of significant others to provide care/be involved in rehabilitation

TEACHING/LEARNING

May report: Nonhealing of oral lesions
Concurrent use of alcohol/history of alcohol abuse

Discharge plan considerations:	**DRG projected mean length of inpatient stay: 5.0–13.0 days**
	Assistance with wound care, treatments, supplies; transportation, shopping; food preparation; self-care, homemaker/maintenance tasks

Refer to section at end of plan for postdischarge considerations.

DIAGNOSTIC STUDIES

Direct/indirect laryngoscopy; laryngeal tomography, biopsy, and needle biopsy: Are the most reliable diagnostic indicators.

Laryngography: May be performed with contrast to study blood vessels and lymph nodes.

Pulmonary function studies, bone scans, or other organ scans: May be indicated if distant metastasis is suspected.

Chest x-ray: Done to establish baseline lung status and/or identify metastases.

CBC: May reveal anemia, which is a common problem.

Immunologic surveys: May be done for patients receiving chemotherapy/immunotherapy.

Biochemical profile: Changes may occur in organ function as a result of cancer, metastasis, and therapies.

ABGs/pulse oximetry: May be done to establish baseline/monitor status of lungs (ventilation).

NURSING PRIORITIES

1. Maintain patent airway, adequate ventilation.
2. Assist patient in developing alternate communication methods.
3. Restore/maintain skin integrity.
4. Re-establish/maintain adequate nutrition.
5. Provide emotional support for acceptance of altered body image.
6. Provide information about disease process/prognosis and treatment.

DISCHARGE GOALS

1. Ventilation/oxygenation adequate for individual needs.
2. Communicating effectively.
3. Complications prevented/minimized.
4. Beginning to cope with change in body image.
5. Disease process/prognosis and therapeutic regimen understood.
6. Plan in place to meet needs after discharge.

NURSING DIAGNOSIS: Airway Clearance, ineffective/Aspiration, risk for

May be related to

Partial/total removal of the glottis, altering ability to breathe, cough, and swallow

Temporary or permanent change to neck breathing (dependent on patent stoma)

Edema formation (surgical manipulation and lymphatic accumulation)

Copious and thick secretions

Possibly evidenced by (Airway Clearance)

Dyspnea/difficulty breathing

Changes in rate/depth of respiration; use of accessory respiratory muscles

Abnormal breath sounds

Cyanosis

DESIRED OUTCOMES/EVALUATION CRITERIA—PATIENT WILL:

Respiratory Status: Ventilation (NOC)

Maintain patent airway with breath sounds clear/clearing.

Expectorate/clear secretions and be free of aspiration.

Demonstrate behaviors to improve/maintain airway clearance within level of ability/situation.

ACTIONS/INTERVENTIONS	RATIONALE

Airway Management (NIC)

Independent

Monitor respiratory rate/depth; note ease of breathing. Auscultate breath sounds. Investigate restlessness, dyspnea, development of cyanosis.	Changes in respirations, use of accessory muscles, and/or presence of rhonchi/wheezes suggests retention of secretions. Airway obstruction (even partial) can lead to ineffective breathing patterns and impaired gas exchange, resulting in complications, e.g., pneumonia, respiratory arrest.
Elevate head of bed 30–45 degrees.	Facilitates drainage of secretions, work of breathing, and lung expansion. *Note:* Increase elevation when oral intake is provided.
Encourage swallowing, if patient is able.	Prevents pooling of oral secretions, reducing risk of aspiration. *Note:* Swallowing is impaired when the epiglottis is removed and/or significant postoperative edema and pain are present.
Encourage effective coughing and deep breathing.	Mobilizes secretions to clear airway and helps prevent respiratory complications.
Suction laryngectomy/tracheostomy tube, oral and nasal cavities. Note amount, color, and consistency of secretions.	Prevents secretions from obstructing airway, especially when swallowing ability is impaired and patient cannot blow nose. Changes in character of secretions may indicate developing problems (e.g., dehydration, infection) and need for further evaluation/treatment.
Demonstrate and encourage patient to begin self-suction procedures as soon as possible. Educate patient in "clean" techniques.	Assists patient to exercise some control in postoperative care and prevention of complications. Reduces anxiety associated with difficulty in breathing or inability to handle secretions when alone.
Maintain proper position of laryngectomy/tracheostomy tube. Check/adjust ties as indicated.	As edema develops/subsides, tube can be displaced, compromising airway. Ties should be snug but not constrictive to surrounding tissue or major blood vessels.
Observe tissue surrounding tube for bleeding. Change patient's position to check for pooling of blood behind neck or on posterior dressings.	Small amount of oozing may be present; however, continued bleeding or sudden eruption of uncontrolled hemorrhage presents a sudden and real possibility of airway obstruction/suffocation.
Change tube/inner cannula as indicated. Instruct patient in cleaning procedures.	Prevents accumulation of secretions and thick mucous plugs from obstructing airway. *Note:* This is a common cause of respiratory distress/arrest in later postoperative period.

Collaborative

Provide supplemental humidification, e.g., compressed air/oxygen mist collar, increased fluid intake.	Normal physiological (nose/nasal passages) means of filtering/humidifying air are bypassed. Supplemental humidity decreases mucous crusting and facilitates coughing/suctioning of secretions through stoma.
Resume oral intake with caution. (Refer to ND: Nutrition: altered, less than body requirements, p. 182.)	Changes in muscle mass/strength and nerve innervation increase likelihood of aspiration.
Monitor serial ABGs/pulse oximetry; chest x-ray.	Pooling of secretions/presence of atelectasis may lead to pneumonia, requiring more aggressive therapeutic measures.

NURSING DIAGNOSIS: Communication, impaired verbal

May be related to

Anatomic deficit (removal of vocal cords)

Physical barrier (tracheostomy tube)

Required voice rest

Possibly evidenced by

Inability to speak

Change in vocal characteristics

DESIRED OUTCOMES/EVALUATION CRITERIA—PATIENT WILL:

Communication Ability (NOC)

Communicate needs in an effective manner.

Identify/plan for appropriate alternate speech methods after healing.

ACTIONS/INTERVENTIONS	RATIONALE
Communication Enhancement: Speech Deficit (NIC)	
Independent	
Review preoperative instructions/discussion of why speech and breathing are altered, using anatomic drawings or models to assist in explanations.	Reinforces teaching at a time when fear of surviving surgery is past.
Determine whether patient has other communication impairments, e.g., hearing, vision, literacy.	Presence of other problems influences plan for alternate communication.
Provide immediate and continual means to summon nurse, e.g., call light/bell. Let the patient know the summons will be answered immediately. Stop by to check on patient periodically without being summoned. Post notice at central answering system/nursing station that patient is unable to speak.	Patient needs assurance that nurse is vigilant and will respond to summons. Trust and self-esteem are fostered when the nurse cares enough to come at times other than when called by the patient.
Prearrange signals for obtaining immediate help.	May decrease patient's anxiety about inability to speak.
Provide alternate means of communication appropriate to patient need, e.g., pad and pencil, magic slate, alphabet/picture board, sign language. Consider placement of IV.	Permits patient to "express" needs/concerns. *Note:* IV positioned in hand/wrist may limit ability to write or sign.
Allow sufficient time for communication.	Loss of speech and stress of alternate communication can cause frustration and block expression, especially when caregivers seem "too busy" or preoccupied.
Provide nonverbal communication, e.g., touching and physical presence. Anticipate needs.	Communicates concern and meets need for contact with others. Touch is believed to generate complex biochemical events, with possible release of endorphins contributing to reduction of anxiety.
Encourage ongoing communication with "outside world," e.g., newspapers, television, radio, calendar, clock.	Maintains contact with "normal lifestyle" and continued communication through other avenues.

ACTIONS/INTERVENTIONS

Independent

Refer to loss of speech as temporary after a partial laryngectomy and/or depending on availability of voice prosthetics/vocal chord transplant.

Caution patient not to use voice until physician gives permission.

Arrange for meeting with other persons who have experienced this procedure, as appropriate.

Collaborative

Consult with appropriate health team members/therapists/rehabilitation agency (e.g., speech pathologist, social services, laryngectomee clubs) for hospital-based rehabilitation and community resources, such as Lost Chord/NewVoice Club, International Association of Laryngectomees, American Cancer Society.

RATIONALE

Provides encouragement and hope for future with the thought that alternate means of communication and speech are available and possible.

Promotes healing of vocal cord and limits potential for permanent cord dysfunction.

Provides role model, enhancing motivation for problem solving and learning new ways to communicate.

Ability to use alternate voice and speech methods (e.g., electrolarynx, tracheosophageal puncture [TEP], voice prosthesis, esophageal speech) varies greatly, depending on extent of surgical procedures, patient's age, emotional state, and motivation to return to an active life. Rehabilitation time may be lengthy and require a number of agencies/resources to facilitate/support learning process. *Note:* Some patients may be candidates for vocal chord transplant at a future date.

NURSING DIAGNOSIS: Skin/Tissue Integrity, impaired

May be related to
Surgical removal of tissues/grafting
Radiation or chemotherapeutic agents
Altered circulation/reduced blood supply
Compromised nutritional status
Edema formation
Pooling/continuous drainage of secretions (oral, lymph, or chyle)

Possibly evidenced by
Disruption of skin/tissue surface
Destruction of skin/tissue layers

DESIRED OUTCOMES/EVALUATION CRITERIA—PATIENT WILL:

Wound Healing: Primary Intention (NOC)

Display timely wound healing without complications.
Demonstrate techniques to promote healing/prevent complications.

ACTIONS/INTERVENTIONS

Skin Surveillance (NIC)

Independent

Assess skin color/temperature and capillary refill in operative and skin graft areas.

RATIONALE

Skin should be pink or similar to color of surrounding skin. Skin graft flaps should be pink and warm and should blanch (when gentle finger pressure is applied), with return to color within seconds. Cyanosis and slow refill may indicate venous congestion, which can lead to tissue ischemia/necrosis.

ACTIONS/INTERVENTIONS

Independent

Keep head of bed elevated 30–45 degrees. Monitor facial edema (usually peaks by third to fifth postoperative day).

Protect skin flaps and suture lines from tension or pressure. Provide pillows/rolls and instruct patient to support head/neck during activity.

Monitor bloody drainage from surgical sites, suture lines, drains. Measure drainage from hemovac device (if used).

Note/report any milky-appearing drainage.

Wound Care (NIC)

Change dressings as indicated.

Cleanse incisions with sterile saline and peroxide (mixed 1:1) after dressings have been removed.

Monitor donor site if graft performed; check dressings as indicated.

Cleanse thoroughly around stoma and neck tubes (if in place), avoiding soap or alcohol. Show patient how to do self-stoma/tube care with clean water and peroxide, using cloth, not tissue or cotton.

Monitor all sites for signs of wound infection, e.g., unusual redness; increasing edema, pain, exudates; and temperature elevation.

Collaborative

Cover donor sites with petroleum gauze or moisture-impermeable dressing

Administer oral, IV, and topical antibiotics as indicated.

RATIONALE

Minimizes postoperative tissue congestion and edema related to excision of lymph channels.

Pressure from tubings and tracheostomy tapes or tension on suture lines can alter circulation/cause tissue injury.

Bloody drainage usually declines steadily after first 24 hr. Steady oozing or frank bleeding indicates problem requiring medical attention.

Milky drainage may indicate thoracic lymph duct leakage (can result in depletion of body fluids and electrolytes). Such a leak may heal spontaneously or require surgical closure.

Damp dressings increase risk of tissue damage/infection. *Note:* Pressure dressings are not used over skin flaps, because blood supply is easily compromised.

Prevents crust formation, which can trap purulent drainage, destroy skin edges, and increase size of wound. Peroxide is not used full strength because it may cauterize wound edges and impair healing.

Donor site may be adjacent to operative site or a distant site (e.g., thigh). Pressure dressings are usually removed within 24–48 hr and wound is left open to air to promote healing.

Keeping area cleansed promotes healing and comfort. Soap and other drying agents can lead to stomal irritation and possible inflammation. Materials other than cloth may leave fibers in stoma that can irritate or be inhaled into lungs.

Impedes healing, which may already be slow because of changes induced by cancer, cancer therapies, and/or malnutrition.

Nonadherent dressing covers exposed sensory nerve endings and protects site from contamination.

Prevents/controls infection.

NURSING DIAGNOSIS: Oral Mucous Membrane, altered

May be related to

Dehydration/absence of oral intake; decreased saliva production secondary to radiation (common) or surgical procedure (rare)

Poor/inadequate oral hygiene

Pathologic condition (oral cancer); mechanical trauma (oral surgery)

Difficulty swallowing and pooling of secretions/drooling

Nutritional deficits

ACTIONS/INTERVENTIONS	RATIONALE
Oral Health Restoration (NIC)	
Independent	
Inspect oral cavity and note changes in:	
Saliva;	Damage to salivary glands may decrease production of saliva, resulting in dry mouth. Pooling and drooling of saliva may occur because of compromised swallowing capability or pain in throat and mouth.
Tongue;	Surgery may have included partial resection of tongue, soft palate, and pharynx. This patient has decreased sensation and movement of tongue, with difficulty swallowing and increased risk of aspiration of secretions, as well as potential for hemorrhage.
Lips;	Surgical removal of part of lip may result in uncontrollable drooling.
Teeth and gums;	Teeth may not be intact (surgical) or may be in poor condition because of malnutrition, chemical therapies, and neglect. Gums may also be surgically altered or inflamed because of poor hygiene, long history of smoking/chewing tobacco, or chemical therapies.
Mucous membranes.	May be excessively dry, ulcerated, erythematous, edematous.
Suction oral cavity gently/frequently. Have patient perform self-suctioning when possible or use gauze wick to drain secretions.	Saliva contains digestive enzymes that may be erosive to exposed tissues. Because drooling may be constant, patient can promote own comfort and enhance oral hygiene.
Show patient how to brush inside of mouth, palate, tongue, and teeth frequently.	Reduces bacteria and risk of infection; promotes tissue healing and comfort.
Apply lubrication to lips; provide oral irrigations as indicated.	Counteracts drying effects of therapeutic measures; negates erosive nature of secretions.
Avoid alcohol-based mouthwashes. Use normal saline or mixture of salt water and baking soda for rinsing. Suggest use of artificial saliva preparations (e.g., pilocarpine hydrochloride [Salagen]) if mucous membranes are dry.	Although drooling is often present and abundant immediately postoperatively, surgical damage to the parotid glands can drastically reduce saliva production on a permanent basis. Cholinergic effect of medication can increase saliva production.

> **NURSING DIAGNOSIS: Pain [acute]**
>
> **May be related to**
> Surgical incisions
> Tissue swelling
> Presence of nasogastric/orogastric feeding tube
>
> **Possibly evidenced by**
> Discomfort in surgical areas/pain with swallowing
> Facial mask of pain
> Distraction behaviors, restlessness; guarding behavior
>
> **DESIRED OUTCOMES/EVALUATION CRITERIA—PATIENT WILL:**
>
> **Pain Level (NOC)**
>
> Report/indicate pain is relieved/controlled.
> Demonstrate relief of pain/discomfort by reduced tension and relaxed manner, sleeping/resting appropriately.

ACTIONS/INTERVENTIONS	RATIONALE
Pain Management (NIC)	
Independent	
Support head and neck with pillows. Show patient how to support neck during activity.	Muscle weakness results from muscle and nerve resection in the structures of the neck and/or shoulders. Lack of support aggravates discomfort and may result in injury to suture areas.
Provide comfort measures (e.g., back rub, position change) and diversional activities (e.g., television, visiting, reading).	Promotes relaxation and helps the patient refocus attention on something besides self/discomfort. May reduce analgesic dosage needs/frequency.
Encourage patient to expectorate saliva or to suction mouth gently if unable to swallow.	Swallowing causes muscle activity that may be painful because of edema/strain on suture lines.
Investigate changes in characteristics of pain. Check mouth, throat suture lines for fresh trauma.	May reflect developing complications requiring further evaluation/intervention. Tissues are inflamed and congested and may be easily traumatized by suction catheter, or feeding tube.
Note nonverbal indicators and autonomic responses to pain. Evaluate effects of analgesics.	Aids in determining presence of pain, need for/effectiveness of medication.
Medicate before activity/treatments as indicated.	May enhance cooperation and participation in therapeutic regimen.
Schedule care activities to balance with adequate periods of sleep/rest.	Prevents fatigue/exhaustion and may enhance coping with stress/discomfort.
Recommend use of stress management behaviors, e.g., relaxation techniques, guided imagery.	Promotes sense of well-being, may reduce analgesic needs and enhance healing.
Collaborative	
Provide oral irrigations, anesthetic sprays, and gargles. Instruct patient in self-irrigations.	Improves comfort, promotes healing, and reduces halitosis. *Note:* Commercial mouthwashes containing alcohol or phenol are to be avoided because of their drying effect.

ACTIONS/INTERVENTIONS

Collaborative

Administer analgesics, e.g., codeine, acetylsalicylic acid (ASA), and propoxyphene (Darvon), as indicated.

RATIONALE

Degree of pain is related to extent and psychological impact of surgery and general body condition. Studies appear to support the idea that many patients experience more pain before than after head and neck surgery.

NURSING DIAGNOSIS: Nutrition: altered, less than body requirements

May be related to

Temporary or permanent alteration in mode of food intake

Altered feedback mechanisms of desire to eat, taste, and smell because of surgical/structural changes, radiation, or chemotherapy

Possibly evidenced by

Inadequate food intake, perceived inability to ingest food

Aversion to eating, lack of interest in food, reported altered taste sensation

Weight loss

Weakness of muscles required for swallowing or mastication

DESIRED OUTCOMES/EVALUATION CRITERIA—PATIENT WILL:

Nutritional Status (NOC)

Indicate understanding of importance of nutrition to healing process and general well-being.

Make dietary choices to meet nutrient needs within individual situation.

Demonstrate progressive weight gain toward goal, with normalization of laboratory values and timely healing of tissues/incisions.

ACTIONS/INTERVENTIONS

Nutrition Therapy (NIC)

Independent

Auscultate bowel sounds.

Maintain feeding tube, e.g., check for tube placement, flush with warm water as indicated.

Monitor intake and weigh as indicated. Show patient how to monitor and record weight on a scheduled basis.

Instruct patient/SO in self-feeding techniques, e.g., bulb syringe, bag and funnel method, and blending soft foods if the patient is to go home with a feeding tube. Make sure patient and SO are able to perform this procedure before discharge and that appropriate food and equipment are available at home.

RATIONALE

Feedings are usually begun after bowel sounds are restored postoperatively. *Note:* In more aggressive therapy, tube feeding may be started earlier if gastric residuals are closely monitored.

Tube is inserted during surgery and usually sutured in place. Initially the tube may be attached to suction to reduce nausea and/or vomiting. Flushing aids in maintaining patency of tube.

Provides information regarding nutritional needs and effectiveness of therapy.

Helps promote nutritional success and preserves dignity in the adult who is now forced to depend on others for very basic needs in the social setting of meals.

ACTIONS/INTERVENTIONS	RATIONALE
Independent	
Begin with small feedings and advance as tolerated. Note signs of gastric fullness, regurgitation, diarrhea.	Content of feeding may result in GI intolerance, requiring change in rate or type of formula.
Provide supplemental water by feeding tube or orally if patient can swallow.	Keeps patient hydrated to offset insensible losses and drainage from surgical areas. Meets free water needs associated with enteral feeding.
Encourage patient when relearning swallowing, e.g., maintain quiet environment, have suction equipment on standby, and demonstrate appropriate breathing techniques.	Helps patient to deal with the frustration and safety concerns involved with swallowing. Provides reassurance that measures are available to prevent/limit aspiration.
Resume oral feedings when feasible. Stay with patient during meals the first few days.	Oral feedings can usually resume after suture lines are healed (8–10 days) unless further reconstruction is required or patient is going home with feeding tube. The patient may experience pain or difficulty with chewing and swallowing initially and may require suctioning during meals, in addition to support and encouragement.
Develop and encourage a pleasant environment for meals.	Promotes socialization and maximizes patient comfort when eating difficulties cause embarrassment.
Help patient/SO develop nutritionally balanced home meal plans.	Promotes understanding of individual needs and significance of nutrition in healing and recovery process.
Collaborative	
Consult with dietitian/nutritional support team as indicated. Incorporate and reinforce dietitian's teaching.	Useful in identifying individual nutritional needs to promote healing and tissue regeneration. Discharge teaching and follow-up by the dietitian may be needed to evaluate patient needs for diet/equipment modifications and meal planning in the home setting.
Provide nutritionally balanced diet (e.g., semisolid/soft foods) or tube feedings (e.g., blended soft food or commercial preparations) as indicated.	Variations can be made to add or limit certain factors, such as fat and sugar, or to provide a food that the patient prefers.
Monitor laboratory studies, e.g., blood urea nitrogen (BUN), glucose, liver function, prealbumin/protein, electrolytes.	Indicators of utilization of nutrients and organ function.

NURSING DIAGNOSIS: Body Image disturbance/Role Performance, altered

May be related to

Loss of voice

Changes in anatomic contour of face and neck (disfigurement and/or severe functional impairment)

Presence of chronic illness

Possibly evidenced by

Report of fear of rejection by/reaction of others; change in social involvement; discomfort in social situations

Negative feelings about body change

Refusal to verify actual change or preoccupation with change/loss, not looking at self in mirror

Change in self/others' perception of role

Anxiety, depression, lack of eye contact

Failure of family members to adapt to change or deal with experience constructively

DESIRED OUTCOMES/EVALUATION CRITERIA—PATIENT WILL:

Body Image (NOC)

Identify feelings and methods for coping with negative perception of self.
Demonstrate initial adaptation to body changes as evidenced by participating in self-care activities and positive interactions with others.

Role Performance (NOC)

Communicate with SO about changes in role that have occurred.
Begin to develop plans for altered lifestyle.
Participate in team efforts toward rehabilitation.

ACTIONS/INTERVENTIONS

Coping Enhancement (NIC)

Independent

Discuss meaning of loss/change with patient, identifying perceptions of current situation/future expectations.

Note nonverbal body language, negative attitudes/self-talk. Assess for self-destructive/suicidal behavior.

Note emotional reactions, e.g., grieving, depression, anger. Allow patient to progress at own rate.

Maintain calm, reassuring manner. Acknowledge and accept expression of feelings of grief, hostility.

Allow but do not participate in patient's use of denial, e.g., when patient is reluctant to participate in self-care (e.g., suctioning stoma). Provide care in a non-judgmental manner.

Set limits on maladaptive behaviors, assisting patient to identify positive behaviors that will aid recovery.

Encourage SO to treat patient normally and not as an invalid.

Alert staff that facial expressions and other nonverbal behaviors need to convey acceptance and not revulsion.

Encourage identification of anticipated personal/work conflicts that may arise.

Recognize behavior indicative of overconcern with future lifestyle/relationship functioning.

Encourage patient to deal with situation in small steps.

RATIONALE

Aids in identifying/defining the problem(s) to focus attention and interventions constructively.

May indicate depression/despair, need for further assessment/more intense intervention.

The patient may experience immediate depression after surgery or react with shock and denial. Acceptance of changes cannot be forced, and the grieving process needs time for resolution.

May help allay patient's fears of dying, suffocation, inability to communicate, or mutilation. Patient and SO need to feel supported and know that all feelings are appropriate for the type of experience they are going through.

Denial may be the most helpful defense for the patient in the beginning, permitting the individual to begin to deal slowly with difficult adjustment.

Acting out can result in lowered self-esteem and impede adjustment to new self-image.

Distortions of body image may be unconsciously reinforced.

The patient is very sensitive to nonverbal communication and may make negative assumptions about others' body language.

Expressions of concern bring problems into the open where they can be examined/dealt with.

Ruminating about anticipated losses/reactions of others is nonproductive and is a block to problem solving.

May feel overwhelmed/have difficulty coping with larger picture but can manage one piece at a time.

ACTIONS/INTERVENTIONS

Independent

Provide positive reinforcement for efforts/progress made.

Encourage patient/SO to communicate feelings to each other.

Collaborative

Refer patient/SO to supportive resources, e.g., psychotherapy, social worker, family counseling, pastoral care.

RATIONALE

Encourages patient to feel a sense of movement toward recovery.

All those involved may have difficulty in this area (because of the loss of voice function and/or disfigurement) but need to understand that they may gain courage and help from one another.

A multifaceted approach is required to assist patient toward rehabilitation and wellness. Families need assistance in understanding the processes that the patient is going through and to help them with their own emotions. The goal is to enable them to guard against the tendency to withdraw from/isolate the patient from social contact.

NURSING DIAGNOSIS: Knowledge Deficit [Learning Need] regarding prognosis, treatment, self care, and discharge needs

May be related to
Lack of information/recall
Misinterpretation of information
Poor assimilation of material presented; lack of interest in learning

Possibly evidenced by
Indications of concern/request for information
Inaccurate follow-through of instructions
Inappropriate or exaggerated behaviors, e.g., hostile, agitated, apathetic

DESIRED OUTCOMES/EVALUATION CRITERIA—PATIENT WILL:

Knowledge: Disease Process (NOC)

Indicate basic understanding of disease process, surgical intervention, prognosis.
Identify symptoms requiring medical evaluation/intervention.

Knowledge: Treatment Regimen (NOC)

Verbalize understanding of treatment regimen and rationale for actions.
Demonstrate ability to provide safe care.
Use resources (e.g., rehabilitation team members) appropriately.
Develop plan for/schedule follow-up appointments.

ACTIONS/INTERVENTIONS

Learning Facilitation (NIC)

Independent

Ascertain amount of preoperative preparation and retention of information. Assess level of anxiety related to diagnosis and surgery.

RATIONALE

Information can provide clues to patient's postoperative reactions. Anxiety may have interfered with understanding of information given before surgery.

ACTIONS/INTERVENTIONS	RATIONALE

Independent

Provide/repeat explanations at patient's level of acceptance.

Overwhelming stressors are present and may be coupled with limited knowledge.

Provide written directions for the patient/SO to read and have available for future reference.

Reinforces proper information and may be used as a home reference.

Teaching: Disease Process (NIC)

Discuss inaccuracies in perception of disease process and therapies with patient and SO.

Misconceptions are inevitable, but failure to explore and correct them can result in the patient's failing to progress toward health.

Educate the patient and SO about basic information regarding stoma, e.g.:

Shower with stoma collar; shampoo by leaning forward; no swimming or water sports;

Although the extra humidity provided by a shower can be beneficial by loosening secretions and enhancing expectoration, excessive water entering airway/stoma is detrimental.

Cover stoma with foam or fiber filter (e.g., cotton or silk);

Prevents dust and particles from being inhaled.

Cover stoma when coughing or sneezing.

Normal airways are bypassed, and mucus will exit from stoma.

Reinforce necessity of not smoking.

Necessary to preserve lung function. *Note:* Patient may need extra support and encouragement to understand that respiratory function and quality of life can be improved by cessation of smoking.

Discuss inability to smell and taste as before surgery.

Safety issues surround the inability to smell (e.g., smoke from fire or odor from infection in stoma). Also the loss of taste affects the desire to resume eating when patient is otherwise able to do so.

Discuss importance of reporting to caregiver/physician immediately such symptoms as stoma narrowing, presence of "lump" in throat, dysphagia, or bleeding.

May be signs of tracheal stenosis, recurrent cancer, or carotid erosion.

Develop a means of emergency communication at home.

Permits patient to summon assistance when needed.

Recommend wearing medical-alert identification tag/bracelet. Encourage family members to become certified in cardiopulmonary resuscitation (CPR) if they are interested/able to do so.

Provides for appropriate care if the patient becomes unconscious or suffers a pulmonary arrest.

Give careful attention to the provision of needed rehabilitative measures, e.g., temporary/permanent prosthesis, dental care, speech therapy, surgical reconstruction; vocational, sexual/marital counseling; financial assistance.

These services can contribute to patient's well-being and have a positive effect on patient's quality of life.

Identify homecare needs and available resources.

Provides support for transition from hospital setting.

POTENTIAL CONSIDERATIONS following acute hospitalization (dependent on patient's age, physical condition/presence of complications, personal resources, and life responsibilities)

Aspiration, risk for—presence of tracheostomy, tube feedings, impaired swallowing, decreased muscle mass/strength (status after neck surgery).

Communication, impaired verbal—anatomic presence of tracheostomy.

Infection, risk for—broken skin/traumatized tissue, stasis of secretions, suppressed inflammatory response, chronic disease, malnutrition.

Nutrition: altered, less than body requirements—temporary alteration in mode of food intake, altered feedback mechanisms relative to senses of taste and smell.

Self-Care deficit—decreased strength/endurance, presence of pain, depression.

VENTILATORY ASSISTANCE (MECHANICAL)

Many patients on ventilators are now being transferred from the intensive care unit (ICU) to medical-surgical units with problems including (1) neuromuscular deficits, such as quadriplegia with phrenic nerve injury or high C-spine injuries, Guillain-Barré syndrome, and amyotrophic lateral sclerosis (ALS); (2) COPD with respiratory muscle atrophy and malnutrition (inability to wean); and (3) restrictive conditions of chest or lungs, such as kyphoscoliosis and interstitial fibrosis.

The expectation is that the majority of patients will be weaned before discharge. That is the focus of this plan of care. However, some patients are either unsuccessful at weaning or are not candidates for weaning. For those patients, portions of this plan of care would need to be modified for the discharge care setting, that is, a long-term facility or home.

Types of Ventilators

Volume-cycled ventilators are the primary choice for long-term ventilation of patients whose permanent changes in lung compliance and resistance require increased pressure to provide adequate ventilation (e.g., COPD).

Pressure-cycled ventilators are desirable for patients with relatively normal lung compliance who cannot initiate or sustain respiration because of muscular/phrenic nerve involvement (e.g., quadriplegics).

CARE SETTING

Patients on ventilators may be cared for in any setting; however, weaning is usually attempted/accomplished in the acute, subacute, or rehabilitation setting.

RELATED CONCERNS

Cardiac surgery: postoperative care, page 102
Chronic obstructive pulmonary disease (COPD), and Asthma, page 126
Hemothorax/Pneumothorax, page 165
Spinal cord injury (acute rehabilitative phase), page 295
Total nutritional support: parenteral/enteral feeding, page 508
Psychosocial aspects of care, page 809

Patient Assessment Database

Gathered data depend on the underlying pathophysiology and/or reason for ventilatory support. Refer to the appropriate plan of care.

Discharge plan considerations:	**DRG projected mean length of inpatient stay: 9.5 days (or more)** If ventilator-dependent, may require changes in physical layout of home, acquisition of equipment/supplies, provision of a backup power source, instruction of SO/caregivers, provision for continuation of plan of care, assistance with transportation, and coordination of resources/support systems

Refer to section at end of plan for postdischarge considerations.

DIAGNOSTIC STUDIES

Pulmonary function studies: Determine the ability of the lungs to exchange oxygen and carbon dioxide and include but are not limited to the following:

  Vital capacity (VC): Is reduced in restrictive chest or lung conditions; is normal or increased in COPD; normal to decreased in neuromuscular diseases (Guillain-Barré syndrome); and decreased in conditions limiting thoracic movement (kyphoscoliosis).

  Forced vital capacity (FVC): Measured by spirometry, is reduced in restrictive conditions and in asthma, and is normal to reduced in COPD.

  Tidal volume (V_T): May be decreased in both restrictive and obstructive processes.

  Negative inspiratory force (NIF): Can be substituted for vital capacity to help determine whether the patient can initiate a breath.

  Minute ventilation (V_E): Measures volume of air inhaled and exhaled in 1 minute of normal breathing. This reflects muscle endurance and is a major determinant of work of breathing.

Inspiratory pressure (Pi$_{max}$): Measures respiratory muscle strength (less than -20 cm H_2O is considered insufficient for weaning).

Forced expiratory volume (FEV): Usually decreased in COPD.

Flow-volume (F-V) loops: Abnormal loops are indicative of large and small airway obstructive disease and restrictive diseases, when far advanced.

ABGs: Assesses status of oxygenation, ventilation, and acid-base balance.

Chest x-ray: Monitors resolution/progression of underlying condition (e.g., adult respiratory distress syndrome [ARDS]) or complications (e.g., atelectasis, pneumonia).

Nutritional assessment: Done to identify nutritional and electrolyte imbalances that might interfere with successful weaning.

NURSING PRIORITIES

1. Promote adequate ventilation and oxygenation.
2. Prevent complications.
3. Provide emotional support for patient/SO.
4. Provide information about disease process/prognosis and treatment needs.

DISCHARGE GOALS

1. Respiratory function maximized/adequate to meet individual needs.
2. Complications prevented/minimized.
3. Effective means of communication established.
4. Disease process/prognosis and therapeutic regimen understood (including home ventilatory support if indicated).
5. Plan in place to meet needs after discharge.

NURSING DIAGNOSIS: Breathing Pattern, ineffective/Spontaneous Ventilation, inability to sustain

May be related to
Respiratory center depression
Respiratory muscle weakness/paralysis
Noncompliant lung tissue (decreased lung expansion)
Alteration of patient's usual O_2/CO_2 ratio

Possibly evidenced by
Changes in rate and depth of respirations
Dyspnea/increased work of breathing, use of accessory muscles
Reduced VC/total lung volume
Tachypnea/bradypnea or cessation of respirations when off the ventilator
Cyanosis
Decreased Po_2 and Sao_2; increased Pco_2
Increased restlessness, apprehension, and metabolic rate

DESIRED OUTCOMES/EVALUATION CRITERIA—PATIENT WILL:

Respiratory Status: Ventilation (NOC)

Re-establish/maintain effective respiratory pattern via ventilator with absence of retractions/use of accessory muscles, cyanosis, or other signs of hypoxia; ABGs/oxygen saturation within acceptable range.
Participate in efforts to wean (as appropriate) within individual ability.

CAREGIVER WILL:
Demonstrate behaviors necessary to maintain patient's respiratory function.

| Mechanical Ventilation (NIC) |

Independent

Investigate etiology of respiratory failure.

Understanding the underlying cause of the patient's particular ventilatory problem is essential to the care of the patient, e.g., decisions about future patient capabilities/ventilation needs and most appropriate type of ventilatory support.

Observe overall breathing pattern. Note respiratory rate, distinguishing between spontaneous respirations and ventilator breaths.

Patients on ventilators can experience hyperventilation/hypoventilation, or dyspnea/"air hunger," and attempt to correct deficiency by overbreathing.

Auscultate chest periodically, noting presence/absence and equality of breath sounds, adventitious breath sounds, and symmetry of chest movement.

Provides information regarding airflow through the tracheobronchial tree and the presence/absence of fluid, mucus obstruction. *Note:* Frequent crackles or rhonchi that do not clear with coughing/suctioning may indicate developing complications (atelectasis, pneumonia, acute bronchospasm, pulmonary edema). Changes in chest symmetry may indicate improper placement of the ET, development of barotrauma.

Count patient's respirations for one full minute and compare to desired/ventilator set rate.

Respirations vary, depending on problem requiring ventilatory assistance, e.g., patient may be totally ventilator-dependent, or be able to take breath(s) on own between ventilator-delivered breaths. Rapid patient respirations can produce respiratory alkalosis and/or prevent desired volume from being delivered by ventilator. Slow patient respirations/hypoventilation increases $PaCO_2$ levels and may cause acidosis.

Verify that patient's respirations are in phase with the ventilator.

Adjustments may be required in tidal volume, respiratory rate, and/or dead space of the ventilator, or the patient may need sedation to synchronize respirations and reduce work of breathing/energy expenditure.

Elevate head of bed or place in orthopedic chair if possible.

Elevation of the patient's head or getting out of bed while still on the ventilator is both physically and psychologically beneficial.

Place in prone position when tolerated.

Prone position relaxes abdominal muscles, improving diaphragmatic excursion, increasing PaO_2.

Inflate tracheal/ET cuff properly using minimal leak/occlusive technique. Check cuff inflation every 4–8 hr and whenever cuff is deflated/reinflated.

The cuff must be properly inflated to ensure adequate ventilation/delivery of desired tidal volume. *Note:* In long-term patients, the cuff may be deflated most of the time or a noncuffed tracheostomy tube used.

Check tubing for obstruction, e.g., kinking or accumulation of water. Drain tubing as indicated, avoiding draining toward the patient or back into the reservoir.

Kinks in tubing prevent adequate volume delivery and increase airway pressure. Water prevents proper gas distribution and predisposes to bacterial growth.

ACTIONS/INTERVENTIONS

RATIONALE

Independent

Check ventilator alarms for proper functioning. Do not turn off alarms, even for suctioning. Remove from ventilator and ventilate manually if source of ventilator alarm cannot be quickly identified and rectified. Ascertain that alarms can be heard in the nurses' station.

Ventilators have a series of visual and audible alarms, e.g., oxygen, low/high pressure, inspiratory : expiratory (I:E) ratio. Turning off/failure to reset alarms places patient at risk for unobserved ventilator failure or respiratory distress/arrest.

Keep resuscitation bag at bedside and ventilate manually whenever indicated.

Provides/restores adequate ventilation when patient or equipment problems require the patient to be temporarily removed from the ventilator.

Assist patient in "taking control" of breathing if weaning is attempted/ventilatory support is interrupted during procedure/activity.

Coaching the patient to take slower, deeper breaths, practice abdominal/pursed-lip breathing, assume position of comfort, and use relaxation techniques can be helpful in maximizing respiratory function.

Collaborative

Assess ventilator settings routinely and readjust as indicated:

Controls/settings are adjusted according to patient's primary disease and results of diagnostic testing to maintain parameters within appropriate limits.

Note operating mode of ventilation, i.e., assist control (ACV), intermittent mandatory (IMV), pressure support (PSV), inverse ratio (IRV);

The patient's respiratory requirements, presence or absence of an underlying disease process, and the extent to which the patient can participate in ventilatory effort determine parameters of each setting. PSV, a relatively new mode, has shown advantages for patients who are on long-term ventilation because it allows the patient to strengthen pulmonary musculature without compromising oxygenation and ventilation during the weaning process. Recent research suggests that intermittent trials of unassisted breathing work faster (for weaning) than methods involving partial ventilatory support.

Observe oxygen concentration percentage (FIO_2); verify that oxygen line is in proper outlet/tank; monitor in-line oxygen analyzer or perform periodic oxygen analysis;

FIO_2 is adjusted (21%–100%) to maintain an acceptable oxygen percentage and saturation for patient's condition. Because machine dials are not always accurate, an oxygen analyzer may be used to ascertain whether patient is receiving the desired concentration of oxygen.

Assess V_E (respiratory rate and V_T);

Respiratory rate of 10–15/min may be appropriate except for patient with COPD and CO_2 retention. In these patients, V_E should be adjusted to achieve patient's baseline $PaCO_2$, not necessarily a "normal" $PaCO_2$.

Assess V_T (10–15 ml/kg). Verify proper function of spirometer, bellows, or computer readout of delivered volume. Note alterations from desired volume delivery;

Monitors amount of air inspired and expired. Changes may indicate alteration in lung compliance or leakage through machine/around tube cuff (if used). *Note:* Smaller tidal volume may be required in patients with decreased lung compliance (e.g., ARDS).

ACTIONS/INTERVENTIONS	RATIONALE
Collaborative	
Note airway pressure;	Airway pressure should remain relatively constant. Increased pressure alarm reading reflects (1) increased airway resistance as may occur with bronchospasm; (2) retained secretions; and/or (3) decreased lung compliance as may occur with obstruction of the ET, development of atelectasis, ARDS, pulmonary edema, worsening COPD, or pneumothorax. Low airway pressure alarms may be triggered by pathophysiological conditions causing hypoventilation, e.g., disconnection from ventilator, low ET cuff pressure, ET displaced above the vocal cords, patient "overbreathing" or out of phase with the ventilator.
Monitor I:E ratio;	Expiratory phase is usually twice the length of the inspiratory rate, but may be longer to compensate for air-trapping to improve gas exchange in the COPD patient.
Check sigh rate intervals (usually $1\frac{1}{2}$ to 2 times V_T);	Sighing promotes maximal ventilation of alveoli to prevent/reduce atelectasis, and enhances movement of secretions.
Note inspired humidity and temperature. Use heat moisture exchanger (HME) as indicated.	Usual warming and humidifying function of nasopharynx is bypassed with intubation. Dehydration can dry up normal pulmonary fluids, cause secretions to thicken, and increase risk of infection. Temperature should be maintained at about body temperature to reduce risk of damage to cilia and hyperthermia reactions. The introduction of a heated wire circuit to the traditional system significantly reduces the problem of "rainout" (condensation in the tubing).

NURSING DIAGNOSIS: Airway Clearance, ineffective

May be related to
Foreign body (artificial airway) in the trachea
Inability to cough/ineffective cough

Possibly evidenced by
Changes in rate or depth of respiration
Cyanosis
Abnormal breath sounds
Anxiety/restlessness

DESIRED OUTCOMES/EVALUATION CRITERIA—PATIENT WILL:

Respiratory Status: Ventilation (NOC)

Maintain patent airway with breath sounds clear.
Be free of aspiration.

CAREGIVER WILL:
Identify potential complications and initiate appropriate actions.

ACTIONS/INTERVENTIONS	RATIONALE

Artificial Airway Management (NIC)

Independent

Assess airway patency.

Obstruction may be caused by accumulation of secretions, mucus plugs, hemorrhage, bronchospasm, and/or problems with the position of tracheostomy/ET.

Evaluate chest movement and auscultate for bilateral breath sounds.

Symmetrical chest movement with breath sounds throughout lung fields indicates proper tube placement/unobstructed airflow. Lower airway obstruction (e.g., pneumonia/atelectasis) produces changes in breath sounds such as rhonchi, wheezing.

Monitor ET placement. Note lip line marking and compare with desired placement. Secure tube carefully with tape or tube holder. Obtain assistance when retaping or repositioning tube.

The ET may slip into the right main-stem bronchus, thereby obstructing airflow to the left lung and putting patient at risk for a tension pneumothorax.

Note excessive coughing, increased dyspnea, high-pressure alarm sounding on ventilator, visible secretions in endotracheal/tracheostomy tube, increased rhonchi.

The intubated patient often has an ineffective cough reflex, or the patient may have neuromuscular or neurosensory impairment, altering ability to cough. These patients are dependent on alternate means such as suctioning to remove secretions.

Suction as needed when patient is coughing or experiencing respiratory distress, limiting duration of suction to 15 sec or less. Choose appropriate suction catheter. Hyperventilate before and after each catheter pass, using 100% oxygen if appropriate (using vent rather than ambu bag, which has an increased risk of barotrauma). Suction continuously or intermittently during withdrawal.

Suctioning should not be routine, and duration should be limited to reduce hazard of hypoxia. Suction catheter diameter should be less than 50% of the internal diameter of the endotracheal/tracheostomy tube for prevention of hypoxia. Hyperoxygenation with ventilator sigh on 100% oxygen may be desired to reduce atelectasis and to reduce accidental hypoxia. *Note:* Instilling normal saline (NS) is no longer recommended, because research reveals that the fluid pools at the distal end of the endotracheal/tracheal tube; this impairs oxygenation and increases bronchospasm and the risk of infection.

Use inline catheter suction when available.

Reduces risk of infection for healthcare workers and helps maintain oxygen saturation and PEEP, when used.

Instruct patient in coughing techniques during suctioning, e.g., splinting, timing of breathing, and "quad cough" as indicated.

Enhances effectiveness of cough effort and secretion clearing.

Reposition/turn periodically.

Promotes drainage of secretions and ventilation to all lung segments, reducing risk of atelectasis.

Encourage/provide fluids within individual capability.

Helps liquefy secretions, enhancing expectoration.

Collaborative

Provide chest physiotherapy as indicated, e.g., postural drainage, percussion.

Promotes ventilation of all lung segments and aids drainage of secretions.

Administer IV and aerosol bronchodilators as indicated, e.g., aminophylline, metaproterenol sulfate (Alupent); isoetharine hydrochloride (Bronkosol).

Promotes ventilation and removal of secretions by relaxation of smooth muscle/bronchospasm.

Assist with fiberoptic broncoscopy, if indicated.

May be performed to remove secretions/mucus plugs.

ACTIONS/INTERVENTIONS	RATIONALE
Communication Enhancement: Speech Deficit (NIC)	
Independent	
Assess patient's ability to communicate by alternate means.	Reasons for long-term ventilatory support are various; patient may be alert and be adept at writing (e.g., chronic COPD with inability to be weaned) or may be lethargic, comatose, or paralyzed. Method of communicating with patient is therefore highly individualized.
Establish means of communication, e.g., maintain eye contact; ask yes/no questions; provide magic slate, paper/pencil, picture/alphabet board; use sign language as appropriate; validate meaning of attempted communications.	Eye contact assures patient of interest in communicating; if patient is able to move head, blink eyes, or is comfortable with simple gestures, a great deal can be done with yes/no questions. Pointing to letter boards or writing is often tiring to patients, who can then become frustrated with the effort needed to attempt conversations. Use of picture boards that express a concept or routine needs may simplify communication. Family members/other caregivers may be able to assist/interpret needs.
Consider form of communication when placing IV.	IV positioned in hand/wrist may limit ability to write or sign.
Place call light/bell within reach, making certain patient is alert and physically capable of using it. Answer call light/bell immediately. Anticipate needs. Tell patient that nurse is immediately available should assistance be required.	Ventilator-dependent patient may be better able to relax, feel safe (not abandoned), and breathe with the ventilator knowing that nurse is vigilant and needs will be met.
Place note at central call station informing staff that patient is unable to speak.	Alerts all staff members to respond to the patient at the bedside instead of over the intercom.
Encourage family/SO to talk with patient, providing information about family and daily happenings.	SO may feel self-conscious in one-sided conversation, but knowledge that he or she is assisting patient to regain/maintain contact with reality and enabling patient to feel part of family unit can reduce feelings of awkwardness.
Collaborative	
Evaluate need for/appropriateness of talking tracheostomy tube.	Patients with adequate cognitive/muscular skills may have the ability to manipulate talking tracheostomy tube.

NURSING DIAGNOSIS: Fear/Anxiety [specify level]

May be related to
Situational crises; threat to self-concept
Threat of death/dependency on mechanical support
Change in health/socioeconomic status/role functioning
Interpersonal transmission/contagion

Possibly evidenced by
Increased muscle/facial tension
Insomnia; restlessness
Hypervigilance
Feelings of inadequacy
Fearfulness, uncertainty, apprehension
Focus on self/negative self-talk
Expressed concern regarding changes in life events

DESIRED OUTCOMES/EVALUATION CRITERIA—PATIENT WILL:

Fear Control/Anxiety Control (NOC)

Verbalize/communicate awareness of feelings and healthy ways to deal with them.
Demonstrate problem-solving skills/behaviors to cope with current situation.
Report anxiety/fear is reduced to manageable level.
Appear relaxed and sleeping/resting appropriately.

ACTIONS/INTERVENTIONS	RATIONALE
Coping Enhancement (NIC)	
Independent	
Identify patient's perception of threat represented by situation.	Defines scope of individual problem and influences choice of interventions.
Observe/monitor physical responses, e.g., restlessness, changes in vital signs, repetitive movements. Note congruency of verbal/nonverbal communication.	Useful in evaluating extent/degree of concerns, especially when compared with "verbal" comments.
Encourage patient/SO to acknowledge and express fears.	Provides opportunity for dealing with concerns, clarifies reality of fears, and reduces anxiety to a more manageable level.
Acknowledge the anxiety and fear of the situation. Avoid meaningless reassurance that everything will be all right.	Validates the reality of the situation without minimizing the emotional impact. Provides opportunity for the patient/SO to accept and begin to deal with what has happened, reducing anxiety.
Identify/review with patient/SO the safety precautions being taken, e.g., backup power and oxygen supplies, emergency equipment at hand for suction. Discuss/review the meanings of alarm system.	Provides reassurance to help allay unnecessary anxiety, reduce concerns of the unknown, and preplan for response in emergency situation.
Note reactions of SO. Provide opportunity for discussion of personal feelings/concerns and future expectations.	Family members have individual responses to what is happening, and their anxiety may be communicated to the patient, intensifying these emotions.
Identify previous coping strengths of patient/SO and current areas of control/ability.	Focuses attention on own capabilities, increasing sense of control.

ACTIONS/INTERVENTIONS	RATIONALE

Independent

Demonstrate/encourage use of relaxation techniques, e.g., focused breathing, guided imagery, progressive relaxation.

Provides active management of situation to reduce feelings of helplessness.

Provide/encourage sedentary diversional activities within individual capabilities, e.g., handicrafts, writing, television.

Although handicapped by dependence on ventilator, activities that are normal/desired by the individual should be encouraged to enhance quality of life.

Collaborative

Refer to support groups and therapy as needed.

May be necessary to provide additional assistance if patient/SO are not managing anxiety or when patient is "identified with the machine."

NURSING DIAGNOSIS: Oral Mucous Membrane, risk for altered

Risk factors may include
Inability to swallow oral fluids
Presence of tube in mouth
Lack of or decreased salivation
Ineffective oral hygiene

Possibly evidenced by
[Not applicable; presence of signs and symptoms establishes an *actual* diagnosis]

DESIRED OUTCOMES/EVALUATION CRITERIA—PATIENT WILL:

Tissue Integrity: Skin and Mucous Membrane (NOC)

Report/demonstrate a decrease in symptoms.

CAREGIVER WILL:
Identify specific interventions to promote healthy oral mucosa as appropriate.

ACTIONS/INTERVENTIONS	RATIONALE

Oral Health Maintenance (NIC)

Independent

Routinely inspect oral cavity, teeth, gums for sores, lesions, bleeding.

Early identification of problems provides opportunity for appropriate intervention/preventive measures.

Administer mouth care routinely and as needed, especially in the patient with an oral intubation tube, e.g., cleanse mouth with water, saline, or preferred mouthwash. Brush teeth with soft toothbrush, Waterpik, or moistened swab.

Prevents drying/ulceration of mucous membrane and reduces medium for bacterial growth. Promotes comfort.

Change position of ET/airway on a regular/prn schedule as appropriate.

Reduces risk of lip and oral mucous membrane ulceration.

Apply lip balm; administer oral lubricant solution.

Maintains moisture, prevents drying.

NURSING DIAGNOSIS: Nutrition: altered, less than body requirements

May be related to

Altered ability to ingest and properly digest food

Increased metabolic demands

Possibly evidenced by

Weight loss; poor muscle tone

Aversion to eating; reported altered taste sensation

Sore, inflamed buccal cavity

Absence of/hyperactive bowel sounds

DESIRED OUTCOMES/EVALUATION CRITERIA—PATIENT WILL:

Nutritional Status (NOC)

Indicate understanding of individual dietary needs.

Demonstrate progressive weight gain toward goal with normalization of laboratory values.

ACTIONS/INTERVENTIONS	RATIONALE
Nutrition Therapy (NIC)	
Independent	
Evaluate ability to eat.	Patients with a tracheostomy tube may be able to eat, but patients with ETs must be tube fed or parenterally nourished.
Observe/monitor for generalized muscle wasting, loss of subcutaneous fat.	These symptoms are indicative of depletion of muscle energy and can reduce respiratory muscle function.
Weigh as indicated.	Significant and recent weight loss (7%–10% body weight) and poor nutritional intake provide clues regarding catabolism, muscle glycogen stores, and ventilatory drive sensitivity.
Document oral intake if/when resumed. Offer foods that patient enjoys.	Appetite is usually poor and intake of essential nutrients may be reduced. Offering favorite foods can enhance oral intake.
Provide small frequent feedings of soft/easily digested foods if able to swallow.	Prevents excessive fatigue, enhances intake, and reduces risk of gastric distress.
Encourage/administer fluid intake of at least 2500 mL/day within cardiac tolerance.	Prevents dehydration that can be exacerbated by increased insensible losses (e.g., ventilator/intubation) and reduces risk of constipation.
Assess GI function: Presence/quality of bowel sounds; note changes in abdominal girth, nausea/vomiting. Observe/document changes in bowel movements, e.g., diarrhea/constipation. Test all stools for occult blood.	A functioning GI system is essential for the proper utilization of enteral feedings. Mechanically ventilated patients are at risk of developing abdominal distension (trapped air or ileus) and gastric bleeding (stress ulcers).
Collaborative	
Adjust diet to meet respiratory needs as indicated.	High carbohydrates, protein, and calories may be desired/needed during ventilation to improve respiratory muscle function. Carbohydrates may be reduced and fat somewhat increased just before weaning attempts to prevent excessive CO_2 production and reduced respiratory drive.

197

ACTIONS/INTERVENTIONS

Collaborative

Administer tube feeding/hyperalimentation as needed. (Refer to CP: Total Nutritional Support: Parenteral/Enteral Feeding, p. 508)

Monitor laboratory studies as indicated, e.g., prealbumin, serum transferrin, BUN/creatinine (Cr), glucose.

RATIONALE

Provides adequate nutrients to meet individual needs when oral intake is insufficient/not appropriate.

Provides information about adequacy of nutritional support/need for change.

NURSING DIAGNOSIS: Infection, risk for

Risk factors may include
Inadequate primary defenses (traumatized lung tissue, decreased ciliary action, stasis of body fluids)
Inadequate secondary defenses (immunosuppression)
Chronic disease, malnutrition
Invasive procedure (intubation)

Possibly evidenced by
[Not applicable; presence of signs and symptoms establishes an *actual* diagnosis.]

DESIRED OUTCOMES/EVALUATION CRITERIA—PATIENT/CAREGIVER WILL:

Knowledge: Infection Control (NOC)

Indicate understanding of individual risk factors.
Identify interventions to prevent/reduce risk of infection.
Demonstrate techniques to promote safe environment.

ACTIONS/INTERVENTIONS

Infection Protection (NIC)

Independent

Note risk factors for occurrence of infection.

Observe color/odor/characteristics of sputum. Note drainage around tracheostomy tube.

Reduce nosocomial risk factors via proper handwashing by all caregivers, maintaining sterile suction techniques, reducing the number of times the ventilator tubes are open, and providing clean nebulizer/tubing changes.

RATIONALE

Intubation, prolonged mechanical ventilation, general debilitation, malnutrition, age, and invasive procedures are factors that potentiate a patient's risk of acquiring infection and prolonging recovery. Awareness of individual risk factors provides opportunity to limit effects.

Yellow/green, purulent odorous sputum is indicative of infection; thick, tenacious sputum suggests dehydration.

These factors may be the simplest but are the most important keys to prevention of hospital-acquired infection. *Note:* Centers for Disease Control and Prevention (CDC) guidelines recommend changing tubing no more often than every 48 hr. Recent research indicates that less frequent tubing changes (every 5–7 days) may even be acceptable.

ACTIONS/INTERVENTIONS	RATIONALE
Independent	
Encourage deep breathing, coughing, and frequent position changes.	Maximizes lung expansion and mobilization of secretions to prevent/reduce atelectasis and accumulation of sticky, thick secretions.
Auscultate breath sounds.	Presence of rhonchi/wheezes suggests retained secretions requiring expectoration/suctioning.
Monitor/screen visitors. Avoid contact with persons with URI.	Individual is already compromised and is at increased risk for development of infections.
Instruct patient/SO in proper secretion disposal, e.g., tissues, soiled tracheostomy dressings.	Reduces transmission of fluid-borne organisms.
Provide respiratory isolation when indicated.	Depending on specific diagnosis, the patient may require protection from others or must prevent transmission of infection to others (e.g., tuberculosis).
Maintain adequate hydration and nutrition. Encourage fluids to 2500 mL/day within cardiac tolerance.	Helps improve general resistance to disease and reduces risk of infection from static secretions.
Measure pH of gastric secretions, and monitor use of antacid medications as indicated.	Maintaining acid level of stomach around 7.2 may help reduce risk of nosocomial infection and stress ulcers.
Encourage self-care/activities to limit of tolerance. Assist with graded exercise program.	Improves general well-being and muscle strength and may stimulate immune system recovery.
Collaborative	
Obtain sputum cultures as indicated.	May be needed to identify pathogens and appropriate antimicrobials.
Administer antimicrobials as indicated.	If infection does occur, one or more agents may be used, depending on identified pathogen(s).

NURSING DIAGNOSIS: Ventilatory Weaning Response (DVWR), risk for dysfunctional

Risk factors may include
Sleep disturbance
Limited/insufficient energy stores
Pain or discomfort
Adverse environment (e.g., inadequate monitoring/support)
Patient-perceived inability to wean; decreased motivation
History of extended weaning

Possibly evidenced by
[Not applicable; presence of signs and symptoms establishes an *actual* diagnosis]

DESIRED OUTCOMES/EVALUATION CRITERIA—PATIENT WILL:

Respiratory Status: Ventilation (NOC)

Actively participate in the weaning process.
Re-establish independent respiration with ABGs within acceptable range and free of signs of respiratory failure.
Demonstrate increased tolerance for activity/participate in self-care within level of ability.

Mechanical Ventilatory Weaning (NIC)

Independent

Assess physical factors involved in weaning, e.g.:

Stable heart rate/rhythm, BP, and clear breath sounds;

The heart has to work harder to meet increased energy needs associated with weaning. Physician may defer weaning if tachycardia, pulmonary crackles, and hypertension are present.

Fever;

Increase of 1°F (0.6°C) in body temperature raises metabolic rate and oxygen demands by 7%.

Nutritional status and muscle strength;

Weaning is hard work. Patient not only must be able to withstand the stress of weaning but also must have the stamina to breathe spontaneously for extended periods.

Respiratory volumes.

Predictors of readiness to wean include (NIP) ≤ -20, (PEP) $\leq +20$, (STV) >5 mL/kg, (MC) $>10–15$ mL/kg, (MV) ≤ 10 L/min.

Determine psychological readiness.

Weaning provokes anxiety for the patient regarding concerns about ability to breathe on own and long-term need of ventilator.

Explain weaning techniques, e.g., T-piece, spontaneous intermittent maximal ventilation (SIMV), continuous positive airway pressure (CPAP), or NIPPV. Discuss individual plan and expectations.

Assists patient to prepare for weaning process, helps limit fear of unknown, promotes cooperation, and enhances likelihood of a successful outcome. *Note:* Pressure support ventilation unloads respiratory muscles, allowing patient to "set" rate and volume and decelerating flow pattern because breath can be shaped to simulate a more normal respiratory pattern with higher gas flow on inspiration then tapering off. This increases patient comfort and is especially beneficial for patients at high risk for DVWR.

Provide undisturbed rest/sleep periods. Avoid stressful procedures/situations or nonessential activities.

Maximizes energy for weaning process; limits fatigue and oxygen consumption. *Note:* It takes approximately 12–14 hr of respiratory rest to rejuvenate tired respiratory muscles. For patients on assist/control, raising the rate to 20 breaths/min can also provide respiratory rest.

Evaluate/document patient's progress. Note restlessness; changes in BP, heart rate, respiratory rate; use of accessory muscles; discoordinated breathing with ventilator; increased concentration on breathing (mild dysfunction); patient's concerns about possible machine malfunction; inability to cooperate/respond to coaching; color changes.

Indicators that patient may require slower weaning/opportunity to stabilize or may need to stop program. *Note:* Moving from pressure/volume (e.g., assist/control) ventilator to T-piece may precipitate a "flash" form of heart failure requiring prompt intervention.

Recognize/provide encouragement for patient's efforts.

Positive feedback provides reassurance and support for continuation of weaning process.

Monitor response to activity.

Excessive oxygen consumption/demand increases the possibility of failure.

Collaborative

Consult with dietitian, nutritional support team for adjustments in composition of diet.

Reduction of carbohydrates/fats may be required to prevent excessive production of CO_2, which could alter respiratory drive.

ACTIONS/INTERVENTIONS

Collaborative

Monitor CBC, serum albumin and prealbumin, transferrin, total iron-binding capacity, and electrolytes (especially potassium, calcium, and phosphorus).

Review chest x-ray and ABGs.

RATIONALE

Verifies that nutrition is adequate to meet energy requirements for weaning.

Chest x-rays should show clear lungs or marked improvement in pulmonary congestion or infiltrates. ABGs should document satisfactory oxygenation on an FIO_2 of 40% or less.

NURSING DIAGNOSIS: Knowledge Deficit [Learning Need] regarding condition, prognosis and therapy, self care and discharge needs

May be related to
Lack of exposure/recall
Misinterpretation of information; unfamiliarity with information resources
Stress of situational crisis

Possibly evidenced by
Questions about care, request for information
Reluctance to learn new skills
Inaccurate follow-through of instructions
Development of preventable complications

DESIRED OUTCOMES/EVALUATION CRITERIA—PATIENT/ SO/CAREGIVER WILL:

Health Seeking Behavior (NOC)

Participate in learning process.
Exhibit increased interest, shown by verbal/nonverbal cues.
Assume responsibility for own learning and begin to look for information and to ask questions.

Knowledge: Treatment Regimen (NOC)

Indicate understanding of mechanical ventilation therapy.
Demonstrate behaviors/new skills to meet individual needs/prevent complications.

ACTIONS/INTERVENTIONS

Learning Facilitation (NIC)

Independent

Determine ability and willingness to learn.

Schedule teaching sessions for quiet, nonstressful times when all participants are well rested.

Arrange information in logical sequence, progressing from simple to more complex material at learners' pace.

RATIONALE

Physical condition may preclude patient involvement in care before and after discharge. SO/caregiver may feel inadequate and afraid of machinery and have reservations about ability to learn or deal with overall situation.

Enhances learners ability to focus on and absorb content provided.

Allows learner to build on information learned in previous sessions, is less threatening/overwhelming.

ACTIONS/INTERVENTIONS	RATIONALE

Independent

Provide material in multiple formats, (e.g., books/pamphlets, audiovisuals, hands-on demonstrations) and take-home instruction sheets as appropriate.

Uses multiple senses to stimulate learning/retention of information. Provides resources for review following discharge.

Knowledge: Disease Process (NIC)

Discuss specific condition requiring ventilatory support, what measures are being tried for weaning, short- and long-term goals of treatment.

Provides knowledge base to aid patient/SO in making informed decisions. Weaning efforts may continue for several weeks (extended period of time). Dependence is evidenced by repeatedly increased Pco_2 and/or decline in Pao_2 during weaning attempts, presence of dypsnea, anxiety, tachycardia, perspiration, cyanosis.

Encourage patient/SO to evaluate impact of ventilatory dependence on their lifestyle and what changes they are willing or unwilling to make. Problem-solve solutions to issues raised.

Quality of life must be resolved by the ventilator-dependent patient and caregivers who need to understand that home ventilatory support is a 24-hour job that affects everyone.

Promote participation in self-care/diversional activities and socialization as appropriate.

Refocuses attention toward more normal life activities, increases endurance, and helps prevent depersonalization.

Review issues of general well-being: role of nutrition; assistance with feeding/meal preparation; graded exercise/specific restrictions; rest periods alternated with activity.

Enhances recuperation and ensures that individual needs will be met.

Recommend that SO/caregivers learn CPR.

Provides sense of security about ability to handle emergency situations that might arise until help can be obtained.

Schedule team conference. Establish in-hospital training for caregivers if patient is to be discharged home on ventilator.

Team approach is needed to coordinate patient's care and teaching program to meet individual needs.

Instruct caregiver and patient in handwashing techniques, use of sterile technique for suctioning, tracheostomy/stoma care, and chest physiotherapy.

Reduces risk of infection and promotes optimal respiratory function.

Provide both demonstration and "hands-on" sessions, as well as written material, about specific type of ventilator to be used, function, and care of equipment.

Enhances familiarity, reducing anxiety and promoting confidence in implementation of new tasks/skills.

Discuss what/when to report to the healthcare provider, e.g., signs of respiratory distress, infection.

Helps to reduce general anxiety while promoting timely/appropriate evaluation and intervention to prevent complications.

Ascertain that all needed equipment is in place and that safety concerns have been addressed, e.g., alternate power source (generator, batteries); backup equipment; patient call/alarm system.

Predischarge preparations can ease the transfer process. Planning for potential problems increases sense of security for patient/SO.

Contact community/hospital-based services.

Suppliers of home equipment, physical therapy, care providers, emergency power provider, social services; financial assistance, aid in procuring equipment/personnel, and facilitating transition to home.

Refer to vocational/occupational therapist.

Some ventilator-dependent patients are able to resume vocations, either while on the ventilator or during the day (while ventilator-dependent at night).

POTENTIAL CONSIDERATIONS following acute hospitalization (dependent on patient's age, physical condition/presence of complications, personal resources, and life responsibilities)

If patient is discharged on ventilator, the patient's needs/concerns remain the same as noted in this plan of care, in addition to:

Self-Care deficit—decreased strength/endurance, inability to perform ADLs, depression, restrictions imposed by therapeutic intervention.

Family Processes, altered—situational crisis.

Caregiver Role Strain, risk for—severity of illness of care receiver, discharge of family member with significant home care needs, presence of situational stressors (economic vulnerability, changes in roles/responsibilities), duration of caregiving required, inexperience in caregiving.

PULMONARY TUBERCULOSIS (TB)

Pulmonary tuberculosis (TB) is on the rise, although many still believe it to be a problem of the past. Although most frequently seen as a pulmonary disease, TB may be extrapulmonary and affect organs and tissues other than the lungs. In the United States, incidence is higher among the homeless, drug-addicted, and impoverished populations, as well as among immigrants from or visitors to countries in which TB is endemic. In addition, persons at highest risk include those who may have been exposed to the bacillus in the past and those who are debilitated or have lowered immunity because of chronic conditions such as AIDS, cancer, advanced age, and malnutrition. When the immune system weakens, dormant TB organisms can reactivate and multiply. When this latent infection develops into active disease, it is known as reactivation TB, which is often drug resistant.

Multidrug-resistant tuberculosis (MDR-TB) can progress from diagnosis to death in as little as 4–6 weeks. MDR tuberculosis can be primary or secondary. Primary is caused by person-to-person transmission of a drug-resistant organism; secondary is usually the result of nonadherence to therapy or inappropriate treatment.

CARE SETTING

Most patients are treated as outpatients, but may be hospitalized for diagnostic evaluation/initiation of therapy, adverse drug reactions, or severe illness/debilitation.

RELATED CONCERNS

Extended care, page 850
Pneumonia: microbial, page 140
Psychosocial aspects of care, page 809

Patient Assessment Database

Data depend on stage of disease and degree of involvement.

ACTIVITY/REST

May report:	Generalized weakness and fatigue
	Shortness of breath with exertion
	Difficulty sleeping with evening or night fever, chills, and/or sweats
	Nightmares
May exhibit:	Tachycardia, tachypnea/dyspnea on exertion
	Muscle wasting, pain, and stiffness (advanced stages)

EGO INTEGRITY

May report:	Recent/long-standing stress factors
	Financial concerns, poverty
	Feelings of helplessness/hopelessness
	Cultural/ethnic populations: Native-American or recent immigrants from Central America, Southeast Asia, Indian subcontinent
May exhibit:	Denial (especially during early stages)
	Anxiety, apprehension, irritability

FOOD/FLUID

May report:	Loss of appetite
	Indigestion
	Weight loss
May exhibit:	Poor skin turgor, dry/flaky skin
	Muscle wasting/loss of subcutaneous fat

PAIN/DISCOMFORT

May report:	Chest pain aggravated by recurrent cough
May exhibit:	Guarding of affected area
	Distraction behaviors, restlessness

RESPIRATION

May report: Cough, productive or nonproductive
Shortness of breath
History of tuberculosis/exposure to infected individual

May exhibit: Increased respiratory rate (extensive disease or fibrosis of the lung parenchyma and pleura)
Asymmetry in respiratory excursion (pleural effusion)
Dullness to percussion and decreased fremitus (pleural fluid or pleural thickening)
Breath sounds diminished/absent bilaterally or unilaterally (pleural effusion/pneumothorax); tubular breath sounds and/or whispered pectoriloquies over large lesions; crackles may be noted over apex of lungs during quick inspiration after a short cough (posttussive crackles)
Sputum characteristics green/purulent, yellowish mucoid, or blood-tinged
Tracheal deviation (bronchogenic spread)
Inattention, marked irritability, change in mentation (advanced stages)

SAFETY

May report: Presence of immunosuppressed conditions, e.g., AIDS, cancer
Positive HIV test/HIV infection
Visit to/immigration from or close contact with persons in countries with high prevalence of TB (e.g., Philippines, Vietnam, Cambodia, Laos, Puerto Rico, Haiti, Russia, Mexico)

May exhibit: Low-grade fever or acute febrile illness

SOCIAL INTERACTION

May report: Feelings of isolation/rejection because of communicable disease
Change in usual patterns of responsibility/change in physical capacity to resume role

TEACHING/LEARNING

May report: Familial history of TB
General debilitation/poor health status
Use/abuse of substances such as IV drugs, alcohol, cocaine, and crack
Failure to improve/reactivation of TB
Nonparticipation in therapy

Discharge plan considerations: **DRG projected mean length of inpatient stay: 6.3–8.3 days.**
May require assistance with/alteration in drug therapy and temporary assistance in self-care and homemaker/maintenance tasks

Refer to section at end of plan for postdischarge considerations.

DIAGNOSTIC STUDIES

Sputum culture: Positive for *Mycobacterium tuberculosis* in the active stage of the disease.

Ziehl-Neelsen (acid-fast stain applied to a smear of body fluid): Positive for acid-fast bacilli (AFB).

Skin tests (purified protein derivative [PPD] or old tuberculin [OT] administered by intradermal injection [Mantoux]; or multipuncture technique [Tine]): A positive reaction (area of induration 10 mm or greater, occurring 48–72 hr after interdermal injection of the antigen) indicates past infection and the presence of antibodies but is not necessarily indicative of active disease. Factors associated with a decreased response to tuberculin include underlying viral or bacterial infection, malnutrition, lymphadenopathy, overwhelming TB infection, insufficient antigen injection, and conscious or unconscious bias. A significant reaction in a patient who is clinically ill means that active TB cannot be dismissed as a diagnostic possibility. A significant reaction in healthy persons usually signifies dormant TB or an infection caused by a different mycobacterium.

Enzyme-linked immunosorbent assay (ELISA)/Western blot: May reveal presence of HIV.

Chest x-ray: May show small infiltrations of early lesions in the upper-lung field, calcium deposits of healed primary lesions, or fluid of an effusion. Changes indicating more advanced TB may include cavitation, fibrous areas.

Histologic or tissue cultures (including gastric washings; urine and CSF; skin biopsy): Positive for *Mycobacterium tuberculosis* and may indicate extrapulmonary involvement.

Needle biopsy of lung tissue: Positive for granulomas of TB; presence of giant cells indicating necrosis.

Electrolytes: May be abnormal depending on the location and severity of infection; e.g., hyponatremia caused by abnormal water retention may be found in extensive chronic pulmonary TB.

ABGs: May be abnormal depending on location, severity, and residual damage to the lungs.

Pulmonary function studies: Decreased vital capacity, increased dead space, increased ratio of residual air to total lung capacity, and decreased oxygen saturation are secondary to parenchymal infiltration/fibrosis, loss of lung tissue, and pleural disease (extensive chronic pulmonary TB).

NURSING PRIORITIES

1. Achieve/maintain adequate ventilation/oxygenation.
2. Prevent spread of infection.
3. Support behaviors/tasks to maintain health.
4. Promote effective coping strategies.
5. Provide information about disease process/prognosis and treatment needs.

DISCHARGE GOALS

1. Respiratory function adequate to meet individual need.
2. Complications prevented.
3. Lifestyle/behavior changes adopted to prevent spread of infection.
4. Disease process/prognosis and therapeutic regimen understood.
5. Plan in place to meet needs after discharge.

NURSING DIAGNOSIS: Infection, risk for [spread/reactivation]

Risk factors may include

Inadequate primary defenses, decreased ciliary action/stasis of secretions

Tissue destruction/extension of infection

Lowered resistance/suppressed inflammatory process

Malnutrition

Environmental exposure

Insufficient knowledge to avoid exposure to pathogens

Possibly evidenced by

[Not applicable; presence of signs and symptoms establishes an *actual* diagnosis]

DESIRED OUTCOMES/EVALUATION CRITERIA—PATIENT WILL:

Risk Control (NOC)

Identify interventions to prevent/reduce risk of spread of infection.

Demonstrate techniques/initiate lifestyle changes to promote safe environment.

ACTIONS/INTERVENTIONS	RATIONALE
Infection Control (NIC)	
Independent	
Review pathology of disease (active/inactive phases; dissemination of infection through bronchi to adjacent tissues or via bloodstream/lymphatic system) and potential spread of infection via airborne droplet during coughing, sneezing, spitting, talking, laughing, singing.	Helps patient realize/accept necessity of adhering to medication regimen to prevent reactivation/complication. Understanding of how the disease is passed and awareness of transmission possibilities help patient/SO take steps to prevent infection of others.
Identify others at risk, e.g., household members, close associates/friends.	Those exposed may require a course of drug therapy to prevent spread/development of infection.

ACTIONS/INTERVENTIONS	RATIONALE

Independent

Instruct patient to cough/sneeze and expectorate into tissue and to refrain from spitting. Review proper disposal of tissue and good handwashing techniques. Encourage return demonstration.

Behaviors necessary to prevent spread of infection.

Review necessity of infection control measures, e.g., temporary respiratory isolation.

May help patient understand need for protecting others while acknowledging patient's sense of isolation and social stigma associated with communicable diseases. *Note:* AFB can pass through standard masks; therefore, particulate respirators are required.

Monitor temperature as indicated.

Febrile reactions are indicators of continuing presence of infection.

Identify individual risk factors for reactivation of tuberculosis, e.g., lowered resistance associated with alcoholism, malnutrition/intestinal bypass surgery; use of immunosuppression drugs/corticosteroids; presence of diabetes mellitus, cancer; postpartum.

Knowledge about these factors helps patient alter lifestyle and avoid/reduce incidence of exacerbation.

Stress importance of uninterrupted drug therapy. Evaluate patient's potential for cooperation.

Contagious period may last only 2–3 days after initiation of chemotherapy, but in presence of cavitation or moderately advanced disease, risk of spread of infection may continue up to 3 months. Compliance with multidrug regimens for prolonged periods is difficult, so directly observed therapy (DOT) should be considered.

Review importance of follow-up and periodic reculturing of sputum for the duration of therapy.

Aids in monitoring the effects and effectiveness of medications and the patient's response to therapy.

Encourage selection/ingestion of well-balanced meals. Provide frequent small "snacks'" in place of large meals as appropriate.

Presence of anorexia and/or preexisting malnutrition lowers resistance to infectious process and impairs healing. Small snacks may enhance overall intake.

Collaborative

Administer anti-infective agents as indicated, e.g.:

Primary drugs: isoniazid (INH), ethambutol (Myambutol), rifampin (RMP/Rifadin), rifampin with isoniazid (Rifamate), pyrazinamide (PZA/Aldinamide), streptomycin (Strycin);

Initial therapy of uncomplicated pulmonary disease usually includes four drugs, e.g., four primary drugs or combination of primary and secondary drugs. INH is usually drug of choice for infected patient and those at risk for developing TB. Short-course chemotherapy, including INH, rifampin (for 6 mo), PZA and ethambutol or streptomycin, is given for at least 2 mo (or until sensitivities are known or until serial sputums are clear) followed by three more months of therapy with INH. Ethambutol should be given if central nervous system (CNS) or disseminated disease is present or if INH resistance is suspected. Extended therapy (up to 24 mo) is indicated for reactivation cases, extrapulmonary reactivated TB, or in the presence of other medical problems, such as diabetes mellitus or silicosis. Prophylaxis with INH for 12 mo should be considered in HIV-positive patients with positive PPD test.

ACTIONS/INTERVENTIONS	RATIONALE

Collaborative

ACTIONS/INTERVENTIONS	RATIONALE
Ethionamide (Trecator-SC), para-amino salicylic (PAS), cycloserine (Seromycin).	These second-line drugs may be required when infection is resistant to or intolerant of primary drugs. *Note:* MDR-TB requires minimum of 18–24 mo therapy with at least three drugs in the regimen known to be effective against the specific infective organism and which the patient has not previously taken. Treatment is often extended to 24 mo in patients with severe symptoms/HIV infection.
Monitor laboratory studies, e.g., sputum smear results;	Patient who has three consecutive negative sputum smears (takes 3–5 mo), is adhering to drug regimen, and is asymptomatic will be classified a nontransmitter.
AST/ALT.	Adverse effects of drug therapy include hepatitis.
Notify local health department.	Helpful in identifying contacts to reduce spread of infection and is required by law in many states. Treatment course is long and usually handled in the community with public health nurse monitoring.

NURSING DIAGNOSIS: Airway Clearance, ineffective

May be related to
Thick, viscous, or bloody secretions
Fatigue, poor cough effort
Tracheal/pharyngeal edema

Possibly evidenced by
Abnormal respiratory rate, rhythm, depth
Abnormal breath sounds (rhonchi, wheezes), stridor
Dyspnea

DESIRED OUTCOMES/EVALUATION CRITERIA—PATIENT WILL:

Respiratory Status: Ventilation (NOC)

Maintain patent airway.
Expectorate secretions without assistance.
Demonstrate behaviors to improve/maintain airway clearance.
Participate in treatment regimen, within the level of ability/situation.
Identify potential complications and initiate appropriate actions.

ACTIONS/INTERVENTIONS	RATIONALE

Airway Management (NIC)

Independent

ACTIONS/INTERVENTIONS	RATIONALE
Assess respiratory function, e.g., breath sounds, rate, rhythm and depth, and use of accessory muscles.	Diminished breath sounds may reflect atelectasis. Rhonchi, wheezes indicate accumulation of secretions/inability to clear airways that may lead to use of accessory muscles and increased work of breathing.

ACTIONS/INTERVENTIONS	RATIONALE

Independent

Note ability to expectorate mucus/cough effectively; document character, amount of sputum, presence of hemoptysis.

Expectoration may be difficult when secretions are very thick as a result of infection and/or inadequate hydration. Blood-tinged or frankly bloody sputum results from tissue breakdown (cavitation) in the lungs or from bronchial ulceration and may require further evaluation/intervention.

Place patient in semi- or high-Fowler's position. Assist patient with coughing and deep-breathing exercises.

Positioning helps maximize lung expansion and decreases respiratory effort. Maximal ventilation may open atelectic areas and promote movement of secretions into larger airways for expectoration.

Clear secretions from mouth and trachea; suction as necessary.

Prevents obstruction/aspiration. Suctioning may be necessary if patient is unable to expectorate secretions.

Maintain fluid intake of at least 2500 mL/day unless contraindicated.

High fluid intake helps thin secretions, making them easier to expectorate.

Collaborative

Humidify inspired air/oxygen.

Prevents drying of mucous membranes; helps thin secretions.

Administer medications as indicated:

Mucolytic agents, e.g., acetylcysteine (Mucomyst);

Reduces the thickness and stickiness of pulmonary secretions to facilitate clearance.

Bronchodilators, e.g., oxtriphylline (Choledyl), theophylline (Theo-Dur);

Increases lumen size of the tracheobronchial tree, thus decreasing resistance to airflow and improving oxygen delivery.

Corticosteroids (prednisone).

May be useful in presence of extensive involvement with profound hypoxemia and when inflammatory response is life-threatening.

Be prepared for/assist with emergency intubation.

Intubation may be necessary in rare cases of bronchogenic TB accompanied by laryngeal edema or acute pulmonary bleeding.

NURSING DIAGNOSIS: Gas Exchange, risk for impaired

Risk factors may include
Decrease in effective lung surface, atelectasis
Destruction of alveolar-capillary membrane
Thick, viscous secretions
Bronchial edema

Possibly evidenced by
[Not applicable; presence of signs and symptoms establishes an *actual* diagnosis]

DESIRED OUTCOMES/EVALUATION CRITERIA—PATIENT WILL:

Respiratory Status: Gas Exchange (NOC)

Report absence of/decreased dyspnea.
Demonstrate improved ventilation and adequate oxygenation of tissues by ABGs within acceptable ranges.
Be free of symptoms of respiratory distress.

Airway Management (NIC)

Independent

Assess for dyspnea, tachypnea, abnormal/diminished breath sounds, increased respiratory effort, limited chest wall expansion, and fatigue.

Pulmonary TB can cause a wide range of effects in the lungs, ranging from a small patch of bronchopneumonia to diffuse intense inflammation, caseous necrosis, pleural effusion, and extensive fibrosis. Respiratory effects can range from mild dyspnea to profound respiratory distress.

Evaluate change in level of mentation. Note cyanosis and/or change in skin color, including mucous membranes and nailbeds.

Accumulation of secretions/airway compromise can impair oxygenation of vital organs and tissues. (Refer to ND: Airway Clearance, ineffective, p. 208.)

Demonstrate/encourage pursed-lip breathing during exhalation, especially for patients with fibrosis or parenchymal destruction.

Creates resistance against outflowing air to prevent collapse/narrowing of the airways, thereby helping distribute air throughout the lungs and relieve/reduce shortness of breath.

Promote bed rest/limit activity and assist with self-care activities as necessary.

Reducing oxygen consumption/demand during periods of respiratory compromise may reduce severity of symptoms.

Collaborative

Monitor serial ABGs/pulse oximetry.

Decreased oxygen content (PaO_2), and/or saturation or increased $PaCO_2$ indicates need for intervention/change in therapeutic regimen.

Provide supplemental oxygen as appropriate.

Aids in correcting the hypoxemia that may occur secondary to decreased ventilation/diminished alveolar lung surface.

NURSING DIAGNOSIS: Nutrition: altered, less than body requirements

May be related to
Fatigue
Frequent cough/sputum production; dyspnea
Anorexia
Insufficient financial resources

Possibly evidenced by
Weight 10%–20% below ideal for frame and height
Reported lack of interest in food, altered taste sensation
Poor muscle tone

DESIRED OUTCOMES/EVALUATION CRITERIA—PATIENT WILL:

Nutritional Status (NOC)

Demonstrate progressive weight gain toward goal with normalization of laboratory values and be free of signs of malnutrition.
Initiate behaviors/lifestyle changes to regain and/or to maintain appropriate weight.

ACTIONS/INTERVENTIONS	RATIONALE

Nutrition Management (NIC)

Independent

Document patient's nutritional status on admission, noting skin turgor, current weight and degree of weight loss, integrity of oral mucosa, ability/inability to swallow, presence of bowel tones, history of nausea/vomiting or diarrhea.

Useful in defining degree/extent of problem and appropriate choice of interventions.

Ascertain patient's usual dietary pattern, likes/dislikes.

Helpful in identifying specific needs/strengths. Consideration of individual preferences may improve dietary intake.

Monitor I&O and weight periodically.

Useful in measuring effectiveness of nutritional and fluid support.

Investigate anorexia and nausea/vomiting and note possible correlation to medications. Monitor frequency, volume, consistency of stools.

May affect dietary choices and identify areas for problem solving to enhance intake/utilization of nutrients.

Encourage and provide for frequent rest periods.

Helps conserve energy, especially when metabolic requirements are increased by fever.

Provide oral care before and after respiratory treatments.

Reduces bad taste left from sputum or medications used for respiratory treatments that can stimulate the vomiting center.

Encourage small, frequent meals with foods high in protein and carbohydrates.

Maximizes nutrient intake without undue fatigue/energy expenditure from eating large meals and reduces gastric irritation.

Encourage SO to bring foods from home and to share meals with patient unless contraindicated.

Creates a more normal social environment during mealtime and helps meet personal, cultural preferences.

Collaborative

Refer to dietitian for adjustments in dietary composition.

Provides assistance in planning a diet with nutrients adequate to meet patient's metabolic requirements, dietary preferences, and financial resources postdischarge.

Consult with respiratory therapy to schedule treatments 1–2 hr before/after meals.

May help to reduce the incidence of nausea and vomiting associated with medications or the effects of respiratory treatments on a full stomach.

Monitor laboratory studies, e.g., BUN, serum protein, and prealbumin/albumin.

Low values reflect malnutrition and indicate need for intervention/change in therapeutic regimen.

Administer antipyretics as appropriate.

Fever increases metabolic needs and therefore calorie consumption.

NURSING DIAGNOSIS: Knowledge Deficit [Learning Need] regarding condition, treatment, prevention, self care, and discharge needs

May be related to

Lack of exposure to/misinterpretation of information

Cognitive limitations

Inaccurate/incomplete information presented

Possibly evidenced by
Request for information
Expressed misconceptions about health status
Lack of or inaccurate follow-through of instructions/behaviors
Expressing or exhibiting feelings of being overwhelmed

DESIRED OUTCOMES/EVALUATION CRITERIA—PATIENT WILL:

Knowledge: Disease Process (NOC)

Verbalize understanding of disease process/prognosis and prevention.
Initiate behaviors/lifestyle changes to improve general well-being and reduce risk of reactivation of TB.
Identify symptoms requiring evaluation/intervention.
Describe a plan for receiving adequate follow-up care.

Knowledge: Treatment Regimen (NOC)

Verbalize understanding of therapeutic regimen and rationale for actions.

ACTIONS/INTERVENTIONS	RATIONALE
Learning Facilitation (NIC)	
Independent	
Assess patient's ability to learn, e.g., level of fear, concern, fatigue, participation level; best environment in which patient can learn; how much content; best media and language; who should be included.	Learning depends on emotional and physical readiness and is achieved at an individual pace.
Provide instruction and specific written information for the patient to refer to, e.g., schedule for medications and follow-up sputum testing for documenting response to therapy.	Written information relieves the patient of the burden of having to remember large amounts of information. Repetition strengthens learning.
Encourage patient/SO to verbalize fears/concerns. Answer questions factually. Note prolonged use of denial.	Provides opportunity to correct misconceptions/alleviate anxiety. Inadequate finances/prolonged denial may affect coping with/managing the tasks necessary to regain/maintain health.
Teaching: Disease Process (NIC)	
Identify symptoms that should be reported to healthcare provider, e.g., hemoptysis, chest pain, fever, difficulty breathing, hearing loss, vertigo.	May indicate progression or reactivation of disease or side effects of medications, requiring further evaluation.
Emphasize the importance of maintaining high-protein and carbohydrate diet and adequate fluid intake. (Refer to ND: Nutrition: altered, less than body requirements, p. 210.)	Meeting metabolic needs helps minimize fatigue and promote recovery. Fluids aid in liquefying/expectorating secretions.
Explain medication dosage, frequency of administration, expected action, and the reason for long treatment period. Review potential interactions with other drugs/substances.	Enhances cooperation with therapeutic regimen and may prevent the patient from discontinuing medication before cure is truly effected. Directly observed therapy (DOT) is the treatment of choice when patient is unable or unwilling to take medications as prescribed.
Review potential side effects of treatment (e.g., dryness of mouth, constipation, visual disturbances, headache, orthostatic hypertension) and problem-solve solutions.	May prevent/reduce discomfort associated with therapy and enhance cooperation with regimen.

ACTIONS/INTERVENTIONS	RATIONALE
Independent	
Stress need to abstain from alcohol while on INH.	Combination of INH and alcohol has been linked with increased incidence of hepatitis.
Refer for eye examination after starting and then monthly while taking ethambutol.	Major side effect is reduced visual acuity; initial sign may be decreased ability to perceive green.
Evaluate job-related risk factors, e.g., working in foundry/rock quarry, sandblasting.	Excessive exposure to silicone dust enhances risk of silicosis, which may negatively affect respiratory function/bronchitis.
Encourage abstaining from smoking.	Although smoking does not stimulate recurrence of TB, it does increase the likelihood of respiratory dysfunction/bronchitis.
Review how TB is transmitted (e.g., primarily by inhalation of airborne organisms but may also spread through stools or urine if infection is present in these systems) and hazards of reactivation.	Knowledge may reduce risk of transmission/reactivation. Complications associated with reactivation include cavitation, abscess formation, destructive emphysema, spontaneous pneumothorax, diffuse interstitial fibrosis, serous effusion, empyema, bronchiectasis, hemoptysis, GI ulceration, bronchopleural fistula, tuberculous laryngitis, and miliary spread.
Refer to public health agency.	DOT by community nurses is often the most effective way to ensure patient adherence to therapy. Monitoring can include pill counts and urine dipstick testing for presence of antitubercular drug. Patients with MDR-TB may be monitored with monthly sputum specimens for AFB smear and culture. *Note:* In some states, there are legal means for involuntary confinement for care if efforts to ensure patient adherence are ineffective.

POTENTIAL CONSIDERATIONS following acute hospitalization (dependent on patient's age, physical condition/presence of complications, personal resources, and life responsibilities)

Therapeutic Regimen: Individual, ineffective management—complexity of therapeutic regimen, economic difficulties, family patterns of health care, perceived seriousness/benefits.
Infection, risk for (secondary)—decrease in ciliary action, stasis of body fluids, suppressed inflammatory response, tissue destruction, chronic disease, malnutrition, increased environmental exposure.
Fatigue—increased energy requirements to perform ADLs, discomfort.
Therapeutic Regimen: Families, ineffective management—complexity of therapeutic regimen, decisional conflicts, economic difficulties, family conflict.

RESPIRATORY ACID-BASE IMBALANCES

The body has the remarkable ability to maintain plasma pH within a narrow range of 7.35–7.45. It does so by means of chemical buffering mechanisms involving the lungs and kidneys. Although simple acid-base imbalances (e.g., respiratory acidosis) do occur, mixed acid-base imbalances are more common (e.g., the respiratory acidosis/metabolic acidosis that occurs with cardiac arrest).

RESPIRATORY ACIDOSIS (PRIMARY CARBONIC ACID EXCESS)

Respiratory acidosis (elevated $PaCO_2$ level) is caused by hypoventilation with resultant excess carbonic acid (H_2CO_3). Acidosis can be due to/associated with primary defects in lung function or changes in normal respiratory pattern. The disorder may be acute or chronic.

Compensatory mechanisms include (1) an increased respiratory rate; (2) hemoglobin (Hb) buffering, forming bicarbonate ions and deoxygenated Hb; and (3) increased renal ammonia acid excretions with reabsorption of bicarbonate.

Acute respiratory acidosis: Associated with acute pulmonary edema, aspiration of foreign body, overdose of sedatives/barbiturate poisoning, smoke inhalation, acute laryngospasm, hemothorax/pneumothorax, atelectasis, ARDS, anesthesia/surgery, mechanical ventilators, excessive CO_2 intake (e.g., use of rebreathing mask, cerebral vascular accident ([CVA]) therapy), Pickwickian syndrome.

Chronic respiratory acidosis: Associated with emphysema, asthma, bronchiectasis; neuromuscular disorders (such as Guillain-Barré syndrome and myasthenia gravis), botulism, spinal cord injuries.

CARE SETTING

This condition does not occur in isolation, but rather is a complication of a broader health problem/disease or condition for which the severely compromised patient requires admission to a medical-surgical or subacute unit.

RELATED CONCERNS

Plans of care specific to predisposing factors/disease or medical condition, e.g.:

Cerebrovascular accident/Stroke, page 257
COPD/Asthma, page 126
Craniocerebral trauma, page 238
Eating disorders: obesity, page 421
Spinal cord injury, page 295
Surgical procedures, page 828
Ventilatory assistance, page 188

OTHER CONCERNS

Fluid and electrolyte imbalances, page 926
Metabolic acidosis, page 523
Metabolic alkalosis, page 527

Patient Assessment Database

Dependent on underlying cause. Findings vary widely.

ACTIVITY/REST

May report:	Fatigue, mild to profound
May exhibit:	Generalized weakness, ataxia/staggering, loss of coordination (chronic), to stupor

CIRCULATION

May exhibit: Low blood pressure/hypotension with bounding pulses, pinkish color, warm skin (reflects vasodilation of severe acidosis)

Tachycardia, irregular pulse (other/various dysrhythmias)

Diaphoresis, pallor, and cyanosis (late stage)

FOOD/FLUID

May report: Nausea/vomiting

NEUROSENSORY

May report: Feeling of fullness in head (acute—associated with vasodilation)

Headache, dizziness, visual disturbances

May exhibit: Confusion, apprehension, agitation, restlessness, somnolence; coma (acute)

Tremors, decreased reflexes (severe)

RESPIRATION

May report: Shortness of breath; dyspnea with exertion

May exhibit: Respiratory rate dependent on underlying cause, i.e., decreased in respiratory center depression/muscle paralysis; otherwise rate is rapid/shallow

Increased respiratory effort with nasal flaring/yawning, use of neck and upper body muscles

Decreased respiratory rate/hypoventilation (associated with decreased function of respiratory center as in head trauma, oversedation, general anesthesia, metabolic alkalosis)

Adventitious breath sounds (crackles, wheezes); stridor, crowing

TEACHING/LEARNING

Refer to specific plans of care reflecting individual predisposing/contributing factors

Discharge plan considerations: **DRG projected mean length of inpatient stay: 4.9 days**

May require assistance with changes in therapies for underlying disease process/condition

Refer to section at end of plan for postdischarge considerations.

DIAGNOSTIC STUDIES

ABGs:

PaO_2: Normal or may be low. Oxygen saturation (SaO_2) decreased.

$PaCO_2$: Increased, greater than 45 mm Hg (primary acidosis).

Bicarbonate (HCO_3): Normal or increased, greater than 26 mEq/L (compensated/chronic stage).

Arterial pH: Decreased, less than 7.35.

Electrolytes:

Serum potassium: May be normal or increased.

Serum chloride: Decreased.

Serum calcium: Increased.

Lactic acid: May be elevated.

Urinalysis: Urine pH decreased.

Other screening tests: As indicated by underlying illness/condition to determine underlying cause.

NURSING PRIORITIES

1. Achieve homeostasis.
2. Prevent/minimize complications.
3. Provide information about condition/prognosis and treatment needs as appropriate.

DISCHARGE GOALS

1. Physiological balance restored.
2. Free of complications.
3. Condition, prognosis, and treatment needs understood.
4. Plan in place to meet needs after discharge.

NURSING DIAGNOSIS: Gas Exchange, impaired

May be related to

Ventilation perfusion imbalance (e.g., altered oxygen-carrying capacity of blood, altered oxygen supply, alveolar-capillary membrane changes, or altered blood flow)

Possibly evidenced by

Dyspnea with exertion, tachypnea

Changes in mentation, irritability

Tachycardia

Hypoxia, hypercapnea

DESIRED OUTCOMES/EVALUATION CRITERIA—PATIENT WILL:

Electrolyte and Acid-Base Balance (NOC)

Demonstrate improved ventilation and adequate oxygenation of tissues as evidenced by ABGs within patient's acceptable limits and absence of symptoms of respiratory distress.

Knowledge: Disease Process (NOC)

Verbalize understanding of causative factors and appropriate interventions.

Participate in treatment regimen within level of ability/situation.

ACTIONS/INTERVENTIONS	RATIONALE
Acid-Base Management: Respiratory Acidosis (NIC)	
Independent	
Monitor respiratory rate, depth, and effort.	Alveolar hypoventilation and associated hypoxemia lead to respiratory distress/failure.
Auscultate breath sounds.	Identifies area(s) of decreased ventilation (e.g., atelectasis) or airway obstruction and changes as patient deteriorates or improves, reflecting effectiveness of treatment, dictating therapy needs.
Note declining level of awareness/consciousness.	Signals severe acidotic state, which requires immediate attention. *Note:* In recovery, sensorium clears slowly because hydrogen ions are slow to cross the blood-brain barrier and clear from cerebrospinal fluid and brain cells.
Monitor heart rate/rhythm.	Tachycardia develops early because the sympathetic nervous system is stimulated, resulting in the release of catecholamines, epinephrine, and norepinephrine, in an attempt to increase oxygen delivery to the tissues. Dysrhythmias that may occur are due to hypoxia (myocardial ischemia) and electrolyte imbalances.
Note skin color, temperature, moisture.	Diaphoresis, pallor, cool/clammy skin are late changes associated with severe or advancing hypoxemia.
Encourage/assist with breathing exercises, turning, and coughing. Suction as necessary. Provide airway adjunct as indicated. Place in semi-Fowler's position.	These measures improve lung ventilation and reduce/prevent airway obstruction associated with accumulation of mucus.
Restrict use of hypnotic sedatives or tranquilizers.	In the presence of hypoventilation, respiratory depression and CO_2 narcosis may develop.

ACTIONS/INTERVENTIONS	RATIONALE
Independent	
Discuss cause of chronic condition (when known) and appropriate interventions/self-care activities.	Promotes participation in therapeutic regimen and may reduce recurrence of disorder.
Collaborative	
Assist with identification/treatment of underlying cause.	Treatment of disorder is directed at improving alveolar ventilation. Addressing the primary condition (e.g., oversedation, lung/respiratory system trauma, pulmonary edema, aspiration) promotes correction of the acid-base disorder.
Monitor/graph serial ABGs, pulse oximetry readings; Hb, serum electrolyte levels.	Evaluates therapy needs/effectiveness. *Note:* Bedside pulse oximetry monitoring is used to show early changes in oxygenation before other signs or symptoms are observed.
Administer oxygen as indicated. Increase respiratory rate or tidal volume of ventilator, if used.	Prevents/corrects hypoxemia and respiratory failure. *Note:* Must be used with caution in presence of emphysema because respiratory depression/failure may result.
Assist with ventilatory aids, e.g., IPPB in conjunction with bronchodilators. Monitor peak flow pressure.	Increases lung expansion and opens airways to improve ventilation, preventing respiratory failure.
Maintain hydration (IV/PO)/provide humidification.	Assists in correction of acidity and thinning/mobilization of respiratory secretions.
Provide appropriate chest physiotherapy, including postural drainage and breathing exercises.	Aids in clearing secretions, which improves ventilation, allowing excess CO_2 to be eliminated.
Administer IV solutions such as lactated Ringer's solution or 0.6 M solution of sodium lactate.	May be useful in nonemergency situations to help control acidosis, until underlying respiratory problem can be corrected.
Administer medications as indicated, e.g.:	
Naloxone hydrochloride (Narcan);	May be useful in arousing patient and stimulating respiratory function in presence of drug overdose/sedation, or acidosis resulting from cardiac arrest.
Sodium bicarbonate ($NaHCO_3$);	May be given in small IV doses in emergency situations to quickly correct acidosis if pH is less than 7.25 and hyperkalemia coexists. *Note:* Rebound alkalosis or tetany may occur.
Potassium chloride (KCl).	Replaces potassium that shifts out of cells during acidotic state. Correction of the acidosis may cause a relative serum hypokalemia as potassium shifts back into cells. Potassium imbalance can impair neuromuscular/respiratory function causing generalized muscle weakness and cardiac dysrhythmias.
Provide low-carbohydrate, high-fat diet (e.g., pulmocare feedings), if indicated.	Helps reduce CO_2 production and improves respiratory muscle function and metabolic homeostasis.

POTENTIAL CONSIDERATIONS following acute hospitalization (dependent on patient's age, physical condition/presence of complications, personal resources, and life responsibilities)

Refer to Potential Considerations relative to underlying cause of acid-base disorder.

RESPIRATORY ALKALOSIS (PRIMARY CARBONIC ACID DEFICIT)

Respiratory alkalosis is a loss of carbon dioxide ($Pco_2 < 35$ mm Hg) with a resultant decrease of carbonic acid (H_2CO_3) due to a marked increase in the rate of respirations. The two primary mechanisms that trigger hyperventilation are (1) hypoxemia and (2) direct stimulation of the central respiratory center of the brain (such as occur with high fever, head trauma/CNS lesions, early salicylate intoxication).

Compensatory mechanisms include decreased respiratory rate (if the body is able to respond to the drop in $Paco_2$), increased renal excretion of bicarbonate, and retention of hydrogen. It is the most frequently occurring acid-base imbalance in hospitalized patients, with the elderly at increased risk because of high incidence of pulmonary disorders and alterations in neurological status.

CARE SETTING

This condition does not occur in isolation but rather is a complication of a broader problem and usually requires inpatient care in a medical/surgical or subacute unit.

RELATED CONCERNS

Plans of care specific to predisposing factors, e.g.:

OTHER CONCERNS

Patient Assessment Database

Dependent on underlying cause.

CIRCULATION

May report:	History/presence of anemia
	Palpitations
May exhibit:	Hypotension
	Tachycardia, irregular pulse/dysrhythmias

EGO INTEGRITY

May exhibit:	Extreme anxiety (most common cause of hyperventilation)

FOOD/FLUID

May report:	Dry mouth
	Nausea/vomiting
May exhibit:	Abdominal distension (elevating diaphragm as with ascites, pregnancy)
	Vomiting

NEUROSENSORY

May report:	Headache, tinnitus
	Numbness/tingling of face, hands, and toes; circumoral paresthesia
	Lightheadedness, syncope, vertigo, blurred vision
May exhibit:	Confusion, restlessness, obtundation, coma
	Hyperactive reflexes, positive Chvostek's sign, tetany, seizures
	Heightened sensitivity to environmental noise and activity
	Muscle weakness, unsteady gait

PAIN/DISCOMFORT

May report:	Muscle spasms/cramps, epigastric pain, precordial pain (tightness)

RESPIRATION

May report:	Dyspnea
	History of asthma, pulmonary fibrosis
	Recent move/visit to location at high altitude
May exhibit:	Tachypnea; rapid, shallow breathing; hyperventilation (often 40 or more respirations/minute)
	Intermittent periods of apnea

SAFETY

May exhibit:	Fever

TEACHING/LEARNING

May report:	Use of salicylates/salicylate overdose, catecholamines, theophylline
Discharge plan considerations:	**DRG projected mean length of inpatient stay: 5.4 days**
	May require change in treatment/therapy of underlying disease process/condition
	Refer to section at end of plan for postdischarge considerations.

DIAGNOSTIC STUDIES

Arterial pH: Greater than 7.45 (may be near normal in chronic stage).
Bicarbonate (HCO_3): Normal or decreased; less than 25 mEq/L (compensatory mechanism).
$Paco_2$: Decreased, less than 35 mm Hg (primary).
Serum potassium: Decreased.
Serum chloride: Increased.
Serum calcium: Decreased.
Urine pH: Increased, greater than 7.0.
Screening tests as indicated to determine underlying cause, e.g.,
   CBC: May reveal severe anemia (decreasing oxygen-carrying capacity).
   Blood cultures: May identify sepsis (usually Gram-negative).
   Blood alcohol: Marked elevation (acute alcoholic intoxication).
   Toxicology screen: May reveal early salicylate poisoning.
   Chest x-ray/lung scan: May reveal multiple pulmonary emboli.

NURSING PRIORITIES

1. Achieve homeostasis.
2. Prevent/minimize complications.
3. Provide information about condition/prognosis and treatment needs as appropriate.

DISCHARGE GOALS

1. Physiological balance restored.
2. Free of complications.
3. Condition, prognosis, and treatment needs understood.
4. Plan in place to meet needs after discharge.

NURSING DIAGNOSIS: Gas Exchange, impaired

May be related to
Ventilation perfusion imbalance (e.g., altered oxygen supply, altered blood flow, altered oxygen-carrying capacity of blood, alveolar-capillary membrane changes)

Possibly evidenced by
Dyspnea, tachypnea
Changes in mentation
Hypocapnea, tachycardia
Hypoxia

ACTIONS/INTERVENTIONS	RATIONALE
Acid-Base Management: Respiratory Alkalosis (NIC)	
Independent	
Monitor respiratory rate, depth, and effort; ascertain cause for hyperventilation if possible, e.g., anxiety, pain, improper ventilator settings.	Identifies alterations from usual breathing pattern and influences choice of intervention.
Encourage patient to breathe slowly and deeply. Speak in a low, calm tone of voice, provide safe environment.	May help reassure and calm the agitated patient, thereby aiding in reduction of respiratory rate. Assists patient to regain control.
Assess level of awareness/cognition and note neuromuscular status, e.g., strength, tone, reflexes, and sensation.	Decreased mentation (mild to severe) and tetany or seizures may occur when alkalosis is severe.
Demonstrate appropriate breathing patterns, if appropriate, and assist with respiratory aids, e.g., rebreathing mask/bag.	Decreasing the rate of respirations can halt the "blowing off" of CO_2, elevating PCO_2 level and normalizing pH.
Provide comfort measures, encourage use of meditation and visualization. Use tepid sponge bath/cool cloths.	Promotes relaxation and reduces stress. Control and reduction of fever reduces potential for seizures and helps reduce respiration rate.
Provide safety/seizure precautions, e.g., bed in low position, padded side rails, frequent observation.	Changes in mentation/CNS and neuromuscular hyperirritability may result in patient harm, especially if tetany/convulsions occur.
Discuss cause of condition (if known) and appropriate interventions/self-care activities.	Promotes participation in therapeutic regimen and may reduce recurrence of disorder.
Collaborative	
Assist with identification/treatment of underlying cause.	Respiratory alkalosis is a complication, not an isolated occurrence; addressing the primary condition (e.g., hyperventilation of panic attack, organ failure, severe anemia; drug effect, such as with paraldehyde or epinephrine) promotes correction of the disorder and reduces likelihood of recurrence.
Monitor/graph serial ABGs, and pulse oximetry.	Identifies therapy needs/effectiveness.
Monitor serum potassium. Replace as indicated.	Hypokalemia may occur as potassium is lost (urine) or shifted into the cell in exchange for hydrogen in an attempt to correct alkalosis.
Provide sedation/pain medication, as indicated.	May be required to reduce psychogenic cause of hyperventilation.

ACTIONS/INTERVENTIONS	RATIONALE
Collaborative	
Administer CO_2, or use rebreathing mask as indicated. Reduce respiratory rate/tidal volume, or add additional dead space (tubing) to mechanical ventilator.	Increasing CO_2 retention may correct carbonic acid deficit.

POTENTIAL CONSIDERATIONS following acute hospitalization (dependent on patient's age, physical condition/presence of complications, personal resources, and life responsibilities)

Refer to Potential Considerations relative to underlying cause of acid-base disorder.

Neurological/
Sensory Disorders

GLAUCOMA

Increased intraocular pressure (IOP) is the result of inadequate drainage of aqueous humor from the anterior chamber of the eye. The increased pressure causes atrophy of the optic nerve and, if untreated, blindness. There are two primary categories of glaucoma: (1) open-angle and (2) closed-angle (or narrow angle). Chronic open-angle glaucoma is the most common type, accounting for 90% of all glaucoma cases. It may be associated with diabetes and myopia and may develop in both eyes simultaneously. Chronic glaucoma has no early warning signs, and the loss of peripheral vision occurs so gradually that substantial optic nerve damage can occur before glaucoma is detected.

Narrow-angle or angle-closure glaucoma is the least common and may be associated with eye trauma, inflammation, and pupillary dilation after the instillation of mydriatic drops. This condition constitutes a medical emergency because blindness may suddenly ensue.

CARE SETTING

Community, unless sudden increase in IOP requires emergency intervention and close monitoring.

RELATED CONCERNS

Psychosocial aspects of care, page 809

Patient Assessment Database

ACTIVITY/REST

May report: Change in usual activities/hobbies due to altered vision

FOOD/FLUID

May report: Nausea/vomiting (acute glaucoma)

NEUROSENSORY

May report: Gradual loss of peripheral vision, frequent change of glasses, difficulty adjusting to darkened room, halos around lights, mild headache (chronic glaucoma)

Cloudy/blurred vision, appearance of halos/rainbows around lights, sudden loss of peripheral vision, photophobia (acute glaucoma)

Glasses/treatment change does not improve vision

May exhibit: Dilated, fixed, cloudy pupils (acute glaucoma)

Fixed pupil and red/hard eye with cloudy cornea (glaucoma emergency)

Increased tearing

Intermescent cataracts, intraocular hemorrhage (glaucoma secondary to trauma)

PAIN/DISCOMFORT

May report: Mild discomfort or aching/tired eyes (chronic glaucoma)

Sudden/persistent severe pain or pressure in and around eye(s), headache (acute glaucoma)

SAFETY

May report: History of hemorrhage, trauma, ocular disease, tumor (secondary to trauma)

Difficulty seeing, managing activities

May exhibit: Inflammatory disease of eye (glaucoma secondary to trauma)

TEACHING/LEARNING

May report: Family history of glaucoma, diabetes, systemic vascular disorders

History of stress, allergies, vasomotor disturbances (e.g., increased venous pressure), endocrine imbalance, diabetes

History of ocular surgery/cataract removal; steroid use

Discharge plan considerations: May require assistance with transportation, meal preparation, self-care, homemaker/maintenance tasks

Refer to section at end of plan for postdischarge considerations.

DIAGNOSTIC STUDIES

Ophthalmoscopy examination: Assesses internal ocular structures, noting optic disc atrophy, papilledema, retinal hemorrhage, and microaneurysms. Slit-lamp examination provides three-dimensional view of eye structures, identifies corneal abnormalities/change in shape, increased IOP, and general vision deficits associated with glaucoma.

Visual acuity tests (e.g., Snellen, Jayer): Vision may be impaired by defects in cornea, lens, aqueous or vitreous humor, refraction, or disease of the nervous or vascular system supplying the retina or optic pathway.

Visual fields (e.g., confrontation, tangent screen, perimetry): Reduction of peripheral vision may be caused by glaucoma or other conditions such as cerebrovascular accident (CVA), pituitary/brain tumor mass, or carotid or cerebral artery pathology.

Tonography measurement: Assesses intraocular pressure (normal: 12–20 mm Hg).

Gonioscopy measurement: Helps differentiate open-angle from angle-closure glaucoma.

Provocative tests: May be useful in establishing presence/type of glaucoma when IOP is normal or only mildly elevated.

Glucose tolerance test/fasting blood sugar (FBS): Determines presence/control of diabetes, which is implicated at times in secondary glaucoma.

NURSING PRIORITIES

1. Prevent further visual deterioration.
2. Promote adaptation to changes in/reduced visual acuity.
3. Prevent complications.
4. Provide information about disease process/prognosis and treatment needs.

DISCHARGE GOALS

1. Vision maintained at highest possible level.
2. Patient coping with situation in a positive manner.
3. Complications prevented/minimized.
4. Disease process/prognosis and therapeutic regimen understood.
5. Plan in place to meet needs after discharge.

NURSING DIAGNOSIS: Sensory-Perceptual alteration: visual

May be related to

Altered sensory reception: altered status of sense organ

Possibly evidenced by

Progressive loss of visual field

Symptom Control Behavior (NOC)

Participate in therapeutic regimen.
Maintain current visual field/acuity without further loss.

ACTIONS/INTERVENTIONS

Coping Enhancement (NIC)

Independent

Ascertain type/degree of visual loss.

Encourage expression of feelings about loss/possibility of loss of vision.

Eye Care (NIC)

Recommend measures to assist patient to manage visual limitations, e.g., reducing clutter, arranging furniture out of travel path; turning head to view subjects; correcting for dim light and problems of night vision.

Demonstrate administration of eyedrops, e.g., counting drops, adhering to schedule, not missing doses.

Collaborative

Assist with administration of medications as indicated:

Chronic, open-angle glaucoma

Pilocarpine hydrochloride (Isopto Carpine, Ocusert [disc], Pilopine HS Gel);

Timolol maleate (Timoptic), betaxalol (Betoptic), carteolol (Ocupress), metipranolol (OptiPranolol), levobunolol (Betagan);

Acetazolamide (Diamox), methazolamide (Neptazane), dorzolamide (Trusopt);

Narrow-angle (angle-closure) type

Myotics (until pupil is constricted);

Carbonic anhydrase inhibitors, e.g., acetazolamide (Diamox);

RATIONALE

Affects choice of interventions and patient's future expectations.

Although early intervention can prevent blindness, the patient faces the possibility or may have already experienced partial or complete loss of vision. Although vision loss cannot be restored (even with treatment), further loss can be prevented.

Reduces safety hazards related to changes in visual fields/loss of vision and papillary accommodation to environmental light.

Controls IOP, preventing further loss of vision.

These direct-acting topical myotic drugs cause pupillary constriction, facilitating the outflow of aqueous humor and lowering IOP. *Note:* Ocusert is a disc (similar to a contact) that is placed in the lower eyelid, where it can remain for up to 1 wk before being replaced.

β-Blockers decrease formation of aqueous humor without changing pupil size, vision, or accommodation. *Note:* These drugs may be contraindicated, or require close monitoring for systemic effects in the presence of bradycardia or asthma.

Carbonic anhydrase inhibitors decrease the rate of production of aqueous humor. *Note:* Systemic adverse effects are common, including mood disturbances, GI upset, and fatigue.

Contracts the sphincter muscles of the iris, deepens anterior chamber, and dilates vessels of outflow tract during acute attack or before surgery.

Decreases secretion of aqueous humor and lowers IOP.

ACTIONS/INTERVENTIONS	RATIONALE
Collaborative	
Sympathomimetics, e.g., Dipivefrin hydrochloride (Propine), brimonidine (Alphagan);	Adrenergic drops also decrease formation of aqueous humor and may be beneficial when patient is unresponsive to other medications. Although free of side effects such as miosis, blurred vision, and night blindness, they have potential for additive adverse cardiovascular effects in combination with other cardiovascular agents. *Note:* Light-colored eyes are more responsive to these drugs than dark-colored eyes, necessitating added considerations when determining appropriate dosage.
Hyperosmotic agents, e.g., mannitol (Osmitrol), glycerine.	Used to decrease circulating fluid volume, which will decrease production of aqueous humor if other treatments have not been successful.
Provide sedation, analgesics as necessary.	Acute glaucoma attack is associated with sudden pain, which can precipitate anxiety/agitation, further elevating IOP. Medical management may require 4–6 hours before IOP decreases and pain subsides.
Prepare for surgical intervention as indicated, e.g.:	
Laser therapy, e.g., argon laser trabeculoplasty (ALT) or trabeculectomy/trephination;	Filtering operations (laser surgery) are highly successful procedures for reducing IOP by creating an opening between the anterior chamber and the subjunctival spaces so that aqueous humor can bypass the trabecular mesh block. *Note:* Apraclonidine (Iopidine) eye drops may be used in conjunction with laser therapy to lessen/prevent postprocedure elevations of IOP.
Iridectomy;	Surgical removal of a portion of the iris facilitates drainage of aqueous humor. Upper iris usually is covered with upper eyelid, and flow of tears washes bacteria downward. *Note:* Bilateral iridectomy is performed because glaucoma usually develops in the other eye.
Malento valve implant;	Experimental ocular implant device corrects or prevents scarring over/closure of drainage sac created by trabeculectomy.
Cyclocryotherapy;	Separates ciliary body from the sclera to facilitate outflow of aqueous humor.
Aqueous-venous shunt;	Used in intractable glaucoma.
Diathermy/cryosurgery.	If other treatments fail, destruction of the ciliary body reduces formation of aqueous humor.

NURSING DIAGNOSIS: Anxiety [specify level]

May be related to
Physiological factors, change in health status; presence of pain; possibility/reality of loss of vision
Unmet needs
Negative self-talk

Possibly evidenced by
Apprehension, uncertainty
Expressed concern regarding changes in life events

DESIRED OUTCOMES/EVALUATION CRITERIA—PATIENT WILL:

> **Anxiety Control (NOC)**

Appear relaxed and report anxiety is reduced to a manageable level.
Demonstrate problem-solving skills.
Use resources effectively.

ACTIONS/INTERVENTIONS	RATIONALE
Anxiety Reduction (NIC)	
Independent	
Assess anxiety level, degree of pain experienced/suddenness of onset of symptoms, and current knowledge of condition.	These factors affect patient perception of threat to self, potentiate the cycle of anxiety, and may interfere with medical attempts to control IOP.
Provide accurate, honest information. Discuss probability that careful monitoring and treatment can prevent additional visual loss.	Reduces anxiety related to unknown/future expectations and provides factual basis for making informed choices about treatment.
Encourage patient to acknowledge concerns and express feelings.	Provides opportunity for patient to deal with reality of situation, clarify misconceptions, and problem-solve concerns.
Identify helpful resources/people.	Provides reassurance that patient is not alone in dealing with problem.

NURSING DIAGNOSIS: Knowledge Deficit [Learning Need] regarding condition, prognosis, treatment, self care, and discharge needs

May be related to
Lack of exposure/unfamiliarity with resources
Lack of recall, information misinterpretation

Possibly evidenced by
Questions; statement of misconception
Inaccurate follow-through of instruction
Development of preventable complications

DESIRED OUTCOMES/EVALUATION CRITERIA—PATIENT WILL:

> **Knowledge: Disease Process (NOC)**

Verbalize understanding of condition, prognosis, and treatment.
Identify relationship of signs/symptoms to the disease process.

> **Knowledge: Treatment Regimen (NOC)**

Verbalize understanding of treatment needs.
Correctly perform necessary procedures and explain reasons for the actions.

ACTIONS/INTERVENTIONS	RATIONALE

Teaching: Disease Process (NIC)

Independent

Review pathology/prognosis of condition and lifelong need for treatment.

Provides opportunity to clarify/dispel misconceptions and present condition as something that is manageable.

Discuss necessity of wearing identification, e.g., Medic-Alert bracelet.

Vital to provide information for caregivers in case of emergency to reduce risk of receiving contraindicated drugs (e.g., atropine).

Demonstrate proper technique for administration of eye drops, gels, or discs. Have patient return demonstration.

Enhances effectiveness of treatment. Provides opportunity for patient to show competence and ask questions.

Review importance of maintaining drug schedule, e.g., eye drops. Discuss medications that should be avoided, e.g., mydriatic drops (atropine/propantheline bromide), overuse of topical steroids.

This disease can be controlled, not cured, and maintaining a consistent medication regimen is vital to control. Some drugs cause pupil dilation, increasing IOP and potentiating additional loss of vision.

Identify potential side effects/adverse reactions of treatment, e.g., decreased appetite, nausea/vomiting, diarrhea, fatigue, "drugged" feeling, decreased libido, impotence, cardiac irregularities, syncope, heart failure (HF).

Drug side/adverse effects range from uncomfortable to severe or health-threatening. Approximately 50% of patients develop sensitivity/allergy to parasympathomimetics (e.g., pilocarpine) or anticholinesterase drugs. These problems require medical evaluation and possible change in therapeutic regimen.

Encourage patient to make necessary changes in lifestyle.

A tranquil lifestyle decreases the emotional response to stress, preventing ocular changes that push the iris forward, which may precipitate an acute attack.

Reinforce avoidance of activities, such as heavy lifting/pushing, snow shoveling, wearing tight/constricting clothing.

May increase IOP, precipitating acute attack. *Note:* If patient is not experiencing pain, cooperation with drug regimen and acceptance of lifestyle changes are often difficult to sustain.

Discuss dietary considerations, e.g., adequate fluid, bulk/fiber intake.

Measures to maintain consistency of stool to avoid constipation/straining during defecation.

Stress importance of routine checkups.

Important to monitor progression/maintenance of disease to allow for early intervention and prevent further loss of vision.

Advise patient to immediately report severe eye pain, inflammation, increased photophobia, increased lacrimation, changes in visual field/veil-like curtain, blurred vision, flashes of light/particles floating in visual field.

Prompt action may be necessary to prevent further vision loss/other complications, e.g., detached retina.

Recommend family members be examined regularly for signs of glaucoma.

Hereditary tendency to shallow anterior chambers places family members at increased risk for developing the condition.

Identify strategies/resources for socialization, e.g., support groups, Visually Impaired Society, local library, and transportation services.

Decreased visual acuity may limit patient's ability to drive/cause patient to withdraw from usual activities.

POTENTIAL CONSIDERATIONS long-term/chronic concerns.

Trauma, risk for—poor vision.
Social Interaction, impaired—limited physical mobility (poor vision), inadequate support system.
Therapeutic Regimen: Individual, ineffective management—complexity of therapeutic regimen, economic difficulties, inadequate number and types of cues to action, perceived seriousness (of condition) or benefit (versus side effects).

SEIZURE DISORDERS

Seizures (convulsions) are the result of uncontrolled electrical discharges from the nerve cells of the cerebral cortex and are characterized by sudden, brief attacks of altered consciousness, motor activity, and/or sensory phenomena. Seizures can be associated with a variety of cerebral or systemic disorders as a focal or generalized disturbance of cortical function. Sensory symptoms arise from the parietal lobe; motor symptoms arise from the frontal lobe.

The phases of seizure activity are prodromal, aural, ictal, and postictal. The *prodromal phase* involves mood or behavior changes that may precede a seizure by hours or days. The *aura* is a premonition of impending seizure activity and may be visual, auditory, or gustatory. The *ictal stage* is characterized by seizure activity, usually musculoskeletal. The *postictal stage* is a period of confusion/somnolence/irritability that occurs after the seizure.

The main causes for seizures can be divided into six categories:

Toxic agents: Poisons, alcohol, overdoses of prescription/nonprescription drugs (with drugs the leading cause).
Chemical imbalances: Hyperkalemia, hypoglycemia, and acidosis.
Fever: Acute infections, heatstroke.
Cerebral pathology: Resulting from head injury, infections, hypoxia, expanding brain lesions, increased intracranial pressure.
Eclampsia: Prenatal hypertension/toxemia of pregnancy.
Idiopathic: Unknown origin.

Seizures can be divided into two major classifications (generalized and partial). Generalized seizure types include tonic-clonic, myoclonic, clonic, tonic, atonic, and absence seizures. Partial (focal) seizures are the most common type and are categorized as either (1) simple (partial motor, partial sensory) or (2) complex.

CARE SETTING

Community; however, may require brief inpatient care on a medical or subacute unit for stabilization/treatment of status epilepticus.

RELATED CONCERNS

Cerebrovascular accident/stroke, page 257
Craniocerebral trauma (acute rehabilitative phase), page 238
Psychosocial aspects of care, page 809
Substance dependence/abuse rehabilitation, page 886

Patient Assessment Database

ACTIVITY/REST

May report:	Fatigue, general weakness
	Limitation of activities/occupation imposed by self/significant other (SO)/healthcare provider or others
May exhibit:	Altered muscle tone/strength
	Involuntary movement/contractions of muscles or muscle groups (generalized tonic-clonic seizures)

CIRCULATION

May exhibit:	Ictal: Hypertension, increased pulse, cyanosis
	Postictal: Vital signs normal or depressed with decreased pulse and respiration

EGO INTEGRITY

May report:	Internal/external stressors related to condition and/or treatment
	Irritability; sense of helplessness/hopelessness
	Changes in relationships
May exhibit:	Wide range of emotional responses

ELIMINATION

May report:	Episodic incontinence
May exhibit:	Ictal: Increased bladder pressure and sphincter tone
	Postictal: Muscles relaxed, resulting in incontinence (urinary/fecal)

FOOD/FLUID

> **May report:**   Food sensitivity nausea/vomiting correlating with seizure activity
>
> **May exhibit:**   Dental/soft tissue damage (injury during seizure)
> Gingival hyperplasia (side effect of long-term phenytoin [Dilantin] use)

NEUROSENSORY

> **May report:**   History of headaches, recurring seizure activity, fainting, dizziness
> History of head trauma, anoxia, cerebral infections
> > Prodromal phase: Vague changes in emotional reactivity or affective response preceding aura in some cases and lasting minutes to hours
> Presence of aura (stimulation of visual, auditory, hallucinogenic areas)
> Postictal: Weakness, muscle pain, areas of paresthesia/paralysis
>
> **May exhibit:**   Seizure characteristics: (ictal, postictal)
> **Generalized seizures:**
> > Tonic-clonic (grand mal): Rigidity and jerking posturing, vocalization, loss of consciousness, dilated pupils, stertorous respiration, excessive salivation (froth), fecal/urinary incontinence, and biting of the tongue may occur and last 2–5 min. Postictal phase: Patient sleeps 30 min to several hours, then may be weak, confused, and amnesic concerning the episode, with nausea and stiff, sore muscles
> > Myoclonic: Short abrupt muscle contractions of arms, legs, torso; may not be symmetrical; lasts seconds
> > Clonic: Muscle contraction with relaxation resembling myoclonic movements but with slower repetitions; may last several minutes
> > Tonic: Abrupt increase in muscle tone of torso/face, flexion of arms, extension of legs; lasts seconds
> > Atonic: Abrupt loss of muscle tone; lasts seconds; patient may fall
> > Absence (petit mal): Periods of altered awareness or consciousness (staring, fluttering of eyes) lasting 5–30 sec, which may occur as many as 100 times a day; minor motor seizures may be akinetic (loss of movement), myoclonic (repetitive motor contractions), or atonic (loss of muscle tone). Postictal phase: Amnesia for seizure events, no confusion, able to resume activity
> > Status epilepticus: Defined as 30 or more minutes of continuous generalized seizure activity or two or more sequential seizures without full recovery of consciousness in between, possibly related to abrupt withdrawal of anticonvulsants and other metabolic phenomena. If absence seizures are the pattern, problem may go undetected for a period of time because the patient does not lose consciousness
> **Partial seizures:**
> > Complex (psychomotor/temporal lobe): Patient generally remains conscious, with reactions such as dream state, staring, wandering, irritability, hallucinations, hostility, or fear. May display involuntary motor symptoms (lip smacking) and behaviors that appear purposeful but are inappropriate (automatism) and include impaired judgment and, on occasion, antisocial acts; lasts 1–3 min. Postictal phase: Absence of memory for these events, mild to moderate confusion
> > Simple (Focal-motor/Jacksonian): Often preceded by aura (may report deja vu or fearful feeling); no loss of consciousness (unilateral) or loss of consciousness (bilateral); convulsive movements and temporary disturbance in part controlled by the brain region involved (e.g., frontal lobe [motor dysfunction], parietal [numbness, tingling], occipital [bright, flashing lights], posterotemporal [difficulty speaking]). Convulsions may march along limb or side of body in orderly progression. If restrained during seizure, patient may exhibit combative and uncooperative behavior; lasts seconds to minutes

PAIN/DISCOMFORT

> **May report:**   Headache, muscle/back soreness postictally
> Paroxysmal abdominal pain during ictal phase (may occur during some partial/focal seizures without loss of consciousness)

May exhibit:	Guarding behavior
	Alteration in muscle tone
	Distraction behavior/restlessness

RESPIRATION

| **May exhibit:** | Ictal: Clenched teeth, cyanosis, decreased or rapid respirations; increased mucous secretions |
| | Postictal: Apnea |

SAFETY

May report:	History of accidental falls/injuries, fractures
	Presence of allergies
May exhibit:	Soft tissue injury/ecchymosis
	Decreased general strength/muscle tone

SOCIAL INTERACTION

| **May report:** | Problems with interpersonal relationships within family/socially |
| | Limitation/avoidance of social contacts |

TEACHING/LEARNING

May report:	Familial history of epilepsy
	Drug (including alcohol) use/misuse
	Increased frequency of episodes/failure to improve
Discharge plan considerations:	**DRG projected mean length of inpatient stay: 4.4 days**
	May require changes in medications, assistance with some homemaker/maintenance tasks relative to issues of safety, and transportation

Refer to section at end of plan for postdischarge considerations.

DIAGNOSTIC STUDIES

Electrolytes: Imbalances may affect/predispose to seizure activity.

Glucose: Hypoglycemia may precipitate seizure activity.

Blood urea nitrogen (BUN): Elevation may potentiate seizure activity or may indicate nephrotoxicity related to medication regimen.

Complete blood count (CBC): Aplastic anemia may result from drug therapy.

Serum drug levels: To verify therapeutic range of antiepileptic drugs (AEDs).

Toxicology screen: Determines potentiating factors such as alcohol or other drug use.

Skull x-rays: Identifies presence of space-occupying lesions, fractures.

Electroencephalogram (EEG) may be done serially: Locates area of cerebral dysfunction; measures brain activity. Brain waves take on characteristic spikes in each type of seizure activity; however, up to 40% of seizure patients have normal EEGs.

Video-EEG monitoring, 24 hours (video picture obtained at same time as EEG): May identify exact focus of seizure activity (advantage of repeated viewing of event with EEG recording).

Computed tomography (CT) scan: Identifies localized cerebral lesions, infarcts, hematomas, cerebral edema, trauma, abscesses, tumor; can be done with or without contrast medium.

Magnetic resonance imaging (MRI): Localizes focal lesions.

Positron emission tomography (PET): Demonstrates metabolic alterations, e.g., decreased metabolism of glucose at site of lesion.

Single photon emission computed tomography (SPECT): May show local areas of brain dysfunction when CT and MRI are normal.

Magnetoencephalogram: Maps the electrical impulses/potential of brain for abnormal discharge patterns.

Lumbar puncture: Detects abnormal cerebrospinal fluid (CSF) pressure, signs of infections or bleeding (i.e., subarachnoid, subdural hemorrhage) as a cause of seizure activity (rarely done).

Wada's test: Determines hemispheric dominance (done as a presurgical evaluation before temporal lobectomy).

NURSING PRIORITIES

1. Prevent/control seizure activity.
2. Protect patient from injury.

3. Maintain airway/respiratory function.
4. Promote positive self-esteem.
5. Provide information about disease process, prognosis, and treatment needs.

DISCHARGE GOALS

1. Seizure activity controlled.
2. Complications/injury prevented.
3. Capable/competent self-image displayed.
4. Disease process/prognosis, therapeutic regimen, and limitations understood.
5. Plan in place to meet needs after discharge.

NURSING DIAGNOSIS: Trauma/Suffocation, risk for

Risk factors may include
Weakness, balancing difficulties
Cognitive limitations/altered consciousness
Loss of large or small muscle coordination
Emotional difficulties

Possibly evidenced by
[Not applicable; presence of signs and symptoms establishes an *actual* diagnosis]

DESIRED OUTCOMES/EVALUATION CRITERIA—PATIENT WILL:

> **Risk Detection (NOC)**

Verbalize understanding of factors that contribute to possibility of trauma and/or suffocation and take steps to correct situation.

> **Risk Control (NOC)**

Demonstrate behaviors, lifestyle changes to reduce risk factors and protect self from injury.
Modify environment as indicated to enhance safety.
Maintain treatment regimen to control/eliminate seizure activity.

CAREGIVERS WILL:

> **Knowledge: Personal Safety (NOC)**

Identify actions/measures to take when seizure activity occurs.

ACTIONS/INTERVENTIONS	RATIONALE

> **Seizure Precautions (NIC)**

Independent

Explore with patient the various stimuli that may precipitate seizure activity.	Alcohol, various drugs, and other stimuli (e.g., loss of sleep, flashing lights, prolonged television viewing) may increase brain activity, thereby increasing the potential for seizure activity.
Discuss seizure warning signs (if appropriate) and usual seizure pattern. Teach SO to recognize warning signs and how to care for patient during and after seizure.	Enables patient to protect self from injury and recognize changes that require notification of physician/further intervention. Knowing what to do when seizure occurs can prevent injury/complications and decrease SO's feelings of helplessness.

ACTIONS/INTERVENTIONS	RATIONALE

Independent

Keep padded side rails up with bed in lowest position, or place bed up against wall and pad floor if rails not available.

Minimizes injury should seizures (frequent/generalized) occur while patient is in bed.

Encourage patient not to smoke except while supervised.

May cause burns if cigarette is accidentally dropped during aura/seizure activity.

Evaluate need for/provide protective headgear.

Use of helmet may provide added protection for individuals who suffer recurrent/severe seizures.

Use tympanic thermometer when necessary to take temperature.

Reduces risk of patient biting and breaking glass thermometer or suffering injury if sudden seizure activity should occur.

Seizure Management (NIC)

Maintain strict bedrest if prodromal signs/aura experienced. Explain necessity for these actions.

Patient may feel restless/need to ambulate or even defecate during aural phase, thereby inadvertently removing self from safe environment and easy observation. Understanding importance of providing for own safety needs may enhance patient cooperation.

Stay with patient during/after seizure.

Promotes patient safety.

Turn head to side/suction airway as indicated. Insert plastic airway/bite block or soft roll between teeth (if jaw relaxed).

Helps maintain airway and reduces risk of oral trauma but should not be "forced" or inserted when teeth are clenched because dental and soft tissue damage may result. *Note:* Wooden tongue blades should not be used because they may splinter and break in patient's mouth. (Refer to ND: Airway Clearance/Breathing Pattern, ineffective, risk for, p. 234.)

Cradle head, place on soft area, or assist to floor if out of bed. Do not attempt to restrain.

Gentle guiding of extremities reduces risk of physical injury when patient lacks voluntary muscle control. *Note:* If attempt is made to restrain patient during seizure, erratic movements may increase, and patient may injure self or others.

Document preseizure activity, presence of aura or unusual behavior, type of seizure activity (e.g., location/duration of motor activity, loss of consciousness, incontinence, eye activity, respiratory impairment/cyanosis), and frequency/recurrence. Note whether patient fell, expressed vocalizations, drooled, or had automatisms (e.g., lip-smacking, chewing, picking at clothes.)

Helps to localize the cerebral area of involvement.

Perform neurological/vital sign check after seizure, e.g., level of consciousness, orientation, ability to comply with simple commands, ability to speak; memory of incident, weakness/motor deficits; blood pressure (BP), pulse/respiratory rate.

Documents postictal state and time/completeness of recovery to normal state. May identify additional safety concerns to be addressed.

Reorient patient following seizure activity.

Patient may be confused, disoriented, and possibly amnesic after the seizure and need help to regain control and alleviate anxiety.

Allow postictal "automatic" behavior without interfering while providing environmental protection.

May display behavior (of motor or psychic origin) that seems inappropriate/irrelevant for time and place. Attempts to control or prevent activity may result in patient becoming aggressive/combative.

ACTIONS/INTERVENTIONS	RATIONALE
Independent	
Investigate reports of pain.	May be result of repetitive muscle contractions or symptom of injury incurred, requiring further evaluation/intervention.
Observe for status epilepticus, i.e., one tonic-clonic seizure after another in rapid succession.	This is a life-threatening emergency that if left untreated could cause metabolic acidosis, hyperthermia, hypoglycemia, arrhythmias, hypoxia, increased intracranial pressure, airway obstruction, and respiratory arrest. Immediate intervention is required to control seizure activity and prevent permanent injury/death. *Note:* Although absence seizures may become static, they are not usually life-threatening.
Collaborative	
Administer medications as indicated:	Specific drug therapy depends on seizure type, with some patients requiring polytherapy or frequent medication adjustments.
Antiepileptic drugs, AEDs, e.g., phenytoin (Dilantin), primidone (Mysoline), carbamazepine (Tegretol), clonazepam (Klonopin), valproic acid (Depakene); divalproex (Depakote);	AEDs raise the seizure threshold by stabilizing nerve cell membranes, reducing the excitability of the neurons, or through direct action on the limbic system, thalamus, and hypothalamus. Goal is optimal suppression of seizure activity with lowest possible dose of drug and with fewest side effects. *Note:* Some patients require polytherapy or frequent medication adjustments to control seizure activity. This increases the risk of adverse reactions and problems with adherence.
Topiramate (Topamax);	Adjunctive therapy for partial seizures or an alternative for patients when seizures are not adequately controlled by other drugs.
Phenobarbital (Luminal);	Potentiates/enhances effects of AEDs and allows for lower dosage to reduce side effects.
Diazepam (Valium), Diastat rectal gel;	May be used alone (or in combination with phenobarbital) as a first-line drug to suppress status seizure activity. Diastat, a gel, may be administered rectally, even in the home setting to reduce frequency of seizures and need for additional medical care.
Glucose, thiamine.	May be given to restore metabolic balance if seizure is induced by hypoglycemia or alcohol.
Monitor/document AED drug levels, corresponding side effects, and frequency of seizure activity.	Standard therapeutic level may not be optimal for individual patient if untoward side effects develop or seizures are not controlled.
Monitor CBC, electrolytes, glucose levels.	Identifies factors that aggravate/decrease seizure threshold.
Prepare for surgery/electrode implantation as indicated.	Vagal nerve stimulator, magnetic beam therapy, or other surgical intervention (e.g., temporal lobectomy) may be done for intractable seizures or well-localized epileptogenic lesions when patient is disabled and at high risk for serious injury.

ACTIONS/INTERVENTIONS	RATIONALE
Airway Management (NIC)	
Independent	
Encourage patient to empty mouth of dentures/foreign objects if aura occurs and to avoid chewing gum/sucking lozenges if seizures occur without warning.	Reduces risk of aspiration/foreign bodies lodging in pharynx.
Place in lying position, flat surface; turn head to side during seizure activity.	Promotes drainage of secretions; prevents tongue from obstructing airway.
Loosen clothing from neck/chest and abdominal areas.	Facilitates breathing/chest expansion.
Insert bite stick/plastic airway or soft roll as indicated and only if jaw is relaxed.	If inserted before jaw is tightened, these devices may prevent biting of tongue and facilitate suctioning/respiratory support if required. Airway adjunct may be indicated after cessation of seizure activity if patient is unconscious and unable to maintain safe position of tongue.
Suction as needed.	Reduces risk of aspiration/asphyxiation.
Collaborative	
Administer supplemental oxygen/bag ventilate as needed postictally.	May reduce cerebral hypoxia resulting from decreased circulation/oxygenation secondary to vascular spasm during seizure. *Note:* Artificial ventilation during general seizure activity is of limited or no benefit because it is not possible to move air in/out of lungs during sustained contraction of respiratory musculature. As seizure abates, respiratory function will return unless a secondary problem exists (e.g., foreign body/aspiration).
Prepare for/assist with intubation, if indicated.	Presence of prolonged apnea postictally may require ventilatory support.

Possibly evidenced by

Verbalization about changed lifestyle

Fear of rejection; negative feelings about body

Change in self-perception of role

Change in usual patterns of responsibility

Lack of follow-through/nonparticipation in therapy

DESIRED OUTCOMES/EVALUATION CRITERIA—PATIENT WILL:

Self-Esteem (NOC)

Identify feelings and methods for coping with negative perception of self.

Verbalize increased sense of self-esteem in relation to diagnosis.

Verbalize realistic perception and acceptance of self in changed role/lifestyle.

ACTIONS/INTERVENTIONS	RATIONALE
Self-Esteem Enhancement (NIC)	
Independent	
Discuss feelings about diagnosis, perception of threat to self. Encourage expression of feelings.	Reactions vary among individuals, and previous knowledge/experience with this condition affects acceptance of therapeutic regimen. Verbalization of fears, anger, and concerns about future implications can help patient begin to accept/deal with situation.
Identify possible/anticipated public reaction to condition. Encourage patient to refrain from concealing problem.	Provides opportunity to problem-solve responses and provides measure of control over situation. Concealment is destructive to self-esteem (potentiates denial), blocking progress in dealing with problem and may actually increase risk of injury/negative response when seizure does occur.
Explore with patient current/past successes and strengths.	Focusing on positive aspects can help alleviate feelings of guilt/self-consciousness and help patient begin to accept manageability of condition.
Avoid overprotecting patient; encourage activities, providing supervision/monitoring when indicated.	Participation in as many experiences as possible can lessen depression about limitations. Observation/supervision may need to be provided for such activities as gymnastics, climbing, and water sports.
Determine attitudes/capabilities of SO. Help individual realize that his/her feelings are normal; however, guilt and blame are not helpful.	Negative expectations from SO may affect patient's sense of competency/self-esteem and interfere with support received from SO, limiting potential for optimal management/personal growth.
Stress importance of staff/SO remaining calm during seizure activity.	Anxiety of caregivers is contagious and can be conveyed to the patient, increasing/multiplying individual's own negative perceptions of situation/self.
Refer patient/SO to support group, e.g., Epilepsy Foundation of America and National Association of Epilepsy Centers.	Provides opportunity to gain information, support, and ideas for dealing with problems from others who share similar experiences.
Discuss referral for psychotherapy with patient/SO.	Seizures have a profound effect on personal self-esteem, and patient/SO may feel guilt over perceived limitations and public stigma. Counseling can help overcome feelings of inferiority/self-consciousness.

NURSING DIAGNOSIS: Knowledge Deficit [Learning Need] regarding condition, prognosis, treatment regimen, self care, and discharge needs

May be related to

Lack of exposure, unfamiliarity with resources

Information misinterpretation

Lack of recall; cognitive limitation

Possibly evidenced by

Questions, statement of concerns

Increased frequency/lack of control of seizure activity

Lack of follow-through of drug regimen

DESIRED OUTCOMES/EVALUATION CRITERIA—PATIENT WILL:

Knowledge: Disease Process (NOC)

Verbalize understanding of disorder and various stimuli that may increase/potentiate seizure activity.

Knowledge: Personal Safety (NOC)

Initiate necessary lifestyle/behavior changes as indicated.

Knowledge: Treatment Regimen (NOC)

Adhere to prescribed drug regimen.

ACTIONS/INTERVENTIONS	RATIONALE
Teaching: Disease Process (NIC)	
Independent	
Review pathology/prognosis of condition and lifelong need for treatment as indicated. Discuss patient's particular trigger factors (e.g., flashing lights, hyperventilation, loud noises, video games, TV viewing)	Provides opportunity to clarify/dispel misconceptions and present condition as something that is manageable within a normal lifestyle.
Review possible effects of hormonal changes.	Alterations in hormonal levels that occur during menstruation and pregnancy may increase risk of seizures.
Discuss significance of maintaining good general health, e.g., adequate diet, rest, moderate exercise, and avoidance of exhaustion, alcohol, caffeine, and stimulant drugs.	Regularity and moderation in activities may aid in reducing/controlling precipitating factors, enhancing sense of general well-being, and strengthening coping ability and self-esteem. *Note:* Too little sleep or too much alcohol can precipitate seizure activity in some people.
Review importance of good oral hygiene and regular dental care.	Reduces risk of oral infections and gingival hyperplasia.
Identify necessity/promote acceptance of actual limitations; discuss safety measures regarding driving, using mechanical equipment, climbing ladders, swimming, and hobbies.	Reduces risk of injury to self or others, especially if seizures occur without warning.
Discuss local laws/restrictions pertaining to persons with epilepsy/seizure disorder. Encourage awareness but not necessarily acceptance of these policies.	Although legal/civil rights of persons with epilepsy have improved during the past decade, restrictions still exist in some states pertaining to obtaining a driver's license, sterilization, worker's compensation, and required reportability to state agencies.

ACTIONS/INTERVENTIONS	RATIONALE

Teaching: Prescribed Medication (NIC)

Independent

Review medication regimen, necessity of taking drugs as ordered, and not discontinuing therapy without physician supervision. Include directions for missed dose.

Lack of cooperation with medication regimen is a leading cause of seizure breakthrough. Patient needs to know risks of status epilepticus resulting from abrupt withdrawal of anticonvulsants. Depending on the drug dose and frequency, patient may be instructed to take missed dose if remembered within a predetermined time frame.

Recommend taking drugs with meals if appropriate.

May reduce incidence of gastric irritation, nausea/vomiting.

Discuss nuisance and adverse side effects of particular drugs, e.g., drowsiness, fatigue, lethargy, hyperactivity, sleep disturbances, gingival hypertrophy, visual disturbances, nausea/vomiting, rashes, syncope/ataxia, birth defects, aplastic anemia.

May indicate need for change in dosage/choice of drug therapy. Promotes involvement/participation in decision-making process, and awareness of potential long-term effects of drug therapy and provides opportunity to minimize/prevent complications.

Provide information about potential drug interactions and necessity of notifying other healthcare providers of drug regimen.

Knowledge of anticonvulsant use reduces risk of prescribing drugs that may interact, thus altering seizure threshold or therapeutic effect. For example, phenytoin (Dilantin) potentiates anticoagulant effect of warfarin (Coumadin), whereas isoniazid (INH) and chloramphenicol (Chloromycetin) increase the effect of phenytoin (Dilantin), and some antibiotics (e.g., erythromycin) can cause elevation of serum level of carbamazepine (Tegretol), possibly to toxic levels.

Encourage patient to wear identification tag/bracelet stating the presence of a seizure disorder.

Expedites treatment and diagnosis in emergency situations.

Stress need for routine follow-up care/laboratory testing as indicated, e.g., CBC should be monitored biannually and in presence of sore throat/fever, signs of other infection.

Therapeutic needs may change and/or serious drug side effects (e.g., agranulocytosis or toxicity) may develop.

POTENTIAL CONSIDERATIONS following acute hospitalization (dependent on patient's age, physical condition/presence of complications, personal resources, and life responsibilities)

Injury, risk for—weakness, balancing difficulties, cognitive limitations/altered consciousness, loss of large or small muscle coordination.

Self-Esteem (specify)—stigma associated with condition, perception of being out of control, personal vulnerability, negative evaluation of self/capabilities.

Therapeutic Regimen: Individual, ineffective management—social support deficits, perceived benefit (versus side effects of medication), perceived susceptibility (possible long periods of remission).

CRANIOCEREBRAL TRAUMA (ACUTE REHABILITATIVE PHASE)

Craniocerebral trauma, also called head or brain injury (open or closed) includes skull fractures, brain concussion, cerebral contusion/laceration, and hemorrhage (subarachnoid, subdural, epidural, intracerebral, brainstem). Primary injury occurs from a direct or indirect blow to the head, causing acceleration/deceleration of the brain. Secondary brain injury results from diffuse intracerebral axonal injury, intracranial hypertension, hypoxemia, hypercapnea, or systemic hypotension. Cerebral concussion is the most common form of head injury.

Consequences of brain injury range from no apparent neurological disturbance to a persistent vegetative state or death. Therefore, every head injury must be considered potentially dangerous.

CARE SETTING

This plan of care focuses on acute care and acute inpatient rehabilitation. Brain injury care for those experiencing moderate to severe trauma progresses along a continuum of care, beginning with acute inpatient hospital care and inpatient rehabilitation to subacute and outpatient rehabilitation, as well as home- and community-based services.

RELATED CONCERNS

Cerebrovascular accident/stroke, page 257
Psychosocial aspects of care, page 809
Seizure disorders/epilepsy, page 228
Surgical intervention, page 828
Thrombophlebitis: deep vein thrombosis, page 115
Total nutritional support: parenteral/enteral feeding, page 508
Upper gastrointestinal/esophageal bleeding, page 333

Patient Assessment Database

Data depend on type, location, and severity of injury and may be complicated by additional injury to other vital organs.

ACTIVITY/REST

May report: Weakness, fatigue, clumsiness, loss of balance

May exhibit: Altered consciousness, lethargy
Hemiparesis, quadriparesis
Unsteady gait (ataxia); balance problems
Orthopedic injuries (trauma)
Loss of muscle tone, muscle spasticity

CIRCULATION

May exhibit: Normal or altered BP (hypotension or hypertension)
Changes in heart rate (bradycardia, tachycardia alternating with bradycardia, other dysrhythmias)

EGO INTEGRITY

May report: Behavior or personality changes (subtle to dramatic)

May exhibit: Anxiety, irritability, delirium, agitation, confusion, depression, impulsivity

ELIMINATION

May exhibit: Bowel/bladder incontinence or dysfunction

FOOD/FLUID

May report: Nausea/vomiting, changes in appetite

May exhibit: Vomiting (may be projectile)
Swallowing problems (coughing, drooling, dysphagia)

NEUROSENSORY

May report:
Loss of consciousness, variable levels of awareness, amnesia surrounding trauma events
Vertigo, syncope, tinnitus, hearing loss
Tingling, numbness in extremity
Visual changes, e.g., decreased acuity, diplopia, photophobia, loss of part of visual field
Loss of/changes in senses of taste or smell

May exhibit:
Alteration in consciousness from lethargy to coma
Mental status changes (orientation, alertness/responsiveness, attention, concentration, problem solving, emotional affect/behavior, memory)
Pupillary changes (response to light, symmetry), deviation of eyes, inability to follow
Loss of senses, e.g., taste, smell, hearing
Facial asymmetry
Unequal, weak handgrip
Absent/weak deep tendon reflexes
Apraxia, hemiparesis, quadriparesis
Posturing (decorticate, decerebrate); seizure activity
Heightened sensitivity to touch and movement
Altered sensation to parts of body
Difficulty in understanding self/limbs in relation to environment (proprioception)

PAIN/DISCOMFORT

May report: Headache of variable intensity and location (usually persistent/long-lasting)
May exhibit: Facial grimacing, withdrawal response to painful stimuli, restlessness, moaning

RESPIRATION

May exhibit:
Changes in breathing patterns (e.g., periods of apnea alternating with hyperventilation)
Noisy respirations, stridor, choking
Rhonchi, wheezes (possible aspiration)

SAFETY

May report: Recent trauma/accidental injuries
May exhibit:
Fractures/dislocations
Impaired vision, visual field disturbances, abnormal eye movements
Skin: Head/facial lacerations, abrasions, discoloration, e.g., raccoon eyes, Battle's sign around ears (trauma signs)
Drainage from ears/nose (CSF)
Impaired cognition
Range-of-motion (ROM) impairment, loss of muscle tone, general strength; paralysis
Fever, instability in internal regulation of body temperature

SOCIAL INTERACTION

May exhibit:
Expressive or receptive aphasia, unintelligible speech, repetitive speech, dysarthria, anomia
Difficulty dealing with noisy environment, interacting with more than one or two individuals at a time
Changes in role/family structure related to illness/condition

TEACHING/LEARNING

May report: Use of alcohol/other drugs
Discharge plan considerations: **DRG projected mean length of inpatient stay: 17.1 days (inclusive/multiple care setting)**
May require assistance with self-care, ambulation, transportation, food preparation, shopping, treatments, medications, homemaker/maintenance tasks; change in physical layout of home or placement in living facility other than home

Refer to section at end of plan for postdischarge considerations.

DIAGNOSTIC STUDIES

CT scan (with/without contrast): Screening image of choice in acute brain injury. Identifies space-occupying lesions, hemorrhage, skull fractures, brain tissue shift.

MRI: Uses similar to those of CT scan but more sensitive than CT for detecting cerebral trauma, determining neurological deficits not explained by CT, evaluating prolonged interval of disturbed consciousness, defining evidence of previous trauma superimposed on acute trauma.

Cerebral angiography: Demonstrates cerebral circulatory anomalies, e.g., brain tissue shifts secondary to edema, hemorrhage, trauma.

Serial EEG: May reveal presence or development of pathological waves. EEG is not generally indicated in the immediate period of emergency response, evaluation, and treatment. If the patient fails to improve, EEG may help in diagnostic evaluation for seizures, focal or diffuse encephalopathy.

X-rays: Detect changes in bony structure (fractures), shifts of midline structures (bleeding/edema), bone fragments.

Brainstem auditory evoked responses (BAER): Determines levels of cortical and brainstem function.

PET/SPECT tomography: Detects changes in metabolic activity in the brain. (These procedures are not in widespread clinical use, but are more often used for research.)

Audiometry, otology, and vestibular function tests: Diagnostic procedures that identify hearing loss reasons for balance problems and/or eighth cranial nerve dysfunction.

Lumbar puncture and CSF analysis: May be performed in patient with suspected or known increased intracranial pressure when CT or MRI is not diagnostic. Generally contraindicated in acute trauma.

ABGs: Determines presence of ventilation or oxygenation problems that may exacerbate/increase intracranial pressure.

Serum chemistry/electrolytes: May reveal imbalances that contribute to increased intracranial pressure (ICP)/changes in mentation.

Toxicology screen: Detects drugs that may be responsible for/potentiate loss of consciousness.

Serum anticonvulsant levels: May be done to ensure that therapeutic level is adequate to prevent seizure activity.

NURSING PRIORITIES

1. Maximize cerebral perfusion/function.
2. Prevent/minimize complications.
3. Promote optimal functioning/return to preinjury level.
4. Support coping process and family recovery.
5. Provide information about condition/prognosis, potential complications, treatment plan, and resources.

DISCHARGE GOALS

1. Cerebral function improved; neurological deficits resolving/stabilized.
2. Complications prevented or minimized.
3. Activities of daily living (ADLs) needs met by self or with assistance of other(s).
4. Family acknowledging reality of situation and involved in recovery program.
5. Condition/prognosis, complications, and treatment regimen understood and available resources identified.
6. Plan in place to meet needs after discharge.

NURSING DIAGNOSIS: Tissue Perfusion, altered cerebral

May be related to

Interruption of blood flow by space-occupying lesions (hemorrhage, hematoma); cerebral edema (localized or generalized response to injury, metabolic alterations, drug/alcohol overdose); decreased systemic BP/hypoxia (hypovolemia, cardiac dysrhythmias)

Possibly evidenced by

Altered level of consciousness; memory loss

Changes in motor/sensory responses, restlessness

Changes in vital signs

Neurological Status (NOC)

Maintain usual/improved level of consciousness, cognition, and motor/sensory function. Demonstrate stable vital signs and absence of signs of increased ICP.

ACTIONS/INTERVENTIONS	RATIONALE

Neurological Monitoring (NIC)

Independent

Determine factors related to individual situation, cause for coma/decreased cerebral perfusion, and potential for increased ICP.

Influences choice of interventions. Deterioration in neurological signs/symptoms or failure to improve after initial insult may reflect decreased intracranial adaptive capacity, requiring the patient be transferred to critical care for monitoring of ICP and/or surgical intervention.

Monitor/document neurological status frequently and compare with baseline, e.g., Glasgow Coma Scale during first 48 hr:

Assesses trends in level of consciousness (LOC) and potential for increased ICP and is useful in determining location, extent, and progression/resolution of central nervous system (CNS) damage.

Evaluate eye opening, e.g., spontaneous (awake), opens only to painful stimuli, keeps eyes closed (coma);

Determines arousal ability/level of consciousness.

Assess verbal response; note whether patient is alert; oriented to person, place, and time; or is confused; uses inappropriate words/phrases that make little sense;

Measures appropriateness of speech and content of consciousness. If minimal damage has occurred in the cerebral cortex, the patient may be aroused by verbal stimuli but may appear drowsy or uncooperative. More extensive damage to the cerebral cortex may be displayed by slow response to commands, lapsing into sleep when not stimulated, disorientation, and stupor. Damage to midbrain, pons, and medulla are manifested by lack of appropriate responses to stimuli.

Assess motor response to simple commands, noting purposeful (obeys command, attempts to push stimulus away) and nonpurposeful (posturing) movement. Note limb movement and document right and left sides separately.

Measures overall awareness and ability to respond to external stimuli and best indicates state of consciousness in the patient whose eyes are closed because of trauma or who is aphasic. Consciousness and involuntary movement are integrated if the patient can both grasp and release the tester's hand, or hold up two fingers on command. Purposeful movement can include grimacing or withdrawing from painful stimuli or movements that the patient desires, e.g., sitting up. Other movements (posturing and abnormal flexion of extremities) usually indicate diffuse cortical damage. Absence of spontaneous movement on one side of the body indicates damage to the motor tracts in the opposite cerebral hemisphere.

Monitor vital signs, e.g.:

BP, noting onset of/continuing systolic hypertension and widening pulse pressure; observe for hypotension in multiple trauma patient;

Normally, autoregulation maintains constant cerebral blood flow despite fluctuations in systemic BP. Loss of autoregulation may follow local or diffuse cerebrovascular damage. Elevating systolic BP accompanied by decreasing diastolic BP (widening pulse pressure) is an ominous sign of increased ICP when accompanied by decreased level of consciousness. Hypovolemia/hypotension (associated with multiple trauma) may also result in cerebral ischemia/damage.

Heart rate/rhythm, noting bradycardia, alternating bradycardia/tachycardia, other dysrhythmias;

Changes in rate (most often bradycardia) and dysrhythmias may develop, reflecting brainstem pressure/injury in the absence of underlying cardiac disease.

Respirations, noting patterns and rhythm, e.g., periods of apnea after hyperventilation, Cheyne-Stokes respiration.

Irregularities can suggest location of cerebral insult/increasing ICP and need for further intervention, including possible respiratory support. (Refer to ND: Breathing Pattern, risk for ineffective, following.)

Evaluate pupils, noting size, shape, equality, light reactivity.

Pupil reactions are regulated by the oculomotor (III) cranial nerve and are useful in determining if the brainstem is intact. Pupil size/equality is determined by balance between parasympathetic and sympathetic enervation. Response to light reflects combined function of optic (II) and oculomotor (III) cranial nerves.

Assess for changes in vision, e.g., double vision (diplopia), blurred vision, alterations in visual field, depth perception.

Visual alterations, which can result from microscopic damage to areas of the brain, have consequent safety concerns and influence choice of interventions.

Assess position/movement of eyes, noting whether in midposition or deviated to side or downward. Note loss of doll's eyes (oculocephalic reflex).

Position and movement of eyes help localize area of brain involvement. An early sign of increased ICP is impaired abduction of eyes, indicating pressure/injury to the fifth cranial nerve. Loss of doll's eyes indicates deterioration in brainstem function and poor prognosis.

Note presence/absence of reflexes (e.g., blink, cough, gag, Babinski).

Altered reflexes reflect injury at level of midbrain or brainstem and have direct implications for patient safety. Loss of blink reflex suggests damage to the pons and medulla. Absence of cough and gag reflexes reflect damage to medulla. Presence of Babinski reflex indicates injury along pyramidal pathways in the brain.

Cerebral Perfusion Promotion (NIC)

Monitor temperature and regulate environmental temperature as indicated. Limit use of blankets; administer tepid sponge bath in presence of fever. Wrap extremities in blankets when hypothermia blanket is used.

Fever may reflect damage to hypothalamus. Increased metabolic needs and oxygen consumption occur (especially with fever and shivering), which can further increase ICP.

Monitor I&O. Weigh as indicated. Note skin turgor, status of mucous membranes.

Useful indicators of total body water, which is an integral part of tissue perfusion. Cerebral trauma/ischemia can result in diabetes insipidus (DI) or syndrome of inappropriate antiduretic hormone (SIADH). Alterations may lead to hypovolemia or vascular engorgement, either of which can negatively affect cerebral pressure.

Maintain head/neck in midline or neutral position, support with small towel rolls and pillows. Avoid placing head on large pillows.

Turning head to one side compresses the jugular veins and inhibits cerebral venous drainage, thereby increasing ICP.

ACTIONS/INTERVENTIONS	RATIONALE
Independent	
Provide rest periods between care activities and limit duration of procedures.	Continual activity can increase ICP by producing a cumulative stimulant effect.
Decrease extraneous stimuli and provide comfort measures, e.g., back massage, quiet environment, soft voice, gentle touch.	Provides calming effect, reduces adverse physiological response, and promotes rest to maintain/lower ICP.
Help patient avoid/limit coughing, vomiting, straining at stool/bearing down when possible. Reposition patient slowly; prevent patient from bending knees and pushing heels against mattress to move up in bed.	These activities increase intrathoracic and intra-abdominal pressures, which can increase ICP.
Avoid/limit use of restraints.	Mechanical restraints may enhance fight response, increasing ICP. *Note:* Cautious use may be indicated to prevent injury to patient.
Hyperventilate/hyperoxygenate patient before and after suctioning bronchial tree. Limit number and duration of suctioning passes (e.g., two passes less than 10 sec each).	Prevents hypoxia and associated vasoconstriction that can impair cerebral perfusion.
Encourage SO to talk to patient.	Familiar voices of family/SO appear to have a relaxing effect on many comatose patients, which can reduce ICP.
Investigate increasing restlessness, moaning, guarding behaviors.	These nonverbal cues may indicate increasing ICP or reflect presence of pain when patient is unable to verbalize complaints. Unrelieved pain can in turn aggravate/potentiate increased ICP.
Palpate for bladder distension, maintain patency of urinary drainage if used. Monitor for constipation.	May trigger autonomic responses potentiating elevation of ICP.
Observe for seizure activity and protect patient from injury.	Seizures can occur as a result of cerebral irritation, hypoxia, or increased ICP; additionally, seizures can further elevate ICP, compounding cerebral damage.
Assess for nuchal rigidity, twitching, increased restlessness, irritability, onset of seizure activity.	Indicative of meningeal irritation, which may occur because of interruption of dura, and/or development of infection during acute or recovery period of brain injury.
Collaborative	
Elevate head of bed gradually to 15–30 degrees as tolerated/indicated.	Promotes venous drainage from head, thereby reducing cerebral congestion and edema/risk of increased ICP.
Restrict fluid intake as indicated. Administer IV fluids with control device.	Fluid restriction may be needed to reduce cerebral edema; minimize fluctuations in vascular load, BP, and ICP.
Administer supplemental oxygen as indicated.	Reduces hypoxemia, which may increase cerebral vasodilation and blood volume, elevating ICP.
Monitor ABGs/pulse oximetry.	Determines respiratory sufficiency (presence of hypoxia/acidosis) and indicates therapy needs.
Administer medications as indicated:	
Diuretics, e.g., mannitol (Osmitrol), furosemide (Lasix);	Diuretics may be used in acute phase to draw water from brain cells, reducing cerebral edema and ICP.
Steroids, e.g., dexamethasone (Decadron), methylprednisolone (Medrol);	Decreases inflammation, reducing tissue edema. *Note:* Use and efficacy of steroids continues to be debated in this diagnosis.

ACTIONS/INTERVENTIONS	RATIONALE

Independent

Anticonvulsant, e.g., phenytoin (Dilantin);

Dilantin is the drug of choice for treatment and prevention of seizure activity in immediate post-traumatic period. Prophylactic anticonvulsive therapy may be continued for an indeterminate period of time.

Chlorpromazine (Thorazine);

Useful in treating posturing and shivering, which can increase ICP. *Note:* This drug can lower the seizure threshold or precipitate Dilantin toxicity.

Mild analgesics, e.g., codeine;

May be indicated to relieve pain and its negative effect on ICP but should be used with caution to prevent respiratory embarrassment.

Sedatives, e.g., diphenhydramine (Benadryl);

May be used to control restlessness, agitation.

Antipyretics, e.g., acetaminophen (Tylenol).

Reduces/controls fever and its deleterious effect on cerebral metabolism/oxygen needs.

Prepare for surgical intervention, if indicated.

Craniotomy or trephination ("burr" holes) may be done to remove bone fragments, elevate depressed fractures, evacuate hematoma, control hemorrhage, and debride necrotic tissue.

NURSING DIAGNOSIS: Breathing Pattern, risk for ineffective

Risk factors may include
Neuromuscular impairment (injury to respiratory center of brain)
Perception or cognitive impairment
Tracheobronchial obstruction

Possibly evidenced by
[Not applicable; presence of signs and symptoms establishes an *actual* diagnosis]

DESIRED OUTCOMES/EVALUATION CRITERIA—PATIENT WILL:

Respiratory status: Ventilation (NOC)

Maintain a normal/effective respiratory pattern, free of cyanosis, with ABGs/pulse oximetry within patient's acceptable range.

ACTIONS/INTERVENTIONS	RATIONALE

Airway Management (NIC)

Independent

Monitor rate, rhythm, depth of respiration. Note breathing irregularities, e.g., apneustic, ataxic, or cluster breathing.

Changes may indicate onset of pulmonary complications (common following brain injury) or indicate location/extent of brain involvement. Slow respiration, periods of apnea (apneustic, ataxic, or cluster breathing patterns) are signs of brainstem injury and warn of impending respiratory arrest.

ACTIONS/INTERVENTIONS	RATIONALE
Independent	
Note competence of gag/swallow reflexes and patient's ability to protect own airway. Insert airway adjunct as indicated.	Ability to mobilize or clear secretions is important to airway maintenance. Loss of swallow or cough reflex may indicate need for artificial airway/intubation. *Note:* Soft nasopharyngeal airways may be preferred to prevent stimulation of the gag reflex caused by hard oropharyngeal airway, which can lead to excessive coughing and increased ICP.
Elevate head of bed as permitted, position on sides as indicated.	Facilitates lung expansion/ventilation and reduces risk of airway obstruction by tongue.
Encourage deep breathing if patient is conscious.	Prevents/reduces atelectasis.
Suction with extreme caution, no longer than 10–15 sec. Note character, color, odor of secretions.	Suctioning is usually required if patient is comatose or immobile and unable to clear own airway. Deep tracheal suctioning should be done with caution, because it can cause or aggravate hypoxia, which produces vasoconstriction, adversely affecting cerebral perfusion.
Auscultate breath sounds, noting areas of hypoventilation and presence of adventitious sounds (crackles, rhonchi, wheezes).	Identifies pulmonary problems such as atelectasis, congestion, and airway obstruction, which may jeopardize cerebral oxygenation and/or indicate onset of pulmonary infection (common complication of head injury).
Monitor use of respiratory depressant drugs, e.g., sedatives.	Can increase respiratory embarrassment/complications.
Collaborative	
Monitor/graph serial ABGs, pulse oximetry.	Determines respiratory sufficiency, acid-base balance, and therapy needs.
Review chest x-rays.	Reveals ventilatory state and signs of developing complications (e.g., atelectasis, pneumonia).
Administer supplemental oxygen.	Maximizes arterial oxygenation and aids in prevention of hypoxia. If respiratory center is depressed, mechanical ventilation may be required.
Assist with chest physiotherapy when indicated.	Although contraindicated in patient with acutely elevated ICP, these measures are often necessary in acute rehabilitation phase to mobilize and clear lung fields and reduce atelectasis/pulmonary complications.

NURSING DIAGNOSIS: Sensory-Perceptual alterations (specify)

May be related to
Altered sensory reception, transmission and/or integration (neurological trauma or deficit)

Possibly evidenced by
Disorientation to time, place, person
Change in usual response to stimuli
Motor incoordination, alterations in posture, inability to tell position of body parts (proprioception)
Altered communication patterns
Visual and auditory distortions
Poor concentration, altered thought processes/bizarre thinking
Exaggerated emotional responses, change in behavior pattern

Cognitive Ability (NOC)

Regain/maintain usual level of consciousness and perceptual functioning.
Acknowledge changes in ability and presence of residual involvement.
Demonstrate behaviors/lifestyle changes to compensate for/overcome deficit.

ACTIONS/INTERVENTIONS

Reality Orientation (NIC)

Independent

Evaluate/continually monitor changes in orientation, ability to speak, mood/affect, sensorium, thought process.

Assess sensory awareness, e.g., response to touch, hot/cold, dull/sharp, and awareness of motion and location of body parts. Note problems with vision, other senses.

Observe behavioral responses, e.g., hostility, crying, inappropriate affect, agitation, hallucinations. (Refer to ND: Thought Processes, altered, following.)

Document specific changes in abilities, e.g., focusing/tracking with both eyes, following simple verbal instructions, answering "yes" or "no" to questions, feeding self with dominant hand.

Eliminate extraneous noise/stimuli as necessary.

Speak in calm, quiet voice. Use short, simple sentences. Maintain eye contact.

Ascertain/validate patient's perceptions, provide feedback. Reorient patient frequently to environment, staff, and procedures, especially if vision is impaired.

Provide meaningful stimulation: verbal (talk to patient), olfactory (e.g., oil of clove, coffee), tactile (touch, hand holding), and auditory (tapes, television, radio, visitors). Avoid physical or emotional isolation of patient.

Provide structured therapies, activities, and environment. Provide written schedule for patient to refer to on a regular basis.

Schedule adequate rest/uninterrupted sleep periods.

RATIONALE

Upper cerebral functions are often the first to be affected by altered circulation/oxygenation. Damage may occur at time of initial injury or develop later because of swelling or bleeding. Motor, perceptual, cognitive, and personality changes may develop and persist, with gradual normalization of responses, or changes may remain permanently to some degree.

Information is essential to patient safety. All sensory systems may be affected, with changes involving increased or decreased sensitivity or loss of sensation and/or the ability to perceive and respond appropriately to stimuli.

Individual responses may be variable but commonalities, such as emotional lability, increased irritability/frustration, apathy, and impulsiveness exist during recovery from brain injury. Documentation of behavior provides information needed for development of structured rehabilitation.

Helps localize areas of cerebral dysfunction and identifies signs of progress toward improved neurological function.

Reduces anxiety, exaggerated emotional responses/confusion associated with sensory overload.

Patient may have limited attention span/understanding during acute and recovery stages, and these measures can help patient attend to communication.

Assists patient to differentiate reality in the presence of altered perceptions. Cognitive dysfunction and/or visual deficits potentiate disorientation and anxiety.

Carefully selected sensory input may be useful for coma stimulation as well as for documenting progress during cognitive retraining.

Promotes consistency and reassurance, reducing anxiety associated with the unknown. Promotes sense of control/cognitive retraining.

Reduces fatigue, prevents exhaustion, and improves sleep. *Note:* Absence of rapid eye movement (REM) sleep is known to aggravate sensory-perceptual deficits.

ACTIONS/INTERVENTIONS

Independent

Use day/night lighting.

Allow adequate time for communication and performance of activities.

Provide patient safety, e.g., padded side rails, assistance with ambulation, protection from hot/sharp objects. Document perceptual deficit and compensatory activities on chart and at bedside.

Identify alternate ways of dealing with perceptual deficits, e.g., arrange bed, personal articles, food to take advantage of functional vision; describe where affected body parts are located.

Collaborative

Refer to physical, occupational, speech, and cognitive therapists.

RATIONALE

Provides for normal sense of passage of time and sleep/wake pattern.

Reduces frustration associated with altered abilities/delayed response pattern.

Agitation, impaired judgment, poor balance, and sensory deficits increase risk of patient injury.

Enables patient to progress toward independence, enhancing sense of control, while compensating for neurological deficits.

Interdisciplinary approach can create an integrated treatment plan based on the individual's unique combination of abilities/disabilities with focus on evaluation and functional improvement in physical, cognitive, and perceptual skills.

NURSING DIAGNOSIS: Thought Processes, altered

May be related to
Physiological changes; psychological conflicts

Possibly evidenced by
Memory deficit/changes in remote, recent, immediate memory
Distractibility, altered attention span/concentration
Disorientation to time, place, person, circumstances, and events
Impaired ability to make decisions, problem-solve, reason, abstract, or conceptualize
Personality changes; inappropriate social behavior

DESIRED OUTCOMES/EVALUATION CRITERIA—PATIENT WILL:

Distorted Thought Control (NOC)

Maintain/regain usual mentation and reality orientation.
Recognize changes in thinking/behavior.
Participate in therapeutic regimen/cognitive retraining.

ACTIONS/INTERVENTIONS

Delirium Management (NIC)

Independent

Assess attention span, distractibility. Note level of anxiety.

RATIONALE

Attention span/ability to attend/concentrate may be severely shortened, which both causes and potentiates anxiety, affecting thought processes.

ACTIONS/INTERVENTIONS	RATIONALE
Independent	
Confer with SO to compare past behaviors/preinjury personality with current responses.	Recovery from head injury includes a phase of agitation, angry responses, and disordered thought sequences/conversation. Hallucinations or altered interpretation of stimuli may have been present before the head injury or be part of developing sequelae of brain injury. *Note:* SOs often have difficulty accepting and dealing with patient's aberrant behavior and may require assistance in coping with situation.
Maintain consistency in staff assigned to patient, to the extent possible.	Provides patient with feelings of stability and control of situation.
Present reality concisely and briefly; avoid challenging illogical thinking.	Patient may be totally unaware of injury (amnesic) or of extent of injury, and therefore deny reality of injury. Structured reality orientation can reduce defensive reactions.
Provide information about injury process in relationship to symptoms. Explain procedures and reinforce explanations given by others.	Loss of internal structure (changes in memory, reasoning, and ability to conceptualize) and fear of the unknown affect processing and retention of information and can compound anxiety, confusion, and disorientation.
Review necessity of recurrent neurological evaluations.	Understanding that assessments are done frequently to prevent/limit complications and do not necessarily reflect seriousness of patient's condition, may help reduce anxiety.
Reduce provocative stimuli, negative criticism, arguments, and confrontations.	Reduces risk of triggering fight/flight response. Severely brain-injured patient may become violent or physically/verbally abusive.
Listen with regard to patient's verbalizations in spite of speech pattern/content.	Conveys interest and worth to individual, enhancing self-esteem and encouraging continued efforts.
Promote socialization within individual limitations.	Reinforcement of positive behaviors (e.g., appropriate interaction with others) may be helpful in relearning internal structure.
Encourage SO to provide current news/family happenings.	Promotes maintenance of contact with usual events, enhancing reality orientation and normalization of thinking.
Instruct in relaxation techniques. Provide diversional activities.	Can help refocus attention and reduce anxiety to manageable levels.
Maintain realistic expectations of patient's ability to control own behavior, comprehend, remember information.	It is important to maintain an expectation of the ability to improve and progress to a higher level of functioning, to maintain hope, and promote continued work of rehabilitation.
Avoid leaving patient alone when agitated, frightened.	Anxiety can lead to loss of control and escalate to panic. Support may provide calming effect, reducing anxiety and risk of injury.
Implement measures to control emotional outbursts/aggressive behavior if needed; e.g., tell patient to "stop," speak in a calm voice, remove patient from the situation, provide distraction, restrain for brief periods of time.	Patient may need help/external control to protect self or others from harm until internal control is regained. Restraints (physical holding, mechanical, pharmacological) should be used judiciously to avoid escalating violent, irrational behavior.

ACTIONS/INTERVENTIONS

Independent

Inform patient/SO that intellectual function, behavior, and emotional functioning will gradually improve but that some effects may persist for months or even be permanent.

Collaborative

Coordinate participation in cognitive retraining or rehabilitation program as indicated.

Refer to support groups, e.g., Brain Injury Association, social services, visiting nurse, and counseling/therapy as needed.

RATIONALE

Most brain-injured patients have persistent problems with concentration, memory, and problem solving. If brain injury was moderate to severe, recovery may be complete or residual effects may remain.

Assists patient with learning methods to compensate for disruption of cognitive skills. Addresses problems in concentration, memory, judgment, sequencing, and problem solving.

Additional long-term assistance may be helpful in supporting/sustaining recovery

---

NURSING DIAGNOSIS: Mobility, impaired physical

May be related to
Perceptual or cognitive impairment
Decreased strength/endurance
Restrictive therapies/safety precautions, e.g., bed rest, immobilization

Possibly evidenced by
Inability to purposefully move within the physical environment, including bed mobility, transfer, ambulation
Impaired coordination, limited range of motion, decreased muscle strength/control

DESIRED OUTCOMES/EVALUATION CRITERIA—PATIENT WILL:

Immobility Consequences: Physiological (NOC)

Maintain/increase strength and function of affected and/or compensatory body part(s).
Regain/maintain optimal position of function, as evidenced by absence of contractures, footdrop.

Mobility Level (NOC)

Demonstrate techniques/behaviors that enable resumption of activities.
Maintain skin integrity, bladder and bowel function.

ACTIONS/INTERVENTIONS

Exercise Therapy: Muscle Control (NIC)

Independent

Review functional ability and reasons for impairment.

Assess degree of immobility, using a scale to rate dependence (0–4).

RATIONALE

Identifies probable functional impairments and influences choice of interventions.

The patient may be completely independent (0), may require minimal assistance/equipment (1), moderate assistance/supervision/teaching (2), extensive assistance/equipment and devices (3), or be completely dependent on caregivers (4). Persons in all categories are at risk for injury, but those in categories 2–4 are at greatest risk.

ACTIONS/INTERVENTIONS	RATIONALE

Independent

Provide/assist with ROM exercises.

Maintains mobility and function of joints/functional alignment of extremities and reduces venous stasis.

Instruct/assist patient with exercise program and use of mobility aids. Increase activity and participation in self-care as tolerated.

Lengthy convalescence often follows brain injury, and physical reconditioning is an essential part of the program. Involving patient in planning and performing activities is important to promote patient cooperation/sustain program.

> ### Bed Rest Care (NIC)

Position patient to avoid skin/tissue pressure damage. Turn at regular intervals, and make small position changes between turns.

Regular turning more normally distributes body weight and promotes circulation to all areas. If paralysis or limited cognition is present, patient should be repositioned frequently.

Provide meticulous skin care, massaging with emollients. Remove wet linen/clothing, keep bedding free of wrinkles.

Promotes circulation and skin elasticity and reduces risk of skin excoriation.

Maintain functional body alignment, e.g., hips, feet, hands. Monitor for proper placement of devices and/or signs of pressure from devices.

Use of high-top tennis shoes, "space boots," and T-bar sheepskin devices can help prevent footdrop. Handsplints are variable and designed to prevent hand deformities and promote optimal function. Use of pillows, bedrolls, and sandbags can help prevent abnormal hip rotation.

Support head and trunk, arms and shoulders, feet and legs when patient is in wheelchair/recliner. Pad chair seat with foam or water-filled cushion, and assist patient to shift weight at frequent intervals.

Maintains comfortable, safe, and functional posture and prevents/reduces risk of skin breakdown.

Provide eye care, artificial tears; patch eyes as indicated.

Protects delicate eye tissues from drying. Patient may require patches during sleep to protect eyes from trauma if unable to keep eyes closed.

Monitor urinary output. Note color and odor of urine. Assist with bladder retraining when appropriate.

Indwelling catheter used during the acute phase of injury may be needed for an extended period of time before bladder retraining is possible. Once the catheter is removed, several methods of continence control may be tried, e.g., intermittent catheterization (for residual and complete emptying), external catheter, planned intervals on commode, incontinence pads.

Provide fluids, including cranberry juice, within individual tolerance (i.e., regarding neurological and cardiac concerns), as indicated.

Once past the acute phase of head injury and if patient has no other contraindicating factors, forcing fluids decreases risk of urinary tract infections/stone formation and provides other positive effects such as normal stool consistency and optimal skin turgor.

Monitor bowel elimination and provide for/assist with a regular bowel routine. Check for impacted stool; use digital stimulation as indicated. Sit patient upright on commode or stool at regular intervals. Add fiber/bulk/fruit juice to diet as appropriate.

A regular bowel routine requires simple but diligent measures to prevent complications. Stimulation of the internal rectal sphincter stimulates the bowel to empty automatically if stool is soft enough to do so. Upright position aids evacuation.

Inspect for localized tenderness, redness, skin warmth, muscle tension, and/or ropy veins in calves of legs. Observe for sudden dyspnea, tachypnea, fever, respiratory distress, chest pain.

Patient is at risk for development of deep vein thrombosis (DVT) and pulmonary embolus (PE), requiring prompt medical evaluation/intervention to prevent serious complications.

ACTIONS/INTERVENTIONS

Collaborative

Provide air/water mattress, kinetic therapy as appropriate.

| Exercise Therapy: Muscle Control (NIC) |

Refer to physical/occupational therapists as indicated.

RATIONALE

Equalizes tissue pressure, enhances circulation, and helps reduce venous stasis to decrease risk of tissue injury.

Useful in determining individual needs, therapeutic activities, and assistive devices.

NURSING DIAGNOSIS: Infection, risk for

Risk factors may include
Traumatized tissues, broken skin, invasive procedures
Decreased ciliary action, stasis of body fluids
Nutritional deficits
Suppressed inflammatory response (steroid use)
Altered integrity of closed system (CSF leak)

Possibly evidenced by
[Not applicable; presence of signs and symptoms establishes an *actual* diagnosis]

DESIRED OUTCOMES/EVALUATION CRITERIA—PATIENT WILL:

| Immune Status (NOC) |

Maintain normothermia, free of signs of infection.
Achieve timely wound healing when present.

ACTIONS/INTERVENTIONS

| Infection Protection (NIC) |

Independent

Provide meticulous/aseptic care, maintain good handwashing techniques.

Observe areas of impaired skin integrity (e.g., wounds, suture lines, invasive line insertion sites), noting drainage characteristics and presence of inflammation.

Monitor temperature routinely. Note presence of chills, diaphoresis, changes in mentation.

Encourage deep breathing, aggressive pulmonary toilet. Observe sputum characteristics.

Provide perineal care. Maintain integrity of closed urinary drainage system if used. Encourage adequate fluid intake.

Observe color/clarity of urine. Note presence of foul odor.

Screen/restrict access of visitors or caregivers with upper respiratory infections (URIs).

RATIONALE

First-line defense against nosocomial infections.

Early identification of developing infection permits prompt intervention and prevention of further complications.

May indicate developing sepsis requiring further evaluation/intervention.

Enhances mobilization and clearing of pulmonary secretions to reduce risk of pneumonia, atelectasis. *Note:* Postural drainage should be used with caution if risk of increased ICP exists.

Reduces potential for bacterial growth/ascending infection.

Indicators of developing urinary tract infection (UTI) requiring prompt intervention.

Reduces exposure of "compromised host."

ACTIONS/INTERVENTIONS

Collaborative

| Infection Control (NIC) |

Obtain specimens as indicated.

RATIONALE

Culture/sensitivity, Gram stain may be done to verify presence of infection and identify causative organism and appropriate treatment choices.

NURSING DIAGNOSIS: Nutrition: altered, risk for less than body requirements

Risk factors may include
Altered ability to ingest nutrients (decreased level of consciousness)
Weakness of muscles required for chewing, swallowing
Hypermetabolic state

Possibly evidenced by
[Not applicable; presence of signs and symptoms establishes an *actual* diagnosis]

DESIRED OUTCOMES/EVALUATION CRITERIA—PATIENT WILL:

| Nutritional Status (NOC) |

Demonstrate maintenance of desired weight/progressive weight gain toward goal.
Experience no signs of malnutrition, with laboratory values within normal range.

ACTIONS/INTERVENTIONS

| Nutrition Therapy (NIC) |

Independent

Assess ability to chew, swallow, cough, handle secretions.

Auscultate bowel sounds, noting decreased/absent or hyperactive sounds.

Weigh as indicated.

Provide for feeding safety, e.g., elevate head of bed while eating or during tube feeding.

Divide feedings into small amounts and give frequently.

Promote pleasant, relaxing environment, including socialization during meals. Encourage SO to bring in food that patient enjoys.

Check stools, gastric aspirant, vomitus for blood.

Collaborative

Consult with dietitian/nutritional support team.

RATIONALE

These factors determine choice of feeding because patient must be protected from aspiration.

GI functioning is usually preserved in brain-injured patients, so bowel sounds help in determining response to feeding or development of complications, e.g., ileus.

Evaluates effectiveness or need for changes in nutritional therapy.

Reduces risk of regurgitation and/or aspiration.

Enhances digestion and patient's tolerance of nutrients and can improve patient cooperation in eating.

Although the recovering patient may require assistance with feeding and/or use of assistive devices, mealtime socialization with SO or friends can improve intake and normalize the life function of eating.

Acute/subacute bleeding may occur (Cushing's ulcer), requiring intervention and alternate method of providing nutrition.

Effective resource for identifying caloric/nutrient needs, depending on age, body size, desired weight, concurrent conditions (trauma, cardiac/metabolic problems).

ACTIONS/INTERVENTIONS

Collaborative

Monitor laboratory studies, e.g., prealbumin/albumin, transferrin, amino acid profile, iron, BUN, nitrogen balance studies, glucose, AST/ALT, electrolytes.

Administer feedings by appropriate means, e.g., IV/tube feeding, oral feedings with soft foods and thick liquids. (Refer to CP: Total Nutritional Support: Parenteral/Enteral Feeding, p. 508.)

Involve speech/occupational/physical therapists when mechanical problem exists, e.g., impaired swallow reflexes, wired jaws, contractures of hands, paralysis.

RATIONALE

Identifies nutritional deficiencies, organ function, and response to nutritional therapy.

Choice of route depends on patient needs/capabilities. Tube feedings (nasogastric, gastric) may be required initially, or parenteral route may be indicated in presence of gastric/intestinal pathology. If the patient is able to swallow, soft foods or semiliquid foods may be more easily managed without aspiration.

Individual strategies/devices may be needed to improve ability to eat.

NURSING DIAGNOSIS: Family Processes, altered

May be related to
Situational transition and crisis
Uncertainty about outcomes/expectations

Possibly evidenced by
Difficulty adapting to change or dealing with traumatic experience constructively
Family not meeting needs of its members
Difficulty accepting or receiving help appropriately
Inability to express or to accept feelings of members

DESIRED OUTCOMES/EVALUATION CRITERIA—FAMILY WILL:

Acceptance: Health Status (NOC)

Begin to express feelings freely and appropriately.
Identify internal and external resources to deal with the situation.
Direct energies in a purposeful manner to plan for resolution of crisis.
Encourage and allow injured member to progress toward independence.

ACTIONS/INTERVENTIONS

Family Integrity Promotion (NIC)

Independent

Note components of family unit, availability/involvement of support systems.

Encourage expression of concerns about seriousness of condition, possibility of death, or incapacitation.

Listen for expressions of helplessness/hopelessness.

RATIONALE

Defines family resources and identifies areas of need.

Verbalization of fears gets concerns out in the open and can decrease anxiety and enhance coping with reality.

Joy of survival of victim is replaced by grief/anger at "loss" and necessity of dealing with "new person that family does not know and may not even like." Prolongation of these feelings may result in depression.

ACTIONS/INTERVENTIONS	RATIONALE
Independent	
Encourage expression of/acknowledge feelings. Do not deny or reassure patient/SO that everything will be all right.	Because it is not possible to predict the outcome, it is more helpful to assist the person to deal with feelings about what is happening instead of giving false reassurance.
Reinforce previous explanations about extent of injury, treatment plan, and prognosis. Provide accurate information at current level of understanding/ability to accept.	Patient/SO are unable to absorb/recall all information, and blocking can occur because of emotional trauma. As time goes by, reinforcement of information can help reduce misconceptions, fear about the unknown/future expectations.
Stress importance of continuous open dialogue between family members.	Provides opportunity to get feelings out in the open. Recognition and awareness promotes resolution of guilt, anger.
Evaluate/discuss family goals and expectations.	Family may believe that if patient is going to live, rehabilitation will bring about a cure. Despite accurate information, expectations may be unrealistic. Also, patient's early recovery may be rapid, then plateau, resulting in disappointment/frustration.
Identify individual roles and anticipated/perceived changes.	Responsibilities/roles may have to be partially or completely assumed by others, which can further complicate family coping.
Assess energy direction, e.g., whether efforts at resolution/problem solving are purposeful or scattered.	May need assistance to focus energies in an effective way/enhance coping.
Identify and encourage use of previously successful coping behaviors.	Focuses on strengths and reaffirms individual's ability to deal with current crisis.
Demonstrate and encourage use of stress management skills, e.g., relaxation techniques, breathing exercises, visualization.	Helps redirect attention toward revitalizing self to enhance coping ability.
Help family recognize needs of all members.	Attention may be so focused on injured member that other members feel isolated/abandoned, which can compromise family growth and unity.
Support family grieving for "loss" of member. Acknowledge normality of wide range of feelings and ongoing nature of process.	Although grief may never be fully resolved and family may vacillate among various stages, understanding that this is typical may help members accept/cope with the situation.
Collaborative	
Include family in rehabilitation team meetings and care planning/placement decisions.	Facilitates communication, enables family to be an integral part of the rehabilitation, and provides sense of control.
Identify community resources, e.g., visiting nurse, homemaker service, day care facility, legal/financial counselor.	Provides assistance with problems that may arise because of altered role function.
Refer to family therapy, support groups.	Cognitive/personality changes are usually very difficult for family to deal with. Decreased impulse control, emotional lability, inappropriate sexual or aggressive/violent behavior can disrupt family and result in abandonment/divorce. Trained therapists and peer role models may assist family to deal with feelings/reality of situation and provide support for decisions that are made.

NURSING DIAGNOSIS: Knowledge Deficit [Learning Need] regarding condition, prognosis, potential complications, treatment, self care, and discharge needs

May be related to

Lack of exposure, unfamiliarity with information/resources

Lack of recall/cognitive limitation

Possibly evidenced by

Request for information, statement of misconception

Inaccurate follow-through of instructions

DESIRED OUTCOMES/EVALUATION CRITERIA—PATIENT/SO WILL:

Knowledge: Disease Process (NOC)

Participate in learning process.

Verbalize understanding of condition, prognosis, potential complications.

Knowledge: Treatment Regimen (NOC)

Verbalize understanding of therapeutic regimen and rationale for actions.

Initiate necessary lifestyle changes and/or involvement in rehabilitation program.

Correctly perform necessary procedures.

ACTIONS/INTERVENTIONS	RATIONALE
Teaching: Disease Process (NIC)	
Independent	
Evaluate capabilities and readiness to learn of both patient and SO.	Permits presentation of material based on individual needs. *Note:* Patient may not be emotionally/mentally capable of assimilating information.
Review information regarding injury process and after-effects.	Aids in establishing realistic expectations and promotes understanding of current situation and needs.
Review/reinforce current therapeutic regimen. Identify ways of continuing program after discharge.	Recommended activities, limitations, medication/therapy needs have been established on the basis of a coordinated interdisciplinary approach, and follow-through is essential to progression of recovery/prevention of complications.
Discuss plans for meeting self-care needs.	Varying levels of assistance may be required/need to be planned based on individual situation.
Provide written instructions and schedules for activity, medication, important facts.	Provides visual reinforcement and reference source after discharge.
Identify signs/symptoms of individual risks, e.g., delayed CSF leak, posttraumatic seizures, headache/chronic pain.	Recognizing developing problems provides opportunity for prompt evaluation and intervention to prevent serious complications.
Discuss with patient/SO development of symptoms, such as re-experiencing traumatic event (flashbacks, intrusive thoughts, repetitive dreams/nightmares); psychic/emotional numbness; changes in lifestyle, including adoption of self-destructive behaviors.	May indicate occurrence/exacerbation of posttrauma response, which can occur months to years after injury, requiring further evaluation and supportive interventions.
Identify community resources, e.g., head injury support groups, social services, rehabilitation facilities, outpatient programs, home care/visiting nurse.	May be needed to provide assistance with physical care, home management, adjustment to lifestyle changes, and emotional and financial concerns.

ACTIONS/INTERVENTIONS	RATIONALE
Independent	
Refer/reinforce importance of follow-up care by rehabilitation team, e.g., physical/occupational/speech/vocational therapists, cognitive retrainers.	With diligent work (often for several years with these providers) the patient may eventually overcome residual neurological deficits and/or be able to resume desired/productive lifestyle.

POTENTIAL CONSIDERATIONS following acute hospitalization (dependent on patient's age, physical condition/presence of complications, personal resources, and life responsibilities)

Memory, impaired—neurological disturbances, anemia, fluid/electrolyte imbalances.

Health/Home Maintenance/Management, impaired—significant alteration in communication skills, lack of ability to make deliberate/thoughtful judgments, perceptual/cognitive impairments, insufficient finances, unfamiliarity with neighborhood resources, inadequate support systems.

Pain [acute]/chronic—tissue injury/neuronal damage, stress/anxiety.

Confusion, chronic—head injury.

CEREBROVASCULAR ACCIDENT (CVA)/STROKE

Cerebrovascular disease refers to any functional or structural abnormality of the brain caused by a pathological condition of the cerebral vessels or of the entire cerebrovascular system. This pathology either causes hemorrhage from a tear in the vessel wall or impairs the cerebral circulation by a partial or complete occlusion of the vessel lumen with transient or permanent effects. Over 700,000 Americans are affected by a CVA annually. CVA is the third leading cause of death after heart disease and cancer and is the leading cause of disability cost to the nation (approximately $30–$40 billion/year.)

Thrombosis, embolism, and hemorrhage are the primary causes for CVA, with thrombosis being the main cause of both CVAs and transient ischemic attacks (TIAs). The most common vessels involved are the carotid arteries and those of the vertebrobasilar system at the base of the brain. A thrombotic CVA causes a slow evolution of symptoms, usually over several hours, and is "completed" when the condition stabilizes. An embolic CVA occurs when a clot is carried into cerebral circulation and causes a localized cerebral infarct. Hemorrhagic CVA is caused by other conditions such as a ruptured aneurysm, hypertension, arteriovenous (AV) malformations, or other bleeding disorders. Symptoms depend on distribution of the cerebral vessel(s) involved. Ischemia may be (1) transient and resolve within 24 hours, (2) reversible with resolution of symptoms over a period of 1 week (reversible ischemic neurological deficit [RIND]), or (3) progress to cerebral infarction with variable effects and degrees of recovery.

CARE SETTING

Although the patient may initially be cared for in the intensive care unit (ICU), this phase of care focuses on the step-down or medical unit and subacute/rehabilitation units to community level.

RELATED CONCERNS

Hypertension: severe, page 33
Craniocerebral trauma (acute rehabilitative phase), page 238
Psychosocial aspects of care, page 809
Seizure disorders/epilepsy, page 228
Total nutritional support: parenteral/enteral feeding, page 508

Patient Assessment Database

Collected data are determined by location, severity, and duration of pathology.

ACTIVITY/REST

May report: Difficulties with activity due to weakness, loss of sensation, or paralysis (hemiplegia)
Tires easily; difficulty resting (pain or muscle twitchings)

May exhibit: Altered muscle tone (flaccid or spastic); paralysis (hemiplegia); generalized weakness
Visual disturbances
Altered level of consciousness

CIRCULATORY

May report: History of postural hypotension, cardiac disease (e.g., myocardial infarction (MI), rheumatic/valvular heart disease, HF, bacterial endocarditis), polycythemia

May exhibit: Arterial hypertension (common unless CVA is due to embolism or vascular malformation)
Pulse rate may vary (preexisting heart conditions, medications, effect of stroke on vasomotor center)
Dysrhythmias, electrocardiogram (ECG) changes
Bruit in carotid, femoral, or iliac arteries, or abdominal aorta

EGO INTEGRITY

May report: Feelings of helplessness, hopelessness
May exhibit: Emotional liability and inappropriate response to anger, sadness, happiness
Difficulty expressing self

ELIMINATION

May exhibit: Change in voiding patterns, e.g., incontinence, anuria
Distended abdomen (overdistended bladder); absent bowel sounds (paralytic ileus)

FOOD/FLUID

May report: Lack of appetite
Nausea/vomiting during acute event (increased ICP)
Loss of sensation in tongue, cheek, and throat; dysphagia
History of diabetes, elevated serum lipids

May exhibit: Mastication/swallowing problems (palatal and pharyngeal reflex involvement)
Obesity (risk factor)

NEUROSENSORY

May report: Dizziness/syncope (before CVA/transient during TIA)
Severe headache (intracerebral or subarachnoid hemorrhage)
Tingling/numbness/weakness (commonly reported during TIAs, found in varying degrees in other types of stroke); involved side seems "dead"
Visual deficits, e.g., blurred vision, partial loss of vision (monocular blindness), double vision (diplopia), or other disturbances in visual fields
Touch: Sensory loss on contralateral side (opposite side) in extremities and sometimes in ipsilateral side (same side) of face
Disturbance in senses of taste, smell
History of TIA, RIND (predisposing factor for subsequent infarction)

May exhibit: Mental status/LOC: Coma usually present in the initial stages of hemorrhagic disturbances; consciousness is usually preserved when the etiology is thrombotic in nature; altered behavior (e.g., lethargy, apathy, combativeness); altered cognitive function (e.g., memory, problem-solving, sequencing)
Extremities: Weakness/paralysis (contralateral with all kinds of stroke), unequal hand grasp; diminished deep tendon reflexes (contralateral)
Facial paralysis or paresis (ipsilateral)
Aphasia: Defect or loss of language function may be expressive (difficulty producing speech); receptive (difficulty comprehending speech); or global (combination of the two)
Loss of ability to recognize or appreciate import of visual, auditory, tactile stimuli (agnosia), e.g., altered body image awareness, neglect or denial of contralateral side of body, disturbances in perception
Loss of ability to execute purposeful motor acts despite physical ability and willingness to do so (apraxia)
Pupil size/reaction: Inequality; dilated and fixed pupil on the ipsilateral side (hemorrhage/herniation)
Nuchal rigidity (common in hemorrhagic etiology); seizures (common in hemorrhagic etiology)

PAIN/DISCOMFORT

May report: Headache of varying intensity (carotid artery involvement)
May exhibit: Guarding/distraction behaviors, restlessness, muscle/facial tension

RESPIRATION

May report: Smoking (risk factor)
May exhibit: Inability to swallow/cough/protect airway
Labored and/or irregular respirations
Noisy respirations/rhonchi (aspiration of secretions)

SAFETY

May exhibit: Motor/sensory: Problems with vision
Changes in perception of body spatial orientation (right CVA)
Difficulty seeing objects on left side (right CVA)
Being unaware of affected side

Inability to recognize familiar objects, colors, words, faces
Diminished response to heat and cold/altered body temperature regulation
Swallowing difficulty, inability to meet own nutritional needs
Impaired judgment, little concern for safety, impatience/lack of insight (right CVA)

SOCIAL INTERACTION

May exhibit: Speech problems, inability to communicate

TEACHING/LEARNING

May report: Family history of hypertension, strokes; African heritage (risk factor)
Use of oral contraceptives, alcohol abuse (risk factor)

Discharge plan considerations: **DRG projected mean length of inpatient stay: 6.4 days**
May require medication regimen/therapeutic treatments
Assistance with transportation, shopping, food preparation, self-care, and homemaker/ maintenance tasks
Changes in physical layout of home; transition placement before return to home setting

Refer to section at end of plan for postdischarge considerations.

DIAGNOSTIC STUDIES

CT scan (with/without enhancement): Demonstrates edema, hematomas, ischemia, and infarctions. *Note:* May not immediately reveal all changes, e.g., ischemic infarcts are not evident on CT for 8–12 hr; however, intracerebral hemorrhage is immediately apparent; therefore, emergency CT is always done before administering tissue plasminogen activator (tPA).

MRI: Shows areas of infarction, hemorrhage, AV malformations; and areas of ischemia.

Cerebral angiography: Helps determine specific cause of stroke, e.g., hemorrhage or obstructed artery, pinpoints site of occlusion or rupture.

Lumbar puncture (LP): Pressure is usually normal and CSF is clear in cerebral thrombosis, embolism, and TIA. Pressure elevation and grossly bloody fluid suggests subarachnoid and intracerebral hemorrhage. CSF total protein level may be elevated in cases of thrombosis because of inflammatory process. LP should be performed if septic embolism from bacterial endocarditis is suspected.

Transcranial Doppler ultrasonography: Identifies AV disease, e.g., problems with carotid system (blood flow/presence of atherosclerotic plaques).

EEG: Identifies problems based on brain waves and may demonstrate specific areas of lesions.

X-rays (skull): May show shift of pineal gland to the opposite side from an expanding mass; calcifications of the internal carotid may be visible in cerebral thrombosis; partial calcification of walls of an aneurysm may be noted in subarachnoid hemorrhage.

Laboratory studies to rule out systemic causes: CBC, platelet and clotting studies, VDRL/RPR, erythrocyte sedimentation rate (ESR), chemistries (glucose, sodium).

ECG, chest x-ray, and echocardiography: To rule out cardiac origin as source of embolus (20% of strokes are the result of blood or vegetative emboli associated with valvular disease, dysrhythmias, or endocarditis).

NURSING PRIORITIES

1. Promote adequate cerebral perfusion and oxygenation.
2. Prevent/minimize complications and permanent disabilities.
3. Assist patient to gain independence in ADLs.
4. Support coping process and integration of changes into self-concept.
5. Provide information about disease process/prognosis and treatment/rehabilitation needs.

DISCHARGE GOALS

1. Cerebral function improved, neurological deficits resolving/stabilized.
2. Complications prevented or minimized.
3. ADL needs met by self or with assistance of other(s).
4. Coping with situation in positive manner, planning for the future.
5. Disease process/prognosis, and therapeutic regimen understood.
6. Plan in place to meet needs after discharge.

ACTIONS/INTERVENTIONS	RATIONALE
Cerebral Perfusion Promotion (NIC)	
Independent	
Determine factors related to individual situation/cause for coma/decreased cerebral perfusion, and potential for increased ICP.	Influences choice of interventions. Deterioration in neurological signs/symptoms or failure to improve after initial insult may reflect decreased intracranial adaptive capacity requiring the patient be transferred to critical care area for monitoring of ICP, other therapies. If the stroke is evolving, the patient can deteriorate quickly and require repeated assessment and progressive treatment. If the stroke is "completed," the neurological deficit is nonprogressive, and treatment is geared toward rehabilitation and preventing recurrence.
Monitor/document neurological status frequently and compare with baseline. (Refer to CP: Craniocerebral Trauma [Acute Rehabilitative Phase], ND: Tissue Perfusion, altered cerebral, p. 238 for complete neurological evaluation.)	Assesses trends in level of consciousness (LOC) and potential for increased ICP and is useful in determining location, extent, and progression/resolution of CNS damage. May also reveal presence of TIA, which may warn of impending thrombotic CVA.
Monitor vital signs, i.e., note:	
Hypertension/hypotension, compare BP readings in both arms;	Fluctuations in pressure may occur because of cerebral pressure/injury in vasomotor area of the brain. Hypertension or postural hypotension may have been a precipitating factor. Hypotension may occur because of shock (circulatory collapse). Increased ICP may occur because of tissue edema or clot formation. Subclavian artery blockage may be revealed by difference in pressure readings between arms.
Heart rate and rhythm; auscultate for murmurs;	Changes in rate, especially bradycardia, can occur because of the brain damage. Dysrhythmias and murmurs may reflect cardiac disease, which may have precipitated CVA (e.g., stroke after MI or from valve dysfunction).

ACTIONS/INTERVENTIONS

Independent

Respirations, noting patterns and rhythm, e.g., periods of apnea after hyperventilation, Cheyne-Stokes respiration.

Evaluate pupils, noting size, shape, equality, light reactivity.

Document changes in vision, e.g., reports of blurred vision, alterations in visual field/depth perception.

Assess higher functions, including speech, if patient is alert. (Refer to ND: Communication, impaired verbal [and/or written], p. 264.)

Position with head slightly elevated and in neutral position.

Maintain bedrest; provide quiet environment; restrict visitors/activities as indicated. Provide rest periods between care activities, limit duration of procedures.

Prevent straining at stool, holding breath.

Assess for nuchal rigidity, twitching, increased restlessness, irritability, onset of seizure activity.

Collaborative

Administer supplemental oxygen as indicated.

Administer medications as indicated:

Alteplase (Activase), tPA;

Anticoagulants, e.g., warfarin sodium (Coumadin), low-molecular-weight heparin (Lovenox); antiplatelet agents, e.g., aspirin (ASA), dipyridamole (Persantine), ticlopidine (Ticlid);

Antifibrolytics, e.g., aminocaproic acid (Amicar);

RATIONALE

Irregularities can suggest location of cerebral insult/increasing ICP and need for further intervention, including possible respiratory support. (Refer to CP: Craniocerebral Trauma [Acute Rehabilitative Phase], ND: Breathing Pattern, risk for ineffective, p. 244.)

Pupil reactions are regulated by the oculomotor (III) cranial nerve and are useful in determining whether the brainstem is intact. Pupil size/equality is determined by balance between parasympathetic and sympathetic enervation. Response to light reflects combined function of the optic (II) and oculomotor (III) cranial nerves.

Specific visual alterations reflect area of brain involved, indicate safety concerns, and influence choice of interventions.

Changes in cognition and speech content are an indicator of location/degree of cerebral involvement and may indicate deterioration/increased ICP.

Reduces arterial pressure by promoting venous drainage and may improve cerebral circulation/perfusion.

Continual stimulation/activity can increase ICP. Absolute rest and quiet may be needed to prevent rebleeding in the case of hemorrhage.

Valsalva maneuver increases ICP and potentiates risk of rebleeding.

Indicative of meningeal irritation, especially in hemorrhagic disorders. Seizures may reflect increased ICP/cerebral injury, requiring further evaluation and intervention.

Reduces hypoxemia, which can cause cerebral vasodilation and increase pressure/edema formation.

Thrombolytic agents are useful in dissolving clot when started within 3 hr of initial symptoms. Thirty percent are likely to recover with little or no disability. Treatment is based on trying to limit the size of the infarct and use requires close monitoring for signs of intracranial hemorrhage. *Note:* These agents are contraindicated in cranial hemorrhage as diagnosed by CT scan.

May be used to improve cerebral blood flow and prevent further clotting when embolus/thrombosis is the problem. Contraindicated in hypertensive patients because of increased risk of hemorrhage.

Used with caution in hemorrhagic disorder to prevent lysis of formed clots and subsequent rebleeding.

Collaborative

Antihypertensives;

Preexisting/chronic hypertension requires cautious treatment because aggressive management increases the risk of extension of tissue damage. Transient hypertension often occurs during acute stroke and resolves often without therapeutic intervention.

Peripheral vasodilators, e.g., cyclandelate (Cyclospasmol), papaverine (Pavabid/Vasospan), isoxsuprine (Vasodilan);

Used to improve collateral circulation or decrease vasospasm.

Steroids, e.g., dexamethasone (Decadron);

Use is controversial in control of cerebral edema.

Neuroprotective agents, e.g., calcium channel blockers, excitatory amino acid inhibitors, gangliosides;

These agents are being researched as a means to protect the brain by interrupting the destructive cascade of biochemical events (e.g., influx of calcium into cells, release of excitatory neurotransmitters, build-up of lactic acid) to limit ischemic injury.

Phenytoin (Dilantin), phenobarbital;

May be used to control seizures and/or for sedative action. *Note:* Phenobarbital enhances action of antiepileptics.

Stool softeners.

Prevents straining during bowel movement and corresponding increase of ICP.

Prepare for surgery, as appropriate, e.g., endarterectomy, microvascular bypass, cerebral angioplasty.

May be necessary to resolve situation, reduce neurological symptoms/risk of recurrent stroke.

Monitor laboratory studies as indicated, e.g., prothrombin time (PT)/activated partial thromboplastin time (aPTT) time, Dilantin level.

Provides information about drug effectiveness/therapeutic level.

NURSING DIAGNOSIS: Mobility, impaired physical

May be related to
Neuromuscular involvement: weakness, paresthesia; flaccid/hypotonic paralysis (initially); spastic paralysis
Perceptual/cognitive impairment

Possibly evidenced by
Inability to purposefully move within the physical environment; impaired coordination; limited range of motion; decreased muscle strength/control

DESIRED OUTCOMES/EVALUATION CRITERIA—PATIENT WILL:

Immobility Consequences: Physiological (NOC)

Maintain/increase strength and function of affected or compensatory body part.
Maintain optimal position of function as evidenced by absence of contractures, foot-drop.

Mobility Level (NOC)

Demonstrate techniques/behaviors that enable resumption of activities.
Maintain skin integrity.

ACTIONS/INTERVENTIONS	RATIONALE

Positioning (NIC)

Independent

Assess functional ability/extent of impairment initially and on a regular basis. Classify according to 0–4 scale. (Refer to CP: Craniocerebral Trauma [Acute Rehabilitative Phase], ND: Mobility, impaired physical, p. 249.)

Identifies strengths/deficiencies and may provide information regarding recovery. Assists in choice of interventions, because different techniques are used for flaccid and spastic paralysis.

Change positions at least every 2 hr (supine, sidelying) and possibly more often if placed on affected side.

Reduces risk of tissue ischemia/injury. Affected side has poorer circulation and reduced sensation and is more predisposed to skin breakdown/decubitus.

Position in prone position once or twice a day if patient can tolerate.

Helps maintain functional hip extension; however, may increase anxiety, especially about ability to breathe.

Prop extremities in functional position, use footboard during the period of flaccid paralysis. Maintain neutral position of head.

Prevents contractures/footdrop and facilitates use when/if function returns. Flaccid paralysis may interfere with ability to support head, whereas spastic paralysis may lead to deviation of head to one side.

Use arm sling when patient is in upright position, as indicated.

During flaccid paralysis, use of sling may reduce risk of shoulder subluxation and shoulder-hand syndrome.

Evaluate use of/need for positional aids and/or splints during spastic paralysis:

Flexion contractures occur because flexor muscles are stronger than extensors.

Place pillow under axilla to abduct arm;

Prevents adduction of shoulder and flexion of elbow.

Elevate arm and hand;

Promotes venous return and helps prevent edema formation.

Place hard hand-rolls in the palm with fingers and thumb opposed;

Hard cones decrease the stimulation of finger flexion, maintaining finger and thumb in a functional position.

Place knee and hip in extended position;

Maintains functional position.

Maintain leg in neutral position with a trochanter roll;

Prevents external hip rotation.

Discontinue use of footboard, when appropriate.

Continued use (after change from flaccid to spastic paralysis) can cause excessive pressure on the ball of the foot, enhance spasticity, and actually increase plantar flexion.

Observe affected side for color, edema, or other signs of compromised circulation.

Edematous tissue is more easily traumatized and heals more slowly.

Inspect skin, particularly over bony prominences, regularly. Gently massage any reddened areas and provide aids such as sheepskin pads as necessary.

Pressure points over bony prominences are most at risk for decreased perfusion/ischemia. Circulatory stimulation and padding helps prevent skin breakdown and decubitus development.

Exercise Therapy: Muscle Control (NIC)

Begin active/passive ROM to all extremities (including splinted) on admission. Encourage exercises such as quadriceps/gluteal exercise, squeezing rubber ball, extension of fingers and legs/feet.

Minimizes muscle atrophy, promotes circulation, helps prevent contractures. Reduces risk of hypercalciuria and osteoporosis if underlying problem is hemorrhage. *Note:* Excessive/imprudent stimulation can predispose to rebleeding.

ACTIONS/INTERVENTIONS	RATIONALE

Independent

Assist to develop sitting balance (e.g., raise head of bed; assist to sit on edge of bed, having patient use the strong arm to support body weight and strong leg to move affected leg; increase sitting time) and standing balance (e.g., put flat walking shoes on patient, support patient's lower back with hands while positioning own knees outside patient's knees, assist in using parallel bars/walkers).

Aids in retraining neuronal pathways, enhancing proprioception and motor response.

Get up in chair as soon as vital signs are stable except following cerebral hemorrhage.

Helps stabilize BP (restores vasomotor tone), promotes maintenance of extremities in a functional position and emptying of bladder/kidneys, reducing risk of urinary stones and infections from stasis. *Note:* If stroke is not completed, activity increases risk of additional bleed/infarction.

Pad chair seat with foam or waterfilled cushion and assist patient to shift weight at frequent intervals.

Prevents/reduces pressure on the coccyx/skin breakdown.

Set goals with patient/SO for participation in activities/exercise and position changes.

Promotes sense of expectation of progress/improvement and provides some sense of control/independence.

Encourage patient to assist with movement and exercises using unaffected extremity to support/move weaker side.

May respond as if affected side is no longer part of body and needs encouragement and active training to "reincorporate" it as a part of own body.

Collaborative

Positioning (NIC)

Provide egg-crate mattress, water bed, flotation device, or specialized beds (e.g., kinetic), as indicated.

Promotes even weight distribution, decreasing pressure on bony points and helping to prevent skin breakdown/decubitus formation. Specialized beds help with positioning, enhance circulation, and reduce venous stasis to decrease risk of tissue injury and complications such as orthostatic pneumonia.

Exercise Therapy: Muscle Control (NIC)

Consult with physical therapist regarding active, resistive exercises and patient ambulation.

Individualized program can be developed to meet particular needs/deal with deficits in balance, coordination, strength.

Assist with electrical stimulation, e.g., transcutaneous electrical nerve stimulator (TENS) unit as indicated.

May assist with muscle strengthening and increase voluntary muscle control.

Administer muscle relaxants, antispasmodics as indicated, e.g., baclofen (Lioresal), dantrolene (Dantrium).

May be required to relieve spasticity in affected extremities.

NURSING DIAGNOSIS: Communication, impaired verbal [and/or written]

May be related to
Impaired cerebral circulation; neuromuscular impairment, loss of facial/oral muscle tone/control; generalized weakness/fatigue

Possibly evidenced by

Impaired articulation; does not/cannot speak (dysarthria)

Inability to modulate speech, find and name words, identify objects; inability to comprehend written/spoken language

Inability to produce written communication

DESIRED OUTCOMES/EVALUATION CRITERIA—PATIENT WILL:

Communication Ability (NOC)

Indicate an understanding of the communication problems.

Establish method of communication in which needs can be expressed.

Use resources appropriately.

ACTIONS/INTERVENTIONS	RATIONALE
Communication Enhancement: Speech Deficit (NIC)	
Independent	
Assess type/degree of dysfunction: e.g., patient does not seem to understand words or has trouble speaking or making self understood;	Helps determine area and degree of brain involvement and difficulty patient has with any or all steps of the communication process. Patient may have trouble understanding spoken words (receptive aphasia/damage to Wernicke's speech area), speaking words correctly (expressive aphasia/damage to Broca's speech areas), or may experience damage to both areas.
Differentiate aphasia from dysarthria;	Choice of interventions depends on type of impairment. Aphasia is a defect in using and interpreting symbols of language and may involve sensory and/or motor components, e.g., inability to comprehend written/spoken words or to write, make signs, speak. A dysarthric person can understand, read, and write language but has difficulty forming/pronouncing words because of weakness and paralysis of oral musculature.
Listen for errors in conversation and provide feedback;	Patient may lose ability to monitor verbal output and be unaware that communication is not sensible. Feedback helps patient realize why caregivers are not understanding/responding appropriately and provides opportunity to clarify content/meaning.
Ask patient to follow simple commands (e.g., "Shut your eyes," "Point to the door"); repeat simple words/sentences;	Tests for receptive aphasia.
Point to objects and ask patient to name them;	Tests for expressive aphasia; e.g., patient may recognize item but not be able to name it.
Have patient produce simple sounds, e.g., "Sh," "Cat";	Identifies dysarthria because motor components of speech (tongue, lip movement, breath control) can affect articulation and may/may not be accompanied by expressive aphasia.
Ask the patient to write name and/or a short sentence. If unable to write, have patient read a short sentence.	Tests for writing disability (agraphia) and deficits in reading comprehension (alexia), which are also part of receptive and expressive aphasia.

Independent

Post notice at nurses' station and patient's room about speech impairment. Provide special call bell if necessary.

Allays anxiety related to inability to communicate and fear that needs will not be met promptly. Call bell that is activated by minimal pressure is useful when patient is unable to use regular call system.

Provide alternative methods of communication, e.g., writing or felt board, pictures. Provide visual clues (gestures, pictures, "needs" list, demonstration).

Provides for communication of needs/desires based on individual situation/underlying deficit.

Anticipate and provide for patient's needs.

Helpful in decreasing frustration when dependent on others and unable to communicate desires.

Talk directly to patient, speaking slowly and distinctly. Use yes/no questions to begin with, progressing in complexity as patient responds.

Reduces confusion/anxiety at having to process and respond to large amount of information at one time. As retraining progresses, advancing complexity of communication stimulates memory and further enhances word/idea association.

Speak in normal tones and avoid talking too fast. Give patient ample time to respond. Talk without pressing for a response.

Patient is not necessarily hearing impaired, and raising voice may irritate or anger the patient. Forcing responses can result in frustration and may cause patient to resort to "automatic" speech, e.g., garbled speech, obscenities.

Encourage SO/visitors to persist in efforts to communicate with patient, e.g., reading mail, discussing family happenings even if patient is unable to respond appropriately.

It is important for family members to continue talking to patient to reduce patient's isolation, promote establishment of effective communication, and maintain sense of connectedness with family.

Discuss familiar topics, e.g., job, family, hobbies.

Promotes meaningful conversation and provides opportunity to practice skills.

Respect patient's preinjury capabilities; avoid "speaking down" to patient or making patronizing remarks.

Enables patient to feel esteemed, because intellectual abilities often remain intact.

Collaborative

Consult with/refer to speech therapist.

Assesses individual verbal capabilities and sensory, motor, and cognitive functioning to identify deficits/ therapy needs.

NURSING DIAGNOSIS: Sensory-Perceptual alterations (specify)

May be related to
Altered sensory reception, transmission, integration (neurological trauma or deficit)
Psychological stress (narrowed perceptual fields caused by anxiety)

Possibly evidenced by
Disorientation to time, place, person
Change in behavior pattern/usual response to stimuli; exaggerated emotional responses
Poor concentration, altered thought processes/bizarre thinking
Reported/measured change in sensory acuity: hypoparesthesia; altered sense of taste/ smell
Inability to tell position of body parts (proprioception)
Inability to recognize/attach meaning to objects (visual agnosia)
Altered communication patterns
Motor incoordination

Cognitive Ability (NOC)

Regain/maintain usual level of consciousness and perceptual functioning.
Acknowledge changes in ability and presence of residual involvement.
Demonstrate behaviors to compensate for/overcome deficits.

ACTIONS/INTERVENTIONS

Environmental Management (NIC)

Independent

Review pathology of individual condition.

Observe behavioral responses, e.g., hostility, crying, inappropriate affect, agitation, hallucination. (Refer to CP: Craniocerebral Trauma [Acute Rehabilitative Phase], ND: Thought Processes, altered, p. 247.)

Eliminate extraneous noise/stimuli as necessary.

Speak in calm, quiet voice, using short sentences. Maintain eye contact.

Ascertain/validate patient's perceptions. Reorient patient frequently to environment, staff, procedures.

Evaluate for visual deficits. Note loss of visual field, changes in depth perception (horizontal/vertical planes), presence of diplopia (double vision).

Approach patient from visually intact side. Leave light on; position objects to take advantage of intact visual fields. Patch affected eye if indicated.

Simplify environment, remove excess equipment/furniture.

Peripheral Sensation Management (NIC)

Assess sensory awareness, e.g., differentiation of hot/cold, dull/sharp; position of body parts/muscle, joint sense.

Stimulate sense of touch; e.g., give patient objects to touch, grasp. Have patient practice touching walls/other boundaries.

Protect from temperature extremes; assess environment for hazards. Recommend testing warm water with unaffected hand.

RATIONALE

Awareness of type/area of involvement aids in assessing for/anticipating specific deficits and planning care.

Individual responses are variable, but commonalities such as emotional lability, lowered frustration threshold, apathy, and impulsiveness may complicate care.

Reduces anxiety and exaggerated emotional responses/confusion associated with sensory overload.

Patient may have limited attention span or problems with comprehension. These measures can help patient to attend to communication.

Assists patient to identify inconsistencies in reception and integration of stimuli and may reduce perceptual distortion of reality.

Presence of visual disorders can negatively affect patient's ability to perceive environment and relearn motor skills and increases risk of accident/injury.

Provides for recognition of the presence of persons/objects; may help with depth perception problems; prevents patient from being startled. Patching may decrease the sensory confusion of double vision.

Decreases/limits amount of visual stimuli that may confuse interpretation of environment; reduces risk of accidental injury.

Diminished sensory awareness and impairment of kinesthetic sense negatively affects balance/positioning and appropriateness of movement, which interferes with ambulation, increasing risk of trauma.

Aids in retraining sensory pathways to integrate reception and interpretation of stimuli. Helps patient orient self spatially and strengthens use of affected side.

Promotes patient safety, reducing risk of injury.

ACTIONS/INTERVENTIONS

Independent

Note inattention to body parts, segments of environment; lack of recognition of familiar objects/persons.

Encourage patient to watch feet when appropriate and consciously position body parts. Make the patient aware of all neglected body parts, e.g., sensory stimulation to affected side, exercises that bring affected side across midline, reminding person to dress/care for affected ("blind") side.

RATIONALE

Presence of agnosia (loss of comprehension of auditory, visual, or other sensations, although sensory sphere is intact) may lead to/result in unilateral neglect, inability to recognize environmental cues/meaning of commonplace objects, considerable self-care deficits, and disorientation or bizarre behavior.

Use of visual and tactile stimuli assists in reintegration of affected side and allows patient to experience forgotten sensations of normal movement patterns.

NURSING DIAGNOSIS: Self-Care deficit (specify)

May be related to
Neuromuscular impairment, decreased strength and endurance, loss of muscle control/coordination
Perceptual/cognitive impairment
Pain/discomfort
Depression

Possibly evidenced by
Impaired ability to perform ADLs, e.g., inability to bring food from receptacle to mouth; inability to wash body part(s), regulate temperature of water; impaired ability to put on/take off clothing; difficulty completing toileting tasks

DESIRED OUTCOMES/EVALUATION CRITERIA—PATIENT WILL:

Self-Care: Activities of Daily Living (ADLs) (NOC)

Demonstrate techniques/lifestyle changes to meet self-care needs.
Perform self-care activities within level of own ability.
Identify personal/community resources that can provide assistance as needed.

ACTIONS/INTERVENTIONS

Self-Care Assistance (NIC)

Independent

Assess abilities and level of deficit (0–4 scale) for performing ADLs.

Avoid doing things for the patient that the patient can do for self, but provide assistance as necessary.

Be aware of impulsive behavior/actions suggestive of impaired judgment.

Maintain a supportive, firm attitude. Allow patient sufficient time to accomplish tasks.

Provide positive feedback for efforts/accomplishments.

RATIONALE

Aids in anticipating/planning for meeting individual needs.

These patients may become fearful and dependent and although assistance is helpful in preventing frustration, it is important for the patient to do as much as possible for self to maintain self-esteem and promote recovery.

May indicate need for additional interventions and supervision to promote patient safety.

Patients need empathy and to know caregivers will be consistent in their assistance.

Enhances sense of self-worth, promotes independence, and encourages patient to continue endeavors.

ACTIONS/INTERVENTIONS

Independent

Create plan for visual deficits that are present, e.g.:

Place food and utensils on the tray related to the patient's unaffected side;

Situate the bed so that the patient's unaffected side is facing the room with the affected side to the wall;

Position furniture against wall/out of travel path.

Provide self-help devices, e.g., button/zipper hook, knife-fork combinations, long-handled brushes, extensions for picking things up from floor; toilet riser, leg bag for catheter; shower chair. Assist and encourage good grooming and makeup habits.

Encourage SO to allow patient to do as much as possible for self.

Assess patient's ability to communicate the need to void and/or ability to use urinal, bedpan. Take patient to the bathroom at frequent/periodic intervals for voiding if appropriate.

Identify previous bowel habits and re-establish normal regimen. Increase bulk in diet; encourage fluid intake, increased activity.

Collaborative

Administer suppositories and stool softeners.

Consult with physical/occupational therapist.

RATIONALE

Patient will be able to see to eat the food.

Will be able to see when getting in/out of bed and observe anyone who comes into the room.

Provides for safety when patient is able to move around the room, reducing risk of tripping/falling over furniture.

Enables patient to manage for self, enhancing independence and self-esteem; reduces reliance on others for meeting own needs; and enables patient to be more socially active.

Re-establishes sense of independence and fosters self-worth and enhances rehabilitation process. *Note:* This may be very difficult and frustrating for the SO/caregiver, depending on degree of disability and time required for patient to complete activity.

Patient may have neurogenic bladder, be inattentive, or be unable to communicate needs in acute recovery phase, but usually is able to regain independent control of this function as recovery progresses.

Assists in development of retraining program (independence) and aids in preventing constipation and impaction (long-term effects).

May be necessary at first to aid in establishing regular bowel function.

Provides expert assistance for developing a therapy plan and identifying special equipment needs.

NURSING DIAGNOSIS: Coping, Individual, ineffective

May be related to
Situational crises, vulnerability, cognitive perceptual changes

Possibly evidenced by
Inappropriate use of defense mechanisms
Inability to cope/difficulty asking for help
Change in usual communication patterns
Inability to meet basic needs/role expectations
Difficulty problem solving

DESIRED OUTCOMES/EVALUATION CRITERIA—PATIENT WILL:

Coping (NOC)

Verbalize acceptance of self in situation.
Talk/communicate with SO about situation and changes that have occurred.
Verbalize awareness of own coping abilities.
Meet psychological needs as evidenced by appropriate expression of feelings, identification of options, and use of resources.

Coping Enhancement (NIC)

Independent

ACTIONS/INTERVENTIONS	RATIONALE
Assess extent of altered perception and related degree of disability.	Determination of individual factors aids in developing plan of care/choice of interventions.
Identify meaning of the loss/dysfunction/change to the patient. Note ability to understand events, provide realistic appraisal of situation.	Some patients accept and manage altered function effectively with little adjustment, while others have considerable difficulty recognizing and adjusting to deficits.
Determine outside stressors, e.g., family, work, social, future nursing/healthcare needs.	Helps identify specific needs, provides opportunity to offer information/support and begin problem-solving.
Encourage patient to express feelings, including hostility or anger, denial, depression.	Demonstrates acceptance of/assists patient in recognizing and beginning to deal with these feelings.
Note whether patient refers to affected side as "it" or denies affected side and says it is "dead."	Suggests rejection of body part/negative feelings about body image and abilities, indicating need for intervention and emotional support.
Acknowledge statement of feelings about betrayal of body; remain matter-of-fact about reality that patient can still use unaffected side and learn to control affected side. Use words (e.g., weak, affected, right-left) that incorporate that side as part of the whole body.	Helps patient to see that the nurse accepts both sides as part of the whole individual. Allows patient to feel hopeful and begin to accept current situation.
Identify previous methods of dealing with life problems. Determine presence/quality of support systems.	Provides opportunity to use behaviors previously effective, build on past successes, and mobilize resources.
Emphasize small gains either in recovery of function or independence.	Consolidates gains, helps reduce feelings of anger and helplessness, and conveys sense of progress.
Support behaviors/efforts such as increased interest/participation in rehabilitation activities.	Suggests possible adaptation to changes and understanding about own role in future lifestyle.
Monitor for sleep disturbance, increased difficulty concentrating, statements of inability to cope, lethargy, withdrawal.	May indicate onset of depression (common after effect of stroke), which may require further evaluation and intervention.
Refer for neuropsychological evaluation and/or counseling if indicated.	May facilitate adaptation to role changes that are necessary for a sense of feeling/being a productive person. *Note:* Depression is common in stroke survivors and may be a direct result of the brain damage and/or an emotional reaction to sudden-onset disability.

NURSING DIAGNOSIS: Swallowing, risk for impaired

Risk factors may include
Neuromuscular/perceptual impairment

Possibly evidenced by
[Not applicable; presence of signs and symptoms establishes an *actual* diagnosis]

DESIRED OUTCOMES/EVALUATION CRITERIA—PATIENT WILL:

Self-Care: Eating (NOC)

Demonstrate feeding methods appropriate to individual situation with aspiration prevented.
Maintain desired body weight.

ACTIONS/INTERVENTIONS	RATIONALE

Swallowing Therapy (NIC)

Independent

Review individual pathology/ability to swallow, noting extent of paralysis; clarity of speech; facial, tongue involvement; ability to protect airway/episodes of coughing or choking; presence of adventitious breath sounds; amount/character of oral secretions. Weigh periodically as indicated.

Nutritional interventions/choice of feeding route is determined by these factors.

Have suction equipment available at bedside, especially during early feeding efforts.

Timely intervention may limit amount/untoward effect of aspiration.

Promote effective swallowing, e.g.:

Schedule activities/medications to provide a minimum of 30 min rest before eating;

Promotes optimal muscle function, helps to limit fatigue.

Provide pleasant environment free of distractions (e.g., TV);

Promotes relaxation and allows patient to focus on task of eating/swallowing.

Assist patient with head control/support;

Counteracts hyperextension, aiding in prevention of aspiration and enhancing ability to swallow.

Place patient in upright position during and after feeding;

Uses gravity to facilitate swallowing and reduces risk of aspiration.

Stimulate lips to close or manually open mouth by light pressure on lips/under chin, if needed;

Aids in sensory retraining and promotes muscular control.

Place room-temperature food in unaffected side of mouth;

Provides sensory stimulation (including taste), which may trigger swallowing efforts and enhance intake. *Note:* Dysphagic patients may be oversensitive to heat/cold.

Touch parts of the cheek with tongue blade/apply ice to weak tongue;

Can improve tongue movement and control (necessary for swallowing) and inhibits tongue protrusion.

Feed slowly allowing 30–45 min, for meals;

Feeling rushed can increase stress/level of frustration, may increase risk of aspiration, and may result in patient terminating meal early.

Begin oral feedings with semiliquid, soft foods when patient can swallow water. Select/assist patient to select foods that require little or no chewing and are easy to swallow, e.g., custard, applesauce, eggs, soft finger foods, or finely chopped foods;

Soft foods/thick fluids are easier to control in mouth, reducing risk of choking/aspiration. *Note:* Pureed food is not recommended because patient may not be able to recognize what is being eaten, and most milk products, peanut butter, syrup, and bananas are avoided because they produce mucus/are sticky.

Offer solid foods and liquids at different times;

Prevents patient from swallowing food before it is thoroughly chewed.

Limit/avoid use of drinking straw for liquids.

Although use may strengthen facial and swallowing muscles, if patient lacks tight lip closure to accommodate straw or if liquid is deposited too far back in mouth, risk of aspiration may be increased.

Encourage SO to bring favorite foods.

Provides familiar tastes and preferences. Stimulates feeding efforts and may enhance swallowing/intake.

Maintain upright position for 45–60 min after eating.

Helps patient manage oral secretions and reduces risk of regurgitation.

ACTIONS/INTERVENTIONS	RATIONALE
Independent	
Maintain accurate I&O; record calorie count.	If swallowing efforts are not sufficient to meet fluid/nutrition needs, alternate methods of feeding must be pursued.
Encourage participation in exercise/activity program.	May increase release of endorphins in the brain, promoting a sense of general well-being and increasing appetite.
Collaborative	
Review results of radiographic studies, e.g., video fluoroscopy.	Aids in determining phase of swallowing difficulties (i.e., oral preparatory, oral, pharyngeal, or esophageal phase).
Administer IV fluids and/or tube feedings.	May be necessary for fluid replacement and nutrition if patient is unable to take anything orally.
Coordinate multidisciplinary approach to develop treatment plan that meets individual needs.	Inclusion of dietitian, speech and occupational therapists can increase effectiveness of long-term plan and significantly reduce risk of silent aspiration.

NURSING DIAGNOSIS: Knowledge Deficit [Learning Need] regarding condition, prognosis, treatment, self care, and discharge needs

May be related to
Lack of exposure; unfamiliarity with information resources
Cognitive limitation, information misinterpretation, lack of recall

Possibly evidenced by
Request for information
Statement of misconception
Inaccurate follow-through of instructions
Development of preventable complications

DESIRED OUTCOMES/EVALUATION CRITERIA—PATIENT/SO WILL:

Knowledge: Disease Process (NOC)

Participate in learning process.
Verbalize understanding of condition/prognosis and potential complications.

Knowledge: Treatment Regimen (NOC)

Verbalize understanding of therapeutic regimen and rationale for actions.
Initiate necessary lifestyle changes.

ACTIONS/INTERVENTIONS	RATIONALE
Teaching: Disease Process (NIC)	
Independent	
Evaluate type/degree of sensory-perceptual involvement.	Deficits affect the choice of teaching methods and content/complexity of instruction.
Discuss specific pathology and individual potentials.	Aids in establishing realistic expectations and promotes understanding of current situation and needs.

ACTIONS/INTERVENTIONS	RATIONALE
Independent	
Identify signs/symptoms requiring further follow-up, e.g., changes/decline in visual, motor, sensory functions; alteration in mentation or behavioral responses; severe headache.	Prompt evaluation and intervention reduces risk of complications/further loss of function.
Review current restrictions/limitations and discuss planned/potential resumption of activities (including sexual relations).	Promotes understanding, provides hope for future, and creates expectation of resumption of more "normal" life.
Review/reinforce current therapeutic regimen, including use of medications to control hypertension, hypercholesterolemia, diabetes, as indicated; aspirin or similar-acting drugs, e.g., ticlopidine (Ticlid), warfarin sodium (Coumadin). Identify ways of continuing program after discharge.	Recommended activities, limitations, and medication/therapy needs are established on the basis of a coordinated interdisciplinary approach. Follow-through is essential to progression of recovery/prevention of complications. *Note:* Long-term anticoagulation may be beneficial for patients over 45 years of age who are prone to clot formation; however, use of these drugs is not effective for CVA resulting from vascular aneurysm/vessel rupture.
Provide written instructions and schedules for activity, medication, important facts.	Provides visual reinforcement and reference source after discharge.
Encourage patient to refer to lists/written communications or notes instead of depending on memory.	Provides aids to support memory and promotes improvement in cognitive skills.
Discuss plans for meeting self-care needs.	Varying levels of assistance may be required/need to be planned for based on individual situation.
Refer to discharge planner/home care supervisor, visiting nurse.	Home environment may require evaluation and modifications to meet individual needs.
Identify community resources, e.g., National Stroke Association, American Heart Associations' Stroke Connection, stroke support clubs, senior services, Meals on Wheels, adult day care/respite program, and visiting nurse.	Enhances coping abilities and promotes home management and adjustment to impairments for both stroke survivors and caregivers. *Note:* Recent innovations include such programs as Menu-Direct, which provides fully-prepared meal programs with nutrition-rich foods. Some entrees have soufflélike consistency to help trigger swallowing response.
Suggest patient reduce/limit environmental stimuli, especially during cognitive activities.	Multiple/concomitant stimuli may aggravate confusion and impair mental abilities.
Recommend patient seek assistance in problem-solving process and validate decisions, as indicated.	Some patients (especially those with right CVA) may display impaired judgment and impulsive behavior, compromising ability to make sound decisions.
Identify individual risk factors (e.g., hypertension, cardiac dysrhythmias, obesity, smoking, heavy alcohol use, atherosclerosis, poor control of diabetes, use of oral contraceptives) and discuss necessary lifestyle changes.	Promotes general well-being and may reduce risk of recurrence. *Note:* Obesity in women has been found to have a high correlation with ischemic stroke.
Review importance of balanced diet, low in cholesterol and sodium if indicated. Discuss role of vitamins and other supplements.	Improves general health and well-being and provides energy for life activities.
Refer to/reinforce importance of follow-up care by rehabilitation team, e.g., physical/occupational/speech/vocational therapists.	Diligent work may eventually overcome/minimize residual deficits.

POTENTIAL CONSIDERATIONS following acute hospitalization (dependent on patient's age, physical condition/presence of complications, personal resources, and life responsibilities)

Injury, risk for—general weakness, visual deficits, balancing difficulties, reduced large/small muscle or hand-eye coordination, cognitive impairment.

Nutrition: altered, less than body requirements—inability to prepare/ingest food, cognitive limitations, limited financial resources.

Self-Care deficit—decreased strength/endurance, perceptual/cognitive impairment, neuromuscular impairment, muscular pain, depression.

Home Maintenance Management, impaired—individual physical limitations, inadequate support systems, insufficient finances, unfamiliarity with neighborhood resources.

Self-Esteem, situational low—cognitive/perceptual impairment, perceived loss of control in some aspect of life, loss of independent functioning.

HERNIATED NUCLEUS PULPOSUS (RUPTURED INTERVERTEBRAL DISC)

A *herniated disc (HNP)* is a major cause of severe, chronic, and recurrent back pain. Herniation, either complete or partial, of the nuclear material in the vertebral areas of L-4 to L-5, L-5 to S-1, or C-5 to C-6, C-6 to C-7 is most common and may be the result of trauma or degenerative changes associated with the aging process.

CARE SETTING

Most disc problems are treated conservatively at the community level, although diagnostics and therapy services may be provided through outpatient facilities. Brief hospitalization is restricted to episodes of severe debilitating pain/neurological deficit.

RELATED CONCERNS

Disc surgery, page 283
Psychosocial aspects of care, page 809

Patient Assessment Database

Data depend on site, severity, whether acute/chronic, effects on surrounding structures, and degree of nerve root compression.

ACTIVITY/REST

May report:	History of occupation requiring heavy lifting, sitting, driving for long periods
	Need to sleep on bedboard/firm mattress, difficulty falling asleep/staying asleep
	Decreased range of motion of affected extremity/extremities
	Inability to perform usual/desired activities
May exhibit:	Atrophy of muscles on the affected side
	Gait disturbances

ELIMINATION

May report:	Constipation, difficulty in defecation
	Urinary incontinence/retention

EGO INTEGRITY

May report:	Fear of paralysis
	Financial, employment concerns
May exhibit:	Anxiety, depression, withdrawal from family/SO

NEUROSENSORY

May report:	Tingling, numbness, weakness of affected extremity/extremities
May exhibit:	Decreased deep tendon reflexes; muscle weakness, hypotonia
	Tenderness/spasm of paravertebral muscles
	Decreased pain perception (sensory)

PAIN/ DISCOMFORT

May report:	Pain knifelike, aggravated by coughing, sneezing, bending, lifting, defecation, straight leg raising; unremitting pain or intermittent episodes of more severe pain; radiation to leg/feet, buttocks area (lumbar) or shoulder or head/face, neck (cervical)
	Heard "snapping" sound at time of initial pain/trauma or felt "back giving way"
	Limited mobility/forward bending
May exhibit:	Stance: Leans away from affected area
	Altered gait, walking with a limp, elevated hip on affected side
	Pain on palpation

SAFETY

May report:	History of previous back problems

TEACHING/LEARNING

May report: Lifestyle sedentary or overactive

Discharge plan considerations: DRG projected mean length of inpatient stay: 4.9–6.5 days

May require assistance with transportation, self-care, and homemaker/maintenance tasks

Refer to section at end of plan for post discharge considerations.

DIAGNOSTIC STUDIES

Spinal x-rays: May show degenerative changes in spine/intervertebral space or rule out other suspected pathology, e.g., tumors, osteomyelitis.

CT scan with/without enhancement: May reveal spinal canal narrowing, disc protrusion.

MRI: Can reveal changes in bone, discs, and soft tissues and can validate disc herniation/surgical decisions.

Provocative tests (discography, nerve root blocks): Determine site of origin of pain by replicating and then relieving symptoms. Can also be used to rule out sacroiliac joint involvement.

Electrophysiologic studies—electromyoneurography (EMG) and nerve conduction studies (NCS): Can localize lesion to level of particular spinal nerve root involved; nerve conduction and velocity study usually done in conjunction with study of muscle response to assist in diagnosis of peripheral nerve impairment and effect on skeletal muscle.

Myelogram: Rarely performed, but when done, may be normal or show "narrowing" of disc space, specific location and size of herniation.

Epidural venogram: May be done for cases where myelogram accuracy is limited.

NURSING PRIORITIES

1. Reduce back stress, muscle spasm, and pain.
2. Promote optimal functioning.
3. Support patient/SO in rehabilitation process.
4. Provide information concerning condition/prognosis and treatment needs.

DISCHARGE GOALS

1. Pain relieved/manageable.
2. Proper lifting, posture, exercises demonstrated.
3. Motor function/sensation restored to optimal level.
4. Disease/injury process, prognosis, and therapeutic regimen understood.
5. Plan in place to meet needs after discharge.

NURSING DIAGNOSIS: Pain [acute]/chronic

May be related to

Physical injury agents: nerve compression, muscle spasm

Possibly evidenced by

Reports of back pain, stiff neck; decreased tolerance for activity

Walking with a limp, inability to walk; preoccupation with pain, self/narrowed focus

Guarding behavior, leans toward affected side when standing

Altered muscle tone

Facial mask of pain; distraction

Autonomic responses (when pain is acute)

Changes in sleep patterns; physical/social withdrawal

DESIRED OUTCOMES/EVALUATION CRITERIA—PATIENT WILL:

Pain Control Behavior (NOC)

Report pain is relieved/controlled.

Verbalize methods that provide relief.

Demonstrate use of therapeutic interventions (e.g., relaxation skills, behavior modification) to relieve pain.

ACTIONS/INTERVENTIONS	RATIONALE

Pain Management (NIC)

Independent

Assess reports of pain, noting location, duration, precipitating/aggravating factors. Ask patient to rate on scale of 0–10 (or other scale as appropriate).

Helps determine choice of interventions and provides basis for comparison and evaluation of therapy.

Maintain bedrest briefly during acute phase. Place patient in semi-Fowler's position with spine, hips, knees flexed; supine with/without head elevated 10–30 degrees; or lateral position.

Bedrest in position of comfort decreases muscle spasm, reduces stress on structures, and facilitates reduction of disc protrusion.

Instruct in logrolling technique for position change if patient requires.

Reduces flexion, twisting, and strain on back, especially when nerve impingement impairs patient's ability to move legs.

Assist with application of brace/corset. Instruct patient in how to self-place brace with assistance, then independently.

Often used briefly during acute phase of ruptured disc or after surgery to provide support and limit flexion/twisting. *Note:* Prolonged use can increase muscle weakness and cause further disc degeneration, nerve impairment.

Limit activity during acute phase as indicated. Intersperse rest periods, shortening rest interval and length as patient improves.

Decreases forces of gravity and motion, which can relieve muscle spasms and reduce edema and stress on structures around affected disc.

Place needed items, call bell within easy reach.

Reduces risk of straining to reach.

Instruct in/assist with relaxation/visualization techniques.

Refocuses attention away from pain, aids in reducing muscle spasm/tension; and promotes tissue oxygenation/healing.

Instruct in/encourage correct body mechanics/body posture.

Alleviates stress on muscles and prevents further aggravation of injury.

Provide opportunities to talk/listen to concerns.

Ventilation of worries can help to decrease stress factors present in illness/hospitalization. Provides opportunity to give information/correct misinformation.

Collaborative

Provide orthopedic bed or firm mattress.

Provides support and reduces spinal flexion, decreasing spasms.

Administer medications as indicated:

Nonsteroidal anti-inflammatory drugs (NSAIDs), e.g., nabumetone (Relafen), ibuprofen (Motrin, Advil), diflunisal (Dolobid), ketoprofen (Orudis), meclofenamate (Meclomen);

Suppresses pain and inflammation, decreases edema and pressure on nerve root(s). *Note:* Epidural or facet joint injection of anti-inflammatory drugs may be tried if other interventions fail to alleviate pain.

Muscle relaxants, e.g., cyclobenzaprine (Flexeril), diazepam (Valium), carisoprodol (Soma), methocarbamol (Robaxin);

Relaxes striated muscles, decreasing pain. *Note:* As these drugs act centrally on the brain, drowsiness, dizziness, and lightheadedness may occur, especially during initial therapy, raising safety concerns.

Analgesics, e.g., acetaminophen (Tylenol) with codeine, meperidine (Demerol), hydrocodone (Vicodin), butorphanol (Stadol), fentanyl (Duragesic); morphine (MS Contin).

May be required for relief of moderate to severe pain usually during periods of exacerbation of symptoms. Used with caution for relief of chronic pain because concerns of dependency must be balanced with patient's functional abilities/quality of life resulting from drug use.

Apply physical supports, e.g., lumbar brace, cervical collar.

Support of structures decreases muscle stress/spasms and reduces pain.

ACTIONS/INTERVENTIONS	RATIONALE
Collaborative	
Maintain traction if indicated.	Sometimes used to remove weight bearing from affected disc area, increasing intravertebral separation and allowing disc bulge to move away from nerve root.
Consult with physical therapist.	Individualized program (including hot and cold packs, ultrasound, massage, therapeutic exercises, and pool therapy) can relieve muscle spasm and strengthen back, extensor, abdominal, and quadriceps muscles to increase support to lumbar area.
Apply/monitor use of cold or moist hot packs, diathermy, ultrasound.	Increases circulation to affected muscles, promotes relief of spasms, and enhances patient's relaxation.
Instruct in postmyelogram/postepidural block care when appropriate, e.g., force fluids and lie flat or at 30-degree elevation, as indicated for specified period of time.	Decreases risk of postprocedure headache/spinal fluid leak.
Assist with/instruct in use of electrical stimulation, e.g., TENS unit.	Decreases stimuli by blocking pain transmission.
Refer to rehabilitation/pain management clinic.	Coordinated team efforts may include physical and psychological therapy to deal with all aspects of chronic pain and allow patient to increase activity and productivity.

NURSING DIAGNOSIS: Mobility, impaired physical

May be related to
Pain and discomfort, muscle spasms
Restrictive therapies, e.g., bedrest, traction
Neuromuscular impairment

Possibly evidenced by
Reports of pain on movement
Reluctance to attempt/difficulty with purposeful movement
Impaired coordination, limited ROM, decreased muscle strength

DESIRED OUTCOMES/EVALUATION CRITERIA—PATIENT WILL:

Immobility Consequences: Physiological (NOC)

Verbalize understanding of situation/risk factors and individual treatment regimen.
Be free of complications.
Demonstrate techniques/behaviors that enable resumption of activities.

Mobility Level (NOC)

Maintain or increase strength and function of affected and/or compensatory body part.

ACTIONS/INTERVENTIONS	RATIONALE
Bed Rest Care (NIC)	
Independent	
Perform/assist with passive and active ROM exercises.	Strengthens abdominal muscles and flexors of spine; promotes good body mechanics.

ACTIONS/INTERVENTIONS

Collaborative

Encourage lower leg/ankle exercises. Evaluate for edema, erythema of lower extremities, calf pain/tenderness, presence of Homan's sign.

Provide good skin care; gently massage pressure points after each position change. Check skin under brace periodically.

Encourage diet high in fiber and adequate fluid intake.

Note emotional/behavioral responses to immobility. Provide diversional activities.

Exercise Therapy: Ambulation (NIC)

Provide for safety measures as indicated by individual situation.

Assist with activity/progressive ambulation.

Demonstrate use of adjunctive devices, e.g., walker, cane.

Collaborative

Administer medication for pain approximately 30 min before turning patient/ambulation, as indicated.

Bed Rest Care (NIC)

Apply antiembolism stockings as indicated.

RATIONALE

Stimulates venous circulation/return, decreasing venous stasis and possible thrombus formation.

Reduces risk of skin irritation/breakdown.

Reduces risk of constipation related to deceased level of activity.

Forced immobility may heighten restlessness, irritability. Diversional activity aids in refocusing attention and enhances coping with limitations.

Depending on area of involvement/type of procedure, imprudent activity increases chance of spinal injury. (Refer to CP: Disc Surgery, ND: Trauma (spinal), risk for, p. 284.)

Activity depends on individual situation but usually progresses slowly according to tolerance.

Provides stability and support to compensate for altered muscle tone/strength and balance.

Anticipation of pain can increase muscle tension. Medication can relax patient, enhance comfort and cooperation during activity.

Promotes venous return, reducing risk of DVT.

NURSING DIAGNOSIS: Anxiety (specify level)/Coping, Individual, ineffective

May be related to
Situational crisis
Threat to/change in health status, socioeconomic status, role functioning
Recurrent disorder with continuing pain
Inadequate relaxation, little or no exercise
Inadequate coping methods

Possibly evidenced by
Apprehension, uncertainty, helplessness
Expressed concerns regarding changes in life events
Verbalization of inability to cope
Muscular tension, general irritability, restlessness; insomnia/fatigue
Inability to meet role expectations

ACTIONS/INTERVENTIONS	RATIONALE
Coping Enhancement (NIC)	
Independent	
Assess level of anxiety. Determine how patient has dealt with problems in the past and how he/she is coping with current situation.	Aids in identifying strengths and skills that may help patient deal with current situation and/or enable others to provide appropriate assistance.
Provide accurate information and honest answers.	Helpful in clarifying misconceptions, identifying actual risk. Enables patient to make decisions based on knowledge.
Provide opportunity for expression of concerns, e.g., possible permanent nerve damage/paralysis, effect on sexual ability, changes in employment/finances, altered role responsibilities.	Most patients have concerns that need to be expressed and responded to with accurate information to promote coping with situation.
Assess presence of secondary gains that may interfere with the wish to recover and may impede recovery.	The patient may unconsciously experience advantages such as attention, control of others, relief from responsibilities. These need to be dealt with positively to promote recovery.
Note behaviors of SO that promote "sick role" for the patient.	SO may unconsciously enable patient to remain dependent by doing things that patient should do for self.
Collaborative	
Refer to community support groups, social services, financial/vocational counselor, marital therapy/psychotherapy, as appropriate.	Provides support for adapting to changes and provides resources to deal with problems.

NURSING DIAGNOSIS: Knowledge Deficit [Learning Need] regarding condition, prognosis, treatment, self care, and discharge needs

May be related to
Misinformation/lack of knowledge
Information misinterpretation, lack of recall
Unfamiliarity with information resources

Possibly evidenced by
Verbalization of problems; statement of misconception
Inaccurate return demonstration
Development of preventable complications

DESIRED OUTCOMES/EVALUATION CRITERIA—PATIENT WILL:

Knowledge: Disease Process (NOC)

Verbalize understanding of condition, prognosis, and treatment.

Knowledge: Treatment Regimen (NOC)

Initiate necessary lifestyle changes.
Participate in therapeutic regimen.

ACTIONS/INTERVENTIONS	RATIONALE
Teaching: Disease Process (NIC)	
Independent	
Review disease/injury process and prognosis. Stress activity restrictions/limitations, e.g., avoid riding in car for long periods, refrain from participation in aggressive sports.	Helpful in clarifying and developing understanding and acceptance of necessary lifestyle modifications. Full knowledge base provides opportunity for patient to make informed choices. May enhance cooperation with treatment program and achievement of optimal recovery.
Give information about and instruct in proper body mechanics and exercises. Include information about proper posture/body mechanics for standing, sitting, and lifting, and use of supportive shoes.	Reduces risk of reinjuring back/neck area by using muscles of thighs/buttocks.
Discuss medications and side effects: e.g., some medications cause drowsiness (analgesics, muscle relaxants); others can irritate gastric mucosa/aggravate ulcer disease (NSAIDs).	Reduces risk of complications/injury.
Recommend use of bedboards/firm mattress, small flat pillow under neck, sleeping on side with knees flexed, avoiding prone position.	May decrease muscle strain through structural support and prevention of hyperextension of spine.
Discuss dietary needs/goals.	High-fiber diet can reduce constipation; calorie restrictions promote weight control/reduction, which can decrease pressure on disc.
Avoid prolonged heat application.	Can increase local tissue congestion; decreased sensitivity to heat can result in thermal injury.
Review use of soft cervical collar.	Maintaining slight flexion of head (allows maximal opening of intervertebral foramina) may be useful for relieving pressure in mild to moderate cervical disc disease. Hyperextension should be avoided.
Encourage regular medical follow-up.	Evaluates resolution/progression of degenerative process; monitors development of side effects/complications of drug therapy; may indicate need for change in therapeutic regimen.
Provide information about what symptoms need to be reported for further evaluation, e.g., sharp pain, loss of sensation/ability to walk, change in bowel/bladder control.	Progression of the process may necessitate further treatment/surgery.
Answer questions about treatment alternatives, e.g.:	

ACTIONS/INTERVENTIONS	RATIONALE
Independent	
Chemonucleolysis;	As an alternative to surgery, the enzyme chymopapain may be injected into the disc (dissolves the mucoprotein disc material without effect on surrounding structure). Although many patients experience relief, the procedure is not widely done because of side effects, including allergic reaction to the enzyme.
Surgical interventions.	Microdiscectomy may be performed to excise fragments of the disc with a comparatively lower risk than more invasive surgery. Laminectomy with/without spinal fusion may be performed when conservative treatment is ineffective or when neurological deficits persist.

POTENTIAL CONSIDERATIONS following acute hospitalization (dependent on patient's age, physical condition/presence of complications, personal resources, and life responsibilities)

Adjustment, impaired—disability requiring change in lifestyle, assault to self-esteem, altered locus of control.
Pain, chronic—prolonged physical/psychosocial disability.
Therapeutic Regimen: Individual, ineffective management—complexity of therapeutic regimen, decisional conflicts, economic difficulties, perceived benefits, powerlessness.
Disuse Syndrome, risk for—severe pain, periods of immobility.

DISC SURGERY

Laminectomy is the excision of a vertebral posterior arch and is commonly performed for injury to the spinal column or to relieve pressure/pain in the presence of a herniated disc. The procedure may be done with or without fusion of vertebrae.

CARE SETTING

Inpatient surgical or orthopedic unit.

RELATED CONCERNS

Psychosocial aspects of care, page 809
Surgical intervention, page 828

Patient Assessment Database

Refer to CP: Herniated Nucleus Pulposus (Ruptured Intervertebral Disc), page 275.

TEACHING/LEARNING

Discharge plan considerations:

DRG projected mean length of inpatient stay: 4.9–6.5 days

May require assistance with ADLs, transportation, homemaker/maintenance tasks, vocational counseling, possible changes in layout of home

Refer to section at end of plan for postdischarge considerations.

DIAGNOSTIC STUDIES

Refer to CP: Herniated Nucleus Pulposus (Ruptured Intervertebral Disc), page 275.

NURSING PRIORITIES

1. Maintain tissue perfusion/neurological function.
2. Promote comfort and healing.
3. Prevent/minimize complications.
4. Assist with return to normal mobility.
5. Provide information about condition/prognosis, treatment needs, and limitations.

DISCHARGE GOALS

1. Neurological function maintained/improved.
2. Complications prevented.
3. Limited mobility achieved with potential for increasing mobility.
4. Condition/prognosis, therapeutic regimen, and behavior/lifestyle changes are understood.
5. Plan in place to meet needs after discharge.

NURSING DIAGNOSIS: Tissue Perfusion, altered (specify)

May be related to
Diminished/interrupted blood flow (e.g., edema of operative site, hematoma formation)
Hypovolemia

Possibly evidenced by
Paresthesia; numbness
Decreased ROM, muscle strength

DESIRED OUTCOMES/EVALUATION CRITERIA—PATIENT WILL:

Neurological Status (NOC)

Report/demonstrate normal sensations and movement as appropriate.

ACTIONS/INTERVENTIONS	RATIONALE

Circulatory Care (NIC)

Independent

Check neurological signs periodically and compare with baseline. Assess movement/sensation of lower extremities and feet (lumbar) and hands/arms (cervical).	Although some degree of sensory impairment is usually present, deterioration/changes may reflect development/resolution of spinal cord edema and/or inflammation of the tissues secondary to damage to motor nerve roots from surgical manipulation; or tissue hemorrhage compressing the spinal cord, requiring prompt medical evaluation/intervention.
Keep patient flat on back for several hours.	Pressure to operative site reduces risk of hematoma.
Monitor vital signs. Note color, warmth, capillary refill.	Hypotension (especially postural) with corresponding changes in pulse rate may reflect hypovolemia from blood loss, restriction of oral intake, nausea/vomiting.
Monitor I&O and Hemovac drainage (if used).	Provides information about circulatory status and replacement needs. Excessive/prolonged blood loss requires further evaluation to determine appropriate intervention.
Palpate operative site for swelling. Inspect dressing for excess drainage and test for glucose if indicated.	Change in contour of operative site suggests hematoma/edema formation. Inspection may reveal frank bleeding or dura leak of CSF (will test glucose-positive), requiring prompt intervention.

Collaborative

Administer IV fluids/blood as indicated.	Fluid replacement depends on the degree of hypovolemia and duration of oozing/bleeding/CSF leaking.
Monitor blood counts, e.g., hemoglobin (Hb), hematocrit (Hct), and red blood cells (RBCs).	Aids in establishing replacement needs and monitors effectiveness of therapy.

NURSING DIAGNOSIS: Trauma, risk for (spinal)

Risk factors may include
Temporary weakness of vertebral column
Balancing difficulties, changes in muscle coordination

Possibly evidenced by
[Not applicable; presence of signs and symptoms establishes an *actual* diagnosis]

DESIRED OUTCOMES/EVALUATION CRITERIA—PATIENT WILL:

Risk Control (NOC)

Maintain proper alignment of spine.
Recognize need for/seek assistance with activity as appropriate.

ACTIONS/INTERVENTIONS	RATIONALE

Positioning: Neurological (NIC)

Independent

Post sign at bedside regarding prescribed position.	Reduces risk of inadvertent strain/flexion of operative area.
Provide bedboard/firm mattress.	Aids in stabilizing back.

ACTIONS/INTERVENTIONS	RATIONALE
Independent	
Maintain cervical collar postoperatively with cervical laminectomy procedure.	Decreases muscle spasm and supports the surrounding structures, allowing normal sensory stimulation to occur.
Limit activities when patient has had a spinal fusion.	Following surgery, spinal movement is restricted to promote healing of fusion, requiring a longer recuperation time.
Logroll patient from side to side. Have patient fold arms across chest, tighten long back muscles, keeping shoulders and pelvis straight. Use pillows between knees during position change and when on side. Use turning sheet and sufficient personnel when turning, especially on the first postoperative day.	Maintains body alignment while turning, preventing twisting motion, which may interfere with healing process.
Assist out of bed: logroll to side of bed, splint back, and raise to sitting position. Avoid prolonged sitting. Move to standing position in single smooth motion.	Avoids twisting and flexing of back while arising from bed/chair, protecting surgical area.
Avoid sudden stretching, twisting, flexing, or jarring of spine.	May cause vertebral collapse, shifting of bone graft, delayed hematoma formation, or subcutaneous wound dehiscence.
Check BP; note reports of dizziness or weakness. Recommend patient change position slowly.	Presence of postural hypotension may result in fainting/falling and possible injury to surgical site.
Have patient wear firm/flat walking shoes when ambulating.	Reduces risk of falls.
Collaborative	
Apply lumbar brace/cervical collar as appropriate.	Brace/corset may be used in and/or out of bed during immediate postoperative phase to support spine and surrounding structures until muscle strength improves. Brace is applied while patient is supine in bed. Spinal fusion generally requires a lengthy recuperation period in a corset/collar.
Refer to physical therapy. Implement program as outlined.	Strengthening exercises may be indicated during the rehabilitative phase to decrease muscle spasm and strain on the vertebral disc area.

NURSING DIAGNOSIS: Breathing Pattern/Airway Clearance, risk for ineffective

Risk factors may include
Tracheal/bronchial obstruction/edema
Decreased lung expansion, pain

Possibly evidenced by
[Not applicable; presence of signs and symptoms establishes an *actual* diagnosis]

DESIRED OUTCOMES/EVALUATION CRITERIA—PATIENT WILL:

Respiratory Status: Ventilation (NOC)

Maintain a normal/effective respiratory pattern free of cyanosis and other signs of hypoxia, with ABGs within acceptable range.

ACTIONS/INTERVENTIONS

Respiratory Status: Ventilation (NIC)	

Independent

Inspect for edema of face/neck (cervical laminectomy) especially first 24–48 hr after surgery.

Listen for hoarseness. Encourage voice rest.

Auscultate breath sounds, note presence of wheezes/rhonchi.

Assist with coughing, turning, and deep breathing.

Collaborative

Administer supplemental oxygen, if indicated.

Monitor/graph ABGs or pulse oximetry.

RATIONALE

Tracheal edema/compression or nerve injury can compromise respiratory function.

May indicate laryngeal nerve injury, which can negatively affect cough (ability to clear airway).

Suggests accumulation of secretions/need to engage in more aggressive therapeutic actions to clear airway.

Facilitates movement of secretions and clearing of lungs; reduces risk of respiratory complications (pneumonia).

May be necessary for periods of respiratory distress or evidence of hypoxia.

Monitors effectiveness of breathing pattern/therapy.

NURSING DIAGNOSIS: Pain [acute]

May be related to
Physical agent: surgical manipulation, edema, inflammation, harvesting of bone graft

Possibly evidenced by
Reports of pain
Autonomic responses: diaphoresis, changes in vital signs, pallor
Alteration in muscle tone
Guarding, distraction behaviors/restlessness

DESIRED OUTCOMES/EVALUATION CRITERIA—PATIENT WILL:

Pain Control Behavior (NOC)	

Report pain is relieved/controlled.
Verbalize methods that provide relief.
Demonstrate use of relaxation skills and diversional activities.

ACTIONS/INTERVENTIONS

Pain Management (NIC)	

Independent

Assess intensity, description, and location/radiation of pain, changes in sensation. Instruct in use of rating scale (e.g., 0–10).

RATIONALE

May be mild to severe with radiation to shoulders/occipital area (cervical) or hips/buttocks (lumbar). If bone graft has been taken from the iliac crest, pain may be more severe at the donor site. Numbness/tingling discomfort may reflect return of sensation after nerve root decompression or result from developing edema causing nerve compression.

ACTIONS/INTERVENTIONS	RATIONALE

Independent

Review expected manifestations/changes in intensity of pain.

Development/resolution of edema and inflammation in the immediate postoperative phase can affect pressure on various nerves and cause changes in degree of pain (especially 3 days after procedure, when muscle spasms/improved nerve root sensation intensify pain).

Encourage patient to assume position of comfort if indicated. Use logroll for position change.

Positioning is dictated by physical preference, type of operation (e.g., head of bed may be slightly elevated after cervical laminectomy). Readjustment of position aids in relieving muscle fatigue and discomfort. Logrolling avoids tension in the operative areas, maintains straight spinal alignment, and reduces risk of displacing epidural patient-controlled analgesia (PCA) when used.

Provide back rub/massage, avoiding operative site.

Relieves/reduces pain by alteration of sensory neurons, muscle relaxation.

Demonstrate/encourage use of relaxation skills, e.g., deep breathing, visualization.

Refocuses attention, reduces muscle tension, promotes sense of well-being, and controls/decreases discomfort.

Provide soft diet, room humidifier; encourage voice rest following anterior cervical laminectomy.

Reduces discomfort associated with sore throat and difficulty swallowing.

Investigate patient reports of return of radicular pain.

Suggests complications (e.g., collapsing of disc space, shifting of bone graft) requiring further medical evaluation and intervention. *Note:* Sciatica and muscle spasms often recur after laminectomy but should resolve within several days or weeks.

Collaborative

Administer analgesics, as indicated:

 Narcotics, e.g., morphine, codeine, meperidine (Demerol), oxycodone (Tylox), hydrocodone (Vicodin), acetaminophen (Tylenol) with codeine;

Narcotics are used during the first few postoperative days, then nonnarcotic agents are incorporated as intensity of pain diminishes. *Note:* Narcotics may be administered via epidural catheter.

 Muscle relaxants, e.g., cyclobenzaprine (Flexeril), diazepam (Valium).

May be used to relieve muscle spasms resulting from intraoperative nerve irritation.

Instruct patient/assist with PCA.

Gives patient control of medication administration (usually narcotics) to achieve a more constant level of comfort, which may enhance healing and sense of well-being.

Provide throat sprays/lozenges, viscous xylocaine.

Sore throat may be a major complaint following cervical laminectomy.

Apply TENS unit as needed.

May be used for incisional pain or when nerve involvement continues after discharge. Decreases level of pain by blocking nerve transmission of pain.

NURSING DIAGNOSIS: Mobility, impaired physical

May be related to
Neuromuscular impairment
Limitations imposed by condition; pain

Possibly evidenced by
Impaired coordination, limited ROM
Reluctance to attempt movement
Decreased muscle strength/control

DESIRED OUTCOMES/EVALUATION CRITERIA—PATIENT WILL:

Knowledge: Personal Safety (NOC)

Demonstrate techniques/behaviors that enable resumption of activities.

Mobility Level (NOC)

Maintain or increase strength and function of affected body part.

ACTIONS/INTERVENTIONS

Body Mechanics Promotion (NIC)

Independent

Schedule activity/procedures with rest periods. Encourage participation in ADLs within individual limitations.

Provide/assist with passive and active ROM exercises depending on surgical procedure.

Assist with activity/progressive ambulation.

Review proper body mechanics/techniques for participating in activities.

RATIONALE

Enhances healing and builds muscle strength and endurance. Patient participation promotes independence and sense of control.

Strengthens abdominal muscles and flexors of spine; promotes good body mechanics.

Until healing occurs, activity is limited and advanced slowly according to individual tolerance.

Reduces risk of muscle strain/injury/pain and increases likelihood of patient involvement in progressive activity.

(Refer to CP: Herniated Nucleus Pulposus (Ruptured Intervertebral Disc), ND: Mobility, impaired physical, p. 278, for further considerations.)

NURSING DIAGNOSIS: Constipation

May be related to
Pain and swelling in surgical area
Immobilization, decreased physical activity
Altered nerve stimulation, ileus
Emotional stress, lack of privacy
Changes/restriction of dietary intake

Possibly evidenced by
Decreased bowel sounds
Increased abdominal girth
Abdominal pain/rectal fullness, nausea
Change in frequency, consistency, and amount of stool

DESIRED OUTCOMES/EVALUATION CRITERIA—PATIENT WILL:

Bowel Elimination (NOC)

Re-establish normal patterns of bowel functioning.
Pass stool of soft/semiformed consistency without straining.

ACTIONS/INTERVENTIONS	RATIONALE

Constipation/Impaction Management (NIC)

Independent

Note abdominal distension and auscultate bowel sounds.	Distension and absence of bowel sounds indicate that bowel is not functioning, possibly because of sudden loss of parasympathetic enervation of the bowel.
Use fracture or child-size bedpan until allowed out of bed.	Promotes comfort, reduces muscle tension.
Provide privacy.	Promotes psychological comfort.
Encourage early ambulation.	Stimulates peristalsis, facilitating passage of flatus.

Collaborative

Begin progressive diet as tolerated.	Solid foods are not started until bowel sounds have returned/flatus has been passed and danger of ileus formation has abated.
Provide rectal tube, suppositories, and enemas as needed.	May be necessary to relieve abdominal distension, promote resumption of normal bowel habits.
Administer laxatives, stool softeners as indicated.	Softens stools, promotes normal bowel habits, decreases straining.

NURSING DIAGNOSIS: Urinary Retention, risk for

Risk factors may include
Pain and swelling in operative area
Need for remaining flat in bed

Possibly evidenced by
[Not applicable; presence of signs and symptoms establishes an *actual* diagnosis]

DESIRED OUTCOMES/EVALUATION CRITERIA—PATIENT WILL:

Urinary Continence (NOC)

Empty bladder adequately according to individual need.

ACTIONS/INTERVENTIONS	RATIONALE

Urinary Retention Care (NIC)

Independent

Observe and record amount/time of voiding.	Determines whether bladder is being emptied and when interventions may be necessary.
Palpate for bladder distension.	May indicate urine retention.
Force fluids.	Maintains kidney function.
Stimulate bladder emptying by running water, pouring warm water over peritoneal area, or having patient put hand in warm water as needed.	Promotes urination by relaxing urinary sphincter.

Collaborative

| Catheterize for bladder residual after voiding when indicated. Insert/maintain indwelling catheter as needed. | Intermittent or continuous catheterization may be necessary for several days postoperatively until swelling is decreased. |

NURSING DIAGNOSIS: Knowledge Deficit [Learning Need] regarding condition, prognosis, treatment, self care, and discharge needs

May be related to
Lack of exposure
Information misinterpretation; lack of recall
Unfamiliarity with information resources

Possibly evidenced by
Request for information; statement of misconception
Inaccurate follow-through of instruction

DESIRED OUTCOMES/EVALUATION CRITERIA—PATIENT WILL:

Knowledge: Disease Process (NOC)

Verbalize understanding of condition, prognosis, and potential complications.
List signs/symptoms requiring medical follow-up.

Knowledge: Treatment Regimen (NOC)

Verbalize understanding of therapeutic regimen.
Initiate necessary lifestyle changes.

ACTIONS/INTERVENTIONS	RATIONALE

Teaching: Disease Process (NIC)

Independent

Review particular condition/prognosis.	Individual needs dictate tolerance levels/limitations of activity.
Discuss possibility of unrelieved/renewed pain.	Some pain may continue for several months as activity level increases and scar tissue stretches. Pain relief from surgical procedure could be temporary if other discs have similar amount of degeneration.
Discuss use of heat, e.g., warm packs, heating pad, or showers.	Increased circulation to the back/surgical area transports nutrients for healing to the area and aids in resolution of pathogens/exudates out of the area. Decreases muscle spasms that may result from nerve root irritation during healing process.
Discuss judicious use of cold packs before/after stretching activity, if indicated.	May decrease muscle spasm in some instances more effectively than heat.
Avoid tub baths for 3–4 wk, depending on physician recommendation.	Tub baths increase risk of falls and flexing/twisting of spine.
Review dietary/fluid needs.	Should be tailored to reduce risk of constipation and avoid excess weight gain while meeting nutrient needs to facilitate healing.
Review/reinforce incisional care.	Correct care promotes healing, reduces risk of wound infection. *Note:* This information is especially critical for the patient's SO/caregiver in this era of early discharge (sometimes 24 hr after surgery).

ACTIONS/INTERVENTIONS	RATIONALE

Independent

Identify signs/symptoms requiring notification of healthcare provider, e.g., fever, increased incisional pain, inflammation, wound drainage, decreased sensation/motor activity in extremities.

Prompt evaluation and intervention may prevent complications/permanent injury.

Discuss necessity of follow-up care.

Long-term medical supervision may be needed to manage problems/complications and to reincorporate individual into desired/altered lifestyle and activities.

Review need for/use of immobilization device, as indicated.

Correct application and wearing time is important to gaining the most benefit from the brace.

Assess current lifestyle/job, finances, activities at home and leisure.

Knowledge of current situation allows nurse to highlight areas for possible intervention, such as referral for occupational/vocational testing and counseling.

Listen/communicate with patient regarding alternatives and lifestyle changes. Be sensitive to patient's needs.

Low back pain is a frequent cause of chronic disability. Many patients may have to stop/modify work, and have long-term/chronic pain creating relationship and financial crises. Often the patient is viewed as being a malingerer, which creates further problems in social/work relationships.

Note overt/covert expressions of concern about sexuality.

Although patient may not ask directly, there may be concerns about the effect of this surgery on both the ability to cope with usual role in the family/community and ability to perform sexually.

Provide written copy of all instructions.

Useful as a reference after discharge.

Identify community resources as indicated, e.g., social services, rehabilitation/vocational counseling services.

A team effort can be helpful in providing support during recuperative period.

Recommend counseling, sex therapy, psychotherapy, as appropriate.

Depression is common in conditions for which a lengthy recuperative time (2–9 mo) is expected. Therapy may alleviate anxiety, assist patient to cope effectively, and enhance healing process. Presence of physical limitations, pain, and depression may negatively impact sexual desire/performance and add additional stress to relationship.

Teaching: Prescribed Activity/Exercise (NIC)

Discuss return to activities, stressing importance of increasing as tolerated.

Although the recuperative period may be lengthy, following prescribed activity program promotes muscle and tissue circulation, healing, and strengthening.

Encourage development of regular exercise program, e.g., walking, stretching.

Promotes healing, strengthens abdominal and erector muscles to provide support to the spinal column, and enhances general physical and emotional well-being.

Discuss importance of good posture and avoidance of prolonged standing/sitting. Recommend sitting in straight-backed chair with feet on a footstool or flat on the floor.

Prevents further injuries/stress by maintaining proper alignment of spine.

Stress importance of avoiding activities that increase the flexion of the spine, e.g., climbing stairs, automobile driving/riding, bending at the waist with knees straight, lifting more than 5 lb, engaging in strenuous exercise/sports. Discuss limitations on sexual relations/positions.

Flexing/twisting of the spine aggravates the healing process and increases risk of injury to spinal cord.

ACTIONS/INTERVENTIONS	RATIONALE
Independent	
Encourage lying-down rest periods, balanced with activity.	Reduces general and spinal fatigue and assists in the healing/recuperative process.
Explore limitations/abilities.	Placing limitations into perspective with abilities allows the patient to understand own situation and exercise choice.

POTENTIAL CONSIDERATIONS following acute hospitalization (dependent on patient's age, physical condition/presence of complications, personal resources, and life responsibilities)

Mobility, impaired physical—decreased strength/endurance, pain, immobilizing device.
Self-Care deficit—decreased strength/endurance, pain, immobilizing device.
Trauma, risk for—weakness, balancing difficulties, decreased muscle coordination, reduced temperature/tactile sensation.
Family Coping ineffective: compromised—temporary family disorganization and role changes.

Sample CP: Cervical Laminectomy with Fusion. ELOS: 3 Days Orthopedic or Surgical Unit

ND and Categories of Care	Day 1 Day of Surgery _____	Day 2 POD #1 _____	Day 3 POD #2 _____
Altered tissue perfusion, R/T to altered blood flow (operative site edema, hematoma formation, hypovolemia)	Goals: Maintain proper alignment of cervical spine Display stable/improved sensation in affected limbs	Display normal sensory/motor response Identify appropriate safety measures	
Diagnostic studies		Hb/Hct, RBC Electrolytes	C–spine–PA/lat
Additional assessments	VS q1hX4 then q4h Neurovascular checks UE, q1hX4 then q4h Dressings/drainage q4h I&O q8h Hemovac (if used) q8h Palpate operative site for swelling, inspect face/neck for edema qhX4	→ qid → qid → → → → q8h	→ → q8h q8h → → bid → D/C →
Medications	IV fluids/blood as indicated	→ D/C or convert to NS lock	→ D/C
Patient education	Purpose/necessity of cervical collar Protocol for position change	Cessation of smoking if indicated	D/C Use of heat Signs/symptoms to be reported to healthcare provider
Additional nursing actions	Position per protocol/HOB elevated 30° Log roll q2h Cervical collar in place BRP w/assistance (tennis shoes—not slippers) Fluids as tolerated	→ → Chair X3 → → → Advance diet as tolerated	→ → Ambulate as tolerated → Per self as tolerated →
Pain R/T to surgical intervention	Report pain controlled	Participate in activities to increase comfort	→ → Verbalize understanding of therapeutic interventions
Additional assessments	Pain characteristics/change Response to interventions	→	→
Medications Allergies: _____	Analgesics–PCA or IM Throat spray/lozenges	→ D/C PCA → PO analgesics →	→ D/C IM → → D/C
Patient education	Orient to unit/room Reporting of pain/effects of interventions Proper use of PCA Recovery/rehabilitation expectations Limitations of movement (e.g., twisting, flexing, pulling) Voice rest (anterior approach)	Relaxation techniques Medication dose, frequency, purpose, side effects	Use of TENS as indicated Signs/symptoms to report to healthcare provider
Additional nursing actions	Provide firm mattress Comfort measures	→ →	→ →
Impaired physical mobility R/T musculoskeletal impairment; pain and therapeutic restriction		Re-establish normal bowel/ bladder elimination	Verbalize understanding of activity program/ restrictions Report plan in place to meet needs postdischarge
Referrals		Social Services Home care	

Sample CP: Cervical Laminectomy with Fusion. ELOS: 3 Days Orthopedic or Surgical Unit *(Continued)*

ND and Categories of Care	Day 1 Day of Surgery _____	Day 2 POD #1 _____	Day 3 POD #2 _____
Additional assessments	General muscle tone/strength Level of functional ability Breath sounds q4h Bowel sounds q4h Amount/time of voids	→ Ability to perform ADLs independently → q8h → q8h → D/C Edema, pain lower extremities, Homans' sign q8h	 → → →
Medications Patient education	Activity level/progression Bed exercises Skin care needs	Stool softener General wellness—diet, exercise, adequate rest Home exercise program Proper body mechanics Use of assistive devices as required	→ Fleets if no BM Activity restrictions e.g., shower instead of tub bath, no lifting, resumption of work, hobbies, sexual activity Provide written copy of instructions
Additional nursing actions	Assist w/passive and active ROM exercises Encourage participation of ADLs w/in level of ability T, C, DB, q2h Incentive spirometry q4h Thigh-high TEDs Skin care per Risk Protocol	→ → → → q4h while awake → Remove q8h →	→ → Per self → Per self → D/C → D/C →

SPINAL CORD INJURY (ACUTE REHABILITATIVE PHASE)

The leading causes of spinal cord injury (SCI) include motor vehicle crashes, falls, acts of violence, and sporting injuries. The mechanism of injury influences the type of SCI and the degree of neurological deficit. Spinal cord lesions are classified as complete (total loss of sensation and voluntary motor function) or incomplete (mixed loss of sensation and voluntary motor function).

Physical findings vary, depending on the level of injury, degree of spinal shock, and phase and degree of recovery, but in general, are classified as follows:

C-1 to C-3: Quadriplegia with total loss of muscular/respiratory function.
C-4 to C-5: Quadriplegia with impairment, poor pulmonary capacity, complete dependency for ADLs.
C-6 to C-7: Quadriplegia with some arm/hand movement allowing some independence in ADLs.
C-7 to C-8: Quadriplegia with limited use of thumb/fingers, increasing independence.
T-1 to L-1: Paraplegia with intact arm function and varying function of intercostal and abdominal muscles.
L-1 to L-2 or below: Mixed motor-sensory loss; bowel and bladder dysfunction.

CARE SETTING

Inpatient medical/surgical and subacute/rehabilitation units.

RELATED CONCERNS

Disc surgery, page 283
Fractures, page 680
Pneumonia: microbial, page 140
Psychosocial aspects of care, page 809
Thrombophlebitis: deep vein thrombosis, page 115
Total nutritional support: parenteral/enteral feeding, page 508
Upper gastrointestinal/esophageal bleeding, page 333
Ventilatory assistance (mechanical), page 188

Patient Assessment Database

ACTIVITY/REST

May exhibit: Paralysis of muscles (flaccid during spinal shock) at/below level of lesion
Muscle/generalized weakness (cord contusion and compression)

CIRCULATION

May report: Palpitations
Dizziness with position changes

May exhibit: Low BP, postural BP changes, bradycardia
Cool, pale extremities
Absence of perspiration in affected area

ELIMINATION

May exhibit: Incontinence of bladder and bowel
Urinary retention
Abdominal distension; loss of bowel sounds
Melena, coffee-ground emesis/hematemesis

EGO INTEGRITY

May report: Denial, disbelief, sadness, anger
May exhibit: Fear, anxiety, irritability, withdrawal

FOOD/FLUID

May exhibit: Abdominal distension; loss of bowel sounds (paralytic ileus)

HYGIENE

May exhibit: Variable level of dependence in ADLs

NEUROSENSORY

May report: Absence of sensation below area of injury, or opposite side sensation
Numbness, tingling, burning, twitching of arms/legs

May exhibit: Flaccid paralysis (spasticity may develop as spinal shock resolves, depending on area of cord involvement)
Loss of sensation (varying degrees may return after spinal shock resolves)
Loss of muscle/vasomotor tone
Loss of/asymmetrical reflexes, including deep tendon reflexes
Changes in pupil reaction, ptosis of upper eyelid
Loss of sweating in affected area

PAIN/DISCOMFORT

May report: Pain/tenderness in muscles
Hyperesthesia immediately above level of injury

May exhibit: Vertebral tenderness, deformity

RESPIRATION

May report: Shortness of breath, "air hunger," inability to breathe

May exhibit: Shallow/labored respirations; periods of apnea
Diminished breath sounds, rhonchi
Pallor, cyanosis

SAFETY

May exhibit: Temperature fluctuations (taking on temperature of environment)

SEXUALITY

May report: Expressions of concern about return to normal functioning

May exhibit: Uncontrolled erection (priapism)
Menstrual irregularities

TEACHING/LEARNING

Discharge plan considerations: **DRG projected mean length of inpatient stay: 17.1–90 days (inclusive of inpatient rehabilitation)**
Will require varying degrees of assistance with transportation, shopping, food preparation, self-care, finances, medications/treatment, and homemaker/maintenance tasks
May require changes in physical layout of home and/or placement in a rehabilitative center

Refer to section at end of plan for postdischarge considerations.

DIAGNOSTIC STUDIES

Spinal x-rays: Locates level and type of bony injury (fracture, dislocation); determines alignment and reduction after traction or surgery.

CT scan: Locates injury, evaluates structural alterations. Useful for rapid screening and providing additional information if x-rays questionable for fracture/cord status.

MRI: Identifies spinal cord lesions, edema, and compression.

Myelogram: May be done to visualize spinal column if pathology is unclear or if occlusion of spinal subarachnoid space is suspected (not usually done after penetrating injuries).

Somatosensory evoked potentials (SEP): Elicited by presenting a peripheral stimulus and measuring degree of latency in cortical response to evaluate spinal cord functioning/potential for recovery.

Chest x-ray: Demonstrates pulmonary status (e.g., changes in level of diaphragm, atelectasis).

Pulmonary function studies (vital capacity, tidal volume): Measures maximum volume of inspiration and expiration; especially important in patients with low cervical lesions or thoracic lesions with possible phrenic nerve and intercostal muscle involvement.

ABGs: Indicates effectiveness of gas exchange and ventilatory effort.

NURSING PRIORITIES

1. Maximize respiratory function.
2. Prevent further injury to spinal cord.
3. Promote mobility/independence.
4. Prevent or minimize complications.
5. Support psychological adjustment of patient/SO.
6. Provide information about injury, prognosis and expectations, treatment needs, possible and preventable complications.

DISCHARGE GOALS

1. Ventilatory effort adequate for individual needs.
2. Spinal injury stabilized.
3. Complications prevented/controlled.
4. Self-care needs met by self/with assistance, depending on specific situation.
5. Beginning to cope with current situation and planning for future.
6. Condition/prognosis, therapeutic regimen, and possible complications understood.
7. Plan in place to meet needs after discharge.

NURSING DIAGNOSIS: Breathing Pattern, risk for ineffective

Risk factors may include

Impairment of innervation of diaphragm (lesions at or above C-5)

Complete or mixed loss of intercostal muscle function

Reflex abdominal spasms; gastric distension

Possibly evidenced by

[Not applicable; presence of signs and symptoms establishes an *actual* diagnosis]

DESIRED OUTCOMES/EVALUATION CRITERIA—PATIENT WILL:

Respiratory Status: Ventilation (NOC)

Maintain adequate ventilation as evidenced by absence of respiratory distress and ABGs within acceptable limits.

Demonstrate appropriate behaviors to support respiratory effort.

ACTIONS/INTERVENTIONS

Respiratory Monitoring (NIC)

Independent

Assess respiratory function by asking patient to take a deep breath. Note presence or absence of spontaneous effort and quality of respirations, e.g., labored, using accessory muscles.

Auscultate breath sounds. Note areas of absent or decreased breath sounds or development of adventitious sounds (e.g., rhonchi).

Note strength/effectiveness of cough.

RATIONALE

C-1 to C-3 injuries result in complete loss of respiratory function. Injuries at C-4 or C-5 can result in variable loss of respiratory function, depending on phrenic nerve involvement and diaphragmatic function, but generally cause decreased vital capacity and inspiratory effort. For injuries below C-6 or C-7, respiratory muscle function is preserved; however, weakness/impairment of intercostal muscles may impair effectiveness of cough and the ability to sigh, deep breathe.

Hypoventilation is common and leads to accumulation of secretions, atelectasis, and pneumonia (frequent complications).

Level of injury determines function of intercostal muscles and ability to cough spontaneously/move secretions.

ACTIONS/INTERVENTIONS	RATIONALE
Independent	
Observe skin color for developing cyanosis, duskiness.	May reveal impending respiratory failure, need for immediate medical evaluation and intervention.
Assess for abdominal distension and muscle spasm.	Abdominal fullness may impede diaphragmatic excursion, reducing lung expansion and further compromising respiratory function.
Monitor/limit visitors as indicated.	General debilitation and respiratory compromise place patient at increased risk for acquiring URIs.
Monitor diaphragmatic movement when phrenic pacemaker is implanted.	Stimulation of phrenic nerve may enhance respiratory effort, decreasing dependency on mechanical ventilator.
Elicit concerns/questions regarding mechanical ventilation devices.	Acknowledges reality of situation. Refer to CP: Ventilatory Assistance, p. 188.)
Provide honest answers.	Future respiratory function/support needs will not be totally known until spinal shock resolves and acute rehabilitative phase is completed. Even though respiratory support may be required, alternative devices/techniques may be used to enhance mobility and promote independence.
Maintain patent airway: keep head in neutral position, elevate head of bed slightly if tolerated, use airway adjuncts as indicated.	Patients with high cervical injury and impaired gag/cough reflexes require assistance in preventing aspiration/maintaining patent airway.
Assist patient in "taking control" of respirations as indicated. Instruct in and encourage deep breathing, focusing attention on steps of breathing.	Breathing may no longer be a totally voluntary activity but require conscious effort, depending on level of injury/involvement of respiratory muscles.
Assist with coughing as indicated for level of injury, e.g., have patient take deep breath and hold for 2 sec before coughing, or inhale deeply, then cough at the end of a slow exhalation. Alternatively, assist by placing hands below diaphragm and pushing upward as patient exhales (quad cough).	Adds volume to cough and facilitates expectoration of secretions or helps move them high enough to be suctioned out. *Note:* Quad cough procedure is generally reserved for patients with stable injuries once they are in the rehabilitation stage.
Suction as necessary. Document quality and quantity of secretions.	If cough is ineffective, suctioning may be needed to remove secretions, enhance gas exchange, and reduce risk of respiratory infections. *Note:* "Routine" suctioning increases risk of hypoxia, bradycardia (vagal response), tissue trauma. Therefore, suctioning needs are based on presence of/inability to move secretions.
Reposition/turn periodically. Avoid/limit prone position when indicated.	Enhances ventilation of all lung segments, mobilizes secretions, reducing risk of complications such as atelectasis and pneumonia. *Note:* Prone position significantly decreases vital capacity, increasing risk of respiratory compromise/failure.
Encourage fluids (at least 2000 mL/day).	Aids in liquefying secretions, promoting mobilization/expectoration.
Measure/graph: Vital capacity (VC), tidal volume (V_T), inspiratory force;	Determines level of respiratory muscle function. Serial measurements may be done to predict impending respiratory failure (acute injury) or determine level of function after spinal shock phase and/or while weaning from ventilatory support.

ACTIONS/INTERVENTIONS

Collaborative

Serial ABGs and/or pulse oximetry.

RATIONALE

Documents status of ventilation and oxygenation, identifies respiratory problems, e.g., hypoventilation (low PaO_2/elevated $PaCO_2$) and pulmonary complications.

Airway Management (NIC)

Administer oxygen by appropriate method, e.g., nasal prongs, mask, intubation/ventilator.

Assist with use of respiratory adjuncts (e.g., incentive spirometer, blow bottles) and aggressive chest physiotherapy (e.g., chest percussion).

Refer to/consult with respiratory and physical therapists.

Method is determined by level of injury, degree of respiratory insufficiency, and amount of recovery of respiratory muscle function after spinal shock phase.

Preventing retained secretions is essential to maximize gas diffusion and to reduce risk of pneumonia.

Helpful in identifying exercises individually appropriate to stimulate and strengthen respiratory muscles/effort. For example, glossopharyngeal breathing uses muscles of mouth, pharynx, and larynx to swallow air into lungs, thereby enhancing VC and chest expansion.

NURSING DIAGNOSIS: Trauma, risk for [additional spinal injury]

Risk factors may include
Temporary weakness/instability of spinal column

Possibly evidenced by
[Not applicable; presence of signs and symptoms establishes an *actual* diagnosis]

DESIRED OUTCOMES/EVALUATION CRITERIA—PATIENT WILL:

Bone Healing (NOC)

Maintain proper alignment of spine without further spinal cord damage.

ACTIONS/INTERVENTIONS

Traction/Immobilization Care (NIC)

Independent

Maintain bedrest and immobilization device(s), e.g., sandbags, traction, halo, hard/soft cervical collars, brace.

Check external stabilization device, e.g., Gardner-Wells tongs or skeletal traction apparatus.

Elevate head of traction frame or bed as indicated. Ensure that traction frames are secure, pulleys aligned, weights hanging free.

Check weights for ordered traction pull (usually 10–20 lb).

RATIONALE

Body rest prevents vertebral column instability and aids healing. *Note:* Traction is used only for cervical spine stabilization.

These devices are used for decompression of spinal fractures and stabilization of vertebral column during the early acute phase of injury to prevent further spinal cord injury.

Creates safe, effective counterbalance to maintain both patient's position and traction pull.

Weight pull depends on patient's size and amount of reduction needed to maintain vertebral column alignment.

ACTIONS/INTERVENTIONS

Independent

Reposition at intervals, using adjuncts for turning and support, e.g., turn sheets, foam wedges, blanket rolls, pillows. Use several staff members when turning/logrolling patient. Follow special instructions for traction equipment, kinetic bed, and frames once halo is in place.

Collaborative

Assist with preparation/maintain skeletal traction via tongs, calipers, halo/vest, as indicated.

Prepare for internal stabilization surgery, e.g., spinal laminectomy or fusion, if indicated.

RATIONALE

Maintains proper spinal column alignment, reducing risk of further trauma. *Note:* Grasping the brace/halo vest to turn or reposition patient may cause additional injury.

Reduces vertebral fracture/dislocation.

Surgery may be indicated for spinal stabilization/cord decompression or removal of bony fragments.

NURSING DIAGNOSIS: Mobility, impaired physical

May be related to
Neuromuscular impairment
Immobilization by traction

Possibly evidenced by
Inability to purposefully move; paralysis
Muscle atrophy; contractures

DESIRED OUTCOMES/EVALUATION CRITERIA—PATIENT WILL:

Immobility Consequences: Physiological (NOC)

Maintain position of function as evidenced by absence of contractures, footdrop.

Muscle Function (NOC)

Increase strength of unaffected/compensatory body parts.
Demonstrate techniques/behaviors that enable resumption of activity.

ACTIONS/INTERVENTIONS

Bedrest Care (NIC)

Independent

Continually assess motor function (as spinal shock/edema resolves) by requesting patient to perform certain actions, e.g., shrug shoulders, spread fingers, squeeze/release examiner's hands.

Provide means to summon help, e.g., special sensitive call light.

Perform/assist with full ROM exercises on all extremities and joints, using slow, smooth movements. Hyperextend hips periodically.

Position arms at 90-degree angle at regular intervals.

Maintain ankles at 90 degrees with footboard, high-top tennis shoes, and so on. Place trochanter rolls along thighs when in bed.

RATIONALE

Evaluates status of individual situation (motor-sensory impairment may be mixed and/or not clear) for a specific level of injury, affecting type and choice of interventions.

Enables patient to have a sense of control and reduces fear of being left alone. *Note:* Quadriplegic on ventilator requires continuous observation in early management.

Enhances circulation, restores/maintains muscle tone and joint mobility, and prevents disuse contractures and muscle atrophy.

Prevents frozen shoulder contractures.

Prevents footdrop and external rotation of hips.

ACTIONS/INTERVENTIONS	RATIONALE

Independent

Elevate lower extremities at intervals when in chair, or raise foot of bed when permitted in individual situation. Assess for edema of feet/ankles.

Loss of vascular tone and "muscle action" results in pooling of blood and venous stasis in the lower abdomen and lower extremities with increased risk of hypotension and thrombus formation.

Plan activities to provide uninterrupted rest periods. Encourage involvement within individual tolerance/ability.

Prevents fatigue, allowing opportunity for maximal efforts/participation by patient.

Measure/monitor BP before and after activity in acute phases or until stable. Change position slowly. Use cardiac bed or tilt table/circoelectric bed as activity level is advanced.

Orthostatic hypotension may occur as a result of venous pooling (secondary to loss of vascular tone). Side-to-side movement or elevation of head can aggravate hypotension and cause syncope.

Reposition periodically even when sitting in chair. Teach patient how to employ weight-shifting techniques.

Reduces pressure areas, promotes peripheral circulation.

Prepare for weight-bearing activities, e.g., use of tilt table for upright position, strengthening/conditioning exercises for unaffected body parts.

Early weight bearing reduces osteoporotic changes in long bones and reduces incidence of urinary infections and kidney stones.

Encourage use of relaxation techniques.

Reduces muscle tension/fatigue, may help limit pain of muscle spasms, spasticity.

Inspect skin daily. Observe for pressure areas, and provide meticulous skin care. Teach patient to inspect skin surfaces and to use a mirror to look at hard-to-see areas.

Altered circulation, loss of sensation, and paralysis potentiate pressure sore formation. This is a lifelong consideration. (Refer to ND: Skin Integrity, risk for impaired, p. 311.)

Assist with/encourage pulmonary hygiene, e.g., deep breathing, coughing, suctioning. (Refer to ND: Breathing Pattern, risk for ineffective, p. 297.)

Immobility and bedrest increase risk of pulmonary infection.

Assess for deep pain, redness, swelling/muscle tension of calf tissues. Record calf and thigh measurements if indicated.

In a high percentage of patients with cervical cord injury, thrombi develop because of altered peripheral circulation, immobilization, and flaccid paralysis.

Investigate sudden onset of dyspnea, cyanosis, and/or other signs of respiratory distress.

Development of pulmonary emboli may be "silent" because pain perception is altered and/or DVT is not readily recognized.

Collaborative

Place patient in kinetic therapy bed when appropriate.

Effectively immobilizes unstable spinal column, and improves systemic circulation, which is thought to decrease complications associated with immobility.

Apply antiembolic hose/leotard or sequential compression devices (SCDs) to legs as appropriate.

Limits pooling of blood in lower extremities or abdomen, thus improving vasomotor tone and reducing incidence of thrombus formation and pulmonary emboli.

Consult with physical/occupational therapists/rehabilitation team.

Helpful in planning and implementing individualized exercise program and identifying/developing assistive devices to maintain function, enhance mobility and independence.

Administer muscle relaxants/antispasticity agents as indicated, e.g.:

Diazepam (Valium), baclofen (Lioresal), dantrolene (Dantrium);

May be useful in limiting or reducing pain associated with spasticity.

Tizanidine (Zanaflex).

Centrally acting α_2-adrenergic agonist reduces spasticity. Short duration of action requires careful dosage monitoring to achieve maximum effect. May have additive effect with baclofen (Lioresal) but needs to be used with caution because both drugs have similar side effects.

ACTIONS/INTERVENTIONS	RATIONALE
Peripheral Sensation Management (NIC)	
Independent	
Assess/document sensory function or deficit (by means of touch, pinprick, hot/cold, etc.), progressing from area of deficit to neurologically intact area.	Changes may not occur during acute phase, but as spinal shock resolves, changes should be documented by dermatome charts or anatomic landmarks, e.g., "2 in above nipple line."
Protect from bodily harm, e.g., falls, burns, positioning of arm or objects.	Patient may not sense pain or be aware of body position.
Assist the patient to recognize and compensate for alterations in sensation.	May help reduce anxiety of the unknown and prevent injury.
Explain procedures before and during care, identifying the body part involved.	Enhances patient perception of "whole" body.
Provide tactile stimulation, touching patient in intact sensory areas, e.g., shoulders, face, head.	Touching conveys caring and fulfills a normal physiological and psychological need.
Position patient to see surroundings and activities. Provide prism glasses when prone on turning frame. Talk to patient frequently.	Provides sensory input, which may be severely limited, especially when patient is in prone position.
Provide diversional activities, e.g., television, radio, music, liberal visitation. Use clocks, calendars, pictures, bulletin boards, and so on. Encourage SO/family to discuss general and personal news.	Aids in maintaining reality orientation and provides some sense of normality in daily passage of time.
Provide uninterrupted sleep and rest periods.	Reduces sensory overload, enhances orientation and coping abilities, and aids in re-establishing natural sleep patterns.
Note presence of exaggerated emotional responses, altered thought processes, e.g., disorientation, bizarre thinking.	Indicative of damage to sensory tracts and/or psychological stress, requiring further assessment and intervention.

> **NURSING DIAGNOSIS: Pain [acute]**
>
> **May be related to**
> Physical injury
> Traction apparatus
>
> **Possibly evidenced by**
> Hyperesthesia immediately above level of injury
> Burning pain below level of injury (paraplegia)
> Muscle spasm/spasticity
> Phantom pain; headaches
>
> **DESIRED OUTCOMES/EVALUATION CRITERIA—PATIENT WILL:**
>
> **Pain Level (NOC)**
>
> Report relief or control of pain/discomfort.
>
> **Pain Control Behavior (NOC)**
>
> Identify ways to manage pain.
> Demonstrate use of relaxation skills and diversional activities as individually indicated.

ACTIONS/INTERVENTIONS	RATIONALE
Pain Management (NIC)	
Independent	
Assess for presence of pain. Help patient identify and quantify pain, e.g., location, type of pain, intensity on scale of 0–10.	Patient usually reports pain above the level of injury, e.g., chest/back or headache possibly from stabilizer apparatus. After spinal shock phase, patient may also report muscle spasms and radicular pain, described as a burning or stabbing pain (associated with injury to peripheral nerves and radiating in a dermatomal pattern). Onset of this pain is within days to weeks after SCI and may become chronic.
Evaluate increased irritability, muscle tension, restlessness, unexplained vital sign (VS) changes.	Nonverbal cues indicative of pain/discomfort requiring intervention.
Assist patient in identifying precipitating factors.	Burning pain and muscle spasms can be precipitated/aggravated by multiple factors, e.g., anxiety, tension, external temperature extremes, sitting for long periods, bladder distension.
Provide comfort measures, e.g., position changes, massage, ROM exercises warm/cold packs, as indicated.	Alternate measures for pain control are desirable for emotional benefit, in addition to reducing pain medication needs/undesirable effects on respiratory function.
Encourage use of relaxation techniques, e.g., guided imagery, visualization, deep-breathing exercises. Provide diversional activities, e.g., television, radio, telephone, unlimited visitors, as appropriate.	Refocuses attention, promotes sense of control, and may enhance coping abilities.
Collaborative	
Administer medications as indicated: muscle relaxants, e.g., dantrolene (Dantrium), baclofen (Lioresal); analgesics; antianxiety agents, e.g., diazepam (Valium).	May be desired to relieve muscle spasm/pain associated with spasticity or to alleviate anxiety and promote rest.

ACTIONS/INTERVENTIONS	RATIONALE
Grief Work Facilitation (NIC)	
Independent	
Identify signs of grieving (e.g., shock, denial, anger, depression).	Patient experiences many emotional reactions to the injury and its actual/potential impact on life. These stages are not static, and the rate at which the patient progresses through them is variable.
Shock	
Note lack of communication or emotional response, absence of questions.	Shock is the initial reaction associated with overwhelming injury. Primary concern is to maintain life, and patient may be too ill to express feelings.
Provide simple, accurate information to patient and SO regarding diagnosis and care. Be honest; do not give false reassurance while providing emotional support.	Patient's awareness of surroundings and activity may be blocked initially, and attention span may be limited. Little is actually known about the final outcome of the patient's injuries during acute phase, and lack of knowledge may add to frustration and grief of family. Therefore, early focus of emotional support may be directed toward SO.
Encourage expressions of sadness, grief, guilt, and fear among patient/SO/friends.	Knowledge that these are appropriate feelings that should be expressed may be very supportive to patient/SO.
Incorporate SO into problem solving and planning for patient's care.	Assists in establishing therapeutic relationships. Provides some sense of control of situation of many losses/forced changes and promotes well-being of patient.
Denial	
Assist patient/SO to verbalize feelings about situation, avoiding judgment about what is expressed.	Important beginning step to deal with what has happened. Helpful in identifying patient's coping mechanisms.
Note comments indicating that patient expects to walk shortly and/or is making a bargain with God. Do not confront these comments in early phases of rehabilitation.	Patient may not deny entire disability but may deny its permanency. Situation is compounded by actual uncertainty of outcome, and denial may be useful for coping at this time.
Focus on present needs (e.g., ROM exercises, skin care).	Attention on "here and now" reduces frustration and hopelessness of uncertain future and may make dealing with today's problems more manageable.

ACTIONS/INTERVENTIONS

Independent

Anger

Identify use of manipulative behavior and reactions to caregivers.

Encourage patient to take control when possible, e.g., establishing care routines, dietary choices, diversional activities.

Accept expressions of anger and hopelessness. Avoid arguing. Show concern for the patient.

Set limits on acting out and unacceptable behavior when necessary (e.g., abusive language, sexually aggressive or suggestive behavior).

Depression

Note loss of interest in living, sleep disturbance, suicidal thoughts, hopelessness. Listen to but do not confront these expressions. Let patient know nurse is available for support.

Arrange visit by individual similarly affected, as appropriate.

Collaborative

Consult with/refer to psychiatric nurse, social worker, psychiatrist, pastor.

RATIONALE

Patient may express anger verbally or physically (e.g., spitting, biting). Patient may say that nothing is done right by caregivers/SO or may pit one caregiver against another.

Helps reduce anger associated with powerlessness and provides patient with some sense of control and expectation of responsibility for own behavior.

Patient is acknowledged as a worthwhile individual, and nonjudgmental care is provided.

Although it is important to express negative feelings, patient and staff need to be protected from violence and embarrassment. This phase is traumatic for all involved, and support of family is essential.

Phase may last weeks, months, or even years. Acceptance of these feelings and consistent support during this phase is important to a satisfactory resolution.

Talking with another person who has shared similar feelings/fears and survived may help patient reach acceptance of reality of condition and deal with perceived/actual losses.

Patient/SO need assistance to work through feelings of alienation, guilt, and resentment concerning lifestyle and role changes. The family (required to make adaptive changes to a member who may be permanently "different") benefit from supportive, long-term assistance and/or counseling in coping with these changes and the future. Patient and SO may suffer great spiritual distress, including feelings of guilt, deprivation of peace, and anger at God, which may interfere with progression through/resolution of grief process.

NURSING DIAGNOSIS: Self-Esteem, situational low

May be related to
Traumatic injury; situational crisis; forced crisis

Possibly evidenced by
Verbalization of forced change in lifestyle
Fear of rejection/reaction by others
Focus on past strength, function, or appearance
Negative feelings about body
Feelings of helplessness, hopelessness, or powerlessness
Actual change in structure and/or function
Lack of eye contact
Change in physical capacity to resume role
Confusion about self, purpose, or direction of life

Psychosocial Adjustment: Life Change (NOC)

Verbalize acceptance of self in situation.
Recognize and incorporate changes into self-concept in accurate manner without negating self-esteem.
Develop realistic plans for adapting to new role/role changes.

ACTIONS/INTERVENTIONS

Self-Esteem Enhancement (NIC)

Independent

Acknowledge difficulty in determining degree of functional incapacity and/or chance of functional improvement.

Listen to patient's comments and responses to situation.

Assess dynamics of patient and SOs (e.g., patient's role in family, cultural factors).

Encourage SO to treat patient as normally as possible (e.g., discussing home situations, family news).

Provide accurate information. Discuss concerns about prognosis and treatment honestly at patient's level of acceptance.

Discuss meaning of loss or change with patient/SO. Assess interactions between patient and SO.

Accept patient, show concern for individual as a person. Encourage patient, identify and build on strengths, give positive reinforcement for progress noted.

Include patient/SO in care, allowing patient to make decisions and participate in self-care activities as possible.

Be alert to sexually oriented jokes/flirting or aggressive behavior. Elicit concerns, fears, feelings about current situation/future expectations.

Be aware of own feelings/reaction to patient's sexual anxiety.

Arrange visit by similarly affected person if patient desires and/or situation allows.

RATIONALE

During acute phase of injury, long-term effects are unknown, which delays the patient's ability to integrate situation into self-concept.

Provides clues to view of self, role changes, and needs and is useful for providing information at patient's level of acceptance.

Patient's previous role in family unit is disrupted or altered by injury, adding to difficulty in integrating self-concept. In addition, issues of independence/dependence need to be addressed.

Involving patient in family unit reduces feelings of social isolation, helplessness, and uselessness and provides opportunity for SO to contribute to patient's welfare.

Focus of information should be on present and immediate needs initially and incorporated into long-term rehabilitation goals. Information should be repeated until patient has assimilated or integrated information.

Actual change in body image may be different from that perceived by patient. Distortions may be unconsciously reinforced by SO.

Establishes therapeutic atmosphere for patient to begin self-acceptance.

Recognizes that patient is still responsible for own life and provides some sense of control over situation. Sets stage for future lifestyle, pattern, and interaction required in daily care. *Note:* Patient may reject all help or may be completely dependent during this phase.

Anxiety develops as a result of perceived loss/change in masculine/feminine self-image and role. Forced dependency is often devastating, especially in light of change in function/appearance.

Behavior may be disruptive, creating conflict between patient/staff, further reinforcing negative feelings and possibly eliminating patient's desire to work through situation/participate in rehabilitation.

May be helpful to patient by providing hope for the future/role model.

ACTIONS/INTERVENTIONS

Collaborative

Refer to counseling/psychotherapy as indicated, e.g., psychiatric nurse/clinical specialist, psychiatrist, social worker, sex therapist.

RATIONALE

May need additional assistance to adjust to change in body image/life.

NURSING DIAGNOSIS: Bowel Incontinence/Constipation

May be related to
Disruption of innervation to bowel and rectum
Perceptual impairment
Altered dietary and fluid intake
Change in activity level

Possibly evidenced by
Loss of ability to evacuate bowel voluntarily
Constipation
Gastric dilation, ileus

DESIRED OUTCOMES/EVALUATION CRITERIA—PATIENT WILL:

> **Bowel Continence (NOC)**

Verbalize behaviors/techniques for individual bowel program.
Re-establish satisfactory bowel elimination pattern.

ACTIONS/INTERVENTIONS

> **Bowel Management (NIC)**

Independent

Auscultate bowel sounds, noting location and characteristics.

Observe for abdominal distension if bowel sounds are decreased or absent.

Note reports of nausea, onset of vomiting. Check vomitus or gastric secretions (if tube in place) and stools for occult blood.

Record frequency, characteristics, and amount of stool.

Recognize signs of/check for presence of impaction, e.g., no formed stool for several days, semiliquid stool, restlessness, increased feelings of fullness in/distension of abdomen.

Establish regular daily bowel program, e.g., digital stimulation, prune juice and/or warm beverage, and use of stool softeners/suppositories at set intervals.

RATIONALE

Bowel sounds may be absent during spinal shock phase. High tinkling sounds may indicate presence of ileus.

Loss of peristalsis (related to impaired innervation) paralyzes the bowel, creating ileus and bowel distention. *Note:* Overdistension of the bowel is a precipitator of autonomic dysreflexia once spinal shock subsides. (Refer to ND: Autonomic Dysreflexia, risk for, p. 309.)

GI bleeding may occur in response to injury (Curling's ulcer) or as a side effect of certain therapies (steroids or anticoagulants).

Identifies degree of impairment/dysfunction and level of assistance required.

Early intervention is necessary to effectively treat constipation/retained stool and reduce risk of complications.

A lifelong program is necessary to routinely evacuate the bowel because the ability to control bowel evacuation is important to the patient's physical independence and social acceptance. *Note:* Bowel movements in patients with upper motor neuron damage are generally regulated with suppositories or digital stimulation. Lower motor neurogenic bowel is more difficult to regulate and usually requires manual disimpaction.

ACTIONS/INTERVENTIONS	RATIONALE

Independent

Encourage well-balanced diet that includes bulk and roughage and increased fluid intake (at least 2000 mL/day), including fruit juices.

Improves consistency of stool for transit through the bowel.

Observe for incontinence and help patient relate incontinence to change in diet or routine.

Patient can eventually achieve fairly normal routine bowel habits, which enhance independence, self-esteem, and socialization.

Provide meticulous skin care.

Loss of sphincter control and innervation in the area potentiates risk of skin irritation/breakdown.

Collaborative

Insert/maintain nasogastric tube and attach to suction if appropriate.

May be used initially to reduce gastric distension and prevent vomiting (reduces risk of aspiration).

Consult with dietitian/nutritional support team.

Aids in creating dietary plan to meet individual nutritional needs with consideration of state of digestion/bowel function.

Insert rectal tube as needed.

Reduces bowel distension, which may precipitate autonomic responses.

Administer medications as indicated, e.g.,

Stool softeners, laxatives, suppositories, enemas;

Stimulates peristalsis and routine bowel evacuation when necessary.

Antacids, cimetidine (Tagamet), ranitidine (Zantac).

Reduces or neutralizes gastric acid to lessen gastric irritation and risk of bleeding.

NURSING DIAGNOSIS: Urinary Elimination, altered

May be related to
Disruption in bladder innervation
Bladder atony

Possibly evidenced by
Bladder distension; incontinence/overflow, retention
Urinary tract infections
Bladder, kidney stone formation
Renal dysfunction

DESIRED OUTCOMES/EVALUATION CRITERIA—PATIENT WILL:

Urinary Continence (NOC)

Verbalize understanding of condition.
Maintain balanced I&O with clear, odor-free urine, free of bladder distension/urinary leakage.
Verbalize/demonstrate behaviors and techniques to prevent retention/urinary infection.

ACTIONS/INTERVENTIONS	RATIONALE

Urinary Elimination Management (NIC)

Independent

Assess voiding pattern, e.g., frequency and amount. Compare urine output with fluid intake. Note specific gravity.

Identifies characteristics of bladder function (e.g., effectiveness of bladder emptying, renal function, and fluid balance).

ACTIONS/INTERVENTIONS	RATIONALE

Independent

Palpate for bladder distension and observe for overflow.

Bladder dysfunction is variable but may include loss of bladder contraction/inability to relax urinary sphincter, resulting in urine retention and reflux incontinence. *Note:* Bladder distension can precipitate autonomic dysreflexia. (Refer to ND: Autonomic Dysreflexia, risk for, following.)

Encourage fluid intake (2–4 L/day), including acid ash juices (e.g., cranberry).

Helps maintain renal function, prevents infection and formation of urinary stones. *Note:* Fluid may be restricted for a period during initiation of intermittent catheterization.

Begin bladder retraining per protocol when appropriate, e.g., fluids between certain hours, digital stimulation of trigger area, contraction of abdominal muscles, Crede's maneuver.

Timing and type of bladder program depend on type of injury (upper or lower neuron involvement). *Note:* Crede's maneuver should be used with caution because it may precipitate autonomic dysreflexia.

Observe for cloudy or bloody urine, foul odor.

Signs of urinary tract or kidney infection that can potentiate sepsis.

Cleanse perineal area and keep dry. Provide catheter care as appropriate.

Decreases risk of skin irritation/breakdown and development of ascending infection.

Collaborative

Urinary Catheterization: [Indwelling/] Intermittent (NIC)

Monitor BUN, creatinine, white blood cell (WBC) count.

Reflects renal function, identifies complications.

Administer medications as indicated, e.g., vitamin C, and/or urinary antiseptics, e.g., methenamine mandelate (Mandelamine).

Maintains acidic environment and discourages bacterial growth.

Refer for further evaluation for bladder/bowel stimulation.

Clinical research is being conducted on the technology of electronic bladder control. The implantable device sends electrical signals to the spinal nerves that control the bladder and bowel. Early results look promising.

Keep bladder deflated by means of indwelling catheter initially. Begin intermittent catheterization program when appropriate.

Indwelling catheter is used during acute phase for prevention of urinary retention and for monitoring output. Intermittent catheterization may be implemented to reduce complications usually associated with long-term use of indwelling catheters. A suprapubic catheter may also be inserted for long-term management.

Measure residual urine via postvoid catheterization or ultrasound.

Helpful in detecting presence of urinary retention/effectiveness of bladder training program. *Note:* Use of ultrasound is noninvasive, reducing risk of colonization of bladder.

NURSING DIAGNOSIS: Autonomic Dysreflexia, risk for

Risk factors may include
Altered nerve function (spinal cord injury at T-8 and above)
Bladder/bowel/skin stimulation (tactile, pain, thermal)

Possibly evidenced by
[Not applicable; presence of signs and symptoms establishes an *actual* diagnosis]

ACTIONS/INTERVENTIONS	RATIONALE

Independent

Dysreflexia Management (NIC)

Identify/monitor precipitating risk factors, e.g., bladder/bowel distension or manipulation; bladder spasms, stones, infection; skin/tissue pressure areas, prolonged sitting position; temperature extremes/drafts.

Visceral distension is the most common cause of autonomic dysreflexia, which is considered an emergency. Treatment of acute episode must be carried out immediately (removing stimulus, treating unresolved symptoms), then interventions must be geared toward prevention.

Observe for signs/symptoms of syndrome, e.g., changes in VS, paroxysmal hypertension, tachycardia/bradycardia; autonomic responses: sweating, flushing above level of lesion, pallor below injury, chills, gooseflesh, nasal stuffiness, diffuse headache. Note associated symptoms, e.g., chest pains, blurred vision, nausea, metallic taste, Horner's syndrome (contraction of pupil, partial stasis of eyelid, enophthalmas [recession of eyeball into the orbit], and sometimes loss of sweating over one side of the face).

Early detection and immediate intervention is essential to prevent serious consequences/complications.

Stay with patient during episode.

This is a potentially fatal complication. Continuous monitoring/intervention may reduce patient's level of anxiety.

Monitor BP frequently (every 3–5 min) during acute autonomic dysreflexia and take action to eliminate stimulus. Continue to monitor BP at intervals after symptoms subside.

Aggressive therapy/removal of stimulus may drop BP rapidly, resulting in a hypotensive crisis, especially in those patients who routinely have low BP. In addition, autonomic dysreflexia may recur, particularly if stimulus is not eliminated.

Elevate head of bed to 45-degree angle or place in sitting position.

Lowers BP to prevent intracranial hemorrhage, seizures, or even death. *Note:* Placing quadriplegic in sitting position automatically lowers BP.

Correct/eliminate causative stimulus as able, e.g., bladder, bowel, skin pressure (including loosening tight leg bands/clothing); temperature extremes.

Removing noxious stimulus usually terminates episode and may prevent more serious autonomic dysreflexia, e.g., in the presence of sunburn, topical anesthetic should be applied. *Note:* Removal of bowel impaction must be delayed until cardiovascular condition is stabilized.

Inform patient/SO of warning signals and how to avoid onset of syndrome, e.g., gooseflesh, sweating, piloerection may indicate full bowel; sunburn may precipitate episode.

This lifelong problem can be largely controlled by avoiding pressure from overdistension of visceral organs or pressure on the skin.

ACTIONS/INTERVENTIONS
Collaborative

Administer medications as indicated and monitor response:

    Ganglion blockers, e.g., trimethaphan camsylate (Arfonad);

    Atropine sulfate;

    Diazoxide (Hyperstat), hydralazine (Apresoline);

    Nifedipine (Procardia);

    Adrenergic blockers, e.g., methysergide maleate (Sansert);

    Antihypertensives, e.g., prazosin (Minipress), phenoxybenzamine (Dibenzyline).

Obtain urinary culture as indicated.

Apply local anesthetic ointment to rectum; remove impaction if indicated after symptoms subside.

Prepare patient for pelvic/pudendal nerve block or posterior rhizotomy if indicated.

RATIONALE

Blocks excessive autonomic nerve transmission.

Increases heart rate if bradycardia occurs.

Reduces BP if severe/sustained hypertension occurs.

Sublingual administration may be effective in absence of IV access for diazoxide (Hyperstat).

May be used prophylactically if problem persists/recurs frequently.

Long-term use may relax bladder neck and enhance bladder emptying, alleviating the most common cause of chronic autonomic dysreflexia.

Presence of infection may trigger autonomic dysreflexia episode.

Ointment blocks further autonomic stimulation and eases later removal of impaction without aggravating symptoms.

Procedures may be considered if autonomic dysreflexia does not respond to other therapies.

NURSING DIAGNOSIS: Skin Integrity, risk for impaired

Risk factors may include
Altered/inadequate peripheral circulation; sensation
Presence of edema; tissue pressure
Altered metabolic state
Immobility, traction apparatus

Possibly evidenced by
[Not applicable; presence of signs and symptoms establishes an *actual* diagnosis]

DESIRED OUTCOMES/EVALUATION CRITERIA—PATIENT WILL:

> **Risk Control (NOC)**

Identify individual risk factors.
Verbalize understanding of treatment needs.
Participate to level of ability to prevent skin breakdown.

ACTIONS/INTERVENTIONS

Independent

> **Skin Surveillance (NIC)**

Inspect all skin areas, noting capillary blanching/refill, redness, swelling. Pay particular attention to back of head, skin under halo frame or vest, and folds where skin continuously touches.

RATIONALE

Skin is especially prone to breakdown because of changes in peripheral circulation, inability to sense pressure, immobility, altered temperature regulation.

ACTIONS/INTERVENTIONS	RATIONALE

Independent

Observe halo and tong insertion sites. Note swelling, redness, drainage.	These sites are prone to inflammation and infection and provide route for pathological microorganisms to enter cranial cavity.
Encourage continuation of regular exercise program.	Stimulates circulation, enhancing cellular nutrition/oxygenation to improve tissue health.
Elevate lower extremities periodically, if tolerated.	Enhances venous return. Reduces edema formation.
Avoid/limit injection of medication below the level of injury.	Reduced circulation and sensation increase risk of delayed absorption, local reaction, and tissue necrosis.

Skin Care: Topical Treatments (NIC)

Massage and lubricate skin with bland lotion/oil. Protect pressure points by use of heel/elbow pads, lamb's wool, foam padding, egg-crate mattress. Use skin hardening agents, e.g., tincture of benzoin, Karaya, Sween cream.	Enhances circulation and protects skin surfaces, reducing risk of ulceration. Quadriplegic and paraplegic patients require lifelong protection from decubiti formation, which can cause extensive tissue necrosis and sepsis.
Reposition frequently, whether in bed or in sitting position. Place in prone position periodically.	Improves skin circulation and reduces pressure time on bony prominences.
Wash and dry skin, especially in high moisture areas such as perineum. Take care to avoid wetting lining of brace/halo vest.	Clean, dry skin is less prone to excoriation/breakdown.
Keep bedclothes dry and free of wrinkles, crumbs.	Reduces/prevents skin irritation.
Cleanse halo/tong insertion sites routinely and apply antibiotic ointment per protocol.	Helpful in preventing local infection and reducing risk of cranial infection.

Collaborative

Provide kinetic therapy or alternating-pressure mattress as indicated.	Improves systemic and peripheral circulation and decreases pressure on skin, reducing risk of breakdown.

NURSING DIAGNOSIS: Knowledge Deficit [Learning Need] regarding condition, prognosis, potential complications, treatment, self care, and discharge needs

May be related to
Lack of exposure/recall
Information misinterpretation
Unfamiliarity with information resources

Possibly evidenced by
Questions; statement of misconception; request for information
Inadequate follow-through of instruction
Inappropriate or exaggerated behaviors, e.g., hostile, agitated, apathetic
Development of preventable complication(s)

DESIRED OUTCOMES/EVALUATION CRITERIA—PATIENT WILL:

Knowledge: Disease Process (NOC)

Verbalize understanding of condition, prognosis, and treatment.

Knowledge: Treatment Regimen (NOC)

Correctly perform necessary procedures and explain reasons for the actions.
Initiate necessary lifestyle changes and participate in treatment regimen.

ACTIONS/INTERVENTIONS	RATIONALE

Teaching: Disease Process (NIC)

Independent

Discuss injury process, current prognosis, and future expectations.

Provides common knowledge base necessary for making informed choices and commitment to the therapeutic regimen.

Provide information and demonstrate:

Positioning;

Promotes circulation; reduces tissue pressure and risk of complications.

Use of pillows/supports, splints.

Keeps spine aligned and prevents/limits contractures, thus improving function and independence.

Encourage continued participation in daily exercise and conditioning program and avoidance of fatigue/chills.

Reduces spasticity, risk of thromboemboli (common complication). Increases mobility, muscle strength and tone for improving organ/body function, e.g., squeezing rubber ball, arm exercises enhance upper body strength to increase independence in transfers/wheelchair mobility; tightening/contracting rectum or vaginal muscles improves bladder control; pushing abdomen up, bearing down, contracting abdomen strengthens trunk and improves GI function (paraplegic).

Have SO/caregivers participate in patient care and demonstrate proper procedures, e.g., applications of splints, braces, suctioning, positioning, skin care, transfers, bowel/bladder program, checking temperature of bath water and food.

Allows home caregivers to become adept and more comfortable with the care tasks they are called on to provide and reduces risk of injury/complications.

Instruct caregiver in techniques to facilitate cough as appropriate.

"Quad coughing" is performed to facilitate expectoration of secretions or to move them high enough to be suctioned out.

Recommend applying abdominal binder before arising (quadriplegic) and remind to change position slowly. Use safety belt and adequate number of people during bed-to-wheelchair transfers.

Reduces pooling of blood in abdomen/pelvis, minimizing postural hypotension. Protects the patient from falls and/or injury to caregivers.

Instruct in proper skin care, inspecting all skin areas daily, using adequate padding (foam, silicone gel, water pads) in bed and chair, and keeping skin dry.

Reduces skin irritation, decreasing incidence of decubitus (patient must manage this throughout life).

Discuss necessity of preventing excessive diaphoresis by using tepid bath water, providing comfortable environment (e.g., fans), removing excess clothes.

Reduces skin irritation/possible breakdown.

Review dietary needs, including adequate bulk and roughage. Problem-solve solutions to alterations in muscular strength/tone and GI function.

Provides adequate nutrition to meet energy needs and promote healing, prevent complications (e.g., constipation, abdominal distension/gas formation).

Review pain management techniques. Discuss the potential for future pain management therapies if pain becomes chronic. Recommend avoidance of over-the-counter (OTC) drugs without approval of healthcare provider.

Enhances patient safety and may improve cooperation with specific regimen. *Note:* Pain often becomes chronic in patients with spinal cord injury and may be mechanical (e.g., overuse syndrome involving joints); radicular (from injury to peripheral nerves); or cervical (burning, aching just below level of injury). Dysesthetic pain (distal to site of injury) is extremely disabling (similar to phantom pain). Treatment for these painful conditions may include a team pain management approach, medications (e.g., Neuromtin, Klonopin, Elavil), or electrical stimulation.

ACTIONS/INTERVENTIONS	RATIONALE
Independent	
Discuss ways to identify and manage autonomic dysreflexia.	Patient may be able to recognize signs, but caregivers need to understand how to prevent precipitating factors and know what to do if autonomic dysreflexia occurs. (Refer to ND: Autonomic Dysreflexia, risk for, p. 309.)
Identify symptoms to report immediately to healthcare provider, e.g., infection of any kind, especially urinary, respiratory; skin breakdown; unresolved autonomic dysreflexia; suspected pregnancy.	Early identification allows for intervention to prevent/ minimize complications.
Stress importance of continuing with rehabilitation team to achieve specific functional goals and continue long-term monitoring of therapy needs.	No matter what the level of injury, individual may ultimately be able to exercise some independence, e.g., manipulating electric wheelchair with mouth stick (C-3/ C-4); being independent for dressing, transfers to bed, car, toilet (C-7); or achieving total wheelchair independence (C-8 to T-4). Over time, new discoveries continue to modify equipment/therapy needs and increase patient's potential.
Evaluate home layout and make recommendations for necessary changes. Identify equipment/medical supply needs and resources.	Physical changes may be required to accommodate patient and support equipment. Prior arrangements facilitate the transfer to the home setting.
Discuss sexual activity and reproductive concerns.	Concerns about individual sexuality/resumption of activity is frequently an unspoken concern that needs to be addressed. Spinal cord injury affects all areas of sexual functioning. In addition, choice of contraception is impacted by level of spinal cord injury and side effects/adverse complications of specific method. Finally, some female patients may develop autonomic dysreflexia during intercourse or labor/delivery.
Identify community resources/supports, e.g., health agencies, visiting nurse, financial counselor; service organizations, Spinal Cord Injury Foundation.	Enhances independence, assisting with home management and providing respite for caregivers.
Coordinate cooperation among community/rehabilitation resources.	Various agencies/therapists/individuals in community may be involved in the long-term care and safety of the patient, and coordination can ensure that needs are not overlooked and optimal level of rehabilitation is achieved.
Arrange for transmitter/emergency call system.	Provides for safety and access to emergency assistance and equipment.
Plan for alternate caregivers as needed.	May be needed to provide respite if regular caregivers are ill or other unplanned emergencies arise.

POTENTIAL CONSIDERATIONS following acute hospitalization (dependent on patient's age, physical condition/presence of complications, personal resources, and life responsibilities)

Disuse Syndrome, risk for—paralysis/mechanical immobilization.
Autonomic Dysreflexia—bladder/bowel distension, skin irritation, lack of caregiver knowledge.
Self-Care deficit—neuromuscular impairment, decreased strength/endurance, pain, depression.
Nutrition: altered, risk for (specify)—dysfunctional eating pattern, excessive/inadequate intake in relation to metabolic need.
Role Performance, altered/Sexual dysfunction—situational crisis and transition, altered body function.
Family Processes, altered—situational crisis and transition.
Caregiver Role Strain—discharge of family member with significant home care needs, situational stressors, such as significant loss, economic vulnerability; duration of caregiving required, lack of respite for caregiver, inexperience with caregiving, caregiver's competing role commitments.

MULTIPLE SCLEROSIS

Multiple sclerosis (MS) is the most common of the demyelinating disorders and the predominant CNS disease among young adults. It is a chronic disorder in which irregular demyelination of the CNS (brain and spinal cord) results in emotional changes and varying degrees of cognitive, motor, and sensory dysfunction at the central and peripheral level. It is a perivascular inflammatory response, possibly to chronic viral infection in genetically susceptible individuals, producing a limited disruption in the blood-brain barrier, allowing β-lymphocyte clones to colonize the CNS. Recent research suggests that in addition to destruction of myelin sheaths (which facilitate the movement of nerve impulses), some underlying nerve fibers are also damaged or severed, which may account for the permanent neurological impairment.

MS is grouped into the following four types:

Relapsing-remitting: Periods of neurological dysfunction followed by partial or full recovery.
Primary-progressive: Steady decline with periods of minimal recovery (fairly uncommon).
Secondary-progressive: Initial pattern of relapse and recovery, which becomes steadily progressive over time.
Progressive-relapsing: Progressive from onset with clear exacerbations (rare).

MS is characterized by periods of exacerbations and remissions and is progressive in approximately 60% of patients. Individual prognosis is variable and unpredictable, presenting complex physical, psychosocial, and rehabilitative issues.

CARE SETTING

Community or long-term care with intermittent hospitalizations for disease-related complications.

RELATED CONCERNS

Extended care, page 850
Pneumonia: microbial, page 140
Psychosocial aspects of care, page 809
Sepsis/Septicemia, page 741

Patient Assessment Database

Degree of symptomatology depends on the stage and extent of disease, areas of neuronal involvement.

ACTIVITY/REST

May report: Extreme fatigue/weakness, exaggerated intolerance to activity, needing to rest after even simple activities such as shaving/showering; increased weakness/intolerance to temperature extremes, especially heat (i.e., summer weather, hot tubs)
Limitation in usual activities, employment, hobbies
Numbness, tingling in the extremities
Sleep disturbances, may awaken early or frequently for multiple reasons (e.g., nocturia, nocturnal spasticity, pain, worry, depression)

May exhibit: Absence of predictable pattern of symptoms
Generalized weakness, decreased muscle tone/mass (disuse), spasticity, tremors
Staggering, dragging of feet, ataxia
Intention tremors, decreased fine motor skills

CIRCULATION

May report: Dependent edema (steroid therapy or inactivity)
May exhibit: Blue/mottled, puffy extremities (inactivity)
Capillary fragility (especially on face)

EGO INTEGRITY

May report: Statements reflecting loss of self-esteem/body image
Expressions of grief
Anxiety/fear of exacerbations/progression of symptoms, pain, disability, rejection, pity
Keeping illness confidential
Feelings of helplessness, hopelessness, powerlessness (loss of control)
Personal tragedies (divorce, abandonment by SO/friends)

May exhibit: Denial, rejection
Mood changes, irritability, restlessness, lethargy, euphoria, depression, anger

ELIMINATION

May report: Nocturia
Incomplete bladder emptying, retention with overflow
Urinary/bowel hesitancy or urgency, incontinence of varying severity
Irregular bowel habits, constipation
Recurrent UTIs

May exhibit: Loss of sphincter control
Kidney stone formation, kidney damage

FOOD/FLUID

May report: Difficulty chewing, swallowing (weak throat muscles), sense of food sticking in throat, coughing after swallowing
Problems getting food to mouth (related to intentional tremors of upper extremities)
Hiccups, possibly lasting extended periods

May exhibit: Difficulty feeding self
Weight loss
Decreased bowel sounds (slowed peristalsis)
Abdominal bloating

HYGIENE

May report: Difficulty with/dependence in some/all ADLs
Use of assistive devices/individual caregiver

May exhibit: Poor personal habits, disheveled appearance, signs of incontinence

NEUROSENSORY

May report: Weakness, nonsymmetrical paralysis of muscles (may affect one, two, or three limbs, usually worse in lower extremities or may be unilateral), numbness, tingling (prickling sensations in parts of the body)
Change in visual acuity (diplopia), scotomas (holes in vision), eye pain (optic neuritis)
Moving head back and forth while watching television, difficulty driving (distorted visual field), blurred vision (difficulty focusing)
Cognitive changes, i.e., attention, comprehension, use of speech, problem solving, difficulty retrieving/recalling, sorting out information (cerebral involvement)
Difficulty making decisions
Communication difficulties, such as coining words
Seizures

May exhibit: Mental status: Mood swings, depression, euphoria, irritability, apathy; lack of judgment; impairment of short-term memory; disorientation/confusion
Scanning speech, slow hesitant speech, poor articulation
Partial/total loss of vision in one eye; vision disturbances
Positional/vibration sense impaired or absent
Impaired touch/pain sensation
Facial/trigeminal nerve involvement, nystagmus, diplopia (brainstem involvement)
Loss of motor skills (major/fine), changes in muscle tone, spastic paresis/total immobility (advanced stages)
Ataxia, decreased coordination, tremors (may be originally misinterpreted as intoxication), intention tremor
Hyperreflexia, positive Babinski's sign, ankle clonus; absent superficial reflexes (especially abdominal)

PAIN/DISCOMFORT

May report: Painful spasms, burning pain along nerve path (some patients do not experience normal pain sensations)

Frequency: varied, may be sporadic/intermittent (possibly once a day) or may be constant

Duration lightning-like, repetitive, intermittent; persistent long-term painful spasms of extremity or back pain

Facial neuralgia

Dull back pain

May exhibit: Distraction behaviors (restlessness, moaning), guarding

Self-focusing

SAFETY

May report: Uneasiness around small children or moving objects, fear of falling (weakness, decreased vision, slowed reflexes, loss of position sense, decreased judgment)

History of falls/accidental injuries

Use of ambulation devices

Vision impairment

Suicidal ideation

May exhibit: Wall/furniture walking

SEXUALITY

May report: Relationship stresses

Enhanced or decreased sexual desire

Problems with positioning

Genital anesthesia/hyperesthesia, decreased lubrication (female)

Impotence/nocturnal erections or ejaculatory difficulties

Disturbances in sexual functioning (affected by nerve impairment, fatigue, bowel and bladder control, sense of vulnerability, and effects of medications)

SOCIAL INTERACTION

May report: Lack of social activities/involvement

Withdrawal from interactions with others/isolation behaviors (e.g., stays at home/in room, watches TV all day)

Feelings of isolation (increased divorce rate/loss of friends)

Difficult time with employment because of excessive fatigue/cognitive dysfunction, physical limitations

May exhibit: Speech impairment

TEACHING/LEARNING

May report: Use of prescription/OTC medications, may forget to take regularly

Difficulty retaining information

Family history of disease (possibly due to common environmental/inherited factors)

Use of "holistic"/natural products/health care practices, "trying out cures," "doctor shopping"

Discharge plan **DRG projected mean length of inpatient stay: 5.7 days.**

considerations: May require assistance in any or all areas, depending on individual situation

May eventually need total care/placement in assisted living/long-term care facility

Refer to section at end of plan for postdischarge considerations.

DIAGNOSTIC STUDIES

Brain MRI: Detects presence of plaques characteristic of MS that are due to nerve sheath demyelination, but is not diagnostic without supporting clinical symptoms.

CT scan: Demonstrates brain lesions, ventricular enlargement or thinning.

Evoked potentials: Visual (VER), brainstem auditory (BAER), and somatosensory (SSER) are abnormal early in a high percentage of patients with definite or suspected MS.

Lumbar puncture: CSF may show elevated levels of IgG and IgM. Protein level normal or only slightly elevated, oligoclonal bands present on electrophoresis; WBC count slightly elevated; elevated concentration of myelin basic protein may be noted during active demyelination process.

EEG: May be mildly abnormal in some cases.

NURSING PRIORITIES

1. Maintain optimal functioning.
2. Assist with/provide for maintenance of ADLs.
3. Support acceptance of changes in body image/self-esteem and role performance.
4. Provide information about disease process/prognosis, therapeutic needs, and available resources.

DISCHARGE GOALS

1. Remains active within limits of individual situation.
2. ADLs are managed by patient/caregivers.
3. Changes in self-concept are acknowledged and being dealt with.
4. Disease process/prognosis, therapeutic regimen are understood and resources identified.
5. Plan in place to meet needs after discharge.

NURSING DIAGNOSIS: Fatigue

May be related to

Decreased energy production, increased energy requirements to perform activities

Psychological/emotional demands

Pain/discomfort

Medication side effects

Possibly evidenced by

Verbalization of overwhelming lack of energy

Inability to maintain usual routines; decreased performance

Impaired ability to concentrate; disinterest in surroundings

Increase in physical complaints

DESIRED OUTCOMES/EVALUATION CRITERIA—PATIENT WILL:

Energy Conservation (NOC)

Identify risk factors and individual actions affecting fatigue.

Identify alternatives to help maintain desired activity level.

Participate in recommended treatment program.

Report improved sense of energy.

ACTIONS/INTERVENTIONS	RATIONALE
Energy Management (NIC)	
Independent	
Note and accept presence of fatigue.	The most persistent and common symptom of MS. Studies indicate that the fatigue encountered by patients with MS occurs with expenditure of minimal energy, is more frequent and severe than "normal" fatigue, has a disproportionate impact on ADLs, has a slower recovery time, and may show no direct relationship between fatigue severity and the patient's clinical neurological status.
Identify/review factors affecting ability to be active, e.g., temperature extremes, inadequate food intake, insomnia, use of medications, time of day.	Provides opportunity to problem-solve to maintain/improve mobility.

ACTIONS/INTERVENTIONS	RATIONALE
Independent	
Accept when patient is unable to do activities.	Ability can vary from moment to moment. Nonjudgmental acceptance of the patient's evaluation of day-to-day variations in capabilities provides opportunity to promote independence while supporting fluctuations in level of required care.
Determine need for walking aids, e.g., Canadian canes, braces, walker, wheelchair, scooter; review safety considerations.	Mobility aids can decrease fatigue, enhancing independence and comfort, as well as safety. However, individual may display poor judgment about ability to safely engage in activity.
Schedule ADLs in the morning if appropriate. Investigate use of cooling vest.	Fatigue commonly worsens in late afternoon (when body temperature rises). Some patients report lessening of fatigue with stabilization of body temperature.
Plan care with consistent rest periods between activities. Encourage afternoon nap.	Reduces fatigue, aggravation of muscle weakness.
Stress need for stopping exercise/activity just short of fatigue.	Pushing self beyond individual physical limits can result in excessive/prolonged fatigue and discouragement. In time, patient can become very adept at knowing limitations.
Collaborative	
Recommend participation in groups involved in fitness/exercise and/or the Multiple Sclerosis Society.	Can help patient to stay motivated to remain active within the limits of the disability/condition. Group activities need to be selected carefully to meet the patient's need(s) and prevent discouragement or anxiety.
Administer medications as indicated, e.g.:	
Amantadine (Symmetrel); pemoline (Cylert);	Useful in treatment of fatigue. Positive antiviral drug effect in 30%–50% of patients. Use may be limited by side effects of increased spasticity, insomnia, paresthesias of hands/feet.
Sertraline (Zoloft), fluoxetine (Prozac);	Antidepressants useful in lifting mood, and "energizing" patient (especially when depression is a factor) and when patient is free of anticholinergic side effects.
Tricyclic antidepressants, e.g., amitriptyline (Elavil), nortriptyline (Pamelor);	Useful in treating emotional lability, neurogenic pain, and associated sleep disorders to enhance willingness to be more active.
Carbamazepine (Tegretol);	Used to treat neurogenic pain and sudden intermittent spasms related to spinal cord irritation.
Steroids, e.g., prednisone (Deltasone), dexamethasone (Decadron); methylprednisolone (SoluMedrol);	May be used during acute exacerbations to reduce/prevent edema formation at the sclerotic plaques; however, long-term therapy seems to have little effect on progression of symptoms.
Vitamin B;	Supports nerve-cell replication, enhances metabolic functions, and may increase sense of well-being/energy level (although reports are more anecdotal than research based).

ACTIONS/INTERVENTIONS

Collaborative

Immunomodulating agents, e.g., cyclophosphamide (Cytoxin), azathioprine (Immuran), methotrexate (Mexate), interferon β-1B (Betaseron); interferon β-1A (Avonex-Rebif), glatiramer (Copaxone).

RATIONALE

May be used to treat acute relapses, reduce the frequency of relapse and promote remission. Interferon β-1B (Betaseron) has been approved for use by ambulatory patients with remitting/relapsing MS and is the first drug found to alter the course of the disease. Current research indicates early treatment with drugs that reduce inflammation and lesion formation may limit permanent damage. Therapy of choice is "A, B, C" drugs: Avonex, Betaseron, and Copaxone. Therapeutic benefits have been reported in patients at all stages of disability with reduction in both steroid use and hospital days. *Note:* Copaxone chemically resembles a component of myelin and may act as a decoy, diverting immune cells away from the myelin target.

NURSING DIAGNOSIS: Self-Care deficit (specify)

May be related to
Neuromuscular/perceptual impairment; intolerance to activity; decreased strength and endurance; motor impairment, tremors
Pain, discomfort, fatigue
Memory loss
Depression

Possibly evidenced by
Frustration; inability to perform tasks of self-care, poor personal hygiene

DESIRED OUTCOMES/EVALUATION CRITERIA—PATIENT WILL:

> **Self-Care Activities of Daily Living (ADLs) (NOC)**

Identify individual areas of weakness/needs.
Demonstrate techniques/lifestyle changes to meet self-care needs.
Perform self-care activities within level of own ability.
Identify personal/community resources that provide assistance.

ACTIONS/INTERVENTIONS

> **Self-Care Assistance (NIC)**

Independent

Determine current activity level/physical condition. Assess degree of functional impairment using 0–4 scale.

Encourage patient to perform self-care to the maximum of ability as defined by the patient. Do not rush patient.

Assist according to degree of disability; allow as much autonomy as possible. Encourage patient input in planning schedule.

RATIONALE

Provides information to develop plan of care for rehabilitation. *Note:* Motor symptoms are less likely to improve than sensory ones.

Promotes independence and sense of control; may decrease feelings of helplessness.

Participation in own care can ease the frustration over loss of independence. Patient's quality of life is enhanced when desires/likes are considered in daily activities.

ACTIONS/INTERVENTIONS	RATIONALE
Independent	
Note presence of/accommodate for fatigue.	Fatigue experienced by patients with MS can be very debilitating and greatly impact ability to participate in ADLs. The subjective nature of reports of fatigue can be misinterpreted by healthcare providers and family, leading to conflict and the belief that the patient is "manipulative" when in fact, this may not be the case.
Encourage scheduling activities early in the day or during the time when energy level is best.	Patients with MS expend a great deal of energy to complete ADLs, increasing the risk of fatigue, which often progresses through the day.
Allot sufficient time to perform task(s), and display patience when movements are slow.	Decreased motor skills/spasticity may interfere with ability to manage even simple activities.
Anticipate hygienic needs and calmly assist as necessary with care of nails, skin, and hair; mouth care; shaving (use electric razor).	Caregiver's example can set a matter-of-fact tone for acceptance of handling mundane needs that may be embarrassing to patient/repugnant to SO.
Provide assistive devices/aids as indicated, e.g., shower chair, elevated toilet seat with arm supports.	Reduces fatigue, enhancing participation in self-care.
Reposition frequently when patient is immobile (bed/chairbound). Provide skin care to pressure points, such as sacrum, ankles, and elbows. Position/encourage to sleep prone as tolerated.	Reduces pressure on susceptible areas, prevents skin breakdown. Minimizes flexor spasms at knees and hips.
Provide massage and active/passive ROM exercises on a regular schedule. Encourage use of splints/footboards as indicated.	Prevents problems associated with muscle dysfunction and disuse. Helps maintain muscle tone/strength and joint mobility and decreases risk of loss of calcium from bones.
Encourage stretching and toning exercises and use of medications, cold packs, and splints and maintenance of proper body alignment, when indicated.	Helps decrease spasticity and its effects.
Problem-solve ways to meet nutritional/fluid needs, e.g., wrap fork handle with tape, cut food, and show patient how to hold cup with both hands.	Provides for adequate intake and enhances patient's feelings of independence/self-esteem.
Collaborative	
Consult with physical/occupational therapist.	Useful in identifying devices/equipment to relieve spastic muscles, improve motor functioning, prevent/reduce muscular atrophy and contractures, promoting independence and increasing sense of self-worth.
Administer medications as indicated, e.g.:	
Tizanidine (Zanaflex); baclofen (Lioresal); carbamazepine (Tegretol);	Newer drugs used for reducing spasticity, promoting muscle relaxation, and inhibiting reflexes at the spinal nerve root level. Enhance mobility and maintenance of activity. Tizanidine (Zanaflex) may have an additive effect with baclofen (Lioresal), but use with caution because both drugs have similar side effects. Short duration of action requires careful individualizing of dosage to maximize therapeutic effect.
Diazepam (Valium); clonazepam (Klonopin); cylobenzaprine (Flexeril); gabapentin (Neurontin); dantrolene (Dantrium);	A variety of medications are used to reduce spasticity. The mechanisms are not well understood, and responses vary in each person. Therefore, it may take a period of medication trials to discover what provides the most effective relief of muscle spasticity and associated pain. *Note:* Adverse effects may be increased muscle weakness, loss of muscle tone, and liver toxicity.

ACTIONS/INTERVENTIONS

Collaborative

Meclizine (Antivert), scopolamine patches (Transderm-Scop);

RATIONALE

Reduces dizziness, allowing patient to be more mobile.

NURSING DIAGNOSIS: Self-Esteem (specify)

May be related to
Changes in structure/function
Disruption in how patient perceives own body
Role reversal; dependence

Possibly evidenced by
Confusion about sense of self, purpose, direction in life
Denial, withdrawal, anger
Negative/self-destructive behavior
Use of ineffective coping methods
Change in self/other's perception of role/physical capacity to resume role

DESIRED OUTCOMES/EVALUATION CRITERIA—PATIENT WILL:

Self-Esteem (NOC)

Verbalize realistic view and acceptance of body as it is.
View self as a capable person.
Participate in and assume responsibility for meeting own needs.
Recognize and incorporate changes in self-concept/role without negating self-esteem.
Develop realistic plans for adapting to role changes.

ACTIONS/INTERVENTIONS

Self-Esteem Enhancement (NIC)

Independent

Establish/maintain a therapeutic nurse-patient relationship, discussing fears/concerns.

Note withdrawn behaviors/use of denial, or overconcern with body/disease process.

Support use of defense mechanisms, allowing patient to deal with information in own time and way.

Acknowledge reality of grieving process related to actual/perceived changes. Help patient deal realistically with feelings of anger and sadness.

Review information about course of disease, possibility of remissions, prognosis.

RATIONALE

Conveys an attitude of caring and develops a sense of trust between patient and caregiver in which the patient is free to express fears of rejection, loss of previous functioning/appearance, feelings of helplessness, powerlessness about changes that may occur. Promotes a sense of well-being for the patient.

Initially may be a normal protective response, but if prolonged, may prevent dealing appropriately with reality and may lead to ineffective coping.

Confronting patient with reality of situation may result in increased anxiety and lessened ability to cope with changed self-concept/role.

Nature of the disease leads to ongoing losses and changes in all aspects of life, blocking resolution of grieving process.

When patient learns about disease and becomes aware that own behavior (including feeling hopeful/maintaining a positive attitude) can significantly improve general well-being and daily functioning, the patient may feel more in control, enhancing sense of self-esteem. *Note:* Some patients may never have a remission.

ACTIONS/INTERVENTIONS	RATIONALE
Independent	
Provide accurate verbal and written information about what is happening and discuss with patient/SO.	Helps patient stay in the "here and now," reduces fear of the unknown, provides reference source for future use.
Explain that labile emotions are not unusual. Problem-solve ways to deal with these feelings.	Relieves anxiety and assists with efforts to manage unexpected emotional displays.
Note presence of depression/impaired thought processes, expressions of suicidal ideation (evaluate on a scale of 1–10).	Adapting to a long-term, progressively debilitating incurable disease is a difficult emotional adjustment. In addition, cognitive impairment may affect adaptation to life changes. A depressed individual may believe that suicide is the best way to deal with what is happening.
Assess interaction between patient and SO. Note changes in relationship.	SO may unconsciously/consciously reinforce negative attitudes and beliefs of the patient, or issues of secondary gain may interfere with progress and ability to manage situation.
Provide open environment for patient/SO to discuss concerns about sexuality, including management of fatigue, spasticity, arousal, and changes in sensation.	Physical and psychological changes often create stressors within the relationship, affecting usual roles/expectations, further impairing self-concept.
Discuss use of medications and adjuncts to improve sexual function.	Patient and partner may want to explore trial of medications (e.g., papaverine [Pavabid], dinoprostone [Prostin UR]) or other avenues of improving sexual relationship.
Collaborative	
Consult with occupational therapist/rehabilitation team.	Identifying assistive devices/equipment enhances level of overall function and participation in activities, enhancing sense of well-being and viewing self as a capable individual.
Refer to psychiatric clinical nurse specialist, social worker, psychologist as indicated.	May require more in-depth/supportive counseling to resolve conflicts, deal with life changes.

NURSING DIAGNOSIS: Powerlessness [specify degree]/Hopelessness

May be related to
Illness-related regimen, unpredictability of disease
Lifestyle of helplessness

Possibly evidenced by
Verbal expressions of having no control or influence over situation
Depression over physical deterioration that occurs despite patient compliance with regimen
Nonparticipation in care or decision making when opportunities are provided
Passivity, decreased verbalization/affect
Verbal cues (despondent content, "I can't," sighing)
Lack of involvement in care/passively allowing care
Isolating behaviors/social withdrawal

DESIRED OUTCOMES/EVALUATION CRITERIA—PATIENT WILL:

Hope (NOC)

Identify and verbalize feelings.
Use coping mechanisms to counteract feelings of hopelessness.
Identify areas over which individual has control.
Participate/monitor and control own self-care and ADLs within limits of the individual situation.

ACTIONS/INTERVENTIONS	RATIONALE

Hope Instillation (NIC)

Independent

Note behaviors indicative of powerlessness/hopelessness, e.g., statements of despair, "They don't care," "It won't make any difference."

The degree to which the patient believes own situation is hopeless, that he or she is powerless to change what is happening, affects how patient handles life situation.

Acknowledge reality of situation, at the same time expressing hope for the patient.

Although the prognosis may be discouraging, remissions may occur, and because the future cannot be predicted, hope for some quality of life should be encouraged. Additionally, research is ongoing and new treatment options are being initiated.

Encourage/assist patient to identify activities he or she would like to be involved in (e.g., volunteer work) within the limits of his or her abilities.

Staying active and interacting with others counteracts feelings of helplessness.

Discuss plans for the future. Suggest visiting alternate care facilities, taking a look at the possibilities for care as condition changes.

When options are considered and plans are made for any eventuality, patient has a sense of control over own circumstances.

Self-Responsibility Facilitation (NIC)

Determine degree of mastery patient has exhibited in life to the present. Note locus of control, i.e., internal/external.

The patient who has assumed responsibility in life previously tends to do the same during difficult times of exacerbation of illness. However, if locus of control has been focused outward, patient may blame others and not take control over own circumstances.

Assist patient to identify factors that are under own control, e.g., list things that can or cannot be controlled.

Knowing and accepting what is beyond individual control can reduce helpless/acting out behaviors, promote focusing on areas individual can control.

Encourage patient to assume control over as much of own care as possible.

Even when unable to do much physical care, individual can help to plan care, having a voice in what is/is not desired.

Discuss needs openly with the patient/SO, setting up agreed-on routines for meeting identified needs.

Helps to deal with manipulative behavior, when patient feels powerless and not listened to.

Incorporate patient's daily routine into home care schedule/hospital stay, as possible.

Maintains sense of control/self-determination and independence.

Collaborative

Refer to vocational rehabilitation as indicated.

Can assist patient to develop and implement a vocational plan incorporating specific interests/abilities.

Identify community resources e.g., adult day enrichment program.

Participation in structured activities can reduce sense of isolation and may enhance feeling of self-worth.

NURSING DIAGNOSIS: Coping, Individual, risk for ineffective

Risk factors may include
Physiological changes (cerebral and spinal lesions)
Psychological conflicts; anxiety; fear
Impaired judgment, short-term memory loss; confusion; unrealistic perceptions/expectations, emotional lability

Personal vulnerability; inadequate support systems
Multiple life changes
Inadequate coping methods

Possibly evidenced by

[Not applicable; presence of signs and symptoms establishes an *actual* diagnosis]

DESIRED OUTCOMES/EVALUATION CRITERIA—PATIENT WILL:

Coping (NOC)

Recognize relationship between disease process (cerebral lesions) and emotional responses, changes in thinking/behavior.
Verbalize awareness of own capabilities/strengths.
Display effective problem-solving skills.
Demonstrate behaviors/lifestyle changes to prevent/minimize changes in mentation and maintain reality orientation.

ACTIONS/INTERVENTIONS	RATIONALE
Coping Enhancement (NIC)	
Independent	
Assess current functional capacity/limitations; note presence of distorted thinking processes, labile emotions, cognitive dissonance. Note how these affect the individual's coping abilities.	Organic or psychological effects may cause patient to be easily distracted; to display difficulties with concentration, problem solving, dealing with what is happening, being responsible for own care.
Determine patient's understanding of current situation and previous methods of dealing with life's problems.	Provides a clue as to how the patient may deal with what is currently happening and helps identify individual resources and need for assistance.
Discuss ability to make decisions, care for children/dependent adults, handle finances. Identify options available to individuals involved.	Impaired judgment, confusion, inadequate support systems may interfere with ability to meet own needs/needs of others. Conservatorship, guardianship, or adult protective services may be required until (if ever) patient is able to manage own affairs.
Maintain an honest, reality-oriented relationship.	Reduces confusion and minimizes painful, frustrating struggles associated with adaptation to altered environment/lifestyle.
Encourage verbalization of feelings/fears, accepting what patient says in a nonjudgmental manner. Note statements reflecting powerlessness, inability to cope. (Refer to ND: Powerlessness/Hopelessness, p. 323.)	May diminish patient's fear, establish trust, and provide an opportunity to identify problems/begin the problem-solving process.
Observe nonverbal communication, e.g., posture, eye contact, movements, gestures, and use of touch. Compare with verbal content and verify meaning with patient as appropriate	May provide significant information about what the patient is feeling; however, verification is important to ensure accuracy of communication. Discrepancy between feelings and what is being said can interfere with ability to cope, problem solve.
Provide clues for orientation, e.g., calendars, clocks, notecards, organizers/date book.	These serve as tangible reminders to aid recognition and permeate memory gaps and enable patient to cope with situation.

ACTIONS/INTERVENTIONS	RATIONALE

Independent

Encourage patient to tape-record important information and listen to it periodically.

Repetition puts information in long-term memory, where it is more easily retrieved and can support decision-making/problem-solving process.

Collaborative

Refer to cognitive retraining program.

Improving cognitive abilities can enhance basic thinking skills when attention span is short; ability to process information is impaired; patient is unable to learn new tasks; or insight, judgment, and problem-solving skills are impaired.

Refer to counseling, psychiatric nurse clinical specialist/psychiatrist, as indicated.

May need additional help to resolve issues of self-esteem and regain effective coping skills.

Administer medications as appropriate, e.g., amitriptyline (Elavil); bupropion (Wellbutrin); imipramine (Tofranil); paroxetine (Paxill).

Medications to improve mood and restful sleep may be useful in combating depression and relieving degree of fatigue interfering with function.

NURSING DIAGNOSIS: Family Coping ineffective: compromised/disabling

May be related to
Situational crisis; temporary family disorganization and role changes
Highly ambivalent family relationships
Prolonged disease/disability progression that exhausts the supportive capacity of SO
Patient providing little support in turn for SO
SO with chronically unexpressed feelings of guilt, anxiety, hostility, despair

Possibly evidenced by
Patient expresses/confirms concern or complaint about SO response to patient's illness
SO withdraws or has limited personal communication with patient or displays protective behavior disproportionate to patient's abilities or need for autonomy
SO preoccupied with own personal reactions
Intolerance, abandonment
Neglectful care of the patient
Distortion of reality regarding patient's illness

DESIRED OUTCOMES/EVALUATION CRITERIA—FAMILY WILL:

> **Coping (NOC)**

Identify/verbalize resources within themselves to deal with the situation.
Express more realistic understanding and expectations of the patient.
Interact appropriately with the patient/healthcare providers providing support and assistance as indicated.
Verbalize knowledge and understanding of disability/disease and community resources.

ACTIONS/INTERVENTIONS	RATIONALE

> **Family Involvement (NIC)**

Independent

Note length/severity of illness. Determine patient's role in family and how illness has changed the family organization.

Chronic/unresolved illness, accompanied by changes in role performance/responsibility, often exhausts supportive capacity and coping abilities of SO/family.

ACTIONS/INTERVENTIONS	RATIONALE
Independent	
Determine SO's understanding of disease process and expectations for the future.	Inadequate information/misconception regarding disease process and/or unrealistic expectations affect ability to cope with current situation. *Note:* A particular area of misconception is the fatigue experienced by patients with MS. Family members may view the patient's inability to perform activities as manipulative behavior rather than an actual physiological deficit.
Discuss with SO/family members their willingness to be involved in care. Identify other responsibilities/factors impacting participation.	Individuals may not have desire/time to assume responsibility for care. If several family members are available, they may be able to share tasks.
Assess other factors that are affecting abilities of family members to provide needed support, e.g., own emotional problems, work concerns.	Individual members' preoccupation with own needs/concerns can interfere with providing needed care/support for stresses of long-term illness. Additionally, caregiver(s) may incur decrease or loss of income/risk losing own health insurance if they alter their work hours.
Discuss underlying reasons for patient's behaviors.	Helps SO understand and accept/deal with behaviors that may be triggered by emotional or physical effects of MS.
Encourage patient/SO to develop and strengthen problem-solving skills to deal with situation.	Family may/may not have handled conflict well before illness, and stress of long-term debilitating condition can create additional problems (including unresolved anger).
Encourage free expression of feelings, including frustration, anger, hostility, and hopelessness.	Individual members may be afraid to express "negative" feelings, believing it will discourage the patient. Free expression promotes awareness and can help with resolution of feelings and problems (especially when done in a caring manner).
Collaborative	
Identify community resources, e.g., local MS organization, support groups, home care agencies, respite programs.	Provides information, opportunities to share with others who are experiencing similar difficulties, and sources of assistance when needed.
Refer to social worker, financial adviser, psychiatric nurse specialist/psychiatrist as appropriate.	May need more in-depth assistance from professional sources.

NURSING DIAGNOSIS: Urinary Elimination, altered

May be related to
Neuromuscular impairment (spinal cord lesions/neurogenic bladder)

Possibly evidenced by
Incontinence; nocturia; frequency
Retention with overflow
Recurrent UTIs

DESIRED OUTCOMES/EVALUATION CRITERIA—PATIENT WILL:

> **Urine Continence (NOC)**

Verbalize understanding of condition.
Demonstrate behaviors/techniques to prevent/minimize infection.
Empty bladder completely and regularly (voluntarily or by catheter as appropriate).
Be free of urine leakage.

ACTIONS/INTERVENTIONS	RATIONALE

Urinary Elimination Management (NOC)

Independent

Note reports of frequency, urgency, burning, incontinence, nocturia, size of/force of urinary stream. Palpate bladder after voiding.

Provides information about degree of interference with elimination or may indicate bladder infection. Fullness over bladder following void is indicative of inadequate emptying and requires intervention.

Institute bladder training program or timed voidings as appropriate.

Helps to restore adequate bladder functioning; lessens occurrence of incontinence and bladder infection.

Encourage adequate fluid intake, avoiding caffeine and limiting intake during late evening and at bedtime. Recommend use of cranberry juice/vitamin C.

Sufficient hydration promotes urinary output and aids in preventing infection. *Note:* When patient is taking sulfa drugs, sufficient fluids are necessary to ensure adequate excretion of drug, reducing risk of cumulative effects.

Promote continued mobility.

Decreases risk of developing bladder and UTI.

Recommend good handwashing/perineal care.

Reduces skin irritation and risk of ascending infection.

Encourage patient to observe for sediment/blood in urine, foul odor, fever, or unexplained increase in MS symptoms (e.g., spasticity, dysarthia).

Indicative of infection requiring further evaluation/treatment.

Collaborative

Urinary Catheterization (NIC)

Refer to urinary continence specialist as indicated.

Helpful for developing individual plan of care to meet patient's specific needs using the latest techniques, continence products.

Administer medications as indicated, e.g.:

Oxybutynin (Ditropan), propantheline (Pro-Banthine), hyoscyamine sulfate (Cytospaz), flavoxate hydrochloride (Urispas), tolterodine (Detrol).

Reduce bladder spasticity and associated symptoms of frequency, urgency, incontinence, nocturia.

Catheterize as indicated.

May be necessary if patient is unable to empty bladder or retains urine.

Teach self-catheterization/instruct in use and care of indwelling catheter.

Helps patient to maintain autonomy and encourages self-care. Indwelling catheter may be required, depending on patient's abilities and degree of urinary problem.

Obtain periodic urinalysis/urine culture and sensitivity as indicated.

Monitors renal status. Colony count over 100,000 indicates presence of infection requiring treatment.

Administer antinfective agents as necessary, e.g.:

Nitrofurantoin macrocrystals (Macrodantin); co-trimoxazole (Bactrim, Septra); ciprofloxacin (Cipro); norfloxacin (Noroxin).

Bacteriostatic agents that inhibit bacterial growth and destroy susceptible bacteria. Prompt treatment of infection is necessary to prevent serious complications of sepsis/shock.

NURSING DIAGNOSIS: Knowledge Deficit [Learning Need] regarding condition, prognosis, complications, treatment, self care, and discharge needs

May be related to

Lack of exposure; information misinterpretation
Unfamiliarity with information resources
Cognitive limitation, lack of recall

Possibly evidenced by

Statement of misconception

Request for information

Inaccurate follow-through of instruction; development of preventable complications

Inappropriate or exaggerated behaviors (e.g., hysterical, hostile, agitated, apathetic)

DESIRED OUTCOMES/EVALUATION CRITERIA—PATIENT WILL:

> **Knowledge: Disease Process (NOC)**

Participate in learning process.

Assume responsibility for own learning and begin to look for information and to ask questions.

Verbalize understanding of condition/disease process and treatment.

Initiate necessary lifestyle changes.

Participate in prescribed treatment regimen.

ACTIONS/INTERVENTIONS

> **Learning Facilitation (NIC)**

Independent

Evaluate desire/readiness of patient and SO/caregiver to learn.

Note signs of emotional lability or if patient is in dissociative state (loss of affect, inappropriate emotional responses).

Provide information in varied formats depending on patient's cognitive/perceptual abilities and considering patient's locus of control.

Encourage active participation of patient/SO in learning process, including use of self-paced instruction as appropriate.

> **Teaching: Disease Process (NIC)**

Review disease process/prognosis, effects of climate, emotional stress, overexertion, fatigue.

Identify signs/symptoms requiring further evaluation.

Discuss importance of daily routine of rest, exercise, activity, and eating, focusing on current capabilities. Instruct in use of appropriate devices to assist with ADLs, e.g., eating utensils, walking aids.

Stress necessity of weight control.

Review possible problems that may arise such as decreased perception of heat and pain, susceptibility to skin breakdown and infections, especially UTI.

RATIONALE

Determines amount/level of information to provide at any given moment.

Patient will not process/retain information and will have difficulty learning during this time.

Changes in cognitive, visual, auditory function impact choice of teaching modalities, e.g., verbal instruction, books/pamphlets, audiovisuals, computer programs. Whether locus of control is internal or external affects patient's attitude toward helpfulness of learning.

Enhances sense of independence and control and may strengthen commitment to therapeutic regimen.

Clarifies patient/SO understanding of individual situation.

Prompt intervention may help limit severity of exacerbation/complications.

Helps patient maintain current level of physical independence and may limit fatigue.

Excess weight can interfere with balance and motor abilities and make care more difficult.

These effects of demyelination and associated complications may compromise patient's safety and/or precipitate an exacerbation of symptoms.

329

ACTIONS/INTERVENTIONS	RATIONALE

Independent

Identify actions that can be taken to avoid injury: e.g., avoid hot baths, inspect skin regularly, take care with transfers and wheelchair/walker mobility, force fluids, and get adequate nutrition. Encourage avoidance of persons with upper respiratory infection.

Review of risk factors can help patient take measures to maintain physical state at optimal level/prevent complications.

Identify bowel elimination concerns. Recommend adequate hydration and intake of fiber; use of stool softeners, bulking agents, suppositories, or possibly mild laxatives; bowel training program.

Constipation is common, and bowel urgency and/or accidents may occur as a result of dietary deficiencies or impaction.

Review specifics of individual medications. Recommend avoidance of OTC drugs.

Reduces likelihood of drug interactions/adverse effects and enhances cooperation with treatment regimen.

Discuss concerns regarding sexual relationships, contraception/reproduction, effects of pregnancy on affected woman. Identify alternate ways to meet individual needs; counsel regarding use of artificial lubrication (females), genitourinary (GU) referral for males regarding available medications/sexual aids.

Pregnancy may be an issue for the young patient relative to issues of genetic predisposition and/or ability to manage pregnancy or parent offspring. Increased libido is not uncommon and may require adjustments within the existing relationship or in the absence of an acceptable partner. Information about different positions and techniques and/or other options for sexual fulfillment (e.g., fondling, cuddling) may enhance personal relationship and feelings of self-worth.

Encourage patient to set goals for the future while focusing on the "here and now," what can be done today.

Having a plan for the future helps retain hope and provides opportunity for patient to see that although today is to be lived, one can plan for tomorrow even in the worst of circumstances.

Identify financial concerns.

Loss or change of employment (for patient and/or SO) impacts income, insurance benefits, and level of independence, requiring additional family/social support.

Refer for vocational rehabilitation as appropriate.

May need assessment of capabilities/job retraining as indicated by individual limitations/disease progression.

Recommend contacting local and national MS organizations, relevant support groups.

Ongoing contact (e.g., mailings) informs patient of programs/services available, and can update patient's knowledge base. Support groups can provide role modeling, sharing of information and enhance problem-solving ability.

NURSING DIAGNOSIS: Caregiver Role Strain, risk for

Risk factors may include
Severity of illness of the care receiver, duration of caregiving required, complexity/amount of caregiving task
Caregiver is female, spouse
Care receiver exhibits deviant, bizarre behavior
Family/caregiver isolation; lack of respite and recreation

Possibly evidenced by
[Not applicable; presence of signs/symptoms establishes an *actual* diagnosis]

DESIRED OUTCOME/EVALUATION CRITERIA—CAREGIVER WILL:

Caregiver Performance: Direct Care (NOC)

Identify individual risk factors and appropriate interventions.
Demonstrate/initiate behaviors or lifestyle changes to prevent development of impaired function.
Use available resources appropriately.
Report satisfaction with plan and support available.

ACTIONS/INTERVENTIONS	RATIONALE
Caregiver Support (NIC)	
Independent	
Note physical/mental condition, therapeutic regimen of care receiver.	Determines individual needs for planning care. Identifies strengths and how much responsibility the patient may be expected to assume, as well as disabilities requiring accommodation.
Determine caregiver's level of commitment, responsibility, involvement in and anticipated length of care. Use assessment tool, such as Burden Interview, to further determine caregiver's abilities, when appropriate.	Progressive debilitation taxes caregiver and may alter ability to meet patient/own needs. (Refer to ND: Family Coping, ineffective: compromised/disabling, p. 326.)
Discuss caregiver's view of and about situation.	Allows ventilation and clarification of concerns, promoting understanding.
Determine available supports and resources currently used.	Organizations (e.g., national MS society, local support groups) can provide information regarding adequacy of supports and identify needs.
Facilitate family conference to share information and develop plan for involvement in care activities as appropriate.	When others are involved in care, the risk of one person becoming overloaded is lessened.
Identify additional resources to include financial, legal assistance.	These areas of concern can add to burden of caregiving if not adequately resolved.
Identify adaptive equipment needs/resources for the home and vehicles.	Enhances independence and safety of both the caregiver and patient.
Provide information and/or demonstrate techniques for dealing with acting-out/violent or disoriented behavior.	Helps caregiver maintain sense of control and competency. Enhances safety for care receiver and caregiver.
Stress importance of self-nurturing, e.g., pursuing self-development interests, personal needs, hobbies, and social activities.	Taking time for self can lessen risk of "burnout"/being overwhelmed by situation.
Identify alternate care sources (such as sitter/day care facility), senior care services, e.g., Meals on Wheels/respite care, home care agency.	As patient's condition worsens, SO may need additional help from several sources to maintain patient at home even on a part-time basis.
Assist caregiver to plan for changes that may be necessary for the care receiver (e.g., eventual placement in long-term care facility).	Planning for this eventuality is important for the time when burden of care becomes too great.
Collaborative	
Refer to supportive services as need indicates.	Medical case manager or social services consultant may be needed to develop ongoing plan to meet changing needs of patient and SO/family.

POTENTIAL CONSIDERATIONS following acute hospitalization (dependent on patient's age, physical condition/presence of complications, personal resources, and life responsibilities)

Trauma, risk for—weakness, poor vision, balancing difficulties, reduced temperature/tactile sensation, reduced muscle, hand/eye coordination, cognitive or emotional difficulties, insufficient finances to purchase necessary equipment.

Home Maintenance Management, impaired—insufficient finances, unfamiliarity with neighborhood resources, inadequate support systems.

Disuse Syndrome, risk for [actual]—paralysis/immobilization, severe pain.

Therapeutic Regimen: Individual, ineffective management—economic difficulties, family conflict, social support deficits.

Gastrointestinal Disorders

UPPER GASTROINTESTINAL/ESOPHAGEAL BLEEDING

Bleeding duodenal ulcer is the most frequent cause of massive upper gastrointestinal (GI) hemorrhage, but bleeding may also occur because of gastric ulcers, gastritis, and esophageal varices. Severe vomiting can precipitate gastric bleeding due to a tear in the mucosa at the gastroesophageal junction (Mallory-Weiss syndrome). Stress ulcers are often associated with severe burns, major trauma/surgery, or severe systemic disease. Esophagitis, esophageal/gastric carcinoma, hiatal hernia, hemophilia, leukemia, and disseminated intravascular coagulation (DIC) are less common causes of upper GI bleeding.

CARE SETTING

Generally, a patient with severe, active bleeding is admitted directly to the critical care unit (CCU); however, a patient may develop GI bleeding on the medical-surgical unit or be admitted there for evaluation/treatment of subacute bleeding.

RELATED CONCERNS

Cirrhosis of the liver, page 484
Fluid and electrolyte imbalances, page 926
Psychosocial aspects of care, page 809
Renal failure: acute, page 575
Subtotal gastrectomy/gastric resection, page 346

Patient Assessment Database

ACTIVITY/REST

May report:	Weakness, fatigue
May exhibit:	Tachycardia, tachypnea/hyperventilation (response to activity)

CIRCULATION

May report:	Palpitations
	Dizziness with position change
May exhibit:	Hypotension (including postural)
	Tachycardia, dysrhythmias (hypovolemia/hypoxemia)
	Weak/thready peripheral pulse
	Capillary refill slow/delayed (vasoconstriction)
	Skin color: pallor, cyanosis (depending on the amount of blood loss)
	Skin/mucous membrane moisture: diaphoresis (reflecting shock state, acute pain, psychological response)

EGO INTEGRITY

May report: Acute or chronic stress factors (financial, relationships, job-related)

Feelings of helplessness

May exhibit: Signs of anxiety, e.g., restlessness, pallor, diaphoresis, narrowed focus, trembling, quivering voice

ELIMINATION

May report: Change in usual bowel patterns/characteristics of stool

May exhibit: Abdominal tenderness, distension

Bowel sounds often hyperactive during bleeding, hypoactive after bleeding subsides

Character of stool: diarrhea; dark bloody, tarry, or occasionally bright red stools; frothy, foul-smelling (steatorrhea); constipation may occur (changes in diet, antacid use)

Urine output may be decreased, concentrated

FOOD/FLUID

May report: Anorexia, nausea, vomiting (protracted vomiting suggests pyloric outlet obstruction associated with duodenal ulcer)

Problems with swallowing; belching, hiccups

Heartburn, indigestion, burping with sour taste

Bloating/distension, flatulence

Food intolerances, e.g., spicy food, chocolate; special diet for preexisting ulcer disease

Weight loss

May exhibit: Vomitus: coffee-ground or bright red, with or without clots

Mucous membranes dry, decreased mucus production, poor skin turgor (chronic bleeding)

Urine specific gravity may be elevated

NEUROSENSORY

May report: Fainting, dizziness/lightheadedness, weakness

Mental status: level of consciousness (LOC) may be altered, ranging from slight drowsiness, disorientation/confusion, to stupor and coma (depending on circulating volume/oxygenation)

PAIN/DISCOMFORT

May report: Pain described as sharp, dull, burning, gnawing; sudden, excruciating (can accompany perforation)

Vague sensation of discomfort/distress following large meals and relieved by food (acute gastritis)

Left to midepigastric pain and/or pain radiating to back, often accompanied by vomiting after eating and relieved by antacids (gastric ulcer)

Localized right to midepigastric pain, gnawing, burning, occurring about 2–3 hr after meals when stomach is empty, and relieved by food or antacids (duodenal ulcers)

Midepigastric pain and burning with regurgitation (chronic gastroesophageal reflux disease [GERD])

Absence of pain (esophageal varices or gastritis)

Precipitating factors may be foods, (e.g., milk, chocolate, caffeine) smoking, alcohol, certain drugs (salicylates, reserpine, antibiotics, ibuprofen), psychological stressors

May exhibit: Facial grimacing, guarding of affected area, pallor, diaphoresis, narrowed focus

SAFETY

May report: Drug allergies/sensitivities, e.g., acetylsalicylic (ASA)

May exhibit: Temperature elevation

Spider angiomas, palmar erythema (reflecting cirrhosis/portal hypertension)

TEACHING/LEARNING

May report: Recent use of prescription/over-the-counter (OTC) drugs containing ASA, alcohol/ recreational drugs, steroids, or nonsteroidal anti-inflammatory drugs (NSAIDs) (leading cause of drug-induced GI bleeding)

Current complaint may reveal admission for related (e.g., anemia) or unrelated (e.g., head trauma) diagnosis, intestinal flu, or severe vomiting episode; long-standing health problems, e.g., cirrhosis, alcoholism, hepatitis, eating disorders.

History of previous hospitalizations for GI bleeding or related GI problems, e.g., peptic/ gastric ulcer, gastritis, gastric surgery, irradiation of gastric area

Discharge plan considerations: **DRG projected mean length of inpatient stay: 5.3 days**
May require changes in therapeutic/medication regimen.

Refer to section at end of plan for postdischarge considerations.

DIAGNOSTIC STUDIES

Esophagogastroduodenoscopy (EGD): Key diagnostic test for upper and lower GI bleeding, done to visualize site of bleeding/degree of tissue ulceration/injury.

Gastrointestinal nuclear scan: Radionuclide uptake at sites of bleeding identifies site (not cause) of bleeding. Test is considered to be more sensitive than EGD, upper GI studies with barium, or angiography in detecting sites of lower GI bleeding or persistent bleeding anywhere in GI tract.

Helicobacter pylori breath test: Patient drinks a carbon-enriched urea solution. If *H. pylori* is present, it breaks down the compound and releases CO_2.

Barium swallow with x-ray: Done after bleeding has ceased for differential diagnosis of cause/site of lesion, presence of structural defects such as strictures.

Gastric aspirate analysis: May be done in suspected peptic ulcer disease as indicated by low to normal pH and/or presence of blood; also in suspected gastric cancer (abnormal acidity, blood and/or abnormal cells on cytological examination).

Gastric cultures: Determine presence of *H. pylori* (Gram-negative urease-producing bacteria), currently accepted as organism responsible for 90% of duodenal and 70%–80% of gastric ulcers.

Angiography: GI vasculature may be reviewed if endoscopy is inconclusive or impractical. Demonstrates collateral circulation and possibly bleeding site.

Stools: Testing for blood will be positive.

Complete blood count (CBC), hemoglobin (Hb)/hematocrit (Hct): Decreased levels occur 6–24 hr after acute bleeding begins. Red blood cells (RBCs) and platelets may also be decreased. White blood cell (WBC) count may be elevated, reflecting body's response to injury.

Prothrombin time (PT) and activated partial thromboplastin time (aPTT); coagulation profile: Prolonged in active bleeding. May indicate need for replacement of coagulation factors (fresh frozen plasma [FFP]). Increased platelets with decreased clotting times may be the body's attempt to restore hemostasis. Severe abnormalities may reveal coagulopathy, e.g., DIC, as cause of bleeding.

Blood urea nitrogen (BUN): Elevates within 24–48 hr as blood proteins are broken down in the GI tract and kidney filtration is decreased.

Creatinine (Cr): Usually not elevated if renal perfusion is maintained.

Ammonia: May be elevated when severe liver dysfunction disrupts the metabolism and proper excretion of urea or when massive whole blood transfusions have been given.

Arterial blood gases (ABGs): May reveal initial respiratory alkalosis (compensating for diminished blood flow through lungs). Later, metabolic acidosis develops in response to sluggish liver flow/accumulation of metabolic waste products.

Sodium: May be elevated as a hormonal compensation to conserve body fluid.

Potassium: May initially be depleted because of massive gastric emptying/vomiting or bloody diarrhea. Elevated potassium levels may occur after multiple transfusions of stored blood or with acute renal impairment.

Serum gastrin analysis: Elevated level suggests Zollinger-Ellison syndrome or possible presence of multiple poorly healed ulcers. Normal or low in type B gastritis.

Serum amylase: Elevated with posterior penetration of duodenal ulcer.

Pepsinogen level: Increased by duodenal ulcer; low level suggestive of gastritis.

Serum parietal cell antibodies: Presence suggestive of chronic gastritis.

NURSING PRIORITIES

1. Control hemorrhage.
2. Achieve/maintain hemodynamic stability.
3. Promote stress reduction.
4. Provide information about disease process/prognosis, treatment needs, and potential complications.

DISCHARGE GOALS

1. Hemorrhage curtailed.
2. Hemodynamically stable.
3. Anxiety/fear reduced to manageable level.
4. Disease process/prognosis, therapeutic regimen, and potential complications understood.
5. Plan in place to meet needs after discharge.

NURSING DIAGNOSIS: Fluid Volume deficit [isotonic]

May be related to
Active fluid volume loss (hemorrhage)

Possibly evidenced by
Hypotension, tachycardia, delayed capillary refill
Changes in mentation, restlessness
Concentrated/decreased urine
Pallor, diaphoresis
Hemoconcentration

DESIRED OUTCOMES/EVALUATION CRITERIA—PATIENT WILL:

Hydration (NOC)

Demonstrate improved fluid balance as evidenced by individually adequate urinary output with normal specific gravity, stable vital signs, moist mucous membranes, good skin turgor, prompt capillary refill.

ACTIONS/INTERVENTIONS

Hypovolemia Management (NIC)

Independent

Note characteristics of vomitus and/or drainage.

Monitor vital signs; compare with patient's normal/previous readings. Take BP in lying, sitting, standing positions when possible.

RATIONALE

May be helpful in differentiating cause of gastric distress. Yellow-green bile content implies that the pylorus is open. Fecal content indicates bowel obstruction. Bright red blood signals recent or acute arterial bleeding, perhaps caused by gastric ulceration; dark red blood may be old blood (retained in intestine) or venous bleeding from varices. Coffee-ground appearance is suggestive of partially digested blood from slowly oozing area. Undigested food indicates obstruction or gastric tumor.

Changes in blood pressure (BP) and pulse may be used for rough estimate of blood loss (e.g., BP less than 90 mm Hg, and pulse greater than 110 suggests a 25% decrease in volume, or approximately 1000 mL). Postural hypotension reflects a decrease in circulating volume. *Note:* Heart rate may not rise above normal until up to 30% of total blood volume is lost.

ACTIONS/INTERVENTIONS

Independent

Note patient's individual physiological response to bleeding, e.g., changes in mentation, weakness, restlessness, anxiety, pallor, diaphoresis, tachypnea, temperature elevation.

Measure central venous pressure (CVP), if available.

Monitor intake and output (I&O), and correlate with weight changes. Measure blood/fluid losses via emesis, gastric suction/lavage, and stools.

Keep accurate record of subtotals of solutions/blood products during replacement therapy.

Maintain bedrest; prevent vomiting and straining at stool. Schedule activities to provide undisturbed rest periods. Eliminate noxious stimuli.

Elevate head of bed during antacid gavage.

Note signs of renewed bleeding after cessation of initial bleeding.

Observe for secondary bleeding, e.g., nose/gums, oozing from puncture sites, appearance of ecchymotic areas following minimal trauma.

Provide clear/bland fluids when intake is resumed. Avoid caffeinated and carbonated beverages.

Collaborative

Administer IV fluids/volume expanders as indicated, e.g., 0.9% sodium chloride, lactated Ringer's solution;

Fresh whole blood/packed RBCs;

Platelets;

RATIONALE

Symptomatology may be useful in gauging severity/length of bleeding episode. Worsening of symptoms may reflect continued bleeding or inadequate fluid replacement.

Reflects circulating volume and cardiac response to bleeding and fluid replacement, e.g., CVP values between 5 and 20 cm H_2O usually reflect adequate volume.

Provides guidelines for fluid replacement.

Potential exists for overtransfusion of fluids, especially when volume expanders are given before blood transfusions.

Activity/vomiting increases intra-abdominal pressure and can predispose to further bleeding.

Prevents gastric reflux and aspiration of antacids, which can cause serious pulmonary complications.

Increased abdominal fullness/distension, nausea or renewed vomiting, and bloody diarrhea may indicate rebleeding.

Loss of/inadequate replacement of clotting factors may precipitate development of DIC.

More easily digested and reduce risk of added irritation to inflamed tissues. Caffeine and carbonated beverages stimulate hydrochloric acid (HCl) production, possibly potentiating rebleeding.

Fluid replacement with isotonic crystalloid solutions depends on degree of hypovolemia and duration of bleeding (acute or chronic). Other volume expanders, such as albumin, may be infused until type and cross-matching can be completed and blood transfusions begun. Approximately 80%–90% of gastric bleeding is controlled by fluid resuscitation and medical management without transfusion of blood products.

Fresh whole blood is indicated only for acute bleeding with severe volume and RBC depletion because stored blood may be deficient in clotting factors. Packed red blood cells (PRCs) are adequate for stable patients with subacute/chronic bleeding to increase oxygen-carrying capability. *Note:* PRCs are preferred for patients with heart failure (HF) to prevent fluid overload.

Transfused more often than any other blood component, platelets are given to correct deficits in platelet number and clotting function. Clotting factors/components are depleted by two mechanisms: hemorrhagic loss and the clotting process at the site of bleeding.

ACTIONS/INTERVENTIONS	RATIONALE
Collaborative	
Fresh frozen plasma.	FFP is an excellent source for clotting factors. Administered to patients with coagulation deficiencies who are bleeding or about to undergo an invasive procedure.
Insert/maintain large-bore nasogastric (NG) tube in acute bleeding.	Provides avenue for removing irritating gastric secretions, blood, and clots; reduces nausea/vomiting; and facilitates diagnostic endoscopy. *Note:* Blood remaining in the stomach/intestines will be broken down into ammonia, which can produce a toxic central nervous system (CNS) effect, e.g., encephalopathy.
Perform gastric lavage with cool or room-temperature saline until aspirate is light pink or clear and free of clots. Simultaneous low pressure gastric suctioning and continuous saline infusion through the air port of a Salem sump tube may also be used.	Flushes out/breaks up clots and may reduce bleeding by local vasoconstriction. Facilitates visualization by endoscopy to locate bleeding source. *Note:* Research suggests that iced saline is no more effective than room temperature solution in controlling bleeding, and it may actually damage gastric mucosa and lower the patient's core temperature, which could prolong bleeding by inhibiting platelet function.
Administer medications, as indicated, e.g.:	
Cimetidine (Tagamet), ranitidine (Zantac), famotidine (Pepcid), nizatidine (Axid);	Histamine (H$_2$)-receptor antagonists may be given parenterally during bleeding to reduce hydrochloric acid production, increase gastric pH, and aid in healing. After bleeding subsides, the patient may begin oral doses with meals.
Sucralfate (Carafate);	Antiulcer agent that coats the stomach, adheres to the ulcer surface and reinforces the mucous barrier. *Note:* Impairs absorption of some drugs, e.g., theophylline, digoxin, phenytoin, tetracycline, amitriptyline.
Cisapride (Propulsid);	Serotonin-4-receptor agonist used to treat peptic ulcer disease (PUD), reflux esophagitis.
Misoprostol (Cytotec);	Aids in mucous production and inhibits acid secretions. Used to prevent gastric ulcers associated with NSAID use.
Antacids: e.g., aluminum-based (Amphojel, Basaljel), magnesium-based (e.g., Mylanta, Riopan);	Antacids (administered orally or by gavage) may be used to reduce total acid load within the gastric lumen. Effectiveness is greatest for duodenal ulcers. Antacids maintain gastric pH level at 4.5 or higher and reduce risk of rebleeding. *Note:* Antacids block the gastric absorption of oral histamine antagonists and therefore should not be administered within 1 hr after oral administration of histamine blockers.
Proton pump inhibitor: omeprazol (Prilosec), lansoprazolel (Prevacid);	Can completely inhibit acid secretion, has a long duration of action. Used for PUD and GERD or short-term therapy for duodenal ulcers (healing duodenal ulcers in 2–4 wk once severe bleeding is controlled). Typically given with antibiotics when *H. pylori* infection is present.

ACTIONS/INTERVENTIONS	RATIONALE
Collaborative	
Belladonna, atropine;	Anticholinergics may be used to decrease gastric motility, particularly in peptic ulcer disease after acute bleeding has subsided.
Octreotide (Sandostatin);	An analogue of the hormone somatstatin thought to help control esophageal bleeding by decreasing blood flow to the gut, thereby lowering pressure to the portal system.
Vasopressin (Pitressin);	Administration of intra-arterial vasocontrictors may be needed in severe, prolonged bleeding (varices). *Note:* Effects of vasopressin (Pitressin) are systemic, whereas octreolide is more regional.
Vitamin K$_1$ (AquaMEPHYTON);	Promotes hepatic synthesis of coagulation factors to support clotting. *Note:* Use of sucralfate may decrease absorption of vitamin K.
Phenobarbital;	Mild sedatives may be given to promote rest, reduce intensity of bleeding, and alleviate pain. *Note:* Use with caution to avoid masking signs of developing hypovolemia.
Antiemetics, e.g., metoclopramide (Reglan), prochlorperazine (Compazine);	Alleviates nausea and prevents vomiting.
Supplemental vitamin B$_{12}$;	In diffuse atrophic gastritis, the intrinsic factor necessary for B$_{12}$ absorption from the GI tract is not secreted, and individual may develop pernicious anemia.
Anti-infectives, e.g., tetracycline (Achromycin), metronidazole (Flagyl), amoxicillin (Amoxil); clarithromycin (Biaxin).	Oral agents may be combined with antacids or histamine blockers to treat infections causing chronic gastritis or peptic ulcers (*H. pylori*). *Note:* Some studies indicate that *H. pylori* is developing widespread resistance to metronidazole (Flagyl).
Monitor laboratory studies, e.g.:	
Hb, Hct, RBC count;	Aids in establishing blood replacement needs and monitoring effectiveness of therapy, e.g., one unit of whole blood should raise Hct two to three points. Levels may initially remain stable, because of loss of both plasma and RBCs. *Note:* Levels may not accurately reflect early/sudden blood loss and low baseline levels may indicate preexisting anemia.
BUN/Cr levels.	BUN greater than 40 with normal Cr level indicates major bleeding. BUN should return to patient's normal level approximately 12 hr after bleeding has ceased.
Assist with/prepare for:	
Sclerotherapy, e.g., ethanolamine, polidocanol, or combination of sodium tetradecyl, alcohol, and sodium chloride;	Injection of an irritating (sclerosing) agent into esophageal varices (to create thrombosis) is standard treatment to stop bleeding and/or prevent recurrence after initial bleeding is controlled. The percentage of rebleeding is still significant (50%–60%) following this therapy in the patient with varices.

ACTIONS/INTERVENTIONS	RATIONALE

Collaborative

Endoscopic variceal ligation (EVL);	This banding technique is used as an effective alternative to sclerotherapy. Active hemorrhage is controlled in a high percentage of patients with fewer complications than with sclerotherapy.
Balloon tamponade;	Short-term intervention technique using Sengstaken-Blakemore tubes when medication or sclerotherapy fail to control esophageal bleed.
Electrocoagulation or photocoagulation (laser) therapy;	Provides direct coagulation of bleeding sites, e.g., gastritis, duodenal ulcer, tumor, esophageal (Mallory-Weiss) tear.
Surgical intervention.	Total/partial gastrectomy, pyloroplasty, and/or vagotomy may be required to control/prevent future gastric bleeding. Shunt procedures (portacaval, splenorenal, mesocaval, or distal splenorenal) may be done to divert blood flow and reduce pressure within esophageal vessels when other measures fail.

NURSING DIAGNOSIS: Tissue Perfusion, risk for altered

Risk factors may include
Hypovolemia

Possibly evidenced by
[Not applicable; presence of signs and symptoms establishes an *actual* diagnosis]

DESIRED OUTCOMES/EVALUATION CRITERIA—PATIENT WILL:

Circulation Status

Maintain/improve tissue perfusion as evidenced by stabilized vital signs, warm skin, palpable peripheral pulses, ABGs within patient norms, adequate urine output.

ACTIONS/INTERVENTIONS	RATIONALE

Shock Prevention

Independent

Investigate changes in level of consciousness, reports of dizziness/headache.	Changes may reflect inadequate cerebral perfusion as a result of reduced arterial blood pressure. *Note:* Changes in sensorium may also reflect elevated ammonia levels/hepatic encephalopathy in patient with liver disease.
Investigate reports of chest pain. Note location, quality, duration, and what relieves pain.	May reflect cardiac ischemia related to decreased perfusion. *Note:* Impaired oxygenation status resulting from blood loss can bring on myocardial infarction (MI) in patient with cardiac disease.
Auscultate apical pulse. Monitor cardiac rate/rhythm if continuous electrocardiogram (ECG) available/indicated.	Dysrhythmias and ischemic changes can occur as a result of hypotension, hypoxia, acidosis, electrolyte imbalance, or cooling near the heart if cold saline lavage is used to control bleeding.
Assess skin for coolness; pallor; diaphoresis; delayed capillary refill; and weak, thready peripheral pulses.	Vasoconstriction is a sympathetic response to lowered circulating volume and/or may occur as a side effect of vasopressin administration.

ACTIONS/INTERVENTIONS

Independent

Note urinary output and specific gravity.

Note reports of abdominal pain, especially sudden, severe pain or pain radiating to shoulder.

Observe skin for pallor, redness. Massage with lotion. Change position frequently.

Collaborative

Monitor ABGs/pulse oximetry.

Provide supplemental oxygen if indicated.

Administer IV fluids as indicated.

RATIONALE

Decreased systemic perfusion may cause kidney ischemia/failure manifested by decreased urine output. Acute tubular necrosis (ATN) may develop if hypovolemic state is prolonged.

Pain caused by gastric ulcer is often relieved after acute bleeding because of buffering effects of blood. Continued severe or sudden pain may reflect ischemia due to vasoconstrictive therapy, bleeding into biliary tract (hematobilia), or perforation/onset of peritonitis.

Compromised peripheral circulation increases risk of skin breakdown.

Identifies hypoxemia, effectiveness of/need for therapy.

Treats hypoxemia and lactic acidosis during acute bleed.

Maintains circulating volume and perfusion. *Note:* Use of lactated Ringer's solution may be contraindicated in presence of hepatic failure because metabolism of lactate is impaired, and lactic acidosis may develop.

NURSING DIAGNOSIS: Fear/Anxiety [specify level]

May be related to
Change in health status, threat of death

Possibly evidenced by
Increased tension, restlessness, irritability, fearfulness
Trembling, tachycardia, diaphoresis
Lack of eye contact, focus on self
Verbalization of specific concern
Withdrawal, panic or attack behavior

DESIRED OUTCOMES/EVALUATION CRITERIA—PATIENT WILL:

Anxiety Control

Discuss fears/concerns recognizing healthy versus unhealthy fears.
Verbalize appropriate range of feelings.
Appear relaxed and report anxiety is reduced to a manageable level.
Demonstrate problem solving and effective use of resources.

ACTIONS/INTERVENTIONS

Anxiety Reduction

Independent

Monitor physiological responses, e.g., tachypnea, palpitations, dizziness, headache, tingling sensations.

Note behavioral cues, e.g., restlessness, irritability, lack of eye contact, combativeness/attack behavior.

RATIONALE

May be indicative of the degree of fear patient is experiencing but may also be related to physical condition/shock state.

Indicators of degree of fear patient is experiencing; e.g., patient may feel out of control of the situation or reach a state of panic.

ACTIONS/INTERVENTIONS	RATIONALE
Independent	
Encourage verbalization of concerns. Assist patient in expressing feelings by Active listening.	Establishes a therapeutic relationship. Assists the patient in dealing with feelings and provides opportunity to clarify misconceptions.
Acknowledge that this is a fearful situation and that others have expressed similar fears.	When patient is expressing own fear, the validation that these feelings are normal can help patient to feel less isolated.
Provide accurate, concrete information about what is being done, e.g., sensations to expect, usual procedures undertaken.	Involves patient in plan of care and decreases unnecessary anxiety about unknowns.
Provide a calm, restful environment.	Removing patient from outside stressors promotes relaxation, may enhance coping skills.
Encourage significant other (SO) to stay with patient as able. Respond to call signal promptly. Use touch and eye contact as appropriate.	Helps reduce fear of going through a frightening experience alone.
Provide opportunity for SO to express feelings/concerns. Encourage SO to project positive, realistic attitude.	Helps SO to deal with own anxiety/fears that can be transmitted to the patient. Promotes a supportive attitude that can facilitate recovery.
Demonstrate/encourage relaxation techniques, e.g., visualization, deep-breathing exercises, guided imagery.	Learning ways to relax can be helpful in reducing fear and anxiety. Because the patient with GI bleeding is often a person who has difficulty relaxing, learning these skills can be important to recovery and prevention of recurrence.
Help the patient identify and initiate positive coping behaviors used successfully in the past.	Successful behaviors can be fostered in dealing with current fear, enhancing patient's sense of self-control and providing reassurance.
Encourage and support patient in evaluation of lifestyle.	Changes may be necessary to avoid recurrence of ulcer condition.
Collaborative	
Administer medications as indicated, e.g.:	
Diazepam (Valium), clorazepate (Tranxene), alprazolam (Xanax).	Sedatives/antianxiety agents may be used on occasion to reduce anxiety and promote rest, particularly in the ulcer patient.
Refer to clinical specialist psychiatric nurse, social services, spiritual advisor.	May need additional assistance during recovery to deal with consequences of emergency situation/adjustments to required/desired changes in lifestyle.

NURSING DIAGNOSIS: Pain [acute]/chronic

May be related to

Chemical burn of gastric mucosa, oral cavity

Physical response, e.g., reflex muscle spasm in the stomach wall

Possibly evidenced by

Communication of pain descriptors

Abdominal guarding, rigid body posture, facial grimacing

Autonomic responses, e.g., changes in vital signs (acute pain)

DESIRED OUTCOMES/EVALUATION CRITERIA—PATIENT WILL:

Pain Level

Verbalize relief of pain.
Demonstrate relaxed body posture and be able to sleep/rest appropriately.

ACTIONS/INTERVENTIONS	RATIONALE
Pain Management	
Independent	
Note reports of pain, including location, duration, intensity (0–10 scale).	Pain is not always present, but if present should be compared with patient's previous pain symptoms. This comparison may assist in diagnosis of etiology of bleeding and development of complications.
Review factors that aggravate or alleviate pain.	Helpful in establishing diagnosis and treatment needs.
Note nonverbal pain cues, e.g., restlessness, reluctance to move, abdominal guarding, tachycardia, diaphoresis. Investigate discrepancies between verbal and nonverbal cues.	Nonverbal cues may be both physiological and psychological and may be used in conjunction with verbal cues to evaluate extent/severity of the problem.
Provide small, frequent meals as indicated for individual patient.	Food has an acid neutralizing effect and dilutes the gastric contents. Small meals prevent distension and the release of gastrin.
Identify and limit foods that create discomfort.	Specific foods that cause distress vary among individuals. Studies indicate pepper is harmful, and coffee (including decaffeinated) can precipitate dyspepsia.
Assist with active/passive range of motion (ROM) exercises.	Reduces joint stiffness, minimizing pain/discomfort.
Provide frequent oral care and comfort measures, e.g., back rub, position change.	Halitosis from stagnant oral secretions is unappetizing and can aggravate nausea. Gingivitis and dental problems may arise.
Collaborative	
Provide and implement prescribed dietary modifications.	Patient may receive nothing by mouth (NPO) initially. When oral intake is allowed, food choices depend on the diagnosis and etiology of the bleeding.
Use regular rather than skim milk, if milk is allowed.	Fat in regular milk may decrease gastric secretions; however, the calcium and protein content (especially in skim milk) increases them.
Administer medications, as indicated, e.g.:	
Analgesics, e.g., morphine sulfate;	May be narcotic of choice to relieve acute/severe pain and reduce peristaltic activity. *Note:* Meperidine (Demerol) has been associated with increased incidence of nausea/vomiting.
Acetaminophen (Tylenol);	Promotes general comfort and rest.
Antacids;	Decreases gastric acidity by absorption or by chemical neutralization. Evaluate choice of antacid in regard to total health picture, e.g., sodium restriction.
Anticholinergics, e.g., belladonna, atropine.	May be given at bedtime to decrease gastric motility, suppress acid production, delay gastric emptying, and alleviate nocturnal pain associated with gastric ulcer.

NURSING DIAGNOSIS: Knowledge Deficit [Learning Need] regarding disease process, prognosis, treatment, self care, and discharge needs

May be related to
Lack of information/recall
Unfamiliarity with information resources
Information misinterpretation

Possibly evidenced by
Verbalization of the problem, request for information, statement of misconceptions
Inaccurate follow-through of instructions
Development of preventable complications

DESIRED OUTCOMES/EVALUATION CRITERIA—PATIENT WILL:

> **Knowledge: Disease Process**

Verbalize understanding of cause of own bleeding episode (if known) and treatment modalities used.
Begin to discuss own role in preventing recurrence.

> **Knowledge: Treatment Regimen**

Identify/implement necessary lifestyle changes.
Participate in treatment regimen.

ACTIONS/INTERVENTIONS	RATIONALE
Teaching: Disease Process	
Independent	
Determine patient perception of cause of bleeding.	Establishes knowledge base and provides some insight into how the teaching plan needs to be constructed for this individual.
Provide/review information regarding etiology of bleeding, cause/effect, relationship of lifestyle behaviors, and ways to reduce risk/contributing factors. Encourage questions.	Provides knowledge base from which patient can make informed choices/decisions about future and control of health problems.
Assist patient to identify relationship of food intake and precipitation of/relief from epigastric pain, including avoidance of gastric irritants, e.g., pepper; caffeine; alcohol; fruit juices; carbonated beverages; and extremely hot, cold, fatty, or spicy foods.	Caffeine stimulates gastric acidity. Alcohol contributes to erosion of gastric mucosa. Although current research indicates that diet does not contribute to the development of PUD, individuals may find that certain foods/fluids increase gastric secretion and pain.
Recommend small, frequent meals/snacks, chewing food slowly, eating at regular time, and avoiding "skipping" meals.	Frequent eating keeps HCl neutralized, dilutes stomach contents to minimize action of acid on gastric mucosa. Small meals prevent gastric overdistension.
Stress importance of reading labels on OTC drugs and either avoiding products containing aspirin or switching to enteric-coated aspirin.	Aspirin damages the protective mucosa, permitting gastric erosion, ulceration, and bleeding to occur.
Review significance of signs/symptoms (S/S) such as coffee-ground emesis, tarry stools, abdominal distension, severe epigastric/abdominal pain radiating to shoulder/back.	Prompt medical evaluation/intervention is required to prevent more serious complications, e.g., perforation, Zollinger-Ellison syndrome.

ACTIONS/INTERVENTIONS	RATIONALE
Independent	
Support use of stress management techniques, avoidance of emotional stress.	Decreases extrinsic stimulation of HCl, reducing risk of recurrence of bleeding.
Review drug regimen, possible side effects, and interaction with other drugs as appropriate.	Helpful to patient's understanding of reason for taking drugs and what symptoms are important to report to healthcare provider. *Note:* Aluminum-containing antacids inhibit the intestinal absorption of some drugs and affect scheduling of drug intake. Some men may incur impotence when using prescription-strength cimetidine (Tagamet). Alternate drug choices are famotidine (Pepcid) and ranitidine (Zantac).
Encourage patient to inform all healthcare providers of bleeding history.	May affect drug choices and/or concomitant prescriptions, e.g., misoprostol (Cytotec) can be given with NSAIDs to inhibit gastric acid secretion and reduce risk of gastric irritability/lesions resulting from NSAID therapy.
Discuss importance of cessation of smoking.	Ulcer healing may be delayed in people who smoke, particularly in those treated with cimetidine (Tagamet). Smoking stimulates gastric acidity and is associated with increased risk of peptic ulcer development/recurrence.
Refer to support groups/counseling for lifestyle/behavior changes/reduction of associated risk factors, e.g., substance abuse/stop-smoking clinics.	Alcohol users have a higher incidence of gastritis/esophageal varices, and cigarette smoking is associated with peptic ulcers and delayed healing.

POTENTIAL CONSIDERATIONS following acute hospitalization (dependent on patient's age, physical condition/presence of complications, personal resources, and life responsibilities)

Therapeutic Regimen: Individual, ineffective management—decisional conflicts (e.g., use of NSAIDs for arthritic/chronic pain condition, perceived benefits (e.g., cessation of smoking), economic difficulties (cost of medication).

SUBTOTAL GASTRECTOMY/GASTRIC RESECTION

Subtotal gastrectomy or gastric resection is indicated for gastric hemorrhage/intractable ulcers, dysfunctional lower esophageal sphincter, pyloric obstruction, perforation, cancer.

CARE SETTING

Inpatient surgical unit.

RELATED CONCERNS

Cancer, page 900
Pancreatitis, page 498
Peritonitis, page 382
Psychosocial aspects of care, page 809
Surgical intervention, page 828
Total nutritional support: parenteral/enteral feeding, page 508
Upper gastrointestinal/Esophageal bleeding, page 333

Patient Assessment Database

Data depends on the underlying condition necessitating surgery.

TEACHING/LEARNING

Discharge plan considerations: **DRG projected mean length of inpatient stay: 3.5 days**
Assistance with administration of enteral feedings/total parenteral nutrition (TPN) (if required) and acquisition of supplies

Refer to section at end of plan for postdischarge considerations.

NURSING PRIORITIES

1. Promote healing and adequate nutritional intake.
2. Prevent complications.
3. Provide information about surgical procedure/prognosis, treatment needs, and concerns.

DISCHARGE GOALS

1. Nutritional intake adequate for individual needs.
2. Complications prevented/minimized.
3. Surgical procedure/prognosis, therapeutic regimen, and long-term needs understood.
4. Plan in place to meet needs after discharge.

(In addition to nursing diagnoses identified in this CP, refer to CP Surgical Intervention, p. 828.)

NURSING DIAGNOSIS: Nutrition: altered, risk for less than body requirements

Risk factors may include
Restriction of fluids and food
Change in digestive process/absorption of nutrients

Possibly evidenced by
[Not applicable; presence of signs and symptoms establishes an *actual* diagnosis]

DESIRED OUTCOMES/EVALUATION CRITERIA—PATIENT WILL:

Nutritional Status

Maintain stable weight/demonstrate progressive weight gain toward goal with normalization of laboratory values.
Be free of signs of malnutrition.

ACTIONS/INTERVENTIONS	RATIONALE
Nutrition Therapy (NIC)	
Independent	
Maintain patency of NG tube. Notify physician if tube becomes dislodged.	Provides rest for GI tract during acute postoperative phase until return of normal function. *Note:* The physician/surgeon may need to reposition the tube endoscopically to prevent injury to the operative area.
Note character and amount of gastric drainage.	Will be bloody for first 12 hr, and then should clear/turn greenish. Continued/recurrent bleeding suggests complications. Decline in output may reflect return of GI function.
Caution the patient to limit the intake of ice chips.	Excessive intake of ice produces nausea and can wash out electrolytes via the NG tube.
Provide oral hygiene on a regular, frequent basis, including petroleum jelly for lips.	Prevents discomfort of dry mouth and cracked lips caused by fluid restriction and the NG tube.
Auscultate for resumption of bowel sounds and note passage of flatus.	Peristalsis can be expected to return about the third postoperative day, signaling readiness to resume oral intake.
Monitor tolerance to fluid and food intake, noting abdominal distension, reports of increased pain/cramping, nausea/vomiting.	Complications of paralytic ileus, obstruction, delayed gastric emptying, and gastric dilation may occur, possibly requiring reinsertion of NG tube.
Avoid milk and high carbohydrate foods in the diet.	May trigger "dumping syndrome." (Refer to ND: Knowledge Deficit [Learning Need], p. 348.)
Note admission weight and compare with subsequent readings.	Provides information about adequacy of dietary intake/determination of nutritional needs.
Collaborative	
Administer IV fluids, TPN, and lipids as indicated.	Meets fluid/nutritional needs until oral intake can be resumed.
Monitor laboratory studies, e.g., Hb/Hct, electrolytes, and total protein/prealbumin.	Indicators of fluid/nutritional needs and effectiveness of therapy and detects developing complications.
Progress diet as tolerated, advancing from clear liquid to bland diet with several small feedings.	Usually NG tube is clamped for specified periods of time when peristalsis returns to determine tolerance. After NG tube is removed, intake is advanced gradually to prevent gastric irritation/distension.
Administer medications as indicated:	
Anticholinergics, e.g., atropine, propantheline bromide (Pro-Banthine);	Controls dumping syndrome, enhancing digestion and absorption of nutrients.
Fat-soluble vitamin supplements, including B_{12}; calcium;	Removal of the stomach prevents absorption of B_{12} (due to loss of intrinsic factor) and can lead to pernicious anemia. In addition, rapid emptying of the stomach reduces absorption of calcium.
Iron preparations;	Corrects/prevents iron deficiency anemia.
Protein supplements;	Additional protein may be helpful for tissue repair and healing.
Pancreatic enzymes, bile salts;	Enhances digestive process.
Medium-chain triglycerides (MCT).	Promotes absorption of fats and fat-soluble vitamins to prevent malabsorption problems.

ACTIONS/INTERVENTIONS	RATIONALE
Teaching: Disease Process (NIC)	
Independent	
Review surgical procedure and long-term expectations.	Provides knowledge base from which informed choices can be made. Recovery following gastric surgery is often slower than may be anticipated with similar types of surgery. Improved strength and partial normalization of dietary pattern may not be evident for at least 3 mo, and full return to usual intake (three "normal" meals/day) may take up to 12 mo. This prolonged convalescence may be difficult for the patient/SO to deal with, especially if he or she has not been prepared.
Discuss and identify stress situations and how to avoid them. Investigate job-related issues.	Can alter gastric motility, interfering with optimal digestion. *Note:* Patient may require vocational counseling if change in employment is indicated.
Review dietary needs/regimen (e.g., low-carbohydrate, low-fat, high-protein) and importance of maintaining vitamin supplementation.	May prevent deficiencies, enhance healing, and promote cooperation with therapy. *Note:* Low-fat diet may be required to reduce risk of alkaline reflux gastritis.
Discuss the importance of eating small, frequent meals slowly and in a relaxed atmosphere; resting after meals; avoiding extremely hot or cold food; restricting high-fiber foods, caffeine, milk products and alcohol, excess sugars and salt; and taking fluids between meals, rather than with food.	These measures can be helpful in avoiding gastric distension/irritation and/or stress on surgical repair, dumping syndrome, and reactive hypoglycemia. *Note:* Ice-cold fluids/foods can cause gastric spasms.
Instruct in avoiding certain fibrous foods and discuss the necessity of chewing food well.	Remaining gastric tissue may have reduced ability to digest such foods as citrus skins/seeds, which can collect, forming a mass (phytobezoar formation) that is not excreted.

ACTIONS/INTERVENTIONS	RATIONALE
Independent	
Recommend foods containing pectin, e.g., citrus fruits, bananas, apples, yellow vegetables, and beans.	Increased intake of these foods may reduce incidence of dumping syndrome.
Identify foods that can cause gastric irritation and increase gastric acid, e.g., chocolate, spicy foods, whole grains, raw vegetables.	Limiting/avoiding these foods reduces risk of gastric bleeding/ulceration in some individuals. *Note:* Ingesting fresh fruits to reduce risk of dumping syndrome should be tempered with adverse effect of gastric irritation.
Identify symptoms that may indicate dumping syndrome, e.g., weakness, profuse perspiration, epigastric fullness, nausea/vomiting, abdominal cramping, faintness, flushing, explosive diarrhea, and palpitations occurring within 15 min to 1 hr after eating.	Can cause severe discomfort or even shock, and reduces absorption of nutrients. Usually self-limiting (1–3 wk after surgery) but can become chronic.
Discuss signs of hypoglycemia and corrective interventions, e.g., ingesting cheese and crackers, orange/ grape juice.	Awareness helps patient take actions to prevent progression of symptoms.
Suggest patient weigh self on a regular basis.	Change in dietary pattern, early satiety, and efforts to avoid dumping syndrome may limit intake, causing weight loss.
Review medication purpose, dosage, and schedule and possible side effects.	Understanding rationale/therapeutic needs can reduce risk of complications, e.g., anticholinergics/ pectin powder may be given to reduce incidence of dumping syndrome; antacids/histamine antagonists reduce gastric irritation.
Caution patient to read labels and avoid products containing ASA, ibuprofen.	Can cause gastric irritation/bleeding.
Discuss reasons and importance of cessation of smoking.	Smoking stimulates gastric acid production and may cause vasoconstriction, compromising mucous membranes and increasing risk of gastric irritation/ ulceration.
Identify signs/symptoms requiring medical evaluation, e.g., persistent nausea/vomiting or abdominal fullness; weight loss; diarrhea; foul-smelling fatty or tarry stools; bloody or coffee-ground vomitus/presence of bile, fever. Instruct patient to report changes in pain characteristics.	Prompt recognition and intervention may prevent serious consequences or potential complications such as pancreatitis, peritonitis, and afferent loop syndrome.
Stress importance of regular checkup with healthcare provider.	Necessary to detect developing complications, e.g., anemia, problems with nutrition, and/or recurrence of disease.

POTENTIAL CONSIDERATIONS following acute hospitalization (dependent on patient's age, physical condition/presence of complications, personal resources, and life responsibilities)

Nutrition: altered, risk for less than body requirements—change in digestive process/absorption of nutrients, early satiety, gastric irritation.

Fatigue—decreased energy production, states of discomfort, increased energy requirements to perform activities of daily living (ADLs).

INFLAMMATORY BOWEL DISEASE: ULCERATIVE COLITIS, REGIONAL ENTERITIS (CROHN'S DISEASE, ILEOCOLITIS)

Inflammatory bowel disease (IBD): Researchers believe that IBD may result from a complex interplay between genetic and environmental factors. Similarities involve (1) chronic inflammation of the alimentary tract and (2) periods of remission interspersed with episodes of acute inflammation.

Ulcerative colitis (UC): A chronic condition of unknown cause usually starting in the rectum and distal portions of the colon and possibly spreading upward to involve the sigmoid and descending colon or the entire colon. It is usually intermittent (acute exacerbation with long remissions), but some individuals (30%–40%) have continuous symptoms. Cure is effected only by total removal of colon and rectum/rectal mucosa.

Regional enteritis (Crohn's disease, ileocolitis): May be found in portions of the alimentary tract from the mouth to the anus but is most commonly found in the small intestine (terminal ileum). It is a slowly progressive chronic disease of unknown cause with intermittent acute episodes and no known cure. UC and regional enteritis share common symptoms but differ in the segment and layer of intestine involved and the degree of severity and complications. Therefore, separate databases are provided.

CARE SETTING

Usually handled at the community level; however, severe exacerbations requiring advanced pain control, nutrition, and rehydration may necessitate short stay in acute care medical unit.

RELATED CONCERNS

Fecal diversions: postoperative care of ileostomy and colostomy, page 364
Fluid and electrolyte imbalances, page 926
Peritonitis, page 382
Psychosocial aspects of care, page 809
Total nutritional support: parenteral/enteral feeding, page 508

Patient Assessment Database—Ulcerative Colitis

ACTIVITY/REST

May report:
Weakness, fatigue, malaise, exhaustion
Insomnia, not sleeping through the night because of diarrhea
Feeling restless
Restriction of activities/work due to effects of disease process

CIRCULATION

May exhibit:
Tachycardia (response to fever, dehydration, inflammatory process, and pain)
Bruising, ecchymotic areas (insufficient vitamin K)
BP: hypotension, including postural changes

EGO INTEGRITY

May report:
Anxiety, apprehension, emotional upsets, e.g., feelings of helplessness/hopelessness
Acute/chronic stress factors, e.g., family/job-related, expense of treatment
Cultural factor—increased prevalence in Jewish population

May exhibit:
Withdrawal, narrowed focus, depression

ELIMINATION

May report:
Stool texture varying from soft-formed to mushy or watery
Unpredictable, intermittent, frequent, uncontrollable episodes of bloody diarrhea (as many as 20–30 stools/day); sense of urgency/cramping (tenesmus); passing blood/pus/mucus with or without passing feces
Rectal bleeding
History of renal stones (dehydration)

May exhibit:	Diminished or hyperactive bowel sounds, absence of peristalsis or presence of visible peristaltic waves
	Hemorrhoids, anal fissures (25%); perianal fistula (more frequently with Crohn's)
	Oliguria

FOOD/FLUID

May report:	Anorexia; nausea/vomiting
	Weight loss
	Dietary intolerances/sensitivities, e.g., raw fruits/vegetables, dairy products, fatty foods
May exhibit:	Decreased subcutaneous fat/muscle mass
	Weakness, poor muscle tone and skin turgor
	Mucous membranes pale; sore, inflamed buccal cavity; dry, cracking of tongue (dehydration/malnutrition)

HYGIENE

May report:	Inability to maintain self-care
May exhibit:	Stomatitis reflecting vitamin deficiency
	Unkempt appearance; body odor

PAIN/DISCOMFORT

May report:	Mild abdominal cramping to severe pain/tenderness in lower-left quadrant (may be relieved with defecation)
	Migratory joint pain, tenderness (arthritis)
	Eye pain, photophobia (iritis)
May exhibit:	Abdominal tenderness, distension, rigidity

SAFETY

May report:	History of lupus erythematosus, hemolytic anemia, vasculitis
	Arthritis (worsening of symptoms with exacerbations in bowel disease)
	Temperature elevation 104°F–105°F (acute exacerbation)
	Blurred vision
	Allergies to foods/milk products (release of histamine into bowel has an inflammatory effect)
May exhibit:	Skin lesions may be present; e.g., erythema nodosum (raised, tender, red, and swollen) on arms, face; pyoderma gangrenosum (purulent pinpoint lesion/boil with a purple border) on trunk, legs, ankles
	Ankylosing spondylitis
	Uveitis, conjunctivitis/iritis

SEXUALITY

| **May report:** | Reduced frequency/avoidance of sexual activity |

SOCIAL INTERACTION

| **May report:** | Relationship/role problems related to condition |
| | Inability to be active socially |

TEACHING/LEARNING

May report:	Family history of IBD, immune disorders
Discharge plan considerations:	**DRG projected mean length of inpatient stay: 4.9 days**
	Assistance with dietary requirements, medication regimen, psychological support
	Refer to section at end of plan for postdischarge considerations.

DIAGNOSTIC STUDIES

Stool specimens (examinations are used in initial diagnosis and in following disease progression): Mainly composed of mucus, blood, pus, and intestinal organisms, especially *Entamoeba histolytica* (active stage).

Proctosigmoidoscopy: Visualizes ulcerations, edema, hyperemia, and inflammation (result of secondary infection of the mucosa and submucosa). Friability and hemorrhagic areas caused by necrosis and ulceration occur in 85% of these patients.

Cytology and rectal biopsy: Differentiates between infectious process and carcinoma (occurs 10–20 times more often than in general population). Neoplastic changes can be detected, as well as characteristic inflammatory infiltrates called crypt abscesses.

Barium enema: May be performed after visual examination has been done, although rarely done during acute, relapsing stage, because it can exacerbate condition.

Colonoscopy: Identifies adhesions, changes in luminal wall (narrowing/irregularity); rules out bowel obstruction.

Abdominal magnetic resonance imaging (MRI)/computed tomography (CT) scan, ultrasound: Detects infections/inflammatory conditions.

CBC: May show hyperchromic anemia (active disease generally present because of blood loss and iron deficiency); leukocytosis may occur, especially in fulminating or complicated cases and in patients on steroid therapy.

Erythrocyte sedimentation rate (ESR): Increased according to severity of disease.

Serum iron level: Lowered because of blood loss.

PT: Prolonged in severe cases from altered factors VII and X caused by vitamin K deficiency.

Thrombocytosis: May occur as a result of inflammatory disease process.

Electrolytes: Decreased potassium and magnesium are common in severe disease.

Prealbumin/Albumin level: Decreased because of loss of plasma proteins/disturbed liver function, decreased dietary intake.

Alkaline phosphatase: Increased, along with serum cholesterol and hypoproteinemia, indicating disturbed liver function (e.g., cholangitis, cirrhosis).

Bone marrow: A generalized depression is common in fulminating types/after a long inflammatory process.

Patient Assessment Database—Regional Enteritis (Crohn's Disease, Ileocolitis)

ACTIVITY/REST

May report:
Weakness, fatigue, malaise, exhaustion
Feeling restless
Restriction of activities/work due to effects of disease process

EGO INTEGRITY

May report:
Anxiety, apprehension, emotional upsets, feelings of helplessness/hopelessness
Acute/chronic stress factors, e.g., family/job-related, expense of treatment
Cultural factor—increased prevalence in Jewish population, frequency increasing in individuals of Northern European and Anglo-Saxon derivation

May exhibit:
Withdrawal, narrowed focus, depression

ELIMINATION

May report:
Unpredictable, intermittent, frequent, uncontrollable episodes of nonbloody diarrhea, soft or semiliquid with flatus; foul-smelling and fatty stools (steatorrhea)
Intermittent constipation
History of renal stones (increased oxalates in the urine)

May exhibit:
Hyperactive bowel sounds with gurgling, splashing sound (borborygmus)
Visible peristalsis

FOOD/FLUID

May report:
Anorexia; nausea/vomiting
Weight loss
Dietary intolerance/sensitivity, e.g., dairy products, fatty foods

May exhibit:
Decreased subcutaneous fat/muscle mass
Weakness, poor muscle tone and skin turgor
Mucous membranes pale

HYGIENE

May report:	Inability to maintain self-care
May exhibit:	Unkempt appearance; body odor

PAIN/DISCOMFORT

May report: Tender abdomen with cramping pain in lower right quadrant (inflammation involving all layers of bowel wall and possibly the mesentery); pain in midlower abdomen (jejunal involvement)

Referred tenderness to periumbilical region

Perineal tenderness/pain

Migratory joint pain, tenderness (arthritis)

Eye pain, photophobia (iritis)

May exhibit: Abdominal tenderness/distension

SAFETY

May report: History of arthritis, systemic lupus erythematosus (SLE), hemolytic anemia, vasculitis

Temperature elevation (low-grade fever)

Blurred vision

May exhibit: Skin lesions may be present: erythema nodosum (raised tender, red swelling) on face, arms; pyoderma gangrenosum (purulent pinpoint lesion/boil with a purple border) on trunk, legs, ankles; perineal lesions/anorectal fistulas

Ankylosing spondylitis

Uveitis, conjunctivitis/iritis

SOCIAL INTERACTION

May report: Relationship/role problems related to condition; inability to be active socially

TEACHING/LEARNING

May report: Family history of IBD, immune disorders

Discharge plan considerations: **DRG projected mean length of inpatient stay: 4.9 days**

Assistance with dietary requirements, medication regimen, psychological support

Refer to section at end of plan for postdischarge considerations.

DIAGNOSTIC STUDIES

Stool examination: Occult blood may be positive (mucosal erosion); steatorrhea and bile salts may be found.

X-rays: Barium swallow may demonstrate luminal narrowing in the terminal ileum, stiffening of the bowel wall, mucosal irritability or ulceration.

Barium enema: Small bowel is nearly always involved, but the rectal area is affected only 50% of the time. Fistulas are common and are usually found in the terminal ileum but may be present in segments throughout the GI tract.

Sigmoidoscopic examination: Can demonstrate edematous hyperemic colon mucosa, transverse fissures, or longitudinal ulcers.

Endoscopy: Provides visualization of involved areas.

Abdominal MRI/CT scan, ultrasound: Detects infections/inflammatory conditions.

CBC: Anemia (hypochromic, occasionally macrocytic) may occur because of malnutrition or malabsorption or depressed bone marrow function (chronic inflammatory process); increased white blood cells (WBCs).

ESR: Increased, reflecting inflammation.

Prealbumin/Albumin/total protein: Decreased.

Cholesterol: Elevated (may have gallstones).

Serum iron-binding folic acid capacity/transferrin levels: Decreased because of chronic infection or secondary to blood loss.

Clotting studies: Alterations may occur because of poor vitamin B_{12} absorption.

Electrolytes: Decreased potassium, calcium, and magnesium, with increased sodium.

Urine: Hyperoxaluria (can cause kidney stones).

Urine culture: If *Escherichia coli* organisms are present, suspect fistula formation into the bladder.

Anticolon antibodies: Suggests autoimmune components in some patients.

NURSING PRIORITIES

1. Control diarrhea/promote optimal bowel function.
2. Minimize/prevent complications.
3. Promote optimal nutrition.
4. Minimize mental/emotional stress.
5. Provide information about disease process, treatment needs, and long-term aspects/potential complications of recurrent disease.

DISCHARGE GOALS

1. Bowel function stabilized.
2. Complications prevented/controlled.
3. Dealing positively with condition.
4. Disease process/prognosis, therapeutic regimen, and potential complications are understood.
5. Plan in place to meet needs after discharge.

NURSING DIAGNOSIS: Diarrhea

May be related to
Inflammation, irritation, or malabsorption of the bowel
Presence of toxins
Segmental narrowing of the lumen

Possibly evidenced by
Increased bowel sounds/peristalsis
Frequent, and often severe, watery stools (acute phase)
Changes in stool color
Abdominal pain; urgency (sudden painful need to defecate), cramping

DESIRED OUTCOMES/EVALUATION CRITERIA—PATIENT WILL:

Bowel Elimination (NOC)

Report reduction in frequency of stools, return to more normal stool consistency.
Identify/avoid contributing factors.

ACTIONS/INTERVENTIONS	RATIONALE
Diarrhea Management (NIC)	
Independent	
Observe and record stool frequency, characteristics, amount, and precipitating factors.	Helps differentiate individual disease and assesses severity of episode.
Promote bedrest, provide bedside commode.	Rest decreases intestinal motility and reduces the metabolic rate when infection or hemorrhage is a complication. Urge to defecate may occur without warning and be uncontrollable, increasing risk of incontinence/falls if facilities are not close at hand.
Remove stool promptly. Provide room deodorizers.	Reduces noxious odors to avoid undue patient embarrassment.
Identify foods and fluids that precipitate diarrhea, e.g., raw vegetables and fruits, whole-grain cereals, condiments, carbonated drinks, milk products.	Avoiding intestinal irritants promotes intestinal rest.

ACTIONS/INTERVENTIONS

Independent

Restart oral fluid intake gradually. Offer clear liquids hourly; avoid cold fluids.

Provide opportunity to vent frustrations related to disease process.

Observe for fever, tachycardia, lethargy, leukocytosis, decreased serum protein, anxiety, and prostration.

Collaborative

Administer medications as indicated:

Antidiarrheals, e.g diphenoxylate (Lomotil); loperamide (Imodium); anodyne suppositories;

Anti-inflammatories, e.g.: 5-aminosalicylates (5-ASA), sulfasalazine (Azulfidine), mesalamine (Pentasa, Asacol, Rowasa);

Antispasmodics, e.g., L-hyoscyamine (Levsin); dicyclomine (Bentyl);

Psyllium (Metamucil);

Cholestyramine (Questran);

Steroids, e.g., adrenocorticotropic hormone (ACTH), hydrocortisone (Cortenema, Cortifoam), prednisolone (Delta-Cortef), prednisone (Deltasone);

Immunosuppressants, e.g., azathioprine (Imuran); mercaptopurine (6-MP) (Purinethol); cyclosporine (Sandimmune);

Antiulcer agents, e.g., antacids; ranitidine (Zantac);

Anti-infectives e.g., metronidazole (Flagyl).

Assist with/prepare for surgical intervention, e.g., ileostomy, total colectomy, percutaneous abscess drainage.

RATIONALE

Provides colon rest by omitting or decreasing the stimulus of foods/fluids. Gradual resumption of liquids may prevent cramping and recurrence of diarrhea; however, cold fluids can increase intestinal motility.

Presence of disease with unknown cause that is difficult to cure and that may require surgical intervention can lead to stress reactions that may aggravate condition.

May signify that toxic megacolon or perforation and peritonitis are imminent/have occurred, necessitating immediate medical intervention.

Decreases GI motility/propulsion (peristalsis) and diminishes digestive secretions to relieve cramping and diarrhea. *Note:* Use with caution in UC because they may precipitate toxic megacolon.

Useful in treating mild/moderate exacerbations because of both anti-inflammatory and antimicrobial properties. Long-term use may prolong remission. *Note:* Available in oral/time-release and pH-dependent forms. Rowasa may be given as an enema in lieu of sulfasalazine (Azulfidine) for patients who are sensitive to oral sulfa drugs.

May be useful to inpatients who do not respond to standard interventions.

Absorbs water to increase bulk in stools, thereby decreasing diarrhea.

Binds bile salts, reducing diarrhea that results from excess bile acid.

Decreases acute inflammatory process. Steroid enemas (Cortenema) may be given in mild/moderate disease to aid absorption of the drug (possibly with atropine sulfate or belladonna suppository). Current research suggests an 8-wk course of time-release steroids may effect remission in Crohn's disease; however, steroids are contraindicated if intra-abdominal abscesses are suspected.

Immunosuppressant may be given to block inflammatory response, decrease steroid requirements, promote healing of fistulas. May be given in conjunction with sulfasalazine.

Decreases gastric irritation, preventing inflammation and reducing risk of infection in colitis.

Treats local suppurative infections, or may be part of long-term treatment regimen.

May be necessary if perforation or bowel obstruction occurs or disease is unresponsive to medical treatment.

ACTIONS/INTERVENTIONS	RATIONALE
Fluid/Electrolyte Management (NIC)	
Independent	
Monitor I&O. Note number, character, and amount of stools; estimate insensible fluid losses, e.g., diaphoresis. Measure urine specific gravity; observe for oliguria.	Provides information about overall fluid balance, renal function, and bowel disease control, as well as guidelines for fluid replacement.
Assess vital signs (BP, pulse, temperature).	Hypotension (including postural), tachycardia, fever can indicate response to and/or effect of fluid loss.
Observe for excessively dry skin and mucous membranes, decreased skin turgor, slowed capillary refill.	Indicates excessive fluid loss/resultant dehydration.
Weigh daily.	Indicator of overall fluid and nutritional status.
Maintain oral restrictions, bed rest; avoid exertion.	Colon is placed at rest for healing and to decrease intestinal fluid losses.
Observe for overt bleeding and test stool daily for occult blood.	Inadequate diet and decreased absorption may lead to vitamin K deficiency and defects in coagulation, potentiating risk of hemorrhage.
Note generalized muscle weakness or cardiac dysrhythmias.	Excessive intestinal loss may lead to electrolyte imbalance, e.g., potassium, which is necessary for proper skeletal and cardiac muscle function. Minor alterations in serum levels can result in profound and/or life-threatening symptoms.
Collaborative	
Administer parenteral fluids, blood transfusions as indicated.	Maintenance of bowel rest requires alternate fluid replacement to correct losses/anemia. *Note:* Fluids containing sodium may be restricted in presence of regional enteritis.
Monitor laboratory studies, e.g., electrolytes (especially potassium, magnesium) and ABGs (acid-base balance).	Determines replacement needs and effectiveness of therapy.
Administer medications as indicated:	
Antidiarrheal (Refer to ND: Diarrhea, p. 354.);	Reduces fluid losses from intestines.
Antiemetics, e.g., trimethobenzamide (Tigan), hydroxyzine (Vistaril), prochlorperazine (Compazine);	Used to control nausea/vomiting in acute exacerbations.

ACTIONS/INTERVENTIONS

Collaborative

Antipyretics, e.g., acetaminophen (Tylenol);

Electrolytes, e.g., potassium supplement (KCl-IV; K-lyte, Slow-K);

Vitamin K (Mephyton).

RATIONALE

Controls fever, reducing insensible losses.

Electrolytes are lost in large amounts, especially in bowel with denuded, ulcerated areas, and diarrhea can also lead to metabolic acidosis through loss of bicarbonate (HCO_3).

Stimulates hepatic formation of prothrombin, stabilizing coagulation and reducing risk of hemorrhage.

NURSING DIAGNOSIS: Nutrition: altered, less than body requirements

May be related to
Altered absorption of nutrients
Hypermetabolic state
Medically restricted intake; fear that eating may cause diarrhea

Possibly evidenced by
Weight loss; decreased subcutaneous fat/muscle mass; poor muscle tone
Hyperactive bowel sounds; steatorrhea
Pale conjunctiva and mucous membranes
Aversion to eating

DESIRED OUTCOMES/EVALUATION CRITERIA—PATIENT WILL:

Nutritional Status (NOC)

Demonstrate stable weight or progressive gain toward goal with normalization of laboratory values and absence of signs of malnutrition.

ACTIONS/INTERVENTIONS

Nutrition Therapy (NIC)

Independent

Weigh daily.

Encourage bedrest and/or limited activity during acute phase of illness.

Recommend rest before meals.

Provide oral hygiene.

Serve foods in well-ventilated, pleasant surroundings, with unhurried atmosphere, congenial company.

Limit foods that might cause/exacerbate abdominal cramping, flatulence (e.g., milk products, foods high in fiber or fat).

Record intake and changes in symptomatology.

Promote patient participation in dietary planning as possible.

RATIONALE

Provides information about dietary needs/effectiveness of therapy.

Decreasing metabolic needs aids in preventing caloric depletion and conserves energy.

Quiets peristalsis and increases available energy for eating.

A clean mouth can enhance the taste of food.

Pleasant environment aids in reducing stress and is more conducive to eating.

Individual tolerance varies, depending on stage of disease and area of bowel affected.

Useful in identifying specific deficiencies and determining GI response to foods.

Provides sense of control for patient and opportunity to select foods desired/enjoyed, which may increase intake.

ACTIONS/INTERVENTIONS	RATIONALE

Independent

Encourage patient to verbalize feelings concerning resumption of diet.

Hesitation to eat may be result of fear that food will cause exacerbation of symptoms.

Collaborative

Keep patient NPO as indicated.

Resting the bowel decreases peristalsis and diarrhea, limiting malabsorption/loss of nutrients.

Resume/advance diet as indicated, e.g., clear liquids progressing to bland, low residue; then high-protein, high-calorie, caffeine-free, nonspicy, and low-fiber as indicated.

Allows the intestinal tract to readjust to the digestive process. Protein is necessary for tissue healing integrity. Low bulk decreases peristaltic response to meal. *Note:* Dietary measures depend on patient's condition, e.g., if disease is mild the patient may do well on low-residue, low-fat diet high in protein and calories with lactose restriction. In moderate disease, elemental enteral products may be given to provide nutrition without overstimulating the bowel. The patient with toxic colitis is NPO and placed on parenteral nutrition.

Provide nutritional support, e.g.,

Enteral feedings, e.g., Ultra Clear Plus via NG, percutaneous endoscopic gastrostomy (PEG), or J-tube;

Many clinical studies have shown early enteral feeding is beneficial in reducing the effects of malabsorption and providing essential nutrients. Although elemental enteral solutions cannot provide all needed nutrients, they can prevent gut atrophy.

Intravenous TPN.

This regimen rests the GI tract completely while providing essential nutrients. Short-term TPN is indicated during periods of disease exacerbation when bowel rest is needed.

Administer medications as indicated, e.g.:

belladonna alkaloids (Donnatal), butabarbital sodium with belladonna (Butibel); propantheline bromide (Pro-Banthine);

Anticholinergics given 15–30 min before eating provide relief from cramping pain and diarrhea, decreasing gastric motility and enhancing time for absorption of nutrients.

Iron (Imferon injectable);

Prevents/treats anemia. Oral route for iron supplement is ineffective because of intestinal alterations that severely reduce absorption.

Vitamin B_{12} (Crystimin, Rubesol);

Malabsorption of B_{12} results from significant loss of functional ileum. Replacement of B_{12} reverses bone marrow depression caused by prolonged inflammatory process, promoting RBC production/correction of anemia.

Folic acid (Folvite);

Folate deficiency is common in presence of Crohn's disease because of decreased intake/absorption, effect of drug therapy sulfasalazine (Azulfidine).

Vitamin C (Ascorbicap).

Promotes tissue healing/regeneration.

NURSING DIAGNOSIS: Anxiety [specify level]

May be related to

Physiological factors/sympathetic stimulation (inflammatory process)

Threat to self-concept (perceived or actual)

Threat to/change in health status, socioeconomic status, role functioning, interaction patterns

Possibly evidenced by
Exacerbation of acute stage of disease
Increased tension, distress, apprehension
Expressed concern regarding changes in life
Somatic complaints
Focus on self

DESIRED OUTCOMES/EVALUATION CRITERIA—PATIENT WILL:

Anxiety control (NOC)

Appear relaxed and report anxiety reduced to a manageable level.
Verbalize awareness of feelings of anxiety and healthy ways to deal with them.

ACTIONS/INTERVENTIONS	RATIONALE
Anxiety Reduction (NIC)	
Independent	
Note behavioral clues, e.g., restlessness, irritability, withdrawal, lack of eye contact, demanding behavior.	Indicators of degree of anxiety/stress, e.g., patient may feel out of control at home/work managing personal problems. Stress may develop as a result of physical symptoms of condition and the reaction of others.
Encourage verbalization of feelings. Provide feedback.	Establishes a therapeutic relationship. Assists the patient/SO in identifying problems causing stress. Patient with severe diarrhea may hesitate to ask for help for fear of becoming a burden to the staff.
Acknowledge that the anxiety and problems are similar to those expressed by others. Active-listen patient's concerns.	Validation that feelings are normal can help reduce stress/isolation and belief that "I am the only one."
Provide accurate, concrete information about what is being done, e.g., reason for bedrest, restriction of oral intake, and procedures.	Involving patient in plan of care provides sense of control and helps decrease anxiety.
Provide a calm, restful environment.	Removing patient from outside stressors promotes relaxation; helps reduce anxiety.
Encourage staff/SO to project caring, concerned attitude.	A supportive manner can help the patient feel less stressed, allowing energy to be directed toward healing/recovery.
Help patient identify/initiate positive coping behaviors used in the past.	Successful behaviors can be fostered in dealing with current problems/stress, enhancing patient's sense of self-control.
Assist patient to learn new coping mechanisms, e.g., stress management techniques, organizational skills.	Learning new ways to cope can be helpful in reducing stress and anxiety, enhancing disease control.
Administer medications as indicated:	
Sedatives, e.g., barbiturates, phenobarbital (Luminal); antianxiety agents, e.g., diazepam (Valium).	May be used to reduce anxiety and to facilitate rest, particularly in the patient with UC.
Refer to clinical specialist psychiatric nurse, social services, spiritual advisor.	May require additional assistance in regaining control and coping with acute episodes/exacerbations, as well as learning to deal with the chronicity and consequences of the disease and therapeutic regimen.

ACTIONS/INTERVENTIONS	RATIONALE
Pain Management (NIC)	
Independent	
Encourage patient to report pain.	May try to tolerate pain rather than request analgesics.
Assess reports of abdominal cramping or pain, noting location, duration, intensity (0–10 scale). Investigate and report changes in pain characteristics.	Colicky intermittent pain occurs with Crohn's. Predefecation pain frequently occurs in UC with urgency, which may be severe and continuous. Changes in pain characteristics may indicate spread of disease/developing complications, e.g., bladder fistula, perforation, toxic megacolon.
Note nonverbal cues, e.g., restlessness, reluctance to move, abdominal guarding, withdrawal, and depression. Investigate discrepancies between verbal and nonverbal cues.	Body language/nonverbal cues may be both physiological and psychological, and may be used in conjunction with verbal cues to determine extent/severity of the problem.
Review factors that aggravate or alleviate pain.	May pinpoint precipitating or aggravating factors (such as stressful events, food intolerance) or identify developing complications.
Encourage patient to assume position of comfort, e.g., knees flexed.	Reduces abdominal tension and promotes sense of control.
Provide comfort measures (e.g., back rub, reposition) and diversional activities.	Promotes relaxation, refocuses attention, and may enhance coping abilities.
Cleanse rectal area with mild soap and water/wipes after each stool and provide skin care, e.g., A&D ointment, Sween ointment, karaya gel, Desitin, petroleum jelly.	Protects skin from bowel acids, preventing excoriation.
Provide sitz bath as appropriate.	Enhances cleanliness and comfort in the presence of perianal irritation/fissures.
Observe for ischiorectal and perianal fistulas.	Fistulas may develop from erosion and weakening of intestinal bowel wall.
Observe/record abdominal distension, increased temperature, decreased BP.	May indicate developing intestinal obstruction from inflammation, edema, and scarring.

ACTIONS/INTERVENTIONS	RATIONALE

Collaborative

Implement prescribed dietary modifications, e.g., commence with liquids and increase to solid foods as tolerated.	Complete bowel rest can reduce pain, cramping.
Administer medications as indicated, e.g. :	
Analgesics;	Pain varies from mild to severe and necessitates management to facilitate adequate rest and recovery. *Note:* Opiates should be used with caution because they may precipitate toxic megacolon.
Anticholinergics;	Relieve spasms of GI tract and resultant colicky pain.
Anodyne suppositories.	Relax rectal muscle, decreasing painful spasms.

NURSING DIAGNOSIS: Coping, Individual, ineffective

May be related to
Multiple stressors, repeated over period of time; situational crisis
Unpredictable nature of disease process
Personal vulnerability; inadequate coping method; lack of support systems
Severe pain
Lack of sleep, rest

Possibly evidenced by
Verbalization of inability to cope, discouragement, anxiety
Preoccupation with physical self, chronic worry, emotional tension, poor self-esteem
Depression and dependency

DESIRED OUTCOMES/EVALUATION CRITERIA—PATIENT WILL:

Coping (NOC)

Assess the current situation accurately.
Identify ineffective coping behaviors and consequences.
Acknowledge own coping abilities.
Demonstrate necessary lifestyle changes to limit/prevent recurrent episodes.

ACTIONS/INTERVENTIONS	RATIONALE

Coping Enhancement (NIC)

Independent

Assess patient's/SO's understanding and previous methods of dealing with disease process.	Enables the nurse to deal more realistically with current problems. Anxiety and other problems may have interfered with previous health teaching/patient learning.
Determine outside stressors, e.g., family, relationships, social or work environment.	Stress can alter autonomic nervous response, affecting the immune system and contributing to exacerbation of disease. Even the goal of independence in the dependent patient can be an added stressor.
Provide opportunity for patient to discuss how illness has affected relationship, including sexual concerns.	Stressors of illness affect all areas of life and patient may have difficulty coping with feelings of fatigue/pain in relation to relationship/sexual needs.

ACTIONS/INTERVENTIONS	RATIONALE
Collaborative	
Help patient identify individually effective coping skills.	Use of previously successful behaviors can help patient deal with current situation/plan for future.
Provide emotional support:	
Active-listen in a nonjudgmental manner;	Aids in communication and understanding the patient's viewpoint. Adds to patient's feelings of self-worth.
Maintain nonjudgmental body language when caring for patient;	Prevents reinforcing patient's feelings of being a burden, e.g., frequent need to empty bedpan/commode.
Assign same staff as much as possible.	Provides a more therapeutic environment and lessens the stress of constant adjustments.
Provide uninterrupted sleep/rest periods.	Exhaustion brought on by the disease tends to magnify problems, interfering with ability to cope.
Encourage use of stress management skills, e.g., relaxation techniques, visualization, guided imagery, deep-breathing exercises.	Refocuses attention, promotes relaxation, and enhances coping abilities.
Collaborative	
Include patient/SO in team conferences to develop individualized program	Promotes continuity of care and enables patient/SO to feel a part of the plan, imparting a sense of control and increasing cooperation with therapeutic regimen.
Administer medications as indicated: antipsychotics, e.g., thioridazine (Mellaril); antianxiety agents, e.g., lorazepam (Ativan), alprazolam (Xanax).	Aids in psychological/physical rest. Conserves energy and may strengthen coping abilities.
Refer to resources as indicated, e.g., local support group, social worker, psychiatric nurse, spiritual advisor.	Additional support and counseling can assist patient/SO in dealing with specific stress/problem areas.

NURSING DIAGNOSIS: Knowledge Deficit [Learning Need] regarding condition, prognosis, treatment, self care, and discharge needs

May be related to
Information misinterpretation, lack of recall
Unfamiliarity with resources

Possibly evidenced by
Questions, request for information, statements of misconceptions
Inaccurate follow-through of instructions
Development of preventable complications/exacerbations

DESIRED OUTCOMES/EVALUATION CRITERIA—PATIENT WILL:

Knowledge: Disease Process (NOC)

Verbalize understanding of disease processes, possible complications.
Identify stress situations and specific action(s) to deal with them.

Knowledge: Treatment Regimen (NOC)

Verbalize understanding of therapeutic regimen.
Participate in treatment regimen.
Initiate necessary lifestyle changes.

Teaching: Disease Process (NIC)

Independent

ACTIONS/INTERVENTIONS	RATIONALE
Determine patient's perception of disease process.	Establishes knowledge base and provides some insight into individual learning needs.
Review disease process, cause/effect relationship of factors that precipitate symptoms and identify ways to reduce contributing factors. Encourage questions.	Precipitating/aggravating factors are individual; therefore, the patient needs to be aware of what foods, fluids, and lifestyle factors can precipitate symptoms. Accurate knowledge base provides opportunity for patient to make informed decisions/choices about future and control of chronic disease. Although most patients know about their own disease process, they may have outdated information or misconceptions.
Review medications, purpose, frequency, dosage, and possible side effects.	Promotes understanding and may enhance cooperation with regimen.
Remind patient to observe for side effects if steroids are given on a long-term basis, e.g., ulcers, facial edema, muscle weakness.	Steroids may be used to control inflammation and to effect a remission of the disease; however, drug may lower resistance to infection and cause fluid retention.
Stress importance of good skin care, e.g., proper handwashing techniques and perineal skin care.	Reduces spread of bacteria and risk of skin irritation/breakdown, infection.
Recommend cessation of smoking.	Can increase intestinal motility, aggravating symptoms.
Emphasize need for long-term follow-up and periodic re-evaluation.	Patients with IBD are at increased risk for colon/rectal cancer, and regular diagnostic evaluations may be required.
Identify appropriate community resources, e.g., Crohn's and Colitis Foundation of America, Inc. (CCFA); Ostomy Association; home healthcare providers/visiting nurse services; dietitian; and social services.	Patient may benefit from the services of these agencies in coping with chronicity of the disease and evaluating treatment options.

POTENTIAL CONSIDERATIONS following acute hospitalization (dependent on patient's age, physical condition/presence of complications, personal resources, and life responsibilities)

Pain [acute]—hyperperistalsis, prolonged diarrhea, skin/tissue irritation, perirectal excoriation, fissures, fistulas.

Coping, Individual, ineffective—multiple stressors, repeated over period of time; unpredictable nature of disease process; personal vulnerability; severe pain, situational crisis.

Infection, risk for—traumatized tissue, change in pH of secretions, altered peristalsis, suppressed inflammatory response, chronic disease, malnutrition.

Therapeutic Regimen: Individual, ineffective management—complexity of therapeutic regimen, perceived benefit, powerlessness.

FECAL DIVERSIONS: POSTOPERATIVE CARE OF ILEOSTOMY AND COLOSTOMY

Within the past 50 years major advances have occurred in ostomy surgery, including continent diversions such as the Kock pouch and the ileoanal reservoir. However, each year in the United States, 100,000 people still undergo surgery to create ostomies. These so-called "incontinent diversions" are the primary focus of this plan of care.

An *ileostomy* is an opening constructed in the terminal ileum to treat regional and ulcerative colitis and to divert intestinal contents in colon cancer, polyps, and trauma. It is usually done when the entire colon, rectum, and anus must be removed, in which case the ileostomy is permanent. A temporary ileostomy is done to provide complete bowel rest in conditions such as chronic colitis and in some trauma cases.

A *colostomy* is a diversion of the effluent of the colon and may be temporary or permanent. Ascending, transverse, and sigmoid colostomies may be performed. Transverse colostomy is usually temporary. A sigmoid colostomy is the most common permanent stoma, usually performed for cancer.

CARE SETTING

Inpatient acute care surgical unit.

RELATED CONCERNS

Cancer, page 900
Fluid and electrolyte imbalances, page 926
Inflammatory bowel disease: ulcerative colitis, regional enteritis, page 350
Psychosocial aspects of care, page 809
Surgical interventions, page 828
Total nutritional support: parenteral/enteral feeding, page 508

Patient Assessment Database

Data depends on the underlying problem, duration, and severity (e.g., obstruction, perforation, inflammation, congenital defects).

TEACHING/LEARNING

Discharge plan considerations: **DRG projected mean length of inpatient stay: 9.4 days**
Assistance with dietary concerns, management of ostomy, and acquisition of supplies may be required

Refer to section at end of plan for postdischarge considerations.

NURSING PRIORITIES

1. Assist patient/SO in psychosocial adjustment.
2. Prevent complications.
3. Support independence in self-care.
4. Provide information about procedure/prognosis, treatment needs, potential complications, and community resources.

DISCHARGE GOALS

1. Adjusting to perceived/actual changes.
2. Complications prevented/minimized.
3. Self-care needs met by self/with assistance depending on specific situation.
4. Procedure/prognosis, therapeutic regimen, potential complications understood and sources of support identified.
5. Plan in place to meet needs after discharge.

NURSING DIAGNOSIS: Skin Integrity, risk for impaired

Risk factors may include
Absence of sphincter at stoma
Character/flow of effluent and flatus from stoma
Reaction to product/chemicals; improper fitting of appliance or removal of adhesive

Possibly evidenced by

[Not applicable; presence of signs and symptoms establishes an *actual* diagnosis]

DESIRED OUTCOMES/EVALUATION CRITERIA—PATIENT WILL:

> **Bowel Elimination (NOC)**

Maintain skin integrity around stoma.
Identify individual risk factors.
Demonstrate behaviors/techniques to promote healing/prevent skin breakdown.

ACTIONS/INTERVENTIONS	RATIONALE

> **Ostomy Care (NIC)**

Independent

Inspect stoma/peristomal skin area with each pouch change. Note irritation, bruises (dark, bluish color), rashes.	Monitors healing process/effectiveness of appliances and identifies areas of concern, need for further evaluation/intervention. Early identification of stomal necrosis/ischemia or fungal infection (from changes in normal bowel flora) provides for timely interventions to prevent serious complications. Stoma should be red and moist. Ulcerated areas on stoma may be from a pouch opening that is too small or a faceplate that cuts into stoma. In patients with an ileostomy, the effluent is rich in enzymes, increasing the likelihood of skin irritation. In the patient with a colostomy, skin care is not as great a concern because the enzymes are no longer present in the effluent.
Clean with warm water and pat dry. Use soap only if area is covered with sticky stool.	Maintaining a clean/dry area helps prevent skin breakdown.
Measure stoma periodically, e.g., at least weekly for first 6 wk, then once a month for 6 mo. Measure both width and length of stoma.	As postoperative edema resolves (during first 6 wk) the stoma shrinks and size of appliance must be altered to ensure proper fit so that effluent is collected as it flows from the ostomy and contact with the skin is prevented.
Verify that opening on adhesive backing of pouch is at least ⅛ in larger than the base of the stoma, with adequate adhesiveness left to apply pouch.	Prevents trauma to the stoma tissue and protects the peristomal skin. Adequate adhesive area is important to maintain a satisfactory seal. *Note:* Too tight a fit may cause stomal edema or stenosis.
Use a transparent, odor-proof drainable pouch.	A transparent appliance during first 4–6 wk allows easy observation of stoma without necessity of removing pouch/irritating skin.
Apply appropriate skin barrier, e.g., hydrocolloid wafer, karaya gum, Durahesive skin barrier, or similar products.	Protects skin from pouch adhesive, enhances adhesiveness of pouch, and facilitates removal of pouch when necessary. *Note:* Sigmoid colostomy may not require use of a skin barrier once stool becomes formed and elimination is regulated through irrigation.
Empty, irrigate, and cleanse ostomy pouch on a routine basis, using appropriate equipment.	Frequent pouch changes are irritating to the skin and should be avoided. Emptying and rinsing the pouch with the proper solution not only removes bacteria and odor-causing stool and flatus but also deodorizes the pouch.

ACTIONS/INTERVENTIONS

Independent

Support surrounding skin when gently removing appliance. Apply adhesive removers as indicated, then wash thoroughly.

Investigate reports of burning/itching/blistering around stoma.

Evaluate adhesive product and appliance fit on ongoing basis.

Collaborative

Consult with enterostomal therapist/nurse.

Apply corticosteroid aerosol spray and nystatin powder as indicated.

RATIONALE

Prevents tissue irritation/destruction associated with "pulling" pouch off.

Indicative of effluent leakage with peristomal irritation, or possibly *Candida* infection, requiring intervention.

Provides opportunity for problem solving. Determines need for further intervention.

Helpful in choosing products appropriate for patient's particular rehabilitation needs, including type of ostomy, physical/mental status, abilities to handle self-care, and financial resources.

Assists in healing if peristomal irritation persists/fungal infection develops. *Note:* These products can have potent side effects and should be used sparingly.

NURSING DIAGNOSIS: Body Image disturbance

May be related to
Biophysical: presence of stoma; loss of control of bowel elimination
Psychosocial: altered body structure
Disease process and associated treatment regimen, e.g., cancer, colitis

Possibly evidenced by
Verbalization of change in body image, fear of rejection/reaction of others, and negative feelings about body
Actual change in structure and/or function (ostomy)
Not touching/looking at stoma, refusal to participate in care

DESIRED OUTCOMES/EVALUATION CRITERIA—PATIENT WILL:

Body Image (NOC)

Verbalize acceptance of self in situation, incorporating change into self-concept without negating self-esteem.
Demonstrate beginning acceptance by viewing/touching stoma and participating in self-care.
Verbalize feelings about stoma/illness; begin to deal constructively with situation.

ACTIONS/INTERVENTIONS

Body Image Enhancement (NIC)

Independent

Ascertain whether support and counseling were initiated when the possibility and/or necessity of ostomy was first discussed.

Encourage patient/SO to verbalize feelings regarding the ostomy. Acknowledge normality of feelings of anger, depression, and grief over loss. Discuss daily "ups and downs" that can occur.

RATIONALE

Provides information about patient's/SO's level of knowledge and anxiety about individual situation.

Helps the patient realize that feelings are not unusual and that feeling guilty about them is not necessary/helpful. Patient needs to recognize feelings before they can be dealt with effectively.

ACTIONS/INTERVENTIONS	RATIONALE
Independent	
Review reason for surgery and future expectations.	Patient may find it easier to accept/deal with an ostomy done to correct chronic/long-term disease than for traumatic injury, even if ostomy is only temporary. Also, the patient who will be undergoing a second procedure (to convert ostomy to a continent or anal reservoir) may possibly encounter less severe self-image problems because body function eventually will be "more normal."
Note behaviors of withdrawal, increased dependency, manipulation, or noninvolvement in care.	Suggestive of problems in adjustment that may require further evaluation and more extensive therapy.
Provide opportunities for patient/SO to view and touch stoma, using the moment to point out positive signs of healing, normal appearance, and so forth. Remind patient that it will take time to adjust, both physically and emotionally.	Although integration of stoma into body image can take months or even years, looking at the stoma and hearing comments (made in a normal, matter-of-fact manner) can help patient with this acceptance. Touching stoma reassures patient/SO that it is not fragile and that slight movements of stoma actually reflect normal peristalsis.
Provide opportunity for patient to deal with ostomy through participation in self-care.	Independence in self-care helps improve self-confidence and acceptance of situation.
Plan/schedule care activities with patient.	Promotes sense of control and gives message that patient can handle situation, enhancing self-concept.
Maintain positive approach during care activities, avoiding expressions of disdain or revulsion. Do not take angry expressions of patient/SO personally.	Assists patient/SO to accept body changes and feel all right about self. Anger is most often directed at the situation and lack of control individual has over what has happened (powerlessness), not with the individual caregiver.
Ascertain patient's desire to visit with a person with an ostomy. Make arrangements for visit, if desired.	A person who is living with an ostomy can be a good support system/role model. Helps reinforce teaching (shared experiences) and facilitates acceptance of change as patient realizes "life does go on" and can be relatively normal.

NURSING DIAGNOSIS: Pain [acute]

May be related to
Physical factors: e.g., disruption of skin/tissues (incisions/drains)
Biological: activity of disease process (cancer, trauma)
Psychological factors: e.g., fear, anxiety

Possibly evidenced by
Reports of pain, self-focusing
Guarding/distraction behaviors, restlessness
Autonomic responses, e.g., changes in vital signs

DESIRED OUTCOMES/EVALUATION CRITERIA—PATIENT WILL:

Pain Level (NOC)

Verbalize that pain is relieved/controlled.
Display relief of pain, able to sleep/rest appropriately.

Pain Control Behavior (NOC)

Demonstrate use of relaxation skills and general comfort measures as indicated for individual situation.

ACTIONS/INTERVENTIONS	RATIONALE

Pain Management (NIC)

Independent

Assess pain, noting location, characteristics, intensity (0–10 scale).	Helps evaluate degree of discomfort and effectiveness of analgesia or may reveal developing complications. Because abdominal pain usually subsides gradually by the third or fourth postoperative day, continued or increasing pain may reflect delayed healing or peristomal skin irritation. *Note:* Pain in anal area associated with abdominal-perineal resection may persist for months.
Encourage patient to verbalize concerns. Active-listen these concerns, and provide support by acceptance, remaining with patient, and giving appropriate information.	Reduction of anxiety/fear can promote relaxation/comfort.
Provide comfort measures, e.g., mouth care, back rub, repositioning (use proper support measures as needed). Assure patient that position change will not injure stoma.	Prevents drying of oral mucosa and associated discomfort. Reduces muscle tension, promotes relaxation, and may enhance coping abilities.
Encourage use of relaxation techniques, e.g., guided imagery, visualization. Provide diversional activities.	Helps patient rest more effectively and refocuses attention, thereby reducing pain and discomfort.
Assist with ROM exercises and encourage early ambulation. Avoid prolonged sitting position.	Reduces muscle/joint stiffness. Ambulation returns organs to normal position and promotes return of usual level of functioning. *Note:* Presence of edema, packing, and drains (if perineal resection has been done) increases discomfort and creates a sense of needing to defecate. Ambulation and frequent position changes reduce perineal pressure.
Investigate and report abdominal muscle rigidity, involuntary guarding, and rebound tenderness.	Suggestive of peritoneal inflammation, which requires prompt medical intervention.
Administer medication as indicated, e.g., narcotics, analgesics, patient-controlled analgesia (PCA).	Relieves pain, enhances comfort, and promotes rest. PCA may be more beneficial, especially following anal-perineal repair.
Provide sitz baths.	Relieves local discomfort, reduces edema, and promotes healing of perineal wound.
Apply/monitor effects of transcutaneous electrical nerve stimulator (TENS) unit.	Cutaneous stimulation may be used to block transmission of pain stimulus.

NURSING DIAGNOSIS: Skin/Tissue Integrity, impaired

May be related to
Invasion of body structure (e.g., perineal resection)
Stasis of secretions/drainage
Altered circulation, edema; malnutrition

Possibly evidenced by
Disruption of skin/tissue: presence of incision and sutures, drains

DESIRED OUTCOMES/EVALUATION CRITERIA—PATIENT WILL:

Wound Healing: Primary Intention (NOC)

Achieve timely wound healing free of signs of infection.

ACTIONS/INTERVENTIONS

Wound Care (NIC)

Independent

Observe wounds, note characteristics of drainage.

Change dressings as needed using aseptic technique.

Encourage side-lying position with head elevated. Avoid prolonged sitting.

Collaborative

Irrigate wound as indicated, using normal saline (NS), diluted hydrogen peroxide, or antibiotic solution.

Provide sitz baths.

RATIONALE

Postoperative hemorrhage is most likely to occur during first 48 hr, whereas infection may develop at any time. Depending on type of wound closure (e.g., first or second intention), complete healing may take 6–8 mo.

Large amounts of serous drainage require that dressings be changed frequently to reduce skin irritation and potential for infection.

Promotes drainage from perineal wound/drains, reducing risk of pooling. Prolonged sitting increases perineal pressure, reducing circulation to wound, and may delay healing.

May be required to treat preoperative inflammation/infection or intraoperative contamination.

Promotes cleanliness and facilitates healing, especially after packing is removed (usually day 3–5).

NURSING DIAGNOSIS: Fluid Volume risk for deficit

Risk factors may include

Excessive losses through normal routes, e.g., preoperative emesis and diarrhea; high-volume ileostomy output

Losses through abnormal routes, e.g., NG/intestinal tube, perineal wound drainage tubes

Medically restricted intake

Altered absorption of fluid, e.g., loss of colon function

Hypermetabolic states, e.g., inflammation, healing process

Possibly evidenced by

[Not applicable; presence of signs and symptoms establishes an *actual* diagnosis]

DESIRED OUTCOMES/EVALUATION CRITERIA—PATIENT WILL:

Hydration (NOC)

Maintain adequate hydration as evidenced by moist mucous membranes, good skin turgor and capillary refill, stable vital signs, and individually appropriate urinary output.

ACTIONS/INTERVENTIONS

Fluid/Electrolyte Management (NIC)

Independent

Monitor intake and output (I&O) carefully, measure liquid stool. Weigh regularly.

RATIONALE

Provides direct indicators of fluid balance. Greatest fluid losses occur with ileostomy, but they generally do not exceed 500–800 mL/day.

ACTIONS/INTERVENTIONS

RATIONALE

Independent

Monitor vital signs, noting postural hypotension, tachycardia. Evaluate skin turgor, capillary refill, and mucous membranes.

Reflects hydration status/possible need for increased fluid replacement.

Limit intake of ice chips during period of gastric intubation.

Ice chips can stimulate gastric secretions and wash out electrolytes.

Collaborative

Monitor laboratory results, e.g., Hct and electrolytes.

Detects homeostasis or imbalance and aids in determining replacement needs.

Administer IV fluid and electrolytes as indicated.

May be necessary to maintain adequate tissue perfusion/organ function.

NURSING DIAGNOSIS: Nutrition: altered, risk for less than body requirements

Risk factors may include
Prolonged anorexia/altered intake preoperatively
Hypermetabolic state (preoperative inflammatory disease; healing process)
Presence of diarrhea/altered absorption
Restriction of bulk and residue-containing foods

Possibly evidenced by
[Not applicable; presence of signs and symptoms establishes an *actual* diagnosis]

DESIRED OUTCOMES/EVALUATION CRITERIA—PATIENT WILL:

Nutritional Status (NOC)

Maintain weight/demonstrate progressive weight gain toward goal with normalization of laboratory values and be free of signs of malnutrition.
Plan diet to meet nutritional needs/limit GI disturbances.

ACTIONS/INTERVENTIONS

RATIONALE

Nutrition Therapy (NIC)

Independent

Obtain a thorough nutritional assessment.

Identifies deficiencies/needs to aid in choice of interventions.

Auscultate bowel sounds.

Return of intestinal function indicates readiness to resume oral intake.

Resume solid foods slowly.

Reduces incidence of abdominal cramps, nausea.

Identify odor-causing foods (e.g., cabbage, fish, beans) and temporarily restrict from diet. Gradually reintroduce one food at a time.

Sensitivity to certain foods is not uncommon following intestinal surgery. Patient can experiment with food several times before determining whether it is creating a problem.

Recommend patient increase use of yogurt, buttermilk, and acidophilus preparations.

May help prevent gas and decrease odor formation.

Suggest patient with ileostomy limit prunes, dates, stewed apricots, strawberries, grapes, bananas, cabbage family, beans, and avoid foods high in cellulose, e.g., peanuts.

These products increase ileal effluent. Digestion of cellulose requires colon bacteria that are no longer present.

ACTIONS/INTERVENTIONS

Independent

Discuss mechanics of swallowed air as a factor in the formation of flatus and some ways the patient can exercise control.

Collaborative

Consult with dietitian.

Advance diet from liquids to low-residue food when oral intake is resumed.

Administer enteral/parenteral feedings when indicated.

RATIONALE

Drinking through a straw, snoring, anxiety, smoking, ill-fitting dentures, and gulping down food increase the production of flatus. Too much flatus not only necessitates frequent emptying, but also can cause leakage from too much pressure within the pouch.

Helpful in assessing patient's nutritional needs in light of changes in digestion and intestinal function, including absorption of vitamins/minerals.

Low-residue diet may be maintained during first 6–8 wk to provide adequate time for intestinal healing.

In the presence of severe debilitation/intolerance of oral intake, parenteral or enteral feedings may be given to supply needed components for healing and prevention of catabolic state.

NURSING DIAGNOSIS: Sleep Pattern disturbance

May be related to
External factors: necessity of ostomy care, excessive flatus/ostomy effluent
Internal factors: psychological stress, fear of leakage of pouch/injury to stoma

Possibly evidenced by
Verbalizations of interrupted sleep, not feeling well rested
Changes in behavior, e.g., irritability, listlessness/lethargy

DESIRED OUTCOMES/EVALUATION CRITERIA—PATIENT WILL:

Sleep (NOC)

Sleep/rest between disturbances.
Report increased sense of well-being and feeling rested.

ACTIONS/INTERVENTIONS

Sleep Enhancement (NIC)

Independent

Explain necessity to monitor intestinal function in early postoperative period.

Provide adequate pouching system. Empty pouch before retiring and, if necessary, on a preagreed schedule.

Let patient know that stoma will not be injured when sleeping.

Restrict intake of caffeine-containing foods/fluids.

RATIONALE

Patient is more apt to be tolerant of disturbances by staff if he or she understands the reasons for/importance of care.

Excessive flatus/effluent can occur despite interventions. Emptying on a regular schedule minimizes threat of leakage.

Patient will be able to rest better if feeling secure about stoma and ostomy function.

Caffeine may delay patient's falling asleep and interfere with REM (rapid eye movement) sleep, resulting in patient not feeling well rested.

ACTIONS/INTERVENTIONS	RATIONALE

Independent

Support continuation of usual bedtime rituals.

Promotes relaxation and readiness for sleep.

Collaborative

Determine cause of excessive flatus or effluent, e.g., confer with dietitian regarding restriction of foods if diet-related.

Identification of cause enables institution of corrective measures that may promote sleep/rest.

Administer analgesics, sedatives at bedtime as indicated.

Pain can interfere with patient's ability to fall/remain asleep. Timely medication can enhance rest/sleep during initial postoperative period. *Note:* Pain pathways in the brain lie near the sleep center and may contribute to wakefulness.

NURSING DIAGNOSIS: Constipation/Diarrhea, risk for

Risk factors may include
Placement of ostomy in descending or sigmoid colon
Inadequate diet/fluid intake

Possibly evidenced by
[Not applicable; presence of signs and symptoms establishes an *actual* diagnosis]

DESIRED OUTCOMES/EVALUATION CRITERIA—PATIENT WILL:

Bowel Elimination (NOC)

Establish an elimination pattern suitable to physical needs and lifestyle with effluent of appropriate amount and consistency.

ACTIONS/INTERVENTIONS	RATIONALE

Bowel Management (NIC)

Independent

Ascertain patient's previous bowel habits and lifestyle.

Assists in formulation of an timely/effective irrigating schedule for the patient with a colostomy.

Investigate delayed onset/absence of effluent. Auscultate bowel sounds.

Postoperative paralytic/adynamic ileus usually resolves within 48–72 hr, and ileostomy should begin draining within 12–24 hr. Delay may indicate persistent ileus or stomal obstruction, which may occur postoperatively because of edema, improperly fitting pouch (too tight), prolapse, or stenosis of the stoma.

Inform the patient with an ileostomy that initially the effluent is liquid. If constipation occurs, it should be reported to enterostomal nurse or physician.

Although the small intestine eventually begins to take on water-absorbing functions to permit a more semi-solid, pasty discharge, constipation may indicate an obstruction. Absence of stool requires emergency medical attention.

Review dietary pattern and amount/type of fluid intake.

Adequate intake of fiber and roughage provides bulk, and fluid is an important factor in determining the consistency of the stool.

ACTIONS/INTERVENTIONS

Independent

Review physiology of the colon and discuss irrigation management of sigmoid ostomy, if appropriate.

Demonstrate use of irrigation equipment to inject NS per protocol until relief is obtained.

Instruct patient in the use of closed-end pouch or a patch, dressing/Band-Aid when irrigation is successful and the sigmoid colostomy effluent becomes more manageable, with stool expelled every 24 hr.

Involve the patient in care of the ostomy on an increasing basis.

Collaborative

Instruct in use of TENS unit if indicated.

RATIONALE

This knowledge helps the patient understand individual care needs.

Irrigations may be done on a daily basis or before special activities. There are differing views on the use of daily irrigations. Many believe cleaning the bowel on a regular basis is helpful. Others believe that this interferes with normal functioning. Most authorities agree that occasional irrigation is useful for emptying the bowel to avoid leakage when special events are planned.

Enables patient to feel more comfortable socially and is less expensive than regular ostomy pouches.

Rehabilitation can be facilitated by encouraging patient independence and control.

Electrical stimulation has been used in some patients to stimulate peristalsis and relieve postoperative ileus.

NURSING DIAGNOSIS: Sexual Dysfunction, risk for

Risk factors may include
Altered body structure/function; radical resection/treatment procedures
Vulnerability/psychological concern about response of SO
Disruption of sexual response pattern, e.g., erectile difficulty

Possibly evidenced by
[Not applicable; presence of signs and symptoms establishes an *actual* diagnosis]

DESIRED OUTCOMES/EVALUATION CRITERIA—PATIENT WILL:

Role Performance (NOC)

Verbalize understanding of relationship of physical condition to sexual problems.
Identify satisfying/acceptable sexual practices and explore alternate methods.
Resume sexual relationship as appropriate.

ACTIONS/INTERVENTIONS

Sexual Counseling (NIC)

Independent

Determine the patient's/SO's sexual relationship before the disease and/or surgery and whether they anticipate problems related to presence of ostomy.

RATIONALE

Identifies future expectations and desires. Mutilation and loss of privacy/control of a bodily function can affect patient's view of personal sexuality. When coupled with the fear of rejection by SO, the desired level of intimacy can be greatly impaired. Sexual needs are very basic, and the patient will be rehabilitated more successfully when a satisfying sexual relationship is continued/developed as desired.

ACTIONS/INTERVENTIONS	RATIONALE
Independent	
Review with the patient/SO sexual functioning in relation to own situation.	Understanding if nerve damage has altered normal sexual functioning (e.g., erection) helps patient/SO to understand the need for exploring alternate methods of satisfaction.
Reinforce information given by the physician. Encourage questions. Provide additional information as needed.	Reiteration of data previously given assists the patient/SO to hear and process the knowledge again, moving toward acceptance of individual limitations/restrictions and prognosis (e.g., that it may take up to 2 yr to regain potency after a radical procedure or that a penile prosthesis may be necessary).
Discuss likelihood of resumption of sexual activity in approximately 6 wk after discharge, beginning slowly and progressing (e.g., cuddling/caressing until both partners are comfortable with body image/function changes). Include alternate methods of stimulation as appropriate.	Knowing what to expect in progress of recovery helps patient avoid performance anxiety/reduce risk of "failure." If the couple is willing to try new ideas, this can assist with adjustment and may help to achieve sexual fulfillment.
Encourage dialogue between partners. Suggest wearing pouch cover, T-shirt, or shortie nightgown.	Disguising ostomy appliance may aid in reducing feelings of self-consciousness, embarrassment during sexual activity.
Stress awareness of factors that might be distracting (e.g., unpleasant odors and pouch leakage). Encourage use of sense of humor.	Promotes resolution of solvable problems. Laughter can help individuals deal more effectively with difficult situation, promote positive sexual experience.
Problem-solve alternative positions for coitus.	Minimizing awkwardness of appliance and physical discomfort can enhance satisfaction.
Discuss/role-play possible interactions or approaches when dealing with new sexual partners.	Rehearsal is helpful in dealing with actual situations when they arise, preventing self-consciousness about "different" body image.
Provide birth control information as appropriate and stress that impotence does not necessarily mean the patient is sterile.	Confusion may exist that can lead to an unwanted pregnancy.
Collaborative	
Arrange meeting with an ostomy visitor if appropriate.	Sharing of how these problems have been resolved by others can be helpful and reduce sense of isolation.
Refer to counseling/sex therapy as indicated.	If problems persist longer than several months after surgery, a trained therapist may be required to facilitate communication between patient and SO.

NURSING DIAGNOSIS: Knowledge Deficit [Learning Need] regarding condition, prognosis, treatment, self care, and discharge needs

May be related to
Lack of exposure/recall information misinterpretation
Unfamiliarity with information resources

Possibly evidenced by
Questions; statement of misconception/misinformation
Inaccurate follow-through of instruction/performance of ostomy care
Inappropriate or exaggerated behaviors (e.g., hostile, agitated, apathetic, withdrawal)

ACTIONS/INTERVENTIONS	RATIONALE
Learning Facilitation (NIC)	
Independent	
Evaluate patient's emotional, cognitive, and physical capabilities.	These factors affect patient's ability to master care-tasks and willingness to assume responsibility for ostomy care.
Include written/picture learning resources.	Provides references for obtaining support, equipment, and additional information after discharge to support patient efforts for independence in self-care.
Teaching: Disease Process (NIC)	
Review anatomy, physiology, and implications of surgical intervention. Discuss future expectations, including anticipated changes in character of effluent.	Provides knowledge base from which patient can make informed choices and offers an opportunity to clarify misconceptions regarding individual situation. (Temporary ileostomy may be converted to ileoanal reservoir at a future date; ileostomy and ascending colostomy cannot be regulated by diet, irrigations, or medications.)
Instruct patient/SO in stomal care. Allot time for return demonstrations and provide positive feedback for efforts.	Promotes positive management and reduces risk of improper ostomy care/development of complications.
Recommend increased fluid intake during warm weather months.	Loss of normal colon function of conserving water and electrolytes can lead to dehydration and constipation.
Discuss possible need to decrease salt intake.	Salt can increase ileal output, potentiating risk of dehydration and increasing frequency of ostomy care needs/patient's inconvenience.
Identify symptoms of electrolyte depletion, e.g., anorexia, abdominal muscle cramps, feelings of faintness or "cold" in arms/legs; general fatigue/weakness, bloating, decreased sensations in arms/legs.	Loss of colon function altering fluid/electrolyte absorption may result in sodium/potassium deficits requiring dietary correction with foods/fluids high in sodium (e.g., bouillon, Gatorade) or potassium (e.g., orange juice, prunes, tomatoes, bananas, or Gatorade).
Discuss need for periodic evaluation/administration of supplemental vitamins and minerals as appropriate.	Depending on portion and amount of bowel resected, lack of absorption may cause deficiencies.
Stress importance of chewing food well, adequate intake of fluids with/following meals, only moderate use of high-fiber foods, avoidance of cellulose.	Reduces risk of bowel obstruction, especially in patient with ileostomy.

ACTIONS/INTERVENTIONS	RATIONALE
Independent	
Review foods that are/may be a source of flatus (e.g., carbonated drinks, beer, beans, cabbage family, onions, fish, and highly seasoned foods) or odor (e.g., onions, cabbage family, eggs, fish, and beans).	These foods may be restricted or eliminated, based on individual reaction, for better ostomy control, or it may be necessary to empty the pouch more frequently if they are ingested.
Identify foods associated with diarrhea, such as green beans, broccoli, highly seasoned foods.	Promotes better bowel control.
Recommend foods used to manage constipation (e.g., bran, celery, raw fruits) and importance of increased fluid intake.	Proper management can prevent/minimize problems of constipation.
Discuss resumption of presurgery level of activity.	Patient should be able to manage same degree of activity as previously enjoyed and in some cases increase activity level.
Talk about the possibility of sleep disturbance, anorexia, loss of interest in usual activities.	"Homecoming depression" may occur, lasting for months after surgery, requiring patience/support and ongoing evaluation as the patient adjusts to living with a stoma.
Explain necessity of notifying healthcare providers and pharmacists of type of ostomy and avoidance of sustained-release medications.	Presence of ostomy may alter rate/extent of absorption of oral medications and increase risk of drug-related complications, e.g., diarrhea/constipation or peristomal excoriation. Liquid, chewable, or injectable forms of medication are preferred for patients with ileostomy to maximize absorption of drug.
Counsel patient concerning medication use and problems associated with altered bowel function. Refer to pharmacist for teaching/advice as appropriate.	The patient with an ostomy has two key problems: altered disintegration and absorption of oral drugs and unusual or pronounced adverse effects. Some of the medications that these patients may respond to differently include laxatives, salicylates, H_2 receptor antagonists, antibiotics, and diuretics.
Discuss effect of medications on effluent, i.e., changes in color, odor, consistency of stool, and need to observe for drug residue indicating incomplete absorption.	Understanding decreases anxiety regarding intestinal function and enhances independence in self-care.
Stress necessity of close monitoring of chronic health conditions requiring routine oral medications.	Monitoring of clinical symptoms and serum blood levels is indicated because of altered drug absorption requiring periodic dosage adjustments.
Identify community resources, e.g., United Ostomy Association, the Crohn's and Colitis Foundation, Ostomy Rehabilitation Program, local ostomy support group, enterostomal therapist, visiting nurse, pharmacy/medical supply house.	Continued support after discharge is essential to facilitate the recovery process and patient's independence in care. Enterostomal nurse can be very helpful in solving appliance problems, identifying alternatives to meet individual patient needs.

POTENTIAL CONSIDERATIONS following acute hospitalization (dependent on patient's age, physical condition/presence of complications, personal resources, and life responsibilities)

Skin Integrity, risk for impaired—absence of sphincter at stoma, character/flow of effluent and flatus from stoma.

Coping, Individual, ineffective—situational crises, vulnerability.

Social Interaction, impaired—self-concept disturbance, concern for loss of control of bodily functions.

APPENDECTOMY

An inflamed appendix may be removed using a laparoscopic approach with laser. However, the presence of multiple adhesions, retroperitoneal positioning of the appendix, or the likelihood of rupture necessitates an open (traditional) procedure.

Recent studies indicate that laparoscopic appendectomy results in significantly less postoperative pain, earlier resumption of solid foods, a shorter hospital stay, lower wound infection rate, and a faster return to normal activities than open appendectomy.

CARE SETTING

Although many of the interventions included here are appropriate for the short-stay patient, this plan of care addresses the traditional appendectomy care provided on a surgical unit.

RELATED CONCERNS

Peritonitis, page 382
Psychosocial aspects of care, page 809
Surgical intervention, page 828

Patient Assessment Database (Preoperative)

ACTIVITY/REST

May report: Malaise

CIRCULATION

May exhibit: Tachycardia

ELIMINATION

May report: Constipation of recent onset
Diarrhea (occasional)

May exhibit: Abdominal distension, tenderness/rebound tenderness, rigidity
Decreased or absent bowel sounds

FOOD/FLUID

May report: Anorexia
Nausea/vomiting

PAIN/DISCOMFORT

May report: Abdominal pain around the epigastrium and umbilicus, which may have an insidious onset and become increasingly severe. Pain may localize at McBurney's point (halfway between umbilicus and crest of right ileum) and be aggravated by walking, sneezing, coughing, or deep respiration. Increasingly severe, generalized pain or the sudden cessation of severe pain suggests perforation or infarction of the appendix
Varied reports of pain/vague symptoms (due to location of appendix [e.g., retrocecally or next to ureter] or due to onset of peritonitis)

May exhibit: Guarding behavior; lying on side or back with knees flexed; increased right lower quadrant (RLQ) pain with extension of right leg/upright position
Rebound tenderness on left side (suggests peritoneal inflammation)

SAFETY

May exhibit: Fever (usually low-grade)

RESPIRATION

May exhibit: Tachypnea; shallow respirations

TEACHING/LEARNING

May report: History of other conditions associated with abdominal pain, e.g., acute pyelitis, ureteral stone, acute salpingitis, regional ileitis
May occur at any age

377

Discharge plan considerations: DRG projected mean length of inpatient stay: 4.2 days/short stay: 24 hours

May need brief assistance with transportation, homemaker tasks

Refer to section at end of plan for postdischarge considerations.

DIAGNOSTIC STUDIES

WBC: Leukocytosis above 12,000/mm³, neutrophil count often elevated to greater than 75%.

Abdominal x-rays: May reveal hardened bit of fecal material in appendix (fecalith), localized ileus.

Ultrasound or CT scan: May be done for differentiation of appendicitis from other causes of abdominal pain (e.g., perforating ulcer, cholecystitis, reproductive organ infections) or to localize drainable abscesses.

NURSING PRIORITIES

1. Prevent complications.
2. Promote comfort.
3. Provide information about surgical procedure/prognosis, treatment needs, and potential complications.

DISCHARGE GOALS

1. Complications prevented/minimized.
2. Pain alleviated/controlled.
3. Surgical procedure/prognosis, therapeutic regimen, and possible complications understood.
4. Plan in place to meet needs after discharge.

NURSING DIAGNOSIS: Infection, risk for

Risk factors may include

Inadequate primary defenses; perforation/rupture of the appendix; peritonitis; abscess formation

Invasive procedures, surgical incision

Possibly evidenced by

[Not applicable; presence of signs and symptoms establishes an *actual* diagnosis]

DESIRED OUTCOMES/EVALUATION CRITERIA—PATIENT WILL:

Wound Healing: Primary Intention (NOC)

Achieve timely wound healing; free of signs of infection/inflammation, purulent drainage, erythema, and fever.

ACTIONS/INTERVENTIONS	RATIONALE
Infection Control (NIC)	
Independent	
Practice/instruct in good handwashing and aseptic wound care. Encourage/provide pericare.	Reduces risk of spread of bacteria.
Inspect incision and dressings. Note characteristics of drainage from wound/drains (if inserted), presence of erythema.	Provides for early detection of developing infectious process, and/or monitors resolution of preexisting peritonitis.
Monitor vital signs. Note onset of fever, chills, diaphoresis, changes in mentation, reports of increasing abdominal pain.	Suggestive of presence of infection/developing sepsis, abscess, peritonitis.
Obtain drainage specimens if indicated.	Gram stain, culture, and sensitivity are useful in identifying causative organism and choice of therapy.

ACTIONS/INTERVENTIONS	RATIONALE
Collaborative	
Administer antibiotics as appropriate.	Antibiotics given before appendectomy are primarily for prophylaxis of wound infection and are not continued postoperatively. Therapeutic antibiotics are administered if the appendix is ruptured/abscessed or peritonitis has developed.
Prepare for/assist with incision and drainage (I&D) if indicated.	May be necessary to drain contents of localized abscess.

NURSING DIAGNOSIS: Fluid Volume risk for deficit

Risk factors may include
Preoperative vomiting, postoperative restrictions (e.g., NPO)
Hypermetabolic state (e.g., fever, healing process)
Inflammation of peritoneum with sequestration of fluid

Possibly evidenced by
[Not applicable; presence of signs and symptoms establishes an *actual* diagnosis]

DESIRED OUTCOMES/EVALUATION CRITERIA—PATIENT WILL:

Hydration (NOC)

Maintain adequate fluid balance as evidenced by moist mucous membranes, good skin turgor, stable vital signs, and individually adequate urinary output.

ACTIONS/INTERVENTIONS	RATIONALE
Fluid Monitoring (NIC)	
Independent	
Monitor BP and pulse.	Variations help identify fluctuating intravascular volumes.
Inspect mucous membranes; assess skin turgor and capillary refill.	Indicators of adequacy of peripheral circulation and cellular hydration.
Monitor I&O; note urine color/concentration, specific gravity.	Decreasing output of concentrated urine with increasing specific gravity suggests dehydration/need for increased fluids.
Auscultate bowel sounds. Note passing of flatus, bowel movement.	Indicators of return of peristalsis, readiness to begin oral intake. *Note:* This may not occur in the hospital if the patient has had a laparoscopic procedure and been discharged in 23 hr.
Provide clear liquids in small amounts when oral intake is resumed, and progress diet as tolerated.	Reduces risk of gastric irritation/vomiting to minimize fluid loss.
Give frequent mouth care with special attention to protection of the lips.	Dehydration results in drying and painful cracking of the lips and mouth.
Collaborative	
Maintain gastric/intestinal suction, as indicated.	An NG tube may be inserted preoperatively and maintained in immediate postoperative phase to decompress the bowel, promote intestinal rest, prevent vomiting.

ACTIONS/INTERVENTIONS	RATIONALE
Collaborative	
Administer IV fluids and electrolytes.	The peritoneum reacts to irritation/infection by producing large amounts of intestinal fluid possibly reducing the circulating blood volume, resulting in dehydration and relative electrolyte imbalances.

NURSING DIAGNOSIS: Pain [acute]

May be related to
Distention of intestinal tissues by inflammation
Presence of surgical incision

Possibly evidenced by
Reports of pain
Facial grimacing, muscle guarding; distraction behaviors
Autonomic responses

DESIRED OUTCOMES/EVALUATION CRITERIA—PATIENT WILL:

Pain Level (NOC)

Report pain is relieved/controlled.
Appear relaxed, able to sleep/rest appropriately.

ACTIONS/INTERVENTIONS	RATIONALE
Pain Management (NIC)	
Independent	
Assess pain, noting location, characteristics, severity (0–10 scale). Investigate and report changes in pain as appropriate.	Useful in monitoring effectiveness of medication, progression of healing. Changes in characteristics of pain may indicate developing abscess/peritonitis, requiring prompt medical evaluation and intervention.
Provide accurate, honest information to patient/SO.	Being informed about progress of situation provides emotional support, helping to decrease anxiety.
Keep at rest in semi-Fowler's position.	Gravity localizes inflammatory exudate into lower abdomen or pelvis, relieving abdominal tension, which is accentuated by supine position.
Encourage early ambulation.	Promotes normalization of organ function, e.g., stimulates peristalsis and passing of flatus, reducing abdominal discomfort.
Provide diversional activities.	Refocuses attention, promotes relaxation, and may enhance coping abilities.
Collaborative	
Keep NPO/maintain NG suction initially.	Decreases discomfort of early intestinal peristalsis and gastric irritation/vomiting.
Administer analgesics as indicated.	Relief of pain facilitates cooperation with other therapeutic interventions, e.g., ambulation, pulmonary toilet.
Place ice bag on abdomen periodically during initial 24–48 hr, as appropriate.	Soothes and relieves pain through desensitization of nerve endings. *Note:* Do not use heat, because it may cause tissue congestion.

NURSING DIAGNOSIS: Knowledge Deficit [Learning Need] regarding condition, prognosis, treatment, self care, and discharge needs

May be related to
Lack of exposure/recall; information misinterpretation
Unfamiliarity with information resources

Possibly evidenced by
Questions; request for information; verbalization of problem/concerns
Statement of misconception
Inaccurate follow-through of instruction
Development of preventable complications

DESIRED OUTCOMES/EVALUATION CRITERIA—PATIENT WILL:

Knowledge: Disease Process (NOC)

Verbalize understanding of disease process and potential complications.

Knowledge: Treatment Regimen (NOC)

Verbalize understanding of therapeutic needs.
Participate in treatment regimen.

ACTIONS/INTERVENTIONS	RATIONALE
Teaching: Disease Process (NIC)	
Independent	
Identify symptoms requiring medical evaluation, e.g., increasing pain; edema/erythema of wound; presence of drainage, fever.	Prompt intervention reduces risk of serious complications, e.g., delayed wound healing, peritonitis.
Review postoperative activity restrictions, e.g., heavy lifting, exercise, sex, sports, driving.	Provides information for patient to plan for return to usual routines without untoward incidence.
Encourage progressive activities as tolerated with periodic rest periods.	Prevents fatigue, promotes healing and feeling of well-being and facilitates resumption of normal activities.
Recommend use of mild laxative/stool softeners as necessary and avoidance of enemas.	Assists with return to usual bowel function; prevents undue straining for defecation.
Discuss care of incision, including dressing changes, bathing restrictions, and return to physician for suture/staple removal.	Understanding promotes cooperation with therapeutic regimen, enhancing healing and recovery process.

POTENTIAL CONSIDERATIONS following acute hospitalization (dependent on patient's age, physical condition/presence of complications, personal resources, and life responsibilities).

Therapeutic Regimen: Individual, ineffective management—perceived seriousness/susceptibility, perceived benefit, demands made on individual (family, work).

PERITONITIS

Inflammation of the peritoneal cavity, caused by either bacteria or chemicals, can be primary or secondary, and acute or chronic. *Primary peritonitis* is a rare condition in which the peritoneum is infected via the blood/lymphatic circulation. Secondary sources of inflammation are the GI tract, ovaries/uterus, urinary system, traumatic injuries, or surgical contaminants. Surgical intervention may be curative in localized peritonitis, as occurs with appendicitis/appendectomy, ulcer plication, and bowel resection. If peritonitis is diffuse, medical management is necessary before or in place of surgical treatment.

CARE SETTING

Inpatient acute medical or surgical unit

RELATED CONCERNS

Appendectomy, page 377
Inflammatory bowel disease, page 350
Pancreatitis, page 498
Renal dialysis: peritoneal, page 612
Psychosocial aspects of care, page 809
Sepsis/septicemia, page 741
Surgical intervention, page 828
Total nutritional support: parenteral/enteral feeding, page 508
Upper gastrointestinal/esophageal bleeding, page 333

Patient Assessment Database

ACTIVITY/REST

May report:	Weakness
May exhibit:	Difficulty ambulating

CIRCULATION

May exhibit:	Tachycardia, diaphoresis, pallor, hypotension (signs of shock)
	Tissue edema

ELIMINATION

May report:	Inability to pass stool or flatus
	Diarrhea (occasionally)
May exhibit:	Hiccups; abdominal distension; quiet abdomen
	Decreased urinary output, dark color
	Decreased/absent bowel sounds (ileus); intermittent loud, rushing bowel sounds (obstruction); abdominal rigidity, distension, rebound tenderness; hyperresonance/tympany (ileus); loss of dullness over liver (free air in abdomen)

FOOD/FLUID

May report:	Anorexia, nausea/vomiting, thirst
May exhibit:	Projectile vomiting
	Dry mucous membranes, swollen tongue, poor skin turgor

PAIN/DISCOMFORT

May report:	Sudden, severe abdominal pain, generalized or localized, referred to shoulder, intensified by movement
May exhibit:	Distention, rigidity, rebound tenderness; distraction behaviors; restlessness; self-focus
	Muscle guarding (abdomen); flexion of knees

RESPIRATION

May exhibit:	Shallow respirations, tachypnea

SAFETY

May report: Fever, chills

SEXUALITY

May report: History of pelvic organ inflammation (salpingitis), puerperal infection, septic abortion, retroperitoneal abscess

TEACHING/LEARNING

May report: History of recent trauma with abdominal penetration, e.g., gunshot/stab wound or blunt trauma to the abdomen; bladder perforation/ruptured gall bladder, perforated carcinoma of the stomach, perforated gastric/duodenal ulcer, gangrenous obstruction of the bowel, perforation of diverticulum, UC, regional ileitis; strangulated hernia

Discharge plan considerations: **DRG projected length of inpatient stay: 4.9 days**
Assistance with homemaker/maintenance tasks

Refer to section at end of plan for postdischarge considerations.

DIAGNOSTIC STUDIES

CBC: WBCs elevated, sometimes greater than 20,000. RBC count may be increased, indicating hemoconcentration.
Serum protein/albumin: May be decreased because of fluid shifts.
Serum amylase: Usually elevated.
Serum electrolytes: Hypokalemia may be present.
ABGs: Respiratory alkalosis and metabolic acidosis may be noted.
Cultures: Causative organism (often *Escherichia coli,* streptococci, staphylococcus, or rarely, pneumococcus) may be identified from blood, exudate/secretions of ascetic fluid.
Abdominal x-ray: May reveal gas distension of bowel/ileus. If a perforated viscera is the cause, free air will be found in the abdomen.
Chest x-ray: May reveal elevation of diaphragm.
Paracentesis: Peritoneal fluid samples may contain blood, pus/exudate, amylase, bile, and creatine.

NURSING PRIORITIES

1. Control infection.
2. Restore/maintain circulating volume.
3. Promote comfort.
4. Maintain nutrition.
5. Provide information about disease process, possible complications, and treatment needs.

DISCHARGE GOALS

1. Infection resolved.
2. Complications presented/minimized.
3. Pain relieved.
4. Disease process, potential complications, and therapeutic regimen understood.
5. Plan in place to meet needs after discharge.

Nursing diagnosis: Infection, risk for (septicemia)

Risk factors may include:
Inadequate primary defenses (broken skin, traumatized tissue, altered peristalsis)
Inadequate secondary defenses (immunosuppression)
Invasive procedures

Possibly evidenced by:
[Not applicable; presence of signs and symptoms establishes an *actual* diagnosis]

ACTIONS/INTERVENTIONS	RATIONALE
Infection control (NIC)	
Independent	
Note individual risk factors, e.g., abdominal trauma, acute appendicitis, peritoneal dialysis.	Influences choice of interventions.
Assess vital signs frequently, noting unresolved or progressing hypotension, decreased pulse pressure, tachycardia, fever, tachypnea.	Signs of impending septic shock. Circulating endotoxins eventually produce vasodilation, shift of fluid from circulation, and a low cardiac output state.
Note changes in mental status (e.g., confusion, stupor).	Hypoxemia, hypotension, and acidosis can cause deteriorating mental status.
Note skin color, temperature, moisture.	Warm, flushed, dry skin is early sign of septicemia. Later manifestations include cool, clammy, pale skin and cyanosis as shock becomes refractory.
Monitor urine output.	Oliguria develops as a result of decreased renal perfusion, circulating toxins, effects of antibiotics.
Maintain strict aseptic technique in care of abdominal drains, incisions/open wounds, dressings, and invasive sites. Cleanse with appropriate solution.	Prevents access or limits spread of infecting organisms/cross-contamination.
Perform/model good handwashing technique. Monitor staff/patient compliance.	Reduces risk of cross-contamination/spread of infection.
Observe drainage from wounds/drains.	Provides information about status of infection.
Maintain sterile technique when catheterizing patient, and provide catheter care/encourage perineal cleansing on a routine basis.	Prevents access, limits bacterial growth in urinary tract.
Monitor/restrict visitors and staff as appropriate. Provide protective isolation if indicated.	Reduces risk of exposure to/acquisition of secondary infection in immunosuppressed patient.
Collaborative	
Obtain specimens/monitor results of serial blood, urine, wound cultures.	Identifies causative microorganisms and helps in assessing effectiveness of antimicrobial regimen.
Assist with peritoneal aspiration, if indicated.	May be done to remove fluid and to identify infecting organisms so appropriate antibiotic therapy can be instituted.
Administer antimicrobials, e.g., gentamicin (Garamycin), amikacin (Amikin), clindamycin (Cleocin), via IV/peritoneal lavage.	Therapy is directed at anaerobic bacteria and aerobic Gram-negative bacilli. Lavage may be used to remove necrotic debris and treat inflammation that is poorly localized/diffuse.
Prepare for surgical intervention if indicated.	Surgery may be treatment of choice (curative) in acute, localized peritonitis, e.g., to drain localized abscess; remove peritoneal exudates, ruptured appendix/gallbladder; plicate perforated ulcer; or resect bowel.

> **NURSING DIAGNOSIS: Fluid Volume deficit [mixed]**
>
> **May be related to**
> Fluid shifts from extracellular, intravascular, and interstitial compartments into intestines and/or peritoneal space
> Vomiting; medically restricted intake, NG/intestinal aspiration
> Fever/hypermetabolic state
>
> **Possibly evidenced by**
> Dry mucous membranes, poor skin turgor, delayed capillary refill, weak peripheral pulses
> Diminished urinary output, dark/concentrated urine
> Hypotension, tachycardia
>
> **DESIRED OUTCOMES/EVALUATION CRITERIA—PATIENT WILL:**
>
> **Fluid Balance (NOC)**
>
> Demonstrate improved fluid balance as evidenced by adequate urinary output with normal specific gravity, stable vital signs, moist mucous membranes, good skin turgor, prompt capillary refill, and weight within acceptable range.

ACTIONS/INTERVENTIONS

Fluid/Electrolyte Management (NIC)

Independent

Monitor vital signs, noting presence of hypotension (including postural changes), tachycardia, tachypnea, fever. Measure central venous pressure (CVP) if available.

Maintain accurate I&O and correlate with daily weights. Include measured/estimated losses, e.g., gastric suction, drains, dressings, hemovacs, diaphoresis, and abdominal girth for third spacing of fluid.

Measure urine specific gravity.

Observe skin/mucous membrane dryness, turgor. Note peripheral/sacral edema.

Eliminate noxious sights/smells from environment. Limit intake of ice chips.

Change position frequently, provide frequent skin care, and maintain dry/wrinkle-free bedding.

Collaborative

Monitor laboratory studies, e.g., Hb/Hct, electrolytes, protein, albumin, BUN, Cr.

RATIONALE

Aids in evaluating degree of fluid deficit/effectiveness of fluid replacement therapy and response to medications.

Reflects overall hydration status. Urine output may be diminished because of hypovolemia and decreased renal perfusion, but weight may still increase, reflecting tissue edema/ascites accumulation. Gastric suction losses may be large, and a great deal of fluid can be sequestered in the bowel and peritoneal space (ascites).

Reflects hydration status and changes in renal function, which may warn of developing acute renal failure in response to hypovolemia and effect of toxins. *Note:* Many antibiotics also have nephrotoxic effects that may further affect kidney function/urine output.

Hypovolemia, fluid shifts, and nutritional deficits contribute to poor skin turgor, taut edematous tissues.

Reduces gastric stimulation and vomiting response. *Note:* Excessive use of ice chips during gastric aspiration can increase gastric washout of electrolytes.

Edematous tissue with compromised circulation is prone to breakdown.

Provides information about hydration, organ function. Varied alterations with significant consequences to systemic function are possible as a result of fluid shifts, hypovolemia, hypoxemia, circulating toxins, and necrotic tissue products.

ACTIONS/INTERVENTIONS	RATIONALE
Collaborative	
Administer plasma/blood, fluids, electrolytes, diuretics as indicated.	Replenishes/maintains circulating volume and electrolyte balance. Colloids (plasma, blood) help move water back into intravascular compartment by increasing osmotic pressure gradient. Diuretics may be used to assist in excretion of toxins and to enhance renal function.
Maintain NPO with nasogastric/intestinal aspiration.	Reduces hyperactivity of bowel and diarrhea losses.

NURSING DIAGNOSIS: Pain [acute]

May be related to
Chemical irritation of the parietal peritoneum (toxins)
Trauma to tissues
Accumulation of fluid in abdominal/peritoneal cavity (abdominal distention)

Possibly evidenced by
Verbalizations of pain
Muscle guarding, rebound tenderness
Facial mask of pain, self-focus
Distraction behavior, autonomic/emotional responses (anxiety)

DESIRED OUTCOMES/EVALUATION CRITERIA—PATIENT WILL:

Pain Control Behavior (NOC)

Report pain is relieved/controlled.
Demonstrate use of relaxation skills, other methods to promote comfort.

ACTIONS/INTERVENTIONS	RATIONALE
Pain Management (NIC)	
Independent	
Investigate pain reports, noting location, duration, intensity (0–10 scale), and characteristics (dull, sharp, constant).	Changes in location/intensity are not uncommon but may reflect developing complications. Pain tends to become constant, more intense, and diffuse over the entire abdomen as inflammatory process accelerates; pain may localize if an abscess develops.
Maintain semi-Fowler's position as indicated.	Facilitates fluid/wound drainage by gravity, reducing diaphragmatic irritation/abdominal tension, and thereby reducing pain.
Move patient slowly and deliberately, splinting painful area.	Reduces muscle tension/guarding, which may help minimize pain of movement.
Provide comfort measures, e.g., massage, back rubs; deep breathing. Instruct in relaxation/visualization exercises. Provide diversional activities.	Promotes relaxation and may enhance patient's coping abilities by refocusing attention.
Provide frequent oral care. Remove noxious environmental stimuli.	Reduces nausea/vomiting, which can increase intra-abdominal pressure/pain.

ACTIONS/INTERVENTIONS

Collaborative

Administer medications as indicated:

Analgesics, narcotics;

Antiemetics, e.g., hydroxyzine (Vistaril);

Antipyretics, e.g., acetaminophen (Tylenol).

RATIONALE

Reduce metabolic rate and intestinal irritation from circulating/local toxins, which aids in pain relief and promotes healing. *Note:* Pain is usually severe and may require narcotic pain control. Analgesics may be withheld during initial diagnostic process because they can mask signs/symptoms.

Reduce nausea and vomiting, which can increase abdominal pain.

Reduce discomfort associated with fever/chills.

NURSING DIAGNOSIS: Nutrition: altered, risk for less than body requirements

Risk factors may include
Nausea/vomiting, intestinal dysfunction
Metabolic abnormalities; increased metabolic needs

Possibly evidenced by
[Not applicable; presence of signs and symptoms establishes an *actual* diagnosis]

DESIRED OUTCOMES/EVALUATION CRITERIA—PATIENT WILL:

Nutritional status (NOC)

Maintain usual weight and positive nitrogen balance.

ACTIONS/INTERVENTIONS

Nutrition Management (NIC)

Independent

Auscultate bowel sounds, noting absent/hyperactive sounds.

Monitor NG tube output. Note presence of vomiting/diarrhea.

Measure abdominal girth.

Assess abdomen frequently for return to softness, reappearance of normal bowel sounds, and passage of flatus.

Weigh regularly.

Collaborative

Monitor BUN, protein, prealbumin/albumin, glucose, nitrogen balance as indicated.

RATIONALE

Although bowel sounds are frequently absent, inflammation/irritation of the intestine may be accompanied by intestinal hyperactivity, diminished water absorption, and diarrhea.

Large amounts of gastric aspirant and vomiting/diarrhea suggest bowel obstruction, requiring further evaluation.

Provides quantitative evidence of changes in gastric/intestinal distension and/or accumulation of ascites.

Indicates return of normal bowel function and ability to resume oral intake.

Initial losses/gains reflect changes in hydration, but sustained losses suggest nutritional deficit.

Reflects organ function and nutritional status/needs.

ACTIONS/INTERVENTIONS	RATIONALE
Collaborative	
Advance diet as tolerated, e.g., clear liquids to soft food.	Careful progression of diet when intake is resumed reduces risk of gastric irritation.
Administer TPN as indicated.	Promotes nutrient utilization and positive nitrogen balance in patients who are unable to assimilate nutrients in a normal fashion.

NURSING DIAGNOSIS: Anxiety [specify level]/Fear

May be related to
Situational crisis
Threat of death/change in health status
Physiological factors, hypermetabolic state

Possibly evidenced by
Increased tension/helplessness
Apprehension, uncertainty, worry, sense of impending doom
Sympathetic stimulation; restlessness; focus on self

DESIRED OUTCOMES/EVALUATION CRITERIA—PATIENT WILL:

Anxiety Control (NOC)

Verbalize awareness of feelings and healthy ways to deal with them.
Report anxiety is reduced to a manageable level.
Appear relaxed.

ACTIONS/INTERVENTIONS	RATIONALE

Anxiety Reduction (NIC)

Independent

Evaluate anxiety level, noting patient's verbal and nonverbal response. Encourage free expression of emotions.	Apprehension may be escalated by severe pain, increasingly ill feeling, urgency of diagnostic procedures, and possibility of surgery.
Provide information regarding disease process and anticipated treatment.	Knowing what to expect can reduce anxiety.
Schedule adequate rest and uninterrupted periods for sleep.	Limits fatigue, conserves energy, and can enhance coping ability.

Refer to CP: Psychosocial Aspects of Care, page 809 for additional interventions.

NURSING DIAGNOSIS: Knowledge Deficit [Learning Need] regarding condition, prognosis, treatment, self-care, and discharge needs

May be related to
Lack of exposure/recall
Information misinterpretation
Unfamiliarity with information resources

Possibly evidenced by
Questions; request for information
Statement of misconception
Inaccurate follow-through of instruction

DESIRED OUTCOMES/EVALUATION CRITERIA—PATIENT WILL:

Knowledge: Disease Process (NOC)

Verbalize understanding of disease process and potential complications.
Identify relationship of signs/symptoms to the disease process and correlate symptoms with causative factors.

Knowledge: Treatment Regimen (NOC)

Verbalize understanding of therapeutic needs.
Correctly perform necessary procedures and explain reasons for actions.

ACTIONS/INTERVENTIONS	RATIONALE
Teaching: Disease Process (NIC)	
Independent	
Review underlying disease process and recovery expectations.	Provides knowledge base from which patient can make informed choices.
Identify signs/symptoms requiring medical evaluation, e.g., recurrent abdominal pain/distension, vomiting, fever, chills, or presence of purulent drainage, swelling/erythema of surgical incision (if present).	Early recognition and treatment of developing complications may prevent more serious illness/injury.
Discuss medication regimen, schedule, and possible side effects.	Antibiotics may be continued after discharge, depending on length of stay.
Recommend gradual resumption of usual activities as tolerated, allowing for adequate rest.	Prevents fatigue, enhances feeling of well-being.
Review activity restrictions/limitations, e.g., avoid heavy lifting, constipation.	Avoids unnecessary increase of intra-abdominal pressure and muscle tension.
Demonstrate aseptic dressing change, wound care.	Reduces risk of contamination. Provides opportunity to evaluate healing process.
Emphasize importance of medical follow-up.	Necessary to monitor resolution of infection and resumption of usual activities.

POTENTIAL CONSIDERATIONS following acute hospitalization (dependent on patient's age, physical condition/presence of complications, personal resources, and life responsibilities)

Fatigue—decreased metabolic energy production, increased energy requirements to perform ADLs, states of discomfort.
Pain [acute]—chemical irritation of the peritoneum, prolonged healing process.

CHOLECYSTITIS WITH CHOLELITHIASIS

Cholecystitis is an acute or chronic inflammation of the gallbladder, usually associated with gallstone(s) impacted in the cystic duct, causing distension of the gallbladder. Stones (calculi) are made up of cholesterol, calcium bilirubinate, or a mixture caused by changes in the bile composition. Gallstones can develop in the common bile duct, the cystic duct, hepatic duct, small bile duct, and pancreatic duct. Crystals can also form in the submucosa of the gallbladder causing widespread inflammation. Acute cholecystitis with cholelithiasis is usually treated by surgery, although several other treatment methods (fragmentation and dissolution of stones) are now being used.

CARE SETTING

Severe acute attacks may require brief hospitalization on a medical unit. This plan of care deals with the acutely ill, hospitalized patient.

RELATED CONCERNS

Cholecystectomy, page 398
Fluid and electrolyte imbalances, page 926
Psychosocial aspects of care, page 809
Total nutritional support: parenteral/enteral feeding, page 508

Patient Assessment Database

ACTIVITY/REST

May report:	Fatigue
May exhibit:	Restlessness

CIRCULATION

May exhibit:	Tachycardia, diaphoresis

ELIMINATION

May report:	Change in color of urine and stools
May exhibit:	Abdominal distension
	Palpable mass in right upper quadrant (RUQ)
	Dark, concentrated urine
	Clay-colored stool, steatorrhea

FOOD/FLUID

May report:	Anorexia, nausea/vomiting
	Intolerance of fatty and "gas-forming" foods; recurrent regurgitation, heartburn, indigestion, flatulence, bloating (dyspepsia)
	Belching (eructation)
May exhibit:	Obesity; recent weight loss
	Normal to hypoactive bowel sounds

PAIN/DISCOMFORT

May report:	Severe epigastric and right upper abdominal pain, may radiate to back or right shoulder
	Midepigastric colicky pain associated with eating
	Pain starting suddenly and usually peaking in 30 min
	Recurring episodes of similar pain
May exhibit:	Rebound tenderness, muscle guarding, or abdominal rigidity when RUQ is palpated; positive Murphy's sign

RESPIRATION

May exhibit:	Increased respiratory rate
	Splinted respiration marked by short, shallow breathing

SAFETY

May exhibit: Fever, chills
Jaundice, with dry, itching skin (pruritus)
Bleeding tendencies (vitamin K deficiency)

TEACHING/LEARNING

May report: Familial tendency for gallstones
Recent pregnancy/delivery; history of diabetes mellitus (DM), IBD, blood dyscrasias

Discharge plan considerations: **DRG projected mean length of inpatient stay: 4.3 days**
May require support with dietary changes/weight reduction

Refer to section at end of plan for postdischarge considerations.

DIAGNOSTIC STUDIES

Biliary ultrasound: Reveals calculi, with gallbladder and/or bile duct distension (frequently the initial diagnostic procedure).

Oral cholecystography (OCG): Preferred method of visualizing general appearance and function of gallbladder, including presence of filling defects, structural defects, and/or stone in ducts/biliary tree. Can be done IV (IVC) when nausea/vomiting prevent oral intake, when the gallbladder cannot be visualized during OCG, or when symptoms persist following cholecystectomy. IVC may also be done perioperatively to assess structure and function of ducts, detect remaining stones after lithotripsy or cholecystectomy, and/or to detect surgical complications. Dye can also be injected via T-tube drain postoperatively.

Endoscopic retrograde cholangiopancreatography (ERCP): Visualizes biliary tree by cannulation of the common bile duct through the duodenum.

Percutaneous transhepatic cholangiography (PTC): Fluoroscopic imaging distinguishes between gallbladder disease and cancer of the pancreas (when jaundice is present).

Cholecystograms (for chronic cholecystitis): Reveals stones in the biliary system. *Note:* Contraindicated in acute cholecystitis because the patient is too ill to take the dye by mouth.

Nonnuclear CT scan: May reveal gallbladder cysts, dilation of bile ducts, and distinguish between obstructive/nonobstructive jaundice.

Hepatobiliary (HIDA, PIPIDA) scan: May be done to confirm diagnosis of cholecystitis, especially when barium studies are contraindicated. Scan may be combined with cholecystokinin injection to demonstrate abnormal gallbladder ejection.

Abdominal x-ray films (multipositional): Reveal radiopaque (calcified) gallstones, calcification of the wall or enlargement of the gallbladder.

Chest x-ray: Rule out respiratory causes of referred pain.

CBC: Moderate leukocytosis (acute).

Serum bilirubin and amylase: Elevated.

Serum liver enzymes—AST; ALT; LDH: Slight elevation; alkaline phosphatase and 5-nucleotidase: markedly elevated in biliary obstruction.

Prothrombin levels: Reduced when obstruction to the flow of bile into the intestine decreases absorption of vitamin K.

NURSING PRIORITIES

1. Relieve pain and promote rest.
2. Maintain fluid and electrolyte balance.
3. Prevent complications.
4. Provide information about disease process, prognosis, and treatment needs.

DISCHARGE GOALS

1. Pain relieved.
2. Homeostasis achieved.
3. Complications prevented/minimized.
4. Disease process, prognosis, and therapeutic regimen understood.
5. Plan in place to meet needs after discharge.

ACTIONS/INTERVENTIONS	RATIONALE
Pain Management (NIC)	
Independent	
Observe and document location, severity (0–10 scale), and character of pain (e.g., steady, intermittent, colicky).	Assists in differentiating cause of pain and provides information about disease progression/resolution, development of complications, and effectiveness of interventions.
Note response to medication, and report to physician if pain is not being relieved.	Severe pain not relieved by routine measures may indicate developing complications/need for further intervention.
Promote bedrest, allowing patient to assume position of comfort.	Bedrest in low-Fowler's position reduces intra-abdominal pressure; however, patient will naturally assume least painful position.
Use soft/cotton linens; calamine lotion, oil (Alpha-Keri) bath; cool/moist compresses as indicated.	Reduces irritation/dryness of the skin and itching sensation.
Control environmental temperature.	Cool surroundings aid in minimizing dermal discomfort.
Encourage use of relaxation techniques, e.g., guided imagery, visualization, deep-breathing exercises. Provide diversional activities.	Promotes rest, redirects attention, may enhance coping.
Make time to listen to and maintain frequent contact with patient.	Helpful in alleviating anxiety and refocusing attention, which can relieve pain.
Collaborative	
Maintain NPO status, insert/maintain NG suction as indicated.	Removes gastric secretions that stimulate release of cholecystokinin and gallbladder contractions.
Administer medications as indicated:	
Anticholinergics, e.g., atropine, propantheline (Pro-Banthine);	Relieves reflex spasm/smooth muscle contraction and assists with pain management.
Sedatives, e.g., phenobarbital;	Promotes rest and relaxes smooth muscle, relieving pain.

ACTIONS/INTERVENTIONS	RATIONALE
Collaborative	
Narcotics, e.g., meperidine hydrochloride (Demerol), morphine sulfate;	Given to reduce severe pain. Morphine is used with caution because it may increase spasms of the sphincter of Oddi, although nitroglycerin may be given to reduce morphine-induced spasms if they occur.
Monoctanoin (Moctanin);	This medication may be used after a cholecystectomy for retained stones, or for newly formed large stones in the bile duct. It is a lengthy treatment (1–3 wk) and is administered via a nasal-biliary tube. A cholangiogram is done periodically to monitor stone dissolution.
Smooth muscle relaxants, e.g., papaverine (Pavabid), nitroglycerin, amyl nitrate;	Relieves ductal spasm.
Chenodeoxycholic acid (Chenix), ursodeoxycholic acid (UCDA, Actigall);	These natural bile acids decrease cholesterol synthesis, dissolving gallstones. Success of this treatment depends on the number and size of gallstones (preferably three or fewer stones under 20 mm in diameter) floating in a functioning gallbladder.
Antibiotics.	To treat infectious process, reducing inflammation.
Prepare for procedures, e.g.:	
Endoscopic papillotomy (removal of ductal stone);	Choice of procedure is dictated by individual situation.
Extracorporeal shock wave lithotripsy (ESWL);	Shock wave treatment is indicated when patient has mild or moderate symptoms, cholesterol stones in gallbladder are 0.5 mm or larger, and there is no biliary tract obstruction. Depending on the machine being used, the patient may sit in a tank of water or lie prone on a water-filled cushion. Treatment takes about 1–2 hr and is 75%–95% successful.
Endoscopic sphincterotomy;	Procedure done to widen the mouth of the common bile duct where it empties into the duodenum. This procedure may also include the manual retrieval of stones from the duct by means of a tiny basket or balloon on the end of the endoscope. Stones must be smaller than 15 mm.
Surgical intervention.	Cholecystectomy may be indicated because of the size of stones and degree of tissue involvement/presence of necrosis. Refer to CP: Cholecystectomy, p. 398.

NURSING DIAGNOSIS: Fluid Volume risk for deficit

Risk factors may include
Excessive losses through gastric suction; vomiting, distention, and gastric hypermotility
Medically restricted intake
Altered clotting process

Possibly evidenced by
[Not applicable; presence of signs and symptoms establishes an *actual* diagnosis]

Hydration (NOC)

Demonstrate adequate fluid balance evidenced by stable vital signs, moist mucous membranes, good skin turgor, capillary refill, individually appropriate urinary output, absence of vomiting.

ACTIONS/INTERVENTIONS	RATIONALE
Fluid/Electrolyte Management (NIC)	
Independent	
Maintain accurate I&O, noting output less than intake, increased urine specific gravity. Assess skin/mucous membranes, peripheral pulses, and capillary refill.	Provides information about fluid status/circulating volume and replacement needs.
Monitor for signs/symptoms of increased/continued nausea or vomiting, abdominal cramps, weakness, twitching, seizures, irregular heart rate, paresthesia, hypoactive or absent bowel sounds, depressed respirations.	Prolonged vomiting, gastric aspiration, and restricted oral intake can lead to deficits in sodium, potassium, and chloride.
Eliminate noxious sights/smells from environment.	Reduces stimulation of vomiting center.
Perform frequent oral hygiene with alcohol-free mouthwash; apply lubricants.	Decreases dryness of oral mucous membranes; reduces risk of oral bleeding.
Use small-gauge needles for injections and apply firm pressure for longer than usual after venipuncture.	Reduces trauma, risk of bleeding/hematoma formation.
Assess for unusual bleeding, e.g., oozing from injection sites, epistaxis, bleeding gums, ecchymosis, petechiae, hematemesis/melena.	Prothrombin is reduced and coagulation time prolonged when bile flow is obstructed, increasing risk of bleeding/hemorrhage.
Collaborative	
Keep patient NPO as necessary	Decreases GI secretions and motility.
Insert NG tube, connect to suction, and maintain patency as indicated.	Provides rest for GI tract.
Administer antiemetics, e.g., prochlorperazine (Compazine).	Reduces nausea and prevents vomiting.
Review laboratory studies, e.g., Hb/Hct, electrolytes, ABGs (pH), clotting times.	Aids in evaluating circulating volume, identifies deficits, and influences choice of intervention for replacement/correction.
Administer IV fluids, electrolytes, and vitamin K.	Maintains circulating volume and corrects imbalances.

NURSING DIAGNOSIS: Nutrition: altered, risk for less than body requirements

Risk factors may include
Self-imposed or prescribed dietary restrictions; nausea/vomiting, dyspepsia, pain
Loss of nutrients; impaired fat digestion due to obstruction of bile flow

Possibly evidenced by
[Not applicable; presence of signs and symptoms establishes an *actual* diagnosis]

DESIRED OUTCOMES/EVALUATION CRITERIA—PATIENT WILL:
Nutritional Status (NOC)
Report relief of nausea/vomiting. Demonstrate progression toward desired weight gain or maintain weight as individually appropriate.

ACTIONS/INTERVENTIONS	RATIONALE

Nutrition Management (NIC)

Independent

ACTIONS/INTERVENTIONS	RATIONALE
Estimate/calculate caloric intake. Keep comments about appetite to a minimum.	Identifies nutritional deficiencies/needs. Focusing on problem creates a negative atmosphere and may interfere with intake.
Weigh as indicated.	Monitors effectiveness of dietary plan.
Consult with patient about likes/dislikes, foods that cause distress, and preferred meal schedule.	Involving patient in planning enables patient to have a sense of control and encourages eating.
Provide a pleasant atmosphere at mealtime; remove noxious stimuli.	Useful in promoting appetite/reducing nausea.
Provide oral hygiene before meals.	A clean mouth enhances appetite.
Offer effervescent drinks with meals, if tolerated.	May lessen nausea and relieve gas. *Note:* May be contraindicated if beverage causes gas formation/gastric discomfort.
Assess for abdominal distension, frequent belching, guarding, reluctance to move.	Nonverbal signs of discomfort associated with impaired digestion, gas pain.
Ambulate and increase activity as tolerated.	Helpful in expulsion of flatus, reduction of abdominal distension. Contributes to overall recovery and sense of well-being and decreases possibility of secondary problems related to immobility (e.g., pneumonia, thrombophlebitis).

Collaborative

ACTIONS/INTERVENTIONS	RATIONALE
Consult with dietitian/nutritional support team as indicated.	Useful in establishing individual nutritional needs and most appropriate route.
Begin low-fat liquid diet after NG tube is removed.	Limiting fat content reduces stimulation of gallbladder and pain associated with incomplete fat digestion and is helpful in preventing recurrence.
Advance diet as tolerated, usually low-fat, high-fiber. Restrict gas-producing foods (e.g., onions, cabbage, popcorn) and foods/fluids high in fats (e.g., butter, fried foods, nuts).	Meets nutritional requirements while minimizing stimulation of the gallbladder.
Administer bile salts, e.g., Bilron, Zanchol, dehydrocholic acid (Decholin), as indicated.	Promotes digestion and absorption of fats, fat-soluble vitamins, cholesterol. Useful in chronic cholecystitis.
Monitor laboratory studies, e.g., BUN, prealbumin, albumin, total protein, transferrin levels.	Provides information about nutritional deficits/effectiveness of therapy.
Provide parenteral/enteral feedings as needed.	Alternate feeding may be required depending on degree of disability/gallbladder involvement and need for prolonged gastric rest.

ACTIONS/INTERVENTIONS	RATIONALE
Teaching: Disease Process (NIC)	
Independent	
Provide explanations of/reasons for test procedures and preparation needed.	Information can decrease anxiety, thereby reducing sympathetic stimulation.
Review disease process/prognosis. Discuss hospitalization and prospective treatment as indicated. Encourage questions, expression of concern.	Provides knowledge base from which patient can make informed choices. Effective communication and support at this time can diminish anxiety and promote healing.
Review drug regimen, possible side effects.	Gallstones often recur, necessitating long-term therapy. Development of diarrhea/cramps during chenodiol therapy may be dose-related/correctable. *Note:* Women of childbearing age should be counseled regarding birth control to prevent pregnancy and risk of fetal hepatic damage.
Discuss weight reduction programs if indicated.	Obesity is a risk factor associated with cholecystitis, and weight loss is beneficial in medical management of chronic condition.
Instruct patient to avoid food/fluids high in fats (e.g., whole milk, ice cream, butter, fried foods, nuts, gravies, pork), gas producers (e.g., cabbage, beans, onions, carbonated beverages), or gastric irritants (e.g., spicy foods, caffeine, citrus).	Prevents/limits recurrence of gallbladder attacks.
Review signs/symptoms requiring medical intervention, e.g., recurrent fever; persistent nausea/vomiting, or pain; jaundice of skin or eyes, itching; dark urine; clay-colored stools; blood in urine, stools; vomitus; or bleeding from mucous membranes.	Indicative of progression of disease process/development of complications requiring further intervention.

ACTIONS/INTERVENTIONS	RATIONALE
Independent	
Recommend resting in semi-Fowler's position after meals.	Promotes flow of bile and general relaxation during initial digestive process.
Suggest patient limit gum chewing, sucking on straw/hard candy, or smoking.	Promotes gas formation, which can increase gastric distension/discomfort.
Discuss avoidance of aspirin-containing products, forceful blowing of nose, straining for bowel movement, contact sports. Recommend use of soft toothbrush, electric razor.	Reduces risk of bleeding related to changes in coagulation time, mucosal irritation, and trauma.

POTENTIAL CONSIDERATIONS following acute hospitalization (dependent on patient's age, physical condition/presence of complications, personal resources, and life responsibilities)

Pain [acute]—recurrence of obstruction/ductal spasm, inflammation, tissue ischemia.

CHOLECYSTECTOMY

Cholecystectomy is performed most frequently by laser through laparoscopic incisions. However, traditional open cholecystectomy is the treatment of choice for many patients with multiple/large gallstones either because of acute symptomatology or to prevent recurrence of stones.

CARE SETTING

This procedure is usually done on a short-stay basis; however, in the presence of suspected complications, e.g., empyema, gangrene, or perforation, an inpatient stay on a surgical unit is indicated.

RELATED CONCERNS

Cholecystitis with cholelithiasis, page 390
Pancreatitis, page 498
Peritonitis, page 382
Psychosocial aspects of care, page 809
Surgical intervention, page 828

Patient Assessment Database/Diagnostic Studies

Refer to CP: Cholecystitis with Cholelithiasis, page 390.

TEACHING/LEARNING

Discharge plan considerations: **DRG projected mean length of inpatient stay: 1 (laparoscopic)–4.3 days**
May require assistance with wound care/supplies, homemaker tasks

Refer to section at end of plan for postdischarge considerations.

NURSING PRIORITIES

1. Promote respiratory function.
2. Prevent complications.
3. Provide information about disease, procedure(s), prognosis, and treatment needs.

DISCHARGE GOALS

1. Ventilation/oxygenation adequate for individual needs.
2. Complications prevented/minimized.
3. Disease process, surgical procedure, prognosis, and therapeutic regimen understood.
4. Plan in place to meet needs after discharge.

NURSING DIAGNOSIS: Breathing Pattern, ineffective

May be related to
Pain
Muscular impairment
Decreased energy/fatigue

Possibly evidenced by
Tachypnea; respiratory depth changes, reduced vital capacity
Holding breath; reluctance to cough

DESIRED OUTCOMES/EVALUATION CRITERIA—PATIENT WILL:

Respiratory Status: Ventilation (NOC)

Establish effective breathing pattern.
Experience no signs of respiratory compromise/complications.

ACTIONS/INTERVENTIONS	RATIONALE
Respiratory Monitoring (NIC)	
Independent	
Observe respiratory rate/depth.	Shallow breathing, splinting with respirations, holding breath may result in hypoventilation/atelectasis.
Auscultate breath sounds.	Areas of decreased/absent breath sounds suggest atelectasis, whereas adventitious sounds (wheezes, rhonchi) reflect congestion.
Assist patient to turn, cough, and deep breathe periodically. Show patient how to splint incision. Instruct in effective breathing techniques.	Promotes ventilation of all lung segments and mobilization and expectoration of secretions.
Elevate head of bed, maintain low-Fowler's position. Support abdomen when coughing, ambulating.	Facilitates lung expansion. Splinting provides incisional support/decreases muscle tension to promote cooperation with therapeutic regimen.
Collaborative	
Assist with respiratory treatments, e.g., incentive spirometer.	Maximizes expansion of lungs to prevent/resolve atelectasis.
Administer analgesics before breathing treatments/therapeutic activities.	Facilitates more effective coughing, deep breathing, and activity.

NURSING DIAGNOSIS: Fluid Volume risk for deficit

Risk factors may include
Losses from NG aspiration, vomiting
Medically restricted intake
Altered coagulation, e.g., reduced prothrombin, prolonged coagulation time

Possibly evidenced by
[Not applicable; presence of signs and symptoms establishes an *actual* diagnosis]

DESIRED OUTCOMES/EVALUATION CRITERIA—PATIENT WILL:

Hydration (NOC)

Display adequate fluid balance as evidenced by stable vital signs, moist mucous membranes, good skin turgor/capillary refill, and individually appropriate urinary output.

ACTIONS/INTERVENTIONS	RATIONALE
Fluid/Electrolyte Management (NIC)	
Independent	
Monitor I&O, including drainage from NG tube, T-tube, and wound. Weigh patient periodically.	Provides information about replacement needs and organ function. Initially, 200–500 mL of bile drainage may be expected via the T-tube, decreasing as more bile enters the intestine. Continuing large amounts of bile drainage may be an indication of unresolved obstruction or, occasionally, a biliary fistula.
Monitor vital signs. Assess mucous membranes, skin turgor, peripheral pulses, and capillary refill.	Indicators of adequacy of circulating volume/perfusion.

ACTIONS/INTERVENTIONS

Independent

Observe for signs of bleeding, e.g., hematemesis, melena; petechiae, ecchymosis.

Use small-gauge needles for injections, and apply firm pressure for longer than usual after venipuncture.

Have the patient use cotton/sponge swabs and mouthwash instead of a toothbrush.

Collaborative

Monitor laboratory studies, e.g., Hb/Hct, electrolytes, prothrombin level/clotting time.

Administer IV fluids, blood products, as indicated;

Electrolytes;

Vitamin K.

RATIONALE

Prothrombin is reduced and coagulation time prolonged when bile flow is obstructed, increasing risk of bleeding/hemorrhage.

Reduces trauma, risk of bleeding/hematoma.

Avoids trauma and bleeding of the gums.

Provides information about circulating volume, electrolyte balance, and adequacy of clotting factors.

Maintains adequate circulating volume and aids in replacement of clotting factors.

Corrects imbalances resulting from excessive gastric/wound losses.

Provides replacement of factors necessary for clotting process.

NURSING DIAGNOSIS: Skin/Tissue Integrity, impaired

May be related to
Chemical substance (bile), stasis of secretions
Altered nutritional state (obesity)/metabolic state
Invasion of body structure (T-tube)

Possibly evidenced by
Disruption of skin/subcutaneous tissues

DESIRED OUTCOMES/EVALUATION CRITERIA—PATIENT WILL:

Wound Healing: Primary/Secondary Intention (NOC)

Achieve timely wound healing without complications.
Demonstrate behaviors to promote healing/prevent skin breakdown.

ACTIONS/INTERVENTIONS

Wound Care (NIC)

Independent

Observe the color and character of the drainage.

Change dressings as often as necessary. Clean the skin with soap and water. Use sterile petroleum jelly gauze, zinc oxide, or karaya powder around the incision.

Apply Montgomery straps.

Use a disposable ostomy bag over a stab wound drain.

RATIONALE

Initially, drainage may contain blood and blood-stained fluid, normally changing to greenish brown (bile color) after the first several hours.

Keeps the skin around the incision clean and provides a barrier to protect skin from excoriation.

Facilitates frequent dressing changes and minimizes skin trauma.

Ostomy appliance may be used to collect heavy drainage for more accurate measurement of output and protection of the skin.

ACTIONS/INTERVENTIONS	RATIONALE

Independent

Place patient in low- or semi-Fowler's position.

Facilitates drainage of bile.

Monitor puncture sites (3–5) if endoscopic procedure is done.

These areas may bleed, or staples and steristrips may loosen at puncture wound sites.

Check the T-tube and incisional drains; make sure they are free flowing.

T-tube may remain in common bile duct for 7–10 days to remove retained stones. Incision site drains are used to remove any accumulated fluid and bile. Correct positioning prevents backup of the bile in the operative area.

Maintain T-tube in closed collection system.

Prevents skin irritation and facilitates measurement of output. Reduces risk of contamination.

Anchor drainage tube, allowing sufficient tubing to permit free turning, and avoid kinks and twists.

Avoids dislodging tube and/or occlusion of the lumen.

Observe for hiccups, abdominal distension, or signs of peritonitis, pancreatitis.

Dislodgment of the T-tube can result in diaphragmatic irritation or more serious complications if bile drains into abdomen or pancreatic duct is obstructed.

Observe skin, sclerae, urine for change in color.

Developing jaundice may indicate obstruction of bile flow.

Note color and consistency of stools.

Clay-colored stools result when bile is not present in the intestines.

Investigate reports of increased/unrelenting RUQ pain; development of fever, tachycardia; leakage of bile drainage around tube/from wound.

Signs suggestive of abscess or fistula formation, requiring medical intervention.

Collaborative

Administer antibiotics as indicated.

Necessary for treatment of abscess/infection.

Clamp the T-tube per schedule.

Tests the patency of the common bile duct before tube is removed.

Prepare for surgical interventions as indicated.

Drainage of blocked duct or fistulectomy may be required to treat abscess or repair fistula.

Monitor laboratory studies, e.g., WBC.

Leukocytosis reflects inflammatory process, e.g., abcess formation or development of peritonitis/pancreatitis.

NURSING DIAGNOSIS: Knowledge Deficit [Learning Need] regarding condition, prognosis, treatment, self care, and discharge needs

May be related to
Lack of exposure; information misinterpretation
Unfamiliarity with information resources
Lack of recall

Possibly evidenced by
Questions; statement of misconception
Request for information
Inaccurate follow-through of instructions

Knowledge: Disease Process (NOC)

Verbalize understanding of disease process, surgical procedure/prognosis, and potential complications.

Knowledge: Treatment Regimen (NOC)

Verbalize understanding of therapeutic needs.
Correctly perform necessary procedures and explain reasons for the actions.
Initiate necessary lifestyle changes and participate in therapeutic regimen.

ACTIONS/INTERVENTIONS	RATIONALE
Teaching: Disease Process (NIC)	
Independent	
Review disease process, surgical procedure/prognosis.	Provides knowledge base on which patient can make informed choices.
Demonstrate care of incisions/dressings and drains.	Promotes independence in care and reduces risk of complications (e.g., infection, biliary obstruction).
Recommend periodic drainage of T-tube collection bag and recording of output.	Reduces risk of reflux, strain on tube/appliance seal. Provides information about resolution of ductal edema/return of ductal function for appropriate timing of T-tube removal.
Emphasize importance of maintaining low-fat diet, eating frequent small meals, gradual reintroduction of foods/fluids containing fats over a 4- to 6-month period.	During initial 6 months after surgery, low-fat diet limits need for bile and reduces discomfort associated with inadequate digestion of fats.
Discuss use of medication such as florantyrone (Sancho) or dehydrocholic acid (Decholin).	Oral replacement of bile salts may be required to facilitate fat absorption.
Discuss avoiding/limiting use of alcoholic beverages.	Minimizes risk of pancreatic involvement.
Inform patient that loose stools may occur for several months.	Intestines require time to adjust to stimulus of continuous output of bile.
Advise patient to note and avoid foods that seem to aggravate the diarrhea.	Although radical dietary changes are not usually necessary, certain restrictions may be helpful; e.g., fats in small amounts are usually tolerated. After a period of adjustment, patient usually will not have problems with most foods.
Identify signs/symptoms requiring notification of healthcare provider, e.g., dark urine; jaundiced color of eyes/skin; clay-colored stools, excessive stools; or recurrent heartburn, bloating.	Indicators of obstruction of bile flow/altered digestion, requiring further evaluation and intervention.
Review activity limitations depending on individual situation.	Resumption of usual activities is normally accomplished within 4–6 wk.

POTENTIAL CONSIDERATIONS following acute hospitalization (dependent on patient's age, physical condition/presence of complications, personal resources, and life responsibilities)

Diarrhea—continuous excretion of bile into bowel, changes in digestive process.
Infection, risk for—invasive procedure (discharge with T-tube in place).

Metabolic and Endocrine Disorders

ANOREXIA NERVOSA/BULIMIA NERVOSA

Anorexia nervosa is an illness of starvation, brought on by severe disturbance of body image and a morbid fear of obesity.

Bulimia nervosa is an eating disorder (binge-purge syndrome) characterized by extreme overeating followed by self-induced vomiting. It may include abuse of laxatives and diuretics.

Although these disorders primarily affect women, approximately 5%–10% of those afflicted are men, and both disorders can be present in the same individual.

CARE SETTING

Acute care is provided through inpatient stay on medical or behavioral unit and for correction of severe nutritional deficits/electrolyte imbalances or initial psychiatric stabilization. Long-term care is provided in outpatient/day treatment program (partial hospitalization) or in the community.

RELATED CONCERNS

Dysrhythmias, page 90
Fluid and electrolyte imbalances, page 926
Metabolic alkalosis (primary base bicarbonate excess), page 527
Total nutritional support: parenteral/enteral feeding, page 508
Psychosocial aspects of care, page 809

Patient Assessment Database

ACTIVITY/REST

May report:	Disturbed sleep patterns, e.g., early morning insomnia; fatigue
	Feeling "hyper" and/or anxious
	Increased activity/avid exerciser, participation in high-energy sports
	Employment in positions/professions that stress/require weight control (e.g., athletics such as gymnasts, swimmers, jockeys; modeling; flight attendants)
May exhibit:	Periods of hyperactivity, constant vigorous exercising

CIRCULATION

May report:	Feeling cold even when room is warm
May exhibit:	Low blood pressure (BP)
	Tachycardia, bradycardia, dysrhythmias

EGO INTEGRITY

May report: Powerlessness/helplessness lack of control over eating (e.g., cannot stop eating/control what or how much is eaten [bulimia]); feeling disgusted with self, depressed or very guilty because of overeating

Distorted (unrealistic) body image, reports self as fat regardless of weight (denial), and sees thin body as fat; persistent overconcern with body shape and weight (fears gaining weight)

High self-expectations

Stress factors, e.g., family move/divorce, onset of puberty

Suppression of anger

May exhibit: Emotional states of depression, withdrawal, anger, anxiety, pessimistic outlook

ELIMINATION

May report: Diarrhea/constipation

Vague abdominal pain and distress, bloating

Laxative/diuretic abuse

FOOD/FLUID

May report: Constant hunger or denial of hunger; normal or exaggerated appetite that rarely vanishes until late in the disorder (anorexia)

Intense fear of gaining weight (female); may have prior history of being overweight (particularly males)

Preoccupation with food, e.g., calorie counting, gourmet cooking

An unrealistic pleasure in weight loss, while denying self pleasure in other areas

Refusal to maintain body weight over minimal norm for age/height (anorexia)

Recurrent episodes of binge eating; a feeling of lack of control over behavior during eating binges; a minimum average of two binge-eating episodes a week for at least 3 mo

Regularly engages in either self-induced vomiting (binge-purge syndrome bulimia) independently or as a complication of anorexia; or strict dieting or fasting

May exhibit: Weight loss/maintenance of body weight 15% or more below that expected (anorexia), or weight may be normal or slightly above or below normal (bulimia)

No medical illness evident to account for weight loss

Cachectic appearance; skin may be dry, yellowish/pale, with poor turgor

Preoccupation with food (e.g., calorie counting, hiding food, cutting food into small pieces, rearranging food on plate)

Irrational thinking about eating, food, and weight

Peripheral edema

Swollen salivary glands; sore, inflamed buccal cavity; continuous sore throat (bulimia)

Vomiting, bloody vomitus (may indicate esophageal tearing [Mallory-Weiss syndrome])

Excessive gum chewing

HYGIENE

May exhibit: Increased hair growth on body (lanugo), hair loss (axillary/pubic), hair is dull/not shiny

Brittle nails

Signs of erosion of tooth enamel, gums in poor condition, ulcerations of mucosa

NEUROSENSORY

May exhibit: Appropriate affect (except in regard to body and eating), or depressive affect

Mental changes: apathy, confusion, memory impairment (brought on by malnutrition/starvation)

Hysterical or obsessive personality style; no other psychiatric illness or evidence of a psychiatric thought disorder present (although a significant number may show evidence of an affective disorder)

PAIN/DISCOMFORT

May report: Headaches, sore throat/mouth, generalized vague complaints

SAFETY

May exhibit: Body temperature below normal
Recurrent infectious processes (indicative of depressed immune system)
Eczema/other skin problems, abrasions/calluses may be noted on back of hands from sticking finger down throat to induce vomiting

SEXUALITY

May report: Absence of at least three consecutive menstrual cycles (decreased levels of estrogen in response to malnutrition)
Promiscuity or denial/loss of sexual interest
History of sexual abuse
Homosexual/bisexual orientation (higher percentage in male patients than in general population)

May exhibit: Breast atrophy, amenorrhea

SOCIAL INTERACTION

May report: Middle-class or upper-class family background
History of being a quiet, cooperative child
Problems of control issues in relationships, difficult communications with others/authority figures, poor communication within family of origin
Engagement in power struggles
An emotional crisis of some sort, such as the onset of puberty or a family move
Altered relationships or problems with relationships (not married/divorced), withdrawal from friends/social contacts
Abusive family relationships
Sense of helplessness
History of legal difficulties (e.g., shoplifting)

May exhibit: Passive father/dominant mother, family members closely fused, togetherness prized, personal boundaries not respected

TEACHING/LEARNING

May report: Family history of higher than normal incidence of depression, other family members with eating disorders (genetic predisposition)
Onset of the illness usually between the ages of 10 and 22
Health beliefs/practice (e.g., certain foods have "too many" calories, use of "health" foods)
High academic achievement
Substance abuse

Discharge plan considerations: **DRG projected mean length of inpatient stay: 6.4 days**
Assistance with maintenance of treatment plan

Refer to section at end of plan for postdischarge considerations.

DIAGNOSTIC STUDIES

Complete blood count (CBC) with differential: Determines presence of anemia, leukopenia, lymphocytosis. Platelets show significantly less than normal activity by the enzyme monoamine oxidase (thought to be a marker for depression).

Electrolytes: Imbalances may include decreased potassium, sodium, chloride, and magnesium.

Endocrine studies:

Thyroid function: Thyroxine (T_4) levels usually normal; however, circulating triiodothyronine (T_3) levels may be low.

Pituitary function: Thyroid-stimulating hormone (TSH) response to thyrotropin-releasing hormone (TRH) is abnormal in anorexia nervosa. Propranolol-glucagon stimulation test studies the response of human growth hormone (GH), which is depressed in anorexia nervosa. Gonadotropic hypofunction is noted.

Cortisol metabolism: May be elevated.

Dexamethasone suppression test (DST): Evaluates hypothalamic-pituitary function. Dexamethasone resistance indicates cortisol suppression, suggesting malnutrition and/or depression.

Luteinizing hormone (LH) secretions test: Pattern often resembles those of prepubertal girls.

Estrogen: Decreased.

MHP 6 levels: Decreased, suggestive of malnutrition/depression.

Serum glucose and basal metabolic rate (BMR): May be low.

Other chemistries: AST elevated. Hypercarotenemia, hypoproteinemia, hypocholesterolemia.

Urinalysis and renal function: Blood urea nitrogen (BUN) may be elevated; ketones present reflecting starvation; decreased urinary 17-ketosteroids, increased specific gravity/dehydration.

Electrocardiogram (ECG): Abnormal tracing with low voltage, T-wave inversion, dysrhythmias.

NURSING PRIORITIES

1. Reestablish adequate/appropriate nutritional intake.
2. Correct fluid and electrolyte imbalance.
3. Assist patient to develop realistic body image/improve self-esteem.
4. Provide support/involve significant other (SO), if available, in treatment program.
5. Coordinate total treatment program with other disciplines.
6. Provide information about disease, prognosis, and treatment to patient/SO.

DISCHARGE GOALS

1. Adequate nutrition and fluid intake maintained.
2. Maladaptive coping behaviors and stressors that precipitate anxiety recognized.
3. Adaptive coping strategies and techniques for anxiety reduction and self-control implemented.
4. Self-esteem increased.
5. Disease process, prognosis, and treatment regimen understood.
6. Plan in place to meet needs after discharge.

NURSING DIAGNOSIS: Nutrition: altered, less than body requirements

May be related to

Inadequate food intake; self-induced vomiting

Chronic/excessive laxative use

Possibly evidenced by

Body weight 15% (or more) below expected, or may be within normal range (bulimia)

Pale conjunctiva and mucous membranes; poor skin turgor/muscle tone; edema

Excessive loss of hair; increased growth of hair on body (lanugo)

Amenorrhea

Hypothermia

Bradycardia; cardiac irregularities; hypotension

DESIRED OUTCOMES/EVALUATION CRITERIA—PATIENT WILL:

> **Knowledge: Diet (NOC)**

Verbalize understanding of nutritional needs.

> **Nutrition Status (NOC)**

Establish a dietary pattern with caloric intake adequate to regain/maintain appropriate weight.

Demonstrate weight gain toward individually expected range.

ACTIONS/INTERVENTIONS	RATIONALE

Eating Disorders Management (NIC)

Independent

Establish a minimum weight goal and daily nutritional requirements.

Malnutrition is a mood-altering condition, leading to depression and agitation and affecting cognitive function/decision making. Improved nutritional status enhances thinking ability, allowing initiation of psychological work.

Use a consistent approach. Sit with patient while eating; present and remove food without persuasion and/or comment. Promote pleasant environment and record intake.

Patient detects urgency and may react to pressure. Any comment that might be seen as coercion provides focus on food. When staff responds in a consistent manner, patient can begin to trust staff responses. The single area in which the patient has exercised power and control is food/eating, and he or she may experience guilt or rebellion if forced to eat. Structuring meals and decreasing discussions about food will decrease power struggles with patient and avoid manipulative games.

Provide smaller meals and supplemental snacks, as appropriate.

Gastric dilation may occur if refeeding is too rapid following a period of starvation dieting. *Note:* Patient may feel bloated for 3–6 wk while body adjusts to food intake.

Make selective menu available, and allow patient to control choices as much as possible.

Patient who gains confidence in self and feels in control of environment is more likely to eat preferred foods.

Be alert to choices of low-calorie foods/beverages; hoarding food; disposing of food in various places, such as pockets or wastebaskets.

Patient will try to avoid taking in what is viewed as excessive calories and may go to great lengths to avoid eating.

Maintain a regular weighing schedule, such as Monday/Friday before breakfast in same attire, and graph results.

Provides accurate ongoing record of weight loss/gain. Also diminishes obsessing about changes in weight.

Weigh with back to scale (depending on program protocols).

Although some programs prefer patient see the results of the weighing, this can force the issue of trust in patient who usually does not trust others.

Avoid room checks and other control devices whenever possible.

External control reinforces feelings of powerlessness and are therefore usually not helpful.

Provide one-to-one supervision and have the patient with bulimia remain in the day-room area with no bathroom privileges for a specified period (e.g., 2 hr) following eating, if contracting is unsuccessful.

Prevents vomiting during/after eating. Patient may desire food and use a binge-purge syndrome to maintain weight. *Note:* A patient may purge for the first time in response to establishment of a weight gain program.

Monitor exercise program and set limits on physical activities. Chart activity/level of work (pacing and so on).

Moderate exercise helps in maintaining muscle tone/weight and combating depression; however, patient may exercise excessively to burn calories.

Maintain matter-of-fact, nonjudgmental attitude if giving tube feedings, hyperalimentation, and so on.

Perception of punishment is counterproductive to patient's self-confidence and faith in own ability to control destiny.

Be alert to possibility of patient disconnecting tube and emptying hyperalimentation if used. Check measurements, and tape tubing snugly.

Sabotage behavior is common in attempt to prevent weight gain.

ACTIONS/INTERVENTIONS	RATIONALE
Collaborative	
Provide nutritional therapy within a hospital treatment program as indicated when condition is life-threatening.	Cure of the underlying problem cannot happen without improved nutritional status. Hospitalization provides a controlled environment in which food intake, vomiting/elimination, medications, and activities can be monitored. It also separates the patient from SO (who may be contributing factor) and provides exposure to others with the same problem, creating an atmosphere for sharing.
Involve patient in setting up/carrying out program of behavior modification. Provide reward for weight gain as individually determined; ignore loss.	Provides structured eating situation while allowing patient some control in choices. Behavior modification may be effective in mild cases or for short-term weight gain.
Provide diet and snacks with substitutions of preferred foods when available.	Having a variety of foods available enables the patient to have a choice of potentially enjoyable foods.
Administer liquid diet and/or tube feedings/hyperalimentation if needed.	When caloric intake is insufficient to sustain metabolic needs, nutritional support can be used to prevent malnutrition/death while therapy is continuing. High-calorie liquid feedings may be given as medication, at preset times separate from meals, as an alternative means of increasing caloric intake.
Blenderize and tube-feed anything left on the tray after a given period of time if indicated.	May be used as part of behavior modification program to provide total intake of needed calories.
Administer supplemental nutrition as appropriate.	Total parenteral nutrition (TPN) may be required for life-threatening situations; however, enteral feedings are preferred because they preserve GI function and reduce atrophy of the gut.
Avoid giving laxatives.	Use is counterproductive because they may be used by patient to rid body of food/calories.
Administer medications as indicated:	
Cypropheptadine (Periactin);	A serotonin and histamine antagonist that may be used in high doses to stimulate the appetite, decrease preoccupation with food, and combat depression. Does not appear to have serious side effects, although decreased mental alertness may occur.
Tricyclic antidepressants, e.g., amitriptyline (Elavil, Endep); imipramine (Tofranil), desipramine (Norpramin); selective serotonin reuptake inhibitors (SSRIs), e.g., fluoxetine (Prozac);	Lifts depression and stimulates appetite. SSRIs reduce binge-purge cycles and may also be helpful in treating anorexia. *Note:* Use must be closely monitored because of potential side effects, although side effects from SSRIs are less significant than those associated with tricyclics.
Antianxiety agents, e.g., alprazolam (Xanax);	Reduces tension, anxiety/nervousness and may help patient to participate in treatment.
Antipsychotic drugs, e.g., chlorpromazine (Thorazine);	Promotes weight gain and cooperation with psychotherapeutic program; however, used only when absolutely necessary because of the possibility of extrapyramidal side effects.
Monoamine oxidase inhibitors (MAOIs), e.g., tranylcypromine sulfate (Parnate).	May be used to treat depression when other drug therapy is ineffective; decreases urge to binge in bulimia.

ACTIONS/INTERVENTIONS

Collaborative

Prepare for/assist with electroconvulsive therapy (ECT) if indicated. Discuss reasons for use and help patient understand this is not punishment.

RATIONALE

In rare and difficult cases in which malnutrition is severe/life-threatening, a short-term ECT series may enable the patient to begin eating and become accessible to psychotherapy.

NURSING DIAGNOSIS: Fluid Volume actual or risk for deficit

May be related to
Inadequate intake of food and liquids
Consistent self-induced vomiting
Chronic/excessive laxative/diuretic use

Possibly evidenced by: (actual)
Dry skin and mucous membranes, decreased skin turgor
Increased pulse rate, body temperature, decreased BP
Output greater than input (diuretic use); concentrated urine/decreased urine output (dehydration)
Weakness
Change in mental state
Hemoconcentration, altered electrolyte balance

DESIRED OUTCOMES/EVALUATION CRITERIA:

Hydration (NOC)

Maintain/demonstrate improved fluid balance, as evidenced by adequate urine output, stable vital signs, moist mucous membranes, good skin turgor.

Risk Control (NOC)

Verbalize understanding of causative factors and behaviors necessary to correct fluid deficit.

ACTIONS/INTERVENTIONS

Fluid/Electrolyte Management (NIC)

Independent

Monitor vital signs, capillary refill, status of mucous membranes, skin turgor.

Monitor amount and types of fluid intake. Measure urine output accurately.

Discuss strategies to stop vomiting and laxative/diuretic use.

Identify actions necessary to regain/maintain optimal fluid balance, e.g., specific fluid intake schedule.

RATIONALE

Indicators of adequacy of circulating volume. Orthostatic hypotension may occur with risk of falls/injury following sudden changes in position.

Patient may abstain from all intake, with resulting dehydration; or substitute fluids for caloric intake, disturbing electrolyte balance.

Helping patient deal with the feelings that lead to vomiting and/or laxative/diuretic use will prevent continued fluid loss. *Note:* The patient with bulimia has learned that vomiting provides a release of anxiety.

Involving patient in plan to correct fluid imbalances improves chances for success.

ACTIONS/INTERVENTIONS	RATIONALE

Collaborative

Review electrolyte/renal function test results.	Fluid/electrolyte shifts, decreased renal function can adversely affect patient's recovery/prognosis and may require additional intervention.
Administer/monitor IV, TPN; electrolyte supplements, as indicated.	Used as an emergency measure to correct fluid/electrolyte imbalance and prevent cardiac dysrhythmias.

NURSING DIAGNOSIS: Thought Processes, altered

May be related to
Severe malnutrition/electrolyte imbalance
Psychological conflicts, e.g., sense of low self-worth, perceived lack of control

Possibly evidenced by
Impaired ability to make decisions, problem-solve
Non–reality-based verbalizations
Ideas of reference
Altered sleep patterns, e.g., may go to bed late (stay up to binge/purge) and get up early
Altered attention span/distractibility
Perceptual disturbances with failure to recognize hunger; fatigue, anxiety, and depression

DESIRED OUTCOMES/EVALUATION CRITERIA—PATIENT WILL:

Distorted Thought Control (NOC)

Verbalize understanding of causative factors and awareness of impairment.
Demonstrate behaviors to change/prevent malnutrition.
Display improved ability to make decisions, problem-solve.

ACTIONS/INTERVENTIONS	RATIONALE

Delusion Management (NIC)

Independent

Be aware of patient's distorted thinking ability.	Allows the caregiver to have more realistic expectations of the patient and provide appropriate information and support.
Listen to/avoid challenging irrational, illogical thinking. Present reality concisely and briefly.	It is not possible to respond logically when thinking ability is physiologically impaired. The patient needs to hear reality, but challenging the patient leads to distrust and frustration. *Note:* Even though patient may gain weight, she or he may continue to struggle with attitudes/behaviors typical of eating disorders, major depression, and/or alcohol dependence for a number of years.
Adhere strictly to nutritional regimen.	Improved nutrition is essential to improved brain functioning. (Refer to ND: Nutrition: altered, less than body requirements, p. 406.)

ACTIONS/INTERVENTIONS

Collaborative

Review electrolyte/renal function tests.

RATIONALE

Imbalances negatively affect cerebral functioning and may require correction before therapeutic interventions can begin.

NURSING DIAGNOSIS: Body Image disturbance/Self-Esteem, chronic low

May be related to
Morbid fear of obesity; perceived loss of control in some aspect of life
Personal vulnerability; unmet dependency needs
Dysfunctional family system
Continual negative evaluation of self

Possibly evidenced by
Distorted body image (views self as fat even in the presence of normal body weight or severe emaciation)
Expresses little concern, uses denial as a defense mechanism, and feels powerless to prevent/make changes
Expressions of shame/guilt
Overly conforming, dependent on others' opinions

DESIRED OUTCOMES/EVALUATION CRITERIA—PATIENT WILL:

Body Image (NOC)

Establish a more realistic body image.

Self-esteem (NOC)

Acknowledge self as an individual.
Accept responsibility for own actions.

ACTIONS/INTERVENTIONS

Body Image Enhancement (NIC)

Independent

Have patient draw picture of self.

Involve in personal development program, preferably in a group setting. Provide information about proper application of makeup and grooming.

Suggest disposing of "thin" clothes as weight gain occurs. Recommend consultation with an image consultant.

Assist patient to confront changes associated with puberty/sexual fears. Provide sex education as necessary.

RATIONALE

Provides opportunity to discuss patient's perception of self/body image and realities of individual situation.

Learning about methods to enhance personal appearance may be helpful to long-range sense of self-esteem/image. Feedback from others can promote feelings of self-worth.

Provides incentive to at least maintain and not lose weight. Removes visual reminder of thinner self. Positive image enhances sense of self-esteem.

Major physical/psychological changes in adolescence can contribute to development of eating disorders. Feelings of powerlessness and loss of control of feelings (in particular sexual sensations) lead to an unconscious desire to desexualize self. Patient often believes that these fears can be overcome by taking control of bodily appearance/development/function.

ACTIONS/INTERVENTIONS	RATIONALE

Self-esteem Enhancement (NIC)

Independent

Establish a therapeutic nurse/patient relationship.

Within a helping relationship, patient can begin to trust and try out new thinking and behaviors.

Promote self-concept without moral judgment.

Patient sees self as weak-willed, even though part of person may feel sense of power and control (e.g., dieting/weight loss).

State rules clearly regarding weighing schedule, remaining in sight during medication and eating times, and consequences of not following the rules. Without undue comment, be consistent in carrying out rules.

Consistency is important in establishing trust. As part of the behavior modification program, patient knows risks involved in not following established rules (e.g., decrease in privileges). Failure to follow rules is viewed as the patient's choice and accepted by staff in matter-of-fact manner so as not to provide reinforcement for the undesirable behavior.

Respond (confront) with reality when patient makes unrealistic statements such as "I'm gaining weight, so there's nothing really wrong with me."

Patient may be denying the psychological aspects of own situation and is often expressing a sense of inadequacy and depression.

Be aware of own reaction to patient's behavior. Avoid arguing.

Feelings of disgust, hostility, and infuriation are not uncommon when caring for these patients. Prognosis often remains poor even with a gain in weight because other problems may remain. Many patients continue to see themselves as fat, and there is also a high incidence of affective disorders, social phobias, obsessive-compulsive symptoms, drug abuse, and psychosexual dysfunction. Nurse needs to deal with own response/feelings so they do not interfere with care of patient.

Assist the patient to assume control in areas other than dieting/weight loss, e.g., management of own daily activities, work/leisure choices.

Feelings of personal ineffectiveness, low self-esteem, and perfectionism are often part of the problem. Patient feels helpless to change and requires assistance to problem-solve methods of control in life situations.

Help the patient formulate goals for self (not related to eating) and create a manageable plan to reach those goals, one at a time, progressing from simple to more complex.

Patient needs to recognize ability to control other areas in life and may need to learn problem-solving skills to achieve this control. Setting realistic goals fosters success.

Note patient's withdrawal from and/or discomfort in social settings.

May indicate feelings of isolation and fear of rejection/judgment by other's. Avoidance of social situations and contact with others can compound feelings of worthlessness.

Encourage patient to take charge of own life in a more healthful way by making own decisions and accepting self as she or he is at this moment (including inadequacies and strengths).

Patient often does not know what she or he may want for self. Parents (mother) often make decisions for patient. Patient may also believe she or he has to be the best in everything and holds self responsible for being perfect.

Let patient know that it is acceptable to be different from family, particularly mother.

Developing a sense of identity separate from family and maintaining sense of control in other ways besides dieting and weight loss is a desirable goal of therapy/program.

412

ACTIONS/INTERVENTIONS	RATIONALE

Independent

Use interpersonal psychotherapy approach, rather than interpretive therapy.	Interaction between persons is more helpful for the patient to discover feelings/impulses/needs from within own self. Patient has not learned this internal control as a child and may not be able to interpret or attach meaning to behavior.
Encourage patient to express anger and acknowledge when it is verbalized.	Important to know that anger is part of self and as such is acceptable. Expressing anger may need to be taught to patient because anger is generally considered unacceptable in the family, and therefore patient does not express it.
Assist patient to learn strategies other than eating for dealing with feelings. Have patient keep a diary of feelings, particularly when thinking about food.	Feelings are the underlying issue, and patient often uses food instead of dealing with feelings appropriately. Patient needs to learn to recognize feelings and how to express them clearly.
Assess feelings of helplessness/hopelessness.	Lack of control is a common/underlying problem for this patient and may be accompanied by more serious emotional disorders. *Note:* Fifty-four percent of patients with anorexia have a history of major affective disorder, and 33% have a history of minor affective disorder.
Be alert to suicidal ideation/behavior.	Intense anxiety/panic about weight gain, depression, hopeless feelings may lead to suicidal attempts, particularly if patient is impulsive.

Collaborative

Involve in group therapy.	Provides an opportunity to talk about feelings and try out new behaviors.
Refer to occupational/recreational therapy.	Can develop interests and skills to fill time that has been occupied by obsession with eating. Involvement in recreational activities encourages social interactions with others and promotes fun and relaxation.
Encourage participation in directed activities, e.g., bicycle tours and wilderness adventures, such as Outward Bound Program.	While exercise is often used negatively by these patients, participation in these directed activities provides an opportunity to learn self-reliance, enhance self-esteem, and realize that food is the fuel required by the body to do its work.
Refer to therapist trained in dealing with sexuality, as indicated.	May need professional assistance to deal with sexuality issues and accept self as a sexual adult.

NURSING DIAGNOSIS: Parenting, altered

May be related to
Issues of control in family
Situational/maturational crises
History of inadequate coping methods

Possibly evidenced by
Dissonance among family members
Family developmental tasks not being met
Focus on "Identified Patient" (IP)
Family needs not being met
Family member(s) acting as "enablers" for IP
Ill-defined family rules, function, and roles

DESIRED OUTCOMES/EVALUATION CRITERIA—FAMILY WILL:

Parenting (NOC)

Demonstrate individual involvement in problem-solving process directed at encouraging patient toward independence.
Express feelings freely and appropriately.
Demonstrate more autonomous coping behaviors with individual family boundaries more clearly defined.
Recognize and resolve conflict appropriately with the individuals involved.

ACTIONS/INTERVENTIONS

RATIONALE

Family Therapy (NIC)

Independent

Identify patterns of interaction. Encourage each family member to speak for self. Do not allow two members to discuss a third without that member's participation.

Helpful information for planning interventions. The enmeshed, overinvolved family members often speak for each other and need to learn to be responsible for their own words and actions.

Discourage members from asking for approval from each other. Be alert to verbal or nonverbal checking with others for approval. Acknowledge competent actions of patient.

Each individual needs to develop own internal sense of self-esteem. Individual often is living up to others' (family's) expectations rather than making own choices. Acknowledgment provides recognition of self in positive ways.

Listen with regard when the patient speaks.

Sets an example and provides a sense of competence and self-worth, in that the patient has been heard and attended to.

Encourage individuals not to answer to everything.

Reinforces individualization and return to privacy.

Communicate message of separation, that it is acceptable for family members to be different from each other.

Individuation needs reinforcement. Such a message confronts rigidity and opens options for different behaviors.

Encourage and allow expression of feelings (e.g., crying, anger) by individuals.

Often these families have not allowed free expression of feelings and need help and permission to learn and accept this.

Prevent intrusion in dyads by other members of the family.

Inappropriate interventions in family subsystems prevent individuals from working out problems successfully.

ACTIONS/INTERVENTIONS

Independent

Reinforce importance of parents as a couple who have rights of their own.

Prevent patient from intervening in conflicts between parents. Assist parents in identifying and solving their marital differences.

Be aware and confront sabotage behavior on the part of family members.

Collaborative

Refer to community resources such as family therapy groups, parents' groups as indicated, and parent effectiveness classes.

RATIONALE

The focus on the child with anorexia is very intense and often is the only area around which the couple interact. The couple needs to explore their own relationship and restore the balance within it to prevent its disintegration.

Triangulation occurs in which a parent-child coalition exists. Sometimes the child is openly pressed to ally self with one parent against the other. The symptom (anorexia) is the regulator in the family system, and the parents deny their own conflicts.

Feelings of blame, shame, and helplessness may lead to unconscious behavior designed to maintain the status quo.

May help reduce overprotectiveness, support/facilitate the process of dealing with unresolved conflicts and change.

NURSING DIAGNOSIS: Skin Integrity, risk for impaired

Risk factors may include:
Altered nutritional/metabolic state; edema
Dehydration/cachectic changes (skeletal prominence)

Possibly evidenced by
[Not applicable; presence of signs and symptoms establishes an *actual* diagnosis]

DESIRED OUTCOMES/EVALUATION CRITERIA—PATIENT WILL:

Risk Control (NOC)

Verbalize understanding of causative factors and absence of itching.
Identify and demonstrate behaviors to maintain soft, supple, intact skin.

ACTIONS/INTERVENTIONS

Skin Surveillance (NIC)

Independent

Observe for reddened, blanched, excoriated areas.

Encourage bathing every other day instead of daily.

Use skin cream twice a day and after bathing.

Massage skin gently, especially over bony prominences.

Discuss importance of frequent position changes, need for remaining active.

Emphasize importance of adequate nutrition/fluid intake. (Refer to ND: Nutrition: altered, less than body requirements, p. 406.)

RATIONALE

Indicators of increased risk of breakdown, requiring more intensive treatment.

Frequent baths contribute to dryness of the skin.

Lubricates skin and decreases itching.

Improves circulation to the skin, enhances skin tone.

Enhances circulation and perfusion to skin by preventing prolonged pressure on tissues.

Improved nutrition and hydration will improve skin condition.

> **NURSING DIAGNOSIS: Knowledge Deficit [Learning Need] regarding condition, prognosis, treatment, self care, and discharge needs**
>
> **May be related to**
>
> Lack of exposure to/unfamiliarity with information about condition
>
> Learned maladaptive coping skills
>
> **Possibly evidenced by**
>
> Verbalization of misconception of relationship of current situation and behaviors
>
> Preoccupation with extreme fear of obesity and distortion of own body image
>
> Refusal to eat; binging and purging; abuse of laxatives and diuretics; excessive exercising
>
> Verbalization of need for new information
>
> Expressions of desire to learn more adaptive ways of coping with stressors
>
> **DESIRED OUTCOMES/EVALUATION CRITERIA—PATIENT WILL:**
>
> **Knowledge: Disease Process (NOC)**
>
> Verbalize awareness of and plan for lifestyle changes to maintain normal weight.
>
> Identify relationship of signs/symptoms (weight loss, tooth decay) to behaviors of not eating/binging-purging.
>
> Assume responsibility for own learning.
>
> Seek out sources/resources to assist with making identified changes.

ACTIONS/INTERVENTIONS	RATIONALE
Learning Facilitation (NIC)	
Independent	
Determine level of knowledge and readiness to learn.	Learning is easier when it begins where the learner is.
Note blocks to learning, e.g., physical/intellectual/emotional.	Malnutrition, family problems, drug abuse, affective disorders, and obsessive-compulsive symptoms can be blocks to learning requiring resolution before effective learning can occur.
Teaching: Disease Process (NIC)	
Provide written information for patient/SO(s).	Helpful as reminder of and reinforcement for learning.
Discuss consequences of behavior.	Sudden death can occur because of electrolyte imbalances; suppression of the immune system and liver damage may result from protein deficiency; or gastric rupture may follow binge-eating/vomiting.
Review dietary needs, answering questions as indicated. Encourage inclusion of high-fiber foods and adequate fluid intake.	Patient/family may need assistance with planning for new way of eating. Constipation may occur when laxative use is curtailed.
Encourage the use of relaxation and other stress-management techniques, e.g., visualization, guided imagery, biofeedback.	New ways of coping with feelings of anxiety and fear help patient manage these feelings in more effective ways, assisting in giving up maladaptive behaviors of not eating/binging-purging.
Assist with establishing a sensible exercise program. Caution regarding overexercise.	Exercise can assist with developing a positive body image and combats depression (release of endorphins in the brain enhances sense of well-being). However, patient may use excessive exercise as a way to control weight.

ACTIONS/INTERVENTIONS

Independent

ACTIONS/INTERVENTIONS	RATIONALE
Discuss need for information about sex and sexuality.	Because avoidance of own sexuality is an issue for this patient, realistic information can be helpful in beginning to deal with self as a sexual being.
Refer to National Association of Anorexia Nervosa and Associated Disorders, Overeaters Anonymous, and other local resources.	May be a helpful source of support and information for patient/SO.

POTENTIAL CONSIDERATIONS following acute hospitalization (dependent on patient's age, physical condition/presence of complications, personal resources, and life responsibilities)

Nutrition: altered, risk for less than body requirements—inadequate food intake, self-induced vomiting, history of chronic laxative use.

Therapeutic Regimen: Individual, ineffective management—complexity of therapeutic regimen, perceived seriousness/benefits, mistrust of regimen and/or health care personnel, excessive demands made on individual, family conflict.

Sample CP: Eating Disorders Program. ELOS: 28 Days Behavioral Unit

ND and Categories of Care	Time Dimension	Goals/Actions	Time Dimension	Goals/Actions	Time Dimension	Goals/Actions
Altered nutrition: less than body requirements R/T inadequate intake, self-induced vomiting, laxative use	Ongoing	Gain 3 lb/wk as indicated	Day 2–28	Consume at least 75% of food provided at each meal	Day 15–28	Demonstrate ability to select foods to meet at least 80% of nutritional needs
Risk for fluid volume deficit R/T inadequate intake, self-induced vomiting, laxative use	Ongoing	Be free of S/S of dehydration	Day 2–28	Ingest at least 1500 mL fluid/day	Day 22–28	Refrain from self-induced vomiting
		Display balanced I&O	Day 3	Vital signs WNL	Day 28	Be free of S/S of malnutrition with all laboratory results WNL
Referral Diagnostic studies	Day 1 & prn Day 1	Dietitian Electrolytes, CBC, BUN/Cr, Thyroid function UA ECG as indicated	Day 14	Repeat selected studies		
Additional assessments	Day 1–2 Day 1 Day 1–28	Vital signs/I&O q shift Weight Types and amount of food/fluid intake Behavior/purging following meals Level of activity	Day 3–7 q AM Day 7, 14	7:30 AM/same clothes	Day 8–28	As indicated
Medications Allergies:	Day 1–28	Periactin Tricyclic antidepressant Vitamin supplement				
Patient education	Day 1 & prn	Orient to unit and schedule Behavior modification program Minimum weight goal and initial nutritional needs	Day 7–14	Principles of nutrition; foods for maintenance of wellness	Day 21–28	Incorporating nutritional plan into lifestyle and home setting
Additional nursing actions	Day 1–3 Day 1–7 Day 1–21 Day 1–28	Assist patient with formulation of behavioral contract and monitoring of cooperation Administer tube feeding/blenderized food as indicated Bathroom locked for 1 hr following meals Provide social setting for meals	Day 7–28	Involve mother/SO as appropriate in nutritional counseling and planning for future		

Sample CP: Eating Disorders Program. ELOS: 28 Days Behavioral Unit (*Continued*)

ND and Categories of Care	Time Dimension	Goals/Actions	Time Dimension	Goals/Actions	Time Dimension	Goals/Actions
Ineffective denial R/T presence of overwhelming anxiety-producing feelings, learned response pattern, personal/family value system	Ongoing Day 2–28	Participate in behavior modification program and adhere to unit policies Cooperate with therapy to restore nutritional well-being	Day 8–28 Day 14	Attend and contribute to group sessions Develop trusting relationship with at least one staff member on each shift	Day 18–28 Day 28	Verbalize acceptance of reality that eating behaviors are maladaptive Demonstrate ability to cope more adaptively Identify ways to gain control in life situation Refrain from use of manipulation of others to achieve control Plan in place to meet needs postdischarge
Referrals	Day 5 (or when physical condition stable)	Psychologist Social worker Psychodramatist	Day 8–28	Group psychotherapy sessions	Day 25	Community resource contact person(s)
Additional assessments	Day 1/ongoing Day 1–17	Degree and stage of denial Perception of situation Ability to trust Use of manipulation to achieve control	Day 5–7 Day 7–28 Day 8–28	Readiness to participate in group sessions Congruence between verbalizations and behaviors (insight) Degree/quality of involvement in group sessions		
Patient education	Day 1 and prn	Privileges and responsibilities of behavior modification Consequences of behaviors	Day 3/ongoing	Eating disorder and consequences of eating behavior	Day 21	Role of support groups/community resources
Additional nursing actions	Day 1/ongoing	Encourage expression of feelings Avoid agreeing with inaccurate statements/perceptions Provide positive feedback for desired insight/behaviors Set limits on maladaptive behavior	Day 5–28 Day 8–28	Promote involvement in unit activities Support interactions with family members Encourage interactions in group sessions	Day 21–28	Involve family (as appropriate) in long range planning for meeting individual needs
Body image disturbance/chronic low self-esteem R/T perceived loss of control, unmet dependency needs, personal vulnerability, negative evaluation of self	Day 7	Acknowledge that attention will not be given to discussion of body image and food	Day 21	Acknowledge misperception of body image as fat Verbalize positive self-attributes	Day 28	Demonstrate realistic body image and self-awareness Verbalize acceptance of self including "imperfections" Acknowledge self as sexual being

Sample CP: Eating Disorders Program. ELOS: 28 Days Behavioral Unit (Continued)

ND and Categories of Care	Time Dimension	Goals/Actions	Time Dimension	Goals/Actions	Time Dimension	Goals/Actions
Referrals	Day 1 (or when physical condition stable)	Therapists: Occupational, recreational, music, art	Day 14	Image consultant	Day 28	Therapist to address issues of sexuality postdischarge as indicated
Additional assessments	Day 1–7	Suicidal ideation/behaviors	Day 8	Individual strengths/weaknesses		
	Day 3	Sexual history including abuse	Day 8–28	Congruency of feelings/perceptions with actions		
	Day 3–28	Perceptions of body image Family patterns of interaction				
Patient education	Day 1–28	Responsibility for self in family setting	Day 8–10	General wellness needs	Day 21–28	Sex education reflecting individual sexuality and needs
	Day 7–28	Clarify misconceptions of body image	Day 8–28	Human behavior and interactions with family/others—transactional analysis (TA)		
			Day 14	Personal appearance and grooming		
			Day 14–28	Alternative coping strategies for dealing with feelings		
Additional nursing actions	Day 1	Develop therapeutic relationship	Day 7	Compare actual measurements of patient's body with patient's perceptions	Day 14–28	Have patient keep diary of feelings, especially when thinking of food Role-play new behaviors for dealing with feelings and conflicts
	Day 1–28	Provide positive feedback for participation and independent decision making	Day 7–9	Assist with planning to meet individual goals		
		Confront sabotage behavior by family members	Day 8–28	Involve in physical activity/exercise program		
	Day 3–5	Encourage control in areas other than diet				
	Day 4–6	Support development of goals not related to eating				

EATING DISORDERS: OBESITY

Obesity is defined as an excess accumulation of body fat at least 20% over average desired weight for age, sex, and height or a body mass index (kg/m^2) of greater than 27.8 for men and greater than 27.3 for women. Obesity is a chronic condition considered by some to be a disability. The general prognosis for achieving and maintaining weight loss is poor; however, the desire for a healthier lifestyle and reduction of risk factors associated with life-threatening illnesses motivate many people toward diets and weight-loss programs.

CARE SETTING

Community level unless morbid obesity requires brief inpatient stay

RELATED CONCERNS

Cerebrovascular accident/stroke, page 257
Cholecystitis with cholelithiasis, page 390
Cirrhosis of the liver, page 484
Diabetes mellitus/Diabetic ketoacidosis, page 440
Heart failure: chronic, page 47
Hypertension: severe, page 33
Myocardial infarction, page 75
Obesity: surgical interventions (gastric partitioning/gastroplasty, gastric bypass), page 430
Psychosocial aspects of care, page 809
Thrombophlebitis: deep vein thrombosis, page 115

Patient Assessment Database

ACTIVITY/REST

May report: Fatigue, constant drowsiness
Inability/lack of desire to be active or engage in regular exercise
Dyspnea with exertion

May exhibit: Increased heart rate/respirations with activity

CIRCULATION

May exhibit: Hypertension, edema

EGO INTEGRITY

May report: History of cultural/lifestyle factors affecting food choices
Weight may/may not be perceived as a problem
Eating relieves unpleasant feelings, e.g., loneliness, frustration, boredom
Perception of body image as undesirable
SOs resistant to weight loss (may sabotage patient's efforts)

FOOD/FLUID

May report: Normal/excessive ingestion of food
Experimentation with numerous types of diets ("yo-yo" dieting) with varied/short-lived results
History of recurrent weight loss and gain

May exhibit: Weight disproportionate to height
Endomorphic body type (soft/round)
Failure to adjust food intake to diminishing requirements (e.g., change in lifestyle from active to sedentary, aging)

PAIN/DISCOMFORT

May report: Pain/discomfort on weight-bearing joints or spine

RESPIRATION

May report: Dyspnea
May exhibit: Cyanosis, respiratory distress (Pickwickian syndrome)

SEXUALITY

May report: Menstrual disturbances, amenorrhea

TEACHING/LEARNING

May report: Problem may be lifelong or related to life event
Family history of obesity
Concomitant health problems may include hypertension, diabetes, gallbladder and cardiovascular disease, hypothyroidism

Discharge plan   **DRG projected mean length of inpatient stay: 5.1 days**
considerations: May require support with therapeutic regimen

Refer to section at end of plan for postdischarge considerations.

DIAGNOSTIC STUDIES

Metabolic/endocrine studies: May reveal abnormalities, e.g., hypothyroidism, hypopituitarism, hypogonadism, Cushing's syndrome (increased insulin levels), hyperglycemia, hyperlipidemia, hyperuricemia, hyperbilirubinemia. It is also suggested that the cause of these disorders may arise from neuroendocrine abnormalities within the hypothalamus, which result in various chemical disturbances.

Anthropometric measurements: Measures fat-to-muscle ratio.

NURSING PRIORITIES

1. Assist patient to identify a workable method of weight control incorporating healthful foods.
2. Promote improved self-concept, including body image, self-esteem.
3. Encourage health practices to provide for weight control throughout life.

DISCHARGE GOALS

1. Healthy patterns for eating and weight control identified.
2. Weight loss toward desired goal established.
3. Positive perception of self verbalized.
4. Plans developed for future weight control.
5. Plan in place to meet needs after discharge.

NURSING DIAGNOSIS: Nutrition: altered, more than body requirements

May be related to
Food intake that exceeds body needs
Psychosocial factors
Socioeconomic status

Possibly evidenced by
Weight of 20% or more over optimum body weight; excess body fat by skinfold/other measurements
Reported/observed dysfunctional eating patterns, intake more than body requirements

DESIRED OUTCOMES/EVALUATION CRITERIA—PATIENT WILL:

Knowledge: Diet (NOC)

Identify inappropriate behaviors and consequences associated with overeating or weight gain.
Demonstrate change in eating patterns and involvement in individual exercise program.

Nutritional Status (NOC)

Display weight loss with optimal maintenance of health.

ACTIONS/INTERVENTIONS	RATIONALE
Weight Reduction Assistance (NIC)	
Independent	
Review individual cause for obesity, e.g., organic or nonorganic.	Identifies/influences choice of some interventions.
Implement/review daily food diary, e.g., caloric intake, types and amounts of food, eating habits.	Provides the opportunity for the individual to focus on/internalize a realistic picture of the amount of food ingested and corresponding eating habits/feelings. Identifies patterns requiring change and/or a base on which to tailor the dietary program.
Discuss emotions/events associated with eating.	Helps identify when patient is eating to satisfy an emotional need, rather than physiological hunger.
Formulate an eating plan with the patient, using knowledge of individual's height, body build, age, gender, and individual patterns of eating, energy, and nutrient requirements. Determine which diets and strategies have been used, results, individual frustrations/factors interfering with success.	Although there is no basis for recommending one diet over another, a good reducing diet should contain foods from all basic food groups with a focus on low-fat intake and adequate protein intake to prevent loss of lean muscle mass. It is helpful to keep the plan as similar to patient's usual eating pattern as possible. A plan developed with and agreed to by the patient is more likely to be successful.
Emphasize the importance of avoiding fad diets.	Elimination of needed components can lead to metabolic imbalances, e.g., excessive reduction of carbohydrates can lead to fatigue, headache, instability/weakness, and metabolic acidosis (ketosis), interfering with effectiveness of weight loss program.
Discuss need to give self permission to include desired/craved food items in dietary plan.	Denying self by excluding desired/favorite foods results in a sense of deprivation and feelings of guilt/failure when individual "succumbs to temptation." These feelings can sabotage weight loss.
Be alert to binge eating and develop strategies for dealing with these episodes, e.g., substituting other actions for eating.	The patient who binges experiences guilt about it, which is also counterproductive because negative feelings may sabotage further weight loss efforts.
Identify realistic increment goals for weekly weight loss.	Reasonable weight loss (1–2 lb/wk) results in more lasting effects. Excessive/rapid loss may result in fatigue and irritability and ultimately lead to failure in meeting goals for weight loss. Motivation is more easily sustained by meeting "stair-step" goals.
Weigh periodically as individually indicated, and obtain appropriate body measurements.	Provides information about effectiveness of therapeutic regimen and visual evidence of success of patient's efforts. (During hospitalization for controlled fasting, daily weighing may be required. Weekly weighing is more appropriate after discharge.)
Determine current activity levels and plan progressive exercise program (e.g., walking) tailored to the individual's goals and choice.	Exercise furthers weight loss by reducing appetite; increasing energy; toning muscles; and enhancing cardiac fitness, sense of well-being, and accomplishment. Commitment on the part of the patient enables the setting of more realistic goals and adherence to the plan.
Develop an appetite reeducation plan with patient.	Signals of hunger and fullness often are not recognized, have become distorted, or are ignored.

ACTIONS/INTERVENTIONS	RATIONALE

Independent

Emphasize the importance of avoiding tension at mealtimes and not eating too quickly.

Reducing tension provides a more relaxed eating atmosphere and encourages more leisurely eating patterns. This is important because a period of time is required for the appestat mechanism to know the stomach is full.

Encourage patient to eat only at a table or designated eating place and to avoid standing while eating.

Techniques that modify behavior may be helpful in avoiding diet failure.

Discuss restriction of salt intake and diuretic drugs if used.

Water retention may be a problem because of increased fluid intake and fat metabolism.

Reassess calorie requirements every 2–4 wk; provide additional support when plateaus occur.

Changes in weight and exercise necessitate changes in plan. As weight is lost, changes in metabolism occur, resulting in plateaus when weight remains stable for periods of time. This can create distrust and lead to accusations of "cheating" on caloric intake, which are not helpful. Patient may need additional support at this time.

Collaborative

Consult with dietitian to determine caloric/nutrient requirements for individual weight loss.

Individual intake can be calculated by several different formulas, but weight reduction is based on the basal caloric requirement for 24 hr, depending on patient's sex, age, current/desired weight, and length of time estimated to achieve desired weight. *Note:* Standard tables are subject to error when applied to individual situations, and circadian rhythms/lifestyle patterns need to be considered.

Provide medications as indicated:

Appetite-suppressant drugs, e.g., diethylpropion (Tenuate), mazindol (Sanorex);

May be used with caution/supervision at the beginning of a weight loss program to support patient during stress of behavioral/lifestyle changes. They are only effective for a few weeks and may cause problems of addiction in some people.

Hormonal therapy, e.g., thyroid (Euthroid);

May be necessary when hypothyroidism is present. When no deficiency is present, replacement therapy is not helpful and may actually be harmful. *Note:* Other hormonal treatments, such as human chorionic gonadrotropin (HCG), although widely publicized, have no documented evidence of value.

Vitamin, mineral supplements.

Obese individuals have large fuel reserves but are often deficient in vitamins and minerals.

Hospitalize for fasting regimen and/or stabilization of medical problems, when indicated.

Aggressive therapy/support may be necessary to initiate weight loss, although fasting is not generally a treatment of choice. Patient can be monitored more effectively in a controlled setting, to minimize complications such as postural hypotension, anemia, cardiac irregularities, and decreased uric acid excretion with hyperuricemia.

Prepare for surgical interventions, e.g., gastric partitioning/bypass, as indicated.

These interventions may be necessary to help the patient lose weight when obesity is life-threatening. (Refer to CP: Obesity: Surgical Interventions, p. 430.)

> **NURSING DIAGNOSIS: Body Image disturbance/Self-Esteem, chronic low**
>
> **May be related to**
>
> Biophysical/psychosocial factors such as patient's view of self (slimness is valued in this society, and mixed messages are received when thinness is stressed)
>
> Family/subculture encouragement of overeating
>
> Control, sex, and love issues
>
> **Possibly evidenced by**
>
> Verbalization of negative feelings about body (mental image often does not match physical reality)
>
> Fear of rejection/reaction by others
>
> Feelings of hopelessness/powerlessness
>
> Preoccupation with change (attempts to lose weight)
>
> Lack of follow-through with diet plan
>
> Verbalization of powerlessness to change eating habits
>
> **DESIRED OUTCOMES/EVALUATION CRITERIA—PATIENT WILL:**
>
> **Body Image (NOC)**
>
> Verbalize a more realistic self-image.
>
> Demonstrate some acceptance of self as is, rather than an idealized image.
>
> **Self-Esteem (NOC)**
>
> Seek information and actively pursue appropriate weight loss.
>
> Acknowledge self as an individual who has responsibility for self.

ACTIONS/INTERVENTIONS	RATIONALE
Body Image Enhancement (NIC)	
Independent	
Determine patient's view of being fat and what it does for the individual.	Mental image includes our ideal and is usually not up-to-date. Fat and compulsive eating behaviors may have deep-rooted psychological implications, (e.g., compensation for lack of love and nurturing or a defense against intimacy).
Provide privacy during care activities.	Individual usually is sensitive/self-conscious about body.
Promote open communication avoiding criticism/judgment about patient's behavior.	Supports patient's own responsibility for weight loss; enhances sense of control, and promotes willingness to discuss difficulties/setbacks and problem-solve. *Note:* Distrust and accusations of "cheating" on caloric intake are not helpful.
Outline and clearly state responsibilities of patient and nurse.	It is helpful for each individual to understand area of own responsibility in the program so that misunderstandings do not arise.
Graph weight on a weekly basis.	Provides ongoing visual evidence of weight changes (reality orientation).
Encourage patient to use imagery to visualize self at desired weight and to practice handling of new behaviors.	Mental rehearsal is very useful in helping the patient plan for and deal with anticipated change in self-image or occasions that may arise (family gatherings, special dinners) where constant decisions about eating many foods will occur.

ACTIONS/INTERVENTIONS	RATIONALE
Independent	
Provide information about the use of makeup, hairstyles, and ways of dressing to maximize figure assets.	Enhances feelings of self-esteem; promotes improved body image.
Encourage buying clothes instead of food treats as a reward for weight loss.	Properly fitting clothes enhance the body image as small losses are made and the individual feels more positive. Waiting until the desired weight loss is reached can become discouraging.
Suggest the patient dispose of "fat clothes."	Removes the "safety valve" of having clothes available "in case" the weight is regained. Retaining fat clothes can convey the message that the weight loss will not occur/be maintained.
Have patient recall coping patterns related to food in family of origin and explore how these may affect current situation.	Parents act as role models for the child. Maladaptive coping patterns (overeating) are learned within the family system and are supported through positive reinforcement. Food may be substituted by the parent for affection and love, and eating is associated with a feeling of satisfaction, becoming the primary defense.
Determine relationship history and possibility of sexual abuse.	May contribute to current issues of self-esteem/patterns of coping.
Identify patient's motivation for weight loss and assist with goal setting.	The individual may harbor repressed feelings of hostility, which may be expressed inward on the self. Because of a poor self-concept, the person often has difficulty with relationships. *Note:* When losing weight for someone else, the patient is less likely to be successful/maintain weight loss.
Be alert to myths the patient/SO may have about weight and weight loss.	Beliefs about what an ideal body looks like or unconscious motivations can sabotage efforts to lose weight. Some of these include the feminine thought of "If I become thin, men will pursue me or rape me"; the masculine counterpart, "I don't trust myself to stay in control of my sexual feelings"; as well as issues of strength, power, or the "good cook" image.
Assist patient to identify feelings that lead to compulsive eating. Encourage journaling.	Awareness of emotions that lead to overeating can be the first step in behavior change (e.g., people often eat because of depression, anger, and guilt).
Develop strategies for doing something besides eating for dealing with these feelings, e.g., talking with a friend.	Replacing eating with other activities helps retrain old patterns and establish new ways to deal with feelings.
Help staff be aware of and deal with own feelings when caring for patient.	Judgmental attitudes, feelings of disgust, anger, and weariness can interfere with care/be transmitted to patient, reinforcing negative self-concept/image.
Collaborative	
Refer to community support and/or therapy group.	Support groups can provide companionship, enhance motivation, decrease loneliness and social ostracism, and give practical solutions to common problems. Group therapy can be helpful in dealing with underlying psychological concerns.

> **NURSING DIAGNOSIS: Social Interaction, impaired**
>
> **May be related to**
> Verbalized or observed discomfort in social situations
> Self-concept disturbance
>
> **Possibly evidenced by**
> Reluctance to participate in social gatherings
> Verbalization of a sense of discomfort with others
>
> **DESIRED OUTCOMES/EVALUATION CRITERIA—PATIENT WILL:**
>
> **Social Involvement (NOC)**
>
> Verbalize awareness of feelings that lead to poor social interactions.
> Become involved in achieving positive changes in social behaviors and interpersonal relationships.

ACTIONS/INTERVENTIONS	RATIONALE
Socialization Enhancement (NIC)	
Independent	
Review family patterns of relating and social behaviors.	Social interaction is primarily learned within the family of origin. When inadequate patterns are identified, actions for change can be instituted.
Encourage patient to express feelings and perceptions of problems.	Helps identify and clarify reasons for difficulties in interacting with others, e.g., may feel unloved/unlovable or insecure about sexuality.
Assess patient's use of coping skills and defense mechanisms.	May have coping skills that will be useful in the process of weight loss. Defense mechanisms used to protect the individual may contribute to feelings of aloneness/isolation.
Have patient list behaviors that cause discomfort.	Identifies specific concerns and suggests actions that can be taken to effect change.
Involve in role-playing new ways to deal with identified behaviors/situations.	Practicing these new behaviors enables the individual to become comfortable with them in a safe situation.
Discuss negative self-concepts and self-talk, e.g., "No one wants to be with a fat person," "Who would be interested in talking to me?"	May be impeding positive social interactions.
Encourage use of positive self-talk such as telling oneself "I am OK," or "I can enjoy social activities and do not need to be controlled by what others think or say."	Positive strategies enhance feelings of comfort and support efforts for change.
Collaborative	
Refer for ongoing family or individual therapy as indicated.	Patient benefits from involvement of SO to provide support and encouragement.

427

> **NURSING DIAGNOSIS: Knowledge Deficit [Learning Need] regarding condition, prognosis, treatment, self care, and discharge needs**
>
> **May be related to**
> Lack of/misinterpretation of information
> Lack of interest in learning, lack of recall
> Inaccurate/incomplete information presented
>
> **Possibly evidenced by**
> Statements of lack of/request for information about obesity and nutritional requirements
> Verbalization of problem with weight reduction
> Inadequate follow-through with previous diet and exercise instructions
>
> **DESIRED OUTCOMES/EVALUATION CRITERIA—PATIENT WILL:**
>
> **Knowledge: Diet (NOC)**
>
> Verbalize understanding of need for lifestyle changes to maintain/control weight.
> Establish individual goal and plan for attaining that goal.
> Begin to look for information about nutrition and ways to control weight.

ACTIONS/INTERVENTIONS

Teaching: Prescribed Diet (NIC)

Independent

Determine level of nutritional knowledge and what patient believes is most urgent need.

Identify individual holistic long-term goals for health (e.g., lowering blood pressure, controlling serum lipid and glucose levels).

Provide information about ways to maintain satisfactory food intake in settings away from home.

Identify other sources of information, e.g., books, tapes, community classes, groups.

Emphasize necessity of continued follow-up care/counseling, especially when plateaus occur.

Identify alternatives to chosen activity program to accommodate weather, travel, and so on. Discuss use of mechanical devices/equipment for reducing.

Determine optimal exercise heart rate. Demonstrate proper technique to monitor pulse.

Discuss necessity of good skin care, especially during summer months/following exercise.

RATIONALE

Necessary to know what additional information to provide. When patient's views are listened to, trust is enhanced.

A high relapse rate at 5-year follow-up suggests obesity cannot be reliably reversed/cured. Shifting the focus from initial weight loss/percentage of body fat to overall wellness may enhance rehabilitation.

"Smart" eating when dining out or when traveling helps individual manage weight while still enjoying social outlets.

Using different avenues of accessing information furthers patient's learning. Involvement with others who are also losing weight can provide support.

As weight is lost, changes in metabolism occur, interfering with further loss by creating a plateau as the body activates a survival mechanism, attempting to prevent "starvation." This requires new strategies and aggressive support to continue weight loss.

Promotes continuation of program. *Note:* Fat loss occurs on a generalized overall basis, and there is no evidence that spot reducing or mechanical devices aid in weight loss in specific areas; however, specific types of exercise or equipment may be useful in toning specific body parts.

Promotes safety as patient exercises to tolerance, not peer pressure.

Prevents skin breakdown in moist skinfolds.

ACTIONS/INTERVENTIONS	RATIONALE
Independent	
Identify alternative ways to "reward" self/family for accomplishments or to provide solace.	Reduces likelihood of relying on food to deal with feelings.
Encourage involvement in social activities that are not centered around food, e.g., bike ride/nature hike, attending musical event, group sporting activities.	Provides opportunity for pleasure and relaxation without "temptation." Activities/exercise may also use calories to help maintain desired weight.

POTENTIAL CONSIDERATIONS following acute hospitalization (dependent on patient's age, physical condition/presence of complications, personal resources, and life responsibilities)

Therapeutic Regimen: Individual, ineffective management—complexity of therapeutic regimen, perceived seriousness/benefits, mistrust of regimen and/or health care personnel, excessive demands made on individual, family conflict.

OBESITY: SURGICAL INTERVENTIONS (GASTRIC PARTITIONING/GASTROPLASTY, GASTRIC BYPASS)

Weight reduction surgery has been reported to improve several co-morbid conditions such as sleep apnea, glucose intolerance and frank diabetes, hypertension, and hyperlipidemia. A number of surgical treatments for morbid obesity have been tried and discarded because of ineffectiveness or complications. The procedure of choice is vertical-banded gastroplasty. On occasion, gastric bypass may be performed.

Gastroplasty (gastric stapling): A small pouch with a restricted outlet is created across the stomach just distal to the gastroesophageal junction. A small opening remains, through which food passes into stomach.

Gastric bypass: Anastomosis of jejunum to upper portion of stomach, bypassing rest of stomach. Use has been generally abandoned because of complications, particularly hepatic failure.

CARE SETTING

Inpatient acute surgical unit

RELATED CONCERNS

Eating disorders: obesity, page 421
Peritonitis, page 382
Psychosocial aspects of care, page 809
Surgical intervention, page 828
Thrombophlebitis: deep vein thrombosis, page 115

Patient Assessment Database

ACTIVITY/REST

May report:	Difficulty sleeping
	Exertional discomfort, inability to participate in desired activity/sports

EGO INTEGRITY

May report:	Motivated to lose weight for oneself (or for gratification of others)
	Repressed feelings of hostility toward authority figures
	History of psychiatric illness/treatment
May exhibit:	Anxiety, depression

FOOD/FLUID

May report:	"Yo-Yo" dieting
	Weight fluctuations
	Dysfunctional eating patterns
May exhibit:	Weight exceeding ideal body weight by 100% or more (morbid obesity)

TEACHING/LEARNING

May report:	Presence of chronic conditions (hypertension, diabetes, arthritis, sleep apnea, Pickwickian syndrome, infertility)
	Adequate trials and failure of other treatment approaches
	Desire to lose weight
Discharge plan considerations:	**DRG projected mean length of inpatient stay: 7.4 days**
	May require support with therapeutic regimen/weight loss, assistance with self-care, homemaker/maintenance tasks
	Refer to section at end of plan for postdischarge considerations.

DIAGNOSTIC STUDIES

Studies depend on individual situation, and are used to rule out underlying disease and provide a preoperative workup, including psychiatric evaluation.

NURSING PRIORITIES

1. Support respiratory function.
2. Prevent/minimize complications.
3. Provide appropriate nutritional intake.
4. Provide information regarding surgical procedure, postoperative expectations, and treatment needs.

DISCHARGE GOALS

1. Ventilation and oxygenation adequate for individual needs.
2. Complications prevented/controlled.
3. Nutritional intake modified for specific procedure.
4. Procedure, prognosis, and therapeutic regimen understood.
5. Plan in place to meet needs after discharge.

NURSING DIAGNOSIS: Breathing Pattern, ineffective

May be related to
Decreased lung expansion
Pain, anxiety
Decreased energy, fatigue
Tracheobronchial obstruction

Possibly evidenced by
Shortness of breath, dyspnea
Tachypnea, respiratory depth changes, reduced vital capacity
Wheezes, rhonchi
Abnormal ABGs

DESIRED OUTCOMES/EVALUATION CRITERIA—PATIENT WILL:

Respiratory Status: Ventilation (NOC)

Maintain adequate ventilation.
Experience no cyanosis or other signs of hypoxia, with ABGs within acceptable range.

ACTIONS/INTERVENTIONS	RATIONALE
Ventilation Assistance (NIC)	
Independent	
Monitor respiratory rate/depth. Auscultate breath sounds. Investigate presence of pallor/cyanosis, increased restlessness, or confusion.	Shallow respirations/effects of anesthesia cause hypoventilation, potentiate atelectasis, and may result in hypoxia. *Note:* Many anesthetic agents are fat-soluble, so that postoperative sedation and the potential for respiratory complications are increased.
Elevate head of bed 30 degrees.	Encourages optimal diaphragmatic excursion/lung expansion and minimizes pressure of abdominal contents on the thoracic cavity. *Note:* When kept recumbent, obese patients are at high risk for severe hypoventilation postoperatively.
Encourage deep-breathing exercises. Assist with coughing and splint incision.	Promotes maximal lung expansion and aids in clearing airways, thus reducing risk of atelectasis, pneumonia.
Turn periodically and ambulate as early as possible.	Promotes aeration of all segments of the lung, mobilizing and aiding in expectoration of secretions.
Pad side rails and teach patient to use them as armrests.	Using the side rail as an armrest allows for greater chest expansion.

ACTIONS/INTERVENTIONS

Independent

Use small pillow under head when indicated.

Avoid use of abdominal binders.

Collaborative

Administer supplemental oxygen.

Assist in use of intermittent positive pressure breathing (IPPB) and/or respiratory adjuncts, e.g., incentive spirometer.

Monitor/graph serial ABGs/pulse oximetry when indicated.

Monitor patient-controlled analgesia (PCA)/administer analgesics as appropriate.

RATIONALE

Many obese patients have large, thick necks, and use of large, fluffy pillows may obstruct the airway.

Can restrict lung expansion.

Maximizes available O_2 for exchange and reduces work of breathing.

Enhances lung expansion; reduces potential for atelectasis.

Reflects ventilation/oxygenation and acid-base status. Used as a basis for evaluating need for/effectiveness of respiratory therapies.

Maintenance of comfort level enhances participation in respiratory therapy, and promotes increased lung expansion.

NURSING DIAGNOSIS: Tissue Perfusion, risk for altered: peripheral

Risk factors may include
Diminished blood flow, hypovolemia
Immobility/bed rest
Interruption of venous blood flow (thrombosis)

Possibly evidenced by
[Not applicable; presence of signs and symptoms establishes an *actual* diagnosis]

DESIRED OUTCOMES/EVALUATION CRITERIA—PATIENT WILL:

Circulation status (NOC)

Maintain perfusion as individually appropriate, e.g., skin warm/dry, peripheral pulses present/strong, vital signs within acceptable range.

Risk Control (NOC)

Identify causative/risk factors.
Demonstrate behaviors to improve/maintain circulation.

ACTIONS/INTERVENTIONS

Circulatory Care (NIC)

Independent

Monitor vital signs. Palpate peripheral pulses routinely; evaluate capillary refill and changes in mentation. Note 24-hr fluid balance.

Encourage frequent range-of-motion (ROM) exercises for legs and ankles.

Assess for Homans' sign, redness, and edema of calf.

Encourage early ambulation; discourage sitting and/or dangling legs at the bedside.

RATIONALE

Indicators of circulatory adequacy. (Refer to ND: Fluid Volume risk for deficit, following.)

Stimulates circulation in the lower extremities; reduces venous stasis.

Indicators of thrombus formation but may not always be present, particularly in obese individuals.

Sitting constricts venous flow, whereas walking encourages venous return.

432

ACTIONS/INTERVENTIONS

Independent

Provide adequate/appropriate equipment and sufficient staff for handling patient.

Collaborative

Administer heparin therapy, as indicated.

Monitor hemoglobin (Hb)/hematocrit (Hct) and coagulation studies.

RATIONALE

Helpful in dealing with the bulky patient for moving, bowel care, and ambulating. Reduces risk of traumatic injury to patient and caregivers.

May be used prophylactically to reduce risk of thrombus formation or to treat thromboemboli.

Provides information about circulatory volume/alterations in coagulation and indicates therapy needs/effectiveness.

NURSING DIAGNOSIS: Fluid Volume, risk for deficit

Risk factors may include
Excessive gastric losses: nasogastric suction, diarrhea
Reduced intake

Possibly evidenced by
[Not applicable; presence of signs and symptoms establishes an *actual* diagnosis.]

DESIRED OUTCOMES/EVALUATION CRITERIA—PATIENT WILL:

> **Hydration (NOC)**

Maintain adequate fluid volume with balanced intake and output (I&O) and be free of signs reflecting dehydration.

ACTIONS/INTERVENTIONS

> **Fluid/Electrolyte Management (NIC)**

Independent

Assess vital signs, noting changes in BP (postural), tachycardia, fever. Assess skin turgor, capillary refill, and moisture of mucous membranes.

Monitor I&O, noting/measuring diarrhea and NG suction losses.

Evaluate muscle strength/tone. Observe for muscle tremors.

Establish individual needs/replacement schedule.

Encourage increased oral intake when able.

Collaborative

Administer supplemental IV fluids as indicated.

RATIONALE

Indicators of dehydration/hypovolemia, adequacy of current fluid replacement. *Note:* Adequately sized cuff must be used to ensure factual measurement of BP. If cuff is too small, reading will be falsely elevated.

Changes in gastric capacity/intestinal motility and nausea greatly influence intake and fluid needs, increasing risk of dehydration.

Large gastric losses may result in decreased magnesium and calcium, leading to neuromuscular weakness/tetany.

Determined by amount of measured losses/estimated insensible losses and dependent on gastric capacity.

Permits discontinuation of invasive fluid support measures and contributes to return of normal bowel functioning.

Replaces fluid losses and restores fluid balance in immediate postoperative phase and/or until patient is able to take sufficient oral fluids.

ACTIONS/INTERVENTIONS

Collaborative

Monitor electrolyte levels and replace as indicated.

RATIONALE

Use of nasogastric (NG) tube and/or vomiting, onset of diarrhea can deplete electrolytes, affecting organ function.

NURSING DIAGNOSIS: Nutrition: altered, risk for less than body requirements

Risk factors may include
Decreased intake, dietary restrictions, early satiety
Increased metabolic rate/healing
Malabsorption of nutrients/impaired absorption of vitamins

Possibly evidenced by
[Not applicable; presence of signs and symptoms establishes an *actual* diagnosis]

DESIRED OUTCOMES/EVALUATION CRITERIA—PATIENT WILL:

> **Knowledge: Diet (NOC)**

Identify individual nutritional needs.

> **Nutritional Status (NOC)**

Display behaviors to maintain adequate nutritional intake.
Demonstrate appropriate weight loss with normalization of laboratory values.

ACTIONS/INTERVENTIONS

> **Weight Reduction Assistance (NIC)**

Independent

Establish hourly intake schedule. Measure/provide food and fluids in amount specified following gastric stapling.

Instruct in how to sip and eat slowly.

Stress importance of being aware of satiety and stopping intake.

Require that patient sit up to drink/eat.

Determine foods that are gas forming and eliminate from diet.

Discuss food preferences with patient and include those foods in pureed diet when possible.

Weigh daily. Establish regular schedule after discharge.

Collaborative

Provide liquid diet, advancing to soft foods that are high in protein and bulk and low in fat, with liquid supplements as needed.

RATIONALE

After partitioning, gastric capacity is reduced to approximately 50 mL, necessitating frequent/small feedings. Management of optimal nutrition depends on reducing the amount of food/fluid (e.g., 1 oz of fluid or 300 calories) passing through the gastrointestinal (GI) system at one time.

Increases satiety and reduces risk of dehydration.

Overeating may cause nausea/vomiting or damage partitioning.

Reduces possibility of aspiration.

May interfere with appetite/digestion and restrict nutritional intake.

May enhance intake, promote sense of participation/control.

Monitors losses and aids in assessing nutritional needs/effectiveness of therapy.

Provides nutrients without exceeding calorie limits
Note: Liquid diet is usually maintained for 8 wk after partitioning procedure.

ACTIONS/INTERVENTIONS

Collaborative

Refer to dietitian.

Administer vitamin supplements and B$_{12}$ injections, folate, and calcium as indicated.

RATIONALE

May need assistance in planning a diet that meets nutritional needs.

Supplements may be needed to prevent anemia because absorption is impaired. Increased intestinal motility following bypass procedure lowers calcium level and increases absorption of oxalates, which can lead to urinary stone formation.

NURSING DIAGNOSIS: Skin Integrity, actual and risk for impaired

May be related to
Trauma/surgery; difficulty in approximation of suture line of fatty tissue
Reduced vascularity, altered circulation
Altered nutritional state: obesity

Possibly evidenced by (actual)
Disruption of skin surface, altered healing

DESIRED OUTCOMES/EVALUATION CRITERIA—PATIENT WILL:

| Wound Healing: Primary Intention (NOC) |

Display timely wound healing without complication.
Demonstrate behaviors to reduce tension on suture line.

ACTIONS/INTERVENTIONS

| Wound Care (NIC)) |

Independent

Support incision when turning, coughing, deep-breathing, and ambulating.

Observe incisions periodically, noting approximation of wound edges, hematoma formation and resolution, presence of bleeding/drainage.

Provide routine incisional care, being careful to keep dressings dry and sterile. Assess patency of drains.

| Skin Surveillance (NIC) |

Encourage frequent position change, inspect pressure points, and massage gently as indicated. Apply transparent skin barrier to elbows/heels.

Provide meticulous skin care; pay particular attention to skin folds.

Provide foam/air mattress or kinetic therapy as indicated.

RATIONALE

Reduces possibility of dehiscence and incisional hernia.

Influences choice of interventions.

Promotes healing. Accumulation of serosanguinous drainage in subcutaneous layers increases tension on suture line, may delay wound healing, and serves as a medium for bacterial growth.

Reduces pressure on skin, promoting peripheral circulation and reducing risk of skin breakdown. Skin barrier reduces risk of shearing injury.

Moisture or excoriation enhances growth of bacteria that can lead to postoperative infection.

Reduces skin pressure and enhances circulation.

ACTIONS/INTERVENTIONS	RATIONALE
Infection Protection (NIC)	
Independent	
Stress/model proper handwashing technique.	Prevents spread of bacteria, cross-contamination.
Maintain aseptic technique in dressing changes, invasive procedures.	Reduces risk of nosocomial infection.
Inspect surgical incisions/invasive sites for erythema, purulent drainage.	Early detection of developing infection provides for prevention of more serious complications.
Encourage frequent position changes; deep breathing, coughing, use of respiratory adjuncts, e.g., incentive spirometer.	Promotes mobilization of secretions, reducing risk of pneumonia.
Provide routine catheter care/encourage good perineal care.	Prevents ascending bladder infections.
Encourage patient to drink acid-ash juices, such as cranberry.	Maintains urine acidity to retard bacterial growth.
Observe for reports of abdominal pain (especially after third postoperative day), elevated temperature, increased white blood cell (WBC) count.	Suggests possibility of developing peritonitis.
Collaborative	
Apply topical antimicrobials/antibiotics as indicated.	Reduces bacterial or fungal colonization on skin; prevents infection in wound.
Administer IV antibiotics as indicated.	A prophylactic antibiotic regimen is usually standard in these patients to reduce risk of perioperative contamination and/or peritonitis.
Obtain specimen of purulent drainage/sputum for culture and sensitivity.	Identifies infectious agent, aids in choice of appropriate therapy.

NURSING DIAGNOSIS: Diarrhea

May be related to
Rapid transit of food through shortened small intestine
Changes in dietary fiber and bulk
Inflammation, irritation, and malabsorption of bowel

Possibly evidenced by
Loose, liquid stools, increased frequency.
Increased/hyperactive bowel sounds

DESIRED OUTCOMES/EVALUATION CRITERIA—PATIENT WILL:

Treatment Behavior: Illness or Injury (NOC)

Verbalize understanding of causative factors and rationale of treatment regimen.
Follow through with treatment recommendations.

Bowel Elimination (NOC)

Regain near-normal bowel function.

ACTIONS/INTERVENTIONS	RATIONALE
Diarrhea Management (NIC)	
Independent	
Observe/record stool frequency, characteristics, and amount.	Diarrhea often develops after resumption of diet.
Encourage diet high in fiber/bulk within dietary limitations, with moderate fluid intake as diet resumes.	Increases consistency of the effluent. Although fluid is necessary for optimal body function, excessive amounts contribute to diarrhea.
Restrict fat intake as indicated.	Low-fat diet reduces risk of steatorrhea and limits laxative effect of decreased fat absorption.
Observe for signs of "dumping syndrome," e.g., instant diarrhea, sweating, nausea, and weakness after eating.	Rapid emptying of food from the stomach may result in gastric distress and alter bowel function.
Assist with frequent perianal care, using ointments as indicated. Provide whirlpool bath.	Anal irritation, excoriation, and pruritus occur because of diarrhea. The patient often cannot reach the area for proper cleansing and may be embarrassed to ask for help.
Collaborative	
Administer medications as indicated, e.g., diphenoxylate with atropine (Lomotil).	May be necessary to control frequency of stools until body adjusts to changes in function brought about by surgery.
Monitor serum electrolytes.	Increased gastric losses potentiate the risk of electrolyte imbalance, which can lead to more serious/life-threatening complications.

ACTIONS/INTERVENTIONS	RATIONALE
Teaching: Disease Process (NIC)	
Independent	
Review specific surgical procedure and postoperative expectations.	Provides knowledge base from which informed choices can be made and goals formulated. Initial weight loss is rapid, with patient often losing half of the total weight loss during the first 6 months. Weight loss then gradually slows over a 2-yr period.
Address concerns about altered body size/image.	Anticipation of problems can be helpful in dealing with situations that arise. (Refer to CP: Eating Disorders: Obesity, ND: Body Image disturbance/Self-Esteem, chronic low, p. 425.) *Note:* Feelings that often occur during more conventional weight loss therapies generally are not encountered in the surgically treated patient.
Review medication regimen, dosage, and side effects.	Knowledge may enhance cooperation with therapeutic regimen and in maintenance of schedule.
Recommend avoidance of alcohol.	May contribute to liver/pancreatic dysfunction.
Discuss responsibility for self-care with patient/SO.	Full cooperation is important for successful outcome after procedure.
Stress importance of regular medical follow-up, including laboratory studies, and discuss possible health problems.	Periodic assessment/evaluation (e.g., over 3–12 mo) promotes early recognition/prevention of such complications as liver dysfunction, malnutrition, electrolyte imbalances, and kidney stones, which may develop after bypass procedure.
Encourage progressive exercise/activity program balanced with adequate rest periods.	Promotes weight loss, enhances muscle tone, and minimizes postoperative complications while preventing undue fatigue.

ACTIONS/INTERVENTIONS	RATIONALE
Independent	
Review proper eating habits, e.g., eat small amounts of food slowly and chew well, sit at table in calm/relaxed environment, eat only at prescribed times, avoid between-meal snacking, do not "make up" skipped feedings.	Focuses attention on eating, increasing awareness of intake and feelings of satiety.
Avoid fluid intake $\frac{1}{2}$ hr before/after meals and use of carbonated beverages.	May cause gastric fullness/gaseous distension, limiting intake of food.
Identify signs of hypokalemia, e.g., diarrhea, muscle cramps/weakness of lower extremities, weak/irregular pulse, dizziness with position changes.	Increasing dietary intake of potassium (e.g., milk, coffee, potatoes, carrots, bananas, oranges) may correct deficit, preventing serious respiratory/cardiac complications.
Discuss symptoms that may indicate dumping syndrome, e.g., weakness, profuse perspiration, nausea, vomiting, faintness, flushing, and epigastric discomfort or palpitations, occurring during or immediately following meals. Problem-solve solutions.	Generally occurring in early postoperative period (1–3 wk), syndrome is usually self-limiting but may become chronic and require medical intervention.
Review symptoms requiring medical evaluation, e.g., persistent nausea/vomiting, abdominal distension/tenderness, change in pattern of bowel elimination, fever, purulent wound drainage, excessive weight loss or plateauing/weight gain.	Early recognition of developing complications allows for prompt intervention, preventing serious outcome.
Refer to community support groups.	Involvement with others who have dealt with same problems enhances coping; may promote cooperation with therapeutic regimen and long-term positive recovery.

POTENTIAL CONSIDERATIONS following acute hospitalization (dependent on patient's age, physical condition/presence of complications, personal resources, and life responsibilities)

Nutrition: altered, risk for more than body requirements—dysfunctional eating patterns, observed use of food as reward/comfort measure, history of morbid obesity.

Refer to Potential Considerations in Surgical Intervention plan of care (p. 828).

DIABETES MELLITUS/DIABETIC KETOACIDOSIS

Diabetes affects 18% of people over the age of 65, and approximately 625,000 new cases of diabetes are diagnosed annually in the general population. Conditions or situations known to exacerbate glucose/insulin imbalance include: (1) previously undiagnosed or newly diagnosed type 1 diabetes; (2) food intake in excess of available insulin; (3) adolescence and puberty; (4) exercise in uncontrolled diabetes; and (5) stress associated with illness, infection, trauma, or emotional distress. Type 1 diabetes can be complicated by instability and diabetic ketoacidosis (DKA). DKA is a life-threatening emergency caused by a relative or absolute deficiency of insulin.

CARE SETTING

Although DKA may be encountered in any setting and mild DKA may be managed at the community level, severe metabolic imbalance requires inpatient acute care on a medical unit.

RELATED CONCERNS

Amputation, page 697
Fluid and electrolyte imbalances, page 926
Metabolic acidosis (primary base bicarbonate deficit), page 523
Psychosocial aspects of care, page 809

Patient Assessment Database

Data depend on the severity and duration of metabolic imbalance, length/stage of diabetic process, and effects on other organ function.

ACTIVITY/REST

May report:	Sleep/rest disturbances Weakness, fatigue, difficulty walking/moving Muscle cramps, decreased muscle strength
May exhibit:	Tachycardia and tachypnea at rest or with activity Lethargy/disorientation, coma Decreased muscle strength/tone

CIRCULATION

May report:	History of hypertension; acute myocardial infarction (MI) Claudication, numbness, tingling of extremities (long-term effects) Leg ulcers, slow healing
May exhibit:	Tachycardia Postural BP changes; hypertension Decreased/absent pulses Dysrhythmias Crackles; jugular venous distention (JVD) (if heart failure [HF] present) Hot, dry, flushed skin; sunken eyeballs

EGO INTEGRITY

May report:	Stress; dependence on others Life stressors including financial concerns related to condition
May exhibit:	Anxiety, irritability

ELIMINATION

May report:	Change in usual voiding pattern (polyuria), nocturia Pain/burning, difficulty voiding (infection), recent/recurrent urinary tract infection (UTI) Abdominal tenderness, bloating Diarrhea
May exhibit:	Pale, yellow, dilute urine; polyuria (may progress to oliguria/anuria if severe hypovolemia occurs) Cloudy, odorous urine (infection)

Abdomen firm, distended
Bowel sounds diminished or hyperactive (diarrhea)

FOOD/FLUID

May report: Loss of appetite; nausea/vomiting
Not following diet; increased intake of glucose/carbohydrates
Weight loss over a period of days/weeks
Thirst
Use of medications exacerbating dehydration, such as diuretics

May exhibit: Dry/cracked skin, poor skin turgor
Abdominal rigidity/distension
Thyroid may be enlarged (increased metabolic needs with increased blood sugar)
Halitosis/sweet, fruity odor (acetone breath)

NEUROSENSORY

May report: Fainting spells/dizziness
Headaches
Tingling, numbness, weakness in muscles
Visual disturbances

May exhibit: Confusion/disorientation; drowsiness, lethargy, stupor/coma (later stages)
Memory impairment (recent, remote)
Deep tendon reflexes (DTRs) decreased (coma)
Seizure activity (late stages of DKA or hypoglycemia)

PAIN/DISCOMFORT

May report: Abdominal bloating/pain (mild/severe)
May exhibit: Facial grimacing with palpation; guarding

RESPIRATION

May report: Air hunger (late stages of DKA)
Cough, with/without purulent sputum (infection)

May exhibit: Increased respiratory rate (tachypnea); deep, rapid (Kussmaul's) respirations (metabolic acidosis)
Rhonchi, wheezes
Yellow or green sputum (infection)

SAFETY

May report: Dry, itching skin; skin ulcerations
Paresthesia (diabetic neuropathy)

May exhibit: Fever, diaphoresis
Skin breakdown, lesions/ulcerations
Decreased general strength/ROM
Weakness/paralysis of muscles, including respiratory musculature (if potassium levels are markedly decreased)

SEXUALITY

May report: Vaginal discharge (prone to infection)
Problems with impotence (men); orgasmic difficulty (women)

TEACHING/LEARNING

May report: Familial risk factors: diabetes mellitus (DM), heart disease, strokes, hypertension
Slow/delayed healing
Use of drugs, e.g., steroids, thiazide diuretics, Dilantin, and phenobarbital (can increase glucose levels)
May/may not be taking diabetic medications as ordered

Discharge plan considerations:	DRG projected mean length of inpatient stay: 5.9 days
	May need assistance with dietary regimen, medication administration/supplies, self-care, glucose monitoring

Refer to section at end of plan for postdischarge considerations.

DIAGNOSTIC STUDIES

Serum glucose: Increased 200–1000 mg/dL or more.

Serum acetone (ketones): Strongly positive.

Fatty acids: Lipids, triglycerides, and cholesterol level elevated.

Serum osmolality: Elevated but usually less than 330 mOsm/L.

Glucagon: Elevated level is associated with conditions that produce (1) actual hypoglycemia, (2) relative lack of glucose (e.g., trauma, infection), or (3) lack of insulin. Therefore, glucagon may be elevated with severe DKA despite hyperglycemia.

Glycosylated hemoglobin (HbA$_{1c}$): Levels 2–4 times normal reflect poor control of DM during past 2–3 mo and is therefore useful in differentiating inadequate control versus incident-related DKA (e.g., current upper respiratory infection [URI]).

Serum insulin: May be decreased/absent (type 1) or normal to high (type 2), indicating insulin insufficiency/improper utilization (endogenous/exogenous). Insulin resistance may develop secondary to formation of antibodies.

Electrolytes:

    Sodium: May be normal, elevated, or decreased.

    Potassium: Normal or falsely elevated (cellular shifts), then markedly decreased.

    Phosphorus: Frequently decreased.

Arterial blood gases (ABGs): Usually reflects low pH and decreased HCO$_3$ (metabolic acidosis) with compensatory respiratory alkalosis.

CBC: Hct may be elevated (dehydration); leukocytosis suggests hemoconcentration, response to stress or infection.

BUN: May be normal or elevated (dehydration/decreased renal perfusion).

Serum amylase: May be elevated, indicating acute pancreatitis as cause of DKA.

Thyroid function tests: Increased thyroid activity can increase blood glucose and insulin needs.

Urine: Positive for glucose and ketones; specific gravity and osmolality may be elevated.

Cultures and sensitivities: Possible UTI, respiratory, or wound infections.

NURSING PRIORITIES

1. Restore fluid/electrolyte and acid/base balance.
2. Correct/reverse metabolic abnormalities.
3. Identify/assist with management of underlying cause/disease process.
4. Prevent complications.
5. Provide information about disease process/prognosis, self-care, and treatment needs.

DISCHARGE GOALS

1. Homeostasis achieved.
2. Causative/precipitating factors corrected/controlled.
3. Complications prevented/minimized.
4. Disease process/prognosis, self-care needs, and therapeutic regimen understood.
5. Plan in place to meet needs after discharge.

NURSING DIAGNOSIS: Fluid Volume deficit [specify]

May be related to

Osmotic diuresis (from hyperglycemia)

Excessive gastric losses: diarrhea, vomiting

Restricted intake: nausea, confusion

Possibly evidenced by

Increased urinary output, dilute urine

Weakness; thirst; sudden weight loss

Dry skin/mucous membranes, poor skin turgor

Hypotension, tachycardia, delayed capillary refill

DESIRED OUTCOMES/EVALUATION CRITERIA—PATIENT WILL:

> **Fluid Balance (NOC)**

Demonstrate adequate hydration as evidenced by stable vital signs, palpable peripheral pulses, good skin turgor and capillary refill, individually appropriate urinary output, and electrolyte levels within normal range.

ACTIONS/INTERVENTIONS	RATIONALE
Fluid/Electrolyte Management (NIC)	
Independent	
Obtain history from patient/SO related to duration/intensity of symptoms such as vomiting, excessive urination.	Assists in estimation of total volume depletion. Symptoms may have been present for varying amounts of time (hours to days). Presence of infectious process results in fever and hypermetabolic state, increasing insensible fluid losses.
Monitor vital signs:	
Note orthostatic BP changes;	Hypovolemia may be manifested by hypotension and tachycardia. Estimates of severity of hypovolemia may be made when patient's systolic BP drops more than 10 mm Hg from a recumbent to a sitting/standing position. *Note:* Cardiac neuropathy may block reflexes that normally increase heart rate.
Respiratory pattern, e.g., Kussmaul's respirations, acetone breath;	Lungs remove carbonic acid through respirations, producing a compensatory respiratory alkalosis for ketoacidosis. Acetone breath is due to breakdown of acetoacetic acid and should diminish as ketosis is corrected.
Respiratory rate and quality; use of accessory muscles, periods of apnea, and appearance of cyanosis;	Correction of hyperglycemia and acidosis will cause the respiratory rate and pattern to approach normal. In contrast, increased work of breathing; shallow, rapid respirations; and presence of cyanosis may indicate respiratory fatigue and/or that patient is losing ability to compensate for acidosis.
Temperature, skin color/moisture.	Although fever, chills, and diaphoresis are common with infectious process, fever with flushed, dry skin may reflect dehydration.
Assess peripheral pulses, capillary refill, skin turgor, and mucous membranes.	Indicators of level of hydration, adequacy of circulating volume.
Monitor I&O; note urine specific gravity.	Provides ongoing estimate of volume replacement needs, kidney function, and effectiveness of therapy.

443

ACTIONS/INTERVENTIONS	RATIONALE
Independent	
Weigh daily.	Provides the best assessment of current fluid status and adequacy of fluid replacement.
Maintain fluid intake of at least 2500 mL/day within cardiac tolerance when oral intake is resumed.	Maintains hydration/circulating volume.
Promote comfortable environment. Cover patient with light sheets.	Avoids overheating, which could promote further fluid loss.
Investigate changes in mentation/sensorium.	Changes in mentation can be due to abnormally high or low glucose, electrolyte abnormalities, acidosis, decreased cerebral perfusion, or developing hypoxia. Regardless of the cause, impaired consciousness can predispose the patient to aspiration.
Note reports of nausea, abdominal pain; presence of vomiting and gastric distension.	Fluid and electrolyte deficits alter gastric motility, frequently resulting in vomiting and potentiating the fluid/electrolyte losses.
Observe for increased fatigue, crackles, edema, increased weight, bounding pulse, vascular distension.	Rapid fluid replacement may potentiate overload and HF.
Collaborative	
Administer fluids as indicated:	
Isotonic (0.9%) or lactated Ringer's solution without additives;	Type and amount of fluid depend on degree of deficit and individual patient response. *Note:* Patients with DKA are often severely dehydrated and commonly need 5–10 L of isotonic saline (2–3 L within first 2 hr of treatment).
Albumin, plasma, dextran.	Plasma expanders may occasionally be needed if the deficit is life-threatening/BP does not normalize with rehydration efforts.
Insert/maintain indwelling urinary catheter.	Provides for accurate/ongoing measurement of urinary output, especially if autonomic neuropathies result in neurogenic bladder (urinary retention/overflow incontinence). May be removed when patient is stable to reduce risk of infection.
Monitor laboratory studies, e.g.:	
Hct;	Assesses level of hydration and is often elevated because of hemoconcentration associated with osmotic diuresis.
BUN/creatinine (Cr);	Elevated values may reflect cellular breakdown from dehydration or signal the onset of renal failure.
Serum osmolality;	Elevated because of hyperglycemia and dehydration.
Sodium;	May be decreased, reflecting shift of fluids from the intracellular compartment (osmotic diuresis). High sodium values reflect severe fluid loss/dehydration, or sodium reabsorption in response to aldosterone secretion.
Potassium.	Initially, hyperkalemia occurs in response to metabolic acidosis, but as this potassium is lost in the urine, the absolute potassium level in the body is depleted. As insulin is replaced and acidosis is corrected, serum potassium deficit becomes apparent.

ACTIONS/INTERVENTIONS

Collaborative

Administer potassium and other electrolytes via IV and/or by oral route as indicated.

Administer bicarbonate if pH is less than 7.1.

Insert NG tube and attach to suction as indicated.

RATIONALE

Potassium should be added to the IV (as soon as urinary flow is adequate) to prevent hypokalemia. *Note:* Potassium phosphate may be drug of choice when IV fluids contain sodium chloride in order to prevent chloride overload.

Given with caution to help correct acidosis in the presence of hypotension or shock, lactic acidosis, or severe hyperkalemia.

Decompresses stomach and may relieve vomiting.

NURSING DIAGNOSIS: Nutrition: altered, less than body requirements

May be related to

Insulin deficiency (decreased uptake and utilization of glucose by the tissues, resulting in increased protein/fat metabolism)

Decreased oral intake: Anorexia, nausea, gastric fullness, abdominal pain; altered consciousness

Hypermetabolic state: Release of stress hormones (e.g., epinephrine, cortisol, and growth hormone), infectious process

Possibly evidenced by

Reported inadequate food intake, lack of interest in food

Recent weight loss; weakness, fatigue, poor muscle tone

Diarrhea

Increased ketones (end products of fat metabolism)

DESIRED OUTCOMES/EVALUATION CRITERIA—PATIENT WILL:

Nutritional Status (NOC)

Ingest appropriate amounts of calories/nutrients.

Display usual energy level.

Demonstrate stabilized weight or gain toward usual/desired range with normal laboratory values.

ACTIONS/INTERVENTIONS

Hyperglycemia Management (NIC)

Independent

Weigh daily or as indicated.

Ascertain patient's dietary program and usual pattern; compare with recent intake.

Auscultate bowel sounds. Note reports of abdominal pain/bloating, nausea, vomiting of undigested food. Maintain nothing by mouth (NPO) status as indicated.

RATIONALE

Assesses adequacy of nutritional intake (absorption and utilization).

Identifies deficits and deviations from therapeutic needs.

Hyperglycemia and fluid and electrolyte disturbances can decrease gastric motility/function (distension or ileus), affecting choice of interventions. *Note:* Long-term difficulties with decreased gastric emptying and poor intestinal motility suggest autonomic neuropathies affecting the GI tract and requiring symptomatic treatment.

ACTIONS/INTERVENTIONS

Independent

Provide liquids containing nutrients and electrolytes as soon as patient can tolerate oral fluids; progress to more solid food as tolerated.

Identify food preferences, including ethnic/cultural needs.

Include SO in meal planning as indicated.

Observe for signs of hypoglycemia, e.g., changes in level of consciousness, cool/clammy skin, rapid pulse, hunger, irritability, anxiety, headache, light-headedness, shakiness.

Collaborative

Perform fingerstick glucose testing.

Monitor laboratory studies, e.g., serum glucose, acetone, pH, HCO₃.

Administer regular insulin by intermittent or continuous IV method, e.g., IV bolus followed by a continuous drip via pump of approximately 5–10 U/hr so that glucose is reduced by 50 mg/dL/hr.

Administer glucose solutions, e.g., dextrose and half-normal saline.

Consult with dietitian for initiation of resumption of oral intake.

RATIONALE

Oral route is preferred when patient is alert and bowel function is restored.

If patient's food preferences can be incorporated into the meal plan, cooperation with dietary requirements may be facilitated after discharge.

Promotes sense of involvement; provides information for SO to understand nutritional needs of the patient. *Note:* Various methods available for dietary planning include exchange list, point system, glycemic index, or preselected menus.

Once carbohydrate metabolism resumes (blood glucose level reduced) and as insulin is being given, hypoglycemia can occur. If patient is comatose, hypoglycemia may occur without notable change in level of consciousness (LOC). This potentially life-threatening emergency should be assessed and treated quickly per protocol. *Note:* Type 1 diabetics of long standing may not display usual signs of hypoglycemia because normal response to low blood sugar may be diminished.

Bedside analysis of serum glucose is more accurate (displays current levels) than monitoring urine sugar, which is not sensitive enough to detect fluctuations in serum levels and can be affected by patient's individual renal threshold or the presence of urinary retention/renal failure. *Note:* Some studies have found that a urine glucose of 20% may be correlated to a blood glucose of 140–360 mg/dL.

Blood glucose will decrease slowly with controlled fluid replacement and insulin therapy. With the administration of optimal insulin dosages, glucose can then enter the cells and be used for energy. When this happens, acetone levels decrease and acidosis is corrected.

Regular insulin has a rapid onset and thus quickly helps move glucose into cells. The IV route is the initial route of choice because absorption from subcutaneous tissues may be erratic. Many believe the continuous method is the optimal way to facilitate transition to carbohydrate metabolism and reduce incidence of hypoglycemia.

Glucose solutions may be added after insulin and fluids have brought the blood glucose to approximately 400 mg/dL. As carbohydrate metabolism approaches normal, care must be taken to avoid hypoglycemia.

Useful in calculating and adjusting diet to meet patient's needs; answer questions and assist patient/SO in developing meal plans.

ACTIONS/INTERVENTIONS

Collaborative

Provide diet of approximately 60% carbohydrates, 20% proteins, 20% fats in designated number of meals/snacks.

Administer other medications as indicated, e.g., metoclopramide (Reglan); tetracycline.

RATIONALE

Complex carbohydrates (e.g., corn, peas, carrots, broccoli, dried beans, oats, apples) decrease glucose levels/insulin needs, reduce serum cholesterol levels, and promote satiation. Food intake is scheduled according to specific insulin characteristics (e.g., peak effect) and individual patient response. *Note:* A snack at bedtime (hs) of complex carbohydrates is especially important (if insulin is given in divided doses) to prevent hypoglycemia during sleep and potential Somogyi response.

May be useful in treating symptoms related to autonomic neuropathies affecting GI tract, thus enhancing oral intake and absorption of nutrients.

NURSING DIAGNOSIS: Infection, risk for [sepsis]

Risk factors may include

High glucose levels, decreased leukocyte function, alterations in circulation
Preexisting respiratory infection, or UTI

Possibly evidenced by

[Not applicable; presence of signs and symptoms establishes an *actual* diagnosis]

DESIRED OUTCOMES/EVALUATION CRITERIA—PATIENT WILL:

Knowledge: Infection Control (NOC)

Identify interventions to prevent/reduce risk of infection.
Demonstrate techniques, lifestyle changes to prevent development of infection.

ACTIONS/INTERVENTIONS

Infection Control (NIC)

Independent

Observe for signs of infection and inflammation, e.g., fever, flushed appearance, wound drainage, purulent sputum, cloudy urine.

Promote good handwashing by staff and patient.

Maintain aseptic technique for IV insertion procedure, administration of medications, and providing maintenance/site care. Rotate IV sites as indicated.

Provide catheter/perineal care. Teach the female patient to clean from front to back after elimination.

Provide conscientious skin care; gently massage bony areas. Keep the skin dry, linens dry and wrinkle-free.

RATIONALE

Patient may be admitted with infection, which could have precipitated the ketoacidotic state, or may develop a nosocomial infection.

Reduces risk of cross-contamination.

High glucose in the blood creates an excellent medium for bacterial growth.

Minimizes risk of UTI. Comatose patient may be at particular risk if urinary retention occurred before hospitalization. *Note:* Elderly female diabetic patients are especially prone to urinary tract/vaginal yeast infections.

Peripheral circulation may be impaired, placing the patient at increased risk for skin irritation/breakdown and infection.

ACTIONS/INTERVENTIONS

Independent

Auscultate breath sounds.

Place in semi-Fowler's position.

Reposition and encourage coughing/deep breathing if patient is alert and cooperative. Otherwise, suction airway, using sterile technique, as needed.

Provide tissues and trash bag in a convenient location for sputum and other secretions. Instruct patient in proper handling of secretions.

Encourage/assist with oral hygiene.

Encourage adequate dietary and fluid intake (approximately 3000 mL/day if not contraindicated by cardiac or renal dysfunction), including 8 oz of cranberry juice per day as appropriate.

Collaborative

Obtain specimens for culture and sensitivities as indicated.

Administer antibiotics as appropriate.

RATIONALE

Rhonchi indicates accumulation of secretions possibly related to pneumonia/bronchitis (may have precipitated the DKA). Pulmonary congestion/edema (crackles) may result from rapid fluid replacement/HF.

Facilitates lung expansion; reduces risk of aspiration.

Aids in ventilating all lung areas and mobilizing secretions. Prevents stasis of secretions with increased risk of infection.

Minimizes spread of infection.

Reduces risk of oral/gum disease.

Decreases susceptibility to infection. Increased urinary flow prevents stasis and aids in maintaining urine pH/acidity, reducing bacteria growth and flushing organisms out of system. *Note:* Use of cranberry juice can help prevent bacteria from adhering to the bladder wall, reducing the risk of recurrent UTI.

Identifies organism(s) so that most appropriate drug therapy can be instituted.

Early treatment may help prevent sepsis.

NURSING DIAGNOSIS: Sensory/Perceptual risk for alterations: (specify)

Risk factors may include
Endogenous chemical alteration: Glucose/insulin and/or electrolyte imbalance

Possibly evidenced by
[Not applicable; presence of signs and symptoms establishes an *actual* diagnosis]

DESIRED OUTCOMES/EVALUATION CRITERIA—PATIENT WILL:

Neurological Status (NOC)

Maintain usual level of mentation.
Recognize and compensate for existing sensory impairments.

ACTIONS/INTERVENTIONS

Neurological Monitoring (NIC)

Independent

Monitor vital signs and mental status.

Address patient by name; reorient as needed to place, person, and time. Give short explanations, speaking slowly and enunciating clearly.

Schedule nursing time to provide for uninterrupted rest periods.

RATIONALE

Provides a baseline from which to compare abnormal findings, e.g., fever may affect mentation.

Decreases confusion and helps maintain contact with reality.

Promotes restful sleep, reduces fatigue, and may improve cognition.

ACTIONS/INTERVENTIONS	RATIONALE
Independent	
Keep patient's routine as consistent as possible. Encourage participation in activities of daily living (ADLs) as able.	Helps keep the patient in touch with reality and maintain orientation to the environment.
Protect patient from injury (use of restraints) when level of consciousness is impaired. Pad bed rails and provide soft airway if patient is prone to seizures.	Disoriented patient is prone to injury, especially at night, and precautions need to be taken as indicated. Seizure precautions need to be taken as appropriate to prevent physical injury, aspiration.
Evaluate visual acuity as indicated.	Retinal edema/detachment, hemorrhage, presence of cataracts or temporary paralysis of extraocular muscles may impair vision, requiring corrective therapy and/or supportive care.
Investigate reports of hyperesthesia, pain, or sensory loss in the feet/legs. Look for ulcers, reddened areas, pressure points, loss of pedal pulses.	Peripheral neuropathies may result in severe discomfort, lack of/distortion of tactile sensation, potentiating risk of dermal injury and impaired balance. *Note:* Mononeuropathy affects a single nerve (most often femoral or cranial), causing sudden pain and loss of motor/sensory function along affected nerve path.
Provide bed cradle. Keep hands/feet warm, avoiding exposure to cool drafts/hot water or use of heating pad.	Reduces discomfort and potential for dermal injury. *Note:* Sudden development of cold hands/feet may reflect hypoglycemia, suggesting need to evaluate serum glucose level.
Assist with ambulation/position changes.	Promotes patient safety, especially when sense of balance is affected.
Collaborative	
Carry out prescribed regimen for correcting DKA as indicated.	Alteration in thought processes/potential for seizure activity is usually alleviated once hyperosmolar state is corrected.
Monitor laboratory values, e.g., blood glucose, serum osmolality, Hb/Hct, BUN/Cr.	Imbalances can impair mentation. *Note:* If fluid is replaced too quickly, excess water may enter brain cells and cause alteration in the level of consciousness (water intoxication).

NURSING DIAGNOSIS: Fatigue

May be related to
Decreased metabolic energy production
Altered body chemistry: Insufficient insulin
Increased energy demands: Hypermetabolic state/infection

Possibly evidenced by
Overwhelming lack of energy, inability to maintain usual routines, decreased performance, accident-prone
Impaired ability to concentrate, listlessness, disinterest in surroundings

DESIRED OUTCOMES/EVALUATION CRITERIA—PATIENT WILL:

> **Endurance (NOC)**

Verbalize increase in energy level.
Display improved ability to participate in desired activities.

ACTIONS/INTERVENTIONS

| RATIONALE |

Energy Management (NIC)

Independent

Discuss with patient the need for activity. Plan schedule with patient and identify activities that lead to fatigue.

Education may provide motivation to increase activity level even though patient may feel too weak initially.

Alternate activity with periods of rest/uninterrupted sleep.

Prevents excessive fatigue.

Monitor pulse, respiratory rate, and BP before/after activity.

Indicates physiological levels of tolerance.

Discuss ways of conserving energy while bathing, transferring, and so on.

Patient will be able to accomplish more with a decreased expenditure of energy.

Increase patient participation in ADLs as tolerated.

Increases confidence level/self-esteem and tolerance level. *Note:* Elderly patients may experience a "lag effect" in which exercise may precipitate hypoglycemia as late as 24 hr after exercising, leading to extensive fatigue and muscle tremors.

NURSING DIAGNOSIS: Powerlessness

May be related to
Long-term/progressive illness that is not curable
Dependence on others

Possibly evidenced by
Reluctance to express true feelings; expressions of having no control/influence over situation
Apathy, withdrawal, anger
Does not monitor progress, nonparticipation in care/decision making
Depression over physical deterioration/complications despite patient cooperation with regimen

DESIRED OUTCOMES/EVALUATION CRITERIA—PATIENT WILL:

Health Beliefs: Perceived Control (NOC)

Acknowledge feelings of helplessness.
Identify healthy ways to deal with feelings.
Assist in planning own care and independently take responsibility for self-care activities.

ACTIONS/INTERVENTIONS

| RATIONALE |

Self-Responsibility Facilitation (NIC)

Independent

Encourage patient/SO to express feelings about hospitalization and disease in general.

Identifies concerns and facilitates problem solving.

Acknowledge normality of feelings.

Recognition that reactions are normal can help the patient problem-solve and seek help as needed. Diabetic control is a full-time job that serves as a constant reminder of both presence of disease and threat to patient's health/life.

ACTIONS/INTERVENTIONS	RATIONALE
Independent	
Assess how patient has handled problems in the past. Identify locus of control.	Knowledge of individual's style helps determine needs for treatment goals. Patient whose locus of control is internal usually looks at ways to gain control over own treatment program. Patient who operates with an external locus of control wants to be cared for by others and may project blame for circumstances onto external factors.
Provide opportunity for SO to express concerns and discuss ways in which they can be helpful to the patient.	Enhances sense of being involved and gives SO a chance to problem-solve solutions to help patient prevent recurrence.
Ascertain expectations/goals of patient and SO.	Unrealistic expectations/pressure from others or self may result in feelings of frustration/loss of control and may impair coping abilities. *Note:* Even with rigid adherence to medical regimen, complications/setbacks may occur.
Determine whether a change in relationship with SO has occurred.	Constant energy and thought required for diabetic control often shifts the focus of a relationship. Development of psychological concerns/visceral neuropathies affecting self-concept (especially sexual role function) may add further stress.
Encourage patient to make decisions related to care, e.g., ambulation, time for activities, and so forth.	Communicates to patient that some control can be exercised over care.
Support participation in self-care and give positive feedback for efforts.	Promotes feeling of control over situation.

NURSING DIAGNOSIS: Knowledge Deficit [Learning Need] regarding disease, prognosis, treatment, self care, and discharge needs

May be related to
Lack of exposure/recall, information misinterpretation
Unfamiliarity with information resources

Possibly evidenced by
Questions/request for information, verbalization of the problem
Inaccurate follow-through of instructions, development of preventable complications

DESIRED OUTCOMES/EVALUATION CRITERIA—PATIENT WILL:

Knowledge: Disease Process (NOC)

Verbalize understanding of disease process, potential complications.
Identify relationship of signs/symptoms to the disease process and correlate symptoms with causative factors.

Knowledge: Treatment Regimen (NOC)

Correctly perform necessary procedures and explain reasons for the actions.
Initiate necessary lifestyle changes and participate in treatment regimen.

ACTIONS/INTERVENTIONS	RATIONALE

Learning Facilitation (NIC)

Independent

Create an environment of trust by listening to concerns, being available.

Work with patient in setting mutual goals for learning.

Select a variety of teaching strategies, e.g., demonstrate needed skills and have patient do return demonstration, incorporate new skills into the hospital routine.

Teaching: Disease Process

Discuss essential elements, e.g.:

What a normal blood glucose level is and how it compares with the patient's level, the type of DM the patient has, the relationship between insulin deficiency and a high glucose level;

Reasons for the ketoacidotic episode;

Acute and chronic complications of the disease, including visual disturbances, neurosensory and cardiovascular changes, renal impairment/hypertension.

Demonstrate fingerstick testing and have patient/SO return demonstration until proficient. Instruct patient to check urine ketones if glucose is greater than 250 mg/dL.

Discuss dietary plan, limiting intake of sugar, fat, salt, and alcohol; eating complex carbohydrates, especially those high in fiber (fruits, vegetables, whole grains), and ways to deal with meals outside the home.

Review medication regimen, including onset, peak, and duration of prescribed insulin, as applicable, with patient/SO.

Review self-administration of insulin and care of equipment. Have patient demonstrate procedure (e.g., drawing up and injecting insulin or use of continuous pump).

Rapport and respect need to be established before patient will be willing to take part in the learning process.

Participation in the planning promotes enthusiasm and cooperation with the principles learned.

Use of different means of accessing information promotes learner retention.

Provides knowledge base from which patient can make informed lifestyle choices.

Knowledge of the precipitating factors may help avoid recurrences.

Awareness helps patient be more consistent with care and may prevent/delay onset of complications.

Self-monitoring of blood glucose four or more times a day allows flexibility in self-care, promotes tighter control of serum levels (e.g., 60–150 mg/dL), and may prevent/delay development of long-term complications.

Awareness of importance of dietary control aids patient in planning meals/sticking to regimen. Fiber can slow glucose absorption, decreasing fluctuations in serum levels, but may cause GI discomfort, increase flatus, and affect vitamin/mineral absorption.

Understanding all aspects of drug usage promotes proper use. Dose algorithms are created, taking into account drug dosages established during inpatient evaluation, usual amount and schedule of physical activity, and meal plan. Including SO provides additional support/resource for patient.

Verifies understanding and correctness of procedure. Identifies potential problems (e.g., vision, memory, and so on) so that alternate solutions can be found for insulin administration. *Note:* If multiple daily injections are required, combinations of regular, intermediate, and long-acting insulin are used. If the pump method is used, the patient programs his/her own basal and bolus settings. Only regular insulin is administered, with a basal dose throughout the day and bolus doses before meals and as needed. An insulin pump more closely mimics normal pancreatic activity because the basal rate may be changed relative to the patient's activity level, presence of stressors/infection or menstrual cycle.

ACTIONS/INTERVENTIONS	RATIONALE

Independent

Discuss timing of insulin injection and mealtime.	One of the many inconveniences people with diabetes cope with is having to decide at least 30–60 min in advance when they are going to have a meal for the timely administration of regular Humulin injections. A newer product, Insulin lispro (Humalog), may be helpful because it works best when taken within 15 min of eating. With the onset twice as fast as regular human insulin and a duration approximately half as long, Humalog closely mimics pancreatic activity. However, hypoglycemia may develop more rapidly and be more severe than with use of regular insulin. A blood glucose level below 80 mg/dL indicates that insulin should be injected after eating rather than before the meal.
Review individual's target blood glucose levels.	Although this range varies per person, the adult ideal range is considered to be 100–160 mg/dL. *Note:* Patients with an insulin pump may maintain blood glucose levels between 120 mg/dL and 200 mg/dL with no urinary ketones.
Stress importance and necessity of maintaining diary of glucose testing, medication dose/time, dietary intake, activity, feelings/sensations, life events.	Aids in creating overall picture of patient situation to achieve better disease control and promotes self-care/independence.
Discuss factors that play a part in diabetic control, e.g., exercise (aerobic versus isometric), stress, surgery, and illness. Review "sick day" rules.	This information promotes diabetic control and can greatly reduce the occurrence of ketoacidosis. *Note:* Aerobic exercise (e.g., walking, swimming) promotes effective use of insulin, lowering glucose levels, and strengthens the cardiovascular system. A "sick day" management plan helps maintain equilibrium during illness, minor surgery, severe emotional stress, or any condition that might send glucose spiraling upward.
Review effects of smoking on insulin use. Encourage cessation of smoking.	Nicotine constricts the small blood vessels, and insulin absorption is delayed for as long as these vessels remain constricted. *Note:* Insulin absorption may be reduced by as much as 30% below normal in the first 30 min after smoking.
Establish regular exercise/activity schedule and identify corresponding insulin concerns.	Exercise times should not coincide with the peak action of insulin. A snack should be ingested before or during exercise as needed, and rotation of injection sites should avoid the muscle group that will be used in the activity (e.g., abdominal site is preferred over thigh/arm before jogging or swimming) to prevent accelerated uptake of insulin.
Identify the symptoms of hypoglycemia (e.g., weakness, dizziness, lethargy, hunger, irritability, diaphoresis, pallor, tachycardia, tremors, headache, changes in mentation) and explain causes.	May promote early detection and treatment, preventing/limiting occurrence. *Note:* Early morning hyperglycemia may reflect the "dawn phenomenon" (indicating need for additional insulin) or a rebound response to hypoglycemia during sleep (Somogyi effect), requiring a decrease in insulin dosage/change in diet (e.g., hs snack). Testing serum levels at 3 AM aids in identifying the specific problem.

ACTIONS/INTERVENTIONS	RATIONALE

Independent

Instruct in importance of routine examination of the feet and proper foot care. Demonstrate ways to examine feet; inspect shoes for fit; and care for toenails, calluses, and corns. Encourage use of natural fiber stockings.	Prevents/delays complications associated with peripheral neuropathies and/or circulatory impairment, especially cellulitis, gangrene, and amputation.
Demonstrate/discuss proper use of transcutaneous electrical nerve stimulator (TENS) unit. Identify safety concerns following local nerve block.	May provide relief of discomfort associated with neuropathies.
Stress importance of regular eye examinations, especially for patients who have had type 1 diabetes for 5 yr or more.	Changes in vision may be gradual and are more pronounced in persons with poorly controlled DM. Problems include changes in visual acuity and may progress to retinopathy and blindness.
Arrange for vision aids when needed, e.g., magnifying sleeve for insulin syringe, large-print instructions, one-touch glucose meters.	Adaptive aids have been developed in recent years to help the visually impaired manage their own DM more effectively.
Discuss sexual functioning and answer questions patient/SO may have.	Impotence may be first symptom of onset of DM. *Note:* Counseling and/or use of penile prosthesis may be of benefit.
Stress importance of use of identification bracelet.	Can promote quick entry into the health system and appropriate care with fewer resultant complications in the event of an emergency.
Recommend avoidance of over-the-counter (OTC) drugs without prior approval of healthcare provider.	These products may contain sugars/interact with prescribed medications.
Discuss importance of follow-up care.	Helps maintain tighter control of disease process and may prevent exacerbations of DM, retarding development of systemic complications.
Review signs/symptoms requiring medical evaluation, e.g., fever; cold or flu symptoms; cloudy, odorous urine, painful urination; delayed healing of cuts/sores; sensory changes (pain or tingling) of lower extremities; changes in blood sugar level, presence of ketones in urine.	Prompt intervention may prevent development of more serious/life-threatening complications.
Demonstrate stress management techniques, e.g., deep-breathing exercises, guided imagery, visualization.	Promotes relaxation and control of stress response, which may help limit incidence of glucose/insulin imbalances.
Identify community resources, e.g., American Diabetic Association, internet resources/online diabetes bulletin boards, visiting nurse, weight-loss/stop-smoking clinic, contact person/diabetic instructor.	Continued support is usually necessary to sustain lifestyle changes and promote well-being.

POTENTIAL CONSIDERATIONS following acute hospitalization (dependent on patient's age, physical condition/presence of complications, personal resources, and life responsibilities)

Therapeutic Regimen: Individual, ineffective management—complexity of therapeutic regimen, economic concerns, perceived susceptibility (recurrence of problem).

Sensory-Perceptual alterations: diabetic neuropathy/visual—endogenous chemical alterations (elevated glucose level).

HYPERTHYROIDISM (THYROTOXICOSIS, GRAVES' DISEASE)

Hyperthyroidism is a metabolic imbalance that results from overproduction of the thyroid hormones triiodothyronine (T_3) and thyroxine (T_4). The most common form is Graves' disease, but other forms of hyperthyroidism include toxic adenoma, TSH-secreting pituitary tumor, subacute or silent thyroiditis, and some forms of thyroid cancer.

Thyroid storm is a rarely encountered manifestation of hyperthyroidism, which can be precipitated by such events as thyroid ablation (surgical or radioiodine), medication overdosage, and trauma. This condition constitutes a medical emergency.

CARE SETTING

Most people with classic hyperthyroidism rarely need hospitalization. Critically ill patients, those with extreme manifestations of thyrotoxicosis plus a significant concurrent illness, require inpatient acute care on a medical unit.

RELATED CONCERNS

Heart failure: chronic, page 47
Psychosocial aspects of care, page 809
Thyroidectomy, page 467

Patient Assessment Database

Data depend on the severity/duration of hormone imbalance and involvement of other organs.

ACTIVITY/REST

May report:	Nervousness, increased irritability, insomnia
	Muscle weakness, incoordination
	Extreme fatigue
May exhibit:	Muscle atrophy

CIRCULATION

May report:	Palpitations
	Chest pain (angina)
May exhibit:	Dysrhythmias (atrial fibrillation); gallop rhythm, murmurs
	Elevated BP with widened pulse pressure
	Tachycardia at rest
	Circulatory collapse, shock (thyrotoxic crisis)

ELIMINATION

May report:	Urinating in large amounts
	Stool changes; diarrhea

EGO INTEGRITY

May report:	Recent stressful experience, e.g., emotional/physical
May exhibit:	Emotional lability (mild euphoria to delirium); anxiety/depression.

FOOD/FLUID

May report:	Recent/sudden weight loss
	Increased appetite; large meals, frequent meals; thirst
	Nausea/vomiting
May exhibit:	Enlarged thyroid; goiter
	Nonpitting edema, especially in pretibial area

NEUROSENSORY

May exhibit:	Rapid and hoarse speech
	Mental status and behavior alterations, e.g., confusion, disorientation, nervousness, irritability, delirium, frank psychosis, stupor, coma
	Fine tremor in hands; purposeless, quick, jerky movements of body parts
	Hyperactive DTRs

PAIN/DISCOMFORT

May report: Orbital pain, photophobia (eye involvement)

RESPIRATION

May report: Difficulty breathing

May exhibit: Increased respiratory rate, tachypnea
Breath sounds: Crackles, wheezes (pulmonary edema associated with thyrotoxic crisis)

SAFETY

May report: Heat intolerance, excessive sweating
Allergy to iodine (may be used in testing)

May exhibit: Elevated temperature (above 100°F), diaphoresis
Skin smooth, warm, and flushed; hair fine, silky, straight
Exophthalmia, lid retraction; conjunctival irritation, tearing
Pruritic, erythematous lesions (often in pretibial area) that become brawny

SEXUALITY

May report: Decreased libido
Hypomenorrhea, amenorrhea
Impotence

TEACHING/LEARNING

May report: Family history of thyroid problems
History of hypothyroidism, thyroid hormone replacement therapy or antithyroid therapy, premature withdrawal of antithyroid drugs, recent partial thyroidectomy
History of insulin-induced hypoglycemia, cardiac disorders or surgery, recent illness (pneumonia), trauma; x-ray contrast studies

Discharge plan considerations: **DRG projected mean length of inpatient stay: 4.3 days**
May require assistance with treatment regimen, self-care activities, homemaker/maintenance tasks

Refer to section at end of plan for postdischarge considerations.

DIAGNOSTIC STUDIES

Radioactive iodine (RAI) uptake test: High in Graves' disease and toxic nodular goiter; low in thyroiditis.
Plasma T_4 and T_3: Increased in hyperthyroidism. Normal T_4 index level with T_3 elevated indicates thyrotoxicosis.
Thyroid-stimulating hormone (TSH): Suppressed and does not respond to thyrotropin-releasing hormone (TRH).
Thyroglobulin: Increased.
TRH stimulation: Hyperthyroidism is indicated if TSH fails to rise after administration of TRH.
Thyroid T_3 uptake: Increased.
Protein-bound iodine: Increased.
Serum glucose: Elevated (related to adrenal involvement).
Plasma cortisol: Low levels (less adrenal reserve).
Alkaline phosphatase and serum calcium: Increased.
Liver function tests: Abnormal.
Electrolytes: Hyponatremia may reflect adrenal response or dilutional effect in fluid replacement therapy. Hypokalemia occurs because of GI losses and diuresis.
Serum catecholamines: Decreased.
Urine creatinine: Increased.
ECG: Atrial fibrillations; shorter systole time; cardiomegaly, heart enlarged with fibrosis and necrosis (late signs or in elderly with masked hyperthyroidism).

NURSING PRIORITIES

1. Reduce metabolic demands and support cardiovascular function.
2. Provide psychological support.
3. Prevent complications.
4. Provide information about disease process/prognosis and therapy needs.

DISCHARGE GOALS

1. Homeostasis achieved.
2. Patient effectively dealing with current situation.
3. Complications prevented/minimized.
4. Disease process/prognosis and therapeutic regimen understood.
5. Plan in place to meet needs after discharge.

NURSING DIAGNOSIS: Cardiac Output, risk for decreased

Risk factors may include

Uncontrolled hyperthyroidism, hypermetabolic state
Increasing cardiac workload
Changes in venous return and systemic vascular resistance
Alterations in rate, rhythm, conduction

Possibly evidenced by

[Not applicable; presence of signs and symptoms establishes an *actual* diagnosis]

DESIRED OUTCOMES/EVALUATION CRITERIA—PATIENT WILL:

Circulatory Status (NOC)

Maintain adequate cardiac output for tissue needs as evidenced by stable vital signs, palpable peripheral pulses, good capillary refill, usual mentation, and absence of dysrhythmias.

ACTIONS/INTERVENTIONS	RATIONALE
Hemodynamic Regulation (NIC)	
Independent	
Monitor BP lying, sitting, and standing, if able. Note widened pulse pressure.	General/orthostatic hypotension may occur as a result of excessive peripheral vasodilation and decreased circulating volume. Widened pulse pressure reflects compensatory increase in stroke volume and decreased systemic vascular resistance (SVR).
Monitor central venous pressure (CVP), if available.	Provides more direct measure of circulating volume and cardiac function.
Investigate reports of chest pain/angina.	May reflect increased myocardial oxygen demands/ischemia.
Assess pulse/heart rate while patient is sleeping.	Provides a more accurate assessment of tachycardia.
Auscultate heart sounds, noting extra heart sounds, development of gallops and systolic murmurs.	Prominent S_1 and murmurs are associated with forceful cardiac output of hypermetabolic state; development of S_3 may warn of impending cardiac failure.
Monitor ECG, noting rate/rhythm. Document dysrhythmias.	Tachycardia (greater than normally expected with fever/increased circulatory demand) may reflect direct myocardial stimulation by thyroid hormone. Dysrhythmias often occur and may compromise cardiac function/output.
Auscultate breath sounds, noting adventitious sounds (e.g., crackles).	Early sign of pulmonary congestion, reflecting developing cardiac failure.

ACTIONS/INTERVENTIONS	RATIONALE

Independent

Monitor temperature; provide cool environment, limit bed linens/clothes, administer tepid sponge baths.	Fever (may exceed 104°F) may occur as a result of excessive hormone levels and can aggravate diuresis/dehydration and cause increased peripheral vasodilation, venous pooling, and hypotension.
Observe signs/symtoms of severe thirst, dry mucous membranes, weak/thready pulse, poor capillary refill, decreased urinary output, and hypotension.	Rapid dehydration can occur, which reduces circulating volume and compromises cardiac output.
Record I&O. Note urine specific gravity.	Significant fluid losses (through vomiting, diarrhea, diuresis, diaphoresis) can lead to profound dehydration, concentrated urine, and weight loss.
Weigh daily. Encourage chair rest/bedrest; limit nonessential activity.	Activity increases metabolic/circulatory demands, which may potentiate cardiac failure.
Note history of asthma/bronchoconstrictive disease, sinus bradycardia/heart blocks, advanced HF; or current pregnancy.	Presence/potential recurrence of these conditions affects choice of therapy; e.g., use of β-adrenergic blocking agents is contraindicated.
Observe for adverse side effects of adrenergic antagonists, e.g., severe decrease in pulse, BP; signs of vascular congestion/HF; cardiac arrest.	Indicates need for reduction/discontinuation of therapy.

Collaborative

Administer IV fluids as indicated.	Rapid fluid replacement may be necessary to improve circulating volume but must be balanced against signs of cardiac failure/need for inotropic support.
Administer medications as indicated:	
β-Blockers, e.g., propranolol (Inderal), atenolol (Tenormin), nadolol (Corgard);	Given to control thyrotoxic effects of tachycardia, tremors, and nervousness and is first drug of choice for acute storm. Decreases heart rate/cardiac work by blocking β-adrenergic receptor sites and blocking conversion of T_4 to T_3. *Note:* If severe bradycardia develops, atropine may be required.
Thyroid hormone antagonists, e.g., propylthiouracil (PTU), methimazole (Tapazole);	Blocks thyroid hormone synthesis and inhibits peripheral conversion of T_4 to T_3. May be definitive treatment or used to prepare patient for surgery; but effect is slow and so may not relieve thyroid storm. *Note:* Once PTU therapy is begun, abrupt withdrawal may precipitate thyroid crisis.
Strong iodine solution (Lugol's solution) or supersaturated potassium iodide (SSKI) PO.	Temporarily acts to prevent release of thyroid hormone into circulation by increasing the amount of thyroid hormone stored within the gland. May interfere with RAI treatment and may exacerbate the disease in some people. May be used as surgical preparation to decrease size and vascularity of the gland or to treat thyroid storm. *Note:* Should be started 1–3 hr after initiation of antithyroid drug therapy to minimize hormone formation from the iodine.

ACTIONS/INTERVENTIONS	RATIONALE
Collaborative	
RAI (Na^{131}I or Na^{125}I) following NRC regulations for radiopharmaceutical;	Radioactive iodine therapy is the treatment of choice for almost all patients with Graves' disease because it destroys abnormally functioning gland tissue. Peak results take 6–12 wk (several treatments may be necessary); however, a single dose controls hyperthyroidism in about 90% of patients. *Note:* This therapy is contraindicated during pregnancy. Also people preparing or administering the dose must have their own thyroid burden measured and contaminated supplies and equipment monitored and stored until decayed.
Corticosteroids, e.g., dexamethasone (Decadron);	Provides glucocorticol support. Decreases hyperthermia; relieves relative adrenal insufficiency; inhibits calcium absorption; and reduces peripheral conversion of T$_3$ from T$_4$. *Note:* May be given before thyroidectomy and discontinued after surgery.
Digoxin (Lanoxin);	Digitalization may be required in patients with HF before β-adrenergic blocking therapy can be considered/safely initiated.
Furosemide (Lasix);	Diuresis may be necessary if HF occurs. *Note:* It also may be effective in reducing calcium level if neuromuscular function is impaired.
Potassium (KCl, K-lyte);	Increased losses of K+ through intestinal/renal routes may result in dysrhythmias if not corrected.
Acetaminophen (Tylenol);	Drug of choice to reduce temperature and associated metabolic demands. Aspirin is contraindicated because it actually increases level of circulating thyroid hormones by blocking binding of T$_3$ and T$_4$ with thyroid-binding proteins.
Sedative, barbiturates;	Promotes rest, thereby reducing metabolic demands/cardiac workload.
Muscle relaxants.	Reduces shivering associated with hyperthermia, which can further increase metabolic demands.
Monitor laboratory/diagnostic studies, as indicated, e.g.:	
Serum potassium (replace as indicated);	Hypokalemia resulting from intestinal losses, altered intake, or diuretic therapy may cause dysrhythmias and compromise cardiac function/output.
Serum calcium;	Elevation may alter cardiac contractility.
Sputum culture;	Pulmonary infection is most frequent precipitating factor of crisis.
Serial ECGs;	May demonstrate effects of electrolyte imbalance or ischemic changes reflecting inadequate myocardial oxygen supply in presence of increased metabolic demands.
Chest x-rays.	Cardiac enlargement may occur in response to increased circulatory demands. Pulmonary congestion may be noted with cardiac decompensation.
Provide supplemental O$_2$ as indicated.	May be necessary to support increased metabolic demands/O$_2$ consumption.

ACTIONS/INTERVENTIONS	RATIONALE
Collaborative	
Provide hypothermia blanket as indicated.	Occasionally used to lower uncontrolled hyperthermia (104°F and greater) to reduce metabolic demands/ O_2 consumption and cardiac workload.
Administer transfusions; assist with plasmapheresis, hemoperfusion, dialysis.	May be done to achieve rapid depletion of extra-thyroidal hormone pool in desperately ill/comatose patient.
Prepare for surgery.	Subtotal thyroidectomy (removal of five-sixths of the gland) may be treatment of choice for hyperthyroidism once euthyroid state is achieved.

NURSING DIAGNOSIS: Fatigue

May be related to
Hypermetabolic state with increased energy requirements
Irritability of central nervous system (CNS); altered body chemistry

Possibly evidenced by
Verbalization of overwhelming lack of energy to maintain usual routine, decreased performance
Emotional lability/irritability; nervousness, tension
Jittery behavior
Impaired ability to concentrate

DESIRED OUTCOMES/EVALUATION CRITERIA—PATIENT WILL:

> **Endurance (NOC)**

Verbalize increase in level of energy.
Display improved ability to participate in desired activities.

ACTIONS/INTERVENTIONS	RATIONALE
Energy Management (NIC)	
Independent	
Monitor vital signs, noting pulse rate at rest and when active.	Pulse is typically elevated and, even at rest, tachycardia (up to 160 bpm) may be noted.
Note development of tachypnea, dyspnea, pallor, and cyanosis.	O_2 demand and consumption are increased in hypermetabolic state, potentiating risk of hypoxia with activity.
Provide for quiet environment; cool room, decreased sensory stimuli, soothing colors, quiet music.	Reduces stimuli that may aggravate agitation, hyperactivity, and insomnia.
Encourage patient to restrict activity and rest in bed as much as possible.	Helps counteract effects of increased metabolism.
Provide comfort measures, e.g., judicious touch/ massage, cool showers.	May decrease nervous energy, promoting relaxation.
Provide for diversional activities that are calming, e.g., reading, radio, television.	Allows for use of nervous energy in a constructive manner and may reduce anxiety.
Avoid topics that irritate or upset the patient. Discuss ways to respond to these feelings.	Increased irritability of the CNS may cause patient to be easily excited, agitated, and prone to emotional outbursts.

ACTIONS/INTERVENTIONS

Independent

Discuss with SO reasons for fatigue and emotional lability.

Collaborative

Administer medications as indicated:

Sedatives, e.g., phenobarbital (Luminal); antianxiety agents, e.g., chlordiazepoxide (Librium).

RATIONALE

Understanding that the behavior is physically based may enhance coping with current situation and encourage SO to respond positively and provide support for the patient.

Combats nervousness, hyperactivity, and insomnia.

NURSING DIAGNOSIS: Nutrition: altered, risk for less than body requirements

Risk factors may include
Increased metabolism (increased appetite/intake with loss of weight)
Nausea/vomiting, diarrhea
Relative insulin insufficiency; hyperglycemia

Possibly evidenced by
[Not applicable; presence of signs and symptoms establishes an *actual* diagnosis]

DESIRED OUTCOMES/EVALUATION CRITERIA—PATIENT WILL:

Nutritional Status (NOC)

Demonstrate stable weight with normal laboratory values and be free of signs of malnutrition.

ACTIONS/INTERVENTIONS

Nutrition Therapy (NIC)

Independent

Auscultate bowel sounds.

Note reports of anorexia, generalized weakness/aches, abdominal pain; presence of nausea/vomiting.

Monitor daily food intake. Weigh daily and report losses.

Encourage patient to eat and increase number of meals and snacks, using high-calorie foods that are easily digested.

Avoid foods that increase peristalsis (e.g., tea, coffee, fibrous and highly seasoned foods) and fluids that cause diarrhea (e.g., apple/prune juice).

Collaborative

Consult with dietitian to provide diet high in calories, protein, carbohydrates, and vitamins.

RATIONALE

Hyperactive bowel sounds reflect increased gastric motility, which can reduce/alter absorption.

Increased adrenergic activity can cause impaired insulin secretion/resistance, resulting in hyperglycemia, polydipsia, polyuria; changes in respiratory rate/depth.

Continued weight loss in face of adequate caloric intake may indicate failure of antithyroid therapy.

Aids in keeping caloric intake high enough to keep up with rapid expenditure of calories caused by hypermetabolic state.

Increased motility of GI tract may result in diarrhea and impair absorption of needed nutrients.

May need assistance to ensure adequate intake of nutrients, identify appropriate supplements.

461

ACTIONS/INTERVENTIONS	RATIONALE
Collaborative	
Administer medications as indicated:	
Glucose, vitamin B complex;	Given to meet energy requirements and prevent or correct hypoglycemia.
Insulin (small doses).	Aids in controlling serum glucose if elevated.

NURSING DIAGNOSIS: Anxiety [specify level]

May be related to
Physiological factors: Hypermetabolic state (CNS stimulation), pseudocatecholamine effect of thyroid hormones

Possibly evidenced by
Increased feelings of apprehension, shakiness, loss of control, panic
Changes in cognition, distortion of environmental stimuli
Extraneous movements, restlessness, tremors

DESIRED OUTCOMES/EVALUATION CRITERIA—PATIENT WILL:

Anxiety Control (NOC)

Appear relaxed.
Report anxiety reduced to a manageable level.
Identify healthy ways to deal with feelings.

ACTIONS/INTERVENTIONS	RATIONALE
Anxiety Reduction (NIC)	
Independent	
Observe behavior indicative of level of anxiety.	Mild anxiety may be displayed by irritability and insomnia. Severe anxiety progressing to panic state may produce feelings of impending doom, terror, inability to speak or move, shouting/swearing.
Monitor physical responses, noting palpitations, repetitive movements, hyperventilation, insomnia.	Increased number of β-adrenergic receptor sites, coupled with effects of excess thyroid hormones, produces clinical manifestations of catecholamine excess even when normal levels of norepinephrine/epinephrine exist.
Stay with patient, maintaining calm manner. Acknowledge fear and allow patient's behavior to belong to the patient.	Affirms to patient/SO that although patient feels out of control, environment is safe. Avoiding personal responses to inappropriate remarks or actions prevents conflicts/overreaction to stressful situation.
Describe/explain procedures, surrounding environment, or sounds that may be heard by the patient.	Provides accurate information, which reduces distortions/misinterpretations, that can contribute to anxiety/fear reactions.
Speak in brief statements, using simple words.	Attention span may be shortened, concentration reduced, limiting ability to assimilate information.
Reduce external stimuli: Place in quiet room; provide soft, soothing music; reduce bright lights; reduce number of persons contacting patient.	Creates a therapeutic environment; shows recognition that unit activity/personnel may increase patient's anxiety.

ACTIONS/INTERVENTIONS

Independent

Discuss with patient/SO reasons for emotional lability/psychotic reaction. (Refer to ND: Thought Processes, risk for altered, following.)

Reinforce expectation that emotional control should return as drug therapy progresses.

Collaborative

Administer antianxiety agents or sedatives and monitor effects.

Refer to support systems as needed, e.g., counseling, social services, pastoral care.

RATIONALE

Understanding that behavior is physically based enhances acceptance of situation and encourages different responses/approaches.

Provides information and reassures patient that the situation is temporary and will improve with treatment.

May be used in conjunction with medical regimen to reduce effects of hyperthyroid secretion.

Ongoing therapy support may be desired/required by patient/SO if crisis precipitates lifestyle alterations.

NURSING DIAGNOSIS: Thought Processes, risk for altered

Risk factors may include
Physiological changes: Increased CNS stimulation/accelerated mental activity
Altered sleep patterns

Possibly evidenced by
[Not applicable; presence of signs and symptoms establishes an *actual* diagnosis]

DESIRED OUTCOMES/EVALUATION CRITERIA—PATIENT WILL:

Distorted Thought Control (NOC)

Maintain usual reality orientation.
Recognize changes in thinking/behavior and causative factors.

ACTIONS/INTERVENTIONS

Delirium Management (NIC)

Independent

Assess thinking processes, e.g., memory, attention span, orientation to person/place/time.

Note changes in behavior.

Assess level of anxiety. (Refer to ND: Anxiety, p. 462.)

Provide quiet environment; decreased stimuli, cool room, dim lights. Limit procedures/personnel.

Reorient to person/place/time as indicated.

Present reality concisely and briefly without challenging illogical thinking.

Provide clock, calendar, room with outside window; alter level of lighting to simulate day/night.

Encourage visits by family/SO. Provide support as needed.

RATIONALE

Determines extent of interference with sensory processing.

May be hypervigilant, restless, extremely sensitive, or crying or may develop frank psychosis.

Anxiety may alter thought processes.

Reduction of external stimuli may decrease hyperactivity/reflexia, CNS irritability, auditory/visual hallucinations.

Helps establish and maintain awareness of reality/environment.

Limits defensive reaction.

Promotes continual orientation cues to assist patient in maintaining sense of normalcy.

Aids in maintaining socialization and orientation. *Note:* Patient's agitation/psychotic behavior may precipitate family quarrels/conflicts.

ACTIONS/INTERVENTIONS

Independent

Provide safety measures, e.g., padded side rails, close supervision, or soft restraints as necessary.

Collaborative

Administer medications as indicated, e.g., sedatives/antianxiety agents/antipsychotic drugs.

RATIONALE

Prevents injury to patient who may be hallucinating/disoriented.

Promotes relaxation, reduces CNS hyperactivity/agitation to enhance thinking ability.

NURSING DIAGNOSIS: Tissue Integrity, risk for impaired

Risk factors may include

Alterations of protective mechanisms of eye: Impaired closure of eyelid/exophthalmos

Possibly evidenced by

[Not applicable; presence of signs and symptoms establishes an *actual* diagnosis]

DESIRED OUTCOMES/EVALUATION CRITERIA—PATIENT WILL:

Tissue Integrity: Skin & Mucous Membranes (NOC)

Maintain moist eye membranes, free of ulcerations.

Risk Control (NOC)

Identify measures to provide protection for eyes and prevent complications.

ACTIONS/INTERVENTIONS

Surveillance (NIC)

Independent

Observe for periorbital edema, lid lag, wide-eyed stare, excessive tearing. Note reports of photophobia, feeling of foreign object in eye; eye pain.

Evaluate visual acuity; note reports of blurred or double vision.

Encourage use of dark glasses when awake and taping the eyelids shut during sleep as needed.

Elevate the head of the bed and restrict salt intake if indicated.

Instruct the patient in extraocular muscle exercises if appropriate.

Provide opportunity for patient to discuss feelings about altered appearance and measures to enhance self-image.

Collaborative

Administer medications as indicated:

Methylcellulose drops;

RATIONALE

Common manifestations of excessive adrenergic stimulation related to thyrotoxicosis, requiring supportive interventions until therapeutic resolution of crisis state relieves symptomatology.

Infiltrative ophthalmopathy (Graves' disease) is the result of increased retro-orbital tissue, creating exophthalmos and lymphocytic infiltration of extraocular muscles, which causes weakness. Corresponding visual impairment may worsen or improve independent of therapy and clinical course of disease.

Protects exposed cornea if patient is unable to close eyelids completely because of edema/fibrosis of fat pads.

Decreases tissue edema when appropriate, e.g., HF, which can aggravate existing exophthalmos.

Improves circulation and maintains mobility of the eyelids.

Protruding eyes may be viewed as unattractive. Appearance can be enhanced with proper use of makeup, overall grooming, and use of shaded glasses.

Lubricates the eyes, reducing risk of lesion formation.

ACTIONS/INTERVENTIONS	RATIONALE
Collaborative	
Adrenocorticotropic hormone (ACTH), prednisone;	Given to decrease rapidly progressive and marked inflammation.
Antithyroid drugs;	May decrease signs/symptoms or prevent worsening of the condition.
Diuretics.	Can decrease edema in mild involvement.
Prepare for surgery as indicated.	Eyelids may need to be sutured shut temporarily to protect the corneas until edema resolves (rare), or increasing space within sinus cavity and adjusting musculature may return eye to a more normal position.

NURSING DIAGNOSIS: Knowledge Deficit [Learning Need] regarding condition, prognosis, treatment, self care, and discharge needs

May be related to
Lack of exposure/recall
Information misinterpretation
Unfamiliarity with information resources

Possibly evidenced by
Questions, request for information, statement of misconception
Inaccurate follow-through of instructions/development of preventable complications

DESIRED OUTCOMES/EVALUATION CRITERIA—PATIENT WILL:

> **Knowledge: Disease Process (NOC)**

Verbalize understanding of disease process and potential complications.
Identify relationship of signs/symptoms to the disease process and correlate symptoms with causative factors.

> **Knowledge: Treatment Regimen (NOC)**

Verbalize understanding of therapeutic needs.
Initiate necessary lifestyle changes and participate in treatment regimen.

ACTIONS/INTERVENTIONS	RATIONALE
Teaching: Disease Process (NIC)	
Independent	
Review disease process and future expectations.	Provides knowledge base from which patient can make informed choices.
Provide information appropriate to individual situation.	Severity of condition, cause, age, and concurrent complications determines course of treatment.
Identify stressors and discuss precipitators of thyroid crises, e.g., personal/social and job concerns, infection, pregnancy.	Psychogenic factors are often of prime importance in the occurrence/exacerbation of this disease.
Provide information about signs/symptoms of hypothyroidism and the need for continuing follow-up care.	The patient who has been treated for hyperthyroidism needs to be aware of possible development of hypothyroidism, which can occur immediately after treatment or as long as 5 yr later.

ACTIONS/INTERVENTIONS	RATIONALE
Independent	
Discuss drug therapy, including need for adhering to regimen, and expected therapeutic and side effects.	Antithyroid medication (either as primary therapy or in preparation for thyroidectomy) requires adherence to a medical regimen over an extended period to inhibit hormone production. Agranulocytosis is the most serious side effect that can occur, and alternative drugs may be given when problems arise.
Identify signs/symptoms requiring medical evaluation, e.g., fever, sore throat, and skin eruptions.	Early identification of toxic reactions (thiourea therapy) and prompt intervention are important in preventing development of agranulocytosis.
Explain need to check with physician/pharmacist before taking other prescribed or OTC drugs.	Antithyroid medications can affect or be affected by numerous other medications, requiring monitoring of medication levels, side effects, and interactions.
Emphasize importance of planned rest periods.	Prevents undue fatigue; reduces metabolic demands. As euthyroid state is achieved, stamina and activity level will increase.
Review need for nutritious diet and periodic review of nutrient needs; avoid caffeine, red/yellow food dyes, artificial preservatives.	Provides adequate nutrients to support hypermetabolic state. As hormonal imbalance is corrected, diet will need to be readjusted to prevent excessive weight gain. Irritants and stimulants should be limited to avoid cumulative systemic effects.
Stress necessity of continued medical follow-up.	Necessary for monitoring effectiveness of therapy and prevention of potentially fatal complications.

POTENTIAL CONSIDERATIONS following acute hospitalization (dependent on patient's age, physical condition/presence of complications, personal resources, and life responsibilities)

Fatigue—hypermetabolic state diminishing body energy reserves, prolonged recovery.
Nutrition: altered, risk for more than body requirements—change in BMR and metabolic needs.

THYROIDECTOMY

Thyroidectomy, although rare, may be performed for patients with thyroid cancer, hyperthyroidism, and drug reactions to antithyroid agents; pregnant women who cannot be managed with drugs; patients who do not want radiation therapy; and patients with large goiters who do not respond to antithyroid drugs. The two types of thyroidectomy include:

Total thyroidectomy: The gland is removed completely. Usually done in the case of malignancy. Thyroid replacement therapy is necessary for life.

Subtotal thyroidectomy: Up to five-sixths of the gland is removed when antithyroid drugs do not correct hyperthyroidism or RAI therapy is contraindicated.

CARE SETTING

Inpatient acute surgical unit

RELATED CONCERNS

Cancer, page 900
Hyperthyroidism (thyrotoxicosis, Graves' disease), page 455
Psychosocial aspects of care, page 809
Surgical intervention, page 828

Patient Assessment Database

Refer to CP: Hyperthyroidism (Thyrotoxicosis, Graves' Disease), page 455 for assessment information.

Discharge plan considerations:

DRG projected mean length of inpatient stay: 2.4 days.

Refer to section at end of plan for postdischarge considerations.

NURSING PRIORITIES

1. Reverse/manage hyperthyroid state preoperatively.
2. Prevent complications.
3. Relieve pain.
4. Provide information about surgical procedure, prognosis, and treatment needs.

DISCHARGE GOALS

1. Complications prevented/minimized.
2. Pain alleviated.
3. Surgical procedure/prognosis and therapeutic regimen understood.
4. Plan in place to meet needs after discharge.

NURSING DIAGNOSIS: Airway Clearance, risk for ineffective

Risk factors may include
Tracheal obstruction; swelling, bleeding, laryngeal spasms

Possibly evidenced by
[Not applicable; presence of signs and symptoms establishes an *actual* diagnosis]

DESIRED OUTCOMES/EVALUATION CRITERIA—PATIENT WILL:

Respiratory Status: Ventilation (NOC)

Maintain patent airway, with aspiration prevented.

ACTIONS/INTERVENTIONS	RATIONALE

Airway Management (NIC)

Independent

Monitor respiratory rate, depth, and work of breathing.

Respirations may remain somewhat rapid, but development of respiratory distress is indicative of tracheal compression from edema or hemorrhage.

Auscultate breath sounds, noting presence of rhonchi.

Rhonchi may indicate airway obstruction/accumulation of copious thick secretions.

Assess for dyspnea, stridor, "crowing," and cyanosis. Note quality of voice.

Indicators of tracheal obstruction/laryngeal spasm, requiring prompt evaluation and intervention.

Caution patient to avoid bending neck; support head with pillows.

Reduces likelihood of tension on surgical wound.

Assist with repositioning, deep-breathing exercises, and/or coughing as indicated.

Maintains clear airway and ventilation. Although "routine" coughing is not encouraged and may be painful, it may be needed to clear secretions.

Suction mouth and trachea as indicated, noting color and characteristics of sputum.

Edema/pain may impair patient's ability to clear own airway.

Check dressing frequently, especially posterior portion.

If bleeding occurs, anterior dressing may appear dry because blood pools dependently.

Investigate reports of difficulty swallowing, drooling of oral secretions.

May indicate edema/sequestered bleeding in tissues surrounding operative site.

Keep tracheostomy tray at bedside.

Compromised airway may create a life-threatening situation requiring emergency procedure.

Collaborative

Provide steam inhalation; humidify room air.

Reduces discomfort of sore throat and tissue edema and promotes expectoration of secretions.

Assist with/prepare for procedures, e.g.:

Tracheostomy;

May be necessary to maintain airway if obstructed by edema of glottis or hemorrhage.

Return to surgery.

May require ligation of bleeding vessels.

NURSING DIAGNOSIS: Communication, impaired verbal

May be related to
Vocal cord injury/laryngeal nerve damage
Tissue edema; pain/discomfort

Possibly evidenced by
Impaired articulation, does not/cannot speak; use of nonverbal cues such as gestures

DESIRED OUTCOMES/EVALUATION CRITERIA—PATIENT WILL:

Communication Ability (NOC)

Establish method of communication in which needs can be understood.

ACTIONS/INTERVENTIONS

RATIONALE

Communication Enhancement: Speech Deficit (NIC)

Independent

Assess speech periodically; encourage voice rest.

Hoarseness and sore throat may occur secondary to tissue edema or surgical damage to recurrent laryngeal nerve and may last several days. Permanent nerve damage can occur (rare) that causes paralysis of vocal cords and/or compression of the trachea.

Keep communication simple; ask yes/no questions.

Reduces demand for response; promotes voice rest.

Provide alternate methods of communication as appropriate, e.g., slate board, letter/picture board. Place IV line to minimize interference with written communication.

Facilitates expression of needs.

Anticipate needs as possible. Visit patient frequently.

Reduces anxiety and patient's need to communicate.

Post notice of patient's voice limitations at central station and answer call bell promptly.

Prevents patient from straining voice to make needs known/summon assistance.

Maintain quiet environment.

Enhances ability to hear whispered communication and reduces necessity for patient to raise/strain voice to be heard.

NURSING DIAGNOSIS: Injury, risk for [tetany]

Risk factors may include
Chemical imbalance: Excessive CNS stimulation

Possibly evidenced by
[Not applicable; presence of signs and symptoms establishes an *actual* diagnosis]

DESIRED OUTCOMES/EVALUATION CRITERIA—PATIENT WILL:

Safety Status: Physical Injury (NOC)

Demonstrate absence of injury with complications minimized/controlled.

ACTIONS/INTERVENTIONS

RATIONALE

Surveillance (NIC)

Independent

Monitor vital signs noting elevating temperature, tachycardia (140–200/min), dysrhythmias, respiratory distress, cyanosis (developing pulmonary edema/HF).

Manipulation of gland during subtotal thyroidectomy may result in increased hormone release, causing thyroid storm.

Evaluate reflexes periodically. Observe for neuromuscular irritability, e.g., twitching, numbness, paresthesias, positive Chvostek's and Trousseau's signs, seizure activity.

Hypocalcemia with tetany (usually transient) may occur 1–7 days postoperatively and indicates hypoparathyroidism, which can occur as a result of inadvertent trauma to/partial-to-total removal of parathyroid gland(s) during surgery.

Keep side rails raised/padded, bed in low position, and airway at bedside. Avoid use of restraints.

Reduces potential for injury if seizures occur. (Refer to CP: Seizure Disorders, ND: Trauma/Suffocation, risk for p. 231.)

ACTIONS/INTERVENTIONS	RATIONALE

Collaborative

Monitor serum calcium levels.	Patients with levels less than 7.5 mg/100 mL generally require replacement therapy.
Administer medications as indicated:	
Calcium (gluconate, lactate);	Corrects deficiency, which is usually temporary but may be permanent. *Note:* Use with caution in patients taking digitalis because calcium increases cardiac sensitivity to digitalis, potentiating risk of toxicity.
Phosphate-binding agents;	Helpful in lowering elevated phosphorus levels associated with hypocalcemia.
Sedatives;	Promotes rest, reducing exogenous stimulation.
Anticonvulsants.	Controls seizure activity until corrective therapy is successful.

NURSING DIAGNOSIS: Pain [acute]

May be related to
Surgical interruption/manipulation of tissues/muscles
Postoperative edema

Possibly evidenced by
Reports of pain
Narrowed focus; guarding behavior; restlessness
Autonomic responses

DESIRED OUTCOMES/EVALUATION CRITERIA—PATIENT WILL:

Pain Control Behavior (NOC)

Report pain is relieved/controlled.
Demonstrate use of relaxation skills and diversional activities appropriate to situation.

ACTIONS/INTERVENTIONS	RATIONALE

Pain Management (NIC)

Independent

Assess verbal/nonverbal reports of pain, noting location, intensity (0–10 scale), and duration.	Useful in evaluating pain, choice of interventions, effectiveness of therapy.
Place in semi-Fowler's position and support head/neck with sandbags or small pillows.	Prevents hyperextension of the neck and protects integrity of the suture line.
Maintain head/neck in neutral position and support during position changes. Instruct patient to use hands to support neck during movement and to avoid hyperextension of neck.	Prevents stress on the suture line and reduces muscle tension.
Keep call bell and frequently needed items within easy reach.	Limits stretching, muscle strain in operative area.
Give cool liquids or soft foods, such as ice cream or popsicles.	Although both may be soothing to sore throat, soft foods may be tolerated better than liquids if patient experiences difficulty swallowing.
Encourage patient to use relaxation techniques, e.g., guided imagery, soft music, progressive relaxation.	Helps refocus attention and assists patient to manage pain/discomfort more effectively.

ACTIONS/INTERVENTIONS

Collaborative

Administer analgesics and/or analgesic throat sprays/lozenges as necessary.

Provide ice collar if indicated.

RATIONALE

Reduces pain and discomfort; enhances rest.

Reduces tissue edema and decreases perception of pain.

NURSING DIAGNOSIS: Knowledge Deficit [Learning Need] regarding condition, prognosis, treatment, self care, and discharge needs

May be related to
Lack of exposure/recall, misinterpretation
Unfamiliarity with information resources

Possibly evidenced by
Questions; request for information; statement of misconception
Inaccurate follow-through of instructions/development of preventable complications

DESIRED OUTCOMES/EVALUATION CRITERIA—PATIENT WILL:

Knowledge: Disease Process (NOC)

Verbalize understanding of surgical procedure and prognosis and potential complications

Knowledge: Treatment Regimen (NOC)

Verbalize understanding of therapeutic needs.
Participate in treatment regimen.
Initiate necessary lifestyle changes.

ACTIONS/INTERVENTIONS

Teaching: Disease Process (NIC)

Independent

Review surgical procedure and future expectations.

Discuss need for well-balanced, nutritious diet and, when appropriate, inclusion of iodized salt.

Recommend avoidance of goitrogenic foods, e.g., excessive ingestion of seafood, soybeans, turnips.

Identify foods high in calcium (e.g., dairy products) and vitamin D (e.g., fortified dairy products, egg yolks, liver).

Encourage progressive general exercise program.

Review postoperative exercises to be instituted after incision heals, e.g., flexion, extension, rotation, and lateral movement of head and neck.

Review importance of rest and relaxation, avoiding stressful situations and emotional outbursts.

RATIONALE

Provides knowledge base from which patient can make informed decisions.

Promotes healing and helps patient regain/maintain appropriate weight. Use of iodized salt is often sufficient to meet iodine needs unless salt is restricted for other health care problems, e.g., HF.

Contraindicated after partial thyroidectomy because these foods inhibit thyroid activity.

Maximizes supply and absorption of calcium if parathyroid function is impaired.

In patients with subtotal thyroidectomy, exercise can stimulate the thyroid gland and production of hormones, facilitating recovery of general well-being.

Regular ROM exercises strengthen neck muscles, enhance circulation and healing process.

Effects of hyperthyroidism usually subside completely, but it takes some time for the body to recover.

ACTIONS/INTERVENTIONS	RATIONALE
Independent	
Instruct in incisional care, e.g., cleansing, dressing application.	Enables patient to provide competent self-care.
Recommend the use of loose-fitting scarves to cover scar, avoiding the use of jewelry.	Covers the incision without aggravating healing or precipitating infections of suture line.
Apply cold cream after sutures have been removed.	Softens tissues and may help minimize scarring.
Discuss possibility of change in voice.	Alteration in vocal cord function may cause changes in pitch and quality of voice, which may be temporary or permanent.
Review drug therapy and the necessity of continuing even when feeling well.	If thyroid hormone replacement is needed because of surgical removal of gland, patient needs to understand rationale for replacement therapy and consequences of failure to routinely take medication.
Identify signs/symptoms requiring medical evaluation, e.g., fever, chills, continued/purulent wound drainage, erythema, gaps in wound edges; sudden weight loss, intolerance to heat, nausea/vomiting, diarrhea, insomnia, weight gain, fatigue, intolerance to cold, constipation, drowsiness.	Early recognition of developing complications such as infection, hyperthyroidism, or hypothyroidism may prevent progression to life-threatening situation. *Note:* As many as 43% of patients with subtotal thyroidectomy will develop hypothyroidism in time.
Stress necessity of continued medical follow-up.	Provides opportunity for evaluating effectiveness of therapy and prevention of complications.

POTENTIAL CONSIDERATIONS following acute hospitalization (dependent on patient's age, physical condition/presence of complications, personal resources, and life responsibilities)

Fatigue—decreased metabolic energy production, altered body chemistry (hypothyroidism).

Refer to Potential Considerations in Surgical Intervention plan of care page 826.

HEPATITIS

Hepatitis is a widespread inflammation of the liver that results in degeneration and necrosis of liver cells. Inflammation of the liver can be due to bacterial invasion, injury by physical or toxic chemical agents (e.g., drugs, alcohol, industrial chemicals), viral infections (hepatitis A, B, C, D, E, G), or autoimmune response. Although most hepatitis is self-limiting, approximately 20% of acute hepatitis B and 50% of hepatitis C cases progress to a chronic state or cirrhosis and can be fatal.

CARE SETTING

Usually community level, although brief inpatient acute care on a medical unit may be required, especially in toxic states.

RELATED CONCERNS

Alcoholism: acute withdrawal, page 873
Substance dependence/abuse rehabilitation, page 886
Cirrhosis of the liver, page 484
Psychosocial aspects of care, page 809
Renal dialysis, page 600
Total nutritional support: parenteral/enteral feeding, page 508

Patient Assessment Database

Data depend on the cause and severity of liver involvement/damage.

ACTIVITY/REST

May report: Fatigue, weakness, general malaise

CIRCULATION

May exhibit: Bradycardia (severe hyperbilirubinemia)
Jaundiced sclera, skin, mucous membranes

ELIMINATION

May report: Dark urine
Diarrhea/constipation; clay-colored stools
Current/recent hemodialysis

FOOD/FLUID

May report: Loss of appetite (anorexia), weight loss or gain (edema)
Nausea/vomiting

May exhibit: Ascites

NEUROSENSORY

May exhibit: Irritability, drowsiness, lethargy, asterixis

PAIN/DISCOMFORT

May report: Abdominal cramping, right upper quadrant (RUQ) tenderness
Myalgias, arthralgias; headache
Itching (pruritus)

May exhibit: Muscle guarding, restlessness

RESPIRATION

May report: Distaste for/aversion to cigarettes (smokers)
Recent flulike URI

SAFETY

May report: Transfusion of blood/blood products in the past
May exhibit: Fever
Urticaria, maculopapular lesions, irregular patches of erythema

Exacerbation of acne

Spider angiomas, palmar erythema, gynecomastia in men (sometimes present in alcoholic hepatitis)

Splenomegaly, posterior cervical node enlargement

SEXUALITY

May report: Lifestyle/behaviors increasing risk of exposure (e.g., sexual promiscuity, sexually active homosexual/bisexual male)

TEACHING/LEARNING

May report: History of known/possible exposure to virus, bacteria, or toxins (contaminated food, water, needles, surgical equipment or blood); carriers (symptomatic or asymptomatic); recent surgical procedure with halothane anesthesia; exposure to toxic chemicals (e.g., carbon tetrachloride, vinyl chloride); prescription drug use (e.g., sulfonamides, phenothiazines, isoniazid)

Travel to/immigration from China, Africa, Southeast Asia, Middle East (hepatitis B [HB] is endemic in these areas)

Street injection drug or alcohol use

Concurrent diabetes, HF, malignancy, or renal disease

Discharge plan considerations: **DRG projected mean length of inpatient stay: 6.1 days**

May require assistance with homemaker/maintenance tasks

Refer to section at end of plan for postdischarge considerations.

DIAGNOSTIC STUDIES

Liver enzymes/isoenzymes: Abnormal (4–10 times normal values). *Note:* Of limited value in differentiating viral from nonviral hepatitis.

AST/ALT: Initially elevated. May rise 1–2 wk before jaundice is apparent, then decline.

Alkaline phosphatase: Slight elevation (unless severe cholestasis present).

Hepatitis A, B, C, D, E panels (antibody/antigen tests): Specify type and stage of disease and determine possible carriers.

CBC: Red blood cells (RBCs) decreased because of shortened life of RBCs (liver enzyme alterations) or hemorrhage.

WBC count and differential: Leukopenia, leukocytosis, monocytosis, atypical lymphocytes, and plasma cells may be present.

Serum albumin: Decreased.

Blood glucose: Transient hyperglycemia/hypoglycemia (altered liver function).

Prothrombin time: May be prolonged (liver dysfunction).

Serum bilirubin: Above 2.5 mg/100 mL. (If above 200 mg/100 mL, poor prognosis is probable because of increased cellular necrosis.)

Stools: Clay-colored, steatorrhea (decreased hepatic function).

Bromsulphalein (BSP) excretion test: Blood level elevated.

Liver biopsy: Defines diagnosis and extent of inflammation/fatty necrosis.

Liver scan: Aids in estimation of severity of parenchymal damage.

Urinalysis: Elevated bilirubin levels; protein/hematuria may occur.

NURSING PRIORITIES

1. Reduce demands on liver while promoting physical well-being.
2. Prevent complications.
3. Enhance self-concept, acceptance of situation.
4. Provide information about disease process, prognosis, and treatment needs.

DISCHARGE GOALS

1. Meeting basic self-care needs.
2. Complications prevented/minimized.
3. Dealing with reality of current situation.
4. Disease process, prognosis, and therapeutic regimen understood.
5. Plan in place to meet needs after discharge.

> **NURSING DIAGNOSIS: Fatigue**
>
> **May be related to**
> Decreased metabolic energy production
> States of discomfort
> Altered body chemistry (e.g., changes in liver function, effect on target organs)
>
> **Possibly evidenced by**
> Reports of lack of energy/inability to maintain usual routines
> Decreased performance
> Increase in physical complaints
>
> **DESIRED OUTCOMES/EVALUATION CRITERIA—PATIENT WILL:**
>
> **Endurance (NOC)**
>
> Report improved sense of energy.
> Perform ADLs and participate in desired activities at level of ability.

ACTIONS/INTERVENTIONS

Energy Management (NIC)

Independent

Promote bedrest/chair (recliner) rest. Provide quiet environment; limit visitors as needed.

Recommend changing position frequently. Provide/instruct caregiver in good skin care.

Do necessary tasks quickly and at one time as tolerated.

Determine and prioritize role responsibilities and alternate providers/possible community resources available, e.g., Meals on Wheels, homemaker/housekeeper services.

Identify energy-conserving techniques, e.g., sitting to shower and brush teeth, planning steps of activity so that all needed materials are at hand, scheduling rest periods.

Increase activity as tolerated, demonstrate passive/active ROM exercises.

Encourage use of stress management techniques, e.g., progressive relaxation, visualization, guided imagery. Discuss appropriate diversional activities, e.g., radio, TV, reading.

Monitor for recurrence of anorexia and liver tenderness/enlargement.

Collaborative

Administer medications as indicated: sedatives, antianxiety agents, e.g., diazepam (Valium), lorazepam (Ativan).

RATIONALE

Promotes rest and relaxation. Available energy is used for healing. Activity and an upright position are believed to decrease hepatic blood flow, which prevents optimal circulation to the liver cells.

Promotes optimal respiratory function and minimizes pressure areas to reduce risk of tissue breakdown.

Allows for extended periods of uninterrupted rest.

Promotes problem solving of most pressing needs of individual/family.

Helps lessen progression of fatigue, allowing patient to accomplish more and feel better about self.

Prolonged bedrest can be debilitating. This can be offset by limited activity alternating with rest periods.

Promotes relaxation and conserves energy, redirects attention, and may enhance coping.

Indicates lack of resolution/exacerbation of the disease, requiring further rest, change in therapeutic regimen.

Assists in managing required rest. *Note:* Use of barbiturates and antianxiety agents, such as prochlorperazine (Compazine) and chlorpromazine (Thorazine), is contraindicated because of hepatotoxic effects.

ACTIONS/INTERVENTIONS	RATIONALE
Collaborative	
Monitor serial liver enzyme levels.	Aids in determining appropriate levels of activity because premature increase in activity potentiates risk of relapse.
Administer antidote or assist with inpatient procedures as indicated (e.g., lavage, catharsis, hyperventilation) depending on route of exposure.	Removal of causative agent in toxic hepatitis may limit degree of tissue involvement/damage.

NURSING DIAGNOSIS: Nutrition: altered, less than body requirements

May be related to
Insufficient intake to meet metabolic demands: anorexia, nausea/vomiting
Altered absorption and metabolism of ingested foods: reduced peristalsis (visceral reflexes), bile stasis
Increased calorie needs/hypermetabolic state

Possibly evidenced by
Aversion to eating/lack of interest in food; altered taste sensation
Abdominal pain/cramping
Loss of weight; poor muscle tone

DESIRED OUTCOMES/EVALUATION CRITERIA—PATIENT WILL:

Treatment Behavior: Illness or Injury (NOC)

Initiate behaviors, lifestyle changes to regain/maintain appropriate weight.

Nutritional Status (NOC)

Demonstrate progressive weight gain toward goal with normalization of laboratory values and no signs of malnutrition.

ACTIONS/INTERVENTIONS	RATIONALE
Weight Gain Assistance (NIC)	
Independent	
Monitor dietary intake/calorie count. Suggest several small feedings and offer "largest" meal at breakfast.	Large meals are difficult to manage when patient is anorexic. Anorexia may also worsen during the day, making intake of food difficult later in the day.
Encourage mouth care before meals.	Eliminating unpleasant taste may enhance appetite.
Recommend eating in upright position.	Reduces sensation of abdominal fullness and may enhance intake.
Encourage intake of fruit juices, carbonated beverages, and hard candy throughout the day.	These supply extra calories and may be more easily digested/tolerated when other foods are not.

ACTIONS/INTERVENTIONS

Collaborative

Consult with dietitian, nutritional support team to provide diet according to patient's needs, with fat and protein intake as tolerated.

Monitor serum glucose as indicated.

Administer medications as indicated:

Antiemetics, e.g., metoclopramide (Reglan), trimethobenzamide (Tigan);

Antacids, e.g., Mylanta, Titralac;

Vitamins, e.g., B complex, C, other dietary supplements as indicated;

Steroid therapy, e.g., prednisone (Deltasone), alone or in combination with azathioprine (Imuran).

Provide supplemental feedings/TPN if needed.

RATIONALE

Useful in formulating dietary program to meet individual needs. Fat metabolism varies according to bile production and excretion and may necessitate restriction of fat intake if diarrhea develops. If tolerated, a normal or increased protein intake helps with liver regeneration. Protein restriction may be indicated in severe disease (e.g., fulminating hepatitis) because the accumulation of the end products of protein metabolism can potentiate hepatic encephalopathy.

Hyperglycemia/hypoglycemia may develop, necessitating dietary changes/insulin administration. Fingerstick monitoring may be done by patient on a regular schedule to determine therapy needs.

Given ½ hr before meals, may reduce nausea and increase food tolerance. *Note:* Prochlorperazine (Compazine) is contraindicated in hepatic disease.

Counteracts gastric acidity, reducing irritation/risk of bleeding.

Corrects deficiencies and aids in the healing process.

Steroids may be contraindicated because they can increase risk of relapse/development of chronic hepatitis in patients with viral hepatitis; however, anti-inflammatory effect may be useful in chronic active hepatitis (especially idiopathic) to reduce nausea/vomiting and enable patient to retain food and fluids. Steroids may decrease serum aminotransferase and bilirubin levels, but they do not affect liver necrosis or regeneration. Combination therapy has fewer steroid-related side effects.

May be necessary to meet caloric requirements if marked deficits are present/symptoms are prolonged.

NURSING DIAGNOSIS: Fluid Volume risk for deficit

Risk factors may include
Excessive losses through vomiting and diarrhea, third-space shift (ascites)
Altered clotting process

Possibly evidenced by
[Not applicable; presence of signs and symptoms establishes an *actual* diagnosis]

DESIRED OUTCOMES/EVALUATION CRITERIA—PATIENT WILL:

Hydration (NOC)

Maintain adequate hydration, as evidenced by stable vital signs, good skin turgor, capillary refill, strong peripheral pulses, and individually appropriate urinary output.

ACTIONS/INTERVENTIONS	RATIONALE

Fluid/Electrolyte Management (NIC)

Independent

Monitor I&O, compare with periodic weight. Note enteric losses, e.g., vomiting and diarrhea.

Provides information about replacement needs/effects of therapy. *Note:* Diarrhea may be due to transient flu-like response to viral infection or may represent a more serious problem of obstructed portal blood flow with vascular congestion in the GI tract, or it may be the intended result of medication use (neomycin, lactulose) to decrease serum ammonia levels in the presence of hepatic encephalopathy.

Assess vital signs, peripheral pulses, capillary refill, skin turgor, and mucous membranes.

Indicators of circulating volume/perfusion.

Bleeding Precautions (NIC)

Check for ascites or edema formation. Measure abdominal girth as indicated.

Useful in monitoring progression/resolution of fluid shifts (edema/ascites).

Use small-gauge needles for injections, applying pressure for longer than usual after venipuncture.

Reduces possibility of bleeding into tissues.

Have patient use cotton/sponge swabs and mouthwash instead of toothbrush.

Avoids trauma and bleeding of the gums.

Observe for signs of bleeding, e.g., hematuria/melena, ecchymosis, oozing from gums/puncture sites.

Prothrombin levels are reduced and coagulation times prolonged when vitamin K absorption is altered in GI tract and synthesis of prothrombin is decreased in affected liver.

Collaborative

Fluid/Electrolyte Management (NIC)

Monitor periodic laboratory values, e.g., Hb/Hct, Na+, albumin, and clotting times.

Reflects hydration and identifies sodium retention/protein deficits, which may lead to edema formation. Deficits in clotting potentiate risk of bleeding/hemorrhage.

Administer antidiarrheal agents, e.g., diphenoxylate with atropine (Lomotil).

Reduces fluid/electrolyte loss from GI tract.

Provide IV fluids (usually glucose), electrolytes.

Provides fluid and electrolyte replacement in acute toxic state.

Protein hydrolysates.

Correction of albumin/protein deficits can aid in return of fluid from tissues to the circulatory system.

Bleeding Precautions (NIC)

Administer medications as indicated, e.g.:

Vitamin K;

Because absorption is altered, supplementation may prevent coagulation problems, which may occur if clotting factors/prothrombin time (PT) is depressed.

Antacids or H$_2$-receptor antagonists, e.g., cimetadine (Tagamet).

Neutralize/reduce gastric secretions to lower risk of gastric irritation/bleeding.

Infuse fresh frozen plasma, as indicated.

May be required to replace clotting factors in the presence of coagulation defects.

NURSING DIAGNOSIS: Self-Esteem, situational low

May be related to

Annoying/debilitating symptoms, confinement/isolation, length of illness/recovery period

Possibly evidenced by

Verbalization of change in lifestyle; fear of rejection/reaction of others, negative feelings about body; feelings of helplessness

Depression, lack of follow-through, self-destructive behavior

DESIRED OUTCOMES/EVALUATION CRITERIA—PATIENT WILL:

Self-Esteem (NOC)

Verbalize feelings.

Identify feelings and methods for coping with negative perception of self.

Verbalize acceptance of self in situation, including length of recovery/need for isolation.

Acknowledge self as worthwhile; be responsible for self.

ACTIONS/INTERVENTIONS	RATIONALE
Self-Esteem Enhancement (NIC)	
Independent	
Contract with patient regarding time for listening. Encourage discussion of feelings/concerns.	Establishing time enhances trusting relationship. Providing opportunity to express feelings allows patient to feel more in control of the situation. Verbalization can decrease anxiety and depression and facilitate positive coping behaviors. Patient may need to express feelings about being ill, length and cost of illness, possibility of infecting others, and (in severe illness) fear of death. May have concerns regarding the stigma of the disease.
Avoid making moral judgments regarding lifestyle (e.g., alcohol use/sexual practices).	Patient may already feel upset/angry and condemn self; judgments from others will further damage self-esteem.
Discuss recovery expectations.	Recovery period may be prolonged (up to 6 mo), potentiating family/situational stress and necessitating need for planning, support, and follow-up.
Assess effect of illness on economic factors of patient/SO.	Financial problems may exist because of loss of patient's role functioning in the family/prolonged recovery.
Offer diversional activities based on energy level.	Enables patient to use time and energy in constructive ways that enhance self-esteem and minimize anxiety and depression.
Suggest patient wear bright reds or blues/blacks instead of yellows or greens.	Enhances appearance, because yellow skin tones are intensified by yellow/green colors. *Note:* Jaundice usually peaks within 1–2 wk, then gradually resolves over 2–4 wk.
Collaborative	
Make appropriate referrals for help as needed, e.g., case manager/discharge planner, social services, and/or other community agencies.	Can facilitate problem solving and help involved individuals cope more effectively with situation.

NURSING DIAGNOSIS: Infection, risk for

Risk factors may include

Inadequate secondary defenses (e.g., leukopenia, suppressed inflammatory response) and immunosuppression

Malnutrition

Insufficient knowledge to avoid exposure to pathogens

Possibly evidenced by

[Not applicable; presence of signs and symptoms establishes an *actual* diagnosis]

DESIRED OUTCOMES/EVALUATION CRITERIA—PATIENT WILL:

Risk Control (NOC)

Verbalize understanding of individual causative/risk factor(s).

Demonstrate techniques; initiate lifestyle changes to avoid reinfection/transmission to others.

ACTIONS/INTERVENTIONS	RATIONALE
Infection Control (NIC)	
Independent	
Establish isolation techniques for enteric and respiratory infections according to infection guidelines/policy. Encourage/model effective handwashing.	Prevents transmission of viral disease to others. Thorough handwashing is effective in preventing virus transmission. Types A and E are transmitted by oral-fecal route, contaminated water, milk, and food (especially inadequately cooked shellfish). Types A, B, C, and D are transmitted by contaminated blood/blood products; needle punctures; open wounds; and contact with saliva, urine, stool, and semen. Incidence of both hepatitis B virus (HBV) and hepatitis C virus (HCV) has increased among healthcare providers and high-risk patients. *Note:* Toxic and alcoholic hepatitis are not communicable and do not require special measures/isolation.
Stress need to monitor/restrict visitors as indicated.	Patient exposure to infectious processes (especially respiratory) potentiates risk of secondary complications.
Explain isolation procedures to patient/SO.	Understanding reasons for safeguarding themselves and others can lessen feelings of isolation and stigmatization. Isolation may last 2–3 wk from onset of illness, depending on type/duration of symptoms.
Give information regarding availability of gammaglobulin, ISG, H-BIG, HB vaccine (Recombivax HB, Engerix-B) through health department or family physician.	Immune globulins may be effective in preventing viral hepatitis in those who have been exposed, depending on type of hepatitis and period of incubation.
Collaborative	
Administer medications as indicated:	
Antiviral drugs: vidarabine (Vira-A), acyclovir (Zovirax);	Useful in treating chronic active hepatitis.
Interferon alfa-2b (Intron-a);	Treats the symptoms of HepC and may lead to temporary improvement in liver function.

ACTIONS/INTERVENTIONS

Collaborative

Ribavirin;

Antibiotics appropriate to causative agents (e.g., Gram-negative, anaerobic bacteria) or secondary process.

RATIONALE

Used in conjunction with interferon to improve the effectiveness of that drug. *Note:* These treatments lead to improvement, not cure of the disease.

Used to treat bacterial hepatitis or to prevent/limit secondary infections.

NURSING DIAGNOSIS: Skin/Tissue Integrity, risk for impaired

Risk factors may include
Chemical substance: Bile salt accumulation in the tissues

Possibly evidenced by
[Not applicable; presence of signs and symptoms establishes an *actual* diagnosis]

DESIRED OUTCOMES/EVALUATION CRITERIA—PATIENT WILL:

Tissue Integrity: Skin and Mucous Membranes (NOC)

Display intact skin/tissues, free of excoriation.
Report absence/decrease of pruritus/scratching.

ACTIONS/INTERVENTIONS

RATIONALE

Skin Surveillance (NIC)

Independent

Encourage use of cool showers and baking soda or starch baths. Avoid use of alkaline soaps. Apply calamine lotion as indicated.

Provide diversional activities.

Suggest use of knuckles if desire to scratch is uncontrollable. Keep fingernails cut short, apply gloves on comatose patient or during hours of sleep. Recommend loose-fitting clothing. Provide soft cotton linens.

Provide a soothing massage at bedtime.

Observe skin for areas of redness, breakdown.

Avoid comments regarding patient's appearance.

Prevents excessive dryness of skin. Provides relief from itching.

Aids in refocusing attention, reducing tendency to scratch.

Reduces potential for dermal injury.

May be helpful in promoting sleep by reducing skin irritation.

Early detection of problem areas allows for additional intervention to prevent complications/promote healing.

Minimizes psychological stress associated with skin changes.

Collaborative

Administer medications as indicated:

Antihistamines, e.g., methidilazine (Tacaryl), diphenhydramine (Benadryl);

Antilipemics, e.g., cholestyramine (Questran).

Relieves itching. *Note:* Use cautiously in severe hepatic disease.

May be used to bind bile acids in the intestine and prevent their absorption. Note side effects of nausea and constipation.

NURSING DIAGNOSIS: Knowledge Deficit [Learning Need] regarding condition, prognosis, treatment, self care, and discharge needs

May be related to
Lack of exposure/recall; information misinterpretation
Unfamiliarity with resources

Possibly evidenced by
Questions or statements of misconception; request for information
Inaccurate follow-through of instructions; development of preventable complications

DESIRED OUTCOMES/EVALUATION CRITERIA—PATIENT WILL:

Knowledge: Disease Process (NOC)

Verbalize understanding of disease process, prognosis, and potential complications.
Identify relationship of signs/symptoms to the disease and correlate symptoms with causative factors.

Knowledge: Treatment Regimen (NOC)

Verbalize understanding of therapeutic needs.
Initiate necessary lifestyle changes and participate in treatment regimen.

ACTIONS/INTERVENTIONS	RATIONALE
Teaching: Disease Process (NIC)	
Independent	
Assess level of understanding of the disease process, expectations/prognosis, possible treatment options.	Identifies areas of lack of knowledge/misinformation and provides opportunity to give additional information as necessary. *Note:* Liver transplantation may be needed in the presence of fulminating disease with liver failure.
Provide specific information regarding prevention/transmission of disease, e.g., contacts may require gamma-globulin; personal items should not be shared; observe strict handwashing and sanitizing of clothes, dishes, and toilet facilities while liver enzymes are elevated. Avoid intimate contact, such as kissing and sexual contact and exposure to infections, especially URI.	Needs/recommendations vary with type of hepatitis (causative agent) and individual situation.
Plan resumption of activity as tolerated with adequate periods of rest. Discuss restriction of heavy lifting, strenuous exercise/contact sports.	It is not necessary to wait until serum bilirubin levels return to normal to resume activity (may take as long as 2 mo), but strenuous activity needs to be limited until the liver returns to normal size. When patient begins to feel better, he or she needs to understand the importance of continued adequate rest in preventing relapse or recurrence. (Relapse occurs in 5%–25% of adults.) *Note:* Energy level may take up to 3–6 mo to return to normal.
Help patient identify appropriate diversional activities.	Enjoyable activities promote rest and help patient avoid focusing on prolonged convalescence.
Encourage continuation of balanced diet.	Promotes general well-being and enhances energy for healing process/tissue regeneration.
Identify ways to maintain usual bowel function, e.g., adequate intake of fluids/dietary roughage, moderate activity/exercise to tolerance.	Decreased level of activity, changes in food/fluid intake, and slowed bowel motility may result in constipation.

482

ACTIONS/INTERVENTIONS	RATIONALE
Independent	
Discuss the side effects and dangers of taking OTC/prescribed drugs (e.g., acetaminophen, aspirin, sulfonamides, some anesthetics) and necessity of notifying future healthcare providers of diagnosis.	Some drugs are toxic to the liver; many others are metabolized by the liver and should be avoided in severe liver diseases because they may cause cumulative toxic effects/chronic hepatitis.
Discuss restrictions on donating blood.	Prevents spread of infectious disease. Most state laws prevent accepting as donors those who have a history of any type of hepatitis.
Emphasize importance of follow-up physical examination and laboratory evaluation.	Disease process may take several months to resolve. If symptoms persist longer than 6 mo, liver biopsy may be required to verify presence of chronic hepatitis.
Review necessity of avoidance of alcohol for a minimum of 6–12 mo or longer based on individual tolerance.	Increases hepatic irritation and may interfere with recovery.
Refer to community resources, drug/alcohol treatment program as indicated.	May need additional assistance to withdraw from substance and maintain abstinence to avoid further liver damage.

POTENTIAL CONSIDERATIONS following acute hospitalization (dependent on patient's age, physical condition/presence of complications, personal resources, and life responsibilities)

Fatigue—generalized weakness, decreased strength/endurance, pain, imposed activity restrictions, depression.

Home Maintenance Management, impaired—prolonged recovery/chronic condition, insufficient finances, inadequate support systems, unfamiliarity with neighborhood resources.

Nutrition: altered, less than body requirements—insufficient intake to meet metabolic demands; anorexia, nausea/vomiting; altered absorption and metabolism of ingested foods; increased calorie needs/hypermetabolic state.

Infection, risk for—inadequate secondary defenses; malnutrition; insufficient knowledge to avoid exposure to pathogens.

CIRRHOSIS OF THE LIVER

Cirrhosis is a chronic disease of the liver characterized by alteration in structure and degenerative changes, impairing cellular function and impeding blood flow through the liver. Causes include malnutrition, inflammation (bacterial or viral), and poisons (e.g., alcohol, carbon tetrachloride, acetaminophen).

CARE SETTING

May be hospitalized on a medical unit during initial or recurrent acute episodes with potentially life-threatening complications. Otherwise, this condition is handled at the community level.

RELATED CONCERNS

Alcoholism: acute withdrawal, page 873
Substance dependence/Abuse rehabilitation, page 886
Fluid and electrolyte imbalances, page 926
Psychosocial aspects of care, page 809
Renal dialysis, page 600
Renal failure: acute, page 575
Total nutritional support: parenteral/enteral feeding, page 508
Upper gastrointestinal/Esophageal bleeding, page 333

Patient Assessment Database

Data depend on underlying cause of the condition.

ACTIVITY/REST

May report:	Weakness, fatigue, exhaustion
May exhibit:	Lethargy
	Decreased muscle mass/tone

CIRCULATION

May report:	History of/recent onset of HF, pericarditis, rheumatic heart disease, or cancer (causing liver impairment leading to failure)
	Easy bruising, nosebleeds, bleeding gums
May exhibit:	Hypertension or hypotension (fluid shifts)
	Dysrhythmias, extra heart sounds (S_3, S_4)
	JVD; distended abdominal veins
	Jaundice, skin, sclera

ELIMINATION

May report:	Flatulence
	Diarrhea or constipation; gradual abdominal enlargement
May exhibit:	Abdominal distention (hepatomegaly, splenomegaly, ascites)
	Decreased/absent bowel sounds
	Clay-colored stools, melena
	Dark, concentrated urine

FOOD/FLUID

May report:	Anorexia, food intolerance/indigestion
	Nausea/vomiting
May exhibit:	Weight loss or gain (fluid)
	Tissue wasting
	Edema generalized in tissues
	Dry skin, poor turgor
	Halitosis/fetor hepaticus, bleeding gums

NEUROSENSORY

May report:	SO(s) may report personality changes, depressed mentation
May exhibit:	Changes in mentation, confusion, hallucinations, coma Slowed/slurred speech Asterixis (hepatic encephalopathy)

PAIN/DISCOMFORT

May report:	Abdominal tenderness/RUQ pain Itching Pins/needles, burning pain in extremities
May exhibit:	Guarding/distraction behaviors Self-focus

RESPIRATION

May report:	Dyspnea
May exhibit:	Tachypnea, shallow respiration, adventitious breath sounds Limited thoracic expansion (ascites) Hypoxia

SAFETY

May report:	Frequent scratching of skin because of itching
May exhibit:	Fever (more common in alcoholic cirrhosis) Jaundice, ecchymosis, petechiae Spider angiomas/telangiectasis, palmar erythema

SEXUALITY

May report:	Menstrual disorders (women), impotence (men)
May exhibit:	Testicular atrophy, gynecomastia, loss of hair (chest, underarm, pubic)

TEACHING/LEARNING

May report:	History of long-term alcohol use/abuse, alcoholic liver disease History of biliary disease, hepatitis, exposure to toxins; liver trauma; upper GI bleeding; episodes of bleeding esophageal varices; use of drugs affecting liver function
Discharge plan considerations:	**DRG projected mean length of inpatient stay: 6.4 days** May need assistance with homemaker/management tasks
	Refer to section at end of plan for postdischarge considerations.

DIAGNOSTIC STUDIES

Liver scans/biopsy: Detects fatty infiltrates, fibrosis, destruction of hepatic tissues, tumors (primary or metastatic), associated ascites.

Percutaneous transhepatic cholangiography (PTHC): May be done to rule out/differentiate causes of jaundice or to perform liver biopsy.

Esophagogastroduodenoscopy (EGD): May demonstrate presence of esophageal varices.

Percutaneous transhepatic portal angiography (PTPA): Visualizes portal venous system circulation.

Serum bilirubin: Elevated because of cellular disruption, inability of liver to conjugate, or biliary obstruction.

Liver enzymes:

    AST/ALT, LDH, and isoenzymes (LDH_5): Increased because of cellular damage and release of enzymes.

    Alkaline phosphatase (ALP) and isoenzyme (LAP1): Elevated because of reduced excretion.

Gamma glutamyl transpeptidase (GTT): Elevated.

Serum albumin: Decreased because of depressed synthesis.

Globulins (IgA and IgG): Increased synthesis.

CBC: Hb/Hct and RBCs may be decreased because of bleeding. RBC destruction and anemia is seen with hypersplenism and iron deficiency. Leukopenia may be present as a result of hypersplenism.

PT/activated partial thromboplastin time (aPTT): Prolonged (decreased synthesis of prothrombin).

Fibrinogen: Decreased.

BUN: Elevation indicates breakdown of blood/protein.

Serum ammonia: Elevated because of inability to convert ammonia to urea.

Serum glucose: Hypoglycemia suggests impaired glycogenesis.

Electrolytes: Hypokalemia may reflect increased aldosterone, although various imbalances may occur. Hypocalcemia may occur because of impaired absorption of vitamin D.

Nutrient studies: Deficiency of vitamins A, B_{12}, C, K; folic acid, and iron may be noted.

Urine urobilinogen: May/may not be present. Serves as guide for differentiating liver disease, hemolytic disease, and biliary obstruction.

Fecal urobilinogen: Decreased.

NURSING PRIORITIES

1. Maintain adequate nutrition.
2. Prevent complications.
3. Enhance self-concept, acceptance of situation.
4. Provide information about disease process/prognosis, potential complications, and treatment needs.

DISCHARGE GOALS

1. Nutritional intake adequate for individual needs.
2. Complications prevented/minimized.
3. Dealing effectively with current reality.
4. Disease process, prognosis, potential complications, and therapeutic regimen understood.
5. Plan in place to meet needs after discharge.

NURSING DIAGNOSIS: Nutrition: altered, less than body requirements

May be related to

Inadequate diet; inability to process/digest nutrients

Anorexia, nausea/vomiting, indigestion, early satiety (ascites)

Abnormal bowel function

Possibly evidenced by

Weight loss

Changes in bowel sounds and function

Poor muscle tone/wasting

Imbalances in nutritional studies

DESIRED OUTCOMES/EVALUATION CRITERIA—PATIENT WILL:

Nutritional Status (NOC)

Demonstrate progressive weight gain toward goal with patient-appropriate normalization of laboratory values.

Experience no further signs of malnutrition.

ACTIONS/INTERVENTIONS	RATIONALE
Nutrition Therapy (NIC)	
Independent	
Measure dietary intake by calorie count.	Provides information about intake, needs/deficiencies.
Weigh as indicated. Compare changes in fluid status, recent weight history, skinfold measurements.	It may be difficult to use weight as a direct indicator of nutritional status in view of edema/ascites. Skinfold measurements are useful in assessing changes in muscle mass and subcutaneous fat reserves.

ACTIONS/INTERVENTIONS

Independent

Assist/encourage patient to eat; explain reasons for the type of diet. Feed patient if tiring easily, or have SO assist patient. Consider preferences in food choices.

Encourage patient to eat all meals/supplementary feedings.

Recommend/provide small, frequent meals.

Provide salt substitutes, if allowed; avoid those containing ammonium.

Restrict intake of caffeine, gas-producing or spicy and excessively hot or cold foods.

Suggest soft foods, avoiding roughage if indicated.

Encourage frequent mouth care, especially before meals.

Promote undisturbed rest periods, especially before meals.

Recommend cessation of smoking.

Collaborative

Monitor laboratory studies, e.g., serum glucose, pre-albumin/albumin, total protein, ammonia.

Maintain NPO status when indicated.

Consult with dietitian to provide diet that is high in calories and simple carbohydrates, low in fat, and moderate to high in protein; limit sodium and fluid as necessary. Provide liquid supplements as indicated.

Provide tube feedings, TPN, lipids if indicated.

RATIONALE

Improved nutrition/diet is vital to recovery. Patient may eat better if family is involved and preferred foods are included as much as possible.

Patient may pick at food or eat only a few bites because of loss of interest in food or because of nausea, generalized weakness, malaise.

Poor tolerance to larger meals may be due to increased intra-abdominal pressure/ascites.

Salt substitutes enhance the flavor of food and aid in increasing appetite; ammonia potentiates risk of encephalopathy.

Aids in reducing gastric irritation/diarrhea and abdominal discomfort that may impair oral intake/digestion.

Hemorrhage from esophageal varices may occur in advanced cirrhosis.

Patient is prone to sore and/or bleeding gums and bad taste in mouth, which contributes to anorexia.

Conserving energy reduces metabolic demands on the liver and promotes cellular regeneration.

Reduces excessive gastric stimulation and risk of irritation/bleeding.

Glucose may be decreased because of impaired glycogenesis, depleted glycogen stores, or inadequate intake. Protein may be low because of impaired metabolism, decreased hepatic synthesis, or loss into peritoneal cavity (ascites). Elevation of ammonia level may require restriction of protein intake to prevent serious complications.

Initially, GI rest may be required in acutely ill patients to reduce demands on the liver and production of ammonia/urea in the GI tract.

High-calorie foods are desired inasmuch as patient intake is usually limited. Carbohydrates supply readily available energy. Fats are poorly absorbed because of liver dysfunction and may contribute to abdominal discomfort. Proteins are needed to improve serum protein levels to reduce edema and to promote liver cell regeneration. *Note:* Protein and foods high in ammonia (e.g., gelatin) are restricted if ammonia level is elevated or if patient has clinical signs of hepatic encephalopathy. In addition, these individuals may tolerate vegetable protein better than meat protein.

May be required to supplement diet or to provide nutrients when patient is too nauseated or anorexic to eat or when esophageal varices interfere with oral intake.

ACTIONS/INTERVENTIONS

RATIONALE

Collaborative

Administer medications as indicated, e.g.:

Vitamin supplements, thiamine, iron, folic acid;

Patient may be vitamin-deficient because of previous poor diet. Also, the injured liver is unable to store vitamins A, B complex, D, and K. Anemia due to iron and folic acid deficiencies may also exist.

Zinc;

Enhances sense of taste/smell, which may stimulate appetite.

Digestive enzymes, e.g., pancrelipase (Viokase);

Promotes digestion of fats and may reduce steatorrhea/diarrhea.

Antiemetics, e.g., trimethobenzamide (Tigan).

Used with caution to reduce nausea/vomiting and increase oral intake.

NURSING DIAGNOSIS: Fluid Volume excess

May be related to

Compromised regulatory mechanism (e.g., syndrome of inappropriate antidiuretic hormone [SIADH], decreased plasma proteins, malnutrition)

Excess sodium/fluid intake

Possibly evidenced by

Edema, anasarca, weight gain

Intake greater than output, oliguria, changes in urine specific gravity

Dyspnea, adventitious breath sounds, pleural effusion

BP changes, altered CVP

JVD, positive hepatojugular reflex

Altered electrolytes

Change in mental status

DESIRED OUTCOMES/EVALUATION CRITERIA—PATIENT WILL:

Fluid Balance (NOC)

Demonstrate stabilized fluid volume, with balanced I&O, stable weight, vital signs within patient's normal range, and absence of edema.

ACTIONS/INTERVENTIONS

RATIONALE

Fluid/Electrolyte Management (NIC)

Independent

Measure I&O, noting positive balance (intake in excess of output). Weigh daily, and note gain greater than 0.5 kg/day.

Reflects circulating volume status, developing/resolution of fluid shifts, and response to therapy. Positive balance/weight gain often reflects continuing fluid retention. *Note:* Decreased circulating volume (fluid shifts) may directly affect renal function/urine output, resulting in hepatorenal syndrome.

Monitor BP (and CVP if available). Note JVD/abdominal vein distension.

BP elevations are usually associated with fluid volume excess but may not occur because of fluid shifts out of the vascular space. Distension of external jugular and abdominal veins is associated with vascular congestion.

ACTIONS/INTERVENTIONS	RATIONALE
Independent	
Assess respiratory status, noting increased respiratory rate, dyspnea.	Indicative of pulmonary congestion/edema.
Auscultate lungs, noting diminished/absent breath sounds and developing adventitious sounds (e.g., crackles).	Increasing pulmonary congestion may result in consolidation, impaired gas exchange, and complications, e.g., pulmonary edema.
Monitor for cardiac dysrhythmias. Auscultate heart sounds, noting development of S_3/S_4 gallop rhythm.	May be caused by HF, decreased coronary arterial perfusion, and electrolyte imbalance.
Assess degree of peripheral/dependent edema.	Fluids shift into tissues as a result of sodium and water retention, decreased albumin, and increased antidiuretic hormone (ADH).
Measure abdominal girth.	Reflects accumulation of fluid (ascites) resulting from loss of plasma proteins/fluid into peritoneal space. *Note:* Excessive fluid accumulation can reduce circulating volume, creating a deficit (signs of dehydration).
Encourage bedrest when ascites is present.	May promote recumbency-induced diuresis.
Provide frequent mouth care; occasional ice chips (if NPO).	Decreases sensation of thirst.
Collaborative	
Monitor serum albumin and electrolytes (particularly potassium and sodium).	Decreased serum albumin affects plasma colloid osmotic pressure, resulting in edema formation. Reduced renal blood flow accompanied by elevated ADH and aldosterone levels and the use of diuretics (to reduce total body water) may cause various electrolyte shifts/imbalances.
Monitor serial chest x-rays.	Vascular congestion, pulmonary edema, and pleural effusions frequently occur.
Restrict sodium and fluids as indicated.	Sodium may be restricted to minimize fluid retention in extravascular spaces. Fluid restriction may be necessary to correct/prevent dilutional hyponatremia.
Administer salt-free albumin/plasma expanders as indicated.	Albumin may be used to increase the colloid osmotic pressure in the vascular compartment (pulling fluid into vascular space), thereby increasing effective circulating volume and decreasing formation of ascites.
Administer medications as indicated:	
Diuretics, e.g., spironolactone (Aldactone), furosemide (Lasix);	Used with caution to control edema and ascites, block effect of aldosterone, and increase water excretion while sparing potassium when conservative therapy with bedrest and sodium restriction do not alleviate problem.
Potassium;	Serum and cellular potassium are usually depleted because of liver disease and urinary losses.
Positive inotropic drugs and arterial vasodilators.	Given to increase cardiac output/improve renal blood flow and function, thereby reducing excess fluid.

> **NURSING DIAGNOSIS: Skin Integrity, risk for impaired**
>
> **Risk factors may include**
> Altered circulation/metabolic state
> Accumulation of bile salts in skin
> Poor skin turgor, skeletal prominence, presence of edema, ascites
>
> **Possibly evidenced by**
> [Not applicable; presence of signs and symptoms establishes an *actual* diagnosis]
>
> **DESIRED OUTCOMES/EVALUATION CRITERIA—PATIENT WILL:**
>
> **Risk Control (NOC)**
>
> Maintain skin integrity.
> Identify individual risk factors and demonstrate behaviors/techniques to prevent skin breakdown.

ACTIONS/INTERVENTIONS

Skin Surveillance (NIC)

Independent

Inspect skin surfaces/pressure points routinely. Gently massage bony prominences or areas of continued stress. Use emollient lotions; limit use of soap for bathing.

Encourage/assist with repositioning on a regular schedule, while in bed/chair; and active/passive ROM exercises as appropriate.

Recommend elevating lower extremities.

Keep linens dry and free of wrinkles.

Suggest clipping fingernails short; provide mittens/gloves if indicated.

Encourage/provide perineal care following urination and bowel movement.

Collaborative

Use alternating pressure mattress, egg carton mattress, waterbed, sheepskins, as indicated.

Apply calamine lotion, provide baking soda baths. Administer medications such as cholestyramine (Questran), hydroxyzine (Atarax), diphenhydramine (Benadryl), if indicated.

RATIONALE

Edematous tissues are more prone to breakdown and to the formation of decubiti. Ascites may stretch the skin to the point of tearing in severe cirrhosis.

Repositioning reduces pressure on edematous tissues to improve circulation. Exercises enhance circulation and improve/maintain joint mobility.

Enhances venous return and reduces edema formation in extremities.

Moisture aggravates pruritus and increases risk of skin breakdown.

Prevents the patient from inadvertently injuring the skin, especially while sleeping.

Prevents skin excoriation breakdown from bile salts.

Reduces dermal pressure, increases circulation, and diminishes risk of tissue ischemia/breakdown.

May be soothing/provide relief of itching associated with jaundice, bile salts in skin.

NURSING DIAGNOSIS: Breathing Pattern, risk for ineffective

Risk factors may include

Intra-abdominal fluid collection (ascites)

Decreased lung expansion, accumulated secretions

Decreased energy, fatigue

Possibly evidenced by

[Not applicable; presence of signs and symptoms establishes an *actual* diagnosis]

DESIRED OUTCOMES/EVALUATION CRITERIA—PATIENT WILL:

Respiratory Status: Ventilation (NOC)

Maintain effective respiratory pattern; be free of dyspnea and cyanosis, with ABGs and vital capacity within acceptable range.

ACTIONS/INTERVENTIONS	RATIONALE
Ventilation Assistance (NIC)	
Independent	
Monitor respiratory rate, depth, and effort.	Rapid shallow respirations/dyspnea may be present because of hypoxia and/or fluid accumulation in abdomen.
Auscultate breath sounds, noting crackles, wheezes, rhonchi.	Indicates developing complications (e.g., presence of adventitious sounds reflects accumulation of fluid/secretions; absent/diminished sounds suggest atelectasis), increasing risk of infection.
Investigate changes in level of consciousness.	Changes in mentation may reflect hypoxemia and respiratory failure, which often accompany hepatic coma.
Keep head of bed elevated. Position on sides.	Facilitates breathing by reducing pressure on the diaphragm and minimizes risk of aspiration of secretions.
Encourage frequent repositioning and deep-breathing exercises/coughing as appropriate.	Aids in lung expansion and mobilizing secretions.
Monitor temperature. Note presence of chills, increased coughing, changes in color/character of sputum.	Indicative of onset of infection, e.g., pneumonia.
Collaborative	
Monitor serial ABGs, pulse oximetry, vital capacity measurements, chest x-rays.	Reveals changes in respiratory status, developing pulmonary complications.
Provide supplemental O_2 as indicated.	May be necessary to treat/prevent hypoxia. If respirations/oxygenation inadequate, mechanical ventilation may be required.
Demonstrate/assist with respiratory adjuncts, e.g., incentive spirometer.	Reduces incidence of atelectasis, enhances mobilization of secretions.
Prepare for/assist with acute care procedures, e.g.:	
Paracentesis;	Occasionally done to remove ascites fluid when respiratory embarrassment is not corrected by other measures.
Peritoneovenous shunt.	Surgical implant of a catheter to return accumulated fluid in the abdominal cavity to systemic circulation via the vena cava; provides long-term relief of ascites and improvement in respiratory function.

ACTIONS/INTERVENTIONS	RATIONALE
Bleeding Precautions (NIC)	
Independent	
Assess for signs/symptoms of GI bleeding; e.g., check all secretions for frank or occult blood. Observe color and consistency of stools, NG drainage, or vomitus.	The GI tract (esophagus and rectum) is the most usual source of bleeding because of its mucosal fragility and alterations in hemostasis associated with cirrhosis.
Observe for presence of petechiae, ecchymosis, bleeding from one or more sites.	Subacute disseminated intravascular coagulation (DIC) may develop secondary to altered clotting factors.
Monitor pulse, BP (and CVP if available).	An increased pulse with decreased BP and CVP can indicate loss of circulating blood volume, requiring further evaluation.
Note changes in mentation/level of consciousness.	Changes may indicate decreased cerebral perfusion secondary to hypovolemia, hypoxemia.
Avoid rectal temperature; be gentle with GI tube insertions.	Rectal and esophageal vessels are most vulnerable to rupture.
Encourage use of soft toothbrush, electric razor, avoiding straining for stool, forceful nose blowing, and so forth.	In the presence of clotting factor disturbances, minimal trauma can cause mucosal bleeding.
Use small needles for injections. Apply pressure to small bleeding/venipuncture sites for longer than usual.	Minimizes damage to tissues, reducing risk of bleeding/hematoma.
Recommend avoidance of aspirin-containing products.	Prolongs coagulation, potentiating risk of hemorrhage.
Collaborative	
Monitor Hb/Hct and clotting factors.	Indicators of anemia, active bleeding, or impending complications (e.g., DIC).
Administer medications as indicated:	
Supplemental vitamins (e.g., vitamins K, D, and C);	Promotes prothrombin synthesis and coagulation if liver is functional. Vitamin C deficiencies increase susceptibility of GI system to irritation/bleeding.
Stool softeners.	Prevents straining for stool with resultant increase in intra-abdominal pressure and risk of vascular rupture/hemorrhage.

ACTIONS/INTERVENTIONS

Collaborative

Provide gastric lavage with room temperature/cool saline solution or water as indicated.

Assist with insertion/maintenance of GI/esophageal tube (e.g., Sengstaken-Blakemore tube).

Prepare for surgical procedures, e.g., direct ligation (banding) of varices, esophagogastric resection, splenorenalportacaval anastomosis.

RATIONALE

In presence of acute bleeding, evacuation of blood from GI tract reduces ammonia production and risk of hepatic encephalopathy.

Temporarily controls bleeding of esophageal varices when control by other means (e.g., lavage) and hemodynamic stability cannot be achieved.

May be needed to control active hemorrhage or to decrease portal and collateral blood vessel pressure to minimize risk of recurrence of bleeding.

NURSING DIAGNOSIS: Confusion, risk for acute

Risk factors may include
Alcohol abuse
Inability of liver to detoxify certain enzymes/drugs

Possibly evidenced by
[Not applicable; presence of signs and symptoms establishes an *actual* diagnosis]

DESIRED OUTCOMES/EVALUATION CRITERIA—PATIENT WILL:

Cognitive Ability (NOC)

Maintain usual level of mentation/reality orientation.
Initiate behaviors/lifestyle changes to prevent or minimize recurrence of problem.

ACTIONS/INTERVENTIONS

Reality Orientation (NIC)

Independent

Observe for changes in behavior and mentation, e.g., lethargy, confusion, drowsiness, slowing/slurring of speech, and irritability (may be intermittent). Arouse patient at intervals as indicated.

Review current medication regimen/schedules.

Evaluate sleep/rest schedule.

Note development/presence of asterixis, fetor hepaticus, seizure activity.

Consult with SO about patient's usual behavior and mentation.

Have patient write name periodically and keep this record for comparison. Report deterioration of ability. Have patient do simple arithmetic computations.

Reorient to time, place, person as needed.

Maintain a pleasant, quiet environment and approach in a slow, calm manner. Encourage uninterrupted rest periods.

RATIONALE

Ongoing assessment of behavior and mental status is important because of fluctuating nature of impending hepatic coma.

Adverse drug reactions or interactions (e.g., cimetidine plus antacids), may potentiate/exacerbate confusion.

Difficulty falling/staying asleep leads to sleep deprivation, resulting in diminished cognition and lethargy.

Suggests elevating serum ammonia levels; increased risk of progression to encephalopathy.

Provides baseline for comparison of current status.

Easy test of neurological status and muscle coordination.

Assists in maintaining reality orientation, reducing confusion/anxiety.

Reduces excessive stimulation/sensory overload, promotes relaxation, and may enhance coping.

ACTIONS/INTERVENTIONS	RATIONALE

Independent

Provide continuity of care. If possible, assign same nurse over a period of time.	Familiarity provides reassurance, aids in reducing anxiety, and provides a more accurate documentation of subtle changes.
Reduce provocative stimuli, confrontation. Refrain from forcing activities. Assess potential for violent behavior.	Avoids triggering agitated, violent responses; promotes patient safety.
Discuss current situation, future expectation.	Patient/SO may be reassured that intellectual (as well as emotional) function may improve as liver involvement resolves.
Maintain bedrest, assist with self-care activities.	Reduces metabolic demands on liver, prevents fatigue, and promotes healing, lowering risk of ammonia buildup.
Identify/provide safety needs, e.g., supervision during smoking, side rails up and pad if necessary. Provide close supervision.	Reduces risk of injury when confusion, seizures, or violent behavior occurs.
Investigate temperature elevations. Monitor for signs of infection.	Infection may precipitate hepatic encephalopathy caused by tissue catabolism and release of nitrogen.
Recommend avoidance of narcotics or sedatives, anti-anxiety agents, and limiting/restricting use of medications metabolized by the liver.	Certain drugs are toxic to the liver, while other drugs may not be metabolized because of cirrhosis, causing cumulative effects that affect mentation, mask signs of developing encephalopathy, or precipitate coma.

Collaborative

Monitor laboratory studies, e.g., ammonia, electrolytes, pH, BUN, glucose, CBC with differential.	Elevated ammonia levels, hypokalemia, metabolic alkalosis, hypoglycemia, anemia, and infection can precipitate or potentiate development of hepatic coma.
Eliminate or restrict protein in diet. Provide glucose supplements, adequate hydration.	Ammonia (product of the breakdown of protein in the GI tract) is responsible for mental changes in hepatic encephalopathy. Dietary changes may result in constipation, which also increases bacterial action and formation of ammonia. Glucose provides a source of energy, reducing need for protein catabolism. *Note:* Vegetable protein may be better tolerated than meat protein.
Administer medications as indicated:	
Electrolytes;	Corrects imbalances and may improve cerebral function/metabolism of ammonia.
Stool softeners, colonic purges (e.g., magnesium sulfate), enemas, lactulose;	Removes protein and blood from intestines. Acidifying the intestine produces diarrhea and decreases production of nitrogenous substances, reducing risk/severity of encephalopathy. *Note:* Long-term use of lactulose may be required for patients with hepatic encephalopathy to reduce ammonia on a daily/regular basis.
Bactericidal agents, e.g., neomycin (Neobiotic), kanamycin (Kantrex).	Destroys intestinal bacteria, reducing production of ammonia, to prevent encephalopathy.
Administer supplemental O_2.	Mentation is affected by O_2 concentration and utilization in the brain.
Assist with procedures as indicated, e.g., dialysis, plasmapheresis, or extracorporeal liver perfusion.	May be used to reduce serum ammonia levels if encephalopathy develops/other measures are not successful.

NURSING DIAGNOSIS: Self-Esteem/Body Image disturbance

May be related to

Biophysical changes/altered physical appearance

Uncertainty of prognosis, changes in role function

Personal vulnerability

Self-destructive behavior (alcohol-induced disease)

Possibly evidenced by

Verbalization of change/restriction in lifestyle

Fear of rejection or reaction by others

Negative feelings about body/abilities

Feelings of helplessness, hopelessness, or powerlessness

DESIRED OUTCOMES/EVALUATION CRITERIA—PATIENT WILL:

Self-Esteem (NOC)

Verbalize understanding of changes and acceptance of self in the present situation.

Identify feelings and methods for coping with negative perception of self.

ACTIONS/INTERVENTIONS	RATIONALE
Self-Esteem Enhancement (NIC)	
Independent	
Discuss situation/encourage verbalization of fears and concerns. Explain relationship between nature of disease and symptoms.	The patient is very sensitive to body changes and may also experience feelings of guilt when cause is related to alcohol (70%) or other drug use.
Support and encourage patient; provide care with a positive, friendly attitude.	Caregivers sometimes allow judgmental feelings to affect the care of the patient and need to make every effort to help the patient feel valued as a person.
Encourage family/SO to verbalize feelings, visit freely/participate in care.	Family members may feel guilty about the patient's condition and may be fearful of impending death. They need nonjudgmental emotional support and free access to the patient. Participation in care helps them feel useful and promotes trust between staff, patient, and SO.
Assist patient/SO to cope with change in appearance; suggest clothing that does not emphasize altered appearance, e.g., use of red, blue, or black clothing.	Patient may present unattractive appearance due to jaundice, ascites, ecchymotic areas. Providing support can enhance self-esteem and promote patient sense of control.
Collaborative	
Refer to support services, e.g., counselors, psychiatric resources, social service, clergy, and/or alcohol treatment program.	Increased vulnerability/concerns associated with this illness may require services of additional professional resources.

NURSING DIAGNOSIS: Knowledge Deficit [Learning Need] regarding condition, prognosis, treatment, self care, and discharge needs

May be related to

Lack of exposure/recall; information misinterpretation

Unfamiliarity with information resources

ACTIONS/INTERVENTIONS	RATIONALE
Teaching: Disease Process (NIC)	
Independent	
Review disease process/prognosis and future expectations.	Provides knowledge base from which patient can make informed choices.
Stress importance of avoiding alcohol. Give information about community services available to aid in alcohol rehabilitation if indicated.	Alcohol is the leading cause in the development of cirrhosis.
Inform the patient of altered effects of medications with cirrhosis and the importance of using only drugs prescribed or cleared by a healthcare provider who is familiar with patient's history.	Some drugs are hepatotoxic (especially narcotics, sedatives, and hypnotics). In addition, the damaged liver has a decreased ability to metabolize all drugs, potentiating cumulative effect and/or aggravation of bleeding tendencies.
Review procedure for maintaining function of peritoneovenous shunt when present.	Insertion of a Denver shunt requires the patient to periodically pump the chamber to maintain patency of the device. Patients with a LeVeen shunt may wear an abdominal binder and/or engage in a Valsalva maneuver to maintain shunt function.
Assist patient in identifying support person(s).	Because of length of recovery, potential for relapses, and slow convalescence, support systems are extremely important in maintaining behavior modifications.
Emphasize the importance of good nutrition. Recommend avoidance of high-protein/salty foods, onions, and strong cheeses. Provide written dietary instructions.	Proper dietary maintenance and avoidance of foods high in sodium and protein aid in remission of symptoms and help prevent ammonia buildup and further liver damage. Written instructions are helpful for patient to refer to at home.
Stress necessity of follow-up care and adherence to therapeutic regimen.	Chronic nature of disease has potential for life-threatening complications. Provides opportunity for evaluation of effectiveness of regimen, including patency of shunt if used.
Discuss sodium and salt substitute restrictions and necessity of reading food and OTC drug labels.	Minimizes ascites and edema formation. Overuse of substitutes may result in other electrolyte imbalances. Food, OTC/personal care products (e.g., antacids, some mouthwashes) may contain sodium or alcohol.

ACTIONS/INTERVENTIONS

Independent

Encourage scheduling activities with adequate rest periods.

Promote diversional activities that are enjoyable to the patient.

Recommend avoidance of persons with infections, especially URI.

Identify environmental dangers, e.g., carbon tetrachloride-type cleaning agents, exposure to hepatitis.

Instruct patient/SO of signs/symptoms that warrant notification of healthcare provider, e.g., increased abdominal girth; rapid weight loss/gain; increased peripheral edema; increased dyspnea, fever; blood in stool or urine; excess bleeding of any kind; jaundice.

Instruct SO to notify healthcare providers of any confusion, untidiness, night wandering, tremors, or personality change.

RATIONALE

Adequate rest decreases metabolic demands on the body and increases energy available for tissue regeneration.

Prevents boredom and minimizes anxiety and depression.

Decreased resistance, altered nutritional status, and immune response (e.g., leukopenia may occur with splenomegaly) potentiate risk of infection.

Can precipitate recurrence.

Prompt reporting of symptoms reduces risk of further hepatic damage and provides opportunity to treat complications before they become life-threatening.

Changes (reflecting deterioration) may be more apparent to SO, although insidious changes may be noted by others with less frequent contact with patient.

POTENTIAL CONSIDERATIONS following acute hospitalization (dependent on patient's age, physical condition/presence of complications, personal resources, and life responsibilities)

Fatigue—decreased metabolic energy production, states of discomfort, altered body chemistry (e.g., changes in liver function, effect on target organs, alcohol withdrawal).
Nutrition: altered, less than body requirements—inadequate diet; inability to process/digest nutrients; anorexia, nausea/vomiting, indigestion, early satiety (ascites); abnormal bowel function.
Family Processes, altered: alcoholism—abuse of alcohol, resistance to treatment, inadequate coping/lack of problem-solving skills, addictive personality/codependency.
Caregiver Role Strain, risk for—addiction or codependency, family dysfunction before caregiving situation, presence of situational stressors, such as economic vulnerability, hospitalization, changes in employment.

PANCREATITIS

Pancreatitis is a painful inflammatory condition in which the pancreatic enzymes are prematurely activated resulting in autodigestion of the pancreas. Pancreatitis may be acute or chronic, with symptoms mild to severe.

CARE SETTING

Inpatient acute medical unit for initial incident or exacerbations with serious complications; otherwise condition is managed at the community level.

RELATED CONCERNS

Alcoholism: acute withdrawal, page 873
Substance dependence/abuse rehabilitation, page 886
Diabetes mellitus/diabetic ketoacidosis, page 440
Peritonitis, page 382
Psychosocial aspects of care, page 809
Renal failure: acute, page 575
Sepsis/Septicemia, page 741
Total nutritional support: parenteral/enteral feeding, page 508

Patient Assessment Database

CIRCULATION

May exhibit: Hypertension (acute pain); hypotension and tachycardia (hypovolemic shock or toxemia)
Edema, ascites
Skin pale, cold, mottled with diaphoresis (vasoconstriction/fluid shifts); jaundiced (inflammation/obstruction of common duct); blue-green-brown discoloration around umbilicus (Cullen's sign) from accumulation of blood (hemorrhagic pancreatitis)

EGO INTEGRITY

May exhibit: Agitation, restlessness, distress, apprehension

ELIMINATION

May report: Diarrhea
May exhibit: Bowel sounds decreased/absent (reduced peristalsis/ileus)
Dark amber or brown, foamy urine (bile)
Frothy, foul-smelling, grayish, greasy, nonformed stool (steatorrhea)
Polyuria (developing DM)

FOOD/FLUID

May report: Food intolerance, anorexia; frequent/persistent vomiting, retching, dry heaves
Weight loss
May exhibit: Diffuse epigastric/abdominal tenderness to palpation, abdominal rigidity, distension
Hypoactive bowel sounds
Urine positive for glucose

NEUROSENSORY

May exhibit: Confusion, agitation
Coarse tremors of extremities (hypocalcemia)

PAIN/DISCOMFORT

May report: Unrelenting severe deep abdominal pain, usually located in the epigastrium and periumbilical regions but may radiate to the back; onset may be sudden and often associated with heavy drinking or a large meal
Radiation to chest and back, may increase in supine position
May exhibit: Abdominal guarding, may curl up on left side with both arms over abdomen and knees/hips flexed
Abdominal rigidity

RESPIRATION

May exhibit: Tachypnea, with/without dyspnea
Decreased depth of respiration with splinting/guarding actions
Bibasilar crackles (pleural effusion)

SAFETY

May exhibit: Fever

SEXUALITY

May exhibit: Current pregnancy (third trimester) with shifting of abdominal contents and compression of biliary tract

TEACHING/LEARNING

May report: Family history of pancreatitis
Diabetic ketoacidosis
History of cholelithiasis with partial or complete common bile duct obstruction; gastritis, duodenal ulcer, duodenitis; diverticulitis; Crohn's disease; recent abdominal surgery (e.g., procedures on the pancreas, biliary tract, stomach, or duodenum); external abdominal trauma
Excessive alcohol intake (90% of cases)
Use of medications, e.g., salicylates, pentamidine, antihypertensives, opiates, thiazides, steroids, some antibiotics, estrogens
Infectious diseases, e.g., mumps, hepatitis B, Coxsackie viral infection

Discharge plan considerations: **DRG projected mean length of inpatient stay: 5.7 days**
May require assistance with dietary program, homemaker/maintenance tasks

Refer to section at end of plan for postdischarge considerations.

DIAGNOSTIC STUDIES

CT scan: Determines extent of edema and necrosis.

Ultrasound of abdomen: May be used to identify pancreatic inflammation, abscess, pseudocysts, carcinoma, or obstruction of biliary tract.

Endoscopy of pancreatic ducts: Useful to diagnose fistulas, obstructive biliary disease, and pancreatic duct strictures/anomalies (procedure is contraindicated in acute phase).

Computed tomography (CT)–guided needle aspiration: Done to determine if infection is present.

Abdominal x-rays: May demonstrate dilated loop of small bowel adjacent to pancreas or other intra-abdominal precipitator of pancreatitis, presence of free intraperitoneal air caused by perforation or abscess formation, pancreatic calcification.

Upper GI series: Frequently exhibits evidence of pancreatic enlargement/inflammation.

Serum amylase: Increased because of obstruction of normal outflow of pancreatic enzymes (normal level does not rule out disease). May be five or more times normal level in acute pancreatitis.

Serum lipase: Usually elevates along with amylase, but stays elevated longer.

Serum bilirubin: Increase is common (may be caused by alcoholic liver disease or compression of common bile duct).

Alkaline phosphatase: Usually elevated if pancreatitis is accompanied by biliary disease.

Serum albumin and protein: May be decreased (increased capillary permeability and transudation of fluid into extracellular space).

Serum calcium: Hypocalcemia may appear 2–3 days after onset of illness (usually indicates fat necrosis and may accompany pancreatic necrosis).

Potassium: Hypokalemia may occur because of gastric losses; hyperkalemia may develop secondary to tissue necrosis, acidosis, renal insufficiency.

Triglycerides: Levels may exceed 1700 mg/dL and may be causative agent in acute pancreatitis.

LDH/AST: May be elevated up to 15 times normal because of biliary and liver involvement.

CBC: WBC count of 10,000–25,000 is present in 80% of patients. Hb may be lowered because of bleeding. Hct is usually elevated (hemoconcentration associated with vomiting or from effusion of fluid into pancreas or retroperitoneal area).

Serum glucose: Transient elevations of greater than 200 mg/dL are common, especially during initial/acute attacks. Sustained hyperglycemia reflects widespread β-cell damage and pancreatic necrosis and is a poor prognostic sign.

Partial thromboplastin time (PTT): Prolonged if coagulopathy develops because of liver involvement and fat necrosis.

Urinalysis: Amylase, myoglobin, hematuria, and proteinuria may be present (glomerular damage).

Urine amylase: Increased within 2–3 days after onset of attack.

Stool: Increased fat content (steatorrhea) indicative of insufficient digestion of fats and protein.

NURSING PRIORITIES

1. Control pain and promote comfort.
2. Prevent/treat fluid and electrolyte imbalance.
3. Reduce pancreatic stimulation while maintaining adequate nutrition.
4. Prevent complications.
5. Provide information about disease process/prognosis and treatment needs.

DISCHARGE GOALS

1. Pain relieved/controlled.
2. Hemodynamically stable.
3. Complications prevented/minimized.
4. Disease process/prognosis, potential complications, and therapeutic regimen understood.
5. Plan in place to meet needs after discharge.

NURSING DIAGNOSIS: Pain [acute]

May be related to
Obstruction of pancreatic, biliary ducts
Chemical contamination of peritoneal surfaces by pancreatic exudate/autodigestion of pancreas
Extension of inflammation to the retroperitoneal nerve plexus

Possibly evidenced by
Reports of pain
Self-focusing, grimacing, distraction/guarding behaviors
Autonomic responses, alteration in muscle tone

DESIRED OUTCOMES/EVALUATION CRITERIA—PATIENT WILL:

Pain Control Behavior (NOC)

Report pain is relieved/controlled.
Follow prescribed therapeutic regimen.
Demonstrate use of methods that provide relief.

ACTIONS/INTERVENTIONS	RATIONALE

Pain Management (NIC)

Independent

Investigate verbal reports of pain, noting specific location and intensity (0–10 scale). Note factors that aggravate and relieve pain.	Pain is often diffuse, severe, and unrelenting in acute or hemorrhagic pancreatitis. Severe pain is often the major symptom in patients with chronic pancreatitis. Isolated pain in the RUQ reflects involvement of the head of the pancreas. Pain in the left upper quadrant (LUQ) suggests involvement of the pancreatic tail. Localized pain may indicate development of pseudocysts or abscesses.
Maintain bedrest during acute attack. Provide quiet, restful environment.	Decreases metabolic rate and GI stimulation/secretions, thereby reducing pancreatic activity.

ACTIONS/INTERVENTIONS	RATIONALE
Independent	
Promote position of comfort, e.g., on one side with knees flexed, sitting up and leaning forward.	Reduces abdominal pressure/tension, providing some measure of comfort and pain relief. *Note:* Supine position often increases pain.
Provide alternate comfort measures (e.g., back rub), encourage relaxation techniques (e.g., guided imagery, visualization), quiet diversional activities (e.g., TV, radio).	Promotes relaxation and enables patient to refocus attention; may enhance coping.
Keep environment free of food odors.	Sensory stimulation can activate pancreatic enzymes, increasing pain.
Administer analgesics in timely manner (smaller, more frequent doses).	Severe/prolonged pain can aggravate shock and is more difficult to relieve, requiring larger doses of medication, which can mask underlying problems/complications and may contribute to respiratory depression.
Maintain meticulous skin care, especially in presence of draining abdominal wall fistulas.	Pancreatic enzymes can digest the skin and tissues of the abdominal wall, creating a chemical burn.
Collaborative	
Administer medications as indicated:	
Narcotic analgesics, e.g., meperidine (Demerol); fentanyl (Sublimaze);	Meperidine is usually effective in relieving pain and may be preferred over morphine, which can have a side effect of biliary-pancreatic spasms. Paravertebral block has been used to achieve prolonged pain control. *Note:* Patients who have recurrent or chronic pancreatitis episodes may be difficult to manage because they may become addicted to the narcotics given for pain control.
Sedatives, e.g., diazepam (Valium); antispasmodics, e.g., atropine;	Potentiates action of narcotic to promote rest and to reduce muscular/ductal spasm, thereby reducing metabolic needs, enzyme secretions.
Antacids, e.g., Mylanta, Maalox, Amphojel, Riopan;	Neutralizes gastric acid to reduce production of pancreatic enzymes and to reduce incidence of upper GI bleeding.
Cimetidine (Tagamet), ranitidine (Zantac).	Decreasing secretion of HCl reduces stimulation of the pancreas and associated pain.
Withhold food and fluid as indicated.	Limits/reduces release of pancreatic enzymes and resultant pain.
Maintain gastric suction when used.	Prevents accumulation of gastric secretions, which can stimulate pancreatic enzyme activity.
Prepare for surgical intervention if indicated.	Surgical exploration may be required in presence of intractable pain/complications involving the biliary tract.

NURSING DIAGNOSIS: Fluid Volume risk for deficit

Risk factors may include

Excessive losses: vomiting, gastric suctioning

Increase in size of vascular bed (vasodilation, effects of kinins)

Third-space fluid transudation, ascites formation

Alteration of clotting process, hemorrhage

ACTIONS/INTERVENTIONS	RATIONALE
Fluid/Electrolyte Management (NIC)	
Independent	
Monitor BP and measure CVP if available.	Fluid sequestration (shifts into third space), bleeding, and release of vasodilators (kinins) and cardiac depressant factor triggered by pancreatic ischemia may result in profound hypotension. Reduced cardiac output/poor organ perfusion secondary to a hypotensive episode can precipitate widespread systemic complications.
Measure I&O including vomiting/gastric aspirate, diarrhea. Calculate 24-hr fluid balance.	Indicators of replacement needs/effectiveness of therapy.
Note decrease in urine output (less than 400 mL/24 hr).	Oliguria may occur, signaling renal impairment/acute tubular necrosis (ATN), related to increase in renal vascular resistance or reduced/altered renal blood flow.
Record color and character of gastric drainage, measure pH, and note presence of occult blood.	Risk of gastric bleeding/hemorrhage is high.
Weigh as indicated. Correlate with calculated fluid balance.	Weight loss may suggest hypovolemia; however, edema, fluid retention, and ascites may be reflected by increased or stable weight, even in the presence of muscle wasting.
Note poor skin turgor, dry skin/mucous membranes, reports of thirst.	Further physiological indicators of dehydration.
Observe/record peripheral and dependent edema. Measure abdominal girth if ascites present.	Edema/fluid shifts occur as a result of increased vascular permeability, sodium retention, and decreased colloid osmotic pressure in the intravascular compartment. *Note:* Fluid loss (sequestration) of greater than 6 L/48 hr is considered a poor prognostic sign.
Investigate changes in sensorium, e.g., confusion, slowed responses.	Changes may be related to hypovolemia, hypoxia, electrolyte imbalance, or impending delirium tremens (in the patient with acute pancreatitis secondary to excessive alcohol intake). Severe pancreatic disease may cause toxic psychosis.

ACTIONS/INTERVENTIONS

Independent

Auscultate heart sounds; note rate and rhythm. Monitor/document rhythm changes.

Inspect skin for petechiae, hematomas, and unusual wound or venipuncture bleeding. Note hematuria, mucous membrane bleeding, and bloody gastric contents.

Observe/report coarse muscle tremors, twitching, positive Chvostek's or Trousseau's sign.

Collaborative

Administer fluid replacement as indicated, e.g., saline solutions, albumin, blood/blood products, dextran.

Monitor laboratory studies, e.g., Hb/Hct, protein, albumin, electrolytes, BUN, creatinine, urine osmolality and sodium/potassium, coagulation studies.

Replace electrolytes, e.g., sodium, potassium, chloride, calcium as indicated.

Prepare for/assist with peritoneal lavage, hemoperitoneal dialysis.

RATIONALE

Cardiac changes/dysrhythmias may reflect hypovolemia and/or electrolyte imbalance, commonly hypokalemia/hypocalcemia. Hyperkalemia may occur related to tissue necrosis, acidosis, and renal insufficiency and may precipitate lethal dysrhythmias if uncorrected. S_3 gallop in conjunction with JVD and crackles suggest HF/pulmonary edema. *Note:* Cardiovascular complications are common and include MI, pericarditis, and pericardial effusion with/without tamponade.

DIC may be initiated by release of active pancreatic proteases into the circulation. The most frequently affected organs are the kidneys, skin, and lungs.

Symptoms of calcium imbalance. Calcium binds with free fats in the intestine and is lost by excretion in the stool.

Choice of replacement solution may be less important than rapidity and adequacy of volume restoration. Saline solutions and albumin may be used to promote mobilization of fluid back into vascular space. Low-molecular-weight dextran is sometimes used to reduce risk of renal dysfunction and pulmonary edema associated with pancreatitis.

Identifies deficits/replacement needs and developing complications, e.g., ATN, DIC.

Decreased oral intake and excessive losses greatly affect electrolyte/acid base balance, which is necessary to maintain optimal cellular/organ function.

Removes toxic chemicals/pancreatic enzymes and allows for more rapid correction of metabolic abnormalities in severe/unresponsive cases of acute pancreatitis.

NURSING DIAGNOSIS: Nutrition: altered, less than body requirements

May be related to
Vomiting, decreased oral intake; prescribed dietary restrictions
Loss of digestive enzymes and insulin (related to pancreatic outflow obstruction or necrosis/autodigestion)

Possibly evidenced by
Reported inadequate food intake
Aversion to eating, reported altered taste sensation, lack of interest in food
Weight loss
Poor muscle tone

ACTIONS/INTERVENTIONS	RATIONALE
Nutrition Management (NIC)	
Independent	
Assess abdomen, noting presence/character of bowel sounds, abdominal distension, and reports of nausea.	Gastric distension and intestinal atony are frequently present, resulting in reduced/absent bowel sounds. Return of bowel sounds and relief of symptoms signal readiness for discontinuation of gastric aspiration (NG tube).
Provide frequent oral care.	Decreases vomiting stimulus and inflammation/irritation of dry mucous membranes associated with dehydration and mouth breathing when NG is in place.
Assist patient in selecting food/fluids that meet nutritional needs and restrictions when diet is resumed.	Previous dietary habits may be unsatisfactory in meeting current needs for tissue regeneration and healing. Use of gastric stimulants, e.g., caffeine, alcohol, cigarettes, gas-producing foods, or ingestion of large meals may result in excessive stimulation of the pancreas/recurrence of symptoms.
Observe color/consistency/amount of stools. Note frothy consistency/foul odor.	Steatorrhea may develop from incomplete digestion of fats.
Hyperglycemia Management (NIC)	
Note signs of increased thirst and urination or changes in mentation and visual acuity.	May warn of developing hyperglycemia associated with increased release of glucagon (damage to α cells), or decreased release of insulin (damage to β cells).
Test urine for sugar and acetone.	Early detection of inadequate glucose utilization may prevent development of ketoacidosis.
Maintain NPO status and gastric suctioning in acute phase.	Prevents stimulation and release of pancreatic enzymes (secretin), released when chyme and HCl enter the duodenum.
Administer hyperalimentation and lipids, if indicated.	IV administration of calories, lipids, and amino acids should be instituted before nutrition/nitrogen depletion is advanced.
Resume oral intake with clear liquids and advance diet slowly to provide high-protein, high-carbohydrate diet, when indicated.	Oral feedings given too early in the course of illness may exacerbate symptoms. Loss of pancreatic function/reduced insulin production may require initiation of a diabetic diet.

ACTIONS/INTERVENTIONS

Collaborative

Provide medium-chain triglycerides (MCTs) (e.g., MCT, Portagen).

Administer medications as indicated:

Vitamins, e.g., A, D, E, K;

Replacement enzymes, e.g., pancreatin (Dizyme), pancrelipase (Viokase, Cotazym).

> **Hyperglycemia Management (NIC)**

Monitor serum glucose.

Provide insulin as appropriate.

RATIONALE

MCTs are elements of enteral feedings (NG or J-tube) that provide supplemental calories/nutrients that do not require pancreatic enzymes for digestion/absorption.

Replacement required because fat metabolism is altered, reducing absorption/storage of fat-soluble vitamins.

Used in chronic pancreatitis to correct deficiencies to promote digestion and absorption of nutrients.

Indicator of insulin needs because hyperglycemia is frequently present, although not usually in levels high enough to produce ketoacidosis.

Corrects persistent hyperglycemia caused by injury to β cells and increased release of glucocorticoids. Insulin therapy is usually short-term unless permanent damage to pancreas occurs.

NURSING DIAGNOSIS: Infection, risk for

Risk factors may include
Inadequate primary defenses: stasis of body fluids, altered peristalsis, change in pH of secretions
Immunosuppression
Nutritional deficiencies
Tissue destruction, chronic disease

Possibly evidenced by:
[Not applicable; presence of signs and symptoms establishes an *actual* diagnosis]

DESIRED OUTCOMES/EVALUATION CRITERIA—PATIENT WILL:

> **Immune Status (NOC)**

Achieve timely healing, be free of signs of infection.
Be afebrile.

> **Risk Control (NOC)**

Participate in activities to reduce risk of infection.

ACTIONS/INTERVENTIONS

> **Infection Protection (NIC)**

Independent

Use strict aseptic technique when changing surgical dressings or working with IV lines, indwelling catheters/tubes, drains. Change soiled dressings promptly.

Stress importance of good handwashing.

RATIONALE

Limits sources of infection, which can lead to sepsis in a compromised patient. *Note:* Studies indicate that infectious complications are responsible for about 80% of deaths associated with pancreatitis.

Reduces risk of cross-contamination.

ACTIONS/INTERVENTIONS

Independent

Observe rate and characteristics of respirations, breath sounds. Note occurrence of cough and sputum production.

Encourage frequent position changes, deep-breathing and coughing. Assist with ambulation as soon as stable.

Observe for signs of infection, e.g.:

Fever and respiratory distress in conjunction with jaundice;

Increased abdominal pain, rigidity/rebound tenderness, diminished/absent bowel sounds;

Increased abdominal pain/tenderness, recurrent fever (greater than 101°F), leukocytosis, hypotension, tachycardia, and chills.

Collaborative

Obtain culture specimens, e.g., blood, wound, urine, sputum, or pancreatic aspirate.

Administer antibiotic therapy as indicated, e.g.: cephalosporins, cefoxitin sodium (Mefoxin); plus aminoglycosides, e.g., gentamicin (Garamycin), tobramycin (Nebcin).

Prepare for surgical intervention as necessary.

RATIONALE

Fluid accumulation and limited mobility predispose to respiratory infections and atelectasis. Accumulation of ascites fluid may cause elevated diaphragm and shallow abdominal breathing.

Enhances ventilation of all lung segments and promotes mobilization of secretions.

Cholestatic jaundice and decreased pulmonary function may be first sign of sepsis involving Gram-negative organisms.

Suggestive of peritonitis.

Abscesses can occur two or more weeks after the onset of pancreatitis (mortality can exceed 50%) and should be suspected whenever the patient is deteriorating despite supportive measures.

Identifies presence of infection and causative organism.

Broad-spectrum antibiotics are generally recommended for sepsis; however, therapy will be based on the specific organisms cultured.

Abscesses may be surgically drained with resection of necrotic tissue. Sump tubes may be inserted for antibiotic irrigation and drainage of pancreatic debris. Pseudocysts (persisting for several weeks) may be drained because of the risk and incidence of infection/rupture.

NURSING DIAGNOSIS: Knowledge Deficit [Learning Need] regarding condition, prognosis, treatment, self care, and discharge needs

May be related to
Lack of exposure/recall
Information misinterpretation; unfamiliarity with information resources

Possibly evidenced by
Questions, request for information; statement of misconception
Inaccurate follow-through of instructions/development of preventable complication

DESIRED OUTCOMES/EVALUATION CRITERIA—PATIENT WILL:

> **Knowledge: Disease Process (NOC)**

Verbalize understanding of condition/disease process and potential complications.

> **Knowledge: Treatment Regimen (NOC)**

Verbalize understanding of therapeutic needs.
Correctly perform necessary procedures and explain reasons for the actions.
Initiate necessary lifestyle changes and participate in treatment regimen.

ACTIONS/INTERVENTIONS	RATIONALE

Teaching: Disease Process (NIC)

Independent

Review specific cause of current episode and prognosis.

Provides knowledge base on which patient can make informed choices.

Discuss other causative/associated factors, e.g., excessive alcohol intake, gallbladder disease, duodenal ulcer, hyperlipoproteinemias, some drugs (e.g., oral contraceptives, thiazides, furosemide [Lasix], isoniazid [INH], glucocorticoids, sulfonamides).

Avoidance may help to limit damage and prevent development of a chronic condition.

Explore availability of treatment programs/rehabilitation of chemical dependency if indicated.

Alcohol abuse is currently the most common cause of recurrence of chronic pancreatitis. Usage of other drugs, whether prescribed or illicit, is increasing as a factor. *Note:* Pain of pancreatitis can be severe and prolonged and may lead to narcotic dependence, requiring need for referral to pain clinic.

Stress the importance of follow-up care, and review symptoms that need to be reported immediately to physician, e.g., recurrence of pain, persistent fever, nausea/vomiting, abdominal distension, frothy/foul-smelling stools, general intolerance of food.

Prolonged recovery period requires close monitoring to prevent recurrence/complications, e.g., infection, pancreatic pseudocysts.

Review importance of initially continuing bland, low-fat diet with frequent small feedings and restricted caffeine, with gradual resumption of a normal diet within individual tolerance.

Understanding the purpose of the diet in maximizing the use of available enzymes while avoiding overstimulation of the pancreas may enhance patient involvement in self-monitoring of dietary needs and responses to foods.

Instruct in use of pancreatic enzyme replacements and bile salt therapy as indicated, avoiding concomitant ingestion of hot foods/fluids.

If permanent damage to the pancreas has occurred, exocrine deficiencies will occur, requiring long-term replacement. Hot foods/fluids can inactivate enzymes.

Recommend cessation of smoking.

Nicotine stimulates gastric secretions and unnecessary pancreatic activity.

Discuss signs/symptoms of diabetes mellitus, i.e., polydipsia, polyuria, weakness, weight loss.

Damage to the β cells may result in a temporary or permanent alteration of insulin production.

POTENTIAL CONSIDERATIONS following acute hospitalization (dependent on patient's age, physical condition/presence of complications, personal resources, and life responsibilities)

Nutrition: altered, less than body requirements—preexisting malnutrition, prescribed dietary restrictions, persistent nausea/vomiting, imbalances in digestive enzymes.

Pain—chemical irritation of peritoneal surfaces by pancreatic enzymes, spasms of biliary ducts, general inflammatory process.

Family Processes, altered: alcoholism—abuse of alcohol, resistance to treatment, inadequate coping/lack of problem-solving skills, addictive personality/codependency.

Therapeutic Regimen: Individual, ineffective management—complexity of therapeutic regimen, economic difficulties, mistrust of regimen, perceived benefit, social support deficits.

TOTAL NUTRITIONAL SUPPORT: PARENTERAL/ENTERAL FEEDING

Nutritional status is a key factor in a patient's overall immune function and a patient's ability to mount a stress response. Underfeeding a patient may lead to increased nosocomial infections, poor wound healing, respiratory muscle dysfunction, and respiratory failure. Overfeeding patients, in contrast, may increase physiological stress and lead to problems such as hyperglycemia, fluid overload, azotemia, and hepatic dysfunction. Therefore, measuring energy expenditure and determining the patient's caloric requirements and feeding status should be included in a thorough nutritional assessment. Specifically designed nutritional therapy can be administered by the parenteral or enteral route when the use of standard diets via the oral route is inadequate or not possible to prevent/correct protein-calorie malnutrition.

Enteral nutrition is preferred for the patient who has a functional GI tract but is unable to consume an adequate nutritional intake or for whom oral intake is contraindicated/impossible. Feeding may be done via NG or orogastric tube, esophagostomy, gastrostomy, duodenostomy, or jejunostomy.

Parenteral nutrition may be chosen because of altered metabolic states or when mechanical or functional abnormalities of the GI tract prevent enteral feeding. Amino acids, fat, carbohydrates, trace elements, vitamins, and electrolytes may be infused via a central or peripheral vein.

CARE SETTING

May be any setting, including community/home care

RELATED CONCERNS

Burns: thermal/chemical/electrical (acute and convalescent phases), page 719
Cancer, page 900
COPD, page 126
Fluid and electrolyte imbalances, page 926
Inflammatory bowel disease, page 350
Pancreatitis, page 498
Renal failure: chronic, page 588
Psychosocial aspects of care, page 809
Surgical intervention, page 828

Patient Assessment DataBase

Clinical signs listed below depend on the degree and duration of malnutrition and include observations indicative of vitamin, mineral, and protein/calorie deficiencies.

ACTIVITY/REST

May exhibit: Muscle wasting (temporal, intercostal, gastrocnemius, dorsum of hand); thin extremities, flaccid muscles, decreased activity tolerance

CIRCULATION

May exhibit: Tachycardia, bradycardia
Diaphoresis, cyanosis

ELIMINATION

May report: Diarrhea or constipation; flatulence associated with food intake
May exhibit: Abdominal distension/increased girth, ascites; tenderness on palpation
Stools may be loose, hard-formed, fatty, or clay-colored

FOOD/FLUID

May report: Recent weight loss/weight loss of 10% or more of body weight within previous 6 months
Problems with chewing, swallowing, choking, or saliva production
Changes in the taste of food; anorexia, nausea/vomiting; inadequate oral intake (NPO) status for 7–10 days, long-term use of 5% dextrose intravenously

May exhibit:	Actual weight (measured) as compared with usual or pre-illness weight is less than 90% of ideal body weight for height, sex, and age or equal to or greater than 120% of ideal/or usual body weight (patient risk in obesity is a tendency to overlook protein and calorie requirements). A distorted actual weight may occur because of the presence of edema, ascites, organomegaly, tumor bulk, anasarca, amputation
	Edentulous or ill-fitting dentures
	Bowel sounds diminished, hyperactive, or absent
	Thyroid, parotid enlargement
	Lips dry, cracked, red, swollen; angular stomatitis
	Tongue may be smooth, pale, slick, coated; color often magenta, beefy red; lingual papillae atrophy/swelling
	Gums swollen/bleeding, multiple caries
	Mucous membranes dry, pale, red, swollen

NEUROSENSORY

May exhibit:	Lethargy, apathy, listlessness, irritability, disorientation, coma
	Gag/swallow reflex may be decreased/absent, e.g., CVA, head trauma, nerve injury

RESPIRATION

May exhibit:	Increased respiratory rate; respiratory distress
	Dyspnea, increased sputum production
	Breath sounds: crackles (protein deficiency/related fluid shifts)

SAFETY

May report:	Recent course of radiation therapy (radiation enteritis)
May exhibit:	Hair may be fragile, coarse, lackluster; alopecia, decreased pigmentation may be present
	Skin dry, scaly, tented; "flaky paint" dermatosis; edema; draining or unhealed wounds, pressure sores; ecchymoses, perifollicular petechiae, subcutaneous fat loss
	Eyes sunken, dull, dry, with pale conjunctiva; Bitot's spots (triangular, shiny, gray spots on the conjunctiva seen in vitamin A deficiency) or scleral icterus
	Nails may be brittle, thin, flattened, ridged, spoon-shaped

SEXUALITY

May report:	Loss of libido
	Amenorrhea

TEACHING/LEARNING

May report:	History of conditions causing protracted protein losses, e.g., malabsorption or short-gut syndrome with increased diarrhea, acute pancreatitis, renal dialysis, fistulas, draining wounds, thermal injuries
	Presence of factors known to alter nutritional requirements/increase energy demands, e.g., single or multiorgan failure; sepsis; fever; trauma; extensive burns; use of steroids, antitumor agents, immunosuppressants
	Use of medications that cause untoward drug/nutrient interactions, e.g., laxatives, anticonvulsants, diuretics, antacids, narcotics, immunosuppressants, high-dose chemotherapy
	Illness of psychiatric origin, e.g., anorexia nervosa/bulimia
	Educational/social factors, e.g., lack of nutrition knowledge, kitchen facilities, reduced/limited financial resources
Discharge plan considerations:	**DRG projected mean length of inpatient stay: 6.1 days,** depending on underlying disease process necessitating therapy
	May require assistance with solution preparation, therapy supplies, and maintenance of feeding device for home nutritional care

Refer to section at end of plan for postdischarge considerations.

DIAGNOSTIC STUDIES

Anthropometrics: Includes measurement of weight-to-height ratio, osseometry, and ratios of lean-to-fat weight:

Triceps skin fold measurement: Estimates subcutaneous fat stores; fat reserves less than tenth percentile suggest advanced depletion; levels less than the thirtieth percentile suggest mild-to-moderate depletion.

Midarm muscle circumference: Measures somatic muscle mass and is used in combination with triceps skin-fold measurement; a decrease of 15–20 percentiles from the expected value suggests a significant reduction.

Visceral proteins: *(Note:* Recent research questions the reliability of serum albumin and transferrin as markers for malnutrition.)

Serum albumin (the classic marker measured): Values of 2.7–3.4 g/dL indicate mild depletion; 2.1–2.7 g/dL, moderate depletion; and less than 2.1 g/dL, severe depletion. Decreased levels are due to poor protein intake, nephrotic syndrome, sepsis, burns, HF, cirrhosis, eclampsia, protein-losing enteropathy; above-normal values (greater than 4.5 g/dL) are seen in dehydration. (Serum prealbumin has a shorter half-life than albumin, so body stores turn over quickly, theoretically making it a more sensitive indicator of improvement/change in protein status.)

Serum transferrin: More sensitive to changes in visceral protein stores than albumin; levels of 150–200 mg/dL reflect mild depletion; 100–150 mg/dL, moderate depletion; and 100 mg/dL, severe depletion. Elevated values are seen with iron deficiency, pregnancy, hypoxia, and chronic blood loss. Decreased values are seen with pernicious anemia, chronic infection, liver disease, iron overload, and protein-losing enteropathy.

Thyroxine-binding prealbumin: Reflects rapid changes in hepatic protein synthesis and thus is a more sensitive indicator of visceral protein depletion. Decreased levels less than 200 mEq/mL are noted with cirrhosis, inflammation, and surgical trauma.

Amino acid profile: Alterations reflect an imbalance of plasma proteins with depressed levels of branched-chain amino acids (common with hepatic encephalopathy or sepsis).

Tests of immune system:

Total lymphocyte count: Less than 1500 cells/mm³ indicates leukopenia and results from decreased generation of T cells, which are very sensitive to malnutrition. Levels are also altered by infection and administration of immunosuppressants.

Tests of micronutrients:

Potassium: Deficiency occurs with inadequate intake and with loss of potassium-containing fluids (e.g., urine, diarrhea, vomiting, fistula drainage, continuous NG suctioning). Potassium is also lost from cells during muscle wasting and is excreted by the kidneys.

Sodium: Levels depend on state of hydration/presence of active loss as may exist in excessive diuresis, GI suctioning, burns.

Phosphorus: May be decreased reflecting inadequate intake or increased cellular uptake; may be elevated in renal failure.

Magnesium: Deficiency is common in alcoholics, chronic vomiting, diarrhea; may be elevated in renal failure.

Calcium: Levels are decreased with conditions associated with hypoalbuminemia, e.g., renal failure (majority of calcium is bound to albumin). Absorption is decreased by fat malabsorption and low-protein diet.

Zinc: Deficiency is seen in alcoholic cirrhosis; or may be secondary to hypoalbuminemia and GI losses (diarrhea).

Tests reflecting protein (nitrogen) loss:

Nitrogen balance studies: Nitrogen (protein) excretion via urine, stool, and insensible losses often exceed nitrogen intake in the acutely ill, reflecting catabolic response to stress and use of endogenous protein stores for energy production (gluconeogenesis). BUN may be severely decreased as a result of chronic malnutrition and depletion of skeletal protein stores.

24-hr creatinine excretion: Because Cr is concentrated in muscle mass, there is a good correlation between lean body mass and 24-hr Cr excretion. Actual values are compared with ideal values (based on height and weight) times 100, known as the Cr height index: 60%–80% indicates moderate depletion; less than 60%, severe depletion.

Tests of GI function (include Schilling test, D-xylose test, 72-hr stool fat, GI series): Determine malabsorption.

Chest x-ray: May be normal or show evidence of pleural effusion; small heart silhouette.

ECG: May be normal or demonstrate low voltage, dysrhythmias/patterns reflective of electrolyte imbalances.

NURSING PRIORITIES

1. Promote consistent intake of adequate calorie and protein requirements.
2. Prevent complications.
3. Minimize energy losses/needs.
4. Provide information about condition, prognosis, and treatment needs.

DISCHARGE GOALS

1. Nutritional intake adequate for individual needs.
2. Complications prevented/minimized.
3. Fatigue alleviated.
4. Condition, prognosis, and therapeutic regimen understood.
5. Plan in place to meet needs after discharge.

NURSING DIAGNOSIS: Nutrition: altered, less than body requirements

May be related to

Conditions that interfere with nutrient intake or increase nutrient need/metabolic demand, e.g., cancer and associated treatments, anorexia, surgical procedures, dysphagia/difficulty swallowing, depressed mental status/level of consciousness

Possibly evidenced by

Body weight 10% or more under ideal
Decreased subcutaneous fat/muscle mass, poor muscle tone
Changes in gastric motility and stool characteristics

DESIRED OUTCOMES/EVALUATION CRITERIA—PATIENT WILL:

| Nutritional Status (NOC) |

Demonstrate stable weight or progressive weight gain toward goal with normalization of laboratory values and no signs of malnutrition.

ACTIONS/INTERVENTIONS	**RATIONALE**
Nutrition Therapy (NIC)	
Independent	
General	
Assess nutritional status continually, during daily nursing care, noting energy level; condition of skin, nails, hair, oral cavity; desire to eat/anorexia.	Provides the opportunity to observe deviations from normals/patient baseline and influences choice of interventions.
Weigh daily and compare with admission weight.	Establishes baseline, aids in monitoring effectiveness of therapeutic regimen, and alerts nurse to inappropriate trends in weight loss/gain.
Document oral intake by use of 24-hour recall, food history, calorie counts as appropriate.	Identifies imbalance between estimated nutritional requirements and actual intake.
Ensure accurate collection of specimens (urine and stool) for nitrogen balance studies.	Inaccurate collection can alter test results, leading to improper interpretation of patient's current status and needs.

ACTIONS/INTERVENTIONS	RATIONALE

Independent

Administer nutritional solutions at prescribed rate via infusion control device as needed. Adjust rate to deliver prescribed hourly intake. Do not increase rate to "catch up" if infusion slows.

Nutrition support prescriptions are based on individually estimated caloric and protein requirements. A consistent rate of nutrient administration ensures proper utilization with fewer side effects, such as hyperglycemia or dumping syndrome. *Note:* Continuous and cyclic infusion of enteral formulas are generally better tolerated than bolus feedings and result in improved absorption.

Be familiar with electrolyte content of nutritional solutions.

Metabolic complications of nutritional support often result from a lack of appreciation of changes that can occur as a result of refeeding, e.g., hyperglycemic, hyperosmotic nonketotic coma (HHNC), electrolyte imbalances.

Schedule activities with adequate rest periods. Promote relaxation techniques.

Conserves energy/reduces calorie needs. (Refer to ND: Fatigue, p. 520.)

Total Parenteral Nutrition (TPN) Administration (NIC)

Observe appropriate "hang" time of parenteral solutions per protocol.

Effectiveness of IV vitamins diminishes and solution degrades after 24 hr.

Monitor fingerstick glucose per protocol (e.g., qid during initiation of therapy).

High glucose content of solutions may lead to pancreatic fatigue, requiring use of supplemental insulin to prevent HHNC. *Note:* Fingerstick determination of glucose level is more accurate than urine testing because of variations in renal glucose threshold.

Enteral Tube Feeding (NIC)

Assess GI function and tolerance to enteral feedings: note bowel sounds; reports of nausea/vomiting, abdominal discomfort; presence of diarrhea/constipation; development of weakness, lightheadedness, diaphoresis, tachycardia, abdominal cramping.

Because protein turnover of the GI mucosa occurs approximately every 3 days, the GI tract is at great risk for early dysfunction and atrophy from disease and malnutrition. Intolerance of formula/presence of dumping syndrome may require alteration of rate of administration/concentration or type of formula, or possibly change to parenteral administration.

Check gastric residuals if bolus feedings are done and as otherwise indicated; hold feeding/return aspirate per protocol for type/rate of feeding used if residual is greater than predetermined level.

Delayed gastric emptying can be caused by a specific disease process, e.g., paralytic ileus/surgery, shock; by drug therapy (especially narcotics); or the protein/fat content of the individual formula. *Note:* Replacement of gastric aspirate reduces loss of gastric acid/electrolytes.

Maintain patency of enteral feeding tubes by flushing with warm water before and after feeding and as indicated, e.g., between multiple doses of medications or when checking gastric residuals.

Enteral formulas contain protein that can clog feeding tubes (more likely with small bore or silicone than with polyurethane tubes) necessitating removal/replacement of tube. *Note:* Cranberry juice or colas are not recommended because they may actually cause an obstruction by promoting formula coagulation. Pancrelipase (a pancreatic enzyme) may be effective in clearing tubing of persistent clog.

Transitional

Stress importance of transition to oral feedings as appropriate.

Although patient may have little interest in food or desire to eat, transition to oral feedings is preferred in view of potential side effects/complications of nutritional support therapy.

ACTIONS/INTERVENTIONS	RATIONALE

Independent

Assess gag reflex, ability to chew/swallow, and motor skills when progressing to transitional feedings.

May require additional interventions, e.g., retraining by dysphagia expert (speech therapist) or long-term nutritional support.

Provide self-help utensils as indicated, e.g., plate guard, utensils with built-up handles, lidded cups.

Patients with neuromuscular deficits, e.g., post-CVA, brain injury, may require use of special aids developed for feeding.

Create optimal environment, e.g., remove noxious stimuli, bedpans, soiled linens. Provide cheerful, attractive tray/table, soft music, companionship.

Encourages patient's attempts to eat, reduces anorexia, and introduces some of the social pleasures usually associated with mealtime.

Allow adequate time for chewing, swallowing, savoring food; provide socialization and feeding assistance as indicated.

Patients need encouragement/assistance to overcome underlying problems such as anorexia, fatigue, muscular weakness.

Offer small, frequent feedings; incorporate patient likes/dislikes in meal planning as much as possible, and include "home foods," as appropriate.

May enhance patient's desire for food and amount of intake.

Provide calorie-containing beverages when oral intake is possible, e.g., juices/jello water, dietary supplements (Sustacal, Ensure), add Polycase to beverages/water.

Maximizes calorie intake when oral intake is limited/restricted.

Collaborative

Refer to nutritional team/registered dietitian.

Aids in identification of nutrient deficits and need for parenteral/enteral nutritional intervention.

Calculate basal energy expenditure (BEE) using formula based on sex, height, weight, age, and estimated energy requirements.

Provides an estimation of calorie and protein needs. *Note:* Although the BEE may more accurately determine individual needs, studies show that BEE is rarely measured and a standard formula for projecting energy requirements is to provide 30 Kcal/kg for weight maintenance, 25 Kcal/kg for weight loss, or 35 Kcal/kg for weight gain.

Review results of indirect calorimetry test if available.

Measures O_2 consumption at basal or resting metabolic rate to aid in estimating calorie/protein requirements.

Enteral Feeding/TPN Administration (NIC)

Assist with insertion and confirm proper placement of infusion/feeding line (e.g., chest x-ray for central venous catheter or aspiration of gastric contents from feeding tube) before administration of solutions.

Reduces risk of feeding-induced complications, including pneumothorax/hemothorax, hydrothorax, air embolus, arterial puncture (central venous line), or aspiration (NG tube).

Administer dextrose-electrolyte or dextrose–amino acid and lipid emulsions (3-in-1) solutions as indicated.

Solutions provide calories, essential amino acids, and micronutrients, usually combined with lipids for complete nutrition known as total nutrient admixtures (TNA). Solutions are modified to meet specific needs, e.g., renal and liver failure (lower protein), respiratory failure (higher fat). *Note:* 3-in-1 solution bags are larger (2–3 L) and can infuse over a 24-hour period, eliminating the need for frequent bag changes and reducing line manipulation/risk of contamination.

ACTIONS/INTERVENTIONS

Collaborative

Co-infuse lipid emulsions if 3-in-1 solutions are not used.

Administer medications, as indicated, e.g.:

Multivitamin preparations;

Insulin;

Diphenoxylate with atropine (Lomotil), camphorated tincture of opium (Paregoric), and metoclopramide (Reglan).

Monitor laboratory studies, e.g., serum glucose, electrolytes, transferrin, prealbumin/albumin, total protein, phosphate, BUN/Cr, liver enzymes, CBC, ABGs.

RATIONALE

Useful in meeting excessive calorie requirements (e.g., burns) or as a source of essential fatty acids during long-term hyperalimentation. *Note:* Lipid solutions may be contraindicated in patients with alterations in fat metabolism or in the presence of pancreatitis, liver damage, anemia, coagulation disorders, pulmonary disease.

Water-soluble vitamins are added to parenteral solutions. Other vitamins may be given for identified deficiencies.

High glucose content of solutions may require exogenous insulin for metabolism, especially in presence of pancreatic insufficiency or disease. *Note:* Insulin is usually now added directly to parenteral solution.

GI side effects of enteral feeding may need to be controlled with antidiarrheal agents (Lomotil/Paregoric) or peristaltic stimulants (Reglan) if more conservative measures such as alteration of rate/strength or type of formula are not successful.

Serum chemistries, blood counts, and lipid profiles are performed before initiation of therapy, providing a baseline for comparison with repeat (monitoring) studies to determine therapy needs/complications. Untoward metabolic effects of TPN include: hypokalemia, hyponatremia and fluid retention, hyperglycemia, hypophosphatemia, increased CO_2 production resulting in respiratory compromise, elevation of liver function tests, renal dysfunction.

NURSING DIAGNOSIS: Infection, risk for

Risk factors may include

Invasive procedures: insertion of venous catheter; surgically placed gastrostomy/jejunostomy feeding tube

Malnutrition; chronic disease

Environmental exposure: access devices in place for extended periods, improper preparation/handling/contamination of the feeding solution

Possibly evidenced by

[Not applicable; presence of signs and symptoms establishes an *actual* diagnosis]

DESIRED OUTCOMES/EVALUATION CRITERIA—PATIENT WILL:

> **Immune Status (NOC)**

Experience no fever or chills.

Demonstrate clean catheter insertion sites, free of drainage and erythema/edema.

ACTIONS/INTERVENTIONS	RATIONALE

Infection Protection (NIC)

Independent

Stress/model proper handwashing technique.

Reduces risk of cross-contamination.

Maintain sterile technique for invasive procedures, e.g., IV, urinary catheter insertion. Provide routine site/wound and perineal care as appropriate.

Prevents entry of bacteria reducing risk of nosocomial infections.

Encourage frequent position changes and out of bed/ambulation as tolerated.

Limits stasis of body fluids, promotes optimal functioning of organ systems, GI tract.

Screen visitors/care providers for infectious processes, especially URI.

Reduces risk of transmission viruses that are difficult to treat.

Monitor/assist with respiratory exercises, use of adjuncts, e.g., incentive spirometer. Auscultate lungs for adventitious sounds.

Promotes deep breathing to clear airways and reduce risk of pneumonia. Presence of wheezes suggests retained secretions, potential complications requiring intervention.

Assess vital signs, including temperature per protocol.

A rise in pulse and temperature may provide warning of infectious process unless patient's immune system is too compromised to respond.

Parenteral TPN Administration (NIC)

Maintain an optimal aseptic environment during bedside insertion of central venous catheters and during changes of TPN bottles and administration tubing.

Catheter-related sepsis may result from entry of pathogenic microorganisms through skin insertion tract or from touch contamination during manipulations of TPN system.

Secure external portion of catheter/administration tubing to dressing with tape. Note intactness of skin suture.

Manipulation of catheter in/out of insertion site can result in tissue trauma (coring) and potentiate entry of skin organisms into catheter tract.

Maintain a sterile occlusive dressing over catheter insertion site. Perform central/peripheral venous catheter dressing care per protocol.

Protects catheter insertion sites from potential sources of contamination. *Note:* Central venous catheter sites can easily become contaminated from tracheostomy/endotracheal secretions or from wounds of the head, neck, and chest.

Inspect insertion site of catheter for erythema, induration, drainage, tenderness.

The catheter is a potential irritant to the surrounding skin and subcutaneous skin tract, and extended use may result in insertion site irritation and infection.

Refrigerate premixed solutions before use; observe a 24-hr hang time for amino acid or total nutrient admixtures solutions and a 12-hr hang time for IV fat emulsions.

TPN solutions and fat emulsions have been shown to support the growth of a variety of pathogenic organisms once contaminated.

Monitor urinary output and serum glucose levels.

A rise in temperature or loss of glucose tolerance (glycosuria, hyperglycemia) are early indications of possible catheter-related sepsis.

Enteral Tube Feeding (NIC)

Keep manipulations of enteral feeding system to a minimum and wash hands before opening system.

Touch contamination of formula is caused by caregiver administration technique.

Alternate nares for tube placement in long-term NG feedings.

Reduces risk of trauma/infection of paranasal tissue (especially important in facial trauma/burns).

ACTIONS/INTERVENTIONS	RATIONALE

Independent

Provide daily/prn site care to abdominally placed feeding tubes.

GI secretions leaking through or around gastrostomy/jejunostomy tube tracts can cause skin breakdown severe enough to require removal of the feeding tube.

Refrigerate reconstituted enteral formulas before use; observe a hang time of 4–8 hr; discard unused formula after 24 hr.

Enteral formulas easily support bacterial growth and can be contaminated during formula preparation. For example, bacterial growth has been shown to occur within 4 hr after contamination.

Collaborative

Infection Protection (NIC)

Aseptically prepare parenteral solutions/enteral formulas for administration.

TPN solutions should be prepared under a laminar flow hood in the pharmacy. Enteral formulas should be mixed in a clean environment in the dietary or pharmacy department, although with the advent of canned/modular formulas, this may not be necessary. *Note:* Additives to TPN solutions, as a rule, should not be made on the unit because of the potential for contamination and drug incompatibilities.

Notify physician if signs of infection present. Follow protocol for obtaining appropriate culture specimens, e.g., blood, solutions, and change bottle/tubing as indicated.

Necessary to identify source of infection and initiate appropriate therapy. May require removal of TPN line and culture of catheter tip.

Administer antibiotics as indicated.

May be given prophylactically or for specifically identified organism.

NURSING DIAGNOSIS: Injury, risk for [multifactor]

Risk factors may include
External environment: catheter-related complications (air emboli and septic thrombophlebitis)
Internal factors: aspiration; effects of therapy/drug interactions

Possibly evidenced by
[Not applicable; presence of signs and symptoms establishes an *actual* diagnosis]

DESIRED OUTCOMES/EVALUATION CRITERIA—PATIENT WILL:

Risk Control (NOC)

Be free of complications associated with nutritional support.
Modify environment/correct hazards to enhance safety for in-home therapy.

ACTIONS/INTERVENTIONS	RATIONALE

Surveillance (NIC)

Independent

Parenteral

Maintain a closed central IV system using Luer-Lok connections/taping of all connections.

Inadvertent disconnection of central IV system can result in lethal air emboli.

ACTIONS/INTERVENTIONS	RATIONALE

Independent

Administer appropriate TPN solution via peripheral or central venous route (including peripherally inserted central catheter [PICC] lines and tunneled catheters).	Solutions containing high concentrations of dextrose (greater than 10%) must be delivered via a central vein because they result in chemical phlebitis when delivered through small peripheral veins.
Monitor for potential drug/nutrient interactions.	Various interactions are possible, for example, digoxin (in conjunction with diuretic therapy) can cause hypomagnesemia; hypokalemia may result from chronic use of laxatives, mineralocorticosteroids, diuretics, or amphotericin.
Assess catheter for signs of displacement out of central venous position, i.e., extended length of catheter on skin surface; leaking of IV solution onto dressing; patient complaints of neck/arm pain, tenderness at catheter site, or swelling of extremity on side of catheter insertion.	Central venous catheter tip may slip out of superior vena cava and migrate into smaller innominate and jugular veins, causing a chemical thrombophlebitis. Incidence of subclavian or superior vena cava thrombosis is increased with extended use of central venous catheters.
Inspect peripheral TPN catheter site routinely and change sites at least every other day, or per protocol.	Peripheral TPN solutions (although less hyperosmolar) can still irritate small veins and cause phlebitis. Peripheral venous access is often limited in malnourished patients, but site should still be changed if signs of irritation develop.
Investigate reports of severe chest pain/coughing in patients with central line. Turn patient to left side in Trendelenburg position if indicated and notify physician.	Suggests presence of air embolus requiring immediate intervention to displace air into apex of heart away from the pulmonary artery.
Maintain an occlusive dressing on catheter insertion sites for 24 hr after subclavian catheter is removed.	Extended catheter use may result in development of catheter skin tract. Once the catheter is removed, air embolus is still a potential risk until skin tract has sealed.

Enteral

Assess gastrostomy or jejunostomy tube sites for evidence of malposition.	Indwelling and mushroom catheters are still frequently used for feeding tubes inserted via the abdomen. Migration of the catheter balloon can result in duodenal or jejunal obstruction. Improperly sutured gastrostomy tubes may easily fall out.

Collaborative

Review chest x-ray as indicated.	Central parenteral line placement is routinely confirmed by x-ray.
Consult with pharmacist in regard to site/time of delivery of drugs that might have action adversely affected by enteral formula.	Absorption of vitamin D is impaired by administration of mineral oil (inhibits micelle formation of bile salts) and by neomycin (inactivates bile salts). Aluminum-containing antacids bind with the phosphorus in the feeding solution, potentiating hypophosphatemia.

NURSING DIAGNOSIS: Aspiration, risk for

Risk factors may include

Presence of GI tube, bolus tube feedings, medication administration

Increased intragastric pressure, delayed gastric emptying

Possibly evidenced by

[Not applicable; presence of signs and symptoms establishes an *actual* diagnosis]

DESIRED OUTCOMES/EVALUATION CRITERIA—PATIENT WILL:

Respiratory Status: Ventilation (NOC)

Maintain clear airway, be free of signs of aspiration.

ACTIONS/INTERVENTIONS

Aspiration Precautions (NIC)

Independent

Confirm placement of nasoenteral feeding tubes. Determine feeding tube position in stomach by x-ray, confirmation of pH of 0 to 5 of the gastric fluid withdrawn through tube, or auscultation of injected air before intermittent feedings. Observe for ability to speak/cough.

Maintain aspiration precautions during enteral feedings, e.g.:

Keep head of bed elevated at 30–45 degrees during feeding and at least 1 hr after feeding;

Inflate tracheostomy cuff during and for 1 hr after intermittent feeding. Interrupt feeding when patient is in prone position;

Add blue food coloring to enteral formula as indicated.

Monitor gastric residuals after bolus feedings (as previously noted in ND: Nutrition: altered, less than body requirements, p. 511).

Note characteristics of sputum/tracheal aspirate. Investigate development of dyspnea, cough, tachypnea, cyanosis. Auscultate breath sounds.

Note indicators of NG tube intolerance, e.g., absence of gag reflex, high risk of aspiration, frequent removal of NG feeding tubes

RATIONALE

Malplacement of nasoenteral feeding tubes may result in aspiration of enteral formula. Patients at particular risk include those who are intubated or obtunded and those who have had a CVA or surgery of the head/neck and upper GI system. *Note:* The reliability of the pH method is reduced if antacids or certain other medications have been given PO/NG in the past 4 hr. Also when using ausculatory method to assess tube placement, air sounds can be transmitted to the epigastrium even if the tube is malpositioned (i.e., in lung or proximal jejunum).

Reduces risk of regurgitation/gastric reflux.

Aspiration of enteral formulas is highly irritating to the lung parenchyma and may result in pneumonia and respiratory compromise.

Helps identify aspiration of enteral formula and/or tracheal esophageal fistula, if discovered in sputum/lung secretions. *Note:* Avoid use of methylene blue dye, which may cause false-positive guaiac test when assessing for GI bleeding.

Presence of large gastric residuals may potentiate an incompetent esophageal sphincter, leading to vomiting and aspiration.

Presence of formula in tracheal secretions or signs/symptoms reflecting respiratory distress suggest aspiration.

May require consideration of surgically placed feeding tube/percutaneous endoscopic gastrostomy (PEG), jejunostomy for patient safety and consistency of enteral formula delivery.

ACTIONS/INTERVENTIONS

Collaborative

Review abdominal x-ray if done.

RATIONALE

Confirmation of placement of gastric feeding tube may be obtained by x-ray.

NURSING DIAGNOSIS: Fluid Volume risk for [fluctuation]

May be related to

Active loss and/or failure of regulatory mechanisms (specific to underlying disease process/trauma); complications of nutrition therapy, e.g., high glucose solutions, hyperglycemia (hyperosmolar nonketotic coma and severe dehydration)
Inability to obtain/ingest fluids

Possibly evidenced by

[Not applicable; presence of signs and symptoms establishes an *actual* diagnosis]

DESIRED OUTCOMES/EVALUATION CRITERIA—PATIENT WILL:

> **Fluid Balance (NOC)**

Display moist skin/mucous membranes, stable vital signs, individually adequate urinary output; be free of edema and excessive weight loss/inappropriate gain.

ACTIONS/INTERVENTIONS

> **Fluid Management (NIC)**

Independent

Assess for clinical signs of dehydration (e.g., thirst, dry skin/mucous membranes, hypotension) or fluid excess (e.g., peripheral edema, tachycardia, adventitious breath sounds).

Incorporate knowledge of caloric density of enteral formulas into assessment of fluid balance.

Provide additional water/flush tubing as indicated.

Record I&O; calculate fluid balance. Measure urine specific gravity.

Weigh daily or as indicated; evaluate changes.

Collaborative

Monitor laboratory studies, e.g.:

Serum potassium/phosphorus;

RATIONALE

Early detection and intervention may prevent occurrence of excessive fluctuation in fluid balance. *Note:* Severely malnourished patients have an increased risk of developing refeeding syndrome, e.g., life-threatening fluid overload, intracellular electrolyte shifts, and cardiac strain occurring during initial 3–5 days of therapy.

Enteric solutions are usually concentrated and do not meet free water needs.

With higher calorie formula, additional water is needed to prevent dehydration/HHNC.

Excessive urinary losses may reflect developing HHNC. Specific gravity is an indicator of hydration and renal function.

Rapid weight gain (reflecting fluid retention) can predispose/potentiate HF or pulmonary edema. Gain of greater than 0.5 lb/day indicates fluid retention and not deposition of lean body mass.

Hypokalemia/phosphatemia can occur because of intracellular shifts during initial refeeding and may compromise cardiac function if not corrected.

ACTIONS/INTERVENTIONS	RATIONALE

Collaborative

Hct;

Reflects hydration/circulating volume.

Serum albumin.

Hypoalbuminemia/decreased colloidal osmotic pressure leads to third spacing of fluid (edema).

Dilute formula or change from hypertonic to isotonic formula as indicated.

May decrease gastric intolerance, reducing occurrence of diarrhea and associated fluid losses.

NURSING DIAGNOSIS: Fatigue

May be related to
Decreased metabolic energy production; increased energy requirements (hypermetabolic states, healing process)
Altered body chemistry: Medications, chemotherapy

Possibly evidenced by
Overwhelming lack of energy, inability to maintain usual routines/accomplish routine tasks
Lethargy, impaired ability to concentrate

DESIRED OUTCOMES/EVALUATION CRITERIA—PATIENT WILL:

Endurance (NOC)

Report increased sense of well-being/energy level.
Demonstrate measurable increase in physical activity.

ACTIONS/INTERVENTIONS	RATIONALE

Energy Management (NIC)

Independent

Monitor physiological response to activity, e.g., changes in BP, or heart/respiratory rate.

Tolerance varies greatly, depending on the stage of the disease process, nutritional state, and fluid balance.

Establish realistic activity goals with patient.

Provides for a sense of control and feelings of accomplishment.

Plan care to allow for rest periods. Schedule activities for periods when patient has most energy. Involve patient/SO in schedule planning.

Frequent rest periods are needed to restore/conserve energy. Planning allows patient to be active during times when energy level is higher, which may restore a feeling of well-being and a sense of control.

Encourage patient to do whatever possible, e.g., self-care, sitting up in chair, walking. Increase activity level as indicated.

Increases strength/stamina and enables patient to become more active without undue fatigue.

Provide passive/active ROM exercises to bedridden patients.

The development of healthy lean muscle mass depends on the provision of both isotonic and isometric exercises.

Keep bed in low position, pathways clear of furniture; assist with ambulation.

Protects patient from injury during activities.

Assist with self-care needs as necessary.

Generalized weakness may make ADLs almost impossible for the patient to complete.

ACTIONS/INTERVENTIONS

Collaborative

Provide supplemental O_2 as indicated.

Refer to physical/occupational therapy.

RATIONALE

Presence of anemia/hypoxemia reduces O_2 available for cellular uptake and contributes to fatigue.

Programmed daily exercises and activities help patient maintain/increase strength and muscle tone and enhance sense of well-being.

NURSING DIAGNOSIS: Knowledge Deficit [Learning Need] regarding condition, prognosis, treatment, self care, and discharge needs

May be related to
Lack of exposure/recall, information misinterpretation
Cognitive limitation

Possibly evidenced by
Request for information, questions/statement of misconception
Inaccurate follow-through of instructions/development of preventable complications

DESIRED OUTCOMES/EVALUATION CRITERIA—PATIENT WILL:

> **Knowledge: Disease Process (NOC)**

Verbalize understanding of condition/disease process and individual nutritional needs.

> **Knowledge: Treatment Procedure (NOC)**

Correctly perform necessary procedures and explain reasons for the actions.

ACTIONS/INTERVENTIONS

> **Teaching: Prescribed Diet (NIC)**

Independent

Assess patient's/SO's knowledge of nutritional state. Review individual situation, signs/symptoms of malnutrition, future expectations, transitional feeding needs.

Discuss reasons for use of parenteral/enteral nutrition support.

Provide adequate time for teaching patient/SO when patient is going home on enteral/parenteral feedings. Document patient's/SO's understanding and ability/competence to deliver safe home therapy.

Discuss proper handling, storage, preparation of nutritional solutions or blenderized feedings; also discuss aseptic or clean techniques for care of insertion sites and use of dressings.

Review use/care of nutritional support devices.

RATIONALE

Provides information from which the patient/SO can make informed choices. Knowledge of the interaction between malnutrition and illness is helpful in understanding need for special therapy.

May experience anxiety regarding inability to eat and may not comprehend the nutritional value of the prescribed TPN/tube feedings.

Generally, 3–4 days is sufficient for patient/SO to become proficient with tube feedings. Parenteral therapy is more complex, and patient/SO may require a week or longer to feel ready for home management; follow-up in the home is required.

Reduces risk of formula-/solution-related problems, metabolic complications, and infection.

Patient understanding and cooperation are key to the safe insertion and maintenance of nutritional support access devices and prevention of complications.

ACTIONS/INTERVENTIONS	RATIONALE

Independent

Review specific precautions depending on type of feeding, e.g., checking placement of tube, sitting upright for enteral feeding, maintaining patency of tube, anchoring of tubing and adequate length of tubing for night-time feeding.	Promotes safe self-care and reduces risk of complications.
Discuss/demonstrate reinsertion of enterostomal feeding tube if appropriate.	Tube may be changed routinely or inserted only for feedings. Intermittent feedings enhance patient mobility and aid in transition to regular feeding pattern.
Identify signs/symptoms requiring medical evaluation, e.g., nausea/vomiting, abdominal cramping or bloating, diarrhea, rapid weight changes; erythema, drainage, foul odor at tube insertion site, fever/chills; coughing/choking or difficulty breathing during enteral feeding.	Early evaluation and treatment of problems (e.g., feeding intolerance, infection, aspiration) may prevent progression to more serious complications.
Instruct patient/SO in glucose monitoring if indicated.	Timely recognition of changes in blood glucose levels reduces risk of hyperglycemic or hypoglycemic reactions in patient on hyperalimentation.
Discuss signs/symptoms and treatment of hyperglycemia/hypoglycemia.	Hyperglycemia is more common for patients receiving parenteral feedings and those who have pancreas or liver disease or are on large doses of corticosteroids. Rebound hypoglycemia can occur when feedings are intentionally/accidentally discontinued.
Encourage use of diary for recording test results, physical feelings/reactions, activity level, oral intake if any, I&O, weekly weight.	Provides resource for review by healthcare providers for optimal management of individual situation.
Recommend daily exercise/activity to tolerance, scheduling of adequate rest periods.	Enhances gastric motility for enteral/transition feedings, promotes feelings of general well-being, and prevents undue fatigue.
Ascertain that all supplies are in place in the home before discharge; make arrangements as needed with suppliers, e.g., hospital, pharmacy, medical equipment company, laboratory.	Provides for successful and competent home therapy.
Refer to nutritional support team, home healthcare agency, and counseling resources. Provide with immediate access phone numbers.	Patient/SO need readily available support persons to assist with nutrition therapy, equipment problems, and emotional adjustments in long-term/home-based therapy.

POTENTIAL CONSIDERATIONS following acute hospitalization (dependent on patient's age, physical condition/presence of complications, personal resources, and life responsibilities)

Fatigue—decreased metabolic energy production; increased energy requirements (hypermetabolic states, healing process); altered body chemistry, e.g., medications, chemotherapy.

Injury, risk for—catheter-related complications (catheter breaks, dislodgement, occlusion), effects of therapy (e.g., electrolyte/fluid shifts, diarrhea)/drug interactions, aspiration.

Infection, risk for—invasive tubes, environmental exposure, malnutrition, chronic disease.

Family Processes, altered—situational crises.

METABOLIC ACID-BASE IMBALANCES

The body has the remarkable ability to maintain plasma pH within the narrow range of 7.35–7.45. It does so by means of chemical buffering mechanisms by the kidneys and the lungs. Although single acid-base (e.g., metabolic acidosis) imbalances do occur, mixed acid-base imbalances are more common (e.g., metabolic acidosis/respiratory acidosis as occurs with cardiac arrest).

METABOLIC ACIDOSIS (PRIMARY BASE BICARBONATE [HCO₃] DEFICIENCY)

Metabolic acidosis (primary base bicarbonate [HCO_3] deficiency) reflects an excess of acid (hydrogen) and a deficit of base (bicarbonate) resulting from acid overproduction, loss of intestinal bicarbonate, inadequate conservation of bicarbonate, and excretion of acid, or anaerobic metabolism. Metabolic acidosis is characterized by normal or high anion gap situations. If the primary problem is direct loss of bicarbonate, gain of chloride, or decreased ammonia production, the anion gap is within normal limits. If the primary problem is the accumulation of organic anions (such as ketones or lactic acid), the condition is known as high anion gap acidosis. Compensatory mechanisms to correct this imbalance include an increase in respirations to blow off excess CO_2, an increase in ammonia formation, and acid excretion (H+) by the kidneys, with retention of bicarbonate and sodium.

High anion gap acidosis occurs in diabetic ketoacidosis; starvational or alcoholic lactic acidosis; renal failure; high-fat diets/lipid administration; poisoning, e.g., salicylate intoxication (after initial stage); paraldehyde intoxication; and drug therapy, e.g., acetazolamide (Diamox), NH_4Cl.

Normal anion gap acidosis is associated with loss of bicarbonate from the body, as may occur in renal tubular acidosis, hyperalimentation, vomiting/diarrhea, small-bowel/pancreatic fistulas, and ileostomy and use of IV sodium chloride in presence of preexisting kidney dysfunction, acidifying drugs (e.g., ammonium chloride).

CARE SETTING

This condition does not occur in isolation but rather is a complication of a broader problem that may require in-patient care in a medical-surgical or subacute unit.

RELATED CONCERNS

Plans of care specific to predisposing factors
Fluid and electrolyte imbalances, page 926
Renal dialysis, page 600
Respiratory acidosis (primary carbonic acid excess), page 214
Respiratory alkalosis (primary carbonic acid deficit), page 218

Patient Assessment Database (Dependent on Underlying Cause)

ACTIVITY/REST

May report: Lethargy, fatigue; muscle weakness

CIRCULATION

May exhibit: Hypotension, wide pulse pressure
Pulse may be weak, irregular (dysrhythmias)
Jaundiced sclera, skin, mucous membranes (liver failure)

ELIMINATION

May report: Diarrhea
May exhibit: Dark/concentrated urine

FOOD/FLUID

May report: Anorexia, nausea/vomiting
May exhibit: Poor skin turgor, dry mucous membranes

NEUROSENSORY

May report: Headache, drowsiness, decreased mental function

May exhibit: Changes in sensorium, e.g., stupor, confusion, lethargy, depression, delirium, coma

RESPIRATION

May report: Dyspnea on exertion

May exhibit: Hyperventilation, Kussmaul's respirations (deep, rapid breathing)

SAFETY

May report: Transfusion of blood/blood products

Exposure to hepatitis virus

May exhibit: Fever, signs of sepsis

TEACHING/LEARNING

History of alcohol abuse

Use of carbonic anhydrase inhibitors or anion-exchange resins, e.g., cholestyramine (Questran)

Discharge plan considerations: **DRG projected mean length of inpatient stay depends on underlying cause**

May require change in therapies for underlying disease process/condition

Refer to section at end of plan for postdischarge considerations.

DIAGNOSTIC STUDIES

Arterial pH: Decreased, less than 7.35.

Bicarbonate (HCO$_3$): Decreased, less than 22 mEq/L.

Paco$_2$: Less than 35 mm Hg.

Base excess: Negative.

Anion gap: Greater than 14 mEq/L (high anion gap) or range of 10 to 14 mEq/L (normal anion gap).

Serum potassium: Increased (except in diarrhea, renal tubular acidosis).

Serum chloride: Increased.

Serum glucose: May be decreased or increased depending on etiology.

Serum ketones: Increased in DM, starvation, alcohol intoxication.

Plasma lactic acid: Elevated in lactic acidosis.

Urine pH: Decreased, less than 4.5 (in absence of renal disease).

ECG: Cardiac dysrhythmias (bradycardia) and pattern changes associated with hyperkalemia, e.g., tall T wave.

NURSING PRIORITIES

1. Achieve homeostasis.
2. Prevent/minimize complications.
3. Provide information about condition/prognosis and treatment needs as appropriate.

DISCHARGE GOALS

1. Physiological balance restored.
2. Free of complications.
3. Condition, prognosis, and treatment needs understood.
4. Plan in place to meet needs after discharge.

Because no current nursing diagnosis speaks clearly to metabolic imbalances, the following interventions are presented in a general format for inclusion in the primary plan of care.

DESIRED OUTCOMES/EVALUATION CRITERIA—PATIENT WILL:

Electrolyte and Acid-Base Balance (NOC)

Display serum bicarbonate and electrolytes within normal limits (WNL).
Be free of symptoms of imbalance, e.g., absence of neurological impairment; vital
signs WNL.

ACTIONS/INTERVENTIONS	RATIONALE
Independent	
Monitor BP.	Arteriolar dilation/decreased cardiac contractility (e.g., sepsis) and hypovolemia (e.g., ketoacidosis) occurs, resulting in systemic shock, evidenced by hypotension and tissue hypoxia.
Assess LOC and note progressive changes in neuromuscular status, e.g., strength, tone, movement.	Decreased mental function, confusion, seizures, weakness, flaccid paralysis can occur because of hypoxia, hyperkalemia, and decreased pH of CNS fluid.
Provide seizure/coma precautions, e.g., bed in low position, use of side rails, frequent observation.	Protects patient from injury resulting from decreased mentation/convulsions.
Monitor heart rate/rhythm.	Acidemia may be manifested by changes in ECG configuration and presence of bradydysrhythmias as well as increased ventricular irritability such as fibrillation (signs of hyperkalemia). Life-threatening cardiovascular collapse may also occur because of vasodilation and decreased cardiac contractility. *Note:* Hypokalemia can occur as acidosis is corrected, resulting in premature ventricular contractions (PVCs)/ventricular tachycardia.
Observe for altered respiratory excursion, rate, and depth.	Deep, rapid respirations (Kussmaul's) may be noted as a compensatory mechanism to eliminate excess acid; however, as potassium shifts out of cell in an attempt to correct acidosis, respirations may become depressed. Transient respiratory depression may be the result of overcorrection of metabolic acidosis with sodium bicarbonate.
Assess skin temperature, color, capillary refill.	Evaluates circulatory status, tissue perfusion, effects of hypotension.
Auscultate bowel sounds; measure abdominal girth as indicated.	In the presence of coexisting hyperkalemia, GI distress (e.g., distension, diarrhea, and colic) may occur.
Monitor I&O closely and weigh daily.	Marked dehydration may be present because of vomiting, diarrhea. Therapy needs are based on underlying cause and fluid balance.
Test/monitor urine pH.	Kidneys attempt to compensate for acidosis by excreting excess hydrogen in the form of weak acids and ammonia. Maximum urine acidity is pH of 4.0.
Provide oral hygiene with sodium bicarbonate washes, lemon/glycerine swabs.	Neutralizes mouth acids and provides protective lubrication.

ACTIONS/INTERVENTIONS	RATIONALE
Collaborative	
Assist with identification/treatment of underlying cause.	Treatment of disorder is directed at mild correction of acidosis until organ(s) function is improved. Addressing the primary condition (e.g., DKA, liver/renal failure, drug poisoning, sepsis) promotes correction of the acid-base disorder.
Monitor/graph serial ABGs.	Evaluates therapy needs/effectiveness. Blood bicarbonate and pH should slowly increase toward normal levels.
Monitor serum electrolytes, e.g., potassium.	As acidosis is corrected, serum potassium deficit may occur as potassium shifts back into the cells.
Replace fluids, as indicated depending on underlying etiology, e.g., D_5W/saline solutions.	Choice of solution varies with cause of acidosis, e.g., DKA. *Note:* Lactate-containing solutions may be contraindicated in the presence of lactic acidosis.
Administer medications as indicated, e.g.:	
Sodium bicarbonate/lactate or saline IV;	Corrects bicarbonate deficit, but is used cautiously to correct severe acidosis (pH less than 7.2) because sodium bicarbonate can cause rebound metabolic alkalosis.
Potassium chloride;	May be required as potassium re-enters the cell, causing a serum deficit.
Phosphate;	May be administered to enhance acid excretion in presence of chronic acidosis with hypophosphatemia.
Calcium.	May be given to improve neuromuscular conduction/function.
Modify diet as indicated, e.g., low-protein, high-carbohydrate diet in presence of renal failure or American Diabetes Association (ADA) diet for the person with diabetes.	Restriction of protein may be necessary to decrease production of acid waste products, whereas addition of complex carbohydrates will correct acid production from the metabolism of fats.
Administer exchange resins and/or assist with dialysis as indicated.	May be desired to reduce acidosis by decreasing excess potassium and acid waste products if pH less than 7.1 and other therapies are ineffective, or HF develops.

POTENTIAL CONSIDERATIONS: Refer to Potential Considerations relative to underlying cause of acid-base disorder.

METABOLIC ALKALOSIS (PRIMARY BASE BICARBONATE EXCESS)

Metabolic alkalosis is characterized by a high pH (loss of hydrogen ions) and high plasma bicarbonate caused by excessive intake of sodium bicarbonate, loss of gastric/intestinal acid, renal excretion of hydrogen and chloride, prolonged hypercalcemia, hypokalemia, and hyperaldosteronism. Compensatory mechanisms include slow, shallow respirations to increase CO_2 level and an increase of bicarbonate excretion and hydrogen reabsorption by the kidneys.

CARE SETTING

This condition does not occur in isolation but rather is a complication of a broader problem that may require inpatient care in a medical-surgical or subacute unit.

RELATED CONCERNS

Plans of care specific to predisposing factors
Fluid and electrolyte imbalances, page 926
Renal dialysis, page 600
Respiratory acidosis (primary carbonic acid excess), page 214
Respiratory alkalosis (primary carbonic acid deficit), page 218

Patient Assessment Database (Dependent on Underlying Cause)

CIRCULATION

May exhibit: Tachycardia, irregularities/dysrhythmias
Cyanosis

ELIMINATION

May report: Diarrhea (with high chloride content)
Use of potassium-losing diuretics (Diuril, Hygroton, Lasix, Edecrin)
Laxative abuse

FOOD/FLUID

May report: Nausea/prolonged vomiting
High salt intake; excessive ingestion of licorice
Recurrent indigestion/heartburn with frequent use of antacids/baking soda

NEUROSENSORY

May report: Tingling of fingers and toes; circumoral paresthesia
Dizziness

May exhibit: Hypertonicity of muscles, tetany, tremors, convulsions
Confusion, irritability, restlessness, belligerence, apathy, coma
Picking at bedclothes

SAFETY

May report: Recent blood transfusions (citrated blood)

RESPIRATION

May exhibit: Hypoventilation (increases P_{CO_2} and conserves carbonic acid), periods of apnea

TEACHING/LEARNING

History of Cushing's syndrome; corticosteroid therapy

Discharge plan considerations: **DRG projected mean length of inpatient stay depends on underlying cause**
May require change in therapy for underlying disease process/condition.

Refer to section at end of plan for postdischarge considerations.

DIAGNOSTIC STUDIES

Arterial pH: Increased, greater than 7.45.

Bicarbonate (HCO₃): Increased, greater than 26 mEq/L (primary).

Paco₂: Slightly increased, greater than 45 mm Hg (compensatory).

Base excess: Increased.

Serum chloride: Decreased, less than 98 mEq/L disproportionately to serum sodium decreases (if alkalosis is hypochloremia).

Serum potassium: Decreased.

Serum calcium: Usually decreased. Prolonged hypercalcemia (nonparathyroid) may be a predisposing factor.

Urine pH: Increased, greater than 7.0.

Urine chloride: Less than 10 mEq/L suggests chloride responsive alkalosis, whereas levels greater than 20 mEq/L suggest chloride resistance.

ECG: May show hypokalemic changes including peaked P waves, flat T waves, depressed ST segment, low T wave merging to P wave, and elevated U waves.

NURSING PRIORITIES

1. Achieve homeostasis.
2. Prevent/minimize complications.
3. Provide information about condition/prognosis and treatment needs as appropriate.

DISCHARGE GOALS

1. Physiological balance restored.
2. Free of complications.
3. Condition, prognosis, and treatment needs understood.
4. Plan in place to meet needs after discharge.

Because no current nursing diagnosis speaks clearly to metabolic imbalances, the following interventions are presented in a general format for inclusion in the primary plan of care.

DESIRED OUTCOMES/EVALUATION CRITERIA—PATIENT WILL:

Electrolyte and Acid-Base Balance (NOC)

Display serum bicarbonate and electrolytes WNL.
Be free of symptoms of imbalance, e.g., absence of neurological impairment/irritability.

ACTIONS/INTERVENTIONS	RATIONALE
Metabolic Alkalosis Management (NIC)	
Independent	
Monitor respiratory rate, rhythm, and depth.	Hypoventilation is a compensatory mechanism to conserve carbonic acid and represents definite risks to the individual, e.g., hypoxemia and respiratory failure.
Assess level of consciousness and neuromuscular status, e.g., strength, tone, movement; note presence of Chvostek's/Trousseau's signs.	The CNS may be hyperirritable (increased pH of CNS fluid), resulting in tingling, numbness, dizziness, restlessness, or apathy and confusion. Hypocalcemia may contribute to tetany (although occurrence is rare).
Monitor heart rate/rhythm.	Atrial/ventricular ectopics and tachydysrhythmias may develop.
Record amount and source of output. Monitor intake and daily weight.	Helpful in identifying source of ion loss; e.g., potassium and HCl are lost in vomiting and GI suctioning.

ACTIONS/INTERVENTIONS	RATIONALE
Independent	
Restrict oral intake and reduce noxious environmental stimuli; use intermittent/low suction during NG suctioning; irrigate gastric tube with isotonic solutions rather than water.	Limits gastric losses of HCl, potassium, and calcium.
Provide seizure/safety precautions as indicated, e.g., padded side rails, airway protection, bed in low position, frequent observation.	Changes in mentation and CNS/neuromuscular hyperirritability may result in patient harm, especially if tetany/convulsions occur.
Encourage intake of foods and fluids high in potassium and possibly calcium (dependent on blood level), e.g., canned grapefruit and apple juices, bananas, cauliflower, dried peaches, figs, and wheat germ.	Useful in replacing potassium losses when oral intake permitted.
Review medication regimen for use of diuretics, such as thiazides (Diuril, Hygroton), furosemide (Lasix), and ethacrynic acid (Edecrin).	Discontinuation of these potassium-losing drugs may prevent recurrence of imbalance.
Instruct patient to avoid use of excessive amounts of sodium bicarbonate.	Ulcer patients can cause alkalosis by taking baking soda and milk of magnesia in addition to prescribed alkaline antacids.
Collaborative	
Assist with identification/treatment of underlying disorder.	Addressing the primary condition (e.g., prolonged vomiting/diarrhea, hyperaldosteronism, Cushing's syndrome) promotes correction of the acid-base disorder.
Monitor laboratory studies as indicated, e.g., ABGs/pH, serum electrolytes (especially potassium), and BUN.	Evaluates therapy needs/effectiveness and monitors renal function.
Administer medications as indicated, e.g.;	
Sodium chloride PO/Ringer's solution IV unless contraindicated;	Correcting sodium, water, and chloride defects may be all that is needed to permit kidneys to excrete bicarbonate and correct alkalosis but must be used with caution in patients with HF or renal insufficiency.
Potassium chloride;	Hypokalemia is frequently present. Chloride is needed so kidney can absorb sodium with chloride, enhancing excretion of bicarbonate.
Ammonium chloride or arginine hydrochloride;	Increases amount of circulating hydrogen ions. Monitor administration closely to prevent too rapid a decrease in pH, hemolysis of RBCs. *Note:* May cause rebound metabolic acidosis and is usually contraindicated in patients with renal/hepatic failure.
Acetazolamide (Diamox);	A carbonic anhydrase inhibitor that increases renal excretion of bicarbonate.
Spironolactone (Aldactone).	Effective in treating chloride-resistant alkalosis, e.g., Cushing's syndrome.
Avoid/limit use of sedatives or hypnotics.	If respirations are depressed, may cause hypoxia/respiratory failure.
Encourage fluids IV/PO.	Replaces extracellular fluid losses, and adequate hydration facilitates removal of pulmonary secretions to improve ventilation.

ACTIONS/INTERVENTIONS	RATIONALE
Independent	
Administer supplemental O_2 as indicated and respiratory treatments to improve ventilation.	Respiratory compensation for metabolic alkalosis is hypoventilation, which may cause decreased PaO_2 levels/hypoxia.
Prepare patient for/assist with dialysis as needed.	Useful when renal dysfunction prevents clearance of bicarbonate.

POTENTIAL CONSIDERATIONS: Refer to Potential Considerations relative to underlying cause of acid/base disorder.

Diseases of the Blood/ Blood-Forming Organs

ANEMIAS (IRON DEFICIENCY, PERNICIOUS, APLASTIC, HEMOLYTIC)

Anemia is a symptom of an underlying condition, such as loss of blood components, inadequate elements, or lack of required nutrients for the formation of blood cells, that results in decreased oxygen-carrying capacity of the blood. There are numerous types of anemias with various causes. The following types of anemia are discussed here: iron deficiency (ID), the result of inadequate absorption or excessive loss of iron; pernicious (PA), the result of a lack of the intrinsic factor essential for the absorption of vitamin B_{12}; aplastic, due to failure of bone marrow; and hemolytic, due to red blood cell (RBC) destruction. Nursing care for the anemic patient has a common theme even though the medical treatments vary widely.

CARE SETTING

Treated at the community level, except in the presence of severe cardiovascular/immune compromise.

RELATED CONCERNS

AIDS, page 765
Burns: thermal/chemical/electrical (acute and convalescent phases), page 791
Cancer, page 900
Cirrhosis of the liver, page 484
Heart failure: chronic, page 47
Psychosocial aspects of care, page 809
Renal failure: acute, page 575
Renal failure: chronic, page 588
Rheumatoid arthritis, page 790
Pulmonary tuberculosis (TB), page 204
Upper gastrointestinal/Esophageal bleeding, page 333

Patient Assessment Database

ACTIVITY/REST

May report: Fatigue, weakness, general malaise
Loss of productivity; diminished enthusiasm for work
Low exercise tolerance
Greater need for rest and sleep

May exhibit:	Tachycardia/tachypnea; dyspnea on exertion or at rest (severe or aplastic anemia)
	Lethargy, withdrawal, apathy, lassitude, and lack of interest in surroundings
	Muscle weakness and decreased strength
	Ataxia, unsteady gait
	Slumping of shoulders, drooping posture, slow walk, and other cues indicative of fatigue

CIRCULATION

May report:	History of chronic blood loss, e.g., chronic gastrointestinal bleeding, heavy menses (ID); angina, heart failure (due to increased cardiac workload)
	History of chronic infective endocarditis
	Palpitations (compensatory tachycardia)
May exhibit:	Blood pressure (BP): Increased systolic with stable diastolic and a widened pulse pressure; postural hypotension
	Dysrhythmias, electrocardiogram abnormalities, e.g., ST-segment depression and flattening or depression of the T wave; tachycardia
	Throbbing carotid pulsations (reflects increased cardiac output as a compensatory mechanism to provide oxygen/nutrients to cells)
	Systolic murmur (ID)
	Extremities (color): Pallor of the skin and mucous membranes (conjunctiva, mouth, pharynx, lips) and nailbeds, or grayish cast in black patients; waxy, pale skin (aplastic, PA) or bright lemon yellow (PA)
	Sclera blue or pearl white (ID); jaundice (PA)
	Capillary refill delayed (diminished blood flow to the periphery and compensatory vasoconstriction)
	Nails brittle, spoon-shaped (koilonychia) (ID)

EGO INTEGRITY

May report:	Negative feelings about self, ability to handle situation/events
May exhibit:	Depression

ELIMINATION

May report:	History of pyelonephritis, renal failure
	Flatulence, malabsorption syndrome (ID)
	Hematemesis, fresh blood in stool, melena
	Diarrhea or constipation
	Diminished urine output
May exhibit:	Abdominal distension

FOOD/FLUID

May report:	Decreased dietary intake, low intake of animal protein/high intake of cereal products (ID)
	Mouth or tongue pain, difficulty swallowing (ulcerations in pharynx)
	Nausea/vomiting, dyspepsia, anorexia
	Recent weight loss
	Insatiable craving or pica for ice, dirt, cornstarch, paint, clay, and so forth (ID)
May exhibit:	Beefy red/smooth appearance of tongue (PA; folic acid and vitamin B_{12} deficiencies)
	Dry, pale mucous membranes
	Skin turgor poor with dry, shriveled appearance/loss of elasticity (ID)
	Stomatitis and glossitis (deficiency states)
	Lips: cheilitis, i.e., inflammation of the lips with cracking at the corners of the mouth (ID)

HYGIENE

May report:	Difficulty maintaining activities of daily living
May exhibit:	Unkempt appearance, poor personal hygiene
	Hair dry, brittle, thinning; premature graying (PA)

NEUROSENSORY

May report: Headaches, fainting, dizziness, vertigo, tinnitus, inability to concentrate
Insomnia, dimness of vision, and spots before eyes
Weakness, poor balance, wobbly legs; paresthesias of hands/feet (PA); claudication
Sensation of being cold

May exhibit: Irritability, restlessness, depression, drowsiness, apathy
Mentation: Notable slowing and dullness in response
Ophthalmic: Retinal hemorrhages (aplastic, PA)
Epistaxis, bleeding from other orifices (aplastic)
Disturbed coordination, ataxia; decreased vibratory and position sense, positive Romberg's sign, paralysis (PA)

PAIN/DISCOMFORT

May report: Vague abdominal pains; headache (ID)
Oral pain

RESPIRATION

May report: History of TB, lung abscesses
Shortness of breath at rest and with activity

May exhibit: Tachypnea, orthopnea, and dyspnea

SAFETY

May report: History of occupational exposure to chemicals, e.g., benzene, lead, insecticides, phenyl-butazone, naphthalene
History of exposure to radiation either as a treatment modality or by accident
History of cancer, cancer therapies
Cold and/or heat intolerance
Previous blood transfusions
Impaired vision
Poor wound healing, frequent infections

May exhibit: Low-grade fever, chills, night sweats
Generalized lymphadenopathy
Petechiae and ecchymosis (aplastic)

SEXUALITY

May report: Changes in menstrual flow, e.g., menorrhagia or amenorrhea in women (ID)
Loss of libido (men and women)
Impotence in men

May exhibit: Pale cervix and vaginal walls

TEACHING/LEARNING

May report: Family tendency for anemia (ID/PA)
Past/present use of anticonvulsants, antibiotics, chemotherapeutic agents (bone marrow failure), aspirin, anti-inflammatory drugs, or anticoagulants
Chronic use of alcohol
Religious/cultural beliefs affecting treatment choices, e.g., refusal of blood transfusions
Recent/current episode of active bleeding (ID)
History of liver, renal disease; hematologic problems; celiac or other malabsorption disease; regional enteritis; tapeworm manifestations; polyendocrinopathies; autoimmune problem (e.g., antibodies to parietal cells, intrinsic factor, thyroid and T-cell antibodies)
Prior surgeries, e.g., splenectomy; tumor excision; prosthetic valve replacement; surgical excision of duodenum or gastric resection, partial/total gastrectomy (ID/PA)
History of problems with wound healing or bleeding; chronic infections (RA), chronic granulomatous disease, or cancer (secondary anemias)

Discharge plan considerations:	**DRG projected mean length of inpatient stay: 4.3 days or depending on type/cause of anemia and severity of complications**

May require assistance with treatment (injections); self-care activities and/or homemaker/ maintenance tasks; changes in dietary plan

Refer to section at end of plan for postdischarge considerations.

DIAGNOSTIC STUDIES

Complete blood count (CBC):

> *Hemoglobin (Hb) and hematocrit (Hct):* Decreased in anemias and overhydration caused by excessive IV fluids, bleeding problems, bone marrow suppression.
>
> *Erythrocyte (RBC) count:* Decreased (PA), severely decreased (aplastic); mean corpuscular volume (MCV) and mean corpuscular hemoglobin (MCH) decreased and microcytic with hypochromic erythrocytes (ID), elevated (PA); pancytopenia (aplastic).
>
> *Stained RBC examination:* Detects changes in color and shape (may indicate particular type of anemia).
>
> *Reticulocyte count:* Varies; helps assess bone marrow function, e.g., decreased (PA), cirrhosis, folic acid deficiency, bone marrow failure, radiation therapy; elevated (blood loss/hemolysis, leukemias, compensated anemias).
>
> *White blood cells (WBCs):* Total cell count and specific WBCs (differential) may be increased (hemolytic) or decreased (aplastic).
>
> *Platelet count:* Decreased (aplastic); elevated (ID); normal or high (hemolytic).
>
> *Erythrocyte sedimentation rate (ESR):* Elevation indicates presence of inflammatory reaction, e.g., increased RBC destruction or malignant disease.

RBC survival time: Useful in the differential diagnosis of anemias because RBCs have shortened life spans in pernicious and hemolytic anemia.

Erythrocyte fragility test: Decreased (ID); increased fragility confirms hemolytic and autoimmune anemias.

Hemoglobin electrophoresis: Identifies type of hemoglobin structure, aids in determining source of hemolytic anemia.

Serum folate and vitamin B_{12}: Aids in diagnosing anemias related to deficiencies in dietary intake/malabsorption.

Serum iron: Absent (ID); elevated (hemolytic, aplastic).

Serum total iron-binding capacity (TIBC): Increased (ID); normal or slightly reduced (AP).

Serum ferritin: Decreased (ID).

Serum bilirubin (unconjugated): Elevated (PA, hemolytic).

Serum lactate dehydrogenase (LDH): May be elevated (PA).

Bleeding time: Prolonged (aplastic).

Schilling test: Decreased urinary excretion of vitamin B_{12} (PA).

Guaiac: May be positive for occult blood in urine, stools, and gastric contents, reflecting acute/chronic bleeding (ID).

Gastric analysis: Decreased secretions with elevated pH and absence of free HCl (PA).

Bone marrow aspiration/biopsy examination: Cells may show changes in number, size and shape, helping to differentiate type of anemia, e.g., increased megaloblasts (PA); fatty marrow with diminished or absence of blood cells at several sites (aplastic).

Endoscopic and radiographic studies: Checks for bleeding sites, e.g., acute/chronic GI bleeding.

NURSING PRIORITIES

1. Enhance tissue perfusion.
2. Provide nutritional/fluid needs.
3. Prevent complications.
4. Provide information about disease process, prognosis, and treatment regimen.

DISCHARGE GOALS

1. ADLs met by self or with assistance of others.
2. Complications prevented/minimized.
3. Disease process/prognosis and therapeutic regimen understood.
4. Plan in place to meet needs after discharge.

> **NURSING DIAGNOSIS: Activity Intolerance**
>
> **May be related to**
> Imbalance between oxygen supply (delivery) and demand
> **Possibly evidenced by**
> Weakness and fatigue
> Reports of decreased exercise/activity tolerance
> Greater need for sleep/rest
> Palpitations, tachycardia, increased BP/respiratory response with minor exertion
> **DESIRED OUTCOMES/EVALUATION CRITERIA—PATIENT WILL:**
>
> **Endurance (NOC)**
>
> Report an increase in activity tolerance (including ADLs).
> Demonstrate a decrease in physiological signs of intolerance, e.g., pulse, respirations, and BP remain within patient's normal range.
> Display laboratory values, e.g., Hb/Hct, within acceptable range.

ACTIONS/INTERVENTIONS

Energy Management (NIC)

Independent

Assess patient's ability to perform normal tasks/ADLs, noting reports of weakness, fatigue, and difficulty accomplishing tasks.

Note changes in balance/gait disturbance, muscle weakness.

Monitor BP, pulse, respirations during and after activity. Note adverse responses to increased levels of activity (e.g., increased heart rate [HR]/BP, dysrhythmias, dizziness, dyspnea, tachypnea, cyanosis of mucous membranes/nailbeds).

Recommend quiet atmosphere; bedrest if indicated. Stress need to monitor and limit visitors, phone calls, and repeated unplanned interruptions.

Elevate head of bed as tolerated.

Suggest patient change position slowly; monitor for dizziness.

Assist patient to prioritize ADLs/desired activities. Alternate rest periods with activity periods. Write out schedule for patient to refer to.

Provide/recommend assistance with activities/ambulation as necessary, allowing patient to do as much as possible.

Plan activity progression with patient, including activities that the patient views as essential. Increase activity levels as tolerated.

RATIONALE

Influences choice of interventions/needed assistance.

May indicate neurological changes associated with vitamin B_{12} deficiency, affecting patient safety/risk of injury.

Cardiopulmonary manifestations result from attempts by the heart and lungs to supply adequate amounts of oxygen to the tissues.

Enhances rest to lower body's oxygen requirements and reduces strain on the heart and lungs.

Enhances lung expansion to maximize oxygenation for cellular uptake. *Note:* May be contraindicated if hypotension is present.

Postural hypotension or cerebral hypoxia may cause dizziness, fainting, and increased risk of injury.

Promotes adequate rest, maintains energy level, and alleviates strain on the cardiac and respiratory systems.

Although help may be necessary, self-esteem is enhanced when patient does some things for self.

Promotes gradual return to normal activity level and improved muscle tone/stamina without undue fatigue. Increases self-esteem and sense of control.

ACTIONS/INTERVENTIONS	RATIONALE

Independent

Identify/implement energy-saving techniques, e.g., shower chair, sitting to perform tasks.

Encourages patient to do as much as possible, while conserving limited energy and preventing fatigue.

Instruct patient to stop activity if palpitations, chest pain, shortness of breath, weakness, or dizziness occur.

Cellular ischemia potentiates risk of infarction and excessive cardiopulmonary strain/stress may lead to decompensation/failure.

Discuss importance of maintaining environmental temperature and body warmth as indicated.

Vasoconstriction (shunting of blood to vital organs) decreases peripheral circulation, impairing tissue perfusion. Patient's comfort/need for warmth must be balanced with need to avoid excessive heat with resultant vasodilation (reduces organ perfusion).

Collaborative

Monitor laboratory studies, e.g., Hb/Hct and RBC count, arterial blood gases (ABGs).

Identifies deficiencies in RBC components affecting oxygen transport and treatment needs/response to therapy.

Provide supplemental oxygen as indicated.

Maximizing oxygen transport to tissues improves ability to function.

Administer as indicated:

Colony-stimulating factors (CSFs), e.g., interleukin-2 (Aldesleukin);

CSFs may be given to stimulate growth of specific blood elements.

Whole blood/packed RBCs (PRCs), blood products as indicated. Monitor closely for transfusion reactions.

Increases number of oxygen-carrying cells; corrects deficiencies to reduce risk of hemorrhage in acutely compromised individuals. *Note:* Transfusions are reserved for severe blood loss anemias with cardiovascular compromise; used after other therapies have failed to restore homeostasis.

Prepare for surgical intervention if indicated.

Bone marrow transplant may be done in presence of bone marrow failure/aplastic anemia.

NURSING DIAGNOSIS: Nutrition: altered, less than body requirements

May be related to
Failure to ingest or inability to digest food/absorb nutrients necessary for formation of normal RBCs

Possibly evidenced by
Weight loss/weight below normal for age, height, and build
Decreased triceps skinfold measurement
Changes in gums, oral mucous membranes
Decreased tolerance for activity, weakness, and loss of muscle tone

DESIRED OUTCOMES/EVALUATION CRITERIA—PATIENT WILL:

Nutritional Status (NOC)

Demonstrate progressive weight gain or stable weight, with normalization of laboratory values.
Experience no signs of malnutrition.
Demonstrate behaviors, lifestyle changes to regain and/or maintain appropriate weight.

ACTIONS/INTERVENTIONS	RATIONALE

Nutrition Therapy (NIC)

Independent

Review nutritional history, including food preferences.

Identifies deficiencies, suggests possible interventions.

Observe and record patient's food intake.

Monitors caloric intake or insufficient quality of food consumption.

Weigh periodically as appropriate (e.g. weekly).

Monitors weight loss and effectiveness of nutritional interventions.

Recommend small, frequent meals and/or between-meal nourishment.

May reduce fatigue and thus enhance intake while preventing gastric distention. Use of Ensure/Isomil or similar product provides additional protein and calories.

Suggest bland diet, low in roughage, avoiding hot, spicy, or very acidic foods as indicated.

When oral lesions are present, pain may restrict type of foods patient can tolerate.

Have patient record and report occurrence of nausea/vomiting, flatus, and other related symptoms such as irritability or impaired memory.

May reflect effects of anemias (hypoxia, vitamin B_{12} deficiency) on organs.

Encourage/assist with good oral hygiene; before and after meals, use soft-bristled toothbrush for gentle brushing. Provide dilute, alcohol-free mouthwash if oral mucosa is ulcerated.

Enhances appetite and oral intake. Diminishes bacterial growth, minimizing possibility of infection. Special mouth-care techniques may be needed if tissue is fragile/ulcerated/bleeding and pain is severe.

Collaborative

Consult with dietitian.

Aids in establishing dietary plan to meet individual needs.

Monitor laboratory studies, e.g., Hb/Hct, blood urea nitrogen (BUN), prealbumin/albumin, protein, transferrin, serum iron, B_{12}, folic acid, TIBC, serum electrolytes.

Evaluates effectiveness of treatment regimen, including dietary sources of needed nutrients.

Administer medications as indicated, e.g.:

Vitamin and mineral supplements, e.g., cyanocobalamin (vitamin B_{12}), folic acid (Folvite); ascorbic acid (vitamin C);

Replacements needed depend on type of anemia and/or presence of poor oral intake and identified deficiencies.

Oral iron supplements, e.g., ferrous sulfate (Feosol, Ferospace, Mol-Iron, Fer-in-Sol), ferrous gluconate (Fergon), ferrous fumarate (Ircon, Femiron);

May be useful in some types of iron deficiency anemias. Oral preparations are taken between meals to enhance absorption and usually correct anemia and replace iron stores over a period of several months.

Iron dextran (INFeD) IM/IV;

Administered until estimated deficit is corrected. Reserved for those who cannot absorb or comply with oral iron therapy or when blood loss is too rapid for oral replacement to be effective.

Antifungal or anesthetic mouthwash, if indicated.

May be needed in the presence of stomatitis/glossitis to promote oral tissue healing and facilitate intake.

NURSING DIAGNOSIS: Constipation/Diarrhea

May be related to

Decreased dietary intake; changes in digestive processes

Drug therapy side effects

ACTIONS/INTERVENTIONS	RATIONALE
Bowel Management (NIC)	
Independent	
Determine stool color, consistency, frequency, and amount.	Assists in identifying causative/contributing factors and appropriate interventions.
Auscultate bowel sounds.	Bowel sounds are generally increased in diarrhea and decreased in constipation.
Monitor intake and output (I&O) with specific attention to food/fluid intake.	May identify dehydration, excessive loss of fluids or aid in identifying dietary deficiencies.
Encourage fluid intake of 2500–3000 mL/day within cardiac tolerance.	Assists in improving stool consistency if constipated. Helps maintain hydration status if diarrhea is present.
Recommend avoiding gas-forming foods.	Decreases gastric distress and abdominal distention.
Assess perianal skin condition frequently, noting changes or beginning breakdown. Encourage/assist with pericare after each bowel movement (BM) if diarrhea is present.	Prevents skin excoriation and breakdown.
Discuss use of stool softeners, mild stimulants, bulk-forming laxatives, or enemas as indicated. Monitor effectiveness.	Facilitates defecation when constipation is present.
Collaborative	
Consult with dietitian to provide well-balanced diet high in fiber and bulk.	Fiber resists enzymatic digestion and absorbs liquids in its passage along the intestinal tract and thereby produces bulk, which acts as a stimulant to defecation.
Administer antidiarrheal medications, e.g., diphenoxylate hydrochloride with atropine (Lomotil) and water-absorbing drugs, e.g., Metamucil.	Decreases intestinal motility when diarrhea is present.

Possibly evidenced by

[Not applicable; presence of signs and symptoms establishes an *actual* diagnosis]

DESIRED OUTCOMES/EVALUATION CRITERIA—PATIENT WILL:

> **Risk Control (NOC)**

Identify behaviors to prevent/reduce risk of infection.

> **Immune status (NOC)**

Be free of signs of infection, achieve timely wound healing (if present).

ACTIONS/INTERVENTIONS

RATIONALE

> **Infection Protection (NIC)**

Independent

ACTIONS/INTERVENTIONS	RATIONALE
Perform/promote meticulous handwashing by caregivers and patient.	Prevents cross-contamination/bacterial colonization. *Note:* Patient with severe/aplastic anemia may be at risk from normal skin flora.
Maintain strict aseptic techniques with procedures/wound care.	Reduces risk of bacterial colonization/infection.
Provide meticulous skin, oral, and perianal care.	Reduces risk of skin/tissue breakdown and infection.
Encourage frequent position changes/ambulation, coughing, and deep-breathing exercises.	Promotes ventilation of all lung segments and aids in mobilizing secretions to prevent pneumonia.
Promote adequate fluid intake.	Assists in liquefying respiratory secretions to facilitate expectoration and prevent stasis of body fluids (e.g., respiratory and renal).
Stress need to monitor/limit visitors. Provide protective isolation if appropriate. Restrict live plants/cut flowers.	Limits exposure to bacteria/infections. Protective isolation may be required in aplastic anemia, when immune response is most compromised.
Monitor temperature. Note presence of chills and tachycardia with/without fever.	Reflective of inflammatory process/infection, requiring evaluation and treatment. *Note:* With bone marrow suppression, leukocytic failure may lead to fulminating infections.
Observe for wound erythema/drainage.	Indicators of local infection. *Note:* Pus formation may be absent if granulocytes are depressed.

Collaborative

ACTIONS/INTERVENTIONS	RATIONALE
Obtain specimens for culture/sensitivity as indicated.	Verifies presence of infection, identifies specific pathogen, and influences choice of treatment.
Administer topical antiseptics; systemic antibiotics.	May be used prophylactically to reduce colonization or used to treat specific infectious process.

> **NURSING DIAGNOSIS: Knowledge Deficit [Learning Need] regarding condition, prognosis, treatment, self care, and discharge needs**
>
> **May be related to**
> Lack of exposure/recall
> Information misinterpretation
> Unfamiliarity with information resources

ACTIONS/INTERVENTIONS	RATIONALE
Teaching: Disease Process (NIC)	
Independent	
Provide information about specific anemia and explain that therapy depends on the type and severity of the anemia.	Provides knowledge base from which patient can make informed choices. Allays anxiety and may promote cooperation with therapeutic regimen.
Discuss effects of anemias on preexisting conditions.	Anemias aggravate heart, lung, and cerebrovascular disease.
Review purpose and preparations for diagnostic studies.	Anxiety/fear of the unknown increases stress level, which in turn increases the cardiac workload. Knowledge of what to expect can diminish anxiety.
Explain that blood taken for laboratory studies will not worsen anemia.	This is often an unspoken concern that can potentiate patient's anxiety.
Review required diet alterations to meet specific dietary needs (determined by type of anemia/deficiency).	Red meat, liver, egg yolks, green leafy vegetables, whole wheat bread, and dried fruits are sources of iron. Green vegetables, whole grains, liver, and citrus fruits are sources of folic acid and vitamin C (enhances absorption of iron).
Assess resources (e.g., financial) and ability to obtain/prepare food).	Inadequate resources may affect ability to purchase/prepare appropriate food items.
Encourage cessation of smoking.	Smoking decreases available oxygen and causes vasonstriction.
Provide information about purpose, dosage, schedule, precautions and potential side effects, interactions, and adverse reactions to all prescribed medications.	Information enhances cooperation with regimen. Recovery from anemias can be slow, requiring lengthy treatment and prevention of secondary complications.
Stress importance of reporting signs of fatigue, weakness, paresthesias, irritability, impaired memory.	Indicates that anemia is progressing or failing to resolve, necessitating further evaluation/treatment changes.
Instruct and demonstrate self-administration of oral iron preparations:	Iron replacement usually takes 3–6 mo, whereas vitamin B_{12} injections may be necessary for the rest of the patient's life.
Discuss importance of taking only prescribed dosages;	Overdose of iron medication can be toxic.

ACTIONS/INTERVENTIONS

Independent

Advise taking with meals or immediately after meals;

Dilute liquid preparations (preferably with orange juice) and administer through a straw;

Caution that BM may appear greenish black/tarry;

Emphasize importance of good oral hygiene measures.

Instruct patient/SO about parenteral iron administration, e.g.:

Z-track administration of medication;

Use separate needles for withdrawing and injecting the medication;

Caution regarding possible systemic reaction, (e.g., flushing, vomiting, nausea, myalgia) and discuss importance of reporting symptoms.

Discuss increased susceptibility to infections, signs/symptoms requiring medical intervention, e.g., fever, sore throat; erythema/draining wound; cloudy urine, burning with urination.

Identify safety concerns, e.g., avoidance of forceful blowing of nose, contact sports, constipation/straining for stool; use of electric razors, soft toothbrush.

Recommend avoiding use of heating pads or hot water bottles; measuring temperature of bath water with a thermometer.

Recommend routine observation of skin, noting changes in turgor, altered color, local warmth, erythema, excoriation.

Identify measures for healthy skin, e.g.:

Reposition periodically and gently massage bony surfaces when sedentary or in bed;

Keep skin surfaces dry and clean, limit use of soap;

Engage regularly in ROM exercises;

Suggest use of protective devices, e.g., sheepskin, egg-crate, alternating air pressure/water mattress, heel/elbow protectors, and pillows as indicated.

Review good oral hygiene, necessity for regular dental care.

Instruct to avoid use of aspirin products.

Refer to appropriate community resources when indicated, e.g., social services for food stamps, meals on wheels.

RATIONALE

Iron is best absorbed on an empty stomach. However, iron salts are gastric irritants and may cause dyspepsia, diarrhea, and abdominal discomfort if taken on an empty stomach.

Undiluted liquid iron preparations may stain the teeth. Ascorbic acid promotes iron absorption.

Excretion of excessive iron changes stool color.

Certain iron supplements (e.g., Feosol) may leave deposits on teeth and gums.

Prevents extravasation (leaking) with accompanying pain and tissue damage.

Medication may stain the skin.

Possible side effects of therapy requiring re-evaluation of drug choice and dosage.

Decreased leukocyte production potentiates risk of infection. *Note:* Purulent drainage may not form in absence of granulocytes (aplastic).

Reduces risk of hemorrhage from fragile tissues and general decrease of coagulation factors.

Thermoreceptors in the dermal tissues may be dulled because of oxygen deprivation, thus increasing the risk of thermal injury.

Condition of the skin is affected by circulation, nutrition, and immobility. Tissues may become fragile and prone to infection and breakdown.

Increases circulation to all skin areas, limiting tissue ischemia/effects of cellular hypoxia.

Moist, contaminated areas provide excellent media for growth of pathogenic organisms. Soap may dry skin excessively and increase irritation.

Promotes circulation to tissues, prevents stasis.

Avoids skin breakdown by preventing/reducing pressure against skin surfaces.

Effects of anemia (oral lesions) and/or iron supplements increase risk of infection/bacteremia.

Increases bleeding tendencies.

May need assistance with groceries/meal preparation.

POTENTIAL CONSIDERATIONS following acute hospitalization (dependent on patient's age, physical condition/presence of complications, personal resources, and life responsibilities)

Activity intolerance—imbalance between oxygen supply (delivery) and demand.

Nutrition: altered, less than body requirements—failure to ingest or inability to digest food/absorb nutrients necessary for formation of normal RBCs.

Infection, risk for—inadequate secondary defenses, e.g., decreased hemoglobin, leukopenia, or decreased granulocytes (suppressed inflammatory response); inadequate primary defenses, e.g., broken skin, stasis of body fluids; invasive procedures; chronic disease, malnutrition.

Therapeutic Regimen: Individual, ineffective management—economic difficulties, perceived benefits.

SICKLE CELL CRISIS

Sickle cell anemia is a genetic disease that primarily affects black populations and people of Mediterranean descent. It renders the individual vulnerable to repeated painful crises that can progressively destroy vital organs. These crises are:

Vaso-occlusive/thrombocytic crisis: Related to infection, dehydration, fever, hypoxia, and characterized by multiple infarcts of bones, joints, and other target organs, with tissue pain and necrosis caused by plugs of sickled cells in the microcirculation.

Hypoplastic/aplastic crisis: May be secondary to severe (usually viral) infection or folic acid deficiency, resulting in cessation of production of RBCs and bone marrow.

Hyperhemolytic crisis: Reticulocytes are increased in peripheral blood; and bone marrow is hyperplastic. Characterized by anemia and jaundice (effects of hemolysis).

Sequestration crisis (more commonly occurs in infants): Massive, sudden erythrostasis with pooling of blood in the viscera (splenomegaly), resulting in hypovolemic shock/possible death. This crisis occurs in patients with intact splenic function.

CARE SETTING

Sickle cell disease is generally managed at the community level, with many of the interventions included here being appropriate for this focus; however, this plan of care addresses sickle cell crisis, which usually requires hospitalization during the acute phase.

RELATED CONCERNS

Cerebrovascular accident/stroke, page 257
Cholecystitis with cholelithiasis, page 390
Chronic obstructive disease and asthma, page 126
Cirrhosis of the liver, page 484
Heart failure: chronic, page 47
Pneumonia: microbial, page 140
Psychosocial aspects of care, page 809
Seizure disorders/Epilepsy, page 228
Sepsis/Septicemia, page 741

Patient Assessment Database

Depends on severity of condition, presence of complications

ACTIVITY/REST

May report:	Lethargy, fatigue, weakness, general malaise
	Loss of productivity; decreased exercise tolerance; greater need for sleep and rest
May exhibit:	Listlessness; severe weakness and increasing pallor (aplastic crisis)
	Gait disturbances (pain, kyphosis, lordosis); inability to walk (pain)
	Poor body posture (slumping of shoulders indicative of fatigue)
	Decreased range of motion (ROM) (swollen, inflamed joints); joint, bone deformities
	Generalized retarded growth; tower-shaped skull with frontal bossing; disproportionately long arms and legs; short trunk; narrowed shoulders/hips; and long, tapered fingers

CIRCULATION

May report:	Palpitations or anginal chest pain (concomitant coronary artery disease [CAD]/myocardial ischemia, acute chest syndrome)
	Intermittent claudication
May exhibit:	Apical pulse: point of maximal impulse (PMI) may be displaced to the left (cardiomegaly)
	Tachycardia, dysrhythmias (hypoxia), systolic murmurs
	BP: Widened pulse pressure
	Generalized symptoms of shock, e.g., hypotension, rapid thready pulse, and shallow respirations (sequestration crisis)

Peripheral pulses throbbing on palpation

Bruits (reflects compensatory mechanisms of anemia; may also be auscultated over the spleen because of multiple splenic infarcts)

Capillary refill delayed (anemia or hypovolemia)

Skin color: Pallor or cyanosis of skin, mucous membranes, and conjunctiva. (*Note:* Pallor may appear as yellowish brown color in brown-skinned patients and as ashen gray in black-skinned patients). Jaundice: Scleral icterus, generalized icteric coloring (excessive RBC hemolysis)

Dry skin/mucous membranes

Diaphoresis (either sequestration or vaso-occlusive crisis; acute pain or shock)

ELIMINATION

May report: Frequent voiding, voiding in large amounts, nocturia

May exhibit: Right upper quadrant (RUQ) abdominal tenderness, enlargement/distension (hepatomegaly); ascites

Left upper quadrant (LUQ) abdominal fullness (spleen may be enlarged or may be atrophic and nonfunctional from repeated splenic infarcts and fibrosis)

Dilute, pale, straw-colored urine; hematuria or smoky appearance (multiple renal infarcts)

Urine specific gravity decreased (may be fixed with progressive renal disease)

EGO INTEGRITY

May report: Resentment and frustration with disease, fear of rejection from others

Negative feelings about self, ability to deal with life/situation

Concern regarding being a burden to significant others (SOs); financial concerns, possible loss of insurance/benefits, lost time at work/school; fear of genetic transmission of disease

May exhibit: Anxiety, restlessness, irritability, apprehension, withdrawal, narrowed focus, self-focusing, unresponsiveness to questions, regression, depression, decreased self-concept

Dependent relationship with whomever can offer security and protection

FOOD/FLUID

May report: Thirst

Anorexia, nausea/vomiting

May exhibit: Height/weight usually in the lower percentiles

Poor skin turgor with visible tenting (crisis, infection, and dehydration)

Dry skin/mucous membranes

Jugular venous distension (JVD) and general peripheral edema (concomitant HF)

HYGIENE

May report: Difficulty maintaining ADLs (pain or severe anemia)

May exhibit: Unkempt appearance, poor personal hygiene

NEUROSENSORY

May report: Headaches or dizziness

Visual disturbances (e.g., hemianopsia, retinopathy, nystagmus)

Tingling in the extremities

Disturbances in pain and position sense

May exhibit: Mental status usually unaffected except in cases of severe sickling (cerebral infarction/intracranial hemorrhage)

Weakness of the mouth, tongue, and facial muscles; aphasia (in cerebral infarction of dominant hemisphere)

Abnormal reflexes, decreased muscle strength/tone; abnormal involuntary movements; hemiplegia or sudden hemiparesis, quadriplegia

Ataxia, seizures

Meningeal irritation (intracranial hemorrhage), e.g., decreasing level of consciousness (LOC), nuchal rigidity, focal neurological deficits, vomiting, severe headache

PAIN/DISCOMFORT

May report: Pain as severe, throbbing, gnawing of varied location (localized, migratory, or generalized)

Recurrent, sharp, transient headaches

Back pain (changes in vertebral column from recurrent infarctions); joint/bone pain accompanied by warmth, tenderness, erythema, and occasional effusions (vaso-occlusive crisis); deep bone infarctions may have no apparent signs of irritation

Gallbladder tenderness and pain (excessive accumulation of bilirubin due to increased erythrocyte destruction)

May exhibit: Sensitivity to palpation over affected areas

Holding joints in position of comfort; decreased ROM (result of pain and swollen joints)

Maladaptive pain behaviors, e.g., guilt for being ill, denial of any aspect of disease, indulgence in precipitating factors (overwork, strenuous exercise)

RESPIRATION

May report: Dyspnea on exertion or at rest

History of repeated pulmonary infections/infarctions, pulmonary fibrosis, pulmonary hypertension or cor pulmonale

May exhibit: Acute respiratory distress, e.g., dyspnea, chest pain, and cyanosis (especially in crisis)

Bronchial/bronchovesicular sounds in lung periphery; diminished breath sounds (pulmonary fibrosis)

Crackles, rhonchi, wheezes, diminished breath sounds (HF)

Increased anteroposterior (AP) diameter of the chest (barrel chest)

SAFETY

May report: History of repeated/frequent transfusions

May exhibit: Low-grade fever

Impaired vision (sickle retinopathy), decreased visual acuity (temporary/permanent blindness)

Leg ulcers (common in adult patients, especially found on the internal and external malleoli and the medial aspect of the tibia)

Lymphadenopathy

SEXUALITY

May report: Loss of libido; amenorrhea; priapism, impotence

May exhibit: Delayed sexual maturity

Pale cervix and vaginal walls (anemia)

TEACHING/LEARNING

May report: History of HF (chronic anemic state); pulmonary hypertension or cor pulmonale (multiple pulmonary infections/infarctions); chronic leg ulcers, delayed healing

Discharge plan considerations: **DRG projected mean length of inpatient stay: 4.3 days**

May need assistance with shopping, transportation, self-care, homemaker/maintenance tasks

Refer to section at end of plan for postdischarge considerations.

DIAGNOSTIC STUDIES

CBC: Reticulocytosis (count may vary from 30%–50%); leukocytosis (especially in vaso-occlusive crisis), with counts over 20,000 indicate infection, decreased Hb (5–10 g/dL) and total RBCs, elevated platelets, and a normal to elevated MCV.

Stained RBC examination: Demonstrates partially or completely sickled, crescent-shaped cells; anisocytosis; poikilocytosis; polychromasia; target cells; Howell-Jolly bodies; basophilic stippling; occasional nucleated RBCs (normoblasts).

Sickle-turbidity tube test (Sickledex): Routine screening test that determines the presence of hemoglobin S (HbS) but does not differentiate between sickle cell anemia and trait.

Hemoglobin electrophoresis: Identifies any abnormal hemoglobin types and differentiates between sickle cell trait and sickle cell anemia. Results may be inaccurate if patient has received a blood transfusion within 3–4 mo before testing.

ESR: Elevated.

Erythrocyte fragility: Decreased (osmotic fragility or RBC fragility); RBC survival time decreased (accelerated breakdown).

ABGs: May reflect decreased PO_2 (defects in gas exchange at the alveolar capillary level); acidosis (hypoxemia and acidic states in vaso-occlusive crisis).

Serum bilirubin (total and indirect): Elevated (increased RBC hemolysis).

Acid phosphatase: Elevated (release of erythrocytic ACP into the serum).

Alkaline phosphatase: Elevated during vaso-occlusive crisis (bone and liver damage).

LDH: Elevated (RBC hemolysis).

Serum potassium and uric acid: Elevated during vaso-occlusive crisis (RBC hemolysis).

Serum iron: May be elevated or normal (increased iron absorption due to excessive RBC destruction).

Total Iron Binding Capacity (TIBC): Normal or decreased.

Urine/fecal urobilinogen: Increased (more sensitive indicators of RBC destruction than serum levels).

Intravenous pyelogram (IVP): May be done to evaluate kidney damage.

Bone radiographs: May demonstrate skeletal changes, e.g., osteoporosis, osteosclerosis, osteomyelitis, or avascular necrosis.

X-rays: May indicate bone thinning, osteoporosis.

NURSING PRIORITIES

1. Promote adequate cellular oxygenation/perfusion.
2. Alleviate pain.
3. Prevent complications.
4. Provide information about disease, process/prognosis, and treatment needs.

DISCHARGE GOALS

1. Oxygenation/perfusion adequate to meet cellular needs.
2. Pain relieved/controlled.
3. Complications prevented/minimized.
4. Disease process, future expectations, potential complications, and therapeutic regimen understood.
5. Plan in place to meet needs after discharge.

NURSING DIAGNOSIS: Gas Exchange, impaired

May be related to

Decreased oxygen-carrying capacity of the blood, reduced RBC life span/premature destruction, abnormal RBC structure; sensitivity to low oxygen tension (strenuous exercise, increase in altitude)

Increased blood viscosity (occlusions created by sickled cells packing together within the capillaries) and pulmonary congestion (impairment of surface phagocytosis)

Predisposition to bacterial pneumonia, pulmonary infarcts

Possibly evidenced by

Dyspnea, use of accessory muscles

Restlessness, confusion

Tachycardia

Cyanosis (hypoxia)

ACTIONS/INTERVENTIONS

Respiratory Monitoring (NIC)

Independent

Monitor respiratory rate/depth, use of accessory muscles, areas of cyanosis.

Auscultate breath sounds, noting presence/absence, and adventitious sounds.

Monitor vital signs; note changes in cardiac rhythm.

Investigate reports of chest pain and increasing fatigue. Observe for signs of increased fever, cough, adventitious breath sounds.

Assess level of consciousness/mentation regularly.

Ventilation Assistance (NIC)

Assist in turning, coughing, and deep-breathing exercises.

Evaluate activity tolerance; limit activities to those within patient tolerance or place patient on bedrest. Assist with ADLs and mobility as needed.

Encourage patient to alternate periods of rest and activity. Schedule rest periods as indicated.

Demonstrate and encourage use of relaxation techniques, e.g., guided imagery and visualization.

Promote adequate fluid intake, e.g., 2–3 L/day within cardiac tolerance.

Screen health status of visitors/staff.

Collaborative

Administer supplemental humidified oxygen as indicated.

RATIONALE

Indicators of adequacy of respiratory function or degree of compromise and therapy needs/effectiveness.

Development of atelectasis and stasis of secretions can impair gas exchange.

Compensatory changes in vital signs and development of dysrhythmias reflect effects of hypoxia on cardiovascular system.

Reflective of developing acute chest syndrome, (i.e., chest pain, dyspnea, fever, and leukocytosis), which increases the workload of the heart and oxygen demand.

Brain tissue is very sensitive to decreases in oxygen and may be an early indicator of developing hypoxia.

Promotes optimal chest expansion, mobilization of secretions, and aeration of all lung fields; reduces risk of stasis of secretions/pneumonia.

Reduction of the metabolic requirements of the body reduces the oxygen requirements/degree of hypoxia.

Protects from excessive fatigue, reduces oxygen demands/degree of hypoxia.

Relaxation decreases muscle tension and anxiety and hence the metabolic demand for oxygen.

Sufficient intake is necessary to provide for mobilization of secretions and to prevent hyperviscosity of blood/capillary occlusion.

Protects from potential sources of respiratory infection.

Maximizes oxygen transport to tissues, particularly in presence of pulmonary insults/pneumonia. *Note:* Oxygen should be given only in the presence of confirmed hypoxemia because oxygen can suppress erythropoietin levels, further reducing the production of RBCs.

ACTIONS/INTERVENTIONS	RATIONALE
Collaborative	
Monitor laboratory studies, e.g., CBC, cultures, ABGs/pulse oximetry, chest x-ray, pulmonary function tests.	Patients are particularly prone to pneumonia, which is potentially fatal because of its hypoxemic effect of increasing sickling.
Perform/assist with chest physiotherapy, intermittent positive pressure breathing (IPPB), and incentive spirometer.	Mobilizes secretions and increases aeration of lung fields.
Administer packed RBCs or exchange transfusions as indicated.	Increases number of oxygen-carrying cells, dilutes the percentage of HbS to prevent sickling, improves circulation, and removes/decreases number of sickled cells. PRCs are usually used because they are less likely to create circulatory overload. *Note:* Partial transfusions are sometimes used prophylactically in high-risk situations, e.g., chronic, severe leg ulcers, preparation for general anesthesia, third trimester of pregnancy.
Administer medications as indicated:	
Antipyretics, e.g., acetaminophen (Tylenol);	Maintains normothermia to reduce metabolic oxygen demands without affecting serum pH, which may occur with aspirin.
Antibiotics.	A broad-spectrum antibiotic is started immediately pending culture results of suspected infections, then may be changed when the specific pathogen is identified.

NURSING DIAGNOSIS: Tissue Perfusion, altered (specify)

May be related to

Vaso-occlusive nature of sickling, inflammatory response

Arteriovenous (AV) shunts in both pulmonary and peripheral circulation

Myocardial damage from small infarcts, iron deposits, and fibrosis

Possibly evidenced by

Changes in vital signs; diminished peripheral pulses/capillary refill; general pallor

Decreased mentation, restlessness

Angina, palpitations

Tingling in extremities, intermittent claudication, bone pain

Transient visual disturbances

Ulcerations of lower extremities, delayed healing

DESIRED OUTCOMES/EVALUATION CRITERIA—PATIENT WILL:

Circulation Status (NOC)

Demonstrate improved tissue perfusion as evidenced by stabilized vital signs, strong/palpable peripheral pulses, adequate urine output, absence of pain; usual mentation; normal capillary refill; skin warm/dry; nailbeds and lips of natural pale, pink color; absence of paresthesias.

ACTIONS/INTERVENTIONS	RATIONALE

Circulatory Care (NIC)

Independent

Monitor vital signs carefully. Assess pulses for rate, rhythm, and volume. Note hypotension; rapid, weak, thready pulse; and increased/shallow respirations.

Sludging and sickling in peripheral vessels may lead to complete or partial obliteration of a vessel with diminished perfusion to surrounding tissues. Sudden massive splenic sequestration of cells can lead to shock.

Assess skin for coolness, pallor, cyanosis, diaphoresis, delayed capillary refill.

Changes reflect diminished circulation/hypoxia potentiating capillary occlusion. (Refer to ND: Gas Exchange, impaired, p. 546.)

Note changes in level of consciousness; reports of headaches, dizziness; development of sensory/motor deficits (e.g., hemiparesis or paralysis), seizure activity.

Changes may reflect diminished perfusion to the central nervous system (CNS) due to ischemia or infarction. Stagnant cells must be mobilized immediately to reduce further ischemia/infarction.

Maintain adequate fluid intake. (Refer to ND: Fluid Volume risk for deficit, following.) Monitor urine output.

Dehydration not only causes hypovolemia but increases sickling and occlusion of capillaries. Decreased renal perfusion/failure may occur because of vascular occlusion.

Assess lower extremities for skin texture, edema, ulcerations (especially of internal and external malleoli).

Reduced peripheral circulation often leads to dermal changes and delayed healing.

Investigate reports of change in character of pain, or development of bone pain, angina, tingling of extremities, eye pain/vision disturbances.

Changes may reflect increased sickling of cells/ diminished circulation with further involvement of organs, e.g., myocardial infarction (MI) or pulmonary infarction, occlusion of vasculature of the eye.

Maintain environmental temperature and body warmth without overheating.

Prevents vasoconstriction; aids in maintaining circulation and perfusion. Excessive body heat may cause diaphoresis adding to insensible fluid losses and risk of dehydration.

Evaluate for developing edema (including genitals in men).

Vaso-occlusion/circulatory stasis may lead to edema of extremities (and priapism in men), potentiating risk of tissue ischemia/necrosis.

Collaborative

Monitor laboratory studies, e.g.:

ABGs, CBC, LDH, AST/ALT, CPK, BUN;

Decreased tissue perfusion may lead to gradual infarction of organ tissues such as the brain, liver, spleen, kidney, skeletal muscle, and so forth with consequent release of intracellular enzymes.

Serum electrolytes. Provide replacements as indicated.

Electrolyte losses (especially sodium) are increased during crisis because of fever, diarrhea, vomiting, diaphoresis.

Administer hypo-osmolar solutions (e.g., 0.45 normal saline) via an infusion pump.

Hydration lowers the HbS concentration within the RBCs, which decreases the sickling tendency and also reduces blood viscosity, which helps to maintain perfusion. Infusion pump may prevent circulatory overload. *Note:* Lactated Ringer's solution or D_5W may cause RBC hemolysis and potentiate thrombus formation.

ACTIONS/INTERVENTIONS	RATIONALE

Independent

Administer experimental antisickling agents (e.g., sodium cyanate) or antineoplastic agents, (e.g., hydroxyurea [Droxia]) carefully. Observe for possible lethal side effects.	Antisickling agents (currently under investigational use) are aimed at prolonging erythrocyte survival and preventing sickling by affecting cell membrane changes. Research indicates that hydroxyurea dramatically decreases the number of sickle cell episodes (by as much as 50%) and reduces the severity of complications such as fever and severe chest pain. *Note:* Use of anticoagulants, plasma expanders, nitrates, vasodilators, and alkylating agents has proven essentially unsuccessful in the management of the vaso-occlusive crisis.
Assist with/prepare for surgical diathermy or photocoagulation.	Direct coagulation of bleeding sites in the eye (resulting from vascular stasis/edema) may prevent progression of proliferative changes if initiated early.
Assist with/prepare for needle aspiration of blood from corpora cavernosa;	Sickling within the penis can cause sustained erection (priapism) and edema. Removal of sludged sickled cells can improve circulation, decreasing psychological trauma and risk of necrosis/infection.
Surgical intervention.	Direct incision and ligation of the dorsal arteries of the penis and saphenocavernous shunting may be necessary in severe cases of priapism to prevent tissue necrosis.

NURSING DIAGNOSIS: Fluid Volume, risk for deficit

Risk factors may include
Increased fluid needs, e.g., hypermetabolic state/fever, inflammatory processes
Renal parenchymal damage/infarctions limiting the kidney's ability to concentrate urine (hyposthenuria)

Possibly evidenced by
[Not applicable; presence of signs and symptoms establishes an *actual* diagnosis]

DESIRED OUTCOMES/EVALUATION CRITERIA—PATIENT WILL:

Hydration (NOC)

Maintain adequate fluid balance as evidenced by individually appropriate urine output with a near-normal specific gravity, stable vital signs, moist mucous membranes, good skin turgor, and prompt capillary refill.

ACTIONS/INTERVENTIONS	RATIONALE

Fluid Monitoring (NIC)

Independent

Maintain accurate I&O. Weigh daily.	Patient may reduce fluid intake during periods of crisis because of malaise, anorexia, and so on. Dehydration from vomiting, diarrhea, fever, may reduce urine output and precipitate a vaso-occlusive crisis.

ACTIONS/INTERVENTIONS	RATIONALE
Independent	
Note urine characteristics and specific gravity.	Kidney can lose its ability to concentrate urine, resulting in excessive losses of dilute urine and fixation of the specific gravity.
Monitor vital signs, comparing with patient's normal/previous readings. Take BP in lying, sitting, and standing positions if possible.	Reduction of circulating blood volume can occur from increased fluid loss, resulting in hypotension and tachycardia.
Observe for fever, changes in level of consciousness, poor skin turgor, dryness of skin and mucous membranes, pain.	Symptoms reflective of dehydration/hemoconcentration with consequent vaso-occlusive state.
Monitor vital signs closely during blood transfusions and note presence of dyspnea, crackles, rhonchi, wheezes, JVD, diminished breath sounds, cough, frothy sputum, and cyanosis.	Patient's heart may already be weakened and prone to failure because of chronic demands placed on it by the anemic state. Heart may be unable to tolerate the added fluid volume from transfusions or rapid IV fluid administered to treat crisis/shock.
Collaborative	
Administer IV fluids as indicated.	Replaces losses/deficits; may reverse renal concentration of RBCs/presence of failure. Fluids must be given immediately (especially in CNS involvement) to decrease hemoconcentration and prevent further infarction.
Monitor laboratory studies, e.g., Hb/Hct, serum and urine electrolytes.	Elevations may indicate hemoconcentration. Kidneys' loss of ability to concentrate urine may result in serum depletions of Na+, K+, and Cl− necessitating replacement.

NURSING DIAGNOSIS: Pain [acute]/chronic

May be related to

Intravascular sickling with localized stasis, occlusion, and infarction/necrosis

Activation of pain fibers due to deprivation of oxygen and nutrients, accumulation of noxious metabolites

Possibly evidenced by

Localized, migratory, or more generalized pain, described as throbbing, gnawing, or severe and incapacitating; affecting peripheral extremities, bones, joints, back, abdomen, or head (headaches recurrent/transient)

Decreased ROM, guarding of the affected areas

Facial grimacing, narrowed/self-focus

DESIRED OUTCOMES/EVALUATION CRITERIA—PATIENT WILL:

Pain Level (NOC)

Verbalize relief/control of pain.

Demonstrate relaxed body posture, have freedom of movement, be able to sleep/rest appropriately.

ACTIONS/INTERVENTIONS	RATIONALE

Pain Management (NIC)

Independent

Assess reports of pain, including location, duration, and intensity (scale of 0–10).

Sickling of cells potentiates cellular hypoxia and may lead to infarction of tissues with resultant pain. Typically pain occurs in the back, ribs, and limbs and lasts 5–7 days.

Observe nonverbal pain cues, e.g., gait disturbances, body positioning, reluctance to move, facial expressions, and physiological manifestations of acute pain (e.g., elevated BP, tachycardia, increased respiratory rate). Explore discrepancies between verbal and nonverbal cues.

Pain is unique to each patient; therefore, one may encounter varying descriptions because of individualized perceptions. Nonverbal cues may aid in evaluation of pain and effectiveness of therapy.

Discuss with the patient/SO what pain relief measures were effective in the past.

Involves patient/SO in care and allows for identification of remedies that have already been found to relieve pain. Helpful in establishing individualized treatment needs.

Explore alternate pain relief measures, e.g., relaxation techniques, biofeedback, yoga, meditation, progressive relaxation techniques, distraction (e.g., visual auditory, tactile, kinesthetic, guided imagery, and breathing techniques).

May reduce reliance on pharmacological therapy and enhance patient's sense of control.

Provide support for and carefully position affected extremities.

Reduces edema, discomfort, and risk of injury, especially if osteomyelitis is present.

Apply local massage gently to affected areas.

Helps reduce muscle tension.

Encourage ROM exercises.

Prevents joint stiffness and possible contracture formation.

Plan activities during peak analgesic effect.

Maximizes movement of joints, enhancing mobility.

Maintain adequate fluid intake.

Dehydration increases sickling/vaso-occlusion and corresponding pain.

Collaborative

Apply warm, moist compresses to affected joints or other painful areas. Avoid use of ice or cold compresses.

Warmth causes vasodilation and increases circulation to hypoxic areas. Cold causes vasoconstriction and compounds the crisis.

Administer medications as indicated: narcotics, e.g., continuous infusion morphine (Astramorph, Duramorph), hydromorphone (Dilaudid); nonnarcotic analgesics, e.g., acetaminophen (Tylenol); or sedatives, e. g., hydroxyzine (Vistaril).

Reduces pain and promotes rest and comfort. *Note:* Acetaminophen (Tylenol) can be used for control of headache, pain, and fever. Aspirin should be avoided because it alters blood pH and can make cells sickle more easily. Meperidine (Demerol) should not be used because its metabolite, normaperidine, can cause seizures.

Administer/monitor RBC transfusion.

Frequency of painful crises may be reduced by routine partial exchange transfusions to maintain population of normal RBCs.

NURSING DIAGNOSIS: Mobility, impaired physical

May be related to

Multiple/recurrent bone infarctions or infections (weight-bearing bones)

Pain/discomfort: Kyphosis of upper back/lordosis of lower back, possible joint effusions

Osteoporosis with fragmentation/collapse of femoral head or vertebra (compression deformities)

Bacterial infections (osteomyelitis)

Possibly evidenced by

Reports of pain

Limited joint ROM, reluctance to move, inability to walk/perform ADLs, guarding of joints, gait disturbances

Generalized weakness, therapeutic restrictions (e.g., bed rest)

DESIRED OUTCOMES/EVALUATION CRITERIA—PATIENT WILL:

Mobility Level (NOC)

Maintain/increase strength and function of affected body parts.

Participate in activities with absence of or improvement in gait disturbances, increased joint ROM, and absence of inflammatory signs.

Refer to CP: Extended Care, ND: Mobility, impaired physical, page 868.

NURSING DIAGNOSIS: Skin Integrity, risk for impaired

Risk factors may include

Impaired circulation (venous stasis and vaso-occlusion); altered sensation

Decreased mobility/bedrest

Possibly evidenced by:

[Not applicable; presence of signs and symptoms establishes an *actual* diagnosis]

DESIRED OUTCOMES/EVALUATION CRITERIA—PATIENT WILL:

Tissue Integrity: Skin and Mucous Membranes (NOC)

Prevent dermal ischemic injury.

Display improvement in wound/lesion healing if present.

Risk Control (NOC)

Participate in behaviors to reduce risk factors/skin breakdown.

ACTIONS/INTERVENTIONS	RATIONALE
Skin Surveillance (NIC)	
Independent	
Reposition frequently, even when sitting in chair.	Prevents prolonged tissue pressure where circulation is already compromised, reducing risk of tissue trauma/ischemia.
Inspect skin/pressure points regularly for redness, provide gentle massage.	Poor circulation may predispose to rapid skin breakdown.

ACTIONS/INTERVENTIONS

Independent

Protect bony prominences with sheepskin, heel/elbow protectors, pillows, as indicated.

Keep skin surfaces dry and clean; linens dry/wrinkle-free.

Monitor ischemic areas, leg bruises, cuts, bumps closely for ulcer formation.

Elevate lower extremities when sitting.

Collaborative

Provide egg-crate, alternating air pressure, or water mattress.

Cleanse open wounds/ulcers with hydrogen peroxide, boric acid, or povidone iodine (Betadine) solutions as indicated. Monitor distribution, size, depth, character, and drainage.

Prepare for/assist with hyperbaric oxygenation to ulcer sites.

ACTIONS/INTERVENTIONS

Independent

Decreases pressure on tissues, preventing skin break-down.

Moist, contaminated areas provide excellent media for growth of pathogenic organisms.

Potential entry sites for pathogenic organisms. In presence of altered immune system, this increases risk of infection/delayed healing.

Enhances venous return, reducing venous stasis/edema formation.

Reduces tissue pressure and aids in maximizing cellular perfusion to prevent dermal injury.

Improvement or delayed healing reflects status of tissue perfusion and effectiveness of interventions. *Note:* These patients are at increased risk of serious complications because of lowered resistance to infection and decreased nutrients for healing.

Maximizes oxygen delivery to tissues, enhancing healing.

NURSING DIAGNOSIS: Infection, risk for

Risk factors may include
Chronic disease process, tissue destruction, e.g., infarction, fibrosis, loss of spleen (autosplenectomy)
Inadequate primary defenses (broken skin, stasis of body fluids, decreased ciliary action)

Possibly evidenced by
[Not applicable; presence of signs and symptoms establishes an *actual* diagnosis]

DESIRED OUTCOMES/EVALUATION CRITERIA—PATIENT WILL:

Knowledge: Infection Control (NOC)

Verbalize understanding of individual causative/risk factors.
Identify interventions to prevent/reduce risk of infection.

Refer to CPs: Pneumonia: Microbial, page 140; Sepsis/Septicemia, page 741; Fractures, ND: Infection, risk for, page 693.

NURSING DIAGNOSIS: Knowledge Deficit [Learning Need] regarding condition, prognosis, treatment, self-care, and discharge needs

May be related to
Lack of exposure/recall
Information misinterpretation
Unfamiliarity with resources

Possibly evidenced by

Questions, request for information, statement of misconceptions

Inaccurate follow-through of instructions; development of preventable complications

Verbal/nonverbal cues of anxiety

DESIRED OUTCOMES/EVALUATION CRITERIA—PATIENT WILL:

Knowledge: Disease Process (NOC)

Verbalize understanding of disease process, including symptoms of crisis, potential complications.

Knowledge: Treatment Regimen (NOC)

Verbalize understanding of therapeutic needs.

Initiate necessary behaviors/lifestyle changes to prevent complications.

Participate in continued medical follow-up; genetic counseling/family planning services.

ACTIONS/INTERVENTIONS	RATIONALE

Teaching : Disease Process (NIC)

Independent

Review disease process and treatment needs.

Provides knowledge base from which patient can make informed choices.

Review precipitating factors, e.g.:

Cold environmental temperatures, failure to dress warmly when engaging in winter activities; wearing tight, restrictive clothing; stressful situations;

Causes peripheral vasoconstriction, which may result in sludging of the circulation, increased sickling, and may precipitate a vaso-occlusive crisis.

Strenuous physical activity/contact-type sports, and extremely warm temperatures;

Increases metabolic demand for oxygen and increases insensible fluid losses (evaporation and perspiration) leading to dehydration, which may increase blood viscosity and tendency to sickle.

Travel to places more than 7000 ft above sea level or flying in unpressurized aircraft;

Decreased oxygen tension present at higher altitudes causes hypoxia and potentiates sickling of cells.

Encourage consumption of at least 4–6 qt of fluid daily, during a steady state of the disease, increasing to 6–8 qt during a painful crisis or while engaging in activities that might precipitate dehydration.

Prevents dehydration and consequent hyperviscosity that can potentiate sickling/crisis.

Encourage ROM exercise and regular physical activity with a balance between rest and activity.

Prevents bone demineralization and may reduce risk of fractures. Aids in maintaining level of resistance and decreases oxygen needs.

Review patient's current diet, reinforcing the importance of diet including liver, green leafy vegetables, citrus fruits, and wheat germ. Provide necessary instruction regarding supplementary vitamins such as folic acid.

Sound nutrition is essential because of increased demands placed on bone marrow (e.g., folate and vitamin B_{12} are used in greater quantities than usual). Folic acid supplements are frequently ordered to prevent aplastic crisis.

Discourage smoking and alcohol consumption; identify appropriate community support groups.

Nicotine induces peripheral vasoconstriction and decreases oxygen tension, which may contribute to cellular hypoxia and sickling. Alcohol increases the possibility of dehydration (precipitating sickling). Maintaining these changes in behavior/lifestyle may require prolonged support.

ACTIONS/INTERVENTIONS	RATIONALE
Independent	
Discuss principles of skin/extremity care and protection from injury. Encourage prompt treatment of cuts, insect bites, sores.	Because of impaired tissue perfusion, especially in the periphery, distal extremities are especially susceptible to altered skin integrity/infection.
Include instructions on care of leg ulcers that might develop.	Fosters independence and maintenance of self-care at home.
Instruct patient to avoid persons with infections such as upper respiratory infections (URIs).	Altered immune response places patient at risk for infections, especially bacterial pneumonia.
Recommend patient avoid cold remedies and decongestants containing ephedrine and large amounts of caffeine. Stress the importance of reading labels on over-the-counter (OTC) drugs and consulting healthcare provider before consuming any drugs.	Those remedies containing vasoconstrictors may decrease peripheral tissue perfusion and cause sludging of sickled cells.
Discuss conditions for which medical attention should be sought, e.g.:	
Urine that appears blood tinged or smoky;	Symptoms suggestive of sickling in the renal medulla.
Indigestion, persistent vomiting, diarrhea, high fever, excessive thirst;	Dehydration may trigger a vaso-occlusive crisis.
Severe joint or bone pain;	May signify a vaso-occlusive crisis due to sickling in the bones or spleen (ischemia or infarction) or onset of osteomyelitis.
Severe chest pain, with or without cough;	May reflect angina, impending MI, or pneumonia.
Abdominal pain; gastric distress following meals;	Cholelithiasis, primarily with bilirubin stones, is present in more than 50% of adults.
Fever, swelling, redness, increasing fatigue/pallor, dizziness, drowsiness, nonhealing leg ulcers.	Suggestive of infections that may precipitate a vaso-occlusive crisis if dehydration develops. *Note:* Severe infections are the most frequent cause of aplastic crisis.
Assist patient to strengthen coping abilities, e.g., deal appropriately with anxiety, get adequate information, use relaxation techniques.	Promotes patient's sense of control, may avert a crisis.
Suggest wearing a medical alert bracelet or carrying a wallet card.	May prevent inappropriate treatment in emergency situation.
Discuss genetic implications of the condition. Encourage SO/family members to seek testing to determine presence of HbS.	Screening may identify other family members with sickle cell trait. Hereditary nature of the disease with the possibility of transmitting the mutation may have a bearing on the decision to have children.
Explore concerns regarding childbearing/family planning and refer to community resources and obstetrician knowledgeable about sickle cell disease, as indicated.	Provides opportunity to correct misconceptions/present information necessary to make informed decisions. Pregnancy can precipitate a vaso-occlusive crisis because the placenta's tortuous blood supply and low oxygen tension potentiate sickling, which in turn can lead to fetal hypoxia.
Encourage patient to have routine follow-ups, e.g.:	
Periodic laboratory studies, e.g., CBC;	Monitors changes in blood components; identifies need for changes in treatment regimen.
Biannual dental examination;	Sound oral hygiene limits opportunity for bacterial invasion/sepsis.

ACTIONS/INTERVENTIONS	RATIONALE

Independent

Annual ophthalmologic examination.	Detects development of sickle retinopathy with either proliferative or nonproliferative ocular changes.
Determine need for vocational/career guidance.	Sedentary career may be necessary because of the decreased oxygen-carrying capacity and diminished exercise tolerance.
Encourage participation in community support groups available to sickle cell patients/SO, such as the Sickle Cell Disease Association of America, March of Dimes, Public Health/visiting nurse.	Helpful in adjustment to long-term situation; reduces feelings of isolation and enhances problem solving through sharing of common experiences. *Note:* Failure to resolve concerns/deal with situation may require more intensive therapy/psychological support.

POTENTIAL CONSIDERATIONS following acute hospitalization (dependent on patient's age, physical condition/presence of complications, personal resources, and life responsibilities)

Pain [acute]/chronic—intravascular sickling with localized stasis, occlusion, and infarction/necrosis; activation of pain fibers due to deprivation of oxygen and nutrients, accumulation of noxious metabolites.

Fluid Volume risk for deficit—increased fluid needs, e.g., hypermetabolic state/fever, inflammatory processes; renal parenchymal damage/infarctions limiting the kidney's ability to concentrate urine (hyposthenuria).

Infection, risk for—chronic disease process, tissue destruction, e.g., infarction, fibrosis, loss of spleen (autosplenectomy); inadequate primary defenses (broken skin, stasis of body fluids, decreased ciliary action).

LEUKEMIAS

The term *leukemia* describes a variety of cancers that arise in the blood-forming organs of the body (spleen, lymphatic system, bone marrow). They are differentiated according to the leukocytic system involved. The common trait of all leukemias is the unregulated proliferation of WBCs in the bone marrow that replace the normal elements. There is an apparent abnormality in the hematopoietic stem cell, which results in its inability to differentiate into normal cells. As the normal cells are replaced by leukemic cells, anemia, neutropenia, and thrombocytopenia occur. In adults, the most common of the acute leukemias is acute myelocytic leukemia, which involves neutrophils, a type of granulocyte. The most common of the chronic leukemias is chronic lymphocytic leukemia, which is characterized by an abnormal increase in lymphocytes.

CARE SETTING

Acute inpatient care on medical unit for initial evaluation and treatment, then at the community level.

RELATED CONCERNS

Cancer, page 900
Psychosocial aspects of care, page 809
Transplantation: postoperative and lifelong needs, page 801

Patient Assessment Database

Data depend on degree/duration of the disease and other organ involvement.

ACTIVITY/REST

May report:	Fatigue, malaise, weakness; inability to engage in usual activities
May exhibit:	Muscle wasting
	Increased need for sleep, somnolence

CIRCULATION

May report:	Palpitations
May exhibit:	Tachycardia, heart murmurs
	Pallor of skin, mucous membranes
	Cranial nerve deficits and/or signs of cerebral hemorrhage

ELIMINATION

May report:	Diarrhea; perianal tenderness, pain
	Bright red blood on tissue paper, tarry stools
	Blood in urine, decreased urine output
May exhibit:	Perianal abscess; hematuria

EGO INTEGRITY

May report:	Feelings of helplessness/hopelessness
May exhibit:	Depression, withdrawal, anxiety, fear, anger, irritability
	Mood changes, confusion

FOOD/FLUID

May report:	Loss of appetite, anorexia, vomiting
	Change in taste/taste distortions
	Weight loss
	Pharyngitis, dysphagia
May exhibit:	Abdominal distension, decreased bowel sounds
	Splenomegaly, hepatomegaly; jaundice
	Stomatitis, oral ulcerations
	Gum hypertrophy (gum infiltration may be indicative of acute monocytic leukemia)

NEUROSENSORY

May report: Lack of coordination/decreased coordination
Mood changes, confusion, disorientation, lack of concentration
Dizziness; numbness, tingling, paresthesias

May exhibit: Muscle irritability, seizure activity

PAIN/DISCOMFORT

May report: Abdominal pain, headaches, bone/joint pain; sternal tenderness, muscle cramping

May exhibit: Guarding/distraction behaviors, restlessness; self-focus

RESPIRATION

May report: Shortness of breath with minimal exertion

May exhibit: Dyspnea, tachypnea
Cough
Crackles, rhonchi
Decreased breath sounds

SAFETY

May report: History of recent/recurrent infections; falls
Visual disturbances/impairment
Spontaneous uncontrollable bleeding with minimal trauma

May exhibit: Fever, infections
Bruises, purpura, retinal hemorrhages, gum bleeding, or epistaxis
Enlarged lymph nodes, spleen, or liver (due to tissue invasion)
Papilledema and exophthalmos
Leukemic infiltrates in the dermis

SEXUALITY

May report: Changes in libido
Changes in menstrual flow, menorrhagia
Impotence

TEACHING/LEARNING

May report: History of exposure to chemicals, e.g., benzene, phenylbutazone, and chloramphenicol; excessive levels of ionizing radiation; previous treatment with chemotherapy, especially alkalating agents
Chromosomal disorder, e.g., Down syndrome or Fanconi's aplastic anemia

Discharge plan considerations: **DRG projected mean length of inpatient stay: 7.4–9.3 days**
May need assistance with therapy and treatment needs/supplies, shopping, food preparation, self-care activities, homemaker/maintenance tasks, transportation

Refer to section at end of plan for postdischarge considerations.

DIAGNOSTIC STUDIES

Carcinoembryonic antigen (CEA): May be elevated.

Cold agglutinins: May be elevated (greater than 1:16) in lymphatic leukemia.

Cryoglobulins: Positive cryoglobulin findings may be present in patients with lymphocytic leukemia.

CBC: Indicates a normocytic, normochromic anemia.

> *Hemoglobin:* May be less than 10 g/100 mL.
> *Reticulocytes:* Count is usually low.
> *Platelet count:* May be very low (less than 50,000/mm).
> *WBC:* May be more than 50,000/cm with increased immature WBCs ("shift to left"). Leukemic blast cells may be present.

Prothrombin time (PT)/activated partial thromboplastin time (aPTT): Prolonged.

LDH: May be elevated.

Serum/urine uric acid: May be elevated.

Serum muramidase (a lysozyme): Elevated in acute monocytic and myelomonocytic leukemias.

Serum copper: Elevated.

Serum zinc: Decreased.

Bence-Jones protein (urine): Increased.

Bone marrow biopsy: Abnormal WBCs usually make up 50% or more of the WBCs in the bone marrow. Often 60%–90% of the cells are blast cells, with erythroid precursors, mature cells, and megakaryocytes reduced.

Chest x-ray and lymph node biopsies: May indicate degree of involvement.

NURSING PRIORITIES

1. Prevent infection during acute phases of disease/treatment.
2. Maintain circulating blood volume.
3. Alleviate pain.
4. Promote optimal physical functioning.
5. Provide psychological support.
6. Provide information about disease process/prognosis and treatment needs.

DISCHARGE GOALS

1. Complications prevented/minimized.
2. Pain relieved/controlled.
3. ADLs met by self or with assistance.
4. Dealing with disease realistically.
5. Disease process/prognosis and therapeutic regimen understood.
6. Plan in place to meet needs after discharge.

Refer to CP: Cancer, page 900, for further discussion/expansion of interventions related to cancer care and for patient teaching.

NURSING DIAGNOSIS: Infection, risk for

Risk factors may include

Inadequate secondary defenses: Alterations in mature WBCs (low granulocyte and abnormal lymphocyte count), increased number of immature lymphocytes; immunosuppression, bone marrow suppression (effects of therapy/transplant)

Inadequate primary defenses (stasis of body fluids, traumatized tissue)

Invasive procedures

Malnutrition; chronic disease

Possibly evidenced by

[Not applicable; presence of signs and symptoms establishes an *actual* diagnosis]

DESIRED OUTCOMES/EVALUATION CRITERIA—PATIENT WILL:

Knowledge: Infection Control (NOC)

Identify actions to prevent/reduce risk of infection.

Demonstrate techniques, lifestyle changes to promote safe environment, achieve timely healing.

ACTIONS/INTERVENTIONS	RATIONALE
Infection Protection (NIC)	
Independent	
Place in private room. Screen/limit visitors as indicated. Prohibit use of live plants/cut flowers. Restrict fresh fruits and vegetables.	Protects patient from potential sources of pathogens/infection. *Note:* Profound bone marrow suppression, neutropenia, and chemotherapy place the patient at great risk for infection.

ACTIONS/INTERVENTIONS

Independent

Require good handwashing protocol for all personnel and visitors.

Monitor temperature. Note correlation between temperature elevations and chemotherapy treatments. Observe for fever associated with tachycardia, hypotension, subtle mental changes.

Prevent chilling. Force fluids, administer tepid sponge bath.

Encourage frequent turning and deep breathing.

Auscultate breath sounds, noting crackles, rhonchi; inspect secretions for changes in characteristics, e.g., increased sputum production or cloudy, foul-smelling urine with urgency or burning.

Handle patient gently. Keep linens dry/wrinkle-free.

Inspect skin for tender, erythematous areas; open wounds. Cleanse skin with antibacterial solutions.

Inspect oral mucous membranes. Provide good oral hygiene. Use a soft toothbrush, sponge or swabs for frequent mouth care.

Promote good perianal hygiene. Provide sitz baths, using Betadine or Hibiclens if indicated. Avoid rectal temperatures, use of suppositories.

Provide uninterrupted rest periods.

Encourage increased intake of foods high in protein and fluids with adequate fiber.

Avoid/limit invasive procedures (e.g., venipuncture and injections) as possible.

Collaborative

Monitor laboratory studies, e.g.:

CBC, noting whether WBC count falls or sudden changes occur in neutrophils;

Gram stain cultures/sensitivity.

Review serial chest x-rays.

RATIONALE

Prevents cross-contamination/reduces risk of infection.

Although fever may accompany some forms of chemotherapy, progressive hyperthermia occurs in some types of infections, and fever (unrelated to drugs or blood products) occurs in most leukemia patients. *Note:* Septicemia may occur without fever.

Helps reduce fever, which contributes to fluid imbalance, discomfort, and CNS complications.

Prevents stasis of respiratory secretions, reducing risk of atelectasis/pneumonia.

Early intervention is essential to prevent sepsis/septicemia in immunosuppressed person.

Prevents sheet burn/skin excoriation.

May indicate local infection. *Note:* Open wounds may not produce pus because of insufficient number of granulocytes.

The oral cavity is an excellent medium for growth of organisms and is susceptible to ulceration and bleeding.

Promotes cleanliness, reducing risk of perianal abscess; enhances circulation and healing.

Conserves energy for healing, cellular regeneration.

Enhances antibody formation and prevents dehydration. *Note:* Constipation potentiates retention of toxins and risk of rectal irritation/tissue injury.

Break in skin could provide an entry for pathogenic/potentially lethal organisms. Use of central venous lines (e.g., tunneled catheter or implanted port) can effectively reduce need for frequent invasive procedures and risk of infection. *Note:* Myelosuppression may be cumulative in nature, especially when multiple drug therapy (including steroids) is prescribed.

Decreased numbers of normal/mature WBCs can result from the disease process or chemotherapy, compromising the immune response and increasing risk of infection.

Verifies presence of infections; identifies specific organisms and appropriate therapy.

Indicator of development/resolution of respiratory complications.

ACTIONS/INTERVENTIONS

Collaborative

Prepare for/assist with leukemia-specific treatments such as chemotherapy, radiation, and/or bone-marrow transplant.

Administer medications as indicated, e.g., antibiotics.

Avoid use of aspirin-containing antipyretics.

Provide nutritious diet, high in protein and calories, avoiding raw fruits, vegetables, or uncooked meats.

RATIONALE

Leukemia is usually treated with a combination of these agents, each requiring specific safety precautions for the patient and care providers.

May be given prophylactically or to treat specific infection.

Aspirin can cause gastric bleeding and further decrease platelet count.

Proper nutrition enhances immune system. Minimizes potential sources of bacterial contamination.

NURSING DIAGNOSIS: Fluid Volume, risk for deficit

Risk factors may include
Excessive losses, e.g., vomiting, hemorrhage, diarrhea
Decreased fluid intake, e.g., nausea, anorexia
Increased fluid need, e.g., hypermetabolic state, fever; predisposition for kidney stone formation/tumor lysis syndrome

Possibly evidenced by
[Not applicable; presence of signs and symptoms establishes an *actual* diagnosis]

DESIRED OUTCOMES/EVALUATION CRITERIA—PATIENT WILL:

Hydration (NOC)

Demonstrate adequate fluid volume, as evidenced by stable vital signs; palpable pulses; urine output, specific gravity, and pH within normal limits.
Identify individual risk factors and appropriate interventions.
Initiate behaviors/lifestyle changes to prevent development of fluid volume deficit.

ACTIONS/INTERVENTIONS

Fluid Management (NIC)

Independent

Monitor I&O. Calculate insensible losses and fluid balance. Note decreased urine in presence of adequate intake. Measure specific gravity and urine pH.

Weigh daily.

Monitor BP and HR.

Evaluate skin turgor, capillary refill, and general condition of mucous membranes.

Note presence of nausea, fever.

Encourage fluids of up to 3–4 L/day when oral intake is resumed.

RATIONALE

Decreased circulation secondary to destruction of RBCs and their precipitation in the kidney tubules and/or development of kidney stones (related to elevated uric acid levels) may lead to urinary retention or renal failure.

Measure of adequacy of fluid replacement and kidney function. Continued intake greater than output may indicate renal insult/obstruction.

Changes may reflect effects of hypovolemia (bleeding/dehydration).

Indirect indicators of fluid status/hydration.

Affects intake, fluid needs, and route of replacement.

Promotes urine flow, prevents uric acid precipitation, and enhances clearance of antineoplastic drugs.

ACTIONS/INTERVENTIONS	RATIONALE

Bleeding Precautions (NIC)

Independent

Inspect skin/mucous membranes for petechiae, ecchymotic areas; note bleeding gums, frank or occult blood in stools and urine; oozing from invasive-line sites.

Suppression of bone marrow and platelet production places the patient at risk for spontaneous/uncontrolled bleeding.

Implement measures to prevent tissue injury/bleeding, e.g., gentle brushing of teeth or gums with soft toothbrush, cotton swab, or sponge-tipped applicator; using electric razor and avoiding sharp razors when shaving; avoid forceful nose blowing and needle sticks when possible; use sustained pressure on oozing puncture sites.

Fragile tissues and altered clotting mechanisms increase the risk of hemorrhage following even minor trauma.

Limit oral care to mouthwash if indicated (a mixture of ¼ tsp baking soda in 4–8 oz water or hydrogen peroxide in water). Avoid mouthwashes with alcohol.

When bleeding is present even gentle brushing may cause more tissue damage. Alcohol has a drying effect and may be painful to irritated tissues.

Provide soft diet.

May help reduce gum irritation.

Collaborative

Fluid Management (NIC)

Administer IV fluids as indicated.

Maintains fluid/electrolyte balance in the absence of oral intake; reduces risk of renal complications.

Administer medications as indicated, e.g.:

Antiemetics: 5-HT$_3$ receptor antagonist drugs such as ondansetron (Zofran) or granisetron (Kytril);

Relieves nausea/vomiting associated with administration of chemotherapy agents.

Allopurinol (Zyloprim);

May be given to reduce the chances of nephropathy as a result of uric acid production.

Potassium acetate or citrate, sodium bicarbonate;

May be used to alkalinize the urine, preventing formation of kidney stones.

Stool softeners.

Helpful in reducing straining at stool with trauma to rectal tissues.

Bleeding Precautions (NIC)

Monitor laboratory studies, e.g., platelets, Hb/Hct, clotting.

When the platelet count is less than 20,000/mm (due to proliferation of WBCs and/or bone marrow suppression secondary to antineoplastic drugs), the patient is prone to spontaneous life-threatening bleeding. Decreasing Hb/Hct is indicative of bleeding (may be occult).

Administer RBCs, platelets, clotting factors.

Restores/normalizes RBC count and oxygen-carrying capacity to correct anemia. Used to prevent/treat hemorrhage.

Maintain external central vascular access device (subclavian or tunneled catheter or implanted port).

Eliminate peripheral venipuncture as source of bleeding.

NURSING DIAGNOSIS: Pain [acute]

May be related to

Physical agents, e.g., enlarged organs/lymph nodes, bone marrow packed with leukemic cells

Chemical agents, e.g., antileukemic treatments

Psychological manifestations, e.g., anxiety, fear

Possibly evidenced by

Reports of pain (bone, nerve, headaches, and so forth)

Guarding/distraction behaviors, facial grimacing, alteration in muscle tone

Autonomic responses

DESIRED OUTCOMES/EVALUATION CRITERIA—PATIENT WILL:

Pain Level (NOC)

Report pain is relieved/controlled.

Appear relaxed and able to sleep/rest appropriately.

Pain Control Behavior (NOC)

Demonstrate behaviors to manage pain.

ACTIONS/INTERVENTIONS	RATIONALE
Pain Management (NIC)	
Independent	
Investigate reports of pain. Note changes in degree (use scale of 0–10) and site.	Helpful in assessing need for intervention; may indicate developing complications.
Monitor vital signs, note nonverbal cues, e.g., muscle tension, restlessness.	May be useful in evaluating verbal comments and effectiveness of interventions.
Provide quiet environment and reduce stressful stimuli, e.g., noise, lighting, constant interruptions.	Promotes rest and enhances coping abilities.
Place in position of comfort and support joints, extremities with pillows/padding.	May decrease associated bone/joint discomfort.
Reposition periodically and provide/assist with gentle ROM exercises.	Improves tissue circulation and joint mobility.
Provide comfort measures (e.g., massage, cool packs), and psychological support (e.g., encouragement, presence).	Minimizes need for/enhances effects of medication.
Review/promote patient's own comfort interventions, position, physical activity/nonactivity, and so forth.	Successful management of pain requires patient involvement. Use of effective techniques provides positive reinforcement, promotes sense of control, and prepares patient for interventions to be used after discharge.
Evaluate and support patient's coping mechanisms.	Using own learned perceptions/behaviors to manage pain can help the patient cope more effectively.
Encourage use of stress management techniques, e.g., relaxation/deep-breathing exercises, guided imagery, visualization; Therapeutic Touch.	Facilitates relaxation, augments pharmacological therapy, and enhances coping abilities.
Assist with/provide diversional activities, relaxation techniques.	Helps with pain management by redirecting attention.
Monitor uric acid level.	Rapid turnover and destruction of leukemic cells during chemotherapy elevates uric acid, causing swollen, painful joints.

ACTIONS/INTERVENTIONS

Collaborative

Administer medications as indicated:

Analgesics, e.g., acetaminophen (Tylenol);

Narcotics, e.g., codeine, meperidine (Demerol), morphine, hydromorphone (Dilaudid);

Antianxiety agents, e.g., diazepam (Valium), lorazepam (Ativan).

RATIONALE

Given for mild pain not relieved by comfort measures. *Note:* Avoid aspirin-containing products because they may potentiate hemorrhage.

Used when pain is severe. Use of patient-controlled analgesia (PCA) may be beneficial in preventing peaks and valleys associated with intermittent drug administration.

May be given to enhance the action of analgesics/narcotics.

NURSING DIAGNOSIS: Activity Intolerance

May be related to

Generalized weakness; reduced energy stores, increased metabolic rate from massive production of leukocytes

Imbalance between oxygen supply and demand (anemia/hypoxia)

Therapeutic restrictions (isolation/bedrest); effect of drug therapy

Possibly evidenced by:

Verbal report of fatigue or weakness

Exertional discomfort or dyspnea

Abnormal heart rate or BP response

DESIRED OUTCOMES/EVALUATION CRITERIA—PATIENT WILL:

Endurance (NOC)

Report a measurable increase in activity tolerance.

Participate in ADLs to level of ability.

Demonstrate a decrease in physiological signs of intolerance; e.g., pulse, respiration, and BP remain within patient's normal range.

ACTIONS/INTERVENTIONS

Energy Management (NIC)

Independent

Evaluate reports of fatigue, noting inability to participate in activities or ADLs.

Encourage patient to keep a diary of daily routines and energy levels, noting activities that increase fatigue.

Provide quiet environment and uninterrupted rest periods. Encourage rest periods before meals.

Implement energy-saving techniques, e.g., sitting, rather than standing, use of shower chair. Assist with ambulation/other activities as indicated.

Schedule meals around chemotherapy. Give oral hygiene before meals and administer antimetics as indicated.

RATIONALE

Effects of leukemia, anemia, and chemotherapy may be cumulative (especially during acute and active treatment phase), necessitating assistance.

Helps patient prioritize activities and arrange them around fatigue pattern.

Restores energy needed for activity and cellular regeneration/tissue healing.

Maximizes available energy for self-care tasks.

May enhance intake by reducing nausea. (Refer to CP: Cancer, ND: Nutrition: altered, less than body requirements, p. 910.)

ACTIONS/INTERVENTIONS	RATIONALE

Independent

Recommend small, nutritious, high-protein meals and snacks throughout the day.

Smaller meals require less energy for digestion than larger meals. Increased intake provides fuel for energy.

Collaborative

Provide supplemental oxygen.

Maximizes oxygen available for cellular uptake, improving tolerance of activity.

NURSING DIAGNOSIS: Knowledge Deficit [Learning Need] regarding disease, prognosis, treatment, self care, and discharge needs

May be related to
Lack of exposure to resources
Information misinterpretation/lack of recall

Possibly evidenced by
Verbalization of problem/request for information
Statement of misconception

DESIRED OUTCOMES/EVALUATION CRITERIA—PATIENT WILL:

Knowledge: Disease Process (NOC)

Verbalize understanding of condition/disease process and potential complications.

Knowledge: Treatment Regimen (NOC)

Verbalize understanding of therapeutic needs.
Initiate necessary lifestyle changes.
Participate in treatment regimen.

ACTIONS/INTERVENTIONS	RATIONALE

Teaching: Disease Process (NIC)

Independent

Review pathology of specific form of leukemia and various treatment options.

Treatments can include various antineoplastic drugs, whole body or liver/spleen radiation, transfusions, peripheral progenitor (stem) cell transplant, and bone marrow transplant.

For additional interventions refer to CP: Cancer, ND: Knowledge deficit, page 923.

POTENTIAL CONSIDERATIONS following acute hospitalization (dependent on patient's age, physical condition/presence of complications, personal resources, and life responsibilities)

Infection, risk for—inadequate secondary defenses: alterations in mature WBCs (low granulocyte and abnormal lymphocyte count), increased number of immature lymphocytes; immunosuppression, bone marrow suppression (effects of therapy/transplant).

Role Performance, altered—situational crisis; health-illness, change in physical capacity.

Therapeutic Regimen: Individual, ineffective management—complexity of therapeutic regimen, decisional conflicts, economic difficulties, excessive demands made on individual or family, perceived benefits, powerlessness.

Family Processes, altered—situational crisis (illness, disabling/expensive treatments).

LYMPHOMAS

Malignant lymphomas are cancers of the lymphoid tissue, classified according to four primary features: cell type, degree of differentiation, type of reaction elicited by tumor cells, and growth patterns. If a nodular growth pattern is observed, the term *nodular* is used after the cell type. If no mention of growth pattern is made, the lymphoma is of a diffuse type.

HODGKIN'S DISEASE

The malignant cell of origin for Hodgkin's is not known, but it is thought to be derived from a B lymphocyte, T lymphocyte, or macrophage cell line.

Hodgkin's disease is divided into four different categories: lymphocyte-predominant, mixed cellularity, lymphocyte-depleted, and nodular sclerosing. The lymphocyte-predominant and nodular sclerosing types usually have a more favorable prognosis than the other two types. Stages I–IV of Hodgkin's disease range from one lymph node region to involvement of multiple systems in the body. All stages have additional classifications, i.e., A (no constitutional symptoms), B (fever greater than 38°C, drenching sweats, weight loss equivalent to 10% of body weight over 6 mo), and C (for States I–III, involvement of a single extranodal site, such as bone marrow or liver). Treatment for Hodgkin's disease depends on its stage and ABC classification and includes radiation, a combination of radiation and chemotherapy, or chemotherapy alone. Long-term survival rates are in the 90% range. Bone marrow transplant or peripheral progenitor (stem) cell transplants with high-dose chemotherapy are recommended for patients who have relapsed/failed primary chemotherapy regimen.

NON-HODGKIN'S LYMPHOMA

Non-Hodgkin's lymphoma is a malignancy of the B lymphocyte and T lymphocyte cell systems. Most patients with non-Hodgkin's lymphoma fall into two broad categories related to their clinical features: the nodular indolent type, and the diffuse, aggressive lymphomas. For treatment purposes, they may also be classified as low-, intermediate-, or high-grade lymphomas. Treatment for non-Hodgkin's lymphomas includes radiation or chemotherapy (usually multiple combinations of antineoplastic agents) and/or peripheral progenitor (stem) cell transplant. With or without treatment, low-grade lymphomas can transform into a more aggressive leukemia/lymphoma-like process, resulting in death soon after. Intermediate- and high-grade lymphomas tend to be more responsive to treatment.

CARE SETTING

Acute inpatient care on a medical unit for initial evaluation and treatment, then at community level. This plan of care addresses potential complications that may be encountered in acute care or hospice settings. (The nurse is referred to other related cancer care plans for nursing interventions related to treatments such as radiation, chemotherapy, and bone marrow transplant.)

RELATED CONCERNS

Anemias (iron deficiency, pernicious, aplastic, hemolytic), page 531
Cancer, page 900
Leukemias, page 558
Psychosocial aspects of care, page 809
Sepsis/Septicemia, page 741
Spinal cord injury (acute rehabilitative phase), page 295 (complication related to spinal cord involvement/ compression)
Transplantation: Postoperative and life-long needs, page 801
Upper gastrointestinal/Esophageal bleeding, page 333

Patient Assessment Database

ACTIVITY/REST

May report:	Fatigue, weakness, or general malaise
	Loss of productivity and decreased exercise tolerance
	Need for more sleep and rest
May exhibit:	Diminished strength, slumping of the shoulders, slow walk, and other cues indicative of fatigue
	Night sweats

CIRCULATION

May report: Palpitations, angina/chest pain

May exhibit: Tachycardia, dysrhythmias

Cyanosis and edema of the face and neck or right arm (superior vena cava syndrome—obstruction of venous drainage from enlarged lymph nodes is a rare occurrence)

Scleral icterus and a generalized jaundice related to liver damage and consequent obstruction of bile ducts by enlarged lymph nodes (may be a late sign)

Pallor (anemia), diaphoresis, night sweats

EGO INTEGRITY

May report: Stress factors, e.g., school, job, family

Fear related to diagnosis and possibility of dying

Anxiety related to diagnostic testing and treatment modalities (chemotherapy and radiation therapy)

Financial concerns: Hospital costs, treatment expenses, fear of losing job-related benefits due to lost time from work

Relationship status: Fear and anxiety related to being a burden on the family

May exhibit: Varied behaviors, e.g., angry, withdrawn, passive

ELIMINATION

May report: Changes in characteristics of urine and/or stool

History of intestinal obstruction, e.g., intussusception or malabsorption syndrome (infiltration from retroperitoneal lymph nodes)

May exhibit: Abdomen: RUQ tenderness and enlargement on palpation (hepatomegaly); LUQ tenderness and enlargement on palpation (splenomegaly)

Decreased output, dark/concentrated urine, anuria (ureteral obstruction/renal failure)

Bowel and bladder dysfunction (spinal cord compression occurs late)

FOOD/FLUID

May report: Anorexia/loss of appetite

Dysphagia (pressure on the esophagus)

Recent unexplained weight loss equivalent to 10% or more of body weight in previous 6 mo with no attempt at dieting

May exhibit: Edema of the lower extremities (inferior vena cava obstruction from intra-abdominal lymph node enlargement associated with non-Hodgkin's)

Ascites (inferior vena cava obstruction related to intra-abdominal lymph node enlargement)

NEUROSENSORY

May report: Nerve pain (neuralgias) reflecting compression of nerve roots by enlarged lymph nodes in the brachial, lumbar, and sacral plexuses

Muscle weakness, paresthesia

May exhibit: Mental status: lethargy, withdrawal, general lack of interest in surroundings

Paraplegia (tumor involvement/spinal cord compression from collapse of vertebral body, disc involvement with compression/degeneration, or compromised blood supply to the spinal cord)

PAIN/DISCOMFORT

May report: Tenderness/pain over involved lymph nodes, e.g., in or around the mediastinum; chest pain, back pain (vertebral compression); generalized bone pain (lymphomatous bone involvement)

Immediate pain in involved areas following ingestion of alcohol

May exhibit: Self-focusing; guarding behaviors

RESPIRATION

May report:	Dyspnea on exertion or at rest; chest pain
May exhibit:	Dyspnea; tachypnea
	Dry, nonproductive cough
	Signs of respiratory distress, e.g., increased respiratory rate and depth, use of accessory muscles, stridor, cyanosis
	Hoarseness/laryngeal paralysis (pressure from enlarged nodes on the laryngeal nerve)

SAFETY

May report:	History of frequent/recurrent infections (abnormalities in cellular immunity predispose the patient to systemic herpes virus infections, TB, toxoplasmosis, or bacterial infections), mononucleosis (higher risk of Hodgkin's disease in patient with high titers of Epstein-Barr virus), AIDS (non-Hodgkins is more prevalent in these patients)
	History/presence of ulcers/perforation, gastric bleeding
	Waxing and waning pattern of lymph node size
	Cyclical pattern of evening temperature elevations lasting a few days to weeks (Pel-Ebstein fever) followed by alternate afebrile periods; drenching night sweats without chills
May exhibit:	Unexplained, persistent fever greater than 38°C (100.4°F) without symptoms of infection
	Asymmetric, painless, yet swollen/enlarged lymph nodes (cervical nodes most commonly involved, left side more than right; then axillary and mediastinal nodes)
	Nodes may feel rubbery and hard, discrete and movable
	Tonsilar enlargement
	Generalized pruritus
	Patchy areas of loss of melanin pigmentation (vitiligo)

SEXUALITY

May report:	Concern about fertility/pregnancy (while disease does not affect either, treatment does)
	Decreased libido

TEACHING/LEARNING

May report:	Familial risk factors (higher incidence among families of Hodgkin's patients than in general population)
	Occupational exposure to herbicides (woodworkers/chemists).
Discharge plan considerations:	**DRG projected mean length of inpatient stay: 7.4 days; with surgical intervention: 9.2 days**
	May need assistance with medical therapies/supplies, self-care activities and/or homemaker/maintenance tasks, transportation, shopping

Refer to section at end of plan for postdischarge considerations.

DIAGNOSTIC STUDIES

These diseases are staged according to the microscopic appearance of involved lymph nodes and the extent and severity of the disorder. Accurate staging is most important in deciding on subsequent treatment regimens and prognosis.

Blood studies may vary from completely normal to marked abnormalities. In stage I, few patients have abnormal blood findings.

CBC:

> *WBC:* Variable, may be normal, decreased, or markedly elevated.
>
> *Differential WBC:* Neutrophilia, monocytosis, basophilia, and eosinophilia may be found. Complete lymphopenia (late symptom).
>
> *RBC and Hb/Hct:* Decreased.
>
> *Erythrocytes:* Stained RBC examination: May demonstrate mild to moderate normocytic, normochromic anemia (hypersplenism).
>
> *Platelets:* Decreased (may be severely depleted; bone marrow replacement by the lymphoma and by hypersplenism).

ESR: Elevated during active stages and indicates inflammatory or malignant disease. Useful to monitor patients in remission and to detect early evidence of recurrence of disease.

Erythrocyte osmotic fragility: Increased.

Coombs' test: Positive reaction (hemolytic anemia) may occur; however, a negative result usually occurs in advanced disease.

C-reactive protein (CRP) serum titer: May be positive in patients with Hodgkin's disease.

Serum cryoglobulins: May be positive in patients with Hodgkin's disease.

Serum haptoglobin: May be elevated in patient's with Hodgkin's disease, and in those with cancer of the lung, large intestine, stomach, breast, and liver.

Serum iron and TIBC: Decreased.

Serum alkaline phosphatase: Elevation may indicate either liver or bone involvement.

Serum copper: Elevation may be seen in exacerbations.

Serum calcium: May be elevated when bone is involved.

Serum uric acid: Elevated related to increased destruction of nucleoproteins and liver and kidney involvement.

BUN: May be elevated when kidney involvement is present.

Serum creatinine, bilirubin, antistreptolysin (ASL); creatinine clearance: May be done to detect organ involvement.

Gamma globulin: Hypergammaglobulinemia is common; may occur in advanced disease.

Chest x-ray: May reveal mediastinal or hilar adenopathy, nodular infiltrates, or pleural effusions.

X-rays of thoracic, lumbar vertebrae, proximal extremities, pelvis, or areas of bone tenderness: Determine areas of involvement and assist in staging.

IVP: May be done to detect renal involvement or ureteral deviation by involved nodes.

Whole lung tomography or chest computed tomography (CT) scan: Done if hilar adenopathy is present to reveal possible involvement of mediastinal lymph nodes.

Abdominal and pelvic CT scan: May be done to rule out diseased nodes in the abdomen and pelvis and associated organs.

Abdominal ultrasound: Evaluates extent of involvement of retroperitoneal lymph nodes.

Bone scans: Done to detect bone involvement.

Gallium-67 scintigraphy (lymphangiography): Proven useful for detecting recurrent nodal disease, especially above the diaphragm.

Bone marrow biopsy: Determines bone marrow involvement, which is seen in advanced stages.

Lymph node biopsy: Establishes the diagnosis of Hodgkin's disease based on the presence of the Reed-Sternberg cell.

Mediastinoscopy: May be performed to establish mediastinal node involvement.

Staging laparoscopy or laparotomy: May be done to obtain specimens of retroperitoneal nodes, of both lobes of the liver, and/or to remove the spleen. (Splenectomy is controversial because it may increase the risk of infection and is currently not usually implemented unless the patient has clinical manifestations of stage IV disease.)

NURSING PRIORITIES

1. Provide physical and psychological support during extensive diagnostic testing and treatment regimen.
2. Prevent complications.
3. Alleviate pain.
4. Provide information about disease process/prognosis and treatment needs.

DISCHARGE GOALS

1. Complications prevented/diminished.
2. Dealing with situation realistically.
3. Pain relieved/controlled.
4. Disease process/prognosis, possible complications, and therapeutic regimen understood.
5. Plan in place to meet needs after discharge.

Refer to CPs: Cancer, page 900, Leukemias, page 558, for general nursing diagnoses and interventions to accomplish corresponding nursing priorities/discharge goals.

> **NURSING DIAGNOSIS: Sexual Dysfunction**
>
> **May be related to:**
> Altered body structure or function (drugs, surgery, disease process, radiation [loss of sexual desire, disruption of sexual response pattern])
>
> **Possibly evidenced by:**
> Verbalization of problem
> Actual or perceived limitation imposed by disease and/or therapy
> Alteration in relationship with SO
>
> **DESIRED OUTCOMES/EVALUATION CRITERIA—PATIENT WILL:**
>
> **Role Performance (NOC)**
>
> Verbalize understanding of individual reasons for sexual problems.
> Identify stressors in lifestyle that may contribute to the dysfunction.
> Discuss concerns about body image, sex role, desirability as a sexual partner with partner/SO.

ACTIONS/INTERVENTIONS	RATIONALE
Sexual Counseling (NIC)	
Independent	
Have patient describe problem in own words.	Provides more accurate picture of patient experience with which to develop plan of care.
Determine importance of sex to individual/partner and patient's motivation for change.	Because lymphomas often affect the relatively young who are in their productive years, these people may be affected more by these problems and may be less knowledgeable about the possibilities of change.
Assess knowledge of patient/SO regarding sexual function and effects of current situation/condition.	Helps identify areas of concern, misconception, and actual problems related to therapy side-effects.
Identify preexisting and current stress factors that may be affecting the relationship.	Patient may be concerned about other issues, such as job, financial, and illness-related problems.
Determine pathophysiology, illness/surgery/trauma involved and impact on (perception of) individual.	Patient's perception of the individual effects of this illness are crucial to planning interventions that will be appropriate to those affected (patient and family).
Assist with treatment of underlying condition.	As illness is treated and patient can see improvement, hope is restored and patient can begin to look to the future.
Provide factual information.	Promotes trust in caregivers.
Encourage and accept expressions of concern, anger, grief, fear.	Helps patient identify feelings and begin to deal with them.
Encourage patient to share thoughts/concerns with partner and to clarify values/impact of condition on relationship.	Helps couple begin to deal with issues that can strengthen or weaken relationship.
Collaborative	
Refer to appropriate community resources/support groups, e.g., CanSurmount.	Provides information about resources that are available to help with individual needs. Meeting with others who are dealing with the effects of devastating illness can help patient/family.

ACTIONS/INTERVENTIONS

Collaborative

Provide written material/bibliotherapy appropriate to age/situation.

Refer to clinical nurse specialist/professional sexual therapist as indicated.

RATIONALE

Reinforces information patient has received.

May need additional in-depth assistance to resolve existing problems.

NURSING DIAGNOSIS: Breathing Pattern/Airway Clearance, risk for ineffective

Risk factors may include:
Tracheobronchial obstruction: Enlarged mediastinal nodes and/or airway edema (Hodgkin's and non-Hodgkin's); superior vena cava syndrome (non-Hodgkin's)

Possibly evidenced by:
[Not applicable; presence of signs and symptoms establishes an *actual* diagnosis]

DESIRED OUTCOMES/EVALUATION CRITERIA—PATIENT WILL:

Respiratory Status: Ventilation (NOC)

Maintain a normal/effective respiratory pattern, free of dyspnea, cyanosis, or other signs of respiratory distress.

ACTIONS/INTERVENTIONS

Ventilation Assistance (NIC)

Independent

Assess/monitor respiratory rate, depth, rhythm. Note reports of dyspnea and/or use of accessory muscles, nasal flaring, altered chest excursion.

Place patient in position of comfort, usually with head of bed elevated or sitting upright leaning forward (weight supported on arms), feet dangling.

Reposition and assist with turning periodically.

Instruct in/assist with deep-breathing techniques and/or pursed-lip or abdominal diaphragmatic breathing if indicated.

Monitor/evaluate skin color, noting pallor, development of cyanosis (particularly in nailbeds, ear-lobes, and lips).

Assess respiratory response to activity. Note reports of dyspnea/"air hunger," increased fatigue. Schedule rest periods between activities.

Identify/encourage energy-saving techniques, e.g., rest periods before and after meals, use of shower chair, sitting for care.

Promote bedrest and provide care as indicated during acute/prolonged exacerbation.

RATIONALE

Changes (such as tachypnea, dyspnea, use of accessory muscles) may indicate progression of respiratory involvement/compromise requiring prompt intervention.

Maximizes lung expansion, decreases work of breathing, and reduces risk of aspiration.

Promotes aeration of all lung segments and mobilizes secretions.

Helps promote gas diffusion and expansion of small airways. Provides patient with some control over respiration, helping to reduce anxiety.

Proliferation of WBCs can reduce oxygen-carrying capacity of the blood, leading to hypoxemia.

Decreased cellular oxygenation reduces activity tolerance. Rest reduces oxygen demands and prevents fatigue and dyspnea.

Aids in reducing fatigue and dyspnea and conserves energy for cellular regeneration and respiratory function.

Worsening respiratory involvement/hypoxia may necessitate cessation of activity to prevent more serious respiratory compromise.

ACTIONS/INTERVENTIONS	RATIONALE
Independent	
Encourage expression of feelings. Acknowledge reality of situation and normality of feelings.	Anxiety increases oxygen demand and hypoxemia potentiates respiratory distress/cardiac symptoms, which in turn escalates anxiety.
Provide calm, quiet environment.	Promotes relaxation, conserving energy and reducing oxygen demand.
Observe for neck vein distension, headache, dizziness, periorbital/facial edema, dyspnea, and stridor.	Non-Hodgkin's patients are at risk for superior vena cava syndrome, which may result in tracheal deviation and airway obstruction, representing an oncologic emergency.
Provide support to family/caregivers. Encourage open expression of feelings.	Development of this complication is very frightening for patient and family because it may indicate end-stage of disease process/approaching death especially in the hospice setting. Keeping family informed may diminish their anxiety and minimize transmission to patient.
Collaborative	
Provide supplemental oxygen.	Maximizes oxygen available for circulatory uptake; aids in reducing hypoxemia.
Monitor laboratory studies, e.g., ABGs, oximetry.	Measures adequacy of respiratory function and effectiveness of therapy.
Administer analgesics and tranquilizers as indicated.	Reducing physiological responses to pain/anxiety decreases oxygen demands and may limit respiratory compromise.
Assist with respiratory treatments/adjuncts, e.g., IPPB, incentive spirometer, if appropriate.	Promotes maximal aeration of all lung segments, preventing atelectasis.
Assist with intubation and mechanical ventilation.	May be necessary to support respiratory function until airway edema is resolved in acutely ill hospitalized patient.
Prepare for emergency radiation therapy when indicated.	Treatment of choice for superior vena cava syndrome.

NURSING DIAGNOSIS: Knowledge Deficit [Learning Need] regarding disease process, prognosis, treatment regimen, self care, and discharge needs

May be related to:
Lack of exposure/recall
Information misinterpretation
Unfamiliarity with information resources
Cognitive limitations

Possibly evidenced by:
Request for information, verbalization of problem, statements reflecting misconceptions
Inaccurate follow-through of instruction, development of preventable complications

DESIRED OUTCOMES/EVALUATION CRITERIA—PATIENT WILL:

Knowledge: Disease Process (NOC)

Verbalize understanding of condition, prognosis, and potential complications.
Identify relationship of signs/symptoms to disease process.
Initiate necessary lifestyle changes.

Refer to CP: Cancer, ND: Knowledge deficit, page 900 for general needs.

ACTIONS/INTERVENTIONS	RATIONALE

Teaching: Disease Process (NIC)

Independent

Discuss potential complications relative to specific therapeutic regimen.	Possible side effects/long-term physical complications of radiation (direct or indirect) and some chemotherapy agents include pneumonitis, hypothyroidism, pericarditis, cardiomyopathy.
Emphasize need for ongoing medical follow-up.	Following treatment, there is increased risk of secondary malignancies in addition to other complications listed.
Identify signs/symptoms requiring further evaluation, e.g., cough, fever, chills, malaise, dyspnea (pneumonitis); weight gain, slow pulse, decreased energy level, intolerance to cold (hypothyroidism); moderate fever, chest pain, dry cough, dyspnea, rapid pulse (pericarditis); dyspnea, fatigue, chest pain, dizziness/syncope (cardiomyopathy).	Prompt intervention can limit progression of complication, reduce debilitating effects.
Recommend regular exercise in moderation, with adequate rest. Discuss energy conservation techniques.	Promotes general well-being. *Note:* Fatigue is associated with disease process and treatment regimen, as well as developing complications. Therefore, balancing activity with rest enhances patients' ability to perform ADLs.
Review infection prevention measures and signs/symptoms requiring further evaluation.	Condition is associated with a complex deficiency in cellular immunity both before and after therapy. *Note: Herpes zoster* is a common occurrence.
Determine financial needs/concerns. Identify community resources, vocational services.	Although survival rates are relatively good, patients often have limitations in physical activities/employment because of dyspnea, chronic fatigue, and difficulties in concentration or memory. Presence of the disease can also impact patient's ability to work or qualify for bank loans or obtain insurance.

POTENTIAL CONSIDERATIONS following acute hospitalization (dependent on patient's age, physical condition/presence of complications, personal resources, and life responsibilities)

Fatigue—decreased metabolic energy production, overwhelming psychological or emotional demands, states of discomfort, altered body chemistry, e.g., chemotherapy.

Family Processes, altered—situational crisis (illness, disabling/expensive treatments).

Renal and Urinary Tract

RENAL FAILURE: ACUTE

Acute renal failure (ARF) has four well-defined stages: onset, oliguric or anuric, diuretic, and convalescent. Treatment depends on stage and severity of renal compromise. ARF can be divided into three major classifications, depending on site:

Prerenal: Prerenal failure is caused by interference with renal perfusion (e.g., blood volume depletion, volume shifts ["third-space" sequestration of fluid], or excessive/too-rapid volume expansion), manifested by decreased glomerular filtration rate (GFR). Disorders that lead to prerenal failure include cardiogenic shock, heart failure (HF), myocardial infarction (MI), burns, trauma, hemorrhage, septic or anaphylactic shock, and renal artery obstruction.

Renal (or intrarenal): Intrarenal causes for renal failure are associated with parenchymal changes caused by ischemia or nephrotoxic substances. Acute tubular necrosis (ATN) accounts for 90% of cases of acute oliguria. Destruction of tubular epithelial cells results from (1) ischemia/hypoperfusion (similar to prerenal hypoperfusion except that correction of the causative factor may be followed by continued oliguria for up to 30 days) and/or (2) direct damage from nephrotoxins.

Postrenal: Postrenal failure occurs as the result of an obstruction in the urinary tract anywhere from the tubules to the urethral meatus. Obstruction most commonly occurs with stones in the ureters, bladder, or urethra; however, trauma, edema associated with infection, prostate enlargement, and strictures also cause postrenal failure.

Note: Iatrogenically induced ARF should be considered when failure develops during or shortly after hospitalization. The most common causative factor is administration of potentially nephrotoxic agents.

CARE SETTING

Inpatient acute medical or surgical unit

RELATED CONCERNS

Metabolic acidosis (primary base bicarbonate deficit), page 523
Fluid and electrolyte imbalances, page 926
Psychosocial aspects of care, page 809
Renal dialysis, page 600
Renal failure: chronic, page 588
Sepsis/Septicemia, page 741
Total nutritional support: parenteral/enteral feeding, page 508
Upper gastrointestinal/Esophageal bleeding, page 333

Patient Assessment Database

ACTIVITY/REST

May report:	Fatigue, weakness, malaise
May exhibit:	Muscle weakness, loss of tone

CIRCULATION

May exhibit: Hypotension or hypertension (including malignant hypertension, eclampsia/pregnancy-induced hypertension)

Cardiac dysrhythmias

Weak/thready pulses, orthostatic hypotension (hypovolemia)

Jugular venous distension (JVD), full/bounding pulses (hypervolemia); flat neck veins (diuretic phase)

Generalized tissue edema (including periorbital area, ankles, sacrum)

Pallor (anemia); bleeding tendencies

ELIMINATION

May report: Change in usual urination pattern: Increased frequency, polyuria (early failure and early recovery), or decreased frequency/oliguria (later phase)

Dysuria, hesitancy, urgency, and retention (inflammation/obstruction/infection)

Abdominal bloating, diarrhea, or constipation

History of benign prostatic hyperplasia (BPH), or kidney/bladder stones/calculi

May exhibit: Change in urinary color, e.g., absence of color, deep yellow, red, brown, cloudy

Oliguria (may last 12–21 days and occurs in 70% of patients); polyuria (2–6 L/day of urine, lacking concentration and regulation of waste products)

FOOD/FLUID

May report: Weight gain (edema), weight loss (dehydration)

Nausea, anorexia, heartburn, vomiting

Use of diuretics

May exhibit: Changes in skin turgor/moisture

Edema (generalized, dependent)

NEUROSENSORY

May report: Headache, blurred vision

Muscle cramps/twitching; "restless leg" syndrome

May exhibit: Altered mental state, e.g., decreased attention span, inability to concentrate, loss of memory, confusion, decreasing level of consciousness (LOC) (azotemia, electrolyte and acid/base imbalance)

Twitching, muscle fasciculations, seizure activity

PAIN/DISCOMFORT

May report: Flank pain, headache

May exhibit: Guarding/distraction behaviors, restlessness

RESPIRATION

May report: Shortness of breath

May exhibit: Tachypnea, dyspnea, increased rate/depth (Kussmaul's respiration); ammonia breath

Cough productive of pink-tinged sputum (pulmonary edema)

SAFETY

May report: Recent transfusion reaction

May exhibit: Fever (sepsis, dehydration)

Petechiae, ecchymotic areas on skin

Pruritus, dry skin

TEACHING/LEARNING

May report: Family history of polycystic disease, hereditary nephritis, urinary calculus, malignancy

History of exposure to toxins, e.g., drugs, environmental poisons

Current/recent use of nephrotoxic drugs, e.g., aminoglycoside antibiotics, amphotericin B; anesthetics; vasodilators

Recent diagnostic testing with radiographic contrast media

Concurrent conditions: Tumors in the urinary tract, Gram-negative sepsis; trauma/crush injuries, hemorrhage, disseminated intravascular coagulation (DIC), burns, electrocution injury; autoimmune disorders (e.g., scleroderma, vasculitis), vascular occlusion/ surgery, diabetes mellitus (DM), cardiac/liver failure

Discharge plan considerations: **DRG projected mean length of inpatient stay: 5.9 days**

May require alteration/assistance with medications, treatments, supplies; transportation, homemaker/maintenance tasks

Refer to section at end of plan for postdischarge considerations.

DIAGNOSTIC STUDIES

Urine:

Volume: Usually less than 100 mL/24 hr (anuric phase) or 400 mL/24 hr (oliguric phase), which occurs within 24–48 hr after renal insult. Nonoliguric (greater than 400 mL/24 hr) renal failure also occurs when renal damage is associated with nephrotoxic agents (e.g., contrast media or antibiotics)

Color: Dirty, brown sediment indicates presence of RBCs, hemoglobin, myoglobin, porphyrins.

Specific gravity: Less than 1.020 reflects kidney disease, e.g., glomerulonephritis, pyelonephritis with loss of ability to concentrate; fixed at 1.010 reflects severe renal damage.

pH: Greater than 7 found in urinary tract infections (UTIs), renal tubular necrosis, and chronic renal failure (CRF).

Osmolality: Less than 350 mOsm/kg is indicative of tubular damage, and urine/serum ratio is often 1:1.

Creatinine (Cr) clearance: Renal function may be significantly decreased before blood urea nitrogen (BUN) and serum Cr show significant elevation.

Sodium: Usually increased if ATN is cause for ARF, greater than 40 mEq/L if kidney is not able to resorb sodium, although it may be decreased in other causes of prerenal failure.

Bicarbonate: Elevated if metabolic acidosis is present.

Red blood cells (RBCs): May be present because of infection, stones, trauma, tumor, or altered glomerular filtration (GF).

Protein: High-grade proteinuria (3–4+) strongly indicates glomerular damage when RBCs and casts are also present. Low-grade proteinuria (1–2+) and white blood cells (WBCs) may be indicative of infection or interstitial nephritis. In ATN, proteinuria is usually minimal.

Casts: Usually signal renal disease or infection. Cellular casts with brownish pigments and numerous renal tubular epithelial cells are diagnostic of ATN. Red casts suggest acute glomerular nephritis.

Blood:

BUN/Cr: Elevated and usually rise in proportion with ratio of 10:1 or greater.

Complete blood count (CBC): Hemoglobin (Hb) decreased in presence of anemia. RBCs often decreased because of increased fragility/decreased survival.

Arterial blood gases (ABGs): Metabolic acidosis (pH less than 7.2) may develop because of decreased renal ability to excrete hydrogen and end products of metabolism. Bicarbonate decreased.

Sodium: Usually increased, but may vary.

Potassium: Elevated related to retention and cellular shifts (acidosis) or tissue release (red cell hemolysis).

Chloride, phosphorus, and magnesium: Usually elevated.

Calcium: Decreased.

Serum osmolality: Greater than 285 mOsm/kg; often equal to urine.

Protein: Decreased serum level may reflect protein loss via urine, fluid shifts, decreased intake, or decreased synthesis because of lack of essential amino acids.

Radionuclide imaging: May reveal calicectasis, hydronephrosis, narrowing, and delayed filling or emptying as a cause of ARF.

Kidneys, ureter, bladder (KUB) x-ray: Demonstrates size of kidneys/ureters/bladder, presence of cysts, tumors, and kidney displacement or obstruction (stones).

Retrograde pyelogram: Outlines abnormalities of renal pelvis and ureters.

Renal arteriogram: Assesses renal circulation and identifies extravascularities, masses.

Voiding cystoureterogram: Shows bladder size, reflux into ureters, retention.

Renal ultrasound: Determines kidney size and presence of masses, cysts, obstruction in upper urinary tract.

Nonnuclear computed tomography (CT) scan: Cross-sectional view of kidney and urinary tract detects presence/extent of disease.

Magnetic resonance imaging (MRI): Provides information about soft tissue damage.

Excretory urography (intravenous urogram or pyelogram): Radiopaque contrast concentrates in urine and facilitates visualization of KUB.

Endourology: Direct visualization may be done of urethra, bladder, ureters, and kidney to diagnose problems, biopsy, and remove small lesions and/or calculi.

Electrocardiogram (ECG): May be abnormal, reflecting electrolyte and acid-base imbalances.

NURSING PRIORITIES

1. Re-establish/maintain fluid and electrolyte balance.
2. Prevent complications.
3. Provide emotional support for patient/significant other (SO).
4. Provide information about disease process/prognosis and treatment needs.

DISCHARGE GOALS

1. Homeostasis achieved.
2. Complications prevented/minimized.
3. Dealing realistically with current situation.
4. Disease process/prognosis and therapeutic regimen understood.
5. Plan in place to meet needs after discharge.

NURSING DIAGNOSIS: Fluid Volume excess

May be related to

Compromised regulatory mechanism (renal failure)

Possibly evidenced by

Intake greater than output, oliguria; changes in urine specific gravity

Venous distension; blood pressure (BP)/central venous pressure (CVP) changes

Generalized tissue edema, weight gain

Changes in mental status, restlessness

Decreased Hb/hematocrit (Hct), altered electrolytes; pulmonary congestion on x-ray

DESIRED OUTCOMES/EVALUATION CRITERIA—PATIENT WILL:

Fluid Balance (NOC)

Display appropriate urinary output with specific gravity/laboratory studies near normal; stable weight, vital signs within patient's normal range; and absence of edema.

ACTIONS/INTERVENTIONS	RATIONALE
Fluid/Electrolyte Management (NIC)	
Independent	
Record accurate intake and output (I&O). Include "hidden" fluids such as IV antibiotic additives, liquid medications, ice chips, frozen treats. Measure gastrointestinal (GI) losses and estimate insensible losses, e.g., diaphoresis.	Low output (less than 400 mL/24 hr) may be first indicator of acute failure, especially in a high-risk patient. Accurate I&O is necessary for determining renal function and fluid replacement needs and reducing risk of fluid overload. *Note:* Hypervolemia occurs in the anuric phase of ARF.
Monitor urine specific gravity.	Measures the kidney's ability to concentrate urine. In intrarenal failure, specific gravity is usually equal to/less than 1.010, indicating loss of ability to concentrate the urine.
Weigh daily on same scale with same equipment and clothing.	Daily body weight is best monitor of fluid status. A weight gain of more than 0.5 kg/day suggests fluid retention.

ACTIONS/INTERVENTIONS	RATIONALE

Independent

Assess skin, face, dependent areas for edema. Evaluate degree of edema (on scale of +1–+4).	Edema occurs primarily in dependent tissues of the body, e.g., hands, feet, lumbosacral area. Patient can gain up to 10 lb (4.5 kg) of fluid before pitting edema is detected. Periorbital edema may be a presenting sign of this fluid shift because these fragile tissues are easily distended by even minimal fluid accumulation.
Monitor heart rate (HR), BP, and JVD/CVP.	Tachycardia and hypertension can occur because of (1) failure of the kidneys to excrete urine, (2) excessive fluid resuscitation during efforts to treat hypovolemia/hypotension or convert oliguric phase of renal failure, and/or (3) changes in the renin-angiotensin system. *Note:* Invasive monitoring may be needed for assessing intravascular volume, especially in patients with poor cardiac function.
Auscultate lung and heart sounds.	Fluid overload may lead to pulmonary edema and HF evidenced by development of adventitious breath sounds, extra heart sounds. (Refer to ND: Cardiac Output, risk for decreased, following.)
Assess level of consciousness; investigate changes in mentation, presence of restlessness.	May reflect fluid shifts, accumulation of toxins, acidosis, electrolyte imbalances, or developing hypoxia.
Plan oral fluid replacement with patient, within multiple restrictions. Intersperse desired beverages throughout 24 hr. Vary offerings, e.g., hot, cold, frozen.	Helps avoid periods without fluids, minimizes boredom of limited choices, and reduces sense of deprivation and thirst.

Collaborative

Correct any reversible cause of ARF, e.g., replace blood loss, maximize cardiac output, discontinue nephrotoxic drug, relieve obstruction via surgery.	Kidneys may be able to return to normal functioning, preventing or limiting residual effects.

Monitor laboratory/diagnostic studies, e.g.:

BUN, Cr;	Assesses progression and management of renal dysfunction/failure. Although both values may be increased, Cr is a better indicator of renal function because it is not affected by hydration, diet, and tissue catabolism. *Note:* Dialysis is indicated if ratio is greater than 10:1 or if therapy fails to correct fluid overload or metabolic acidosis.
Urine sodium and Cr;	In ATN, tubular functional integrity is lost and sodium resorption is impaired, resulting in increased sodium excretion. Urine creatinine is usually decreased as serum creatinine elevates.
Serum sodium;	Hyponatremia may result from fluid overload (dilutional) or kidney's inability to conserve sodium. Hypernatremia indicates total body water deficit.
Serum potassium;	Lack of renal excretion and/or selective retention of potassium to excrete excess hydrogen ions leads to hyperkalemia, requiring prompt intervention.
Hb/Hct;	Decreased values may indicate hemodilution (hypervolemia); however, during prolonged failure, anemia frequently develops as a result of RBC loss/decreased production. Other possible causes (active or occult hemorrhage) should also be evaluated.

ACTIONS/INTERVENTIONS	RATIONALE
Collaborative	
Serial chest x-rays.	Increased cardiac size, prominent pulmonary vascular markings, pleural effusion, infiltrates/congestion indicate acute responses to fluid overload or chronic changes associated with renal and heart failure.
Administer/restrict fluids as indicated.	Fluid management is usually calculated to replace output from all sources plus estimated insensible losses (metabolism, diaphoresis). Prerenal failure (azotemia) is treated with volume replacement and/or vasopressors. The oliguric patient with adequate circulating volume or fluid overload who is unresponsive to fluid restriction and diuretics requires dialysis.
Administer medications as indicated:	
Diuretics, e.g., furosemide (Lasix); bumetanide (Bumex); torsemide (Demadex); mannitol (Osmitrol);	Given early in oliguric phase of ARF in an effort to convert to nonoliguric phase, to flush the tubular lumen of debris, reduce hyperkalemia, and promote adequate urine volume.
Antihypertensives, e.g., clonidine (Catapres), methyldopa (Aldomet), prazosin (Minipress).	May be given to treat hypertension by counteracting effects of decreased renal blood flow and/or circulating volume overload.
Insert/maintain indwelling catheter, as indicated.	Catheterization excludes lower tract obstruction and provides means of accurate monitoring of urine output during acute phase; however, indwelling catheterization may be contraindicated because of increased risk of infection.
Prepare for dialysis as indicated, e.g., hemodialysis, peritoneal dialysis, or continuous renal replacement therapy (CRRT).	Done to correct volume overload, electrolyte and acid-base imbalances, and to remove toxins. The type of dialysis chosen for ARF depends on the degree of hemodynamic compromise and the patient's ability to withstand the procedure. (Refer to CP: Renal Dialysis, p. 600.)

NURSING DIAGNOSIS: Cardiac Output, risk for decreased

Risk factors may include
Fluid overload (kidney dysfunction/failure, overzealous fluid replacement)
Fluid shifts, fluid deficit (excessive losses)
Electrolyte imbalance (potassium, calcium); severe acidosis
Uremic effects on cardiac muscle/oxygenation

Possibly evidenced by
[Not applicable; presence of signs and symptoms establishes an *actual* diagnosis]

DESIRED OUTCOMES/EVALUATION CRITERIA—PATIENT WILL:

Circulatory Status (NOC)

Maintain cardiac output as evidenced by BP and HR/rhythm within patient's normal limits; peripheral pulses strong and equal with adequate capillary refill time.

ACTIONS/INTERVENTIONS	RATIONALE

Hemodynamic Regulation (NIC)

Independent

Monitor BP and HR.

Fluid volume excess, combined with hypertension (often occurs in renal failure) and effects of uremia, increases cardiac workload and can lead to cardiac failure. In ARF, cardiac failure is usually reversible.

Observe ECG or telemetry for changes in rhythm.

Changes in electromechanical function may become evident in response to progressing renal failure/accumulation of toxins and electrolyte imbalance. For example, hyperkalemia is associated with peaked T wave, wide QRS, prolonged PR interval, flattened/absent P wave. Hypokalemia is associated with flat T wave, peaked P wave, and appearance of U waves. Prolonged QT interval may reflect calcium deficit.

Auscultate heart sounds.

Development of S_3/S_4 are indicative of failure. Pericardial friction rub may be only manifestation of uremic pericarditis, requiring prompt intervention/possibly acute dialysis.

Assess color of skin, mucous membranes, and nailbeds. Note capillary refill time.

Pallor may reflect vasoconstriction or anemia. Cyanosis is a late sign and is related to pulmonary congestion and/or cardiac failure.

Note occurrence of slow pulse, hypotension, flushing, nausea/vomiting, and depressed level of consciousness (central nervous system [CNS] depression).

Using drugs (e.g., antacids) containing magnesium can result in hypermagnesmia, potentiating neuromuscular dysfunction and risk of respiratory/cardiac arrest.

Investigate reports of muscle cramps, numbness/tingling of fingers, with muscle twitching, hyperreflexia.

Neuromuscular indicators of hypocalcemia, which can also affect cardiac contractility and function.

Maintain bedrest or encourage adequate rest and provide assistance with care and desired activities.

Reduces oxygen consumption/cardiac workload.

Collaborative

Monitor laboratory studies, e.g.:

  Potassium;

During oliguric phase, hyperkalemia is present but often shifts to hypokalemia in diuretic or recovery phase. Any potassium value associated with ECG changes requires intervention. *Note:* A serum level of 6.5 mEq or greater constitutes a medical emergency.

  Calcium;

In addition to its own cardiac effects, calcium deficit enhances the toxic effects of potassium.

  Magnesium.

Dialysis or calcium administration may be necessary to combat the CNS-depressive effects of an elevated serum magnesium level.

Administer/restrict fluids as indicated (Refer to NDs: Fluid Volume excess, p. 578, and Fluid Volume, risk for deficit, p. 585.)

Cardiac output depends on circulating volume (affected by both fluid excess and deficit) and myocardial muscle function.

Provide supplemental oxygen if indicated.

Maximizes available oxygen for myocardial uptake to reduce cardiac workload and cellular hypoxia.

581

ACTIONS/INTERVENTIONS	RATIONALE

Collaborative

Administer medications as indicated:

ACTIONS/INTERVENTIONS	RATIONALE
Inotropic agents, e.g., digoxin (Lanoxin);	May be used to improve cardiac output by increasing myocardial contractility and stroke volume. Dosage depends on renal function and potassium balance to obtain therapeutic effect without toxicity.
Calcium gluconate;	Serum calcium is often low but usually does not require specific treatment in ARF. Calcium gluconate may be given to treat hypocalcemia and to offset the effects of hyperkalemia by modifying cardiac irritability.
Aluminum hydroxide gels (Amphojel, Basalgel);	Increased phosphate levels may occur as a result of failure of glomerular filtration and require use of phosphate-binding antacids to limit phosphate absorption from the GI tract.
Glucose/insulin solution;	Temporary measure to lower serum potassium by driving potassium into cells when cardiac rhythm is endangered.
Sodium bicarbonate or sodium citrate;	May be used to correct acidosis or hyperkalemia (by increasing serum pH) if patient is severely acidotic and not suffering from fluid overload.
Sodium polystyrene sulfonate (Kayexalate) with/without sorbitol.	Exchange resin trades sodium for potassium in the GI tract to lower serum potassium level. Sorbitol may be included to cause osmotic diarrhea to help excrete potassium.
Prepare for/assist with dialysis as necessary.	May be indicated for persistent dysrhythmias, progressive HF unresponsive to other therapies.

NURSING DIAGNOSIS: Nutrition: altered, risk for less than body requirements

Risk factors may include
Protein catabolism; dietary restrictions to reduce nitrogenous waste products
Increased metabolic needs
Anorexia, nausea/vomiting; ulcerations of oral mucosa

Possibly evidenced by
[Not applicable; presence of signs and symptoms establishes an *actual* diagnosis]

DESIRED OUTCOMES/EVALUATION CRITERIA—PATIENT WILL:

Nutritional Status (NOC)

Maintain/regain weight as indicated by individual situation, free of edema.

ACTIONS/INTERVENTIONS	RATIONALE

Nutrition Therapy (NIC)

Independent

ACTIONS/INTERVENTIONS	RATIONALE
Assess/document dietary intake.	Aids in identifying deficiencies and dietary needs. General physical condition, uremic symptoms (e.g., nausea, anorexia, altered taste), and multiple dietary restrictions affect food intake.

ACTIONS/INTERVENTIONS	RATIONALE
Independent	
Provide frequent, small feedings.	Minimizes anorexia and nausea associated with uremic state/diminished peristalsis.
Give patient/SO a list of permitted foods/fluids and encourage involvement in menu choices.	Provides patient with a measure of control within dietary restrictions. Food from home may enhance appetite.
Offer frequent mouth care/rinse with dilute (0.25%) acetic acid solution; provide gum, hard candy, breath mints between meals.	Mucous membranes may become dry and cracked. Mouth care soothes, lubricates, and helps freshen mouth taste, which is often unpleasant because of uremia and restricted oral intake. Rinsing with acetic acid helps neutralize ammonia formed by conversion of urea.
Weigh daily.	The fasting/catabolic patient normally loses 0.2–0.5 kg/day. Changes in excess of 0.5 kg may reflect shifts in fluid balance.
Collaborative	
Monitor laboratory studies, e.g., BUN, prealbumin/albumin, transferrin, sodium, and potassium.	Indicators of nutritional needs, restrictions, and necessity for/effectiveness of therapy.
Consult with dietitian/nutritional support team.	Determines individual calorie and nutrient needs within the restrictions and identifies most effective route and product, e.g., oral supplements, enteral or parenteral nutrition.
Provide high-calorie, low-/moderate-protein diet. Include complex carbohydrates and fat sources to meet caloric needs (avoiding concentrated sugar sources) and essential amino acids.	The amount of needed exogenous protein is less than normal unless the patient is on dialysis. Carbohydrates meet energy needs and limit tissue catabolism, preventing ketoacid formation from protein and fat oxidation. Carbohydrate intolerance mimicking DM may occur in severe renal failure. Essential amino acids improve nitrogen balance and nutritional status.
Restrict potassium, sodium, and phosphorus intake as indicated.	Restriction of these electrolytes may be needed to prevent further renal damage, especially if dialysis is not part of treatment, and/or during recovery phase of ARF.
Administer medications as indicated:	
Iron preparations;	Iron deficiency may occur if protein is restricted, patient is anemic, or GI function is impaired.
Calcium carbonate;	Restores normal serum levels to improve cardiac and neuromuscular function, blood clotting, and bone metabolism. *Note:* Low serum calcium is often corrected as phosphate absorption is decreased in the GI system. Calcium may be substituted as a phosphate binder.
Vitamin D;	Necessary to facilitate absorption of calcium from the GI tract.

ACTIONS/INTERVENTIONS	RATIONALE

Collaborative

B complex vitamins;

Vital as coenzyme in cell growth and actions. Intake is decreased because of protein restrictions.

Antiemetics, e.g., prochlorperazine (Compazine), trimethobenzamide (Tigan).

Given to relieve nausea/vomiting and may enhance oral intake.

NURSING DIAGNOSIS: Infection, risk for

Risk factors may include
Depression of immunologic defenses (secondary to uremia)
Invasive procedures/devices (e.g., urinary catheter)
Changes in dietary intake/malnutrition

Possibly evidenced by
[Not applicable; presence of signs and symptoms establishes an *actual* diagnosis]

DESIRED OUTCOMES/EVALUATION CRITERIA—PATIENT WILL:

Immune Status (NOC)

Experience no signs/symptoms of infection.

ACTIONS/INTERVENTIONS	RATIONALE

Infection Protection (NIC)

Independent

Promote good handwashing by patient and staff.

Reduces risk of cross-contamination.

Avoid invasive procedures, instrumentation, and manipulation of indwelling catheters whenever possible. Use aseptic technique when caring for/manipulating IV/invasive lines. Change site/dressings per protocol. Note edema, purulent drainage.

Limits introduction of bacteria into body. Early detection/treatment of developing infection may prevent sepsis.

Provide routine catheter care and promote meticulous perianal care. Keep urinary drainage system closed and remove indwelling catheter as soon as possible.

Reduces bacterial colonization and risk of ascending UTI.

Encourage deep breathing, coughing, frequent position changes.

Prevents atelectasis and mobilizes secretions to reduce risk of pulmonary infections.

Assess skin integrity. (Refer to CP: Renal Failure: Chronic; ND: Skin Integrity, risk for impaired, p. 595.)

Excoriations from scratching may become secondarily infected.

Monitor vital signs.

Fever with increased pulse and respirations is typical of increased metabolic rate resulting from inflammatory process, although sepsis can occur without a febrile response.

Collaborative

Monitor laboratory studies, e.g., WBC count with differential.

Although elevated WBCs may indicate generalized infection, leukocytosis is commonly seen in ARF and may reflect inflammation/injury within the kidney. A shifting of the differential to the left is indicative of infection.

ACTIONS/INTERVENTIONS

Collaborative

Obtain specimen(s) for culture and sensitivity and administer appropriate antibiotics as indicated.

RATIONALE

Verification of infection and identification of specific organism aids in choice of the most effective treatment. *Note:* A number of anti-infective agents require adjustments of dose and/or time while renal clearance is impaired.

NURSING DIAGNOSIS: Fluid Volume, risk for deficit

Risk factors may include

Excessive loss of fluid (diuretic phase of ARF, with rising urinary volume and delayed return of tubular reabsorption capabilities)

Possibly evidenced by

[Not applicable; presence of signs and symptoms establishes an *actual* diagnosis]

DESIRED OUTCOMES/EVALUATION CRITERIA—PATIENT WILL:

Fluid Balance (NOC)

Display I&O near balance; good skin turgor, moist mucous membranes, palpable peripheral pulses, stable weight and vital signs, electrolytes within normal range.

ACTIONS/INTERVENTIONS

Fluid Monitoring (NIC)

Independent

Measure I&O accurately. Weigh daily. Calculate insensible fluid losses.

Provide allowed fluids throughout 24-hr period.

Monitor BP (noting postural changes) and heart rate.

Note signs/symptoms of dehydration, e.g., dry mucous membranes, thirst, dulled sensorium, peripheral vasoconstriction.

Control environmental temperature; limit bed linens as indicated.

Collaborative

Monitor laboratory studies, e.g., sodium.

RATIONALE

Helps estimate fluid replacement needs. Fluid intake should approximate losses through urine, nasogastric/wound drainage, and insensible losses (e.g., diaphoresis and metabolism). *Note:* Some sources believe that fluid replacement should not exceed two-thirds of the previous day's output to prevent prolonging the diuresis.

Diuretic phase of ARF may revert to oliguric phase if fluid intake is not maintained or nocturnal dehydration occurs.

Orthostatic hypotension and tachycardia suggests hypovolemia.

In diuretic or postobstructive phase of renal failure, urine output can exceed 3 L/day. Extracellular fluid volume depletion activates the thirst center, and sodium depletion causes persistent thirst, unrelieved by drinking water. Continued fluid losses/inadequate replacement may lead to hypovolemic state.

May reduce diaphoresis, which contributes to overall fluid losses.

In nonoliguric ARF or in diuretic phase of ARF, large urine losses may result in sodium wasting while elevated urinary sodium acts osmotically to increase fluid losses. Restriction of sodium may be indicated to break the cycle.

585

NURSING DIAGNOSIS: Knowledge Deficit [Learning Need] regarding condition, prognosis, treatment, self care, and discharge needs

May be related to
Lack of exposure/recall
Information misinterpretation
Unfamiliarity with information resources

Possibly evidenced by
Questions/request for information, statement of misconception
Inaccurate follow-through of instructions/development of preventable complications

DESIRED OUTCOMES/EVALUATION CRITERIA—PATIENT WILL:

Knowledge: Disease Process (NOC)

Verbalize understanding of condition/disease process, prognosis, and potential complications.
Identify relationship of signs/symptoms to the disease process and correlate symptoms with causative factors.

Knowledge: Treatment Regimen (NOC)

Verbalize understanding of therapeutic needs.
Initiate necessary lifestyle changes and participate in treatment regimen.

ACTIONS/INTERVENTIONS	RATIONALE
Teaching: Disease Process (NIC)	
Independent	
Review disease process, prognosis, and precipitating factors if known.	Provides knowledge base from which patient can make informed choices.
Explain level of renal function after acute episode is over.	Patient may experience residual defects in kidney function, which may/may not be permanent.
Discuss renal dialysis or transplantation if these are likely options for the future.	Although these options would have been previously presented by the physician, the patient may now be at a point when options need to be considered/decisions made and may desire additional input.
Review dietary plan/restrictions. Include fact sheet listing food restrictions.	Adequate nutrition is necessary to promote healing/tissue regeneration while adherence to restrictions may prevent complications.
Encourage patient to observe characteristics of urine and amount/frequency of output.	Changes may reflect alterations in renal function/need for dialysis.
Establish regular schedule for weighing.	Useful tool for monitoring fluid and dietary status/needs.
Review fluid intake/restriction. Remind patient to spread fluids over entire day and to include all fluids (e.g., ice) in daily fluid counts.	Depending on the cause/stage of ARF, patient may need to either restrict or increase intake of fluids.
Discuss activity restriction and gradual resumption of desired activity. Encourage use of energy-saving, relaxation, and diversional techniques.	Patient with severe ARF may need to restrict activity and/or may feel weak for an extended period during lengthy recovery phase, requiring measures to conserve energy and reduce boredom/depression.

ACTIONS/INTERVENTIONS	RATIONALE
Independent	
Discuss reality of continued presence of fatigue.	Decreased metabolic energy production, presence of anemia, and states of discomfort commonly result in fatigue.
Determine/prioritize ADLs and personal responsibilities. Identify available resources/support systems.	Helps patient manage lifestyle changes and meet personal/family needs.
Recommend scheduling activities with adequate rest periods.	Prevents excessive fatigue and conserves energy for healing, tissue regeneration.
Discuss/review medication use. Encourage patient to discuss all medications (including over-the-counter [OTC] drugs) with physician.	Medications that are concentrated in/excreted by the kidneys can cause toxic cumulative reactions and/or permanent damage to kidneys.
Stress necessity of follow-up care, laboratory studies.	Renal function may be slow to return following acute failure (up to 12 mo) and deficits may persist, requiring changes in therapy to avoid recurrence/complications.
Identify symptoms requiring medical intervention, e.g., decreased urinary output, sudden weight gain, presence of edema, lethargy, bleeding, signs of infection; altered mentation.	Prompt evaluation and intervention may prevent serious complications/progression to CRF.

POTENTIAL CONSIDERATIONS following acute hospitalization (dependent on patient's age, physical condition/presence of complications, personal resources, and life responsibilities)

Fluid Volume deficit (specify)—dependent on cause, duration, and stage of recovery.

Fatigue—decreased metabolic energy production/dietary restriction, anemia, increased energy requirements, e.g., fever/inflammation, tissue regeneration.

Infection, risk for—depression of immunologic defenses (secondary to uremia), changes in dietary intake/malnutrition, increased environmental exposure.

Therapeutic Regimen: Individuals, ineffective management—complexity of therapeutic regimen, economic difficulties, perceived benefit.

RENAL FAILURE: CHRONIC

Chronic renal failure (CRF) is the end result of a gradual, progressive loss of kidney function. Causes include chronic infections (glomerulonephritis, pyelonephritis), vascular diseases (hypertension, nephrosclerosis), obstructive processes (renal calculi), collagen diseases (systemic lupus), nephrotoxic agents (drugs, such as aminoglycosides), and endocrine diseases (diabetes, hyperparathyroidism). This syndrome is generally progressive and produces major changes in all body systems. The final stage of renal dysfunction, end-stage renal disease (ESRD), is demonstrated by a glomeruler filtration rate (GFR) of 15%–20% of normal or less.

CARE SETTING

Primary focus is at the community level, although inpatient acute hospitalization may be required for life-threatening complications.

RELATED CONCERNS

Anemias (iron deficiency, pernicious, aplastic, hemolytic), page 531
Fluid and electrolyte imbalances, page 926
Heart failure: chronic, page 47
Hypertension: severe, page 33
Metabolic acidosis (primary base bicarbonate deficit), page 523
Psychosocial aspects of care, page 809
Upper gastrointestinal/Esophageal bleeding, page 333

Additional associated nursing diagnoses are found in:
Renal dialysis, page 600
Renal failure: acute, page 575
Seizure disorders/Epilepsy, page 228

Patient Assessment Database

ACTIVITY/REST

May report:	Extreme fatigue, weakness, malaise
	Sleep disturbances (insomnia/restlessness or somnolence)
May exhibit:	Muscle weakness, loss of tone, decreased range of motion (ROM)

CIRCULATION

May report:	History of prolonged or severe hypertension
	Palpitations; chest pain (angina)
May exhibit:	Hypertension; JVD, full/bounding pulses, generalized tissue and pitting edema of feet, legs, hands
	Cardiac dysrhythmias, distant heart sounds
	Weak thready pulses, orthostatic hypotension reflects hypovolemia (rare in end-stage disease)
	Pericardial friction rub
	Pallor; bronze-gray, yellow skin
	Bleeding tendencies

EGO INTEGRITY

May report:	Stress factors, e.g., financial, relationship, and so on
	Feelings of helplessness, hopelessness, powerlessness
May exhibit:	Denial, anxiety, fear, anger, irritability, personality changes

ELIMINATION

May report:	Decreased urinary frequency; oliguria, anuria (advanced failure)
	Abdominal bloating, diarrhea, or constipation
May exhibit:	Change in urine color, e.g., deep yellow, red, brown, cloudy
	Oliguria, may become anuric

FOOD/FLUID

May report: Rapid weight gain (edema), weight loss (malnutrition)
Anorexia, heartburn, nausea/vomiting; unpleasant metallic taste in the mouth (ammonia breath)
Use of diuretics

May exhibit: Abdominal distension/ascites, liver enlargement (end-stage)
Changes in skin turgor/moisture
Edema (generalized, dependent)
Gum ulcerations, bleeding of gums/tongue
Muscle wasting, decreased subcutaneous fat, debilitated appearance

HYGIENE

May report: Difficulty performing ADLs

NEUROSENSORY

May report: Headache, blurred vision
Muscle cramps/twitching, "restless leg" syndrome; burning numbness of soles of feet
Numbness/tingling and weakness, especially of lower extremities (peripheral neuropathy)

May exhibit: Altered mental state, e.g., decreased attention span, inability to concentrate, loss of memory, confusion, decreasing level of consciousness, stupor, coma
Gait abnormalities
Twitching, muscle fasciculations, seizure activity
Thin, dry, brittle nails and hair

PAIN/DISCOMFORT

May report: Flank pain; headache; muscle cramps/leg pain (worse at night)
May exhibit: Guarding/distraction behaviors, restlessness

RESPIRATION

May report: Shortness of breath; paroxysmal nocturnal dyspnea; cough with/without thick, tenacious sputum

May exhibit: Tachypnea, dyspnea, increased rate/depth (Kussmaul's respiration)
Cough productive of pink-tinged sputum (pulmonary edema)

SAFETY

May report: Itching skin, frequent scratching
Recent/recurrent infections

May exhibit: Scratch marks, petechiae, ecchymotic areas on skin
Fever (sepsis, dehydration); normothermia may actually represent an elevation in the patient who has developed a lower-than-normal body temperature (effect of CRF/depressed immune response)
Bone fractures; calcium phosphate deposits (metastatic calcifications) in skin, soft tissues, joints; limited joint movement

SEXUALITY

May report: Decreased libido; amenorrhea; infertility

SOCIAL INTERACTION

May report: Difficulties imposed by condition, e.g., unable to work, maintain social contacts or usual role function in family

TEACHING/LEARNING

May report: Family history of polycystic disease, hereditary nephritis, urinary calculus, malignancy

History of DM (high risk for renal failure); exposure to toxins, e.g., nephrotoxic drugs, drug overdose, environmental poisons

Current/recent use of nephrotoxic antibiotics, angiotensin-converting enzyme (ACE) inhibitors, chemotherapy agents, heavy metals, nonsteroidal anti-inflammatory drugs (NSAIDs), radiocontrast agents

Discharge plan considerations:

DRG projected mean length of inpatient stay: 5.9 days

May require alteration/assistance with medications, treatments, supplies; transportation, homemaker/maintenance tasks

Refer to section at end of plan for postdischarge considerations.

DIAGNOSTIC STUDIES

Urine:

Volume: Usually less than 400 mL/24 hr (oliguria) or urine is absent (anuria).

Color: Abnormally cloudy urine may be caused by pus, bacteria, fat, colloidal particles, phosphates, or urates. Dirty, brown sediment indicates presence of RBCs, hemoglobin, myoglobin, porphyrins.

Specific gravity: Less than 1.015 (fixed at 1.010 reflects severe renal damage).

Osmolality: Less than 350 mOsm/kg is indicative of tubular damage, and urine/serum ratio is often 1:1.

Creatinine clearance: May be significantly decreased (less than 80 mL/min early failure; less than 10 mL/min in ESRD).

Sodium: Greater than 40 mEq/L because kidney is not able to reabsorb sodium.

Protein: High-grade proteinuria (3–4+) strongly indicates glomerular damage when RBCs and casts are also present.

Blood:

BUN/Cr: Elevated, usually in proportion. Creatinine level of 12 mg/dL suggests ESRD. A BUN of >25 mg/dL is indicative of renal damage.

CBC: Hb decreased because of anemia, usually less than 7–8 g/dL.

RBCs: Life span decreased because of erythropoietin deficiency, and azotemia.

ABGs: pH decreased. Metabolic acidosis (less than 7.2) occurs because of loss of renal ability to excrete hydrogen and ammonia or end products of protein catabolism. Bicarbonate and Pco_2 decreased.

Serum sodium: May be low (if kidney "wastes sodium") or normal (reflecting dilutional state of hypernatremia).

Potassium: Elevated related to retention and cellular shifts (acidosis) or tissue release (RBC hemolysis). In end-stage disease, ECG changes may not occur until potassium is 6.5 mEq or greater. Potassium may also be decreased if the patient is on potassium-wasting diuretics or when the patient is being dialyzed.

Magnesium, phosphorus: Elevated.

Calcium/phosphorus: Decreased.

Proteins (especially albumin): Decreased serum level may reflect protein loss via urine, fluid shifts, decreased intake, or decreased synthesis because of lack of essential amino acids.

Serum osmolality: Greater than 285 mOsm/kg; often equal to urine.

KUB x-rays: Demonstrates size of kidneys/ureters/bladder and presence of obstruction (stones).

Retrograde pyelogram: Outlines abnormalities of renal pelvis and ureters.

Renal arteriogram: Assesses renal circulation and identifies extravascularities, masses.

Voiding cystourethrogram: Shows bladder size, reflux into ureters, retention.

Renal ultrasound: Determines kidney size and presence of masses, cysts, obstruction in upper urinary tract.

Renal biopsy: May be done endoscopically to examine tissue cells for histological diagnosis.

Renal endoscopy, nephroscopy: Done to examine renal pelvis; flush out calculi, hematuria; and remove selected tumors.

ECG: May be abnormal, reflecting electrolyte and acid/base imbalances.

X-ray of feet, skull, spinal column, and hands: May reveal demineralization/calcifications resulting from electrolyte shifts associated with CRF.

NURSING PRIORITIES

1. Maintain homeostasis.
2. Prevent complications.
3. Provide information about disease process/prognosis and treatment needs.
4. Support adjustment to lifestyle changes.

DISCHARGE GOALS

1. Fluid/electrolyte balance stabilized.
2. Complications prevented/minimized.
3. Disease process/prognosis and therapeutic regimen understood.
4. Dealing realistically with situation; initiating necessary lifestyle changes.
5. Plan in place to meet needs after discharge.

NURSING DIAGNOSIS: Cardiac Output, risk for decreased

Risk factors may include

Fluid imbalances affecting circulating volume, myocardial workload, and systemic vascular resistance (SVR)

Alterations in rate, rhythm, cardiac conduction (electrolyte imbalances, hypoxia)

Accumulation of toxins (urea), soft-tissue calcification (deposition of calcium phosphate)

Possibly evidenced by

[Not applicable; presence of signs and symptoms establishes an *actual* diagnosis]

DESIRED OUTCOMES/EVALUATION CRITERIA—PATIENT WILL:

Circulatory Status (NOC)

Maintain cardiac output as evidenced by BP and heart rate within patient's normal range; peripheral pulses strong and equal with prompt capillary refill time.

ACTIONS/INTERVENTIONS	RATIONALE
(In addition to those in CP: Renal Failure: Acute; ND: Cardiac Output, risk for decreased, p. 580.)	

Hemodynamic Regulation (NIC)

Independent

ACTIONS/INTERVENTIONS	RATIONALE
Auscultate heart and lung sounds. Evaluate presence of peripheral edema/vascular congestion and reports of dyspnea.	S_3/S_4 heart sounds with muffled tones, tachycardia, irregular heart rate, tachypnea, dyspnea, crackles, wheezes, and edema/jugular distension suggest HF.
Assess presence/degree of hypertension: monitor BP; note postural changes, e.g., sitting, lying, standing.	Significant hypertension can occur because of disturbances in the renin-angiotensin-aldosterone system (caused by renal dysfunction). Although hypertension is common, orthostatic hypotension may occur because of intravascular fluid deficit, response to effects of antihypertensive medications, or uremic pericardial tamponade.
Investigate reports of chest pain, noting location, radiation, severity (0–10 scale), and whether or not it is intensified by deep inspiration and supine position.	Although hypertension and chronic HF may cause MI, approximately half of CRF patients on dialysis develop pericarditis, potentiating risk of pericardial effusion/tamponade.
Evaluate heart sounds (note friction rub), BP, peripheral pulses, capillary refill, vascular congestion, temperature, and sensorium/mentation.	Presence of sudden hypotension, paradoxic pulse, narrow pulse pressure, diminished/absent peripheral pulses, marked jugular distension, pallor, and a rapid mental deterioration indicate tamponade, which is a medical emergency.
Assess activity level, response to activity.	Weakness can be attributed to HF and anemia.

591

ACTIONS/INTERVENTIONS	RATIONALE

Collaborative

ACTIONS/INTERVENTIONS	RATIONALE
Monitor laboratory/diagnostic studies, e.g.:	
Electrolytes (potassium, sodium, calcium, magnesium), BUN/Cr;	Imbalances can alter electrical conduction and cardiac function.
Chest x-rays.	Useful in identifying developing cardiac failure or soft-tissue calcification.
Administer antihypertensive drugs, e.g., prazosin (Minipress), captopril (Capoten), clonidine (Catapres), hydralazine (Apresoline).	Reduces systemic vascular resistance and/or renin release to decrease myocardial workload and aid in prevention of HF and/or MI.
Prepare for dialysis.	Reduction of uremic toxins and correction of electrolyte imbalances and fluid overload may limit/prevent cardiac manifestations, including hypertension and pericardial effusion.
Assist with pericardiocentesis as indicated.	Accumulation of fluid within pericardial sac can compromise cardiac filling and myocardial contractility, impairing cardiac output and potentiating risk of cardiac arrest.

NURSING DIAGNOSIS: Protection, risk for altered

Risk factors may include
Abnormal blood profile (suppressed erythropoietin production/secretion; decreased RBC production and survival; altered clotting factors; increased capillary fragility)

Possibly evidenced by
[Not applicable; presence of signs and symptoms establishes an *actual* diagnosis]

DESIRED OUTCOMES/EVALUATION CRITERIA—PATIENT WILL:

Risk Control (NOC)

Experience no signs/symptoms of bleeding/hemorrhage.
Maintain/demonstrate improvement in laboratory values.

ACTIONS/INTERVENTIONS	RATIONALE

Bleeding Precautions (NIC)

Independent

ACTIONS/INTERVENTIONS	RATIONALE
Note reports of increasing fatigue, weakness. Observe for tachycardia, pallor of skin/mucous membranes, dyspnea, and chest pain. Plan patient activities to avoid fatigue.	May reflect effects of anemia and cardiac response necessary to keep cells oxygenated.
Monitor level of consciousness and behavior.	Anemia may cause cerebral hypoxia manifested by changes in mentation, orientation, and behavioral responses.
Evaluate response to activity, ability to perform tasks. Assist as needed and develop schedule for rest.	Anemia decreases tissue oxygenation and increases fatigue, which may require intervention, changes in activity, and rest.
Limit vascular sampling, combine laboratory tests when possible.	Recurrent/excessive blood sampling can worsen anemia.

ACTIONS/INTERVENTIONS	RATIONALE
Independent	
Observe for oozing from venipuncture sites, bleeding/ecchymotic areas following slight trauma, petechiae; joint swelling or mucous membrane involvement, e.g., bleeding gums, recurrent epistaxis, hematemesis, melena, and hazy/red urine.	Bleeding can occur easily because of capillary fragility/altered clotting functions and may worsen anemia.
Hematest GI secretions/stool for blood.	Mucosal changes and altered platelet function due to uremia may result in gastric mucosal erosion/GI hemorrhage.
Provide soft toothbrush, electric razor; use smallest needle possible and apply prolonged pressure following injections/vascular punctures.	Reduces risk of bleeding/hematoma formation.
Collaborative	
Monitor laboratory studies, e.g.:	
RBCs, Hb/Hct;	Uremia (e.g., elevated ammonia, urea, other toxins) decreases production of erythropoietin and depresses RBC production and survival time. In CRF, Hb and Hct are usually low but tolerated; e.g., patient may not be symptomatic until Hb is below 7.
Platelet count, clotting factors;	Suppression of platelet formation and inadequate levels of factors III and VIII impair clotting and potentiate risk of bleeding. *Note:* Bleeding may become intractable in end-stage disease.
Prothrombin time (PT) level.	Abnormal prothrombin consumption lowers serum levels and impairs clotting.
Administer fresh blood, packed RBCs (PRCs) as indicated.	May be necessary when patient is symptomatic with anemia. PRCs are usually given when patient is experiencing fluid overload or being dialyzed. Washed RBCs are used to prevent hyperkalemia associated with stored blood.
Administer medications, as indicated, e.g.:	
Erythropoietin preparations, (Epogen, EPO, Procrit);	Corrects many of the symptoms of CRF resulting from anemia by stimulating the production and maintenance of RBCs, thus decreasing the need for transfusion.
Iron preparations: folic acid (Folvite), cyanocobalamin (Betalin);	Useful in managing symptomatic anemia related to nutritional/dialysis-induced deficits. *Note:* Iron should not be given with phosphate binders because they may decrease iron absorption.
Cimetidine (Tagamet), ranitidine (Zantac); antacids;	May be given prophylactically to reduce/neutralize gastric acid and thereby reduce the risk of GI hemorrhage.
Hemastatics/fibrinolysis inhibitors, e.g., aminocaproic acid (Amicar);	Inhibits bleeding that does not subside spontaneously/respond to usual treatment.
Stool softeners (e.g., Colace); bulk laxative (e.g., Metamucil).	Straining to pass hard-formed stool increases likelihood of mucosal/rectal bleeding.

ACTIONS/INTERVENTIONS	RATIONALE
Reality Orientation (NIC)	
Independent	
Assess extent of impairment in thinking ability, memory, and orientation. Note attention span.	Uremic syndrome's effect can begin with minor confusion/irritability and progress to altered personality or inability to assimilate information and participate in care. Awareness of changes provides opportunity for evaluation and intervention.
Ascertain from SO patient's usual level of mentation.	Provides comparison to evaluate progression/resolution of impairment.
Provide SO with information about patient's status.	Some improvement in mentation may be expected with restoration of more normal levels of BUN, electrolytes, and serum pH.
Provide quiet/calm environment and judicious use of television, radio, and visitation.	Minimizes environmental stimuli to reduce sensory overload/increased confusion while preventing sensory deprivation.
Reorient to surroundings, person, and so forth. Provide calendars, clocks, outside window.	Provides clues to aid in recognition of reality.
Present reality concisely, briefly, and do not challenge illogical thinking.	Confrontation potentiates defensive reactions and may lead to patient mistrust and heightened denial of reality.
Communicate information/instructions in simple, short sentences. Ask direct, yes/no questions. Repeat explanations as necessary.	May aid in reducing confusion and increases possibility that communications will be understood/remembered.
Establish a regular schedule for expected activities.	Aids in maintaining reality orientation and may reduce fear/confusion.
Promote adequate rest and undisturbed periods for sleep.	Sleep deprivation may further impair cognitive abilities.
Collaborative	
Monitor laboratory studies, e.g., BUN/Cr, serum electrolytes, glucose level, and ABGs (Po_2, pH).	Correction of elevations/imbalances can have profound effects on cognition/mentation.

ACTIONS/INTERVENTIONS

Collaborative

Provide supplemental O_2 as indicated.

Avoid use of barbiturates and opiates.

Prepare for dialysis.

RATIONALE

Correction of hypoxia alone can improve cognition.

Drugs normally detoxified in the kidneys will have increased half-life/cumulative effects, worsening confusion.

Marked deterioration of thought processes may indicate worsening of azotemia and general condition, requiring prompt intervention to regain homeostasis.

NURSING DIAGNOSIS: Skin Integrity, risk for impaired

Risk factors may include

Altered metabolic state, circulation (anemia with tissue ischemia), and sensation (peripheral neuropathy)

Alterations in skin turgor (edema/dehydration)

Reduced activity/immobility

Accumulation of toxins in the skin

Possibly evidenced by

[Not applicable; presence of signs and symptoms establishes an *actual* diagnosis]

DESIRED OUTCOMES/EVALUATION CRITERIA—PATIENT WILL:

Tissue Integrity: Skin and Mucous Membranes (NOC)

Maintain intact skin.

Risk Management (NOC)

Demonstrate behaviors/techniques to prevent skin breakdown/injury.

ACTIONS/INTERVENTIONS

Skin Surveillance (NIC)

Independent

Inspect skin for changes in color, turgor, vascularity. Note redness, excoriation. Observe for ecchymosis, purpura.

Monitor fluid intake and hydration of skin and mucous membranes.

Inspect dependent areas for edema. Elevate legs as indicated.

Change position frequently; move patient carefully; pad bony prominences with sheepskin, elbow/heel protectors.

Provide soothing skin care. Restrict use of soaps. Apply ointments or creams (e.g., lanolin, Aquaphor).

Keep linens dry, wrinkle-free.

RATIONALE

Indicates areas of poor circulation/breakdown that may lead to decubitus formation/infection.

Detects presence of dehydration or overhydration that affect circulation and tissue integrity at the cellular level.

Edematous tissues are more prone to breakdown. Elevation promotes venous return, limiting venous stasis/edema formation.

Decreases pressure on edematous, poorly perfused tissues to reduce ischemia.

Baking soda, cornstarch baths decrease itching and are less drying than soaps. Lotions and ointments may be desired to relieve dry, cracked skin.

Reduces dermal irritation and risk of skin breakdown.

ACTIONS/INTERVENTIONS	RATIONALE
Independent	
Investigate reports of itching.	Although dialysis has largely eliminated skin problems associated with uremic frost, itching can occur because the skin is an excretory route for waste products, e.g., phosphate crystals (associated with hyperparathyroidism in end-stage disease).
Recommend patient use cool, moist compresses to apply pressure (rather than scratch) pruritic areas. Keep fingernails short; encourage use of gloves during sleep if needed.	Alleviates discomfort and reduces risk of dermal injury.
Suggest wearing loose-fitting cotton garments.	Prevents direct dermal irritation and promotes evaporation of moisture on the skin.
Collaborative	
Provide foam/flotation mattress.	Reduces prolonged pressure on tissues, which can limit cellular perfusion, potentiating ischemia/necrosis.

NURSING DIAGNOSIS: Oral Mucous Membrane, risk for altered

Risk factors may include
Lack of/or decreased salivation, fluid restrictions
Chemical irritation, conversion of urea in saliva to ammonia

Possibly evidenced by
[Not applicable; presence of signs and symptoms establishes an *actual* diagnosis]

DESIRED OUTCOMES/EVALUATION CRITERIA—PATIENT WILL:

Oral Health (NOC)

Maintain integrity of mucous membranes.
Identify/initiate specific interventions to promote healthy oral mucosa.

ACTIONS/INTERVENTIONS	RATIONALE
Oral Health Maintenance (NIC)	
Independent	
Inspect oral cavity; note moistness, character of saliva, presence of inflammation, ulcerations, leukoplakia.	Provides opportunity for prompt intervention and prevention of infection.
Provide fluids throughout 24-hr period within prescribed limit.	Prevents excessive oral dryness from prolonged period without oral intake.
Offer frequent mouth care/rinse with 0.25% acetic acid solution; provide gum, hard candy, breath mints between meals.	Mucous membranes may become dry and cracked. Mouth care soothes, lubricates, and helps freshen mouth taste, which is often unpleasant because of uremia and restricted oral intake. Rinsing with acetic acid helps neutralize ammonia formed by conversion of urea.
Encourage good dental hygiene after meals and at bedtime. Recommend avoidance of dental floss.	Reduces bacterial growth and potential for infection. Dental floss may cut gums, potentiating bleeding.
Recommend patient stop smoking and avoid lemon/glycerine products or mouthwash containing alcohol.	These substances are irritating to the mucosa and have a drying effect, potentiating discomfort.
Provide artificial saliva as needed, e.g., Ora-Lube.	Prevents dryness, buffers acids, and promotes comfort.

ACTIONS/INTERVENTIONS

Collaborative

Administer medications as indicated, e.g., antihistamines: cyproheptadine (Periactin).

RATIONALE

May be given for relief of itching.

NURSING DIAGNOSIS: Knowledge Deficit [Learning Need] regarding condition, prognosis, treatment, self care, and discharge needs

May be related to
Lack of exposure/recall, information misinterpretation
Cognitive limitation

Possibly evidenced by
Questions/request for information, statement of misconception
Inaccurate follow-through of instructions/development of preventable complications

DESIRED OUTCOMES/EVALUATION CRITERIA—PATIENT WILL:

Knowledge: Disease Process (NOC)

Verbalize understanding of condition/disease process and potential complications.

Knowledge: Treatment Regimen (NOC)

Verbalize understanding of therapeutic needs.
Correctly perform necessary procedures and explain reasons for the actions.
Demonstrate/initiate necessary lifestyle changes.
Participate in treatment regimen.

ACTIONS/INTERVENTIONS

RATIONALE

(In addition to interventions outlined in CP: Renal Failure: Acute; Knowledge deficit, p. 586.)

Teaching: Disease Process (NIC)

Independent

Review disease process/prognosis and future expectations.

Provides knowledge base from which patient can make informed choices.

Review dietary restrictions, including:

Phosphorus (e.g., carbonated drinks, processed foods, poultry, corn, peanuts) and magnesium (e.g., whole grain products, legumes);

Retention of phosphorus stimulates the parathyroid glands to shift calcium from bones (renal osteodystrophy), and accumulation of magnesium can impair neuromuscular function and mentation.

Fluid and sodium restrictions when indicated.

If fluid retention is a problem, the patient may need to restrict intake of fluid to 1100 cc (or less) and restrict dietary sodium. If fluid overload is present, diuretic therapy or dialysis will be part of the regimen. (Refer to CP: Renal Failure, Acute, ND: Fluid Volume excess, p. 578.)

Discuss other nutritional concerns, e.g., regulating protein intake according to level of renal function (generally 0.6–0.7 g/k of body weight per day of good quality protein, such as meat, eggs).

Metabolites that accumulate in blood derive almost entirely from protein catabolism; as renal function declines proteins may be restricted proportionately. Too little protein can result in malnutrition. *Note:* The patient on dialysis may not need to be as vigilant with protein intake.

ACTIONS/INTERVENTIONS	RATIONALE

Independent

Encourage adequate calorie intake, especially from carbohydrates in the nondiabetic patient.	Spares protein, prevents wasting, and provides energy. *Note:* Use of special glucose polymer powders can add calories to enhance energy level without extra food or fluid intake.
Discuss drug therapy, including use of calcium supplements and phosphate binders, e.g., aluminum hydroxide antacids (Amphojel, Basalgel) and avoidance of magnesium antacids (Mylanta, Maalox, Gelusil); vitamin D.	Prevents serious complications, e.g., reducing phosphate absorption from the GI tract and supplying calcium to maintain normal serum levels, reducing risk of bone demineralization/fractures, tetany; however, use of aluminum-containing products should be monitored because accumulation in the bones potentiates osteodystrophy. Magnesium products potentiate risk of hypermagnesemia. *Note:* Supplemental vitamin D may be required to facilitate calcium absorption.
Stress importance of reading all product labels (drugs and food) and not taking medications without prior approval of healthcare provider.	It is difficult to maintain electrolyte balance when exogenous intake is not factored into dietary restrictions, e.g., hypercalcemia can result from routine supplement use in combination with increased dietary intake of calcium-fortified foods and medications containing calcium.
Review measures to prevent bleeding/hemorrhage, e.g., use of soft toothbrush, electric razor; avoidance of constipation, forceful blowing of nose, strenuous exercise/contact sports.	Reduces risks related to alteration of clotting factors/ decreased platelet count.
Instruct in self-observation and self-monitoring of BP, including scheduling rest period before taking BP, using same arm/position.	Incidence of hypertension is increased in CRF, often requiring management with antihypertensive drugs, necessitating close observation of treatment effects, e.g., vascular response to medication.
Caution against exposure to external temperature extremes, e.g., heating pad/snow.	Peripheral neuropathy may develop, especially in lower extremities (effects of uremia, electrolyte/acid-base imbalances), impairing peripheral sensation and potentiating risk of tissue injury.
Establish routine exercise program within limits of individual ability; intersperse adequate rest periods with activities.	Aids in maintaining muscle tone and joint flexibility. Reduces risks associated with immobility (including bone demineralization), while preventing fatigue.
Address sexual concerns.	Physiological effects of uremia/antihypertensive therapy may impair sexual desire/performance.
Identify available resources as indicated. Stress necessity of medical and laboratory follow-up.	Close monitoring of renal function and electrolyte balance is necessary to adjust dietary prescription, treatment and/or make decisions about possible options such as dialysis/transplantation.
Identify signs/symptoms requiring immediate medical evaluation, e.g.:	
Low-grade fever, chills, changes in characteristics of urine/sputum, tissue swelling/drainage, oral ulcerations;	Depressed immune system, anemia, malnutrition all contribute to increased risk of infection.
Numbness/tingling of digits, abdominal/muscle cramps, carpopedal spasms;	Uremia and decreased absorption of calcium may lead to peripheral neuropathies.

ACTIONS/INTERVENTIONS	RATIONALE

Independent

Joint swelling/tenderness, decreased ROM, reduced muscle strength;	Hyperphosphatemia with corresponding calcium shifts from the bone may result in deposition of the excess calcium phosphate as calcifications in joints and soft tissues. Symptoms of skeletal involvement are often noted before impairment in organ function is evident.
Headaches, blurred vision, periorbital/sacral edema, "red eyes";	Suggestive of development/poor control of hypertension, and/or changes in eyes caused by calcium.
Review strategies to prevent constipation, including stool softeners (Colace) and bulk laxatives (Metamucil) but avoiding magnesium products (Milk of Magnesia).	Reduced fluid intake, changes in dietary pattern, and use of phosphate-binding products often result in constipation that is not responsive to nonmedical interventions. Use of products containing magnesium increases risk of hypermagnesemia.

POTENTIAL CONSIDERATIONS following acute hospitalization (dependent on patient's age, physical condition/presence of complications, personal resources, and life responsibilities)

Fluid Volume excess—compromised regulatory mechanism.

Fatigue—decreased metabolic energy production/dietary restriction, anemia, increased energy requirements, e.g., fever/inflammation, tissue regeneration.

Therapeutic Regimen: Individual, ineffective management—complexity of therapeutic regimen, decisional conflicts: patient value system; health beliefs, cultural influences; powerlessness; economic difficulties; family conflict; lack of/refusal of support systems.

Hopelessness—deteriorating physiological condition, long-term stress, prolonged activity limitations.

RENAL DIALYSIS

Dialysis is a process that substitutes for renal function by removing excess fluid and/or accumulated endogenous or exogenous toxins. Dialysis is most often used for patients with ARF and chronic (end-stage) renal disease. The two most common types are hemodialysis and peritoneal dialysis. Dialysis therapies include intermittent hemodialysis (IHD), continuous arteriovenous hemodialysis (CAVHD), continuous venovenous hemodialysis (CVVHD), and peritoneal dialysis.

Patients with ARF are sometimes so hemodynamically unstable that they cannot tolerate conventional hemodialysis. These patients may benefit from continuous renal replacement therapy (CRRT), which more slowly removes plasma water and compensates for the loss of intravascular volume. Ultrafiltration methods include continuous arteriovenous hemofiltration (CAVH) and continuous venovenous hemofiltration (CVVH).

The chosen type of fluid and or solute removal depends on the patient's cause for renal failure, current hemodynamic status, vascular access, and healthcare providers' equipment and training.

CARE SETTING

Community level/dialysis center, although inpatient acute stay may be required during initiation of therapy.

RELATED CONCERNS

Anemias (Iron deficiency, pernicious, aplastic, hemolytic), page 531
Heart failure: chronic, page 47
Peritonitis, page 382
Psychosocial aspects of care, page 809
Sepsis/Septicemia, page 741
Total nutritional support: parenteral/enteral feeding, page 508
Transplantation: postoperative and lifelong needs, page 801

Patient Assessment Database

Refer to CPs: Renal Failure: Acute, page 575; Renal Failure: Chronic, page 588 for assessment information.

Discharge plan considerations: **DRG projected mean length of inpatient stay: 2.2 days to initiate therapy**
May require assistance with treatment regimen, transportation, activities of daily living (ADLs), homemaker/maintenance tasks

Refer to section at end of plan for postdischarge considerations.

DIAGNOSTIC STUDIES

Studies and results are variable, depending on reason for dialysis (e.g., removal of excess fluid or toxins/drugs), degree of renal involvement, and patient considerations (e.g., distance from treatment center, cognition, available support).

NURSING PRIORITIES

1. Promote homeostasis.
2. Maintain comfort.
3. Prevent complications.
4. Support patient independence/self-care.
5. Provide information about disease process/prognosis and treatment needs.

DISCHARGE GOALS

1. Fluid and electrolyte balance maximized.
2. Complications prevented/minimized.
3. Discomfort alleviated.
4. Dealing realistically with current situation; independent within limits of condition.
5. Disease process/prognosis and therapeutic regimen understood.
6. Plan in place to meet needs after discharge.

GENERAL CONSIDERATIONS

This section addresses the general nursing management issues of the patient receiving some form of dialysis.

NURSING DIAGNOSIS: Nutrition: altered, less than body requirements

May be related to

GI disturbances (result of uremia/medication side effects): anorexia, nausea/vomiting, and stomatitis

Sensation of feeling full (abdominal distension during continuous ambulatory peritoneal dialysis [CAPD])

Dietary restrictions (bland, tasteless food); lack of interest in food

Loss of peptides and amino acids (building blocks for proteins) during dialysis

Possibly evidenced by

Inadequate food intake, aversion to eating, altered taste sensation

Poor muscle tone/weakness

Sore, inflamed buccal cavity; pale conjunctiva/mucous membranes

DESIRED OUTCOMES/EVALUATION CRITERIA—PATIENT WILL:

Nutritional Status (NOC)

Demonstrate stable weight/gain toward goal with normalization of laboratory values and no signs of malnutrition.

ACTIONS/INTERVENTIONS	RATIONALE
Nutrition Therapy (NIC)	
Independent	
Monitor food/fluid ingested and calculate daily caloric intake.	Identifies nutritional deficits/therapy needs.
Recommend patient/SO keep a food diary, including estimation of ingested calories, electrolytes of individual concern (e.g., sodium, potassium, chloride, magnesium), and protein.	Helps patient realize "big picture" and allows opportunity to alter dietary choices to meet individual desires within identified restriction.
Measure muscle mass via triceps skinfold or similar procedure. Determine muscle-to-fat ratio.	Assesses adequacy of nutrient utilization by measuring changes in fat deposits that may suggest presence/absence of tissue catabolism.
Note presence of nausea/anorexia.	Symptoms accompany accumulation of endogenous toxins that can alter/reduce intake and require intervention.
Encourage patient to participate in menu planning.	May enhance oral intake and promote sense of control/responsibility.
Recommend small, frequent meals. Schedule meals according to dialysis needs.	Smaller portions may enhance intake. Type of dialysis influences meal patterns, e.g., patients receiving hemodialysis might not be fed directly before/during procedure because this can alter fluid removal, and patients undergoing peritoneal dialysis may be unable to ingest food while abdomen is distended with dialysate.

ACTIONS/INTERVENTIONS	RATIONALE

Independent

Encourage use of herbs/spices, e.g., garlic, onion, pepper, parsley, cilantro, and lemon.	Adds zest to food to help reduce boredom with diet. *Note:* Some salt substitutes are high in K+ and regular soy sauce is high in Na+ and therefore are to be avoided.
Suggest socialization during meals.	Provides diversion and promotes social aspects of eating.
Encourage frequent mouth care.	Reduces discomfort of oral stomatitis and undesirable/metallic taste in mouth, which can interfere with food intake.

Collaborative

Refer to dietitian.	Necessary to develop complex and highly individual dietary program to meet cultural/lifestyle needs within specific kilocalories, protein restrictions while controlling phosphorus, sodium, potassium. *Note:* Dietary allowances tend to be somewhat more liberal for patients receiving peritoneal dialysis because of the frequency of exchanges.
Provide a balanced diet of complex carbohydrates and ordered amount of high-quality protein and essential amino acids.	Provides sufficient nutrients to improve energy and prevent muscle wasting (catabolism); promotes tissue regeneration/healing, and electrolyte balance. *Note:* Fifty percent of protein intake should be derived from protein sources with high biological value, such as red meat, poultry, fish, eggs.
Restrict sodium/potassium as indicated, e.g., avoid bacon, ham, other processed meats and foods, orange juice, tomato soup.	These electrolytes can quickly accumulate, causing fluid retention, weakness, and potentially lethal cardiac dysrhythmias. *Note:* Peritoneal dialysis is not as effective in lowering elevated Na+ level, necessitating tighter control of Na+ intake.
Administer multivitamins, including ascorbic acid (vitamin C), folic acid, vitamins B_6 and D, and iron supplements, as indicated.	Replaces vitamin/mineral deficits resulting from malnutrition/anemia or lost during dialysis.
Administer parenteral supplements as indicated.	Hyperalimentation may be needed to enhance renal tubular regeneration/resolution of underlying disease process and to provide nutrients if oral/enteral feeding is contraindicated.
Monitor laboratory studies, e.g.:	
Serum protein, prealbumin/albumin levels;	Indicator of protein needs. *Note:* Peritoneal dialysis is associated with significant protein loss.
Hb, RBC, and iron levels.	Anemia is the most pervasive complication affecting energy levels in ESRD.
Administer medications as appropriate:	
Antiemetics, e.g., prochlorperazine (Compazine);	Reduces stimulation of the vomiting center.
Histamine blockers, e.g., famotidine (Pepcid);	Gastric distress is common and may be a neuropathy-induced gastric paresis. Hypersecretion can cause persistent gastric distress and digestive dysfunction.

ACTIONS/INTERVENTIONS

Collaborative

Hormones and supplements as indicated, e.g., erythropoietin (EPO, Epogen) and iron supplement (Niferex).

Insert/maintain nasogastric (NG) tube if indicated.

RATIONALE

Although EPO is given to increase numbers of RBCs, it is not effective without iron supplementation. Niferex is preferred because it can be given once daily and has fewer side effects than many iron preparations.

May be necessary when persistent vomiting occurs or when enteral feeding is desired.

NURSING DIAGNOSIS: Mobility, impaired physical

May be related to
Restrictive therapies, e.g., lengthy dialysis procedure
Fear of/real danger of dislodging dialysis lines/catheter
Decreased strength/endurance; musculoskeletal impairment
Perceptual/cognitive impairment

Possibly evidenced by
Reluctance to attempt movement
Inability to move within physical environment
Decreased muscle mass/tone and strength
Impaired coordination
Pain, discomfort

DESIRED OUTCOMES/EVALUATION CRITERIA—PATIENT WILL:

Mobility Level (NOC)

Maintain optimal mobility/function.
Display increased strength and be free of associated complications (contractures, decubiti).

ACTIONS/INTERVENTIONS

Bed Rest Care (NIC)

Independent

Assess activity limitations, noting presence/degree of restriction/ability.

Encourage frequent change of position when on bedrest or chair rest; support affected body parts/joints with pillows, rolls, sheepskin, elbow/heel pads as indicated.

Provide gentle massage. Keep skin clean and dry. Keep linens dry and wrinkle-free.

Encourage deep breathing and coughing. Elevate head of bed as appropriate.

Suggest/provide diversion as appropriate to patient's condition, e.g., visitors, radio/television, books. Take time to interact with patient, showing interest in their lives.

RATIONALE

Influences choice of interventions.

Decreases discomfort, maintains muscle strength/joint mobility, enhances circulation, and prevents skin breakdown.

Stimulates circulation; prevents skin irritation.

Mobilizes secretions, improves lung expansion, and reduces risk of respiratory complications, e.g., atelectasis, pneumonia.

Decreases boredom; promotes relaxation. *Note:* Recent studies indicate that patients on dialysis do feel bored and that caregivers/dialysis staff do not tend to talk with them, resulting in patients feeling like they are "just part of the scenery."

ACTIONS/INTERVENTIONS	RATIONALE
Independent	
Instruct in and assist with active/passive ROM exercises.	Maintains joint flexibility, prevents contractures, and aids in reducing muscle tension.
Institute a planned activity/exercise program as appropriate, with patient's input.	Increases patient's energy and sense of well-being/control. Studies have shown that regular exercise programs have benefited patients with ESRD both physically and emotionally. Stable patients have not been shown to have adverse effects.
Collaborative	
Provide foam/flotation mattress or soft chair cushion.	Reduces tissue pressure and may enhance circulation, thereby reducing risk of dermal ischemia/breakdown.

NURSING DIAGNOSIS: Self-Care deficit (specify)

May be related to
Intolerance to activity; decreased strength and endurance; pain/discomfort
Perceptual/cognitive impairment (accumulated toxins)

Possibly evidenced by
Reported inability to carry out ADLs
Disheveled/unkempt appearance, strong body odor

DESIRED OUTCOMES/EVALUATION CRITERIA—PATIENT WILL:

Self-Care: Activities of Daily Living (ADLs) (NOC)

Participate in ADLs within level of own ability/constraints of the illness.

ACTIONS/INTERVENTIONS	RATIONALE
Self-Care Assistance (NIC)	
Independent	
Determine patient's ability to participate in self-care activities (scale of 0–4).	Underlying condition dictates level of deficit/needs affecting choice of interventions.
Provide assistance with activities as necessary.	Meets needs while supporting patient participation and independence.
Encourage/use energy-saving techniques, e.g., sitting, not standing; using shower chair; doing tasks in small increments.	Conserves energy, reduces fatigue, and enhances patient ability to perform tasks.
Recommend scheduling activities to allow patient sufficient time to accomplish tasks to fullest extent of ability.	Unhurried approach reduces frustration, promotes patient participation, enhancing self-esteem.

NURSING DIAGNOSIS: Constipation, risk for

Risk factors may include
Decreased fluid intake, altered dietary pattern
Reduced intestinal motility, compression of bowel (peritoneal dialysate); electrolyte imbalances; decreased mobility

Possibly evidenced by
[Not applicable; presence of signs and symptoms establishes an *actual* diagnosis]

DESIRED OUTCOMES/EVALUATION CRITERIA—PATIENT WILL:

Bowel Elimination (NOC)

Maintain usual/improved bowel function.

ACTIONS/INTERVENTIONS

Constipation/Impaction Management (NIC)

Independent

Auscultate bowel sounds. Note consistency/frequency of bowel movements (BMs), presence of abdominal distension.

Review current medication regimen.

Ascertain usual dietary pattern/food choices.

Suggest adding fresh fruits, vegetables, and fiber to diet (within restrictions) when indicated.

Encourage/assist with ambulation when able.

Provide privacy at bedside commode/bathroom.

Collaborative

Administer stool softeners (e.g., Colace), bulk-forming laxatives (e.g., Metamucil) as indicated.

Keep patient NPO; insert NG tube as indicated.

RATIONALE

Decreased bowel sounds, passage of hard-formed/dry stools suggests constipation and requires ongoing intervention to manage.

Side effects of some drugs (e.g., iron products, some antacids) may compound problem.

Although restrictions may be present, thoughtful consideration of menu choices can aid in controlling problem.

Provides bulk, which improves stool consistency.

Activity may stimulate peristalsis, promoting return to normal bowel activity.

Promotes psychological comfort needed for elimination.

Produces a softer/more easily evacuated stool.

Decompresses stomach when recurrent episodes of unrelieved vomiting occur. Large gastric output suggests ileus (common early complication of peritoneal dialysis) with accumulation of gas and intestinal fluid that cannot be passed rectally.

NURSING DIAGNOSIS: Thought Processes, altered

May be related to
Physiological changes, e.g., presence of uremic toxins, electrolyte imbalances, hypervolemia/fluid shifts; hyperglycemia (infusion of a dialysate with a high glucose concentration)

Possibly evidenced by
Changes in mentation/behavior, e.g., decreased concentration, memory; disorientation; altered sleep patterns; lethargy, confusion, stupor, dementia

Cognitive Ability (NOC)

Regain usual/improved level of mentation.
Recognize changes in thinking/behavior and demonstrate behaviors to prevent/minimize changes.

ACTIONS/INTERVENTIONS	RATIONALE

Delirium Management (NIC)

Independent

Assess for behavioral change/change in level of consciousness, e.g., orientation to time, place, and person.	May indicate level of uremic toxicity, response to or developing complication of dialysis (e.g., "dialysis dementia" secondary to accumulation of aluminum) and requires further assessment/intervention.
Keep explanations simple, reorient frequently. Provide "normal" day/night lighting patterns, clock, calendar.	Improves reality orientation.
Provide a safe environment, restrain as indicated, pad side rails during procedure as appropriate.	Prevents patient trauma and/or inadvertent removal of dialysis lines/catheter.
Drain peritoneal dialysate promptly at end of specified equilibration period.	Prompt outflow will decrease risk of hyperglycemia/hyperosmolar fluid shifts affecting cerebral function.
Investigate reports of headache, associated with onset of nausea/vomiting, confusion/agitation, hypertension, tremors, or seizure activity.	May reflect development of disequilibrium syndrome, which can occur near completion of/following hemodialysis and is thought to be caused by ultrafiltration or by the too-rapid removal of urea from the bloodstream not accompanied by equivalent removal from brain tissue. The hypertonic cerebrospinal fluid (CSF) causes a fluid shift into the brain, resulting in cerebral edema.
Monitor changes in speech pattern, development of dementia, myoclonus activity during hemodialysis.	Occasionally, accumulation of aluminum may cause dialysis dementia, progressing to death if untreated.

Collaborative

Monitor BUN/Cr, serum glucose; alternate/change dialysate concentrations or add insulin as indicated.	Follows progression/resolution of azotemia. Hyperglycemia may develop secondary to glucose crossing peritoneal membrane and entering circulation. May require initiation of insulin therapy.
Obtain aluminum level as indicated.	Elevation may warn of impending cerebral involvement/dialysis dementia.
Administer medication, as indicated, e.g., phenytoin (Dilantin).	If disequilibrium syndrome occurs during dialysis, medication may be needed to control seizures in addition to a change in dialysis prescription or discontinuation of therapy.

NURSING DIAGNOSIS: Anxiety [specify level]/Fear

May be related to
Situational crisis, threat to self-concept; change in health status/role functioning, socioeconomic status
Threat of death, unknown consequences/outcome

Possibly evidenced by

Increased tension, apprehension, uncertainty, fear

Expressed concerns

Sympathetic stimulation; focus on self

DESIRED OUTCOMES/EVALUATION CRITERIA—PATIENT WILL:

Anxiety or Fear Control (NOC)

Verbalize awareness of feelings and reduction of anxiety/fear to a manageable level.

Demonstrate problem-solving skills and effective use of resources.

Appear relaxed, able to rest/sleep appropriately.

ACTIONS/INTERVENTIONS	RATIONALE
Anxiety Reduction (NIC)	
Independent	
Assess level of fear of both patient and SO. Note signs of denial, depression, or narrowed focus of attention.	Helps determine the kind of interventions required.
Explain procedures/care as delivered. Repeat explanations frequently/as needed. Provide information in multiple formats, including pamphlets and films.	Fear of unknown is lessened by information/knowledge and may enhance acceptance of permanence of ESRD and necessity for dialysis. Alteration in thought processes and high levels of anxiety/fear may reduce comprehension, requiring repetition of important information. *Note:* Uremia can impair short-term memory, requiring repetition/reinforcement of information provided.
Acknowledge normalcy of feelings in this situation.	Knowing feelings are normal can allay fear that patient is losing control.
Provide opportunities for patient/SO to ask questions and verbalize concerns.	Creates feeling of openness and cooperation and provides information that will assist in problem identification/solving.
Encourage SO to participate in care, as able/desired.	Involvement promotes sense of sharing, strengthens feelings of usefulness, provides opportunity to acknowledge individual capabilities, and may lessen fear of the unknown.
Acknowledge concerns of patient/SO.	Prognosis/possibility of need for long-term dialysis and resultant lifestyle changes are a major concern for this patient and those who may be involved in future care.
Point out positive indicators of treatment, e.g., improvement in laboratory values, stable BP, lessened fatigue.	Promotes sense of success/progress in an otherwise chronic process that seems endless while patient still is experiencing physical deterioration and depression.
Collaborative	
Arrange for visit to dialysis center/meeting with another dialysis patient as appropriate.	Interaction with others who have encountered similar problems may assist patient/SO to work toward acceptance of chronic condition/focus on problem-solving activities.

May be related to

Situational crisis, chronic illness with changes in usual roles/body image

Possibly evidenced by

Verbalization of changes in lifestyle; focus on past function, negative feelings about body; feelings of helplessness, powerlessness

Continuous physical deterioration, premature aging, disfigurement

Extension of body boundary to incorporate environmental objects (e.g., dialysis equipment)

Change in social involvement

Overdependence on others for care, not taking responsibility for self-care/lack of follow-through, self-destructive behavior

DESIRED OUTCOMES/EVALUATION CRITERIA—PATIENT WILL:

Self-Esteem (NOC)

Identify feelings and methods for coping with negative perception of self.

Verbalize acceptance of self in situation.

Demonstrate adaptation to changes/events that have occurred, as evidenced by setting realistic goals and active participation in care/life.

ACTIONS/INTERVENTIONS	RATIONALE
Body Image or Self-Esteem Enhancement (NIC)	
Independent	
Assess level of patient's knowledge about condition and treatment and anxiety related to current situation.	Identifies extent of problem/concern and necessary interventions.
Support active information seeking by patient/SO.	Concern/belief that sharing of information may be "controlled" by healthcare providers perpetuates sense of a "power differential," potentiating dependence/mistrust.
Discuss meaning of loss/change to the patient.	Some patients may view situation as a challenge, though many have difficulty dealing with changes in life/role performance and loss of ability to control own body.
Note withdrawn behavior, ineffective use of denial, or behaviors indicative of overconcern with body and its functions. Investigate reports of feelings of depersonalization or the bestowing of humanlike qualities on machinery.	Indicators of developing difficulty handling stress of what is happening. *Note:* Some patients may feel tied to/controlled by technology central to their survival, even to the point of extending body boundary to incorporate dialysis equipment.
Assess use of addictive substances (e.g., alcohol), self-destructive/suicidal behavior.	May reflect dysfunctional coping and attempt to handle problems in an ineffective manner.
Determine stage of grieving. Note signs of severe/prolonged depression.	Identification of stage patient is experiencing provides guide to recognizing and dealing appropriately with behavior as patient/SO works to come to terms with loss and limitations associated with condition. Prolonged depression may indicate need for further intervention.

ACTIONS/INTERVENTIONS	RATIONALE

Independent

Acknowledge normalcy of feelings.	Recognition that feelings are to be expected helps patient to accept and deal with them more effectively.
Encourage verbalization of personal and work conflicts that may arise. Active-listen concerns.	Helps patient identify problems and problem-solve solutions.
Determine patient's role in family constellation and patient's perception of expectation of self and others.	Long-term/permanent illness and disability alter patient's ability to fulfill usual role(s) in family/work setting. Unrealistic expectations can undermine self-esteem and affect outcome of illness.
Recommend SO treat patient normally and not as an invalid.	Conveys expectation that patient is able to manage situation and helps maintain sense of self-worth and purpose in life.
Assist patient to incorporate disease management into lifestyle.	Necessities of treatment assume a more normal aspect when they are a part of the daily routine.
Identify strengths, past successes, previous methods patient has used to deal with life stressors.	Focusing on these reminders of own ability to deal with problems can help patient deal with current situation.
Help patient identify areas over which they have some measure of control. Provide opportunity to participate in decision-making process.	Provides sense of control over uncontrollable situation, fostering independence.

Collaborative

Recommend participation in local support group.	Reduces sense of isolation as patient learns that others have been where patient is now. Provides role models for dealing with situation, problem solving and "getting on with life." Reinforces that therapeutic regimen can be beneficial.
Refer to healthcare/community resources, e.g., social service, vocational counselor, psychiatric nurse specialist.	Provides additional assistance for long-term management of chronic illness/change in lifestyle.

NURSING DIAGNOSIS: Knowledge Deficit [Learning Need] regarding condition, prognosis, treatment, self care, and discharge needs

May be related to
Lack of exposure/recall
Unfamiliarity with information resources
Cognitive limitations

Possibly evidenced by
Questions/request for information; statement of misconception
Inaccurate follow-through of instruction/development of preventable complications

DESIRED OUTCOMES/EVALUATION CRITERIA—PATIENT WILL:

Knowledge: Disease Process (NOC)

Verbalize understanding of condition and relationship of signs/symptoms of the disease process, and potential complications.

Knowledge: Treatment Regimen (NOC)

Verbalize understanding of therapeutic needs.
Correctly perform necessary procedures and explain reasons for actions.

ACTIONS/INTERVENTIONS	RATIONALE

Teaching: Disease Process (NIC)

Independent

Note level of anxiety/fear and alteration of thought processes.

These factors directly affect ability to participate/access and use knowledge. In addition, studies indicate that during the dialysis procedure, the patient's cognitive function may be impaired, and patients themselves state that they feel "fuzzy." Therefore, learning may not be optimal during this time.

Review particular disease process, procedures, and purpose of dialysis in terms understandable to the patient. Repeat explanations as required.

Providing information at the level of the patient's/SO's understanding will reduce anxiety and misconceptions about what the patient is experiencing.

Acknowledge that certain feelings/patterns of response are normal during course of therapy.

Patient/SO may initially be hopeful and positive about the future, but as treatment continues and progress is less dramatic, they can become discouraged/depressed, and conflicts of dependence/independence may develop.

Encourage and provide opportunity for questions.

Enhances learning process, promotes informed decision making, and reduces anxiety associated with the unknown.

Stress necessity of reading all product labels (food/beverage and OTC drugs) and not taking medications/herbal supplements without prior approval of healthcare provider.

It is difficult to maintain electrolyte balance when exogenous intake is not factored into dietary restriction, e.g., hypercalcemia can result from routine supplement use in combination with increased dietary intake of calcium-fortified foods and medicines.

Discuss significance of maintaining nutritious eating habits; preventing wide fluctuation of fluid/electrolyte balance; avoidance of crowds/people with infectious processes.

Depressed immune system, presence of anemia, invasive procedures, and malnutrition potentiate risk of infection.

Instruct patient/SO in home dialysis as indicated:

Purpose of dialysis;

Provides knowledge base from which patient can make informed observations/choices.

Operation and maintenance of equipment (including vascular shunt); sources of supplies;

Information diminishes anxiety of the unknown and provides opportunity for patient to be knowledgeable about own care.

Aseptic/clean technique;

Prevents contamination and reduces risk of infection.

Self-monitoring of effectiveness of procedure;

Provides information necessary to evaluate effects of therapy/need for change.

Management of potential complications;

Reduces concerns regarding personal well-being; supports efforts at self-care.

Contact person.

Readily available support person can answer questions, troubleshoot problems, and facilitate timely medical intervention when indicated.

Instruct patient about Epoetin (Epogen) when indicated. Have patient/SO demonstrate ability to administer and state adverse side effects and healthcare practices associated with this therapy.

Epogen is used for the management of the anemia associated with CRF. The drug is given to increase and maintain RBC production, which can allow the patient to feel better and stronger. Contraindications may include adverse side effects such as polycythemia/increased clotting, failure to administer correctly or have appropriate follow-up.

ACTIONS/INTERVENTIONS

Independent

Identify healthcare/community resources, e.g., dialysis support group, social services, mental health clinic.

RATIONALE

Knowledge and use of these resources assist patient/SO to manage care more effectively. Interaction with others in similar situation provides opportunity for discussion of options and making informed choices, e.g., stopping dialysis, renal transplantation.

(Refer to Renal Dialysis: Peritoneal, following, or Hemodialysis, page 618, to complete the plan of care.)

POTENTIAL CONSIDERATIONS following acute hospitalization (dependent on patient's age, physical condition/presence of complications, personal resources, and life responsibilities)

Fatigue—decreased metabolic energy production, states of discomfort, overwhelming psychologic or emotional demands, altered body chemistry.

Fluid Volume excess—fluid retention/excessive intake, inadequate therapeutic regimen.

Infection, risk for—invasive procedures, decreased hemoglobin, chronic disease, malnutrition.

Caregiver Role Strain, risk for—severity of illness of care receiver, discharge of family member with significant home care needs, caregiver is female/spouse, presence of situational stressors.

RENAL DIALYSIS: PERITONEAL

The peritoneum serves as the semipermeable membrane permitting transfer of nitrogenous wastes/toxins and fluid from the blood into a dialysate solution. Peritoneal dialysis is sometimes preferred because it uses a simpler technique and provides more gradual physiological changes than hemodialysis.

The manual single-bag method is usually done as an inpatient procedure with short dwell times of only 30–60 minutes and is repeated until desired effects are achieved. The most commonly used type of peritoneal dialysis is continuous ambulatory peritoneal dialysis (CAPD), which permits the patient to manage the procedure at home with bag and gravity flow, using a prolonged dwell time at night and a total of 3–5 cycles daily, 7 days a week. No machinery is required.

Continuous cycling peritoneal dialysis (CCPD) mechanically cycles shorter dwell times during night (3–6 cycles) with one 8-hr dwell time during daylight hours, increasing the patient's independence. An automated machine is required to infuse and drain dialysate at preset intervals.

NURSING DIAGNOSIS: Fluid Volume risk for excess

Risk factors may include
Inadequate osmotic gradient of dialysate
Fluid retention (malpositioned or kinked/clotted catheter, bowel distension; peritonitis, scarring of peritoneum)
Excessive PO/IV intake

Possibly evidenced by
[Not applicable; presence of signs and symptoms establishes an *actual* diagnosis]

DESIRED OUTCOMES/EVALUATION CRITERIA—PATIENT WILL:

Fluid Balance (NOC)

Demonstrate dialysate outflow exceeding/approximating infusion.
Experience no rapid weight gain, edema, or pulmonary congestion.

ACTIONS/INTERVENTIONS

Peritoneal Dialysis Therapy (NIC)

Independent

Maintain a record of inflow/outflow volumes and cumulative fluid balance.

Record serial weights, compare with I&O balance. Weigh patient when abdomen is empty of dialysate (consistent reference point).

Assess patency of catheter, noting difficulty in draining. Note presence of fibrin strings/plugs.

Check tubing for kinks; note placement of bottles/bags. Anchor catheter so that adequate inflow/outflow is achieved.

Turn from side to side, elevate the head of the bed, apply gentle pressure to the abdomen.

Note abdominal distension associated with decreased bowel sounds, changes in stool consistency, reports of constipation.

RATIONALE

In most cases, the amount drained should equal or exceed the amount instilled. A positive balance indicates need of further evaluation.

Serial body weights are an accurate indicator of fluid volume status. A positive fluid balance with an increase in weight indicates fluid retention.

Slowing of flow rate/presence of fibrin suggests partial catheter occlusion requiring further evaluation/intervention.

Improper functioning of equipment may result in retained fluid in abdomen and insufficient clearance of toxins.

May enhance outflow of fluid when catheter is malpositioned/obstructed by the omentum.

Bowel distension/constipation may impede outflow of effluent. (Refer to CP: Renal Dialysis; ND: Constipation, risk for, p. 604.)

ACTIONS/INTERVENTIONS

Independent

Monitor BP and pulse, noting hypertension, bounding pulses, neck vein distension, peripheral edema; measure CVP if available.

Evaluate development of tachypnea, dyspnea, increased respiratory effort. Drain dialysate, and notify physician.

Assess for headache, muscle cramps, mental confusion, disorientation.

Collaborative

Alter dialysate regimen as indicated.

Monitor serum sodium.

Add heparin to initial dialysis runs, assist with irrigation of catheter with heparinized saline.

Maintain fluid restriction as indicated.

RATIONALE

Elevations indicate hypervolemia. Assess heart and breath sounds, noting S_3 and/or crackles, rhonchi. Fluid overload may potentiate HF/pulmonary edema.

Abdominal distension/diaphragmatic compression may cause respiratory distress.

Symptoms suggest hyponatremia or water intoxication.

Changes may be needed in the glucose or sodium concentration to facilitate efficient dialysis.

Hypernatremia may be present, although serum levels may reflect dilutional effect of fluid volume overload.

May be useful in preventing fibrin clot formation, which can obstruct peritoneal catheter.

Fluid restrictions may have to be continued to decrease fluid volume overload.

NURSING DIAGNOSIS: Fluid Volume, risk for deficit

Risk factors may include
Use of hypertonic dialysate with excessive removal of fluid from circulating volume.

Possibly evidenced by
[Not applicable; presence of signs and symptoms establishes an *actual* diagnosis]

DESIRED OUTCOMES/EVALUATION CRITERIA—PATIENT WILL:

Hydration (NOC)

Achieve desired alteration in fluid volume and weight with BP and electrolyte levels within acceptable range.
Experience no symptoms of dehydration.

ACTIONS/INTERVENTIONS

Peritoneal Dialysis Therapy (NIC)

Independent

Maintain record of inflow/outflow volumes and individual/cumulative fluid balance.

Adhere to schedule for draining dialysate from abdomen.

Weigh when abdomen is empty, following initial 6–10 runs, then as indicated.

Monitor BP (lying and sitting) and pulse. Note level of jugular pulsation.

Note reports of dizziness, nausea, increasing thirst.

RATIONALE

Provides information about the status of the patient's loss or gain at the end of each exchange.

Prolonged dwell times, especially when 4.5% glucose solution is used, may cause excessive fluid loss.

Detects rate of fluid removal by comparison with baseline body weight.

Decreased BP, postural hypotension, and tachycardia are early signs of hypovolemia.

May indicate hypovolemia/hyperosmolar syndrome.

613

ACTIONS/INTERVENTIONS	RATIONALE

ACTIONS/INTERVENTIONS

Independent

Inspect mucous membranes, evaluate skin turgor, peripheral pulses, capillary refill.

Collaborative

Monitor laboratory studies as indicated, e.g.:

Serum sodium and glucose levels;

Serum potassium levels.

RATIONALE

Dry mucous membranes, poor skin turgor and diminished pulses/capillary refill are indicators of dehydration and need for increased intake/changes in strength of dialysate.

Hypertonic solutions may cause hypernatremia by removing more water than sodium. In addition, dextrose may be absorbed from the dialysate, thereby elevating serum glucose.

Hypokalemia may occur and can cause cardiac dysrhythmias.

NURSING DIAGNOSIS: Trauma, risk for

Risk factors may include
Catheter inserted into peritoneal cavity
Site near the bowel/bladder with potential for perforation during insertion or by manipulation of the catheter

Possibly evidenced by
[Not applicable; presence of signs and symptoms establishes an *actual* diagnosis]

DESIRED OUTCOMES/EVALUATION CRITERIA—PATIENT WILL:

> **Risk Control (NOC)**

Experience no injury to bowel or bladder.

ACTIONS/INTERVENTIONS

RATIONALE

> **Peritoneal Dialysis Therapy (NIC)**

Independent

Have patient empty bladder before peritoneal catheter insertion if indwelling catheter not present.

Anchor catheter/tubing with tape. Stress importance of patient avoiding pulling/pushing on catheter. Restrain hands if indicated.

Note presence of fecal material in dialysate effluent or strong urge to defecate, accompanied by severe, watery diarrhea.

Note reports of intense urge to void, or large urine output following initiation of dialysis run. Test urine for sugar as indicated.

Stop dialysis if there is evidence of bowel/bladder perforation, leaving peritoneal catheter in place.

An empty bladder is more distant from insertion site and reduces likelihood of being punctured during catheter insertion.

Reduces risk of trauma by manipulation of the catheter.

Suggests bowel perforation with mixing of dialysate and bowel contents.

Suggests bladder perforation with dialysate leaking into bladder. Presence of glucose-containing dialysate in the bladder will elevate glucose level of urine.

Prompt action will prevent further injury. Immediate surgical repair may be required. Leaving catheter in place facilitates diagnosing/locating the perforation.

> **NURSING DIAGNOSIS: Pain [acute]**
>
> **May be related to**
>
> Insertion of catheter through abdominal wall/catheter irritation, improper catheter placement
>
> Irritation/infection within the peritoneal cavity
>
> Infusion of cold or acidic dialysate, abdominal distension, rapid infusion of dialysate
>
> **Possibly evidenced by**
>
> Reports of pain
>
> Self-focusing
>
> Guarding/distraction behaviors, restlessness
>
> **DESIRED OUTCOMES/EVALUATION CRITERIA—PATIENT WILL:**
>
> **Pain Level (NOC)**
>
> Verbalize decrease of pain/discomfort.
>
> Demonstrate relaxed posture/facial expression, be able to sleep/rest appropriately.

ACTIONS/INTERVENTIONS	RATIONALE
Pain Management (NIC)	
Independent	
Investigate patient's reports of pain; note intensity (0–10), location, and precipitating factors.	Assists in identification of source of pain and appropriate interventions.
Explain that initial discomfort usually subsides after the first few exchanges.	Information may reduce anxiety and promote relaxation during procedure.
Monitor for pain that begins during inflow and continues during equilibration phase. Slow infusion rate as indicated.	Pain occurs at these times if acidic dialysate causes chemical irritation of peritoneal membrane.
Note reports of discomfort that is most pronounced near the end of inflow and instill no more than 2000 mL of solution at a single time.	Likely the result of abdominal distension from dialysate. Amount of infusion may have to be decreased initially.
Prevent air from entering peritoneal cavity during infusion. Note report of pain in area of shoulder blade.	Inadvertent introduction of air into the abdomen irritates the diaphragm and results in referred pain to shoulder blade. This type of discomfort may also be reported during initiation of therapy/during infusions and usually is related to stretching/irritation of the diaphragm with abdominal distension. Smaller exchange volumes may be required until patient adjusts.
Elevate head of bed at intervals. Turn patient from side to side. Provide back care and tissue massage.	Position changes and gentle massage may relieve abdominal and general muscle discomfort.
Warm dialysate to body temperature before infusing.	Warming the solution increases the rate of urea removal by dilating peritoneal vessels. Cold dialysate causes vasoconstriction, which can cause discomfort and/or excessively lower the core body temperature, precipitating cardiac arrest.
Monitor for severe/continuous abdominal pain and temperature elevation (especially after dialysis has been discontinued).	May indicate developing peritonitis. (Refer to ND: Infection, risk for [peritonitis], following.)
Encourage use of relaxation techniques, e.g., deep-breathing exercises, guided imagery, visualization. Provide diversional activities.	Redirects attention, promotes sense of control.

615

ACTIONS/INTERVENTIONS	RATIONALE
Collaborative	
Administer analgesics.	Relieves pain and discomfort.
Add sodium hydroxide to dialysate, if indicated.	Occasionally used to alter pH if patient is not tolerating acidic dialysate.

NURSING DIAGNOSIS: Infection, risk for [peritonitis]

Risk factors may include
Contamination of the catheter during insertion, periodic changing of tubings/bags
Skin contaminants at catheter insertion site
Sterile peritonitis (response to the composition of dialysate)

Possibly evidenced by
[Not applicable; presence of signs and symptoms establishes an *actual* diagnosis]

DESIRED OUTCOMES/EVALUATION CRITERIA—PATIENT WILL:

Risk Control (NOC)

Identify interventions to prevent/reduce risk of infection.
Experience no signs/symptoms of infection.

ACTIONS/INTERVENTIONS	RATIONALE
Infection Protection (NIC)	
Independent	
Observe meticulous aseptic techniques and wear masks during catheter insertion, dressing changes, and whenever the system is opened. Change tubings per protocol.	Prevents the introduction of organisms and airborne contamination that may cause infection.
Change dressings as indicated, being careful not to dislodge the catheter. Note character, color, odor, or drainage from around insertion site.	Moist environment promotes bacterial growth. Purulent drainage at insertion site suggests presence of local infection. *Note:* Polyurethane adhesive film (e.g., blister film) dressings have been found to decrease amount of pressure on catheter and exit site, as well as incidence of site infections.
Observe color and clarity of effluent.	Cloudy effluent is suggestive of peritoneal infection.
Apply povidone-iodine (Betadine) barrier in distal, clamped portion of catheter when intermittent dialysis therapy used.	Reduces risk of bacterial entry through catheter between dialysis treatments when catheter is disconnected from closed system.
Investigate reports of nausea/vomiting, increased/severe abdominal pain; rebound tenderness, fever, and leukocytosis.	Signs/symptoms suggesting peritonitis, requiring prompt intervention.
Collaborative	
Monitor WBC count of effluent.	Presence of WBCs initially may reflect normal response to a foreign substance; however, continued/new elevation suggests developing infection.
Obtain specimens of blood, effluent, and/or drainage from insertion site as indicated for culture/sensitivity.	Identifies types of organism(s) present, choice of interventions.

ACTIONS/INTERVENTIONS	RATIONALE
Collaborative	
Monitor renal clearance/BUN, Cr.	Choice and dosage of antibiotics are influenced by level of renal function.
Administer antibiotics systemically or in dialysate as indicated.	Treats infection, prevents sepsis.

NURSING DIAGNOSIS: Breathing Pattern, risk for ineffective

Risk factors may include
Abdominal pressure/restricted diaphragmatic excursion; rapid infusion of dialysate; pain
Inflammatory process (e.g., atelectasis/pneumonia)

Possibly evidenced by
[Not applicable; presence of signs and symptoms establishes an *actual* diagnosis]

DESIRED OUTCOMES/EVALUATION CRITERIA—PATIENT WILL:

Respiratory Status: Ventilation (NOC)

Display an effective respiratory pattern with clear breath sounds, ABGs within patient's normal range.
Experience no signs of dyspnea/cyanosis.

ACTIONS/INTERVENTIONS	RATIONALE
Respiratory Monitoring (NIC)	
Independent	
Monitor respiratory rate/effort. Reduce infusion rate if dyspnea is present.	Tachypnea, dyspnea, shortness of breath, and shallow breathing during dialysis suggests diaphragmatic pressure from distended peritoneal cavity or may indicate developing complications.
Auscultate lungs, noting decreased, absent, or adventitious breath sounds, e.g., crackles/wheezes/rhonchi.	Decreased areas of ventilation suggest presence of atelectasis, whereas adventitious sounds may suggest fluid overload, retained secretions, or infection.
Note character, amount, and color of secretions.	Patient is susceptible to pulmonary infections as a result of depressed cough reflex and respiratory effort, increased viscosity of secretions, as well as altered immune response and chronic/debilitating disease.
Elevate head of bed or have patient up in chair. Promote deep-breathing exercises and coughing.	Facilitates chest expansion/ventilation and mobilization of secretions.
Collaborative	
Review ABGs/pulse oximetry and serial chest x-rays.	Changes in PaO_2/$PaCO_2$ and appearance of infiltrates/congestion on chest x-ray suggests developing pulmonary problems.
Administer supplemental O_2 as indicated.	Maximizes oxygen for vascular uptake, preventing/lessening hypoxia.
Administer analgesics as indicated.	Alleviates pain, promotes comfortable breathing, maximal cough effort.

HEMODIALYSIS

In hemodialysis (HD), blood is shunted through an artificial kidney (dialyzer) for removal of toxins/excess fluid and then returned to the venous circulation. Hemodialysis is a fast and efficient method for removing urea and other toxic products and correcting fluid and electrolyte imbalances, but requires permanent arteriovenous access. Procedure is usually performed three times per week for 4 hours. HD may be done in the hospital, outpatient dialysis center, or at home.

NURSING DIAGNOSIS: Injury, risk for [loss of vascular access]

Risk factors may include
Clotting; hemorrhage related to accidental disconnection; infection

Possibly evidenced by
[Not applicable; presence of signs and symptoms establishes an *actual* diagnosis]

DESIRED OUTCOMES/EVALUATION CRITERIA—PATIENT WILL:

Risk Control (NOC)

Maintain patent vascular access, be free of infection.

ACTIONS/INTERVENTIONS	RATIONALE

Hemodialysis Therapy (NIC)

Independent

Clotting

Monitor internal AV shunt patency at frequent intervals:

Palpate for distal thrill;

Thrill is caused by turbulence of high-pressure arterial blood flow entering low-pressure venous system and should be palpable above venous exit site.

Auscultate for a bruit;

Bruit is the sound caused by the turbulence of arterial blood entering venous system and should be audible by stethoscope, although may be very faint.

Note color of blood and/or obvious separation of cells and serum;

Change of color from uniform medium red to dark purplish red suggests sluggish blood flow/early clotting. Separation in tubing is indicative of clotting. Very dark reddish-black blood next to clear yellow fluid indicates full clot formation.

Palpate skin around shunt for warmth.

Diminished blood flow results in "coolness" of shunt.

Notify physician and/or initiate declotting procedure if there is evidence of loss of shunt patency.

Rapid intervention may save access; however, declotting must be done by experienced personnel.

Evaluate reports of pain, numbness/tingling; note extremity swelling distal to access.

May indicate inadequate blood supply.

Avoid trauma to shunt; e.g., handle tubing gently, maintain cannula alignment. Limit activity of extremity. Avoid taking BP or drawing blood samples in shunt extremity. Instruct patient not to sleep or carry packages, books, purse on affected extremity.

Decreases risk of clotting/disconnection.

ACTIONS/INTERVENTIONS	RATIONALE
Independent	
Hemorrhage	
Attach two cannula clamps to shunt dressing. Have tourniquet available. If cannulas separate, clamp the arterial cannula first, then the venous. If tubing comes out of vessel, clamp cannula that is still in place and apply direct pressure to bleeding site. Place tourniquet above site or inflate BP cuff to pressure just above patient's systolic BP.	Prevents massive blood loss while awaiting medical assistance if cannula separates or shunt is dislodged.
Infection	
Assess skin around vascular access, noting redness, swelling, local warmth, exudate, tenderness.	Signs of local infection, which can progress to sepsis if untreated.
Avoid contamination of access site. Use aseptic technique and masks when giving shunt care, applying/changing dressings, and when starting/completing dialysis process.	Prevents introduction of organisms that can cause infection.
Monitor temperature. Note presence of fever, chills, hypotension.	Signs of infection/sepsis requiring prompt medical intervention.
Collaborative	
Culture the site/obtain blood samples as indicated.	Determines presence of pathogens.
Monitor PT, activated partial thromboplastin time (aPTT) as appropriate.	Provides information about coagulation status, identifies treatment needs and evaluates effectiveness.
Administer medications as indicated, e.g.:	
Heparin (low-dose);	Infused on arterial side of filter to prevent clotting in the filter without systemic side effects.
Antibiotics (systemic and/or topical).	Prompt treatment of infection may save access, prevent sepsis.
Discuss use of acetylsalicylic acid (ASA), warfarin sodium (Coumadin) as appropriate.	Ongoing low-dose anticoagulation may be useful in maintaining patency of shunt.

NURSING DIAGNOSIS: Fluid Volume, risk for deficit

Risk factors may include

Ultrafiltration

Fluid restrictions; actual blood loss (systemic heparinization or disconnection of the shunt)

Possibly evidenced by

[Not applicable; presence of signs and symptoms establishes an *actual* diagnosis]

DESIRED OUTCOMES/EVALUATION CRITERIA—PATIENT WILL:

Hydration (NOC)

Maintain fluid balance as evidenced by stable/appropriate weight and vital signs, good skin turgor, moist mucous membranes, absence of bleeding.

ACTIONS/INTERVENTIONS	RATIONALE

Hemodialysis Therapy (NIC)

Independent

Measure all sources of I&O. Have patient keep diary.

Aids in evaluating fluid status, especially when compared with weight. *Note:* Urine output is an inaccurate evaluation of renal function in dialysis patients. Some individuals have water output with little renal clearance of toxins while others have oliguria or anuria.

Weigh daily before/after dialysis run.

Weight loss over precisely measured time is a measure of ultrafiltration and fluid removal.

Monitor BP, pulse, and hemodynamic pressures if available during dialysis.

Hypotension, tachycardia, falling hemodynamic pressures suggest volume depletion.

Note/ascertain whether diuretics and/or antihypertensives are to be withheld.

Dialysis potentiates hypotensive effects if these drugs have been administered.

Verify continuity of shunt/access catheter.

Disconnected shunt/open access permits exsanguination.

Apply external shunt dressing. Permit no puncture of shunt.

Minimizes stress on cannula insertion site to reduce inadvertent dislodgement and bleeding from site.

Place patient in a supine/Trendelenburg's position as necessary.

Maximizes venous return if hypotension occurs.

Assess for oozing or frank bleeding at access site or mucous membranes, incisions/wounds. Hematest/guaiac stools, gastric drainage.

Systemic heparinization during dialysis increases clotting times and places patient at risk for bleeding, especially during the first 4 hr after procedure.

Collaborative

Monitor laboratory studies as indicated:

Hb/Hct;

May be reduced because of anemia, hemodilution, or actual blood loss.

Serum electrolytes and pH;

Imbalances may require changes in the dialysate solution or supplemental replacement to achieve balance.

Clotting times, e.g., PT/aPTT, and platelet count.

Use of heparin to prevent clotting in blood lines and hemofilter alters coagulation and potentiates active bleeding.

Administer IV solutions (e.g., normal saline [NS])/volume expanders (e.g., albumin) during dialysis as indicated;

Saline/dextrose solutions, electrolytes, and $NaHCO_3$ may be infused in the venous side of continuous arteriovenous (CAV) hemofilter when high ultrafiltration rates are used for removal of extracellular fluid and toxic solutes. Volume expanders may be required during/following hemodialysis if sudden/marked hypotension occurs.

Blood/PRCs if needed.

Destruction of RBCs (hemolysis) by mechanical dialysis, hemorrhagic losses, decreased RBC production may result in profound/progressive anemia requiring corrective action.

Reduce rate of ultrafiltration during dialysis as indicated.

Reduces the amount of water being removed and may correct hypotension/hypovolemia.

Administer protamine sulfate if indicated.

May be needed to return clotting times to normal or if heparin rebound occurs (up to 16 hr after hemodialysis).

NURSING DIAGNOSIS: Fluid Volume risk for excess

Risk factors may include
Rapid/excessive fluid intake: IV, blood, plasma expanders, saline given to support BP during dialysis

Possibly evidenced by
[Not applicable; presence of signs and symptoms establishes an *actual* diagnosis]

DESIRED OUTCOMES/EVALUATION CRITERIA—PATIENT WILL:

Fluid Balance (NOC)

Maintain "dry weight" within patient's normal range; be free of edema; have clear breath sounds and serum sodium levels within normal limits.

ACTIONS/INTERVENTIONS	RATIONALE
Fluid Management (NIC)	
Independent	
Measure all sources of I&O. Weigh routinely.	Aids in evaluating fluid status, especially when compared with weight. Weight gain between treatments should not exceed 0.5 kg/day.
Monitor BP, pulse.	Hypertension and tachycardia between hemodialysis runs may result from fluid overload and/or HF.
Note presence of peripheral/sacral edema, respiratory rales, dyspnea, orthopnea, distended neck veins, ECG changes indicative of ventricular hypertrophy.	Fluid volume excess due to inefficient dialysis or repeated hypervolemia between dialysis treatments may cause/exacerbate HF, as indicated by signs/symptoms of respiratory and/or systemic venous congestion.
Note changes in mentation. (Refer to CP: Renal Dialysis; ND: Thought Processes, altered, p. 605.)	Fluid overload/hypervolemia may potentiate cerebral edema (disequilibrium syndrome).
Collaborative	
Monitor serum sodium levels. Restrict sodium intake as indicated.	High sodium levels are associated with fluid overload, edema, hypertension, and cardiac complications.
Restrict PO/IV fluid intake as indicated, spacing allowed fluids throughout a 24-hr period.	The intermittent nature of hemodialysis results in fluid retention/overload between procedures and may require fluid restriction. Spacing fluids helps reduce thirst.

URINARY DIVERSIONS/ UROSTOMY (POSTOPERATIVE CARE)

Incontinent urinary diversions: These ostomies require permanent stoma care and external collecting devices.

> *Ileal conduit:* Ureters are anastomosed to a segment of ileum, resected with the blood supply intact (usually 15–20 cm long). The proximal section is closed, and the distal end brought to skin opening to form a stoma (a passageway, not a storage reservoir).
>
> *Colonic conduit:* This is a similar procedure using a segment of colon.
>
> *Ureterostomy:* The ureter(s) is brought directly through the abdominal wall to form its own stoma.

Continent urinary diversions (CURs): CURs have become one of the major options for patients requiring urinary diversion to improve their quality of life regarding stoma care and the ability to sleep and travel.

> *Kock reservoir or Indiana (ileocecal) pouch:* A section of intestine is used to form a pouch inside the patient's abdomen, creating a reservoir that the patient periodically drains by inserting a catheter through the stoma, thus negating the need for an external collecting device.

CARE SETTING:

Inpatient acute surgical unit.

RELATED CONCERNS

Cancer, page 900
Peritonitis, page 382
Psychosocial aspects of care, page 809
Surgical intervention, page 828

Patient Assessment Database

Data depends on underlying problem, duration, and severity, e.g., malignant bladder tumor, congenital malformations, trauma, chronic infections, or intractable incontinence due to injury/disease of other body systems (e.g., multiple sclerosis). (Refer to appropriate CP.)

TEACHING/LEARNING

Discharge plan considerations: **DRG projected mean length of inpatient stay: 5.5 days**
May require assistance with management of ostomy and acquisition of supplies.

Refer to section at end of plan for postdischarge considerations.

DIAGNOSTIC STUDIES

Intravenous pyelogram (IVP): Visualizes size/location of kidneys and ureters and rules out presence of tumors elsewhere in urinary tract.

Cystoscopy with biopsy: Determines tumor location/stage of malignancy. Ultraviolet cystoscopy outlines bladder lesion.

Bone scan: Determines presence of metastatic disease.

Bilateral pedal lymphangiogram: Determines involvement of pelvic nodes, where bladder tumor easily seeds because of close proximity.

CT scan: Defines size of tumor mass, degree of pelvic spread.

Urine cystoscopy: Detects tumor cells in urine (for determining presence and type of tumor).

Endoscopy: Evaluates intestines for use as conduit.

Conduitogram: Assesses length and emptying ability of the conduit and presence of stricture, obstruction, reflux, angulation, calculi, or tumor (may complicate or contraindicate use as a urinary diversion).

NURSING PRIORITIES

1. Prevent complications.
2. Assist patient/SO in physical and psychosocial adjustment.
3. Support independence in self-care.
4. Provide information about procedure/prognosis, treatment needs, potential complications, and resources.

DISCHARGE GOALS

1. Complications prevented/minimized.
2. Adjusting to perceived/actual changes.
3. Self-care needs met by self/with assistance as necessary.
4. Procedure/prognosis, therapeutic regimen, potential complications understood and sources of support identified.
5. Plan in place to meet needs after discharge.

NURSING DIAGNOSIS: Skin Integrity, risk for impaired

Risk factors may include

Absence of sphincter at stoma [actual] with continuous flow of urine

Character/flow of urine from stoma

Reaction to product/chemicals; improper fitting of appliance or removal of adhesive

Possibly evidenced by

[Not applicable; presence of signs and symptoms establishes an *actual* diagnosis]

DESIRED OUTCOMES/EVALUATION CRITERIA—PATIENT WILL:

Tissue Integrity: Skin and Mucous Membranes (NOC)

Maintain skin integrity.

Risk Control (NOC)

Identify individual risk factors.

Demonstrate behaviors/techniques to promote healing/prevent skin breakdown.

ACTIONS/INTERVENTIONS	RATIONALE
Ostomy Care (NIC)	
Independent	
Inspect stoma/peristomal skin. Note irritation, bruises (dark, bluish color), rashes, status of sutures.	Monitors healing process/effectiveness of appliance and identifies areas of concern, need for further evaluation/intervention. Stoma should be pink or reddish, similar to mucous membranes. Color changes may be temporary, but persistent changes may require surgical intervention. Early identification of stomal necrosis/ischemia or fungal infection provides for timely interventions to prevent skin necrosis.
Clean with water and pat dry (or use hair dryer on cool setting).	Maintaining a clean/dry area helps prevent skin breakdown.
Handle stoma gently to prevent irritation.	Mucosa has good blood supply and bleeds easily with rubbing or trauma.
Measure stoma periodically, e.g., each appliance change for first 6 wk, then monthly times six.	As postoperative edema resolves (during first 6 wk), size of appliance must be altered to ensure proper fit so that urine is collected as it flows from the stoma and contact with the skin is prevented.
Apply effective sealant barrier, e.g., Skin Prep or similar product.	Protects skin from pouch adhesive, enhances adhesiveness of pouch, and facilitates removal of pouch when necessary.

ACTIONS/INTERVENTIONS	RATIONALE

Independent

Make sure opening for adhesive backing of pouch is at least $\frac{1}{16}$ in larger than the base of the stoma (Wound Ostomy Continence Nursing [WOCN] standard), with adequate adhesiveness left to apply pouch.

Prevents trauma to the stoma tissue and protects the peristomal skin. Adequate adhesive area is important to maintain a seal. Note: Too tight a fit may cause stomal edema or stenosis.

Use a transparent, odor-proof drainable pouch. Keep gauze square/wick over stoma while cleansing area, and have patient cough or strain before applying pouch.

A transparent appliance during first 4–6 wk allows easy observation of stoma and stents (when used) without necessity of removing pouch and irritating skin. Covering stoma prevents urine from wetting the peristomal area during pouch changes. Coughing empties distal portion of conduit, followed by a brief pause in drainage to facilitate application of pouch.

Avoid use of karaya-type appliances.

Will not protect skin because urine melts karaya.

Apply waterproof tape around pouch edges if desired.

Reinforces anchoring.

Connect collecting pouch to continuous bedside drainage system, when necessary.

May be needed during times when rate of urine formation is increased, e.g., while IV fluids are administered. Weight of the urine can cause pouch to pull loose/leak when pouch becomes more than half full.

Cleanse ostomy pouch on a routine basis, using vinegar solution.

Frequent pouch changes are irritating to the skin and should be avoided. Emptying and rinsing the pouch with vinegar not only removes bacteria but also deodorizes the pouch.

Change pouch every 3–5 days or as needed for leakage. Remove appliance gently while supporting skin. Use adhesive removers as indicated and wash off completely.

Prevents tissue irritation/destruction associated with "pulling" pouch off.

Investigate reports of burning/itching around stoma.

Suggests peristomal irritation or possibly Candida infections, both requiring intervention. Note: Continuous exposure of skin to urine can cause hyperplasia around stoma, affecting pouch fit and increasing risk of infection.

Evaluate adhesive product and appliance fit on ongoing basis.

Provides opportunity for problem solving. Determines need for further intervention.

Monitor for distension of lower abdomen (with ileal conduit); assess bowel sounds.

Intestinal distension can cause tension on new suture lines with possibility of rupture.

Collaborative

Consult with enterostomal nurse.

Helpful in problem solving and choosing products appropriate for patient needs, considering stoma characteristics, patient's physical/mental status, and financial resources. In the presence of persistent or recurring problems, the ostomy nurse has a wider range of knowledge and resources. Note: WOCN standards mandate that a patient be capable of changing an ostomy appliance before discharge, or receive home care until such time as the patient or caregivers are competent.

Apply antifungal spray or powder, as indicated.

Assists in healing if peristomal irritation is caused by fungal infection. Note: These products can have potent side effects and should be used sparingly. Creams/ointments are to be avoided, because they interfere with adhesion of the appliance.

NURSING DIAGNOSIS: Body Image disturbance

May be related to

Biophysical: Presence of stoma; loss of control of urine elimination

Psychosocial: Altered body structure

Disease process and associated treatment regimen, e.g., cancer

Possibly evidenced by

Verbalization of change in body image, fear of rejection/reaction of others, and negative feelings about body

Actual change in structure and/or function (ostomy)

Not touching/looking at stoma, refusal to participate in care

DESIRED OUTCOMES/EVALUATION CRITERIA—PATIENT WILL:

> **Body Image (NOC)**

Demonstrate beginning acceptance by viewing/touching stoma and participating in self-care.

Verbalize feelings about stoma/illness; begin to deal constructively with situation.

Verbalize acceptance of self in situation, incorporating change into self-concept without negating self-esteem.

ACTIONS/INTERVENTIONS	RATIONALE

> **Body Image Enhancement (NIC)**

Independent

Review reason for surgery and future expectations.	Patient may find it easier to accept/deal with an ostomy done for chronic/long-term disease (e.g., intractable incontinence, infections) than for traumatic injury.
Ascertain whether counseling was initiated when the possibility and/or necessity of urinary diversion was first discussed.	Provides information about patient's/SO's level of knowledge about individual situation and process of acceptance.
Answer all questions concerning urostomy and its function.	Establishes rapport and conveys interest/concern of caregiver. Provides additional information for patient to consider.
Encourage the patient/SO to verbalize feelings. Acknowledge normality of feelings of anger, depression, and grief over loss. Discuss daily "ups and downs" that can occur after discharge.	Provides opportunity to deal with issues/misconceptions. Helps the patient/SO to realize that feelings experienced are not unusual and that feeling guilty for them is not necessary/helpful. Patient needs to recognize feelings before they can be dealt with effectively.
Note behaviors of withdrawal, increased dependency, manipulation, or noninvolvement in care.	Suggestive of problems in adjustment that may require further evaluation and more extensive therapy. May reflect grief response to loss of body part/function and worry over acceptance by others and fear of further disability/loss of life from cancer.
Provide opportunities for patient/SO to view and touch stoma, using the moment to point out positive signs of healing, normal appearance, and so forth.	Although integration of stoma into body image can take months or even years, looking at the stoma and hearing comments (made in a normal, matter-of-fact manner) can help patient with this acceptance. Touching stoma reassures patient/SO that it is not fragile and that slight movements of stoma actually reflect normal peristalsis.

625

ACTIONS/INTERVENTIONS	RATIONALE

Independent

Provide opportunity for patient to deal with ostomy through participation in self-care.	Independence in self-care helps improve self-esteem. In the case of a continent diversion, the patient needs the energy, ability, and time to intubate the stoma four times a day.
Maintain positive approach during care activities, avoiding expressions of disdain or revulsion. Do not take patient's angry expressions personally.	Assists patient/SO to accept body changes and feel all right about self. Anger is most often directed at the situation and lack of control individual has over what has happened (powerlessness), not the individual caregiver.
Plan/schedule care activities with patient.	Promotes sense of control and gives message that the patient can handle this situation, enhancing self-esteem.
Discuss possibility of contacting ostomy/urostomy visitor and make arrangements for visit if desired.	Can provide a good support system. Helps reinforce teaching (shared experiences) and facilitates acceptance of change as patient realizes "life does go on" and can be relatively normal.
Discuss sexual functioning, medications that promote erection, and penile implant, if applicable, and alternate ways for sexual pleasuring. (Refer to ND: Sexual Dysfunction, risk for, p. 631.)	Patient may experience anticipatory anxiety, fear of failure in relation to sex after surgery, usually because of ignorance, lack of knowledge. Surgery that removes the bladder and prostate (removed with the bladder) may disrupt parasympathetic nerve fibers that control erection in men, although newer techniques are available that may be used in individual cases to preserve nerve function.

NURSING DIAGNOSIS: Pain [acute]

May be related to
Physical factors, e.g., disruption of skin/tissues (incisions/drains)
Biological: activity of disease process (cancer, trauma)
Psychological factors, e.g., fear, anxiety

Possibly evidenced by
Reports of pain
Guarding/distraction behaviors, restlessness
Self-focusing
Autonomic responses, e.g., changes in vital signs

DESIRED OUTCOMES/EVALUATION CRITERIA—PATIENT WILL:

Pain Level (NOC)

Verbalize relief/control of pain.
Appear relaxed, able to sleep/rest appropriately.

Pain Control Behavior (NOC)

Perform general comfort measures.

ACTIONS/INTERVENTIONS	RATIONALE

Pain Management (NIC)

Independent

Assess pain, noting location, characteristics, intensity (0–10 scale).	Helps evaluate degree of discomfort and effectiveness of analgesia or may reveal developing complications, e.g., because abdominal pain usually subsides gradually by the third or fourth postoperative day, continued or increasing pain may reflect delayed healing, peristomal skin irritation, infection, intestinal obstruction.
Auscultate bowel sounds; note passage of flatus.	Indicates re-establishment of bowel function. Lack of return of bowel sounds/function within 72 hr may indicate presence of complication, e.g., peritonitis, hypokalemia, mechanical obstruction.
Note urine flow and characteristics.	Decreased flow may reflect urinary retention (due to edema) with increased pressure in upper urinary tract or leakage into peritoneal cavity (failure of anastomosis). Cloudy urine may be normal (presence of mucus) or indicate infectious process.
Encourage patient to verbalize concerns. Active-listen these concerns and provide support by acceptance, remaining with patient and giving appropriate information.	Reduction of anxiety/fear can promote relaxation and comfort.
Provide comfort measures, e.g., back rub, repositioning (using body support measures as needed). Assure patient that position change will not injure stoma.	Reduces muscle tension, promotes relaxation, and may enhance coping abilities.
Encourage use of relaxation techniques, e.g., guided imagery, visualization, diversional activities.	Helps patient rest more effectively and refocuses attention, which may enhance coping ability, reducing pain and discomfort.
Assist with ROM exercises and encourage early ambulation.	Reduces muscle/joint stiffness. Ambulation returns organs to normal position and promotes return of peristalsis/passage of flatus and feelings of general well-being.
Investigate and report abdominal muscle rigidity, involuntary guarding, and rebound tenderness.	Suggestive of peritoneal inflammation, requiring prompt medical intervention.

Collaborative

Administer medications as indicated, e.g., narcotics, analgesics; patient-controlled analgesia (PCA).	Relieves pain, enhances comfort, and promotes rest. PCA may be more beneficial than intermittent analgesia, especially following radical resection.
Provide sitz baths, if indicated.	Relieves local discomfort, reduces edema, and promotes healing of perineal wound associated with radical procedure.
Apply/monitor effects of transcutaneous electrical nerve stimulator (TENS) unit.	Cutaneous stimulation may be used to block transmission of pain stimulus.
Maintain patency of NG tube.	Decompresses stomach/intestines; prevents abdominal distension when intestinal function is impaired.

ACTIONS/INTERVENTIONS	RATIONALE
Infection Protection (NIC)	
Independent	
Empty ostomy pouch when it becomes one-third full, once IV fluids and continuous pouch drainage have been discontinued.	Reduces risk of urinary reflux and maintains integrity of appliance seal if pouch does not have an antireflux valve.
Document urine characteristics, and note whether changes are associated with reports of flank pain.	Cloudy odorous urine indicates infection (possibly pyelonephritis); however, urine normally contains mucus after a conduit procedure.
Test urine pH with Nitrazine paper (use fresh specimen, not from pouch); notify physician if greater than 6.5.	Urine is normally acidic, which discourages bacterial growth/UTIs. *Note:* Presence of alkaline urine also creates favorable environment for stone formation in presence of hypercalciuria.
Report sudden cessation of urethral drainage.	Constant drainage usually subsides within 10 days; however, abrupt cessation may indicate plugging and lead to abscess formation.
Note red rash around stoma.	Rash is most commonly caused by yeast. Urine leakage or allergy to appliance or products may also cause red, irritated areas.
Inspect incision line around stoma. Observe and document wound drainage, signs of incisional inflammation, systemic indicators of sepsis.	Provides baseline reference. Complications may include interrupted anastomosis of intestine/bowel or ureteral conduit, with leakage of bowel contents into abdomen or urine into peritoneal cavity.
Change dressings as indicated when used.	Moist dressings act as a wick to the wound and provide media for bacterial growth.
Assess skinfold areas in groin, perineum, under arms and breasts.	Use of antibiotics and trapping of moisture in skinfold areas increases risk of *Candida* infections.
Monitor vital signs.	An elevated temperature suggests incisional infection or UTI and/or respiratory complications.

ACTIONS/INTERVENTIONS

Independent

Auscultate breath sounds.

Collaborative

Use pouch with antireflux valve, if available.

Obtain specimens of exudates, urine, sputum, blood as indicated.

Administer medications as indicated, e.g.:

Cephalosporins, e.g., cefoxitin (Mefoxin), cefazolin (Ancef);

Antifungal powder;

Ascorbic acid/vitamin C.

Assist with injection of IV methylene blue.

RATIONALE

Patient is at high risk for development of respiratory complications because of length of time under anesthesia. Often this patient is older and may already have a compromised immune system. Also, painful abdominal incisions cause patient to breathe more shallowly than normal and to limit coughing effort. Accumulation of secretions in respiratory system predisposes to atelectasis and infections.

Prevents backflow of urine into stoma, reducing risk of infection.

Identifies source of infection/most effective treatment. Infected urine may cause pyelonephritis. *Note:* Urine specimen must be obtained from the conduit because the pouch is considered contaminated.

Given to treat identified infection or may be given prophylactically, especially with history of recurrent pyelonephritis.

Used to treat yeast infections around stoma.

Given to acidify urine, reduce bacterial growth/risk of infection. *Note:* Large doses of vitamin C can impair GI absorption of B_{12}, potentiating pernicious anemia.

Dye appearing in wound drainage signifies urine leakage into peritoneal cavity and need for surgical repair.

NURSING DIAGNOSIS: Urinary Elimination, altered

May be related to
Surgical diversion; tissue trauma, postoperative edema

Possibly evidenced by
Loss of continence
Changes in amount, character of urine; urinary retention

DESIRED OUTCOMES/EVALUATION CRITERIA—PATIENT WILL:

> **Urinary Elimination (NOC)**

Display continuous flow of urine, with output adequate for individual situation.

ACTIONS/INTERVENTIONS

> **Urinary Elimination Management (NIC)**

Independent

Assess for presence of stents/ureteral catheters. Label "right" and "left" and observe urine flow through each.

RATIONALE

Maintains patency of ureters and assists in healing of anastomosis by keeping it urine-free.

ACTIONS/INTERVENTIONS	RATIONALE
Independent	
Record urinary output; investigate sudden reduction/cessation of urine flow.	Sudden decrease in urine flow may indicate obstruction/dysfunction, (e.g., blockage by edema or mucus) or dehydration. *Note:* Reduced urinary output (not related to hypovolemia) associated with abdominal distension, fever, and clear/watery discharge from incision suggests urinary fistula, also requiring prompt intervention.
Observe and record color of urine. Note hematuria and/or bleeding from stoma.	Urine may be slightly pink, which should clear up in 2–3 days. Rubbing/washing stoma may cause temporary oozing due to vascular nature of tissues. Continued bleeding, frank blood in the pouch, or oozing around the base of stoma requires medical evaluation/intervention.
Position tubing and drainage pouch so that it allows unimpeded flow of urine. Monitor/protect placement of stents.	Blocked drainage allows pressure to build within urinary tract, risking anastomosis leakage and damage to renal parenchyma. *Note:* Stents inserted to maintain patency of ureters during period of postoperative edema may be inadvertently dislodged, compromising urine flow.
Demonstrate self-catheterization techniques and reservoir irrigations as appropriate.	Patients with continent diversions do not require an external collection device. Periodic catheterization empties the internal reservoir and reduces risk of injury from overdistention. Daily irrigations remove accumulated mucus from the reservoir. *Note:* Patients with Kock pouches connected to the urethra are instructed to void every 2 hr during the day and every 3 hr during the night. This is done by bearing down and applying hand pressure on the lower abdomen to aid in emptying the reservoir.
Encourage increased fluids and maintain accurate intake.	Maintains hydration and good urine flow.
Monitor vital signs. Assess peripheral pulses, skin turgor, capillary refill, and oral mucosa. Weigh daily.	Indicators of fluid balance. Reflects level of hydration and effectiveness of fluid replacement therapy.
Collaborative	
Administer IV fluids as indicated.	Assists in maintaining hydration/adequate circulating volume and urinary flow.
Monitor electrolytes, ABGs, calcium.	Impaired renal function in patient with intestinal conduit increases risk of severe electrolyte and/or acid-base problems, e.g., hyperchloremic acidosis. Elevated calcium levels increase risk of crystal/stone formation, affecting both urinary flow and tissue integrity.
Prepare for diagnostic testing, procedures as indicated.	Retrograde ileogram may be done to evaluate patency of conduit; nephrostomy tube or stents may be inserted to maintain urine flow until edema/obstruction is resolved.

NURSING DIAGNOSIS: Sexual Dysfunction, risk for

Risk factors may include

Altered body structure/function; radical resection/treatment procedures

Vulnerability/psychological concern about response of SO

Disruption of sexual response pattern, e.g., erection difficulty

Possibly evidenced by

[Not applicable; presence of signs and symptoms establishes an *actual* diagnosis]

DESIRED OUTCOMES/EVALUATION CRITERIA—PATIENT WILL:

Self-Esteem (NOC)

Verbalize understanding of relationship of physical condition to sexual problems.

Identify satisfying/acceptable sexual practices and explore alternate methods.

Resume sexual relationship as appropriate.

ACTIONS/INTERVENTIONS

Sexual Counseling (NIC)

Independent

Ascertain the patient's/SO's sexual relationship before the disease and/or surgery. Identify future expectations and desires.

Review with the patient/SO anatomy and physiology of sexual functioning in relation to own situation.

Reinforce information given by the physician. Encourage questions. Provide additional information as needed.

Discuss resumption of sexual activity approximately 6 wk after discharge, beginning slowly and progressing (e.g., cuddling/caressing until both partners are comfortable with body image/function changes). Include alternate methods of stimulation as appropriate.

Encourage dialogue between patient/SO. Suggest wearing pouch cover, T-shirt, or shortie nightgown.

Stress awareness of factors that might be distracting (e.g., unpleasant odors and pouch leakage).

Encourage use of sense of humor.

Problem-solve alternative positions for coitus.

RATIONALE

Mutilation and loss of privacy/control of a bodily function can affect patient's view of personal sexuality. When coupled with the fear of rejection by SO, the desired level of intimacy can be greatly impaired. Sexual needs are very basic, and the patient will be rehabilitated more successfully when a satisfying sexual relationship is continued/developed.

Understanding normal physiology helps patient/SO understand the mechanisms of nerve damage and need for exploring alternative methods of satisfaction.

Reiteration of previously given information assists the patient/SO to hear and process the knowledge again, moving toward acceptance of individual limitations/restrictions and prognosis (e.g., that it may take up to 2 yr to regain potency after a radical procedure or that a penile prosthesis may be necessary).

Knowing what to expect in progress of recovery helps patient avoid performance anxiety/reduce risk of "failure." If the couple is willing to try new ideas, this can assist with adjustment and may help achieve sexual fulfillment.

Disguising urostomy appliance may aid in reducing feelings of self-consciousness, embarrassment during sexual activity.

Promotes resolution of solvable problems.

Laughter can help individuals deal more effectively with difficult situation and promote a positive sexual experience.

Minimizing awkwardness of appliance and physical discomfort can enhance satisfaction.

ACTIONS/INTERVENTIONS	RATIONALE

Independent

| Discuss/role-play possible interactions or approaches when dealing with new sexual partners. | Rehearsal helps deal with actual situations when they arise, preventing self-consciousness about "different" body image. |
| Provide birth control information as appropriate and stress that impotence does not mean the patient is necessarily sterile. | Confusion about impotency and sterility can lead to an unwanted pregnancy. |

Collaborative

| Arrange meeting with an ostomy visitor if appropriate. | Sharing of how these problems have been resolved by others can be helpful and reduce sense of isolation. |
| Refer to counseling/sex therapy as indicated. | If problems persist longer than several months after surgery, a trained therapist may be required to facilitate communication between patient and SO. |

NURSING DIAGNOSIS: Knowledge Deficit [Learning Need] regarding condition, prognosis, treatment, self care, and discharge needs

May be related to
Lack of exposure/recall; information misinterpretation
Unfamiliarity with information resources

Possibly evidenced by
Questions; statement of misconception/misinformation
Inaccurate follow-through of instruction/performance of urostomy care
Inappropriate or exaggerated behaviors (e.g., hostile, agitated, apathetic, withdrawn)

DESIRED OUTCOMES/EVALUATION CRITERIA—PATIENT WILL:

Knowledge: Disease Process (NOC)

Verbalize understanding of condition/disease process, prognosis, and potential complications.

Knowledge: Treatment Regimen (NOC)

Verbalize understanding of therapeutic needs.
Correctly perform necessary procedures, explain reasons for the action.
Initiate necessary lifestyle changes.

ACTIONS/INTERVENTIONS	RATIONALE

Teaching: Disease Process (NIC)

Independent

Evaluate patient's emotional and physical capabilities.	These factors affect patient's ability to master tasks and willingness to assume responsibility for ostomy care.
Review anatomy, physiology, and implications of surgical intervention. Discuss future expectations.	Provides knowledge base from which patient can make informed choices and an opportunity to clarify misconceptions regarding individual situation.
Include written/picture resources.	Provides references after discharge to support patient efforts for independence in self-care.
Instruct patient/SO in stomal care as appropriate. Allot time for return demonstrations and provide positive feedback for efforts.	Promotes positive management and reduces risk of improper ostomy care.

ACTIONS/INTERVENTIONS	RATIONALE
Independent	
Ensure that stoma and appliance are odorless, non-leaking.	When patient feels confident about urostomy, energy/attention can be focused on other tasks.
Demonstrate padding to absorb urethral drainage; ask patient to report changes in amount, odor, character.	Small amount of leakage may continue for several weeks after prostate surgery with bladder left in place (temporary diversion procedure).
Recommend routine clipping/trimming of hair around stoma to edges of pouch adhesive.	Hair can be pulled out when the pouch is changed, causing irritation of hair follicles and increasing risk of local infection.
Encourage patients with Kock pouch to lengthen voiding interval by 1 hr each week unless discomfort noted.	Increases capacity of reservoir to achieve a more normal voiding pattern. Presence of discomfort suggests reservoir is full, necessitating prompt emptying.
Instruct patient in a progressive exercise program to include Kegel exercises and stop/start of urinary stream.	Improves tone of pelvic muscles and the external sphincter to enhance continence when patient voids through urethra.
Encourage optimal nutrition.	Promotes wound healing, increases utilization of energy to facilitate tissue repair. Anorexia may be present for several months postoperatively, requiring conscious effort to meet nutritional needs.
Discuss use of acid-ash diet (e.g., cranberries, prunes, plums, cereals, rice, peanuts, noodles, cheese, poultry, fish); avoidance of salt substitutes, sodium bicarbonate, and antacids; and cautious use of products containing calcium.	May be useful in acidifying urine to decrease risk of infection and crystal/stone formation. Products containing bicarbonate/calcium potentiate risk of crystal/stone formation affecting both urinary flow and tissue integrity *Note:* Use of sulfa drugs requires alkaline urine for optimal absorption, so acid-ash diet/vitamin C supplements should be withheld.
Discuss importance of maintaining normal weight.	Changes in weight can affect size of stoma/appliance fit. *Note:* Weight loss of 10–20 lb is not uncommon because of intestinal involvement and anorexia.
Stress necessity of increased fluid intake of at least 2–3 L/day; of cranberry juice or ascorbic acid/vitamin C tablets; avoidance of citrus fruits as indicated.	Maintains urinary output and promotes acidic urine to reduce risk of infection and stone formation. *Note:* Oranges/citrus fruits make urine alkaline and are therefore contraindicated. Large doses of vitamin C can inhibit vitamin B_{12} absorption requiring periodic monitoring of vitamin B_{12} levels.
Discuss resumption of presurgery level of activity and possibility of sleep disturbance, anorexia, loss of interest in usual activities.	Patient should be able to manage same degree of activity as previously enjoyed and in some cases increase activity level except for contact sports. "Homecoming depression" may occur, lasting for up to 3 mo after surgery, requiring patience/support and ongoing evaluation.
Encourage regular activity/exercise program.	Immobility/inactivity increases urinary stasis and calcium shift out of bones, potentiating risk of stone formation and resultant urinary obstruction, infection.
Identify signs/symptoms requiring medical evaluation, e.g., changes in character, amount and flow of urine, unusual drainage from wound; fatigue/muscle weakness, anorexia, abdominal distension, confusion.	Early detection and prompt intervention of developing problems such as UTI, stricture, intestinal fistula may prevent more serious complications. Urinary electrolytes (especially chloride) are resorbed in the intestinal conduit, which leads to compensatory bicarbonate loss, lowered serum pH (metabolic acidosis), and potassium deficit.

ACTIONS/INTERVENTIONS	RATIONALE
Independent	
Stress importance of follow-up appointments.	Monitors healing, disease process; provides opportunity for discussion of appliance fitting problems, generalized health, and adaptation to condition. *Note:* Extensive surgery requires prolonged recuperation for regaining strength and endurance.
Identify community resources, e.g., United Ostomy Association, and local ostomy support group, enterostomal therapist, visiting nurse, pharmacy/medical supply house.	Continued support after discharge is essential to facilitate the recovery process and patient's independence in care. Enterostomal nurse can be very helpful in solving appliance problems and identifying alternatives to meet individual patient needs.

POTENTIAL CONSIDERATIONS following acute hospitalization (dependent on patient's age, physical condition/presence of complications, personal resources, and life responsibilities)

In addition to postsurgical concerns:
Urinary Elimination, altered—anatomic diversion.
Self-Esteem, situational low—loss of/altered control of body function.

BENIGN PROSTATIC HYPERPLASIA (BPH)

Benign prostatic hyperplasia is characterized by progressive enlargement of the prostate gland (commonly seen in men over age 50), causing varying degrees of urethral obstruction and restriction of urinary flow.

CARE SETTING

Community level, with more acute care provided during outpatient procedures.

RELATED CONCERNS

Renal failure: acute, page 575
Psychosocial aspects of care, page 809
Prostatectomy, page 643

Patient Assessment Database

CIRCULATION

May exhibit: Elevated BP (renal effects of advanced enlargement)

ELIMINATION

May report: Decreased force/caliber of urinary stream; dribbling
Hesitancy in initiating voiding
Inability to empty bladder completely; urgency and frequency of urination
Nocturia, dysuria, hematuria
Sitting to void
Recurrent UTIs, history of calculi (urinary stasis)
Chronic constipation (protrusion of prostate into rectum)

May exhibit: Firm mass in lower abdomen (distended bladder), bladder tenderness
Inguinal hernia; hemorrhoids (result of increased abdominal pressure required to empty bladder against resistance)

FOOD/FLUID

May report: Anorexia; nausea, vomiting
Recent weight loss

PAIN/DISCOMFORT

May report: Suprapubic, flank, or back pain; sharp, intense (in acute prostatitis)
Low back pain

SAFETY

May report: Fever

SEXUALITY

May report: Concerns about effects of condition/therapy on sexual abilities
Fear of incontinence/dribbling during intimacy
Decrease in force of ejaculatory contractions

May exhibit: Enlarged, tender prostate

TEACHING/LEARNING

May report: Family history of cancer, hypertension, kidney disease
Use of antihypertensive or antidepressant medications, OTC cold/allergy medications containing sympathomimetics, urinary antibiotics or antibacterial agents

Discharge plan considerations: **DRG projected mean length of stay: 3.7 days**
May need assistance with management of therapy, e.g., catheter

Refer to section at end of plan for postdischarge considerations.

DIAGNOSTIC STUDIES

Urinalysis: Color yellow, dark brown, dark or bright red (bloody); appearance may be cloudy; pH 7 or greater (suggests infection); bacteria, WBCs, RBCs may be present microscopically.

Urine culture: May reveal *Staphylococcus aureus*, *Proteus*, *Klebsiella*, *Pseudomonas*, or *Escherichia coli*.

Urine cytology: To rule out bladder cancer.

BUN/Cr: Elevated if renal function is compromised.

Prostate-specific antigen (PSA): Glycoprotein contained in the cytoplasm of prostatic epithelial cells, detected in the blood of adult men. Level is greatly increased in prostatic cancer but can also be elevated in BPH. *Note:* Research suggests elevated PSA levels with a low percentage of free PSA are more likely associated with prostate cancer than with a benign prostate condition.

WBC: May be greater than 11,000, indicating infection if patient is not immunosuppressed.

Uroflowmetry: Assesses degree of bladder obstruction.

IVP with postvoiding film: Shows delayed emptying of bladder, varying degrees of urinary tract obstruction, and presence of prostatic enlargement, bladder diverticuli, and abnormal thickening of bladder muscle.

Voiding cystourethrography: May be used instead of IVP to visualize bladder and urethra because it uses local dyes.

Cystometrogram: Measures pressure and volume in the bladder to identify bladder dysfunction unrelated to BPH.

Cystourethroscopy: To view degree of prostatic enlargement and bladder-wall changes (bladder diverticulum).

Cystometry: Evaluates detrusor muscle function and tone.

Transrectal prostatic ultrasound: Measures size of prostate and amount of residual urine; locates lesions unrelated to BPH.

NURSING PRIORITIES

1. Relieve acute urinary retention.
2. Promote comfort.
3. Prevent complications.
4. Help patient deal with psychosocial concerns.
5. Provide information about disease process/prognosis and treatment needs.

DISCHARGE GOALS

1. Voiding pattern normalized.
2. Pain/discomfort relieved.
3. Complications prevented/minimized.
4. Dealing with situation realistically.
5. Disease process/prognosis and therapeutic regimen understood.
6. Plan in place to meet needs after discharge.

NURSING DIAGNOSIS: Urinary Retention [acute/chronic]

May be related to
Mechanical obstruction; enlarged prostate
Decompensation of detrusor musculature
Inability of bladder to contract adequately

Possibly evidenced by
Frequency, hesitancy, inability to empty bladder completely; incontinence/dribbling
Bladder distension, residual urine

DESIRED OUTCOMES/EVALUATION CRITERIA—PATIENT WILL:

> **Urinary Elimination (NOC)**

Void in sufficient amounts with no palpable bladder distention.
Demonstrate postvoid residuals of less than 50 mL, with absence of dribbling/overflow.

ACTIONS/INTERVENTIONS	RATIONALE
Urinary Retention Care (NIC)	

Independent

Encourage patient to void every 2–4 hr and when urge is noted.	May minimize urinary retention/overdistension of the bladder.
Ask patient about stress incontinence when moving, sneezing, coughing, laughing, lifting objects.	High urethral pressure inhibits bladder emptying or can inhibit voiding until abdominal pressure increases enough for urine to be involuntarily lost.
Observe urinary stream, noting size and force.	Useful in evaluating degree of obstruction and choice of intervention.
Have patient document time and amount of each voiding. Note diminished urinary output. Measure specific gravity as indicated.	Urinary retention increases pressure within the ureters and kidneys, which may cause renal insufficiency. Any deficit in blood flow to the kidney impairs its ability to filter and concentrate substances.
Percuss/palpate suprapubic area.	A distended bladder can be felt in the suprapubic area.
Encourage oral fluids up to 3000 mL daily, within cardiac tolerance, if indicated.	Increased circulating fluid maintains renal perfusion and flushes kidneys, bladder, and ureters of "sediment and bacteria." *Note:* Initially, fluids may be restricted to prevent bladder distension until adequate urinary flow is re-established.
Monitor vital signs closely. Observe for hypertension, peripheral/dependent edema, changes in mentation. Weigh daily. Maintain accurate I&O.	Loss of kidney function results in decreased fluid elimination and accumulation of toxic wastes; may progress to complete renal shutdown.
Provide/encourage meticulous catheter and perineal care.	Reduces risk of ascending infection.
Recommend sitz bath as indicated.	Promotes muscle relaxation, decreases edema, and may enhance voiding effort.

Collaborative

Administer medications as indicated:	
Androgen inhibitors, e.g., finasteride (Proscar).	Reduces the size of the prostate and decreases symptoms if taken long-term; however, side effects such as decreased libido and ejaculatory dysfunction may influence patient's choice for long-term use.
Alpha-adrenergic antagonists, e.g., tamsulosin (Flomax), prazosin (Minipress), terazosin (Hytrin), doxazosin mesylate (Cardura);	Studies indicate that these drugs may be as effective as Proscar for outflow obstruction and may have fewer side effects in regard to sexual function.
Antispasmodics, e.g., oxybutynin (Ditropan);	Relieves bladder spasms related to irritation by the catheter.
Rectal suppositories (B&O);	Suppositories are absorbed easily through mucosa into bladder tissue to produce muscle relaxation/relieve spasms.
Antibiotics and antibacterials.	Given to combat infection. May be used prophylactically.

ACTIONS/INTERVENTIONS	RATIONALE
Collaborative	
Catheterize for residual urine and leave indwelling catheter as indicated.	Relieves/prevents urinary retention and rules out presence of ureteral stricture. Coudé catheter may be required because the curved tip eases passage of the tube through the prostatic urethra. *Note:* Bladder decompression should be done in increments of 200 mL to prevent hematuria (rupture of blood vessels in the mucosa of the overdistended bladder) and syncope (excessive autonomic stimulation).
Irrigate catheter as indicated.	Maintains patency/urinary flow.
Monitor laboratory studies, e.g.:	
BUN, Cr, electrolytes;	Prostatic enlargement (obstruction) eventually causes dilation of upper urinary tract (ureters and kidneys), potentially impairing kidney function and leading to uremia.
Urinalysis and culture.	Urinary stasis potentiates bacterial growth, increasing risk of UTI.
Prepare for/assist with urinary drainage, e.g., Cystostomy.	May be indicated to drain bladder during acute episode with azotemia or when surgery is contraindicated because of patient's health status.
Prepare for surgical intervention, e.g.:	
Balloon urethroplasty/transurethral dilation of the prostatic urethra;	Inflation of a balloon-tipped catheter within the obstructed area stretches the urethra and displaces prostatic tissue, thus improving urinary flow.
Transurethral incision of the prostate (TUIP);	A procedure of almost equivalent efficacy to transurethral resection of the prostate (TURP) used for prostates with estimated resected tissue weight of 30 g or less. It may be performed instead of balloon dilation with better outcomes. Procedure can be done in ambulatory or short-stay settings. *Note:* Open prostate resection procedures (TURP) are typically performed on patients with very large prostates.
Transurethral microwave thermotherapy (TUMT).	Heating the central portion of the prostate by the insertion of a heating element through the urethra destroys prostate cells. Treatment is usually completed in a one-time procedure carried out in the physician's office. Note: This procedure was approved by the Food and Drug Administration (FDA) in 1996.

NURSING DIAGNOSIS: Pain [acute]

May be related to

Mucosal irritation: bladder distension, renal colic; urinary infection; radiation therapy

Possibly evidenced by

Reports of pain (bladder/rectal spasm)

Narrowed focus; altered muscle tone, grimacing; distraction behaviors, restlessness

Autonomic responses

DESIRED OUTCOMES/EVALUATION CRITERIA—PATIENT WILL:

Pain Level (NOC)

Report pain relieved/controlled.
Appear relaxed.
Be able to sleep/rest appropriately.

ACTIONS/INTERVENTIONS

Pain Management (NIC)

Independent

Assess pain, noting location, intensity (scale of 0–10), duration.

Tape drainage tube to thigh and catheter to the abdomen (if traction not required).

Recommend bedrest as indicated.

Provide comfort measures, e.g., back rub, helping patient assume position of comfort. Suggest use of relaxation/deep-breathing exercises, diversional activities.

Encourage use of sitz baths, warm soaks to perineum.

Collaborative

Insert catheter and attach to straight drainage as indicated.

Instruct in prostatic massage.

Administer medications as indicated:

  Narcotics, e.g., meperidine (Demerol);

  Antibacterials, e.g., methenamine hippurate (Hiprex);

  Antispasmodics and bladder sedatives, e.g., flavoxate (Urispas); oxybutynin (Ditropan).

RATIONALE

Provides information to aid in determining choice/effectiveness of interventions.

Prevents pull on the bladder and erosion of the penile-scrotal junction.

Bedrest may be needed initially during acute retention phase; however, early ambulation can help restore normal voiding patterns and relieve colicky pain.

Promotes relaxation, refocuses attention, and may enhance coping abilities.

Promotes muscle relaxation.

Draining bladder reduces bladder tension and irritability.

Aids in evacuation of ducts of gland to relieve congestion/inflammation. Contraindicated if infection is present.

Given to relieve severe pain, provide physical and mental relaxation.

Reduces bacteria present in urinary tract and those introduced by drainage system.

Relieves bladder irritability.

NURSING DIAGNOSIS: Fluid Volume, risk for deficit

Risk factors may include
Postobstructive diuresis from rapid drainage of a chronically overdistended bladder
Endocrine, electrolyte imbalances (renal dysfunction)

Possibly evidenced by
[Not applicable; presence of signs and symptoms establishes an *actual* diagnosis]

| Hydration (NOC) |

Maintain adequate hydration as evidenced by stable vital signs, palpable peripheral pulses, good capillary refill, and moist mucous membranes.

ACTIONS/INTERVENTIONS	RATIONALE

| Fluid Management (NIC) |

Independent

Monitor output carefully. Note outputs of 100–200 mL/hr.	Rapid/sustained diuresis could cause the patient's total fluid volume to become depleted and limits sodium reabsorption in renal tubules.
Encourage increased oral intake based on individual needs.	Patient may have restricted oral intake in an attempt to control urinary symptoms, reducing homeostatic reserves and increasing risk of dehydration/hypovolemia.
Monitor BP, pulse. Evaluate capillary refill and oral mucous membranes.	Enables early detection of and intervention for systemic hypovolemia.
Promote bedrest with head elevated.	Decreases cardiac workload, facilitating circulatory homeostasis.

Collaborative

| Monitor electrolyte levels, especially sodium. | As fluid is pulled from extracellular spaces, sodium may follow the shift, causing hyponatremia. |
| Administer IV fluids (hypertonic saline) as needed. | Replaces fluid and sodium losses to prevent/correct hypovolemia following outpatient procedures. |

NURSING DIAGNOSIS: Fear/Anxiety [specify level]

May be related to
Change in health status: possibility of surgical procedure/malignancy
Embarrassment/loss of dignity associated with genital exposure before, during, and
    after treatment; concern about sexual ability

Possibly evidenced by
Increased tension, apprehension, worry
Expressed concerns regarding perceived changes
Fear of unspecific consequences

DESIRED OUTCOMES/EVALUATION CRITERIA—PATIENT WILL:

| Anxiety or Fear Control (NOC) |

Appear relaxed.
Verbalize accurate knowledge of the situation.
Demonstrate appropriate range of feelings and lessened fear.
Report anxiety is reduced to a manageable level.

ACTIONS/INTERVENTIONS

Anxiety Reduction (NIC)

Independent

Be available to the patient. Establish trusting relationship with patient/SO.

Provide information about specific procedures and tests and what to expect afterward, e.g., catheter, bloody urine, bladder irritation. Be aware of how much information the patient wants.

Maintain matter-of-fact attitude in doing procedures/dealing with patient. Protect patient's privacy.

Encourage patient/SO to verbalize concerns and feelings.

Reinforce previous information patient has been given.

RATIONALE

Demonstrates concern and willingness to help. Helpful in discussing sensitive subjects.

Helps patient understand purpose of what is being done and reduces concerns associated with the unknown, including fear of cancer. However, overload of information is not helpful and may increase anxiety.

Communicates acceptance and eases patient's embarrassment.

Defines the problem, providing opportunity to answer questions, clarify misconceptions, and problem-solve solutions.

Allows the patient to deal with reality and strengthens trust in caregivers and information presented.

NURSING DIAGNOSIS: Knowledge Deficit [Learning Need] regarding condition, prognosis, treatment, self care, and discharge needs

May be related to
Lack of exposure/recall, information misinterpretation
Unfamiliarity with information resources
Concern about sensitive area

Possibly evidenced by
Questions, request for information; verbalization of the problem
Inappropriate behaviors, e.g., apathetic, withdrawn
Inaccurate follow-through of instructions, development of preventable complications

DESIRED OUTCOMES/EVALUATION CRITERIA—PATIENT WILL:

Knowledge: Disease Process (NOC)

Verbalize understanding of disease process/prognosis, and potential complications.
Identify relationship of signs/symptoms to the disease process.

Knowledge: Treatment Regimen (NOC)

Verbalize understanding of therapeutic needs.
Initiate necessary lifestyle/behavior changes.
Participate in treatment regimen.

ACTIONS/INTERVENTIONS

Teaching: Disease Process (NIC)

Independent

Review disease process, patient expectations.

Encourage verbalization of fears/feelings and concerns.

RATIONALE

Provides knowledge base from which patient can make informed therapy choices.

Helping patient work through feelings can be vital to rehabilitation.

ACTIONS/INTERVENTIONS	RATIONALE
Independent	
Give information that the condition is not sexually transmitted.	May be an unspoken fear.
Recommend avoiding spicy foods, coffee, alcohol, long automobile rides, rapid intake of fluids (particularly alcohol).	May cause prostatic irritation with resulting congestion. Sudden increase in urinary flow can cause bladder distension and loss of bladder tone, resulting in episodes of acute urinary retention.
Address sexual concerns, e.g., during acute episodes of prostatitis, intercourse is avoided, but may be helpful in treatment of chronic condition.	Sexual activity can increase pain during acute episodes but may serve as massaging agent in presence of chronic disease. *Note:* Medications such as finasteride (Proscar) are known to interfere with libido and erections. Alternatives include terazosin (Hytrin), doxazosin mesylate (Cardura), and tamsulosin (Flomax), which do not affect testosterone levels.
Provide information about basic sexual anatomy. Encourage questions and promote a dialogue about concerns.	Having information about anatomy involved helps patient understand the implications of proposed treatments because they might affect sexual performance.
Review signs/symptoms requiring medical evaluation, e.g., cloudy, odorous urine; diminished urinary output, inability to void; presence of fever/chills.	Prompt interventions may prevent more serious complications.
Discuss necessity of notifying other healthcare providers of diagnosis.	Reduces risk of inappropriate therapy; e.g., use of decongestants, anticholinergics, and antidepressants, which can increase urinary retention and may precipitate an acute episode.
Reinforce importance of medical follow-up for at least 6 mo to 1 yr, including rectal examination, urinalysis.	Recurrence of hypertrophy and/or infection (caused by same or different organisms) is not uncommon and requires changes in therapeutic regimen to prevent serious complications.

POTENTIAL CONSIDERATIONS following acute hospitalization (dependent on patient's age, physical condition/presence of complications, personal resources, and life responsibilities)

Urinary Retention [acute/chronic]—urethral obstruction, decompensation of detrusor musculature, loss of bladder tone.
Infection, risk for—urinary stasis, invasive procedure (periodic catheterization).

PROSTATECTOMY

Many males over age 75 have small, slow-growing prostate tumors that cause little harm. However, surgical resection of the portion of the prostate gland encroaching on the urethra may be required to improve urinary flow and relieve acute urinary retention regardless of the patient's age. *Note:* Laser prostatectomy is being done in routine practice; however, published data relative to the efficacy of the procedure is currently insufficient.

Transurethral resection of the prostate (TURP): Obstructive prostatic tissue of the medial lobe surrounding the urethra is removed by means of a cystoscope/resectoscope introduced through the urethra.

Suprapubic/open prostatectomy: Indicated for masses exceeding 60 g (2 oz). Obstructing prostatic tissue is removed through a low midline incision made through the bladder. This approach is preferred if bladder stones are present.

Retropubic prostatectomy: Hypertrophied prostatic tissue mass (located high in the pelvic region) is removed through a low abdominal incision without opening the bladder.

Perineal prostatectomy: Large prostatic masses low in the pelvic area are removed through an incision between the scrotum and the rectum. This radical procedure is done for cancer and may result in impotence.

CARE SETTING

Inpatient acute surgical unit.

RELATED CONCERNS

Surgical intervention, page 828
Cancer, page 900
Psychosocial aspects of care, page 809

Patient Assessment Datebase

Refer to CP: Benign Prostatic Hyperplasia (BPH), page 635, for assessment information.

Discharge plan considerations: DRG projected mean length of inpatient stay: 3.3–7.1 days

Refer to section at end of plan for postdischarge considerations

NURSING PRIORITIES

1. Maintain homeostasis/hemodynamic stability.
2. Promote comfort.
3. Prevent complications.
4. Provide information about surgical procedure/prognosis, treatment, and rehabilitation needs.

DISCHARGE GOALS

1. Urinary flow restored/enhanced.
2. Pain relieved/controlled.
3. Complications prevented/minimized.
4. Procedure/prognosis, therapeutic regimen, and rehabilitation needs understood.
5. Plan in place to meet needs after discharge.

NURSING DIAGNOSIS: Urinary Elimination, altered

May be related to

Mechanical obstruction: Blood clots, edema, trauma, surgical procedure

Pressure and irritation of catheter/balloon

Loss of bladder tone due to preoperative overdistension or continued decompression

Possibly evidenced by
Frequency, urgency, hesitancy, dysuria, incontinence, retention
Bladder fullness; suprapubic discomfort

DESIRED OUTCOMES/EVALUATION CRITERIA—PATIENT WILL:

Urinary Elimination (NOC)

Void normal amounts without retention.
Demonstrate behaviors to regain bladder/urinary control.

ACTIONS/INTERVENTIONS	RATIONALE

Urinary Elimination Management (NIC)

Independent

Assess urine output and catheter/drainage system, especially during bladder irrigation.	Retention can occur because of edema of the surgical area, blood clots, and bladder spasms.
Assist patient to assume normal position to void, e.g., stand, walk to bathroom at frequent intervals after catheter is removed.	Encourages passage of urine and promotes sense of normality.
Note time, amount of voiding, and size of stream after catheter is removed. Note reports of bladder fullness; inability to void, urgency.	The catheter is usually removed 2–5 days after surgery, but voiding may continue to be a problem for some time because of urethral edema and loss of bladder tone.
Encourage patient to void when urge is noted but not more than every 2–4 hr per protocol.	Voiding with urge prevents urinary retention. Limiting voids to every 4 hr (if tolerated), increases bladder tone and aids in bladder retraining.
Measure residual volumes via suprapubic catheter if present, or with Doppler ultrasound.	Monitors effectiveness of bladder emptying. Residuals greater than 50 mL suggest need for continuation of catheter until bladder tone improves.
Encourage fluid intake to 3000 mL as tolerated. Limit fluids in the evening, once catheter is removed.	Maintains adequate hydration and renal perfusion for urinary flow. "Scheduling" fluid intake reduces need to void/interrupt sleep during the night.
Instruct patient in perineal exercises, e.g., tightening buttocks, stopping and starting urine stream.	Helps to regain bladder/sphincter/urinary control, minimizing incontinence.
Advise patient that "dribbling" is to be expected after catheter is removed and should resolve as recuperation progresses.	Information helps patient deal with the problem. Normal functioning may return in 2–3 wk but can take up to 8 months following perineal approach.

Collaborative

Maintain continuous bladder irrigation (CBI), as indicated in early postoperative period.	Flushes bladder of blood clots and debris to maintain patency of the catheter/urinary flow.

NURSING DIAGNOSIS: Fluid Volume, risk for deficit

Risk factors may include
Vascular nature of surgical area; difficulty controlling bleeding
Restricted intake preoperatively
Postobstructive diuresis

Possibly evidenced by

[Not applicable; presence of signs and symptoms establishes an *actual* diagnosis]

DESIRED OUTCOMES/EVALUATION CRITERIA—PATIENT WILL:

Hydration (NOC)

Maintain adequate hydration as evidenced by stable vital signs, palpable peripheral pulses, good capillary refill, moist mucous membranes, and appropriate urinary output.

Display no active bleeding.

ACTIONS/INTERVENTIONS	RATIONALE
Fluid Management (NIC)	
Independent	
Monitor I&O.	Indicator of fluid balance and replacement needs. With bladder irrigations, monitoring is essential for estimating blood loss and accurately assessing urine output. *Note:* Following release of urinary tract obstruction, marked diuresis may occur during initial recovery period.
Monitor vital signs, noting increased pulse and respiration, decreased BP, diaphoresis, pallor, delayed capillary refill, and dry mucous membranes.	Dehydration/hypovolemia requires prompt intervention to prevent impending shock. *Note:* Hypertension, bradycardia, nausea/vomiting suggests "TURP syndrome," requiring immediate medical intervention.
Investigate restlessness, confusion, changes in behavior.	May reflect decreased cerebral perfusion (hypovolemia) or indicate cerebral edema from excessive solution absorbed into the venous sinusoids during TUR procedure ("TURP syndrome").
Encourage fluid intake to 3000 mL/day unless contraindicated.	Flushes kidneys/bladder of bacteria and debris but may result in water intoxication/fluid overload if not monitored closely.
Bleeding Reduction (NIC)	
Anchor catheter, avoid excessive manipulation.	Movement/pulling of catheter may cause bleeding or clot formation and plugging of the catheter, with bladder distension.
Observe catheter drainage, noting excessive/continued bleeding.	Bleeding is not unusual during first 24 hr for all but the perineal approach. Continued/heavy bleeding or recurrence of active bleeding requires medical evaluation/intervention.
Evaluate color, consistency of urine, e.g.:	
Bright red with bright red clots;	Usually indicates arterial bleeding and requires aggressive therapy.
Dark burgundy with dark clots, increased viscosity;	Suggests venous source (the most common type of bleeding), which usually subsides on its own.
Bleeding with absence of clots.	May indicate blood dyscrasias or systemic clotting problems.

ACTIONS/INTERVENTIONS	RATIONALE
Independent	
Inspect dressings/wound drains. Weigh dressings if indicated. Note hematoma formation.	Bleeding may be evident or sequestered within tissues of the perineum.
Avoid taking rectal temperatures and use of rectal tubes/enemas.	May result in referred irritation to prostatic bed and increased pressure on prostatic capsule with risk of bleeding.
Collaborative	
Monitor laboratory studies as indicated, e.g.:	
Hb/Hct, RBCs;	Useful in evaluating blood losses/replacement needs.
Coagulation studies, platelet count.	May indicate developing complications, e.g., depletion of clotting factors, DIC.
Administer IV therapy/blood products as indicated.	May need additional fluids, if oral intake inadequate, or blood products, if losses are excessive.
Maintain traction on indwelling catheter; tape catheter to inner thigh.	Traction on the 30-mL balloon positioned in the prostatic urethral fossa creates pressure on the arterial supply of the prostatic capsule to help prevent/control bleeding.
Release traction within 4–5 hr. Document period of application and release of traction, if used.	Prolonged traction may cause permanent trauma/problems with urinary control.
Administer stool softeners, laxatives as indicated.	Prevention of constipation/straining for stool reduces risk of rectal-perineal bleeding.

NURSING DIAGNOSIS: Infection, risk for

Risk factors may include
Invasive procedures: instrumentation during surgery, catheter, frequent bladder irrigation
Traumatized tissue, surgical incision (e.g., perineal)

Possibly evidenced by
[Not applicable; presence of signs and symptoms establishes an *actual* diagnosis]

DESIRED OUTCOMES/EVALUATION CRITERIA—PATIENT WILL:

Wound Healing: Primary Intention (NOC)

Achieve timely healing.
Experience no signs of infection.

ACTIONS/INTERVENTIONS	RATIONALE
Infection Protection (NIC)	
Independent	
Maintain sterile catheter system; provide regular catheter/meatal care with soap and water, applying antibiotic ointment around catheter site.	Prevents introduction of bacteria and resultant infection/sepsis.
Ambulate with drainage bag dependent.	Avoids backward reflux of urine, which may introduce bacteria into the bladder.
Monitor vital signs, noting low-grade fever, chills, rapid pulse and respiration, restlessness, irritability, disorientation.	Patient who has had cystoscopy and/or TURP is at increased risk for surgical/septic shock related to manipulation/instrumentation.

646

ACTIONS/INTERVENTIONS

Independent

Observe drainage from wounds, around suprapubic catheter.

Change dressings frequently (suprapubic/retropubic and perineal incisions), cleaning and drying skin thoroughly each time.

Use ostomy-type skin barriers.

Collaborative

Administer antibiotics as indicated.

RATIONALE

Presence of drains, suprapubic incision increases risk of infection, as indicated by erythema, purulent drainage.

Wet dressings cause skin irritation and provide media for bacterial growth, increasing risk of wound infection.

Provides protection for surrounding skin, preventing excoriation and reducing risk of infection.

May be given prophylactically because of increased risk of infection with prostatectomy.

NURSING DIAGNOSIS: Pain [acute]

May be related to
Irritation of the bladder mucosa; reflex muscle spasm associated with surgical procedure and/or pressure from bladder balloon (traction)

Possibly evidenced by
Reports of painful bladder spasms
Facial grimacing, guarding, restlessness
Autonomic responses

DESIRED OUTCOMES/EVALUATION CRITERIA—PATIENT WILL:

Pain Level (NOC)

Report pain is relieved/controlled.
Appear relaxed, sleep/rest appropriately.

Pain Control Behavior (NOC)

Demonstrate use of relaxation skills and diversional activities as indicated for individual situation.

ACTIONS/INTERVENTIONS

Pain Management (NIC)

Independent

Assess pain, noting location, intensity (0–10 scale).

Maintain patency of catheter and drainage system. Keep tubings free of kinks and clots.

Promote intake of up to 3000 mL/day as tolerated.

Give patient accurate information about catheter, drainage, and bladder spasms.

RATIONALE

Sharp, intermittent pain with urge to void/passage of urine around catheter suggests bladder spasms, which tend to be more severe with suprapubic or TUR approaches (usually decrease by the end of 48 hr).

Maintaining a properly functioning catheter and drainage system decreases risk of bladder distension/spasm.

Decreases irritation by maintaining a constant flow of fluid over the bladder mucosa.

Allays anxiety and promotes cooperation with necessary procedures.

ACTIONS/INTERVENTIONS

Independent

Provide comfort measures, e.g., position changes/back rub, Therapeutic Touch, and diversional activities. Encourage use of relaxation techniques, including deep-breathing exercises, visualization, guided imagery.

Provide sitz baths or heat lamp if indicated.

Collaborative

Administer antispasmodics, e.g.:

Oxybutynin (Ditropan), B&O suppositories;

Propantheline bromide (Pro-Banthine).

RATIONALE

Reduces muscle tension, refocuses attention, and may enhance coping abilities.

Promotes tissue perfusion and resolution of edema, and enhances healing (perineal approach).

Relaxes smooth muscle to provide relief of spasms and associated pain.

Relieves bladder spasms by anticholinergic action. Usually discontinued 24–48 hr before anticipated removal of catheter to promote normal bladder contraction.

NURSING DIAGNOSIS: Sexual Dysfunction, risk for

Risk factors may include
Situational crisis (incontinence, leakage of urine after catheter removal, involvement of genital area)
Threat to self-concept/change in health status

Possibly evidenced by
[Not applicable; presence of signs and symptoms establishes an *actual* diagnosis]

DESIRED OUTCOMES/EVALUATION CRITERIA—PATIENT WILL:

Role Performance (NOC)

Reports understanding of sexual function and alterations that may occur with surgery in individual situation
Discuss concerns about possible changes in body image, sexual functioning with partner/SO and caregiver.
Demonstrate problem-solving skills regarding solutions to problems that occur.

ACTIONS/INTERVENTIONS

Sexual Counseling (NIC)

Independent

Provide openings for patient/SO to talk about concerns of incontinence and sexual functioning.

Discuss basic anatomy. Be honest in answers to patient's questions.

RATIONALE

May have anxieties about the effects of surgery and may be hesitant about asking necessary questions. Anxiety may have affected ability to access information given previously.

The nerve plexus that controls erection runs posteriorly to the prostate through the capsule. In procedures that do not involve the prostatic capsule, impotence and sterility usually are not consequences. Surgical procedure may not provide a permanent cure, and hypertrophy may recur.

ACTIONS/INTERVENTIONS

Independent

Give accurate information about expectation of return of sexual function.

Discuss retrograde ejaculation if transurethral/suprapubic approach is used.

Instruct in perineal and interruption/continuation of urinary stream exercises.

Collaborative

Refer to sexual counselor as indicated.

RATIONALE

Physiological impotence occurs when the perineal nerves are cut during radical procedures; with other approaches, sexual activity can usually be resumed in 6–8 wk. *Note:* Penile prosthesis may be recommended to facilitate erection and correct impotence following radical perineal procedure.

Seminal fluid goes into the bladder and is excreted with the urine. This does not interfere with sexual functioning but will decrease fertility and cause urine to be cloudy.

Kegel exercises promote regaining muscular control of urinary continence and sexual function.

Persistent/unresolved problems may require professional intervention.

NURSING DIAGNOSIS: Knowledge Deficit [Learning Need] regarding condition, prognosis, treatment, self care, and discharge needs

May be related to
Lack of exposure/recall; information misinterpretation
Unfamiliarity with information resources

Possibly evidenced by
Questions, request for information, statement of misconception
Verbalization of the problem
Inaccurate follow-through of instruction/development of preventable complications

DESIRED OUTCOMES/EVALUATION CRITERIA—PATIENT WILL:

Knowledge: Disease Process (NOC)

Verbalize understanding of surgical procedure and potential complications.

Knowledge: Treatment Regimen (NOC)

Verbalize understanding of therapeutic needs.
Correctly perform necessary procedures and explain reasons for actions.
Initiate necessary lifestyle changes.
Participate in therapeutic regimen.

ACTIONS/INTERVENTIONS

Teaching: Disease Process (NIC)

Independent

Review implications of procedure and future expectations.

Stress necessity of good nutrition; encourage inclusion of fruits, increased fiber in diet.

RATIONALE

Provides knowledge base from which patient can make informed choices.

Promotes healing and prevents constipation, reducing risk of postoperative bleeding.

ACTIONS/INTERVENTIONS	RATIONALE
Independent	
Discuss initial activity restrictions, e.g., avoidance of heavy lifting, strenuous exercise, prolonged sitting/long automobile trips, climbing more than two flights of stairs at a time.	Increased abdominal pressure/straining places stress on the bladder and prostate, potentiating risk of bleeding.
Encourage continuation of perineal exercises.	Facilitates urinary control and alleviation of incontinence.
Instruct in urinary catheter care if present. Identify source for supplies/support.	Promotes independence and competent self-care.
Instruct patient to avoid tub baths after discharge.	Decreases the possibility of infection, introduction of bacteria.
Review signs/symptoms requiring medical evaluation, e.g., erythema, purulent drainage from wound sites; changes in character/amount of urine, presence of urgency/frequency; heavy bleeding, fever, or chills.	Prompt intervention may prevent serious complications. *Note:* Urine may appear cloudy for several weeks until postoperative healing occurs and may appear cloudy after intercourse because of retrograde ejaculation.

POTENTIAL CONSIDERATIONS following acute hospitalization (dependent on patient's age, physical condition/presence of complications, personal resources, and life responsibilities)

In addition to postsurgical concerns:

Urinary Elimination, altered—loss of bladder tone, possible discharge with catheter in place.
Sexual dysfunction—leakage of urine; loss of erectile function following radical procedure.

Sample CP: TURP, hospital, ELOS: 3 Days Urology or Surgical Unit

ND and Categories of Care	Day 1 _____ Day of Surgery	Day 2 _____ POD #1	Day 3 _____ POD #2
Altered urinary elimination R/T mechanical obstruction, loss of bladder tone, therapeutic intervention	Display urine output individually appropriate, few clots and catheter free-flowing	Verbalize understanding of home care needs, S/S to report to healthcare provider	Void normal amounts w/o retention Demonstrate behaviors to regain bladder/urinary control Plan in place to meet postdischarge needs
Referrals		Home care	
Additional assessments	Characteristics of urinary drainage → Urinary output q8h → Presence of spontaneous voiding →		Voiding frequency, character of urine Amount per void →
Patient education	Foley catheter function, hygiene	Perineal exercises Home care needs, activity/dietary restrictions, sexual concerns S/S to report to healthcare provider	Provide written instructions, schedule for follow-up visits
Additional nursing actions	Foley catheter to straight drain, → DC irrigate/CBI per protocol Bedrest if CBI Bed flat X 8 hr if epidural anesthesia	Stand to void q2–4h → Ambulate as tolerated → Encourage fluids to 3 L/day as → indicated	Per self q4h Ad lib
Pain R/T increased frequency/force of ureteral contractions, tissue trauma, edema	Report pain relieved/controlled →		→ Verbalize understanding of pain management postdischarge

Sample CP: TURP, hospital, ELOS: 3 Days Urology or Surgical Unit *(Continued)*

ND and Categories of Care	Day 1 Day of Surgery		Day 2 POD #1	Day 3 POD #2	
Additional assessments	Pain characteristics/changes, presence of bladder spasms	→		→	
	Response to interventions	→		→	
			Return of bowel function	→	
Medications Allergies:	Analgesic of choice IM/PO q4h	→	PO analgesic	→	
	Antispasmotic prn	→	D/C		
			Stool softener/laxative	→	
Patient education	Reporting of pain/effects of intervention				
	Relaxation techniques				
Additional nursing actions	Routine comfort measures	→		→	
	Anchor catheter, avoid manipulation				
	Maintain potency of catheter				
			Sitz bath as indicated	→	
Risk for fluid volume deficit, R/T nausea and vomiting, postobstructive diuresis	Maintain adequate hydration with VS stable, palpable pulses, good capillary refill, adequate urinary output	→		→	
	Free of active bleeding	→		→	
Diagnostic studies			Hb/Hct, RBC		
Additional assessments	Characteristics of catheter drainage	→	Characteristics of urine	→	
	VS per postoperative protocol	→	q8h	→	
	Peripheral pulses, capillary refill, status of skin q8h	→		→	D/C
	I&O q8h	→		→	D/C
	Mental status/restlessness q4h	→	q8h	→	D/C
	Temperature q8h	→		→	
Medications	IV therapy/blood products as indicated	→	DC		
Patient education	Fluid needs/restrictions				
Additional nursing actions	Maintain catheter traction as indicated, release q4h per protocol	→	D/C		
	Begin PO fluids as tolerated	→	Advance diet/fluids as tolerated	→	

UROLITHIASIS (RENAL CALCULI)

Kidney stones (calculi) are formed of mineral deposits, most commonly calcium oxalate and calcium phosphate; however, uric acid, struvite, and cystine are also calculus formers. Although renal calculi can form anywhere in the urinary tract, they are most commonly found in the renal pelvis and calyces. Renal calculi can remain asymptomatic until passed into a ureter and/or urine flow is obstructed, when the potential for renal damage is acute.

CARE SETTING

Acute episodes may require inpatient treatment on a medical or surgical unit.

RELATED CONCERNS

Metabolic acidosis (primary base bicarbonate deficit), page 523
Metabolic alkalosis (primary base bicarbonate excess), page 527
Fluid and electrolyte imbalances, page 926
Psychosocial aspects of care, page 809
Renal failure: acute, page 575

Patient Assessment Database

Dependent on size, location, and etiology of calculi

ACTIVITY/REST

May report: Sedentary occupation or occupation in which patient is exposed to high environmental temperatures
Activity restrictions/immobility due to a preexisting condition (e.g., debilitating disease, spinal cord injury)

CIRCULATION

May exhibit: Elevated BP/pulse (pain, anxiety, kidney failure)
Warm, flushed skin; pallor

ELIMINATION

May report: History of recent/chronic UTI; previous obstruction (calculi)
Decreased urinary output, bladder fullness
Burning, urgency with urination
Diarrhea

May exhibit: Oliguria, hematuria, pyuria
Alterations in voiding pattern

FOOD/FLUID

May report: Nausea/vomiting, abdominal tenderness
Diet high in purines, calcium oxalate, and/or phosphates
Insufficient fluid intake; does not drink fluids well

May exhibit: Abdominal distention; decreased/absent bowel sounds
Vomiting

PAIN/DISCOMFORT

May report: Acute episode of excruciating, colicky pain with location depending on stone location, e.g., in the flank in the region of the costovertebral angle; may radiate to back, abdomen, and down to the groin/genitalia. Constant dull pain suggests calculi located in the renal pelvis or calyces
Pain may be described as acute, severe, not relieved by positioning or any other measures

May exhibit: Guarding; distraction behaviors; self-focusing
Tenderness in renal areas on palpation

SAFETY

May report: Use of alcohol
Fever; chills

TEACHING/LEARNING

May report: Family history of calculi, kidney disease, hypertension, gout, chronic UTI
History of small-bowel disease, previous abdominal surgery, hyperparathyroidism
Use of antibiotics, antihypertensives, sodium bicarbonate, allopurinol, phosphates, thiazides, excessive intake of calcium or vitamin D

Discharge plan considerations: **DRG projected mean length of inpatient stay: 2.9 days**

Refer to section at end of plan for postdischarge considerations.

DIAGNOSTIC STUDIES

Urinalysis: Color may be yellow, dark brown, bloody. Commonly shows RBCs, WBCs, crystals (cystine, uric acid, calcium oxalate), casts, minerals, bacteria, pus, pH may be less than 5 (promotes cystine and uric acid stones) or greater than 7.5 (promotes magnesium, struvite, phosphate, or calcium phosphate stones).

Urine (24-hr): Cr, uric acid, calcium, phosphorus, oxalate, or cystine may be elevated.

Urine culture: May reveal UTI *(Staphylococcus aureus, Proteus, Klebsiella, Pseudomonas).*

Biochemical survey: Elevated levels of magnesium, calcium, uric acid, phosphates, protein, electrolytes.

Serum and urine BUN/Cr: Abnormal (high in serum/low in urine) secondary to high obstructive stone in kidney causing ischemia/necrosis.

Serum chloride and bicarbonate levels: Elevation of chloride and decreased levels of bicarbonate suggest developing renal tubular acidosis.

CBC:

     Hb/Hct: Abnormal if patient is severely dehydrated or polycythemia is present (encourages precipitation of solids), or patient is anemic (hemorrhage, kidney dysfunction/failure).

     RBCs: Usually normal.

     WBCs: May be increased indicating infection/septicemia.

Parathyroid hormone (PTH): May be increased if kidney failure present. (PTH stimulates reabsorption of calcium from bones, increasing circulating serum and urine calcium levels.)

KUB x-ray: Shows presence of calculi and/or anatomic changes in the area of the kidneys or along the course of the ureter.

IVP: Provides rapid confirmation of urolithiasis as a cause of abdominal or flank pain. Shows abnormalities in anatomic structures (distended ureter) and outline of calculi.

Cystoureteroscopy: Direct visualization of bladder and ureter may reveal stone and/or obstructive effects.

CT scan: Identifies/delineates calculi and other masses; kidney, ureteral, and bladder distension.

Ultrasound of kidney: To determine obstructive changes, location of stone; without the risk of failure induced by contrast medium.

NURSING PRIORITIES

1. Alleviate pain.
2. Maintain adequate renal functioning.
3. Prevent complications.
4. Provide information about disease process/prognosis and treatment needs.

DISCHARGE GOALS

1. Pain relieved/controlled.
2. Fluid/electrolyte balance maintained.
3. Complications prevented/minimized.
4. Disease process/prognosis and therapeutic regimen understood.
5. Plan in place to meet needs after discharge.

> **NURSING DIAGNOSIS: Pain [acute]**
>
> **May be related to**
> Increased frequency/force of ureteral contractions
> Tissue trauma, edema formation; cellular ischemia
>
> **Possibly evidenced by**
> Reports of colicky pain
> Guarding/distraction behaviors, restlessness, moaning, self-focusing, facial mask of pain, muscle tension
> Autonomic responses
>
> **DESIRED OUTCOMES/EVALUATION CRITERIA—PATIENT WILL:**
>
> **Pain Level (NOC)**
>
> Report pain is relieved with spasms controlled.
> Appear relaxed, able to sleep/rest appropriately.

ACTIONS/INTERVENTIONS	RATIONALE
Pain Management (NIC)	
Independent	
Document location, duration, intensity (0–10 scale), and radiation. Note nonverbal signs, e.g., elevated BP and pulse, restlessness, moaning, thrashing about.	Helps evaluate site of obstruction and progress of calculi movement. Flank pain suggests that stones are in the kidney area, upper ureter. Flank pain radiates to back, abdomen, groin, genitalia because of proximity of nerve plexus and blood vessels supplying other areas. Sudden, severe pain may precipitate apprehension, restlessness, severe anxiety.
Explain cause of pain and importance of notifying caregivers of changes in pain occurrence/characteristics.	Provides opportunity for timely administration of analgesia (helpful in enhancing the patient's coping ability and may reduce anxiety) and alerts caregivers to possibility of passing of stone/developing complications. Sudden cessation of pain usually indicates stone passage.
Provide comfort measures, e.g., back rub, restful environment.	Promotes relaxation, reduces muscle tension, and enhances coping.
Assist with/encourage use of focused breathing, guided imagery, diversional activities.	Redirects attention and aids in muscle relaxation.
Encourage/assist with frequent ambulation as indicated and increased fluid intake of at least 3–4 L/day within cardiac tolerance.	Vigorous hydration promotes passing of stone, prevents urinary stasis, and aids in prevention of further stone formation.
Note reports of increased/persistent abdominal pain.	Complete obstruction of ureter can cause perforation and extravasation of urine into perirenal space. This represents an acute surgical emergency.
Collaborative	
Administer medications as indicated:	
Narcotics, e.g., meperidine (Demerol), morphine;	Usually given during acute episode to decrease ureteral colic and promote muscle/mental relaxation.
Antispasmodics, e.g., flavoxate (Urispas), oxybutynin (Ditropan);	Decreasing reflex spasm may decrease colic and pain.

ACTIONS/INTERVENTIONS	RATIONALE
Collaborative	
Corticosteroids.	May be used to reduce tissue edema to facilitate movement of stone.
Apply warm compresses to back.	Relieves muscle tension and may reduce reflex spasms.
Maintain patency of catheters when used.	Prevents urinary stasis/retention, reduces risk of increased renal pressure and infection.

NURSING DIAGNOSIS: Urinary Elimination, altered

May be related to
Stimulation of the bladder by calculi, renal or ureteral irritation
Mechanical obstruction, inflammation

Possibly evidenced by
Urgency and frequency; oliguria (retention)
Hematuria

DESIRED OUTCOMES/EVALUATION CRITERIA—PATIENT WILL:

Urinary Elimination (NOC)

Void in normal amounts and usual pattern.
Experience no signs of obstruction.

ACTIONS/INTERVENTIONS	RATIONALE
Urinary Elimination Enhancement (NIC)	
Independent	
Monitor I&O and characteristics of urine.	Provides information about kidney function and presence of complications, e.g., infection and hemorrhage. Bleeding may indicate increased obstruction or irritation of ureter. *Note:* Hemorrhage due to ureteral ulceration is rare.
Determine patient's normal voiding pattern and note variations.	Calculi may cause nerve excitability, which causes sensations of urgent need to void. Usually frequency and urgency increase as calculus nears ureterovesical junction.
Encourage increased fluid intake.	Increased hydration flushes bacteria, blood, and debris and may facilitate stone passage.
Strain all urine. Document any stones expelled and send to laboratory for analysis.	Retrieval of calculi allows for identification of type of stone and influences choice of therapy.
Investigate reports of bladder fullness; palpate for suprapubic distension. Note decreased urine output, presence of periorbital/dependent edema.	Urinary retention may develop, causing tissue distension (bladder/kidney) and potentiates risk of infection, renal failure.
Observe for changes in mental status, behavior, or level of consciousness.	Accumulation of uremic wastes and electrolyte imbalances can be toxic to the CNS.
Collaborative	
Monitor laboratory studies, e.g., electrolytes, BUN, Cr.	Elevated BUN, Cr, and certain electrolytes indicate presence/degree of kidney dysfunction.
Obtain urine for culture and sensitivities.	Determines presence of UTI, which may be causing/complicating symptoms.

655

ACTIONS/INTERVENTIONS	RATIONALE

Collaborative

Administer medications as indicated, e.g.:

Acetazolamide (Diamox), allopurinol (Zyloprim);	Increases urine pH (alkalinity) to reduce formation of acid stones. Antigout agents such as allopurinol (Zyloprim) also lower uric acid production and potential of stone formation.
Hydrochlorothiazide (Esidrix, Hydrodiuril), chlorthalidone (Hygroton);	May be used to prevent urinary stasis and decrease calcium stone formation if not caused by underlying disease process such as primary hyperthyroidism or vitamin D abnormalities.
Ammonium chloride; potassium or sodium phosphate (Sal-Hepatica);	Reduces phosphate stone formation.
Antibiotics;	Presence of UTI/alkaline urine potentiates stone formation.
Sodium bicarbonate;	Replaces losses incurred during bicarbonate wasting and/or alkalinization of urine; may reduce/prevent formation of some calculi.
Ascorbic acid.	Acidifies urine to prevent recurrence of alkaline stone formation.
Maintain patency of indwelling catheters (ureteral, urethral, or nephrostomy) when used.	May be required to facilitate urine flow/prevent retention and corresponding complications. *Note:* Tubes may be occluded by stone fragments.
Irrigate with acid or alkaline solutions as indicated.	Changing urine pH may help dissolve stones and prevent further stone formation.

Prepare patient for/assist with endoscopic procedures, e.g.:

Basket procedure;	Calculi in the distal and midureter may be removed by endoscopic cystoscope with capture of the stone in a basketing catheter.
Ureteral stents;	Catheters are positioned above the stone to promote urethral dilation/stone passage. Continuous or intermittent irrigation can be carried out to flush kidneys/ureters and adjust pH of urine to permit dissolution of stone fragments following lithotripsy.
Percutaneous or open pyelolithotomy, nephrolithotomy, ureterolithotomy;	Surgery may be necessary to remove stone that is too large to pass through ureters.
Percutaneous ultrasonic lithotripsy;	Invasive shock wave treatment for stones in renal pelvis/calyx or upper ureters.
Extracorporeal shock-wave lithotripsy (ESWL).	Noninvasive procedure in which kidney stones are pulverized by shock waves delivered from outside the body.

NURSING DIAGNOSIS: Fluid Volume, risk for deficit

Risk factors may include
Nausea/vomiting (generalized abdominal and pelvic nerve irritation from renal or ureteral colic)
Postobstructive diuresis

Possibly evidenced by

[Not applicable; presence of signs or symptoms establishes an *actual* diagnosis]

DESIRED OUTCOMES/EVALUATION CRITERIA—PATIENT WILL:

Hydration (NOC)

Maintain adequate fluid balance as evidenced by vital signs and weight within patient's normal range, palpable peripheral pulses, moist mucous membranes, good skin turgor.

ACTIONS/INTERVENTIONS	RATIONALE
Fluid/Electrolyte Management (NIC)	
Independent	
Monitor I&O.	Comparing actual and anticipated output may aid in evaluating presence/degree of renal stasis/impairment. *Note:* Impaired kidney functioning and decreased urinary output can result in higher circulating volumes with signs/symptoms of HF.
Document incidence and note characteristics and frequency of vomiting and diarrhea, as well as accompanying or precipitating events.	Nausea/vomiting and diarrhea are commonly associated with renal colic because celiac ganglion serves both kidneys and stomach. Documentation may help rule out other abdominal occurrences as a cause for pain or pinpoint calculi.
Increase fluid intake to 3–4 L/day within cardiac tolerance.	Maintains fluid balance for homeostasis and "washing" action that may flush the stone(s) out. Dehydration and electrolyte imbalance may occur secondary to excessive fluid loss (vomiting and diarrhea).
Monitor vital signs. Evaluate pulses, capillary refill, skin turgor, and mucous membranes.	Indicators of hydration/circulating volume and need for intervention. *Note:* Decreased GFR stimulates production of renin, which acts to raise BP in an effort to increase renal blood flow.
Weigh daily.	Rapid weight gain may be related to water retention.
Collaborative	
Monitor Hb/Hct, electrolytes.	Assesses hydration and effectiveness of/need for interventions.
Administer IV fluids.	Maintains circulating volume (if oral intake is insufficient), promoting renal function.
Provide appropriate diet, clear liquids, bland foods as tolerated.	Easily digested foods decrease GI activity/irritation and help maintain fluid and nutritional balance.
Administer medications as indicated: antiemetics, e.g., prochlorperazine (Compazine).	Reduces nausea/vomiting.

NURSING DIAGNOSIS: Knowledge Deficit [Learning Need] regarding condition, prognosis, treatment, self care, and discharge needs

May be related to

Lack of exposure/recall; information misinterpretation
Unfamiliarity with information resources

> **Possibly evidenced by**
> Questions; request for information; statement of misconception
> Inaccurate follow-through of instructions, development of preventable complications
> **DESIRED OUTCOMES/EVALUATION CRITERIA—PATIENT WILL:**
>
> **Knowledge: Disease Process (NOC)**
>
> Verbalize understanding of disease process and potential complications.
> Correlate symptoms with causative factors.
>
> **Knowledge: Treatment Regimen (NOC)**
>
> Verbalize understanding of therapeutic needs.
> Initiate necessary lifestyle changes and participate in treatment regimen.

ACTIONS/INTERVENTIONS

Teaching: Disease Process (NIC)

Independent

Review disease process and future expectations.

Stress importance of increased fluid intake, e.g., 3–4 L/day or as much as 6–8 L/day. Encourage patient to notice dry mouth and excessive diuresis/diaphoresis and to increase fluid intake whether or not feeling thirsty.

Review dietary regimen, as individually appropriate:

Low-purine diet, e.g., limited lean meat, turkey, legumes, whole grains, alcohol;

Low-calcium diet, e.g., limited milk, cheese, green leafy vegetables, yogurt;

Low-oxalate diet, e.g., restrict chocolate, caffeine-containing beverages, beets, spinach.

Shorr regimen: low-calcium/phosphorus diet with aluminum carbonate gel 30–40 mL, 30 min pc/hs.

Discuss medication regimen; avoidance of OTC drugs and reading all product/food ingredient labels.

Encourage regular activity/exercise program.

RATIONALE

Provides knowledge base from which patient can make informed choices.

Flushes renal system, decreasing opportunity for urinary stasis and stone formation. Increased fluid losses/dehydration require additional intake beyond usual daily needs.

Diet depends on the type of stone. Understanding reason for restrictions provides opportunity for patient to make informed choices, increases cooperation with regimen, and may prevent recurrence.

Decreases oral intake of uric acid precursors.

Reduces risk of calcium stone formation. *Note:* Recent research suggests that restricting dietary calcium is not helpful in reducing calcium-stone formation, and researchers, although not advocating high calcium diets, are urging that calcium limitation be re-examined.

Reduces calcium oxalate stone formation.

Prevents phosphatic calculi by forming an insoluble precipitate in the GI tract, reducing the load to the kidney nephron. Also effective against other forms of calcium calculi. *Note:* May cause constipation.

Drugs will be given to acidify or alkalize urine, depending on underlying cause of stone formation. Ingestion of products containing individually contraindicated ingredients (e.g., calcium, phosphorus) potentiates recurrence of stones.

Inactivity contributes to stone formation through calcium shifts and urinary stasis.

ACTIONS/INTERVENTIONS	RATIONALE
Independent	
Active-listen concerns about therapeutic regimen/lifestyle changes.	Helps patient work through feelings and gain a sense of control over what is happening.
Identify signs/symptoms requiring medical evaluation, e.g., recurrent pain, hematuria, oliguria.	With increased probability of recurrence of stones, prompt interventions may prevent serious complications.
Demonstrate proper care of incisions/catheters if present.	Promotes competent self-care and independence.

POTENTIAL CONSIDERATIONS following acute hospitalizations (dependent on patient's age, physical condition/presence of complications, personal resources, and life responsibilities)

Urinary Elimination, altered—recurrence of calculi.

Women's Reproductive

HYSTERECTOMY

Hysterectomy is the surgical removal of the uterus, most commonly performed for malignancies and certain nonmalignant conditions (e.g., endometriosis/tumors), to control life-threatening bleeding/hemorrhage, and in the event of intractable pelvic infection or irreparable rupture of the uterus. A less radical procedure (myeomectomy) is sometimes performed for removing fibroids while sparing the uterus.

Abdominal hysterectomy types include the following:

Subtotal (partial): Body of the uterus is removed; cervical stump remains.
Total: Removal of the uterus and cervix.
Total with bilateral salpingo-oophorectomy: Removal of uterus, cervix, fallopian tubes, and ovaries is the treatment of choice for invasive cancer (11% of hysterectomies), fibroid tumors that are rapidly growing or produce severe abnormal bleeding (about one-third of all hysterectomies), and endometriosis invading other pelvic organs.

Vaginal hysterectomy or laparoscopically assisted vaginal hysterectomy (LAVH) may be done in certain conditions, such as uterine prolapse, cystocele/rectocele, carcinoma in situ, and high-risk obesity. These procedures offer the advantages of less pain, no visible (or much smaller) scars, and a shorter hospital stay and about half the recovery time, but are contraindicated if the diagnosis is obscure.

CARE SETTING

Inpatient acute surgical unit, or short-stay unit, depending on type of procedure.

RELATED CONCERNS

Surgical intervention (for general considerations and interventions)
Cancer, page 900
Psychosocial aspects of care, page 809
Surgical intervention, page 828
Thrombophlebitis: deep vein thrombosis, page 115

Patient Assessment Database

Data depends on the underlying disease process/need for surgical intervention (e.g., cancer, prolapse, dysfunctional uterine bleeding, severe endometriosis, or pelvic infections unresponsive to medical management) and associated complications (e.g., anemia).

TEACHING/LEARNING

Discharge plan considerations:	**DRG projected mean length of inpatient stay: 2.9–5.9 days**
	May need temporary help with transportation; homemaker/maintenance tasks
	Refer to section at end of plan for postdischarge considerations.

DIAGNOSTIC STUDIES

Pelvic examination: May reveal uterine/other pelvic organ irregularities such as masses, tender nodules, visual changes of cervix, requiring further diagnostic evaluation.

Pap smear: Cellular dysplasia reflects possibility of/presence of cancer.

Ultrasound or computed tomography (CT) scan: Aids in identifying size/location of pelvic mass.

Laparoscopy: Done to visualize tumors, bleeding, known or suspected endometriosis. Biopsy may be performed or laser treatment for endometriosis. Rarely, exploratory laparotomy may be done for staging cancer or to assess effects of chemotherapy.

Dilation and curettage (D&C) with biopsy (endometrial/cervical): Permits histopathologic study of cells to determine presence/location of cancer.

Schiller's test (staining of cervix with iodine): Useful in identifying abnormal cells.

Complete blood count (CBC): Decreased hemoglobin (Hb) may reflect chronic anemia, while decreased hematocrit (Hct) suggests active blood loss. Elevated white blood cell (WBC) count may indicate inflammation/infectious process.

NURSING PRIORITIES

1. Support adaptation to change.
2. Prevent complications.
3. Provide information about procedure/prognosis and treatment needs.

DISCHARGE GOALS

1. Dealing realistically with situation.
2. Complications prevented/minimized.
3. Procedure/prognosis and therapeutic regimen understood.
4. Plan in place to meet needs after discharge.

NURSING DIAGNOSIS: Self-Esteem, situational low

May be related to

Concerns about inability to have children, changes in femininity, effect on sexual relationship

Religious conflicts

Possibly evidenced by

Expressions of specific concerns/vague comments about result of surgery; fear of rejection or reaction of significant other (SO)

Withdrawal, depression

DESIRED OUTCOMES/EVALUATION CRITERIA—PATIENT WILL:

Self-Esteem (NOC)

Verbalize concerns and indicate healthy ways of dealing with them.

Verbalize acceptance of self in situation and adaptation to change in body/self-image.

ACTIONS/INTERVENTIONS

Self-Esteem Enhancement (NIC)

Independent

Provide time to listen to concerns and fears of patient and SO. Discuss patient's perceptions of self related to anticipated changes and her specific lifestyle.

RATIONALE

Conveys interest and concern; provides opportunity to correct misconceptions, e.g., women may fear loss of femininity and sexuality, weight gain, and menopausal body changes.

ACTIONS/INTERVENTIONS

Independent

Assess emotional stress the patient is experiencing. Identify meaning of loss for patient/SO. Encourage patient to vent feelings appropriately.

Provide accurate information, reinforcing information previously given.

Ascertain individual strengths and identify previous positive coping behaviors.

Provide open environment for patient to discuss concerns about sexuality.

Note withdrawn behavior, negative self-talk, use of denial, or over-concern with actual/perceived changes.

Collaborative

Refer to professional counseling as necessary.

RATIONALE

Nurses need to be aware of what this operation means to the patient to avoid inadvertent casualness or over-solicitude. Depending on the reason for the surgery (e.g., cancer or long-term heavy bleeding), the woman can be frightened or relieved. She may fear loss of ability to fulfill her reproductive role and may experience grief.

Provides opportunity for patient to question and assimilate information.

Helpful to build on strengths already available for patient to use in coping with current situation.

Promotes sharing of beliefs/values about sensitive subject and identifies misconceptions/myths that may interfere with adjustment to situation. (Refer to ND: Sexual dysfunction, risk for, p. 665.)

Identifies stage of grief/need for interventions.

May need additional help to resolve feelings about loss.

NURSING DIAGNOSIS: Urinary Elimination, altered/Urinary Retention [acute]

May be related to
Mechanical trauma, surgical manipulation, presence of local tissue edema, hematoma
Sensory/motor impairment: nerve paralysis

Possibly evidenced by
Sensation of bladder fullness, urgency
Small, frequent voiding or absence of urinary output
Overflow incontinence
Bladder distension

DESIRED OUTCOMES/EVALUATION CRITERIA—PATIENT WILL:

Urinary Elimination (NOC)

Empty bladder regularly and completely.

ACTIONS/INTERVENTIONS

Urinary Elimination Management (NIC)

Independent

Note voiding pattern and monitor urinary output.

Palpate bladder. Investigate reports of discomfort, fullness, inability to void.

Provide routine voiding measures, e.g., privacy, normal position, running water in sink, pouring warm water over perineum.

RATIONALE

May indicate urinary retention if voiding frequently in small/insufficient amounts (<100 mL).

Perception of bladder fullness, distension of bladder above symphysis pubis indicates urinary retention.

Promotes relaxation of perineal muscles and may facilitate voiding efforts.

ACTIONS/INTERVENTIONS	RATIONALE
Independent	
Provide/encourage good perianal cleansing and catheter care (when present).	Promotes cleanliness, reducing risk of ascending urinary tract infection (UTI).
Assess urine characteristics, noting color, clarity, odor.	Urinary retention, vaginal drainage, and possible presence of intermittent/indwelling catheter increase risk of infection, especially if patient has perineal sutures.
Collaborative	
Catheterize when indicated/per protocol if patient is unable to void or is uncomfortable.	Edema or interference with nerve supply may cause bladder atony/urinary retention requiring decompression of the bladder. *Note:* Indwelling urethral or suprapubic catheter may be inserted intraoperatively if complications are anticipated.
Decompress bladder slowly.	When large amount of urine has accumulated, rapid bladder decompression releases pressure on pelvic arteries, promoting venous pooling.
Maintain patency of indwelling catheter; keep drainage tubing free of kinks.	Promotes free drainage of urine, reducing risk of urinary stasis/retention and infection.
Check residual urine volume after voiding as indicated.	May not be emptying bladder completely; retention of urine increases possibility for infection and is uncomfortable/painful.

NURSING DIAGNOSIS: Constipation/Diarrhea, risk for

Risk factors may include
Physical factors: abdominal surgery, with manipulation of bowel, weakening of abdominal musculature
Pain/discomfort in abdomen or perineal area
Changes in dietary intake

Possibly evidenced by
[Not applicable; presence of signs and symptoms establishes an *actual* diagnosis]

DESIRED OUTCOMES/EVALUATION CRITERIA—PATIENT WILL:

Bowel Elimination (NOC)

Display active bowel sounds/peristaltic activity.
Maintain usual pattern of elimination.

ACTIONS/INTERVENTIONS	RATIONALE
Bowel Management (NIC)	
Independent	
Auscultate bowel sounds. Note abdominal distension, presence of nausea/vomiting.	Indicators of presence/resolution of ileus, affecting choice of interventions.
Assist patient with sitting on edge of bed and walking.	Early ambulation helps stimulate intestinal function and return of peristalsis.
Encourage adequate fluid intake, including fruit juices, when oral intake is resumed.	Promotes softer stool; may aid in stimulating peristalsis.
Provide sitz baths.	Promotes muscle relaxation, minimizes discomfort.

ACTIONS/INTERVENTIONS	RATIONALE
Collaborative	
Restrict oral intake as indicated.	Prevents nausea/vomiting until peristalsis returns (1–2 days).
Maintain nasogastric (NG) tube, if present.	May be inserted in surgery to decompress stomach.
Provide clear/full liquids and advance to solid foods as tolerated.	When peristalsis begins, food and fluid intake promote resumption of normal bowel elimination.
Use rectal tube; apply heat to the abdomen, if appropriate.	Promotes the passage of flatus.
Administer medications, e.g., stool softeners, mineral oil, laxatives as indicated.	Promotes formation/passage of softer stool.

NURSING DIAGNOSIS: Tissue Perfusion, risk for altered (specify)

Risk factors may include
Hypovolemia
Reduction/interruption of blood flow: Pelvic congestion, postoperative tissue inflammation, venous stasis
Intraoperative trauma or pressure on pelvic/calf vessels: lithotomy position during vaginal hysterectomy

Possibly evidenced by
[Not applicable; presence of signs and symptoms establishes an *actual* diagnosis]

DESIRED OUTCOMES/EVALUATION CRITERIA—PATIENT WILL:

Tissue Perfusion: (Specify) (NOC)

Demonstrate adequate perfusion, as evidenced by stable vital signs, palpable pulses, good capillary refill, usual mentation, individually adequate urinary output.
Be free of edema, signs of thrombus formation.

ACTIONS/INTERVENTIONS	RATIONALE
Circulatory Care (NIC)	
Independent	
Monitor vital signs; palpate peripheral pulses, and note capillary refill; assess urinary output/characteristics. Evaluate changes in mentation.	Indicators of adequacy of systemic perfusion, fluid/blood needs, and developing complications.
Inspect dressings and perineal pads, noting color, amount, and odor of drainage. Weigh pads and compare with dry weight if patient is bleeding heavily.	Proximity of large blood vessels to operative site and/or potential for alteration of clotting mechanism (e.g., cancer) increases risk of postoperative hemorrhage.
Turn patient and encourage frequent coughing and deep-breathing exercises.	Prevents stasis of secretions and respiratory complications.
Avoid high-Fowler's position and pressure under the knees or crossing of legs.	Creates vascular stasis by increasing pelvic congestion and pooling of blood in the extremities, potentiating risk of thrombus formation.
Assist with/instruct in foot and leg exercises and ambulate as soon as able.	Movement enhances circulation and prevents stasis complications.
Check for Homans' sign. Note erythema, swelling of extremity, or reports of sudden chest pain with dyspnea.	May be indicative of development of thrombophlebitis/pulmonary embolus.

ACTIONS/INTERVENTIONS	RATIONALE
Collaborative	
Administer IV fluids, blood products as indicated.	Replacement of blood losses maintains circulating volume and tissue perfusion.
Apply antiembolus stockings.	Aids in venous return; reduces stasis and risk of thrombosis.
Assist with/encourage use of incentive spirometer.	Promotes lung expansion/minimizes atelectasis.

NURSING DIAGNOSIS: Sexual dysfunction, risk for

Risk factors may include

Altered body structure/function, e.g., shortening of vaginal canal; changes in hormone levels, decreased libido

Possible change in sexual response pattern, e.g., absence of rhythmic uterine contractions during orgasm; vaginal discomfort/pain (dyspareunia)

Possibly evidenced by

[Not applicable; presence of signs and symptoms establishes an *actual* diagnosis]

DESIRED OUTCOMES/EVALUATION CRITERIA—PATIENT WILL:

Role Performance (NOC)

Verbalize understanding of changes in sexual anatomy/function.
Discuss concerns about body image, sex role, desirability as a sexual partner with SO.
Identify satisfying/acceptable sexual practices and some alternative ways of dealing with sexual expression.

ACTIONS/INTERVENTIONS	RATIONALE
Sexual Counseling (NIC)	
Independent	
Listen to comments of patient/SO.	Sexual concerns are often disguised as humor and/or offhand remarks.
Assess patient's/SO's information regarding sexual anatomy/function and effects of surgical procedure.	May have misinformation/misconceptions that can affect adjustment. Negative expectations are associated with poor overall outcome. Changes in hormone levels can affect libido and/or decrease suppleness of the vagina. Although a shortened vagina can eventually stretch, intercourse initially may be uncomfortable/painful.
Identify cultural/value factors and conflicts present.	May affect return to satisfying sexual relationship.
Assist patient to be aware of/deal with stage of grieving.	Acknowledging normal process of grieving for actual/perceived changes may enhance coping and facilitate resolution.
Encourage patient to share thoughts/concerns with partner.	Open communication can identify areas of agreement/problems and promote discussion and resolution.
Problem-solve solutions to potential problems, e.g., postponing sexual intercourse when fatigued, substituting alternate means of expression, using positions that avoid pressure on abdominal incision, using vaginal lubricant.	Helps patient return to desired/satisfying sexual activity.

ACTIONS/INTERVENTIONS	RATIONALE

Independent

Discuss expected physical sensations/discomforts, changes in response as appropriate to the individual.

Vaginal pain may be significant following vaginal procedure, or sensory loss may occur because of surgical trauma. Although sensory loss is usually temporary, it may take weeks/months to resolve. In addition, changes in vaginal size, altered hormone levels, and loss of sensation of rhythmic contractions of the uterus during orgasm can impair sexual satisfaction. *Note:* Many women experience few negative effects because fear of pregnancy is gone, and relief from symptoms often improves enjoyment of intercourse.

Collaborative

Refer to counselor/sex therapist as needed.

May need additional assistance to promote a satisfactory outcome.

NURSING DIAGNOSIS: Knowledge Deficit [Learning Need] regarding condition, prognosis, treatment, self care, and discharge needs

May be related to
Lack of exposure/recall
Information misinterpretation
Unfamiliarity with information resources

Possibly evidenced by
Questions/request for information; statement of misconception
Inaccurate follow-through of instructions, development of preventable complications

DESIRED OUTCOMES/EVALUATION CRITERIA—PATIENT WILL:

> **Knowledge: Disease Process (NOC)**

Verbalize understanding of condition and potential complications.
Identify relationship of signs/symptoms related to surgical procedure and actions to deal with them.

> **Knowledge: Treatment Regimen (NOC)**

Verbalize understanding of therapeutic needs.

ACTIONS/INTERVENTIONS	RATIONALE

> **Teaching: Disease Process (NIC)**

Independent

Review effects of surgical procedure and future expectations; e.g., patient needs to know she will no longer menstruate or bear children, whether surgical menopause will occur, and the possible need for hormonal replacement.

Provides knowledge base from which patient can make informed choices.

Discuss complexity of problems anticipated during recovery, e.g., emotional lability and expectation of feelings of depression/sadness; excessive fatigue, sleep disturbances, urinary problems.

Physical, emotional, and social factors can have a cumulative effect, which may delay recovery, especially if hysterectomy was performed because of cancer. Providing an opportunity for problem solving may facilitate the process. Patient/SO may benefit from the knowledge that a period of emotional lability is normal and expected during recovery.

ACTIONS/INTERVENTIONS	RATIONALE
Independent	
Discuss resumption of activity. Encourage light activities initially, with frequent rest periods and increasing activities/exercise as tolerated. Stress importance of individual response in recuperation.	Patient can expect to feel tired when she goes home and needs to plan a gradual resumption of activities, with return to work an individual matter. Prevents excessive fatigue; conserves energy for healing/tissue regeneration. *Note:* Some studies suggest that recovery from hysterectomy (especially when oophorectomy is done) may take up to four times as long as recovery from other major surgeries (12 mo versus 3 mo).
Identify individual restrictions, e.g., avoiding heavy lifting and strenuous activities (such as vacuuming, straining at stool); prolonged sitting/driving. Avoid tub baths/douching until physician allows.	Strenuous activity intensifies fatigue and may delay healing. Activities that increase intra-abdominal pressure can strain surgical repairs, and prolonged sitting potentiates risk of thrombus formation. Showers are permitted, but tub baths/douching may cause vaginal or incisional infections and are a safety hazard.
Review recommendations of resumption of sexual intercourse. (Refer to ND: Sexual dysfunction, risk for, p. 665.)	When sexual activity is cleared by the physician, it is best to resume activity easily and gently, expressing sexual feelings in other ways or using alternate coital positions.
Identify dietary needs, e.g., high protein, additional iron.	Facilitates healing/tissue regeneration and helps correct anemia when present.
Review hormone replacement therapy (HRT).	Total hysterectomy with bilateral salpingo-oophorectomy (surgically induced menopause) requires replacement hormones. The long-term benefits of HRT (particularly estrogen) include a decreased incidence of cardiovascular disease, protection against osteoporosis, improved mood and cognition.
Encourage taking prescribed drug(s) routinely (e.g., with meals).	Taking hormones with meals establishes routine for taking drug and reduces potential for initial nausea.
Discuss potential side effects, e.g., weight gain, increased skin pigmentation or acne, breast tenderness, headaches, photosensitivity.	Development of some side effects is expected but may require problem solving such as change in dosage or use of sunscreen.
Recommend cessation of smoking when receiving estrogen therapy.	Some studies suggest an increased risk of thrombophlebitis, myocardial infarction (MI), cerebrovascular accident (CVA), and pulmonary emboli associated with smoking and concurrent estrogen therapy.
Review incisional care when appropriate.	Facilitates competent self-care, promoting independence.
Stress importance of follow-up care.	Provides opportunity to ask questions, clear up misunderstandings, and detect developing complications.
Identify signs/symptoms requiring medical evaluation, e.g., fever/chills, change in character of vaginal/wound drainage; bright bleeding.	Early recognition and treatment of developing complications such as infection/hemorrhage may prevent life-threatening situations. *Note:* Hemorrhage may occur as late as 2 wk postoperatively.

POTENTIAL CONSIDERATIONS following acute hospitalization (dependent on patient's age, physical condition/presence of complications, personal resources, and life responsibilities)

In addition to surgical and cancer concerns (if appropriate):

Sexual dysfunction—altered body structure/function; changes in hormone levels, decreased libido; possible change in sexual response pattern; vaginal discomfort/pain (dyspareunia).

Self-Esteem, situational low—concerns about inability to have children, changes in femininity, effect on sexual relationship; religious conflicts.

MASTECTOMY

The choice of treatment for breast cancer depends on tumor type, size, and location, as well as clinical characteristics (staging). Therapy may include surgical intervention with/without radiation, chemotherapy, and hormone therapy. The use of gene therapy and stem cell rescue (autologous bone marrow transplantation) is under investigation. Breast reconstruction is now often done at the time of cancer surgery because it does not compromise adjuvant treatment or interfere with cure of the cancer, and it improves the patient's adjustment and acceptance

Types of surgery are generally grouped into three categories: radical mastectomy, total mastectomy, and more limited procedures (e.g., segmental, lumpectomy). *Total (simple) mastectomy* removes all breast tissue, but all or most axillary lymph nodes and chest muscles are left intact. *Modified radical mastectomy* (now the most common surgical option) removes the entire breast, some or most lymph nodes, and sometimes the pectoralis minor chest muscles. Major chest muscles are left intact. *Radical (Halsted's) mastectomy* is a procedure that is rarely performed because it requires removal of the entire breast, skin, major and minor pectoral muscles, axillary lymph nodes, and sometimes internal mammary or supraclavicular lymph nodes. Limited procedures (i.e., lumpectomy) may be done on an outpatient basis because only the tumor and some surrounding tissue are removed. Lumpectomy is reserved for well-defined nonmetastatic tumors of less than 5 cm in size that do not involve the nipple. The procedure may be diagnostic (determines cell type) and/or curative when combined with radiation therapy.

CARE SETTING

Inpatient acute surgical unit.

RELATED CONCERNS

Cancer, page 900 (for additional nursing interventions regarding cancer treatment)
Psychosocial aspects of care, page 809
Surgical intervention, page 828

Patient Assessment Database

ACTIVITY/REST

May report: Work, activity involving frequent/repetitive arm movements
Sleep style (e.g., sleeping on stomach)

CIRCULATION

May exhibit: Unilateral engorgement in affected arm (invaded lymph system)

FOOD/FLUID

May report: Loss of appetite, recent weight loss

EGO INTEGRITY

May report: Constant stressors in work/home life
Stress/fear involving diagnosis, prognosis, future expectations

PAIN/DISCOMFORT

May report: Pain in advanced/metastatic disease (localized pain rarely occurs in early malignancy)
Some experience discomfort or "funny feeling" in breast tissue
Heavy, painful breasts premenstrually usually indicate fibrocystic disease

SAFETY

May exhibit: Nodular axillary masses
Edema, erythema of involved skin

SEXUALITY

May report: Presence of a breast lump (usually painless); changes in breast symmetry or size
Changes in breast skin (pitting, dumpling), color or temperature (redness); unusual nipple discharge (watery, clear or bloody, sticky); itching, burning, or retracted nipple or changes in vein pattern

History of early menarche (younger than age 12); late menopause (after age 50); late first pregnancy (after age 35)

Concerns about sexuality/intimacy

May exhibit: Change in breast contour/mass, asymmetry

Dimpling, puckering of skin; changes in skin color/texture, swelling, redness or heat in breast

Retraction of nipple; discharge from nipple (serous, serosanguinous, sanguinous, watery discharge increase likelihood of cancer, especially when accompanied by lump)

TEACHING/LEARNING

May report: Family history of genetically transmitted breast cancer includes those with multiple relatives with breast cancer (maternal and paternal), family history of ovarian cancer along with breast cancer, family history of bilateral or early-onset breast cancer, or breast cancer in a male relative. *Note:* Most breast cancer patients have no relatives with the disease, with only 5–10% now thought to be attributable to hereditary factors

Previous unilateral breast cancer, endometrial or ovarian cancer

Discharge plan considerations: **DRG projected mean length of inpatient stay: 4.1 days**

May need assistance with treatments/rehabilitation, decisions, self-care activities, homemaker/maintenance tasks

Refer to section at end of plan for postdischarge considerations.

DIAGNOSTIC STUDIES

Mammography: Visualizes internal structure of the breast, is capable of detecting nonpalpable cancers or tumors that are in early stages of development.

Galactography (ductography): Contrast mammograms obtained by injecting dye into a draining duct.

Ultrasound: May be helpful in distinguishing between solid masses and cysts and in women whose breast tissue is dense; complements findings of mammography.

Xeroradiography: Reveals increased circulation around tumor site.

Thermography: Identifies rapidly growing tumors as "hot spots" because of increased blood supply and corresponding higher skin temperature.

Diaphanography (transillumination): Identifies tumor or mass by differentiating the way that tissues transmit and scatter light. Procedure remains experimental and is considered less accurate than mammography.

CT scan and magnetic resonance imaging (MRI): Scanning techniques can detect breast disease, especially larger masses, or tumors in small, dense breasts that are difficult to examine by mammography. These techniques are not suitable for routine screening and are not a substitute for mammography.

Positron emission tomography (PET) scintimammography: Helps detect malignant tissue outside the breast: may help determine status of lymph nodes to reduce the need for biopsy. Also can provide information regarding makeup of malignant tumors to guide treatment choices.

Breast biopsy (fine-needle aspiration, core sampling needle biopsy, or excisional): Provides definitive diagnosis of mass and is useful for histological classification, staging, and selection of appropriate therapies.

Sentinel node biopsy: May eliminate need for axillary dissection in small breast tumors, limiting damage to lymph ducts and nerves

Hormone receptor assays: Reveal whether cells of excised tumor or biopsy specimens contain hormone receptors (estrogen and progesterone). In malignant cells, the estrogen-plus receptor complex stimulates cell growth and division. About two-thirds of all women with breast cancer are estrogen-receptor positive and tend to respond favorably to the addition of hormone therapy, which extends the disease-free period and increases survival time.

Chest x-ray, liver function studies, CBC, and bone scan: Done to assess for presence of metastasis.

Breast cancer genes: Researchers have now discovered BRCA-1 and BRCA-2. It is believed that if these genes are mutated, they may cause a high percentage of inherited–type breast cancers. The tests are not widely performed at this time.

NURSING PRIORITIES

1. Assist patient/SO in dealing with stress of situation/prognosis.
2. Prevent complications.
3. Establish individualized rehabilitation program.
4. Provide information about disease process, procedure, prognosis, and treatment needs.

DISCHARGE GOALS

1. Dealing realistically with situation.
2. Complications prevented/minimized.
3. Exercise regimen initiated.
4. Disease process, surgical procedure, prognosis, and therapeutic regimen understood.
5. Plan in place to meet needs after discharge.

PREOPERATIVE

NURSING DIAGNOSIS: Fear/Anxiety [specify level]

May be related to
Threat of death, e.g., extent of disease
Threat to self-concept: change of body image; scarring, loss of body part, sexual attractiveness
Change in health status

Possibly evidenced by
Increased tension; apprehension; feelings of helplessness/inadequacy
Decreased self-assurance
Self-focus; restlessness; sympathetic stimulation
Expressed concerns regarding actual/anticipated changes in life

DESIRED OUTCOMES/EVALUATION CRITERIA—PATIENT WILL:

| Fear or Anxiety Control (NOC) |

Acknowledge and discuss concerns.
Demonstrate appropriate range of feelings.
Report fear and anxiety are reduced to a manageable level.

ACTIONS/INTERVENTIONS	RATIONALE

| Anxiety Reduction (NIC) |

Independent

Ascertain what information patient has about diagnosis, expected surgical intervention, and future therapies. Note presence of denial or extreme anxiety.	Provides knowledge base for the nurse to enable reinforcement of needed information and helps identify patient with high anxiety, low capacity for information processing, and need for special attention. *Note:* Denial may be useful as a coping method for a time, but extreme anxiety needs to be dealt with immediately.
Explain purpose and preparation for diagnostic tests.	Clear understanding of procedures and what is happening increases feelings of control and lessens anxiety.
Provide an atmosphere of concern, openness, and availability, as well as privacy for the patient/SO. Suggest that SO be present as much as possible/desired.	Time and privacy are needed to provide support, discuss feelings of anticipated loss and other concerns. Therapeutic communication skills, open questions, listening, and so forth facilitate this process.
Encourage questions and provide time for expression of fears. Tell patient that stress related to breast cancer can persist for many months and to seek help/support.	Provides opportunity to identify and clarify misconceptions and offer emotional support.
Assess degree of support available to the patient. Give information about community resources, such as Reach to Recovery, YWCA Encore program. Encourage/provide for visit with a woman who has recovered from a mastectomy.	Can be a helpful resource when patient is ready. A peer who has experienced the same process serves as a role model and can provide validity to the comments, hope for recovery/normal future.

ACTIONS/INTERVENTIONS

Independent

Discuss role of rehabilitation after surgery.

RATIONALE

Rehabilitation is an essential component of therapy intended to meet physical, social, emotional, and vocational needs so that the patient can achieve the best possible level of physical and emotional functioning.

POSTOPERATIVE

NURSING DIAGNOSIS: Skin/Tissue Integrity, impaired

May be related to

Surgical removal of skin/tissue; altered circulation, presence of edema, drainage; changes in skin elasticity, sensation; tissue destruction (radiation)

Possibly evidenced by

Disruption of skin surface, destruction of skin layers/subcutaneous tissues

DESIRED OUTCOMES/EVALUATION CRITERIA—PATIENT WILL:

Wound Healing: Primary Intention (NOC)

Achieve timely wound healing, free of purulent drainage or erythema.
Demonstrate behaviors/techniques to promote healing/prevent complications.

ACTIONS/INTERVENTIONS

Incision Site Care (NIC)

Independent

Assess dressings/wound for characteristics of drainage. Monitor amount of edema, redness, and pain in the incision.

Perform routine assessment of involved arm. Elevate hand/arm with shoulder positioned at appropriate angles (no greater than 65 degrees of flexion, 45 degrees to 65 degrees of abduction, 45 degrees to 60 degrees of internal rotation) and forearm resting on wedge or pillow, as indicated.

Monitor temperature.

Place in semi-Fowler's position on back or unaffected side, avoid letting the affected arm dangle.

Avoid measuring blood pressure (BP), injecting medications, or inserting IVs in affected arm.

Inspect donor/graft site (if done) for color, blister formation; note drainage from donor site.

RATIONALE

Use of dressings depends on the extent of surgery and the type of wound closure. (Pressure dressings are usually applied initially and are reinforced, not changed.) Drainage occurs because of the trauma of the procedure and manipulation of the numerous blood vessels and lymphatics in the area.

Preventing or minimizing edema reduces the discomfort and complications associated with it. Elevation of affected arm facilitates drainage and resolution of edema. *Note:* Lymphedema is present in about 25% of patients and may develop immediately after surgery or years later.

Early recognition of developing infection can enable rapid institution of treatment.

Assists with drainage of fluid through use of gravity.

Increases potential of constriction, infection, and lymphedema on affected side.

Color will be affected by availability of circulatory supply. Blister formation provides a site for bacterial growth/infection.

ACTIONS/INTERVENTIONS	RATIONALE

Independent

| Assess wound drains, periodically noting amount and characteristics of drainage. | Drainage of accumulated fluids (e.g., lymph, blood) enhances healing and reduces the susceptibility to infection. Suction devices (e.g., Hemovac, Jackson-Pratt) are often inserted during surgery to maintain negative pressure in wound. Tubes are usually removed around the third day or when drainage ceases. |
| Encourage wearing of loose-fitting/nonconstrictive clothing. Tell patient not to wear wristwatch or other jewelry on affected arm. | Reduces pressure on compromised tissues, which may improve circulation/healing and minimize lymphedema. |

Collaborative

| Administer antibiotics as indicated. | May be given prophylactically or to treat specific infection and enhance healing. |

NURSING DIAGNOSIS: Pain [acute]

May be related to
Surgical procedure; tissue trauma, interruption of nerves, dissection of muscles

Possibly evidenced by
Reports of stiffness, numbness in chest area, shoulder/arm pain; alteration of muscle tone
Self-focusing; distraction/guarding behaviors

DESIRED OUTCOMES/EVALUATION CRITERIA—PATIENT WILL:

> **Pain Level (NOC)**

Express reduction in pain/discomfort.
Appear relaxed, able to sleep/rest appropriately.

ACTIONS/INTERVENTIONS	RATIONALE

> **Pain Management (NIC)**

Independent

Assess reports of pain and stiffness, noting location, duration, and intensity (0–10 scale). Note reports of numbness and swelling. Be aware of verbal and non-verbal cues.	Aids in identifying degree of discomfort and need for/effectiveness of analgesia. The amount of tissue, muscle, and lymphatic system removed can affect the amount of pain experienced. Destruction of nerves in axillary region causes numbness in upper arm and scapular region, which may be more intolerable than surgical pain. *Note:* Pain in chest wall can occur from muscle tension, be affected by extremes in heat and cold, and continue for several months.
Discuss normality of phantom breast sensations.	Provides reassurance that sensations are not imaginary and that relief can be obtained.
Assist patient to find position of comfort.	Elevation of arm, size of dressings, and presence of drains affects patient's ability to relax and rest/sleep effectively.

ACTIONS/INTERVENTIONS

Independent

Provide basic comfort measures (e.g., repositioning on back or unaffected side, backrub) and diversional activities. Encourage early ambulation and use of relaxation techniques, guided imagery, therapeutic touch.

Splint/support chest during coughing and deep-breathing exercises.

Give appropriate pain medication on a regular schedule before pain is severe and before activities are scheduled.

Collaborative

Administer narcotics/analgesics as indicated.

RATIONALE

Promotes relaxation, helps refocus attention, and may enhance coping abilities.

Facilitates participation in activity without undue discomfort.

Maintains comfort level and permits patient to exercise arm and to ambulate without pain hindering efforts.

Provides relief of discomfort/pain and facilitates rest, participation in postoperative therapy.

NURSING DIAGNOSIS: Self-Esteem, situational low

May be related to:
Biophysical: Disfiguring surgical procedure
Psychosocial: Concern about sexual attractiveness

Possibly evidenced by:
Actual change in structure/body contour
Verbalization of fear of rejection or of reaction by others, change in social involvement
Negative feelings about body, preoccupation with change or loss, not looking at body, nonparticipation in therapy

DESIRED OUTCOMES/EVALUATION CRITERIA—PATIENT WILL:

Self-Esteem (NOC)

Demonstrate movement toward acceptance of self in situation.
Recognize and incorporate change into self-concept without negating self-esteem.
Set realistic goals and actively participate in therapy program.

ACTIONS/INTERVENTIONS

Self-Esteem Enhancement (NIC)

Independent

Encourage questions about current situation and future expectations. Provide emotional support when surgical dressings are removed.

Identify role concerns as woman, wife, mother, career woman, and so forth.

Encourage patient to express feelings, e.g., anger, hostility, and grief.

Discuss signs/symptoms of depression with patient/SO.

RATIONALE

Loss of the breast causes many reactions, including feeling disfigured, fear of viewing scar, and fear of partner's reaction to change in body.

May reveal how patient's self-view has been altered.

Loss of body part, disfigurement, and perceived loss of sexual desirability engender grieving process that needs to be dealt with so that patient can make plans for the future. *Note:* Grief may resurface when subsequent procedures are done (e.g., fitting for prosthesis, reconstructive procedure) if postponed.

Common reaction to this type of procedure that needs to be recognized and acknowledged to seek timely intervention as indicated.

ACTIONS/INTERVENTIONS	RATIONALE

Independent

Provide positive reinforcement for gains/improvement and participation in self-care/treatment program.

Encourages continuation of healthy behaviors.

Review possibilities for reconstructive surgery and/or prosthetic augmentation.

If feasible, reconstruction provides less disfiguring/ "near-normal" cosmetic result. Variations in skin flap may be done for facilitation of reconstructive procedure, which is often performed at the same time as the mastectomy. The associated emotional boost may help the patient get through the more complex surgical recovery process and adjunctive therapies. *Note:* On occasion, reconstruction may not be done for 3–6 mo. A prolonged delay may result in increased tension in relationships and impair patient's incorporation of changes into self-concept

Ascertain feelings/concerns of partner regarding sexual aspects, and provide information and support.

Negative responses directed at the patient may actually reflect partner's concern about hurting patient, fear of cancer/death, difficulty in dealing with personality/behavior changes in patient, or inability to look at operative area.

Discuss and refer to support groups, including "Men in Our Lives" for SO as appropriate.

Provides a place to exchange concerns and feelings with others who have had a similar experience and identifies ways SO can facilitate patient's recovery.

Collaborative

Provide temporary soft prosthesis, if indicated.

Prosthesis of nylon and Dacron fluff may be worn in bra until incision heals if reconstructive surgery is not performed at the time of mastectomy. This may promote social acceptance and allow patient to feel more comfortable about body image at the time of discharge.

NURSING DIAGNOSIS: Mobility, impaired physical

May be related to
Neuromuscular impairment; pain/discomfort; edema formation

Possibly evidenced by
Reluctance to attempt movement
Limited range of motion (ROM); decreased muscle mass/strength

DESIRED OUTCOMES/EVALUATION CRITERIA—PATIENT WILL:

> **Muscle Function (NOC)**

Display willingness to participate in therapy.
Demonstrate techniques that enable resumption of activities.
Increase strength of affected body parts.

ACTIONS/INTERVENTIONS	RATIONALE

> **Exercise Therapy: Muscle Control (NIC)**

Independent

Elevate affected arm as indicated.

Promotes venous return, lessening possibility of lymphedema.

ACTIONS/INTERVENTIONS	RATIONALE

Independent

Begin passive ROM (e.g., flexion/extension of elbow, pronation/supination of wrist, clenching/extending fingers) as soon as possible.

Early postoperative exercises are usually started in the first 24 hr to prevent joint stiffness that can further limit movement/mobility.

Have patient move fingers, noting sensations and color of hand on affected side.

Lack of movement may reflect problems with the intercostal brachial nerve, and discoloration can indicate impaired circulation.

Encourage patient to use affected arm for personal hygiene, e.g., feeding, combing hair, washing face.

Increases circulation, helps minimize edema, and maintains strength and function of the arm and hand. These activities use the arm without abduction, which can stress the suture line in the early postoperative period.

Help with self-care activities as necessary.

Conserves patient's energy, prevents undue fatigue.

Assist with ambulation and encourage correct posture.

Patient will feel unbalanced and may need assistance until accustomed to change. Keeping back straight prevents shoulder from moving forward, avoiding permanent limitation in movement and posture.

Advance exercise as indicated, e.g., active extension of arm and rotation of shoulder while lying in bed, pendulum swings, rope turning, elevating arms to touch fingertips behind head.

Prevents joint stiffness, increases circulation, and maintains muscle tone of the shoulders and arm.

Progress to hand climbing (walking fingers up wall), clasping hands behind head, and full abduction exercises as soon as patient can manage.

Because this group of exercises can cause excessive tension on the incision, they are usually delayed until healing process is well-established.

Evaluate presence/degree of exercise-related pain and changes in joint mobility. Measure upper arm and forearm if edema develops.

Monitors progression/resolution of complications. May need to postpone increasing exercises and wait until further healing occurs.

Discuss types of exercises to be done at home to regain strength and enhance circulation in the affected arm.

Exercise program needs to be continued to regain optimal function of the affected side.

Coordinate exercise program into self-care and homemaker activities, e.g., dressing self, washing, dusting, mopping; and leisure activities, such as swimming.

Patient is usually more willing to participate or finds it easier to maintain an exercise program that fits into lifestyle and accomplishes tasks as well.

Assist patient to identify signs/symptoms of shoulder tension, e.g., inability to maintain posture, burning sensation in postscapular region. Instruct patient to avoid sitting or holding arm in dependent position for extended periods.

Altered weight and support put tension on surrounding structures.

Collaborative

Administer medications as indicated, e.g.:

Analgesics;

Pain needs to be controlled before exercise or patient may not participate optimally and incentive to exercise may be lost.

Diuretics.

May be useful in treating and preventing fluid accumulation/lymphedema.

Maintain integrity of elastic bandages or custom-fitted pressure-gradient elastic sleeve.

Promotes venous return and decreases risk/effects of edema formation.

Refer to physical/occupational therapist.

Provides individual exercise program. Assesses limitations/restrictions regarding employment requirements.

ACTIONS/INTERVENTIONS

RATIONALE

Teaching: Disease Process (NIC)

Independent

Review disease process, surgical procedure, and future expectations.

Provides knowledge base from which patient can make informed choices, including participation in radiation/chemotherapy programs.

Review/have patient demonstrate care of drains/wound sites.

Shorter hospital stays may result in discharge with drains in place, requiring more complex care by patient/caregivers. Drains may be removed 7–10 days after surgery.

Recommend continuation of exercises, increasing program as healing progresses, for at least a year.

Enhances development of collateral lymphatic channels, reduces the tightening of scar tissue and maintains muscle strength and function.

Discuss necessity for well-balanced, nutritious meals and adequate fluid intake.

Provides optimal nutrition and maintains circulating volume to enhance tissue regeneration/healing process.

Suggest alternating schedule of frequent rest and activity periods, especially in situations when sitting/standing is prolonged.

Prevents/limits fatigue, promotes healing, and enhances feelings of general well-being. Positions in which arm is dangling/extended intensify stress on affected structures, creating muscle tension/stiffness, and may interfere with healing.

Instruct patient to protect hands and arms by wearing long sleeves and gloves when gardening; use thimble when sewing; use potholders when handling hot items; use plastic gloves when doing dishes; avoid lifting or moving heavy objects; and do not carry purse or wear jewelry/wristwatch on affected side.

Compromised lymphatic system causes tissues to be more susceptible to infection and/or injury, which may lead to lymphedema.

Demonstrate holding affected arm appropriately, e.g., not dangling the arm, swinging arms with elbows bent when walking, placing arm above heart level when sitting/lying down.

Helps prevent/minimize lymphedema and "frozen shoulder."

ACTIONS/INTERVENTIONS	RATIONALE
Independent	
Warn against having blood withdrawn or receiving IV fluids/medications or BP measurements on the affected side.	May restrict the circulation and increase risk of infection when the lymphatic system is compromised.
Recommend wearing of a medical identification device.	Prevents unnecessary trauma (e.g., BPs, injections) to affected arm in emergency situations.
Demonstrate use of intermittent sequential pumping or low-stretch compression custom-made garments, as appropriate.	Occasionally used in managing lymphedema by promoting circulation and venous return.
Suggest gentle massage of healed incision with emollients.	Stimulates circulation, promotes elasticity of skin, and reduces discomfort associated with phantom breast sensations.
Recommend use of sexual positions that avoid pressure on chest wall. Encourage alternate forms of sexual expression (cuddling, touching) during initial healing process/while operative area is still tender.	Promotes feelings of femininity and sense of ability to resume sexual activities.
Encourage regular self-examination of remaining breast. Determine recommended schedule for mammography.	Identifies changes in breast tissue indicative of recurrent/new tumor development.
Stress importance of regular medical follow-up.	Other treatment may be required as adjunctive therapy, such as radiation. Recurrence of malignant breast tumors also can be identified and managed by oncologist.
Identify signs/symptoms requiring medical evaluation, e.g., breast or arm red, warm, and swollen; edema, purulent wound drainage; fever/chills.	Lymphangitis can occur as a result of infection, causing lymphedema.
Address additional concerns as indicated, e.g., ongoing therapies and expected and/or adverse side effects.	Medications, such as tamoxifen (Nolvadex) used as follow-up to surgery/radiation require ongoing involvement in care.

POTENTIAL CONSIDERATIONS following acute hospitalization (dependent on patient's age, physical condition/presence of complications, personal resources, and life responsibilities)

In addition to surgical and cancer concerns:

Skin/Tissue Integrity, impaired—surgical removal of skin/tissue; altered circulation, presence of edema, drainage; changes in skin elasticity, sensation, tissue destruction (radiation).

Self-Esteem, situational low—biophysical; disfiguring surgical procedure; concern about sexual attractiveness.

Self-Care deficit (specify)—decreased strength/endurance, pain, muscular impairment.

Sample CP: Mastectomy (Modified Radical), Hospital. ELOS: 3 Days Surgical Unit

ND and Categories of Care	Day 1 _____ Day of Surgery	Day 2 _____ POD #1	Day 3 _____ POD #2
Impaired skin/tissue integrity R/T therapeutic interventions	Display wound drainage w/in established limits (___ mL) Maintain usual color, sensation, motion in fingers/hand	Participate in self-care activities/beginning exercise program Identify ways to maximize healing/minimize risk of injury to art	Display early signs of healing w/minimal erythema, absence of purulent drainage, edema resolving Report plan in place to meet postdischarge needs
Referrals		Physical therapist Occupational therapist Home care	
Additional assessments	Dressing/drainage q2hX4 → q4h	→ q8h	→
	Presence/degree of edema q8h	→	Wound characteristics
	Donor/graft site if used q4h	→ q8h	→
	VS q1hX4 → q4h	→ q8h	→ q12h
	Neurovascular check affected UE q1hX8	→ q8h	→ D/C
	I&O q8h	→	→ D/C
	JP drainage q8h	→	→ D/C if less that 30 mL/24hr
		Measure upper arm/forearm if edema present qd	→
Medications	Diuretic if edema present	→	→
Patient teaching	Protection of affected arm: shaving, use of deodorant/ creams, activity limitations, avoidance of heat/cold, proper posture/positioning of arm, sexual positions to prevent pressure on chest wall, wearing loose-fitting clothing	Graduated exercise program incorporating ADLs/homemaking activities General healthcare needs to promote healing, dietary fluids, rest/pacing self	Wound care Management of JP drain if not removed S/S to report to healthcare provider Gentle massage of healed incision Breast self-examination Use of medical alert device Provide written instructions, schedule for follow-up visits/additional treatment modalities
Additional nursing actions	Position per protocol; HOB elevated 30° or more	→ HOB elevated 30°	→
	BRP/chair w/assist	→ Chair, ambulate as tolerated	→ Up ad lib
	Elevate affected arm	→	→
	Turn C, DB, Incentive spirometry q2h	→ DB, IS q2hWA	→
	Maintain elastic bandages/ custom fitted pressure-gradient sleeve is used	→	→
	Reinforce dressing PRN	→	→ D/C dressing/assist
	Encourage progressive exercises	→	→ w/dressing change
	Advance diet as tolerated	→	→
Pain R/T tissue trauma, muscle dissection	Report pain reduced to manageable level	→	Verbalize understanding of therapeutic regimen
	Participate in activities to manage pain	→	→
Additional assessments	Pain characteristics/changes	→	→
	Response to interventions	→	→
Medications: Allergies:	Analgesic of choice IM/PO	→ PO analgesic	→

Sample CP: Mastectomy (Modified Radical), Hospital. ELOS: 3 Days Surgical Unit (Continued)

ND and Categories of Care	Day 1 _____ Day of Surgery	Day 2 _____ POD #1	Day 3 _____ POD #2
Patient education	Orient to unit/room Reporting of pain/effects of interventions Initial exercises of fingers/wrist of affected arm; ROM exercises of unaffected limbs Relaxation techniques Splinting of chest w/cough, DB exercise	S/S of shoulder tension; possibility of phantom breast pain Progression of exercises as tolerated	Home exercise program Medication: dose, time/frequency, purpose, side effects
Additional nursing actions	Routine comfort measures Passive ROM/exercises per protocol Assist w/self-care	→ → Advance exercises as tolerated →	→ → →
Self-Esteem, situational low	Verbalize feelings, verbal/ nonverbal communication congruent	→ Participate in care/planning for future	→ → View incision, verbalize acceptance of self Plan in place to meet postdischarge needs
Referrals		Social Services Reach to Recovery	
Additional assessments	Response to surgical procedure by patient and SO Availability/effectiveness of support systems	Future expectations, role concerns, usual coping strategies, past coping successes Understanding of diagnosis	
Patient education	Postoperative routines Extent/outcome of surgical procedure Future treatment needs	Community resources for patient and SO Use of/sources for temporary prosthesis Possibilities for reconstructive surgery/ prosthetic augmentation Healthcare needs for general well-being (diet, rest, exercise)	S/S to report to healthcare provider (depression) Written information regarding diagnosis/ treatment options
Additional nursing actions	Discuss normalcy of feelings Encourage participation in self-care at level of ability	Provide positive reinforcement for participation in self-care/treatment program Role-play ways of handling responses of others	Identify options for managing home/work responsibilities; importance of taking time for self Provide support/answer questions when dressing removed

Orthopedic

FRACTURES

A *fracture* is a discontinuity or break in a bone. There are more than 150 fracture classifications. Five major ones are as follow:

1. *Incomplete:* Fracture involves only a portion of the cross-section of the bone. One side breaks; the other usually just bends (greenstick).
2. *Complete:* Fracture line involves entire cross-section of the bone, and bone fragments are usually displaced.
3. *Closed:* The fracture does not extend through the skin.
4. *Open:* Bone fragments extend through the muscle and skin, which is potentially infected.
5. *Pathological:* Fracture occurs in diseased bone (such as cancer, osteoporosis), with no or only minimal trauma.

Stable fractures are usually treated with casting. Unstable fractures that are unlikely to reduce may require surgical fixation.

CARE SETTING

Most fractures are managed at the community level. Although a number of the interventions listed here are appropriate for this population, this plan of care addresses more complicated injuries encountered on an inpatient acute medical-surgical unit.

RELATED CONCERNS

Craniocerebral trauma (acute rehabilitative phase), page 238
Pneumonia: microbial, page 140
Psychosocial aspects of care, page 809
Renal failure, acute, page 575
Spinal cord injury (acute rehabilitative phase), page 295
Surgical intervention, page 828
Thrombophlebitis: deep vein thrombosis, page 115

Patient Assessment Database

Symptoms of fracture depend on the site, severity, type, and amount of damage to other structures.

ACTIVITY/REST

May report: Weakness, fatigue
Gait and/or mobility problems

May exhibit: Restricted/loss of function of affected part (may be immediate, because of the fracture, or develop secondarily from tissue swelling, pain)

Weakness (e.g., affected extremity or generalized)

CIRCULATION

May exhibit: Hypertension (occasionally seen as a response to acute pain/anxiety) or hypotension (severe blood loss)

Tachycardia (stress response, hypovolemia)

Pulse diminished/absent distal to injury in extremity

Delayed capillary refill, pallor of affected part

Tissue swelling, bruising, or hematoma mass at site of injury

ELIMINATION

May exhibit: Hematuria, sediment in urine, changes in output, acute renal failure (ARF) (with major skeletal muscle damage)

NEUROSENSORY

May report: Loss of/impaired motion or sensation

Muscle spasms, worsening over time

Numbness/tingling (paresthesias)

May exhibit: Local musculoskeletal deformities, e.g., abnormal angulation, posture changes, shortening of limbs, rotation, crepitation (grating sound with movement or touch), muscle spasms, visible weakness/loss of function

Giving way/collapse or locking of joints; dislocations

Agitation (may be related to pain/anxiety or other trauma)

Range-of-motion (ROM) deficits

PAIN/DISCOMFORT

May report: Sudden severe pain at the time of injury (may be localized to the area of tissue/skeletal damage and then become more diffuse; can diminish on immobilization); absence of pain suggests nerve damage

Muscle aching pain, spasms/cramping (after immobilization)

May exhibit: Guarding/distraction behaviors, restlessness

Self-focus

SAFETY

May report: Circumstances of incident that do not support type of injury incurred (suggestive of abuse)

May exhibit: Skin lacerations, tissue avulsion, bleeding, color changes

Localized swelling (may increase gradually or suddenly)

Use of alcohol or other drugs

Presence of fall-risk factors, e.g., age, osteoporosis, dementia, arthritis, other chronic conditions

TEACHING/LEARNING

May report: Use of multiple medications (prescribed and over-the-counter [OTC]) with interactive effects

Discharge plan considerations: **DRG projected mean length of inpatient stay: Femur 9.0 days; hip/pelvis, 6.7 days; all other, 2.5–5.0 days if hospitalization required**

May require temporary assistance with transportation, self-care activities, and homemaker/maintenance tasks

May require additional therapy/rehabilitation postdischarge, or possible placement in assisted-living/extended-care facility for a period of time

Refer to section at end of plan for postdischarge considerations.

DIAGNOSTIC STUDIES

X-ray examinations: Determines location and extent of fractures/trauma.

Bone scans, tomograms, computed tomography (CT)/magnetic resonance imaging (MRI) scans: Visualizes fractures; bleeding and soft-tissue damage, differentiates between stress/trauma fractures and bone neoplasms.

Arteriograms: May be done when occult vascular damage is suspected.

Complete blood count (CBC): Hematocrit (Hct) may be increased (hemoconcentration) or decreased (signifying hemorrhage at the fracture site or at distant organs in multiple trauma). Increased white blood cell (WBC) count is a normal stress response after trauma.

Urine creatinine (Cr) clearance: Muscle trauma increases load of Cr for renal clearance.

Coagulation profile: Alterations may occur because of blood loss, multiple transfusions, or liver injury.

NURSING PRIORITIES

1. Prevent further bone/tissue injury.
2. Alleviate pain.
3. Prevent complications.
4. Provide information about condition/prognosis and treatment needs.

DISCHARGE GOALS

1. Fracture stabilized.
2. Pain controlled.
3. Complications prevented/minimized.
4. Condition, prognosis, and therapeutic regimen understood.
5. Plan in place to meet needs after discharge.

NURSING DIAGNOSIS: Trauma, risk for [additional]

Risk factors may include

Loss of skeletal integrity (fractures)/movement of bone fragments

Possibly evidenced by

[Not applicable; presence of signs and symptoms establishes an *actual* diagnosis]

DESIRED OUTCOMES/EVALUATION CRITERIA—PATIENT WILL:

> **Bone Healing (NOC)**

Maintain stabilization and alignment of fracture(s).
Display callus formation/beginning union at fracture site as appropriate.

> **Risk Control (NOC)**

Demonstrate body mechanics that promote stability at fracture site.

ACTIONS/INTERVENTIONS	RATIONALE
Independent	
Maintain bedrest/limb rest as indicated. Provide support of joints above and below fracture site, especially when moving/turning.	Provides stability, reducing possibility of disturbing alignment/muscle spasms, which enhances healing.
Place a bedboard under the mattress or place patient on orthopedic bed.	Soft or sagging mattress may deform a wet (green) plaster cast, crack a dry cast, or interfere with pull of traction.
Cast Care: Wet (NIC)	
Support fracture site with pillows/folded blankets. Maintain neutral position of affected part with sandbags, splints, trochanter roll, footboard.	Prevents unnecessary movement and disruption of alignment. Proper placement of pillows also can prevent pressure deformities in the drying cast.

ACTIONS/INTERVENTIONS	RATIONALE

Independent

Use sufficient personnel for turning. Avoid using abduction bar for turning patient with spica cast.

Hip/body or multiple casts can be extremely heavy and cumbersome. Failure to properly support limbs in casts may cause the cast to break.

Evaluate splinted extremity for resolution of edema.

Coaptation splint (e.g., Jones-Sugar tong) may be used to provide immobilization of fracture while excessive tissue swelling is present. As edema subsides, readjustment of splint or application of plaster/fiberglass cast may be required for continued alignment of fracture.

Traction/Immobilization Care (NIC)

Maintain position/integrity of traction (e.g., Buck's, Dunlop, Pearson, Russell).

Traction permits pull on the long axis of the fractured bone and overcomes muscle tension/shortening to facilitate alignment and union. Skeletal traction (pins, wires, tongs) permits use of greater weight for traction pull than can be applied to skin tissues.

Ascertain that all clamps are functional. Lubricate pulleys and check ropes for fraying. Secure and wrap knots with adhesive tape.

Assures that traction setup is functioning properly to avoid interruption of fracture approximation.

Keep ropes unobstructed with weights hanging free; avoid lifting/releasing weights.

Optimal amount of traction weight is maintained. *Note:* Assuring free movement of weights during repositioning of patient avoids sudden excess pull on fracture with associated pain and muscle spasm.

Assist with placement of lifts under bed wheels if indicated.

Helps maintain proper patient position and function of traction by providing counterbalance.

Position the patient so that appropriate pull is maintained on the long axis of the bone.

Promotes bone alignment and reduces risk of complications (e.g., delayed healing/nonunion).

Review restrictions imposed by therapy, e.g., not bending at waist/sitting up with Buck's traction or not turning below the waist with Russell traction.

Maintains integrity of pull of traction.

Assess integrity of external fixation device.

Hoffman traction provides stabilization and rigid support for fractured bone without use of ropes, pulleys, or weights, thus allowing for greater patient mobility/comfort and facilitating wound care. Loose or excessively tightened clamps/nuts can alter the compression of the frame, causing misalignment.

Collaborative

Review follow-up/serial x-rays.

Provides visual evidence of proper alignment or beginning callus formation/healing process to determine level of activity and need for changes in/additional therapy.

Administer alendronate (Fosamax) as indicated.

Acts as a specific inhibitor of osteoclast-mediated bone resorption, allowing bone formation to progress at a greater ratio, promoting healing of fractures/decreasing rate of bone turnover in presence of osteoporosis.

Initiate/maintain electrical stimulation if used.

May be indicated to promote bone growth in presence of delayed healing/nonunion.

NURSING DIAGNOSIS: Pain [acute]

May be related to
Muscle spasms
Movement of bone fragments, edema, and injury to the soft tissue
Traction/immobility device
Stress, anxiety

Possibly evidenced by
Reports of pain
Distraction; self-focusing/narrowed focus; facial mask of pain
Guarding, protective behavior; alteration in muscle tone; autonomic responses

DESIRED OUTCOMES/EVALUATION CRITERIA—PATIENT WILL:

Pain Level (NOC)

Verbalize relief of pain.
Display relaxed manner; able to participate in activities, sleep/rest appropriately.

Pain Control Behavior (NOC)

Demonstrate use of relaxation skills and diversional activities as indicated for individual situation.

ACTIONS/INTERVENTIONS	RATIONALE
Pain Management (NIC)	
Independent	
Maintain immobilization of affected part by means of bedrest, cast, splint, traction. (Refer to ND: Trauma, risk for [additional], p. 682.)	Relieves pain and prevents bone displacement/extension of tissue injury.
Elevate and support injured extremity.	Promotes venous return, decreases edema, and may reduce pain.
Avoid use of plastic sheets/pillows under limbs in cast.	Can increase discomfort by enhancing heat production in the drying cast.
Elevate bed covers; keep linens off toes.	Maintains body warmth without discomfort due to pressure of bedclothes on affected parts.
Evaluate/document reports of pain/discomfort, noting location and characteristics, including intensity (0–10 scale), relieving and aggravating factors. Note nonverbal pain cues (changes in vital signs and emotions/behavior). Listen to reports of family member/SO regarding patient's pain.	Influences choice of/monitors effectiveness of interventions. Many factors, including level of anxiety, may affect perception of/reaction to pain. *Note:* Absence of pain expression does not necessarily mean lack of pain.
Encourage patient to discuss problems related to injury.	Helps alleviate anxiety. Patient may feel need to relive the accident experience.
Explain procedures before beginning them.	Allows patient to prepare mentally for activity and to participate in controlling level of discomfort.
Medicate before care activities. Let patient know it is important to request medication before pain becomes severe.	Promotes muscle relaxation and enhances participation.

ACTIONS/INTERVENTIONS	RATIONALE

Independent

Perform and supervise active/passive ROM exercises.

Maintains strength/mobility of unaffected muscles and facilitates resolution of inflammation in injured tissues.

Provide alternate comfort measures, e.g., massage, backrub, position changes.

Improves general circulation; reduces areas of local pressure and muscle fatigue.

Provide emotional support and encourage use of stress management techniques, e.g., progressive relaxation, deep-breathing exercises, visualization/guided imagery, provide Therapeutic Touch.

Refocuses attention, promotes sense of control, and may enhance coping abilities in the management of the stress of traumatic injury and pain, which is likely to persist for an extended period.

Identify diversional activities appropriate for patient age, physical abilities, and personal preferences.

Prevents boredom, reduces muscle tension, and can increase muscle strength; may enhance coping abilities.

Investigate any reports of unusual/sudden pain or deep, progressive, and poorly localized pain unrelieved by analgesics.

May signal developing complications; e.g., infection, tissue ischemia, compartmental syndrome. (Refer to ND: Peripheral Neurovascular, risk for dysfunction, following.)

Collaborative

Apply cold/ice pack first 24–72 hr and as necessary.

Reduces edema/hematoma formation, decreases pain sensation.

Administer medications as indicated: narcotic and nonnarcotic analgesics e.g., morphine, meperidine (Demerol), hydrocodone (Vicodin); injectable and oral nonsteroidal anti-inflammatory drugs (NSAIDs), e.g., ketorolac (Toradol) ibuprofen (Motrin); and/or muscle relaxants, e.g., cyclobenzaprine (Flexeril), carisoprodol (Soma), diazepam (Valium). Administer analgesics around the clock for 3–5 days;

Given to reduce pain and/or muscle spasms. Studies of ketorolac (Toradol) have proven it to be effective in alleviating bone pain, with longer action and fewer side effects than narcotic agents.

Maintain/monitor IV patient-controlled analgesia (PCA) using peripheral, epidural, or intrathecal routes of administration. Maintain safe and effective infusions/equipment.

Routinely administered or PCA maintains adequate blood level of analgesia, preventing fluctuations in pain relief with associated muscle tension/spasms.

NURSING DIAGNOSIS: Peripheral Neurovascular, risk for dysfunction

Risk factors may include
Reduction/interruption of blood flow
Direct vascular injury, tissue trauma, excessive edema, thrombus formation
Hypovolemia

Possibly evidenced by
[Not applicable; presence of signs and symptoms establishes an *actual* diagnosis]

DESIRED OUTCOMES/EVALUATION CRITERIA—PATIENT WILL:

Tissue Perfusion: Peripheral (NOC)

Maintain tissue perfusion as evidenced by palpable pulses, skin warm/dry, normal sensation, usual sensorium, stable vital signs, and adequate urinary output for individual situation.

ACTIONS/INTERVENTIONS	RATIONALE

Circulatory Care (NIC)

Independent

Remove jewelry from affected limb.	May restrict circulation when edema occurs.
Evaluate presence/quality of peripheral pulse distal to injury via palpation/Doppler. Compare with uninjured limb.	Decreased/absent pulse may reflect vascular injury and necessitates immediate medical evaluation of circulatory status. Be aware that occasionally a pulse may be palpated even though circulation is blocked by a soft clot through which pulsations may be felt. In addition, perfusion through larger arteries may continue after increased compartment pressure has collapsed the arteriole/venule circulation in the muscle.
Assess capillary return, skin color, and warmth distal to the fracture.	Return of color should be rapid (3–5 sec). White, cool skin indicates arterial impairment. Cyanosis suggests venous impairment. *Note:* Peripheral pulses, capillary refill, skin color, and sensation may be normal even in presence of compartmental syndrome because superficial circulation is usually not compromised.
Maintain elevation of injured extremity(ies) unless contraindicated by confirmed presence of compartment syndrome.	Promotes venous drainage/decreases edema. *Note:* In presence of increased compartment pressure, elevation of the extremity actually impedes arterial flow, decreasing perfusion.
Assess entire length of injured extremity for swelling/edema formation. Measure injured extremity and compare with uninjured extremity. Note appearance/spread of hematoma.	Increasing circumference of injured extremity may suggest general tissue swelling/edema but may reflect hemorrhage. *Note:* A 1-inch increase in an adult thigh can equal approximately 1 unit of sequestered blood.
Note reports of pain extreme for type of injury or increasing pain on passive movement of extremity, development of paresthesia, muscle tension/tenderness with erythema, and change in pulse quality distal to injury. Do not elevate extremity. Report symptoms to physician at once.	Continued bleeding/edema formation within a muscle enclosed by tight fascia can result in impaired blood flow and ischemic myositis or compartmental syndrome, necessitating emergency interventions to relieve pressure/restore circulation. *Note:* This condition constitutes a medical emergency and requires immediate intervention.
Investigate sudden signs of limb ischemia, e.g., decreased skin temperature, pallor, and increased pain.	Fracture dislocations of joints (especially the knee) may cause damage to adjacent arteries, with resulting loss of distal blood flow.
Encourage patient to routinely exercise digits/joints distal to injury. Ambulate as soon as possible.	Enhances circulation and reduces pooling of blood, especially in the lower extremities.
Investigate tenderness, swelling, pain on dorsiflexion of foot (positive Homans' sign).	There is an increased potential for thrombophlebitis and pulmonary emboli in patients immobile for several days. *Note:* The absence of a positive Homan's sign is not a reliable indicator in many people, especially the elderly because they often have reduced pain sensation.
Monitor vital signs. Note signs of general pallor/cyanosis, cool skin, changes in mentation.	Inadequate circulating volume compromises systemic tissue perfusion.
Test stools/gastric aspirant for occult blood. Note continued bleeding at trauma/injection site(s) and oozing from mucous membranes.	Increased incidence of gastric bleeding accompanies fractures/trauma and may be related to stress or occasionally reflects a clotting disorder requiring further evaluation.

ACTIONS/INTERVENTIONS	RATIONALE

Pressure Management (NIC)

Independent

Perform neurovascular assessments, noting changes in motor/sensory function. Ask patient to localize pain/discomfort.

Impaired feeling, numbness, tingling, increased/diffuse pain occurs when circulation to nerves is inadequate or nerves are damaged.

Test sensation of peroneal nerve by pinch/pinprick in the dorsal web between the first and second toe, and assess ability to dorsiflex toes if indicated.

Length and position of peroneal nerve increases risk of its injury in the presence of leg fracture, edema/compartmental syndrome, or malposition of traction apparatus.

Assess tissues around cast edges for rough places/pressure points. Investigate reports of "burning sensation" under cast.

These factors may be the cause of or be indicative of tissue pressure/ischemia, leading to breakdown/necrosis.

Monitor position/location of supporting ring of splints or sling.

Traction apparatus can cause pressure on vessels/nerves, particularly in the axilla and groin, resulting in ischemia and possible permanent nerve damage.

Circulatory Care (NIC)

Collaborative

Apply ice bags around fracture site for short periods of time on an intermittent basis for 24–72 hr.

Reduces edema/hematoma formation, which could impair circulation.

Monitor hemoglobin (Hb)/Hematocrit (Hct), coagulation studies, e.g., prothrombin time (PT) levels.

Assists in calculation of blood loss and needs/effectiveness of replacement therapy. Coagulation deficits may occur secondary to major trauma, presence of fat emboli, or anticoagulant therapy.

Administer IV fluids/blood products as needed.

Maintains circulating volume, enhancing tissue perfusion.

Administer sodium warfarin (Coumadin) if indicated.

May be given prophylactically to reduce threat of deep venous thrombus.

Apply antiembolic hose/sequential pressure hose as indicated.

Decreases venous pooling and may enhance venous return, thereby reducing risk of thrombus formation.

Pressure Management (NIC)

Split/bivalve cast as needed.

May be done on an emergency basis to relieve restriction and improve impaired circulation resulting from compression and edema formation in injured extremity.

Assist with/monitor intracompartmental pressures as appropriate.

Elevation of pressure (usually to 30 mm Hg or more) indicates need for prompt evaluation and intervention. *Note:* This is not a widespread diagnostic tool, so special interventions and training may be required.

Review electromyography (EMG)/nerve conduction velocity (NCV) studies.

May be performed to differentiate between true nerve dysfunction/muscle weakness and reduced use due to secondary pain.

Prepare for surgical intervention (e.g., fibulectomy/fasciotomy) as indicated.

Failure to relieve pressure/correct compartmental syndrome within 4–6 hr of onset can result in severe contractures/loss of function and disfigurement of extremity distal to injury or even necessitate amputation.

ACTIONS/INTERVENTIONS	RATIONALE
Respiratory Monitoring (NIC)	
Independent	
Monitor respiratory rate and effort. Note stridor, use of accessory muscles, retractions, development of central cyanosis.	Tachypnea, dyspnea, and changes in mentation are early signs of respiratory insufficiency and may be the only indicator of developing pulmonary emboli in the early stage. Remaining signs/symptoms reflect advanced respiratory distress/impending failure.
Auscultate breath sounds, noting development of unequal, hyperresonant sounds; also note presence of crackles/rhonchi/wheezes and inspiratory crowing or croupy sounds.	Changes in/presence of adventitious breath sounds reflects developing respiratory complications, e.g., atelectasis, pneumonia, emboli, adult respiratory distress syndrome (ARDS). Inspiratory crowing reflects upper airway edema and is suggestive of fat emboli.
Handle injured tissues/bones gently, especially during first several days.	This may prevent the development of fat emboli (usually seen in first 12–72 hr), which are closely associated with fractures, especially of the long bones and pelvis.
Instruct and assist with deep-breathing and coughing exercises. Reposition frequently.	Promotes alveolar ventilation and perfusion. Repositioning promotes drainage of secretions and decreases congestion in dependent lung areas.
Note increasing restlessness, confusion, lethargy, stupor.	Impaired gas exchange/presence of pulmonary emboli can cause deterioration in the patient's level of consciousness as hypoxemia/acidosis develops.
Observe sputum for signs of blood.	Hemoptysis may occur with pulmonary emboli.
Inspect skin for petechiae above nipple line; in axilla, spreading to abdomen/trunk; buccal mucosa, hard palate; conjunctival sacs and retina.	This is the most characteristic sign of fat emboli, which may appear within 2–3 days after injury.
Collaborative	
Assist with incentive spirometry.	Maximizes ventilation/oxygenation and minimizes atelectasis.
Administer supplemental oxygen if indicated.	Increases available O_2 for optimal tissue oxygenation.
Monitor laboratory studies, e.g.:	
Serial ABGs;	Decreased PaO_2 and increased $PaCO_2$ indicate impaired gas exchange/developing failure.

688

ACTIONS/INTERVENTIONS

Collaborative

Hb, calcium, erythrocyte sedimentation rate (ESR), serum lipase, fat screen, platelets, as appropriate.

Administer medications as indicated:

Low-molecular-weight heparin or heparinoids, e.g., enoxaparin (Lovenox), dalteparin (Fragmin), ardeparin (Normiflow);

Corticosteroids.

RATIONALE

Anemia, hypocalcemia, elevated ESR and lipase levels, fat globules in blood/urine/sputum, and decreased platelet count (thrombocytopenia) are often associated with fat emboli.

Used for prevention of thromboembolic phenomena, including deep vein thrombosis and pulmonary emboli.

Steroids have been used with some success to prevent/treat fat embolus.

NURSING DIAGNOSIS: Mobility, impaired physical

May be related to
Neuromuscular skeletal impairment; pain/discomfort; restrictive therapies (limb immobilization)
Psychological immobility

Possibly evidenced by
Inability to move purposefully within the physical environment, imposed restrictions
Reluctance to attempt movement; limited ROM
Decreased muscle strength/control

DESIRED OUTCOMES/EVALUATION CRITERIA—PATIENT WILL:

Mobility Level (NOC)

Regain/maintain mobility at the highest possible level.
Maintain position of function.
Increase strength/function of affected and compensatory body parts.
Demonstrate techniques that enable resumption of activities.

ACTIONS/INTERVENTIONS

Bed Rest Care (NIC)

Independent

Assess degree of immobility produced by injury/treatment and note patient's perception of immobility.

Encourage participation in diversional/recreational activities. Maintain stimulating environment, e.g., radio, TV, newspapers, personal possessions/pictures, clock, calendar, visits from family/friends.

Instruct patient in/assist with active/passive ROM exercises of affected and unaffected extremities.

Encourage use of isometric exercises starting with the unaffected limb.

RATIONALE

Patient may be restricted by self-view/self-perception out of proportion with actual physical limitations, requiring information/interventions to promote progress toward wellness.

Provides opportunity for release of energy, refocuses attention, enhances patient's sense of self-control/self-worth, and aids in reducing social isolation.

Increases blood flow to muscles and bone to improve muscle tone, maintain joint mobility; prevent contractures/atrophy, and calcium resorption from disuse.

Isometrics contract muscles without bending joints or moving limbs and help maintain muscle strength and mass. *Note:* These exercises are contraindicated while acute bleeding/edema is present.

ACTIONS/INTERVENTIONS	RATIONALE

Independent

Provide footboard, wrist splints, trochanter/hand rolls as appropriate.

Useful in maintaining functional position of extremities, hands/feet, and preventing complications (e.g., contractures/footdrop).

Place in supine position periodically if possible, when traction is used to stabilize lower limb fractures.

Reduces risk of flexion contracture of hip.

Instruct in/encourage use of trapeze and "post position" for lower limb fractures.

Facilitates movement during hygiene/skin care and linen changes; reduces discomfort of remaining flat in bed. "Post position" involves placing the uninjured foot flat on the bed with the knee bent while grasping the trapeze and lifting the body off the bed.

Assist with/encourage self-care activities (e.g., bathing, shaving).

Improves muscle strength and circulation, enhances patient control in situation, and promotes self-directed wellness.

Provide/assist with mobility by means of wheelchair, walker, crutches, canes as soon as possible. Instruct in safe use of mobility aids.

Early mobility reduces complications of bed rest (e.g., phlebitis) and promotes healing and normalization of organ function. Learning the correct way to use aids is important to maintain optimal mobility and patient safety.

Monitor blood pressure (BP) with resumption of activity. Note reports of dizziness.

Postural hypotension is a common problem following prolonged bedrest and may require specific interventions (e.g., tilt table with gradual elevation to upright position).

Reposition periodically and encourage coughing/deep-breathing exercises.

Prevents/reduces incidence of skin and respiratory complications (e.g., decubitus, atelectasis, pneumonia).

Auscultate bowel sounds. Monitor elimination habits and provide for regular bowel routine. Place on bedside commode, if feasible, or use fracture pan. Provide privacy.

Bedrest, use of analgesics, and changes in dietary habits can slow peristalsis and produce constipation. Nursing measures that facilitate elimination may prevent/limit complications. Fracture pan limits flexion of hips and lessens pressure on lumbar region/lower extremity cast.

Encourage increased fluid intake to 2000–3000 mL/day (within cardiac tolerance), including acid/ash juices.

Keeps the body well hydrated, decreasing risk of urinary infection, stone formation, and constipation.

Provide diet high in proteins, carbohydrates, vitamins, and minerals, limiting protein content until after first bowel movement.

In the presence of musculoskeletal injuries, nutrients required for healing are rapidly depleted, often resulting in a weight loss of as much as 20–30 lb during skeletal traction. This can have a profound effect on muscle mass, tone, and strength. *Note:* Protein foods increase contents in small bowel, resulting in gas formation and constipation. Therefore, gastrointestinal (GI) function should be fully restored before protein foods are increased.

Increase the amount of roughage/fiber in the diet. Limit gas-forming foods.

Adding bulk to stool helps prevent constipation. Gas-forming foods may cause abdominal distension, especially in presence of decreased intestinal motility.

Collaborative

Consult with physical/occupational therapist and/or rehabilitation specialist.

Useful in creating individualized activity/exercise program. Patient may require long-term assistance with movement, strengthening, and weight-bearing activities, as well as use of adjuncts, e.g., walkers, crutches, canes; elevated toilet seats; pickup sticks/reachers; special eating utensils.

ACTIONS/INTERVENTIONS

Collaborative

Initiate bowel program (stool softeners, enemas, laxatives) as indicated.

Refer to psychiatric nurse, clinical specialist/therapist as indicated.

RATIONALE

Done to promote regular bowel evacuation.

Patient/SO may require more intensive treatment to deal with reality of current condition/prognosis, prolonged immobility, perceived loss of control.

NURSING DIAGNOSIS: Skin/Tissue Integrity, impaired: actual/risk for

May be related to

Puncture injury; compound fracture; surgical repair; insertion of traction pins, wires, screws

Altered sensation, circulation; accumulation of excretions/secretions

Physical immobilization

Possibly evidenced by (actual)

Reports of itching, pain, numbness, pressure in affected/surrounding area

Disruption of skin surface; invasion of body structures; destruction of skin layers/tissues

DESIRED OUTCOMES/EVALUATION CRITERIA—PATIENT WILL:

Tissue Integrity: Skin & Mucous Membranes (NOC)

Verbalize relief of discomfort.

Demonstrate behaviors/techniques to prevent skin breakdown/facilitate healing as indicated.

Achieve timely wound/lesion healing if present.

ACTIONS/INTERVENTIONS

Skin Surveillance (NIC)

Independent

Examine the skin for open wounds, foreign bodies, rashes, bleeding, discoloration, duskiness, blanching.

Massage skin and bony prominences. Keep the bed linens dry and free of wrinkles. Place water pads/other padding under elbows/heels as indicated.

Reposition frequently. Encourage use of trapeze if possible.

Assess position of splint ring of traction device.

Cast Care: Wet (NIC)

Plaster cast application and skin care:

Cleanse skin with soap and water. Rub gently with alcohol and/or dust with small amount of a borate or stearate of zinc powder;

RATIONALE

Provides information regarding skin circulation and problems that may be caused by application and/or restriction of cast/splint or traction apparatus; or edema formation that may require further medical intervention.

Reduces pressure on susceptible areas and risk of abrasions/skin breakdown.

Lessens constant pressure on same areas and minimizes risk of skin breakdown. Use of trapeze may reduce risk of abrasions to elbows/heels.

Improper positioning may cause skin injury/breakdown.

Provides a dry, clean area for cast application. *Note:* Excess powder may cake when it comes in contact with water/perspiration.

ACTIONS/INTERVENTIONS	RATIONALE
Independent	
Cut a length of stockinette to cover the area and extend several inches beyond the cast;	Useful for padding bony prominences, finishing cast edges, and protecting the skin.
Use palm of hand to apply, hold, or move cast and support on pillows after application;	Prevents indentations/flattening over bony prominences and weight-bearing areas (e.g., back of heels), which would cause abrasions/tissue trauma. An improperly shaped or dried cast is irritating to the underlying skin and may lead to circulatory impairment.
Trim excess plaster from edges of cast as soon as casting is completed;	Uneven plaster is irritating to the skin and may result in abrasions.
Promote cast drying by removing bed linen, exposing to circulating air;	Prevents skin breakdown caused by prolonged moisture trapped under cast.
Observe for potential pressure areas, especially at the edges of and under the splint/cast;	Pressure can cause ulcerations, necrosis, and/or nerve palsies. These problems may be painless when nerve damage is present.
Pad (petal) the edges of the cast with waterproof tape;	Provides an effective barrier to cast flaking and moisture. Helps prevent breakdown of cast material at edges and reduces skin irritation/excoriation.
Cleanse excess plaster from skin while still wet, if possible;	Dry plaster may flake into completed cast and cause skin damage.
Protect cast and skin in perineal area. Provide frequent pericare;	Prevents tissue breakdown and infection by fecal contamination.
Instruct patient/SO to avoid inserting objects inside casts;	"Scratching an itch" may cause tissue injury.
Massage the skin around the cast edges with alcohol;	Has a drying effect, which toughens the skin. Creams and lotions are not recommended because excessive oils can seal cast perimeter, not allowing the cast to "breathe." Powders are not recommended because of potential for excessive accumulation inside the cast.
Turn frequently to include the uninvolved side, back, and prone positions (as tolerated) with patient's feet over the end of the mattress.	Minimizes pressure on feet and around cast edges.

Traction/Immobilization Care (NIC)	
Skin traction application and skin care:	
Cleanse the skin with warm, soapy water;	Reduces level of contaminants on skin.
Apply tincture of benzoin;	"Toughens" the skin for application of skin traction.
Apply commercial skin traction tapes (or make some with strips of moleskin/adhesive tape) lengthwise on opposite sides of the affected limb;	Traction tapes encircling a limb may compromise circulation.
Extend the tapes beyond the length of the limb;	Traction is inserted in line with the free ends of the tape.
Mark the line where the tapes extend beyond the extremity;	Allows for quick assessment of slippage.
Place protective padding under the leg and over bony prominences;	Minimizes pressure on these areas.
Wrap the limb circumference, including tapes and padding, with elastic bandages, being careful to wrap snugly but not too tightly;	Provides for appropriate traction pull without compromising circulation.

ACTIONS/INTERVENTIONS

Independent

Palpate taped tissues daily and document any tenderness or pain;

Remove skin traction every 24 hr, per protocol; inspect and give skin care.

Skeletal traction/fixation application and skin care:

Bend wire ends or cover ends of wires/pins with rubber or cork protectors or needle caps;

Pad slings/frame with sheepskin, foam.

Collaborative

Pressure Management (NIC)

Provide foam mattress, sheepskins, flotation pads, or air mattress as indicated.

Monovalve, bivalve, or cut a window in the cast, per protocol.

RATIONALE

If area under tapes is tender, suspect skin irritation, and prepare to remove the bandage system.

Maintains skin integrity.

Prevents injury to other body parts.

Prevents excessive pressure on skin and promotes moisture evaporation that reduces risk of excoriation.

Because of immobilization of body parts, bony prominences other than those affected by the casting may suffer from decreased circulation.

Allows the release of pressure and provides access for wound/skin care.

NURSING DIAGNOSIS: Infection, risk for

Risk factors may include
Inadequate primary defenses: broken skin, traumatized tissues; environmental exposure
Invasive procedures, skeletal traction

Possibly evidenced by
[Not applicable; presence of signs and symptoms establishes an *actual* diagnosis]

DESIRED OUTCOMES/EVALUATION CRITERIA—PATIENT WILL:

Infection Status (NOC)

Achieve timely wound healing, be free of purulent drainage or erythema, and be afebrile.

ACTIONS/INTERVENTIONS

Infection Prevention (NIC)

Independent

Inspect the skin for preexisting irritation or breaks in continuity.

Assess pin sites/skin areas noting reports of increased pain/burning sensation or presence of edema, erythema, foul odor, or drainage.

Provide sterile pin/wound care according to protocol, and exercise meticulous handwashing.

Instruct patient not to touch the insertion sites.

Line perineal cast edges with plastic wrap.

RATIONALE

Pins or wires should not be inserted through skin infections, rashes, or abrasions (may lead to bone infection).

May indicate onset of local infection/tissue necrosis, which can lead to osteomyelitis.

May prevent cross-contamination and possibility of infection.

Minimizes opportunity for contamination.

Damp, soiled casts can promote growth of bacteria.

ACTIONS/INTERVENTIONS	RATIONALE
Independent	
Observe wounds for formation of bullae, crepitation, bronze discoloration of skin, frothy/fruity-smelling drainage.	Signs suggestive of gas gangrene infection.
Assess muscle tone, reflexes, and ability to speak.	Muscle rigidity, tonic spasms of jaw muscles, and dysphagia reflect development of tetanus.
Monitor vital signs. Note presence of chills, fever, malaise, changes in mentation.	Hypotension, confusion may be seen with gas gangrene; tachycardia and chills/fever reflect developing sepsis.
Investigate abrupt onset of pain/limitation of movement with localized edema/erythema in injured extremity.	May indicate development of osteomyelitis.
Institute prescribed isolation procedures.	Presence of purulent drainage requires wound/linen precautions to prevent cross-contamination.
Collaborative	
Monitor laboratory/diagnostic studies, e.g.:	
Complete blood count (CBC);	Anemia may be noted with osteomyelitis; leukocytosis is usually present with infective processes.
ESR;	Elevated in osteomyelitis.
Cultures and sensitivity of wound/serum/bone;	Identifies infective organism.
Radioisotope scans.	Hot spots signify increased areas of vascularity, indicative of osteomyelitis.
Administer medications as indicated, e.g.:	
IV/topical antibiotics;	Wide-spectrum antibiotics may be used prophylactically or may be geared toward a specific microorganism.
Tetanus toxoid.	Given prophylactically because the possibility of tetanus exists with any open wound. *Note:* Risk increases when injury/wound(s) occur in "field conditions" (outdoor/rural areas, work environment).
Provide wound/bone irrigations and apply warm/moist soaks as indicated.	Local debridement/cleansing of wounds reduces microorganisms and incidence of systemic infection. Continuous antimicrobial drip into bone may be necessary to treat osteomyelitis, especially if blood supply to bone is compromised.
Assist with procedures, e.g., incision/drainage, placement of drains, hyperbaric oxygen therapy.	Numerous procedures may be carried out in treatment of local infections, osteomyelitis, gas gangrene.
Prepare for surgery, as indicated.	Sequestrectomy (removal of necrotic bone) is necessary to facilitate healing and prevent extension of infectious process.

NURSING DIAGNOSIS: Knowledge Deficit [Learning Need] regarding condition, prognosis, treatment, self care, and discharge needs

May be related to

Lack of exposure/recall

Information misinterpretation/unfamiliarity with information resources

Possibly evidenced by
Questions/request for information, statement of misconception
Inaccurate follow-through of instructions/development of preventable complications

DESIRED OUTCOMES/EVALUATION CRITERIA—PATIENT WILL:

Knowledge: Disease Process (NOC)

Verbalize understanding of condition, prognosis, and potential complications.
Correctly perform necessary procedures and explain reasons for actions.

ACTIONS/INTERVENTIONS	RATIONALE

Teaching: Disease Process (NIC)

Independent

Review pathology, prognosis, and future expectations.	Provides knowledge base from which patient can make informed choices. *Note:* Internal fixation devices can ultimately compromise the bone's strength, and intramedullary nails/rods or plates may be removed at a future date.
Discuss dietary needs.	A low-fat diet with adequate quality protein and rich in calcium promotes healing and general well-being.
Discuss individual drug regimen as appropriate.	Proper use of pain medication and antiplatelet agents can reduce risk of complications. Long-term use of alendronate (Fosamax) may reduce risk of stress fractures. *Note:* Fosamax should be taken on an empty stomach with plain water because absorption of drug may be altered by food and some medications (e.g., antacids, calcium supplements).
Reinforce methods of mobility and ambulation as instructed by physical therapist when indicated.	Most fractures require casts, splints, or braces during the healing process. Further damage and delay in healing could occur secondary to improper use of ambulatory devices.
Suggest use of a backpack.	Provides place to carry necessary articles and leaves hands free to manipulate crutches; may prevent undue muscle fatigue when one arm is casted.
List activities the patient can perform independently and those that require assistance.	Organizes activities around need and who is available to provide help.
Identify available community services, e.g., rehabilitation teams, home nursing/homemaker services.	Provides assistance to facilitate self-care and support independence. Promotes optimal self-care and recovery.
Encourage patient to continue active exercises for the joints above and below the fracture.	Prevents joint stiffness, contractures, and muscle wasting, promoting earlier return to independence in activities of daily living (ADLs).
Discuss importance of clinical and therapy follow-up appointments.	Fracture healing may take as long as a year for completion, and patient cooperation with the medical regimen facilitates proper union of bone. Physical therapy (PT)/occupational therapy (OT) may be indicated for exercises to maintain/strengthen muscles and improve function. Additional modalities such as low-intensity ultrasound may be used to stimulate healing of lower-forearm or lower-leg fractures.
Review proper pin/wound care.	Reduces risk of bone/tissue trauma and infection, which can progress to osteomyelitis.

695

ACTIONS/INTERVENTIONS	RATIONALE

Independent

Recommend cleaning external fixator regularly.	Keeping device free of dust/contaminants reduces risk of infection.
Identify signs/symptoms requiring medical evaluation, e.g., severe pain, fever/chills, foul odors; changes in sensation, swelling, burning, numbness, tingling, skin discoloration, paralysis, white/cool toes or fingertips; warm spots, soft areas, cracks in cast.	Prompt intervention may reduce severity of complications such as infection/impaired circulation. *Note:* Some darkening of the skin (vascular congestion) may occur normally when walking on the casted extremity or using casted arm; however, this should resolve with rest and elevation.
Discuss care of "green" or wet cast.	Promotes proper curing to prevent cast deformities and associated misalignment/skin irritation. *Note:* Placing a "cooling" cast directly on rubber or plastic pillows traps heat and increases drying time.
Suggest the use of a blow-dryer to dry small areas of dampened casts.	Cautious use can hasten drying.
Demonstrate use of plastic bags to cover plaster cast during wet weather or while bathing. Clean soiled cast with a slightly dampened cloth and some scouring powder.	Protects from moisture, which softens the plaster and weakens the cast. *Note:* Fiberglass casts are being used more frequently because they are not affected by moisture. In addition, their light weight may enhance patient participation in desired activities.
Emphasize importance of not adjusting clamps/nuts of external fixator.	Tampering may alter compression and misalign fracture.
Recommend use of adaptive clothing.	Facilitates dressing/grooming activities.
Suggest ways to cover toes, if appropriate, e.g., stockinette or soft socks.	Helps to maintain warmth/protect from injury.
Discuss postcast removal instructions:	
Instruct the patient to continue exercises as permitted;	Reduces stiffness and improves strength and function of affected extremity.
Inform the patient that the skin under the cast is commonly mottled and covered with scales or crusts of dead skin;	It will be several weeks before normal appearance returns.
Wash the skin gently with soap, povidone-iodine (Betadine), or pHisoDerm, and water. Lubricate with a protective emollient;	New skin is extremely tender because it has been protected beneath a cast.
Inform the patient that muscles may appear flabby and atrophied (less muscle mass). Recommend supporting the joint above and below the affected part and the use of mobility aids, e.g., elastic bandages, splints, braces, crutches, walkers, or canes;	Muscle strength will be reduced and new or different aches and pains may occur for awhile secondary to loss of support.
Elevate the extremity as needed.	Swelling and edema tend to occur after cast removal.

POTENTIAL CONSIDERATIONS following acute hospitalization (dependent on patient's age, physical condition/presence of complications, personal resources, and life responsibilities)

In addition to surgical considerations:

Trauma, risk for—loss of skeletal integrity, weakness, balancing difficulties, reduced muscle coordination, lack of safety precautions, history of previous trauma.

Mobility, impaired physical—neuromuscular skeletal impairment; pain/discomfort, restrictive therapies (limb immobilization); psychological immobility.

Self-Care deficit—musculoskeletal impairment, decreased strength/endurance, pain.

Infection, risk for—inadequate primary defenses: broken skin, traumatized tissues; environmental exposure; invasive procedures, skeletal traction.

AMPUTATION

In general, amputation of limbs is the result of trauma, peripheral vascular disease, tumors, and congenital disorders. For the purpose of this plan of care, amputation refers to the surgical/traumatic removal of a limb. Upper-extremity amputations are generally due to trauma from industrial accidents. Reattachment surgery may be possible for fingers, hands, and arms. Lower-extremity amputations are performed much more frequently than upper-extremity amputations. Five levels are currently used in lower-extremity amputation: foot and ankle, below knee (BKA), knee disarticulation and above (thigh), knee-hip disarticulation; and hemipelvectomy and translumbar amputation. There are two types of amputations: (1) open (provisional), which requires strict aseptic techniques and later revisions, and (2) closed, or "flap."

CARE SETTING

Inpatient acute surgical unit and subacute or rehabilitation unit.

RELATED CONCERNS

Cancer, page 900
Diabetes mellitus/Diabetic ketoacidosis, page 440
Surgical intervention, page 828
Psychosocial aspects of care, page 809

Patient Assessment Database

Data depends on underlying reason for surgical procedure, e.g., severe trauma, peripheral vascular/arterial occlusive disease, diabetic neuropathy, osteomyelitis, cancer.

ACTIVITY/REST

May report: Actual/anticipated limitations imposed by condition/amputation

CIRCULATION

May exhibit: Presence of edema; absent/diminished pulses in affected limb/digits

EGO INTEGRITY

May report: Concern about negative effects/anticipated changes in lifestyle, financial situation, reaction of others
Feelings of helplessness, powerlessness

May exhibit: Anxiety, apprehension, irritability, anger, fearfulness, withdrawal, grief, false cheerfulness

NEUROSENSORY

May report: Loss of sensation in affected area

SAFETY

May exhibit: Necrotic/gangrenous area
Nonhealing wound, local infection

SEXUALITY

May report: Concerns about intimate relationships

SOCIAL INTERACTION

May report: Problems related to illness/condition
Concern about role function, reaction of others

TEACHING/LEARNING

Discharge plan considerations: **DRG projected mean length of inpatient stay: 5.8–12.7 days.**
May require assistance with wound care/supplies, adaptation to prosthesis/ambulatory devices, transportation, homemaker/maintenance tasks, possibly self-care activities and vocational retraining

Refer to section at end of plan for postdischarge considerations.

DIAGNOSTIC STUDIES

Studies depend on underlying condition necessitating amputation and are used to determine the appropriate level for amputation.

X-rays: Identify skeletal abnormalities.

CT scan: Identifies soft tissue and bone destruction, neoplastic lesions, osteomyelitis, hematoma formation.

Angiography and blood flow studies: Evaluate circulation/tissue perfusion problems and help predict potential for tissue healing after amputation.

Doppler ultrasound, laser Doppler flowmetry: Performed to assess and measure blood flow.

Transcutaneous oxygen pressure: Maps out areas of greater and lesser perfusion in the involved extremity.

Thermography: Measures temperature differences in an ischemic limb at two sites, at the skin and center of the bone. The lower the difference between the two readings, the greater the chance for healing.

Plethysmography: Segmental systolic BP measurements evaluate arterial blood flow.

ESR: Elevation indicates inflammatory response.

Wound cultures: Identify presence of infection and causative organism.

White blood cell (WBC) count/differential: Elevation and "shift to left" suggest infectious process.

Biopsy: Confirms diagnosis of benign/malignant mass.

NURSING PRIORITIES

1. Support psychological and physiological adjustment.
2. Alleviate pain.
3. Prevent complications.
4. Promote mobility/functional abilities.
5. Provide information about surgical procedure/prognosis and treatment needs.

DISCHARGE GOALS

1. Dealing with current situation realistically.
2. Pain relieved/controlled.
3. Complications prevented/minimized.
4. Mobility/function regained or compensated for.
5. Surgical procedure, prognosis, and therapeutic regimen understood.
6. Plan in place to meet needs after discharge.

NURSING DIAGNOSIS: Self-Esteem, situational low

May be related to

Loss of body part/change in functional abilities

Possibly evidenced by

Anticipated changes in lifestyle; fear of rejection/reaction by others

Negative feelings about body, focus on past strength, function, or appearance

Feelings of helplessness, powerlessness

Preoccupation with missing body part, not looking at or touching stump

Perceived change in usual patterns of responsibility/physical capacity to resume role

DESIRED OUTCOMES/EVALUATION CRITERIA—PATIENT WILL:

Grief Resolution (NOC)

Begin to show adaptation and verbalize acceptance of self in situation (amputee).

Recognize and incorporate changes into self-concept in accurate manner without negating self-esteem.

Develop realistic plans for adapting to new role/role modifications.

ACTIONS/INTERVENTIONS	RATIONALE

Grief Work Facilitation (NIC)

Independent

Assess/consider the patient's preparation for and view of amputation.

Research shows that amputation poses serious threats to the patient's psychological and psychosocial adjustment. The patient who views amputation as lifesaving or reconstructive may be able to accept the new self more quickly. The patient with sudden traumatic amputation or who considers amputation to be the result of failure in other treatments is at greater risk for self-concept disturbances.

Encourage expression of fears, negative feelings, and grief over loss of body part.

Venting emotions helps patient begin to deal with the fact and reality of life without a limb.

Reinforce preoperative information including type/location of amputation, type of prosthetic fitting if appropriate (immediate, delayed), expected postoperative course, including pain control and rehabilitation.

Provides opportunity for patient to question and assimilate information and begin to deal with changes in body image and function, which can facilitate postoperative recovery.

Assess degree of support available to the patient.

Sufficient support by SO and friends can facilitate rehabilitation process.

Discuss patient's perceptions of self related to change and how patient sees self in usual lifestyle/role functioning.

Aids in defining concerns in relation to previous lifestyle and facilitates problem solving. For example, the patient likely fears loss of independence, may lose ability to work, express sexuality, and may experience role/relationship changes.

Ascertain individual strengths and identify previous positive coping behaviors.

Helpful to build on strengths that are already available for patient to use in coping with current situation.

Self-Esteem Enhancement (NIC)

Encourage participation in ADLs. Provide opportunities to view/care for stump, using the moment to point out positive signs of healing.

Promotes independence and enhances feelings of self-worth. Although integration of stump into body image can take months or even years, looking at the stump and hearing positive comments (made in a normal, matter-of-fact manner) can help patient with this acceptance.

Encourage/provide for visit by another amputee, especially one who is successfully rehabilitating.

A peer who has been through a similar experience serves as a role model and can provide validity to comments and hope for recovery and a normal future.

Provide open environment for patient to discuss concerns about sexuality.

Promotes sharing of beliefs/values about sensitive subject and identifies misconceptions/myths that may interfere with adjustment to situation.

Note withdrawn behavior, negative self-talk, use of denial, or overconcern with actual/perceived changes.

Identifies stage of grief/need for interventions.

Collaborative

Discuss availability of various resources, e.g., psychiatric/sexual counseling, occupational therapist.

May need assistance for these concerns to facilitate optimal adaptation and rehabilitation.

699

NURSING DIAGNOSIS: Pain [acute]

May be related to

Physical injury/tissue and nerve trauma

Psychological impact of loss of body part

Possibly evidenced by

Reports of pain

Narrowed self-focus

Autonomic responses, guarding/protective behavior

DESIRED OUTCOMES/EVALUATION CRITERIA—PATIENT WILL:

Pain Level (NOC)

Report pain is relieved/controlled.

Appear relaxed and able to rest/sleep appropriately.

Verbalize understanding of phantom pain and methods to provide relief.

ACTIONS/INTERVENTIONS	RATIONALE
Pain Management (NIC)	
Independent	
Document location and intensity of pain (0–10 scale). Investigate changes in pain characteristics, e.g., numbness, tingling.	Aids in evaluating need for and effectiveness of interventions. Changes may indicate developing complications, e.g., necrosis/infection.
Elevate affected part by raising foot of bed slightly or use of pillow/sling for upper-limb amputation.	Lessens edema formation by enhancing venous return; reduces muscle fatigue and skin/tissue pressure. *Note:* After initial 24 hr and in absence of edema, stump may be extended and kept flat.
Acknowledge reality of phantom-limb sensations, that they are usually self-limiting, and that various modalities will be tried for pain relief.	Knowing about these sensations allows the patient to understand this is a normal phenomenon that may develop immediately or several weeks postoperatively. Although the sensations usually resolve on their own, some individuals continue to experience the discomfort for several months/years. *Note:* Phantom pain is not well relieved by traditional pain medications. A transcutaneous electrical nerve stimulator (TENS) has proven to offer short-term relief, when used in addition to managing stump tissue and prosthesis problems.
Provide/promote general comfort measures (e.g., frequent turning, backrub) and diversional activities. Encourage use of stress management techniques (e.g., deep-breathing exercises, visualization, guided imagery) and Therapeutic Touch.	Refocuses attention, promotes relaxation, may enhance coping abilities and may decrease occurrence of phantom-limb pain.
Provide gentle massage to stump as tolerated once dressings are discontinued.	Enhances circulation; reduces muscle tension.
Investigate reports of progressive/poorly localized pain unrelieved by analgesics.	May indicate developing compartmental syndrome, especially following traumatic injury. (Refer to CP: Fractures; ND: Peripheral Neurovascular risk for dysfunction, p. 685.)

ACTIONS/INTERVENTIONS

Collaborative

Administer medications, as indicated, e.g.: analgesics, muscle relaxants. Instruct in/monitor use of PCA.

Maintain electrical stimulating device (e.g., TENS), if used.

Provide topical heat as indicated.

RATIONALE

Reduces pain/muscle spasms. PCA provides for timely drug administration, preventing fluctuations in pain with associated muscle tension/spasms.

Provides continuous low-level nerve stimulation, blocking transmission of pain sensation. *Note:* There is some evidence that abnormal nerve stimuli and feedback mechanisms are present, possibly because of actual interrupted nerve pathways and partly because of abnormal activity of the remaining nerve fibers. Electrical stimulation offers a short-term rerouting or stimulation of different nerve pathways, thus reducing the activity of the usual pain patterns.

May be used to promote muscle relaxation, enhance circulation, and facilitate resolution of edema.

NURSING DIAGNOSIS: Tissue Perfusion, risk for altered: peripheral

Risk factors may include:
Reduced arterial/venous blood flow; tissue edema, hematoma formation
Hypovolemia

Possibly evidenced by:
[Not applicable; presence of signs and symptoms establishes an *actual* diagnosis]

DESIRED OUTCOMES/EVALUATION CRITERIA—PATIENT WILL:

Tissue Perfusion: Peripheral (NOC)

Maintain adequate tissue perfusion as evidenced by palpable peripheral pulses, warm/dry skin, and timely wound healing.

ACTIONS/INTERVENTIONS

Circulatory Care (NIC)

Independent

Monitor vital signs. Palpate peripheral pulses, noting strength and equality.

Perform periodic neurovascular assessments, e.g., sensation, movement, pulse, skin color, and temperature.

Inspect dressings/drainage device, noting amount and characteristics of drainage.

Apply direct pressure to bleeding site if hemorrhage occurs. Contact physician immediately.

Investigate reports of persistent/unusual pain in operative site.

Evaluate nonoperated lower limb for inflammation, positive Homans' sign.

RATIONALE

General indicators of circulatory status and adequacy of perfusion.

Postoperative tissue edema, hematoma formation, or restrictive dressings may impair circulation to stump, resulting in tissue necrosis.

Continued blood loss may indicate need for additional fluid replacement and evaluation for coagulation defect or surgical intervention to ligate bleeder.

Direct pressure to bleeding site may be followed by application of a bulk dressing secured with an elastic wrap once bleeding is controlled.

Hematoma can form in muscle pocket under flap, compromising circulation and intensifying pain.

Increased incidence of thrombus formation in patients with preexisting peripheral vascular disease/diabetic changes.

ACTIONS/INTERVENTIONS	RATIONALE

Independent

Encourage/assist with early ambulation.	Enhances circulation, helps prevent stasis and associated complications. Promotes sense of general well-being.

Collaborative

Administer IV fluids/blood products as indicated.	Maintains circulating volume to maximize tissue perfusion.
Apply antiembolic/sequential compression hose to nonoperated leg, as indicated.	Enhances venous return, reducing venous pooling and risk of thrombophlebitis.
Administer low-dose anticoagulant as indicated.	May be useful in preventing thrombus formation without increasing risk of postoperative bleeding/hematoma formation.
Monitor laboratory studies, e.g.:	
Hb/Hct;	Indicators of hypovolemia/dehydration that can impair tissue perfusion.
PT/activated partial thromboplastin time (aPTT).	Evaluates need for/effectiveness of anticoagulant therapy and identifies developing complication, e.g., posttraumatic disseminated intravascular coagulation (DIC).

NURSING DIAGNOSIS: Infection, risk for

Risk factors may include
Inadequate primary defenses (broken skin, traumatized tissue)
Invasive procedures; environmental exposure
Chronic disease, altered nutritional status

Possibly evidenced by
[Not applicable; presence of signs and symptoms establishes an *actual* diagnosis]

DESIRED OUTCOMES/EVALUATION CRITERIA—PATIENT WILL:

Wound Healing: Primary Intention (NOC)

Achieve timely wound healing; be free of purulent drainage or erythema; and be afebrile.

ACTIONS/INTERVENTIONS	RATIONALE

Wound Care (NIC)

Independent

Maintain aseptic technique when changing dressings/caring for wound.	Minimizes opportunity for introduction of bacteria.
Inspect dressings and wound; note characteristics of drainage.	Early detection of developing infection provides opportunity for timely intervention and prevention of more serious complications (e.g., osteomyelitis).
Maintain patency and routinely empty drainage device.	Hemovac, Jackson-Pratt drains facilitate removal of drainage, promoting wound healing and reducing risk of infection.
Cover dressing with plastic when using the bedpan or if incontinent.	Prevents contamination in lower-limb amputation.

ACTIONS/INTERVENTIONS	RATIONALE
Independent	
Expose stump to air; wash with mild soap and water after dressings are discontinued.	Maintains cleanliness, minimizes skin contaminants, and promotes healing of tender/fragile skin.
Monitor vital signs.	Temperature elevation/tachycardia may reflect developing sepsis.
Collaborative	
Obtain wound/drainage cultures as appropriate.	Identifies presence of infection/specific organisms and appropriate therapy.
Administer antibiotics as indicated.	Wide-spectrum antibiotics may be used prophylactically, or antibiotic therapy may be geared toward specific organisms.

NURSING DIAGNOSIS: Mobility, impaired physical

May be related to
Loss of a limb (particularly a lower extremity); pain/discomfort; perceptual impairment (altered sense of balance)

Possibly evidenced by
Reluctance to attempt movement
Impaired coordination; decreased muscle strength, control, and mass

DESIRED OUTCOMES/EVALUATION CRITERIA—PATIENT WILL:

Risk Control (NOC)

Verbalize understanding of individual situation, treatment regimen, and safety measures.
Maintain position of function as evidenced by absence of contractures.

Mobility Level (NOC)

Demonstrate techniques/behaviors that enable resumption of activities.
Display willingness to participate in activities.

ACTIONS/INTERVENTIONS	RATIONALE
Amputation Care (NIC)	
Independent	
Provide stump care on a routine basis, e.g., inspect area, cleanse and dry thoroughly, and rewrap stump with elastic bandage or air splint, or apply a stump shrinker (heavy stockinette sock), for "delayed" prosthesis.	Provides opportunity to evaluate healing and note complications (unless covered by immediate prosthesis). Wrapping stump controls edema and helps form stump into conical shape to facilitate fitting of prosthesis. *Note:* Air splint may be preferred, because it permits visual inspection of the wound.
Measure circumference periodically.	Measurement is done to estimate shrinkage to ensure proper fit of sock and prosthesis.
Rewrap stump immediately with an elastic bandage, elevate if "immediate/early" cast is accidentally dislodged. Prepare for reapplication of cast.	Edema will occur rapidly, and rehabilitation can be delayed.

ACTIONS/INTERVENTIONS	RATIONALE

Independent

Assist with specified ROM exercises for both the affected and unaffected limbs beginning early in postoperative stage.	Prevents contracture deformities, which can develop rapidly and could delay prosthesis usage.
Encourage active/isometric exercises for upper torso and unaffected limbs.	Increases muscle strength to facilitate transfers/ambulation and promote mobility and more normal lifestyle.
Provide trochanter rolls as indicated.	Prevents external rotation of lower-limb stump.
Instruct patient to lie in prone position as tolerated at least twice a day with pillow under abdomen and lower-extremity stump.	Strengthens extensor muscles and prevents flexion contracture of the hip, which can begin to develop within 24 hr of sustained malpositioning.
Caution against keeping pillow under lower-extremity stump or allowing BKA limb to hang dependently over side of bed or chair.	Use of pillows can cause permanent flexion contracture of hip; a dependent position of stump impairs venous return and may increase edema formation.
Demonstrate/assist with transfer techniques and use of mobility aids, e.g., trapeze, crutches, or walker.	Facilitates self-care and patient's independence. Proper transfer techniques prevent shearing abrasions/dermal injury related to "scooting."
Assist with ambulation.	Reduces potential for injury. Ambulation after lower-limb amputation depends on timing of prosthesis placement. For example: (1) Immediate postoperative fitting: A rigid plaster-of-paris dressing is applied to the stump and a pylon and artificial foot are attached. Weight bearing begins within 24–48 hr. (2) Early postoperative fitting: Weight bearing does not occur until 10–30 days postoperatively. (3) Delayed fitting: More common in areas that do not have facilities available for immediate/early application of prosthesis or when the condition of the stump and/or the patient precludes these choices. *Note:* Amputation of an upper extremity can affect the patient's sense of balance, necessitating monitoring/assistance with ambulation.
Help patient continue preoperative muscle exercises as able/when allowed out of bed; e.g., patient should (while holding on to chair for balance) perform abdominal-tightening exercises and knee bends; hop on foot; stand on toes.	Contributes to gaining improved sense of balance and strengthens compensatory body parts.
Instruct patient in stump-conditioning exercises, e.g., pushing the stump against a pillow initially, then progressing to harder surface.	Hardens the stump by toughening the skin and altering feedback of resected nerves to facilitate use of prosthesis.

Collaborative

Refer to rehabilitation team, e.g., physical and occupational therapy, prosthetic specialists.	Provides for creation of exercise/activity program to meet individual needs and strengths, and identifies mobility functional aids to promote independence. Early use of a temporary prosthesis promotes activity and enhances general well-being/positive outlook. *Note:* Vocational counseling/retraining also may be indicated.
Provide foam/flotation mattress.	Reduces pressure on skin/tissues that can impair circulation, potentiating risk of tissue ischemia/breakdown.

NURSING DIAGNOSIS: Knowledge Deficit [Learning Need] regarding condition, prognosis, treatment, self care, and discharge needs

May be related to
Lack of exposure/recall
Information misinterpretation

Possibly evidenced by
Questions/request for information, verbalization of the problem
Inaccurate follow-through of instructions/development of preventable complications

DESIRED OUTCOMES/EVALUATION CRITERIA—PATIENT WILL:

Knowledge: Disease Process (NOC)

Verbalize understanding of condition/disease process and potential complications.

Knowledge: Treatment Regimen (NOC)

Verbalize understanding of therapeutic needs.
Correctly perform necessary procedures and explain reasons for the actions.
Initiate necessary lifestyle changes and participate in treatment regimen.

ACTIONS/INTERVENTIONS	RATIONALE

Teaching: Disease Process (NIC)

Independent

Review disease process/surgical procedure and future expectations.	Provides knowledge base from which patient can make informed choices.
Instruct in dressing/wound care, inspection of stump using mirror to visualize all areas, skin massage, and appropriate wrapping of the stump.	Promotes competent self-care; facilitates healing and fitting of prosthesis and reduces potential for complications.
Discuss general stump care, e.g.:	
Massaging the stump after dressings are discontinued and suture line is healed;	Massage softens scar and prevents adherence to the bone, decreases tenderness, and stimulates circulation.
Avoiding use of lotions/powders;	Although a small amount of lotion may be indicated if skin is dry, emollients/creams soften skin and may cause maceration when a prosthesis is worn. Powder may cake, potentiating skin irritation.
Wearing only properly fitted, clean, wrinkle-free limb sock;	Stump may continue to shrink for up to 2 yr, and an improperly fitting sock or one that is mended or dirty can cause skin irritation/breakdown.
Using clean cotton T-shirt under harness for upper-limb prosthesis.	Absorbs perspiration; prevents skin irritation from harness.
Demonstrate care of prosthetic device. Stress importance of routine maintenance/periodic refitting.	Ensures proper fit, reduces risk of complications, and prolongs life of prosthesis.
Encourage continuation of postoperative exercise program.	Enhances circulation/healing and function of affected part, facilitating adaptation to prosthetic device.
Identify techniques to manage phantom pain, e.g., good stump care, properly fitted prosthesis, gentle massage/pressure to stump. Emphasize stress management and relaxation training, and discuss various medications that may be used for pain management.	Reduces muscle tension and enhances control of situation and coping abilities.

705

ACTIONS/INTERVENTIONS	RATIONALE
Independent	
Stress importance of well-balanced diet and adequate fluid intake.	Provides needed nutrients for tissue regeneration/healing, aids in maintaining circulating volume and normal organ function, and aids in maintenance of proper weight (weight changes affect fit of prosthesis).
Recommend cessation of smoking. Offer referral resources for smoking cessation.	Smoking potentiates peripheral vasoconstriction, impairing circulation and tissue oxygenation.
Identify signs/symptoms requiring medical evaluation, e.g., edema, erythema, increased/odorous drainage from incision; changes in sensation, movement, skin color; persistent phantom pain.	Prompt intervention may prevent serious complication and/or loss of function. *Note:* Chronic phantom-limb pain may indicate neuroma, requiring surgical resection.
Identify community support and rehabilitation, e.g., certified prosthetist-orthotist, amputee groups, home care service, homemaker services, as needed.	Facilitates transfer to home, supports independence, and enhances coping.

POTENTIAL CONSIDERATIONS following acute hospitalization (dependent on patient's age, physical condition/presence of complications, personal resources, and life responsibilities)

In addition to considerations in Surgical Intervention plan of care:

Trauma, risk for—balancing difficulties/altered gait, muscle weakness, reduced muscle coordination, lack of safety precautions, hazards associated with use of assistive devices.

Self-Esteem, situational low—loss of body part, change in functional abilities.

Self-Care deficit/Home Maintenance Management, impaired (dependent on location of amputation)—musculoskeletal impairment, decreased strength/endurance, pain, depression.

TOTAL JOINT REPLACEMENT

Joint replacement is indicated for irreversibly damaged joints with loss of function and unremitting pain (e.g., degenerative and rheumatoid arthritis [RA]), selected fractures (e.g., hip/femoral neck), joint instability, and congenital hip disorders. The surgery can be performed on any joint except the spine. Hip and knee replacements are the most common procedures. The prosthesis may be metallic or polyethylene (or a combination) implanted with a methylmethacrylate cement, or it may be a porous, coated implant that encourages bony ingrowth.

CARE SETTING

Inpatient acute surgical unit and subacute or rehabilitation unit.

RELATED CONCERNS

Fractures, page 680
Psychosocial aspects of care, page 809
Rheumatoid arthritis, page 790
Sepsis/Septicemia, page 741
Surgical intervention, page 828
Thrombophlebitis: deep vein thrombosis, page 115

Patient Assessment Database

ACTIVITY/REST

May report:	History of occupation/participation in sports activities that wears on particular joint
	Difficulty walking; stiffness in joints (worse in the morning or after period of inactivity)
	Fatigue, generalized and muscle weakness
	Inability to participate in occupational/recreational activities at desired level
	Interruption of sleep, delayed falling asleep/awakened by pain; does not feel well-rested
May exhibit:	Decreased ROM and muscle strength/tone

HYGIENE

May report:	Difficulty performing ADLs
	Use of special equipment/mobility devices
	Need for assistance with some/all activities

NEUROSENSORY

May exhibit:	Soft tissue swelling, nodules
	Muscle spasm, stiffness, deformity
	Impaired ROM of affected joints

PAIN/DISCOMFORT

May report:	Pain (dull, aching, persistent) in affected joint(s), worsened by movement

SAFETY

May report:	Traumatic injury/fractures affecting the joint
	Congenital deformities
	History of inflammatory, debilitating arthritis (RA or osteoarthritis); aseptic necrosis of the joint head
May exhibit:	Distorted joints
	Joint/tissue swelling, decreased ROM, changes in gait

TEACHING/LEARNING

May report:	Current medication use, e.g., anti-inflammatory, analgesics/narcotics, steroids
Discharge plan considerations:	**DRG projected mean length of inpatient stay: 3–5 days (depending on joint replaced)**
	May need assistance with transportation, self-care activities, homemaker/maintenance tasks, possible placement in extended-care facility for continued rehabilitation/assistance

Refer to section at end of plan for postdischarge considerations.

DIAGNOSTIC STUDIES

X-rays: May reveal destruction of articular cartilage, bony demineralization, fractures, soft tissue swelling; narrowing of joint space, joint subluxations or deformity.

Bone Scan, CT/MRI: Determine extent of degeneration and rule out malignancy.

NURSING PRIORITIES

1. Prevent complications.
2. Promote optimal mobility.
3. Alleviate pain.
4. Provide information about diagnosis, prognosis, and treatment needs.

DISCHARGE GOALS

1. Complications prevented/minimized.
2. Mobility increased.
3. Pain relieved/controlled.
4. Diagnosis, prognosis, and therapeutic regimen understood.
5. Plan in place to meet needs after discharge.

NURSING DIAGNOSIS: Infection, risk for

Risk factors may include
Inadequate primary defenses (broken skin, exposure of joint)
Inadequate secondary defenses/immunosuppression (long-term corticosteroid use, cancer)
Invasive procedures; surgical manipulation; implantation of foreign body
Decreased mobility

Possibly evidenced by
[Not applicable; presence of signs and symptoms establishes an *actual* diagnosis]

DESIRED OUTCOMES/EVALUATION CRITERIA—PATIENT WILL:

Infection Status (NOC)

Achieve timely wound healing, be free of purulent drainage or erythema, and be afebrile.

ACTIONS/INTERVENTIONS	RATIONALE
Infection Protection (NIC)	
Independent	
Promote good handwashing by staff and patient.	Reduces risk of cross-contamination.
Use strict aseptic or clean techniques as indicated to reinforce/change dressings and when handling drains. Instruct patient not to touch/scratch incision.	Prevents contamination and risk of wound infection, which could require removal of prosthesis.
Maintain patency of drainage devices (e.g., Hemovac/Jackson-Pratt) when present. Note characteristics of wound drainage.	Reduces risk of infection by preventing accumulation of blood and secretions in the joint space (medium for bacterial growth). Purulent, nonserous, odorous drainage is indicative of infection, and continuous drainage from incision may reflect developing skin tract, which can potentiate infectious process.
Assess skin/incision color, temperature, and integrity; note presence of erythema/inflammation, loss of wound approximation.	Provides information about status of healing process and alerts staff to early signs of infection.

ACTIONS/INTERVENTIONS

Independent

Investigate reports of increased incision area pain, changes in characteristics of pain.

Monitor temperature. Note presence of chills.

Encourage fluid intake, high-protein diet with roughage.

Collaborative

Maintain reverse/protective isolation, if appropriate.

Administer antibiotics as indicated.

RATIONALE

Deep, dull, aching pain in operative area may indicate developing infection in joint. *Note:* Infection is devastating because joint cannot be saved once infection sets in and prosthetic loss will occur.

Although temperature elevations are common in early postoperative phase, elevations occurring 5 or more days postoperatively and/or presence of chills usually requires intervention to prevent more serious complications, e.g., sepsis, osteomyelitis, tissue necrosis, and prosthetic failure.

Maintains fluid and nutritional balance to support tissue perfusion and provide nutrients necessary for cellular regeneration and tissue healing.

May be done initially to reduce contact with sources of possible infection, especially in elderly, immunosuppressed, or diabetic patient.

Used prophylactically in the operating room and first 24 hr to prevent infection.

NURSING DIAGNOSIS: Mobility, impaired physical

May be related to
Pain and discomfort, musculoskeletal impairment
Surgery/restrictive therapies

Possibly evidenced by
Reluctance to attempt movement, difficulty purposefully moving within the physical environment
Reports of pain/discomfort on movement
Limited ROM; decreased muscle strength/control

DESIRED OUTCOMES/EVALUATION CRITERIA—PATIENT WILL:

Mobility Level (NOC)

Maintain position of function, as evidenced by absence of contracture.
Display increased strength and function of affected joint and limb.
Participate in ADLs/rehabilitation program.

ACTIONS/INTERVENTIONS

Positioning (NIC)

Independent

Maintain affected joint in prescribed position and body in alignment when in bed.

Medicate before procedures/activities.

RATIONALE

Provides for stabilization of prosthesis and reduces risk of injury during recovery from effects of anesthesia.

Muscle relaxants, narcotics/analgesics decrease pain, reduce muscle tension/spasm, and facilitate participation in therapy.

ACTIONS/INTERVENTIONS	RATIONALE

Independent

Turn on unoperated side using adequate number of personnel and maintaining operated extremity in prescribed alignment. Support position with pillows/wedges.

Prevents dislocation of hip prosthesis and prolonged skin/tissue pressure, reducing risk of tissue ischemia/breakdown.

Demonstrate/assist with transfer techniques and use of mobility aids, e.g., trapeze, walker.

Facilitates self-care and patient's independence. Proper transfer techniques prevent shearing abrasions of skin and falls.

Determine upper body strength as appropriate. Involve in exercise program.

Replacement of lower extremity joint requires increased use of upper extremities for transfer activities and use of ambulation devices.

Inspect skin, observe for reddened areas. Keep linens dry and wrinkle-free. Massage skin/bony prominences routinely. Protect operative heel, elevating whole length of leg with pillow and placing heel on water glove if burning sensation reported.

Prevents skin irritation/breakdown.

Exercise Therapy: Joint Mobility (NIC)

Perform/assist with ROM to unaffected joints.

Patient with degenerative joint disease can quickly lose joint function during periods of restricted activity.

Medicate before procedures/activities.

Muscle relaxants, narcotics/analgesics decrease pain, reduce muscle tension/spasm, and facilitate participation in therapy.

Promote participation in rehabilitative exercise program, e.g.:

Total hip: Quadriceps and gluteal muscle setting, isometrics, leg lifts, dorsiflexion, plantar flexion of the foot;

Total knee: Quadriceps setting, gluteal contraction, flexion/extension exercises, isometrics;

Strengthens muscle groups, increasing muscle tone and mass; stimulates circulation; prevents decubitus. Active use of the joint may be painful but will not injure the joint. Continuous passive motion (CPM) exercise may be initiated on the knee joint postoperatively.

Other joints: Exercises are individually designed, e.g., toes and knee movements; arm and unaffected fingers (for finger-joint replacement), exercise fingers/wrist of affected arm (for shoulder replacement).

Meets specific needs of the replaced joint.

Observe appropriate limitations based on specific joint; e.g., avoid marked flexion/rotation of hip and flexion or hyperextension of leg; adhere to weight-bearing restrictions; wear knee immobilizer as indicated.

Joint stress is to be avoided at all times during stabilization period to prevent dislocation of new prosthesis.

Investigate sudden increase in pain and shortening of limb, as well as changes in skin color, temperature, and sensation.

Indicative of slippage of prosthesis, requiring medical evaluation/intervention.

Encourage participation in ADLs.

Enhances self-esteem; promotes sense of control and independence.

Provide positive reinforcement for efforts.

Promotes a positive attitude and encourages involvement in therapy.

Collaborative

Consult with physical/occupational therapists and rehabilitation specialist.

Useful in creating individualized activity/exercise program. Patient may require ongoing assistance with movement, strengthening, and weight-bearing activities, as well as use of adjuncts, e.g., walkers, crutches, canes, elevated toilet seat, pickup sticks, and so on.

ACTIONS/INTERVENTIONS

Collaborative

Provide foam/flotation mattress.

RATIONALE

Reduces skin/tissue pressure; limits feelings of fatigue and general discomfort.

NURSING DIAGNOSIS: Peripheral Neurovascular, risk for dysfunction

Risk factors may include

Orthopedic surgery; mechanical compression (e.g., dressing, brace, cast), vascular obstruction, immobilization

Possibly evidenced by

[Not applicable; presence of signs and symptoms establishes an *actual* diagnosis]

DESIRED OUTCOMES/EVALUATION CRITERIA—PATIENT WILL:

Tissue Perfusion: Peripheral (NOC)

Maintain function as evidenced by sensation, movement within normal limits (WNL) for individual situation.

Demonstrate adequate tissue perfusion as evidenced by palpable pulses, brisk capillary refill, skin warm/dry, and normal color.

ACTIONS/INTERVENTIONS

Circulatory Care (NIC)

Independent

Palpate pulses. Evaluate capillary refill and skin color and temperature. Compare with nonoperated limb.

Assess motion and sensation of operated extremity.

Test sensation of peroneal nerve by pinch/pinprick in the dorsal web between first and second toe, and assess ability to dorsiflex toes after hip/knee replacement.

Monitor vital signs.

Monitor amount and characteristics of drainage on dressings/from suction device. Note swelling in operative area.

RATIONALE

Diminished/absent pulses, delayed capillary refill time, pallor, blanching, cyanosis, and coldness of skin reflect diminished circulation/perfusion. Comparison with unoperated limb provides clues as to whether neurovascular problem is localized or generalized.

Increasing pain, numbness/tingling, inability to perform expected movements (e.g., flex foot) suggest nerve injury, compromised circulation, or dislocation of prosthesis, requiring immediate intervention.

Position and length of peroneal nerve increase risk of direct injury or compression by tissue edema/hematoma.

Tachycardia and decreasing BP may reflect response to hypovolemia/blood loss or suggest anaphylaxis related to absorption of methylmethacrylate into systemic circulation. *Note:* This occurs less often because of the advent of prosthetics with a porous layer that fosters ingrowth of bone instead of total reliance on adhesives to internally fix the device.

May indicate excessive bleeding/hematoma formation, which can potentiate neurovascular compromise. *Note:* Drainage following hip replacement may reach 1000 cc in early postoperative period, potentially impacting circulating volume.

ACTIONS/INTERVENTIONS	RATIONALE
Independent	
Ensure that stabilizing devices (e.g., abduction pillow, splint device) are in correct position and are not exerting undue pressure on skin and underlying tissue. Avoid use of pillow or knee gatch under knees.	Reduces risk of pressure on underlying nerves or compromised circulation to extremities.
Evaluate for calf tenderness, positive Homans' sign, and inflammation.	Early identification of thrombus development and intervention may prevent embolus formation.
Observe for signs of continued bleeding, oozing from puncture sites/mucous membranes, or ecchymosis following minimal trauma.	Depression of clotting mechanisms/sensitivity to anticoagulants may result in bleeding episodes that can affect red blood cell (RBC) level and circulating volume.
Observe for restlessness, confusion, sudden chest pain, dyspnea, tachycardia, fever, development of petechiae.	Fat emboli can occur (usually in first 72 hr postoperatively) because of surgical trauma and manipulation of bone during implantation of prosthesis.
Collaborative	
Administer IV fluids, blood/plasma expanders as needed.	Restores circulating volume to maintain perfusion. *Note:* Drainage collected from operative site during first 6–10 hr following procedure may be reinfused per protocol, reducing need for transfusion from unknown donor.
Monitor laboratory studies, e.g.:	
Hct;	Usually done 24–48 hr postoperatively for evaluation of blood loss, which can be quite large because of high vascularity of surgical site in hip replacement. *Note:* Monitoring of CBC/repeated count may be indicated for patients' receiving enoxaparin (Lovenox).
Coagulation studies.	Evaluates presence/degree of alteration in clotting mechanisms and effects of anticoagulant/antiplatelet agents when used. *Note:* Not necessary for patients receiving enoxaparin (Lovenox); however, stool occult blood tests may be indicated.
Administer medications as indicated, e.g.: sodium warfarin (Coumadin), heparin, aspirin, low-molecular-weight heparin, e.g., enoxaparin (Lovenox).	Anticoagulants/antiplatelet agents may be used to reduce risk of thrombophlebitis and pulmonary emboli.
Apply cold/heat as indicated.	Ice packs are used initially to limit edema/hematoma formation. Heat may then be used to enhance circulation, facilitating resolution of tissue edema.
Maintain intermittent compression stocking/foot pumps when used.	Promotes venous return and prevents venous stasis, reducing risk of thrombus formation.
Prepare for surgical procedure as indicated.	Evacuation of hematoma or revision of prosthesis may be required to correct compromised circulation.

NURSING DIAGNOSIS: Pain [acute]
May be related to
Injuring agents: biological, physical/psychological (e.g., muscle spasms, surgical procedure, preexisting chronic joint diseases, elderly age, anxiety)

Possibly evidenced by
Reports of pain; distraction/guarding behaviors
Narrowed focus/self-focusing
Alteration in muscle tone; autonomic responses

DESIRED OUTCOMES/EVALUATION CRITERIA—PATIENT WILL:

Pain Level (NOC)

Report pain relieved/controlled.
Appear relaxed, able to rest/sleep appropriately.

Pain Control Behavior (NOC)

Demonstrate use of relaxation skills and diversional activities as indicated by individual situation.

ACTIONS/INTERVENTIONS

Pain Management (NIC)

Independent

Assess reports of pain, noting intensity (scale of 0–10), duration, and location.

Maintain proper position of operated extremity.

Provide comfort measures (e.g., frequent repositioning, backrub) and diversional activities. Encourage stress management techniques (e.g., progressive relaxation, guided imagery, visualization, meditation). Provide Therapeutic Touch as appropriate.

Medicate on a regular schedule and before activities/procedures.

Investigate reports of sudden, severe joint pain with muscle spasms and changes in joint mobility; sudden, severe chest pain with dyspnea and restlessness.

Collaborative

Administer narcotics, analgesics, and muscle relaxants as needed. Instruct in/monitor use of PCA/epidural administration.

Apply ice packs as indicated.

RATIONALE

Provides information on which to base and monitor effectiveness of interventions.

Reduces muscle spasm and undue tension on new prosthesis and surrounding tissues.

Reduces muscle tension, refocuses attention, promotes sense of control, and may enhance coping abilities in the management of discomfort/pain, which can persist for an extended period.

Reduces muscle tension; improves comfort, and facilitates participation.

Early recognition of developing problems, such as dislocation of prosthesis or pulmonary emboli (blood/fat), provides opportunity for prompt intervention and prevention of more serious complications.

Relieves surgical pain and reduces muscle tension/spasm, which contributes to overall discomfort. Narcotic infusion (including epidural) may be given during first 24–48 hr, with oral analgesics added to pain management program as patient progresses. *Note:* Use of ketorolac (Toradol) or other NSAIDs is contraindicated when patient is receiving enoxaparin (Lovenox) therapy.

Promotes vasoconstriction to reduce bleeding/tissue edema in surgical area and lessens perception of discomfort.

ACTIONS/INTERVENTIONS	RATIONALE
Collaborative	
Initiate/maintain extremity mobilization: e.g., ambulation, physical therapy, exerciser/CPM device.	Increases circulation to affected muscles. Minimizes joint stiffness; relieves muscle spasms related to disuse.

NURSING DIAGNOSIS: Knowledge Deficit [Learning Need] regarding condition, prognosis, treatment, self care, and discharge needs

May be related to
Lack of exposure/recall
Information misinterpretation

Possibly evidenced by
Questions/request for information, statement of misconception
Inaccurate follow-through of instructions/development of preventable complications

DESIRED OUTCOMES/EVALUATION CRITERIA—PATIENT WILL:

> **Knowledge: Disease Process (NOC)**

Verbalize understanding of surgical procedure and prognosis.
Correctly perform necessary procedures and explain reasons for the actions.

ACTIONS/INTERVENTIONS	RATIONALE
Teaching: Disease Process (NIC)	
Independent	
Review disease process, surgical procedure, and future expectations.	Provides knowledge base from which patient can make informed choices.
Encourage alternating rest periods with activity.	Conserves energy for healing and prevents undue fatigue, which can increase risk of injury/fall.
Stress importance of continuing prescribed exercise/rehabilitation program within patient's tolerance: crutch/cane walking, weight-bearing exercises, stationary bicycling, or swimming.	Increases muscle strength and joint mobility. Most patients will be involved in formal rehabilitation/outpatient homecare programs or be followed in extended-care facilities by physical therapists. Muscle aching indicates too much weight bearing or activity, signaling a need to cut back.
Review/instruct in home use of CPM exercise program.	CPM therapy may be continued for some patients after discharge. *Note:* CPM therapy is used in only about 50% of patients at this time.
Review activity limitations, depending on joint replaced, e.g., for hip/knee—sitting for long periods or in low chair/toilet seat/recliner, jogging, jumping, excessive bending, lifting, twisting or crossing legs.	Prevents undue stress on implant. Long-term restrictions depend on individual situation/physician protocol.
Discuss need for safe environment in home (e.g., removing scatter rugs and unnecessary furniture) and use of assistive devices (e.g., handrails in tub/toilet, raised toilet seat, cane for long walks).	Reduces risk of falls and excessive stress on joints.
Review/have patient or caregiver demonstrate incisional/wound care.	Promotes independence in self-care, reducing risk of complications.

ACTIONS/INTERVENTIONS	RATIONALE

Independent

Identify signs/symptoms requiring medical evaluation, e.g., fever/chills, incisional inflammation, unusual wound drainage, pain in calf or upper thigh, or development of "strep" throat/dental infections.

Bacterial infections require prompt treatment to prevent progression to osteomyelitis in the operative area and prosthesis failure, which could occur at any time, even years later.

Review drug regimen, e.g., anticoagulants or antibiotics for invasive procedures (e.g., tooth extraction).

Prophylactic therapy may be necessary for a prolonged period after discharge to limit risk of thromboemboli/infection. Procedures known to cause bacteremia can result in osteomyelitis and prosthesis failure.

Identify bleeding precautions, (e.g., use of soft toothbrush, electric razor, avoidance of trauma/forceful blowing of nose), and necessity of routine laboratory follow-up.

Reduces risk of therapy-induced bleeding/hemorrhage.

Encourage intake of balanced diet, including roughage and adequate fluids.

Enhances healing and feeling of general well-being. Promotes bowel and bladder function during period of altered activity.

POTENTIAL CONSIDERATIONS following acute hospitalization (dependent on patient's age, physical condition/presence of complications, personal resources, and life responsibilities)

In addition to considerations in Surgical Intervention plan of care:

Trauma, risk for—balancing difficulties/altered gait, weakness, lack of safety precautions, hazards associated with use of assistive devices.

Self-Care deficit/Home Maintenance Management, impaired—musculoskeletal impairment, decreased strength/endurance, pain in operative site or other joints.

Sample CP: Total Hip Replacement, Hospital. ELOS: 6 Days Orthopedic or Surgical Unit

ND and Categories of Care	Day 1 Day of Surgery	Day 2 POD 1	Day 3 POD 2	Day 4 POD 3	Day 5 POD 4
Risk for infection R/T broken skin, exposure of joint, long-term steroid use, decreased mobility	Goals: Participate in activities to reduce risk of post-operative infection	Free of purulent drainage → Be afrebile	→ →	→ →	Display early signs of wound healing, free of erythema or drainage
				Verbalize understanding of healthcare needs to enhance healing, promote wellness	Plan in place to meet postdischarge needs, self-care
Diagnostics	Hb/Hct Pulse oximetry	→ D/C if stable	Electrolytes if indicated		
Additional assessments	VS/Temp-per post-operative protocol Breath sounds q8h Amount/characteristics of Hemovac drainage q8h	→ q4h → →	→ q8h → → D/C Characteristics of wound/drainage qd and prn	→ bid unless elevated → bid →	→ →
Medications Allergies:	IV antibiotics IV fluids/blood products Tylenol—Temp ≥ 101°F	→ D/C → →	→ NS lock or D/C →	→ D/C lock → D/C	
Patient education	Disease process/surgical procedure Handwashing technique, avoid touching of dressing/wound Respiratory exercises, incentive spirometry		Dietary needs S/S to report to healthcare provider	Wound care Balancing rest/activity	Provide written instructions for home care
Additional nursing actions	Aseptic/clean technique Protective isolation as indicated Reinforce dressing Encourage PO fluids as tolerated T, C, B, DB, q2h Incentive spirometry q2h Supplemental O₂ as indicated	→ → → → → q2hWA → D/C if stable	→ → D/C → Change dressing qd and prn → Per self → q4hWA High calorie/protein diet	→ → D/C if incision dry → Clean incision bid → →	→ → → →

Sample CP: Total Hip Replacement, Hospital. ELOS: 6 Days Orthopedic or Surgical Unit (Continued)

ND and Categories of Care	Day 1 Day of Surgery	Day 2 POD 1	Day 3 POD 2	Day 4 POD 3	Day 5 POD 4
Impaired physical mobility R/T musculoskeletal impairment/discomfort, therapeutic restrictions	Maintain proper alignment and position of function	→	→	Independent in transfers	Independent in ambulation
	Participate in rehabilitation/exercise program	→	→	Display increased strength/function of operated limb	→ Free of DT/thromboembolic complications Establish regular bladder/bowel elimination
Referrals		PT-assistive devices if not done preop	PT-exercises/ambulation	OT/Rehabilitation specialist Social Services if placement indicated	Home care
Diagnostic studies		PT (coumadin use)	→	→	→ CBC w/platelets (if Lovenox used)
Additional assessments	Neurovascular status/ alignment of operated leg per postoperative protocol	→ q4h	→ q8h	→ bid	→
	Skin (especially heels) q8h or per protocol	→	→	→ qd	→
	Voiding/urinary output q8h	→	→	→ D/C	
	Bowel sounds q8h	→	→ bid	→ qd	→ D/C
		Stool characteristics			
Medications Allergies: _____	Coumadin (if Lovenox not ordered)	Daily order Lovenox q12h	→	→	→
		Stool softener qhs	Laxative if no BM	Suppository/Fleets if no BM	→
Patient education	Hip precautions Use of trapeze Initial exercises—ankle pumps, quad/gluteal sets	Transfer techniques	Use of mobility aids S/S to report to healthcare provider Self-administer Lovenox	Ambulation/weight-bearing exercises Activity level/restrictions postdischarge Sexual concerns	Provide written instructions Home exercise program Coumadin dose, time, purpose, side effects, precautions, monitoring (if used)
Additional nursing actions	Bedrest/HOB elevated 30°	→ Chair/commode elevate operated leg	→ Chair ×3/ambulate with assistance	→ Ambulate ×3 with assistance as needed	→
	Pillow between knees	→	→	→ prn	→
	Turn per protocol q2h	→	→	→	→

Sample CP: Total Hip Replacement, Hospital. ELOS: 6 Days Orthopedic or Surgical Unit (Continued)

ND and Categories of Care	Day 1 Day of Surgery	Day 2 POD 1	Day 3 POD 2	Day 4 POD 3	Day 5 POD 4
	ROM to nonoperated side q2h	→	→ Per self	→	→
	Initial exercises q1hWA	→	→	→	→
			Knee exercise X5 q1hWA	Leg strengthening	→
				D/C if PT 1.3 or above	Shower as indicated
	SCDs to calves	While in bed	Self-care	→	→
	Total care	Assist w/care	→	→	→
	Fracture pan	Elevated toilet seat	→ D/C Foley-male	D/C Foley-female	→ Send home
	Straight catheter if no void q8h prn X2	Insert Foley on #3 if no void			
	Foam/special mattress	→	→	→	→
Pain R/T therapeutic interventions, preexisting chronic joint disease	Verbalize pain within manageable level	→	→	→	→
		Participate in actions to decrease pain	→	→	Verbalize understanding of medications/modalities for pain management; Demonstrates proper use adjunct comfort measures
Additional assessments	Pain characteristics/changes	→	→	→	→
	Response to interventions	→	→	→	→
Medications Allergies:	PCA—narcotic of choice	→ D/C, begin IM/PO	→ D/C IM if tolerated	→	→
	Antiemetic prn	→ D/C	Acetaminophen prn for breakthrough pain	→	→
	Muscle relaxant	→		→	→
Patient education	Orient to unit/room	Relaxation techniques, guided imagery, breathing exercises		Medications: dose, time, route, purpose, side effects	Written instructions for home care needs, equipment resources
	Proper use of PCA				→
	Reporting of pain/effects of interventions	→		→	
Additional nursing actions	Maintain position/alignment of leg per protocol	→	→	→	→
	Ice pack to operated site	→ prn	→ D/C		
	Routine comfort measures prn	→	→	→	→

Integumentary

BURNS: THERMAL/CHEMICAL/ELECTRICAL (ACUTE AND CONVALESCENT PHASES)

Each year, more than 2 million burn injuries occur in the United States; approximately 100,000 people require hospital care. Thermal burns, which are the most common type, occur because of fires, motor vehicle crashes, home fires, hot liquid spills, electrical malfunctions, and war. Survival rates have risen in recent years because of newer treatments and skin barrier development; however, moderate and severe burns account for many dollars spent on physical and psychological rehabilitation.

Thermal burns: Injuring agent can be flame, hot liquid, or contact with hot object. Flame burns are associated with smoke/inhalation injury.

Chemical burns: Occur from type/content of injuring agent, as well as concentration and temperature of agent.

Electrical burns: Occur from type/voltage of current that generates heat in proportion to resistance offered and travels the pathway of least resistance (i.e., nerves offer the least resistance and bones the greatest resistance). Underlying injury is more severe than visible injury.

Superficial partial-thickness (first-degree) burns: Involve only the epidermis. Wounds appear bright pink to red with minimal edema and no blisters. The skin is often warm/dry.

Moderate partial-thickness (second-degree) burns: Involve the epidermis and dermis. Wounds appear red to pink with moderate edema and moist, weeping blisters.

Deep partial-thickness (second-degree) burns: Involve the deep dermis. Wounds appear pink to pale ivory with moderate edema and blisters. These wounds are dryer than the moderate partial-thickness burns.

Full-thickness (third-degree) burns: Involve all layers of skin, subcutaneous fat, and may involve the muscle, nerves, and blood supply. Wound appearance varies from white to cherry red to brown or black, with blistering uncommon. These wounds have a dry, leathery texture.

Full-thickness (fourth-degree) burns: Involve all skin layers plus muscle, organ tissue, and bone. Charring occurs.

CARE SETTING

The following adult patients are admitted for acute care and during the rehabilitation phase may be cared for in a subacute or rehabilitation unit: those with partial-thickness burns greater than 15% total body surface area (TBSA) or whose age is considered high risk (over 65 years of age); full-thickness burns more than 2% of TBSA; burns of face, both hands, perineum, or both feet; or inhalation and all electrical burns.

RELATED CONCERNS

Fluid and electrolyte imbalances, page 926
Metabolic acidosis (primary base bicarbonate deficit), page 523
Psychosocial aspects of care, page 809

Patient Assessment Database

Data depends on type, severity, and body surface area involved.

ACTIVITY/REST

May exhibit: Decreased strength, endurance
Limited ROM of involved areas
Impaired muscle mass, altered tone

CIRCULATION

May exhibit (with burn injury involving more than 20% TBSA):
Hypotension (shock)
Peripheral pulses diminished distal to extremity injury; generalized peripheral vasocon-
striction with loss of pulses, mottling of skin, and coolness (electrical shock)
Tachycardia (shock/anxiety/pain)
Dysrhythmias (electrical shock)
Tissue edema formation (all burns)

EGO INTEGRITY

May report: Feeling scared, self-conscious, conspicuous, angry, embarrassed, different
Concerns about family, job, finances, disfigurement
May exhibit: Anxiety, crying, dependency, denial, withdrawal, hostility, aggressive behavior

ELIMINATION

May exhibit: Urinary output decreased/absent during emergent phase; color may be pink (hemo-
chromogens from damaged red blood cells [RBCs]) or reddish black if myoglobin
present, indicating deep-muscle damage
Diuresis (after capillary leak sealed and fluids mobilized back into circulation)
Bowel sounds decreased/absent, especially in cutaneous burns of greater than 20%, because stress reduces gastric motility/peristalsis

FOOD/FLUID

May exhibit: Generalized tissue edema (swelling is rapid and may be extreme in early hours after injury)
Anorexia, nausea/vomiting

NEUROSENSORY

May report: Mixed areas of numbness, tingling, burning pain
Changes in vision, decreased visual acuity (electrical shock)
May exhibit: Changes in orientation, affect, behavior
Decreased deep tendon reflexes (DTRs), reflexes and sensation in injured extremities
Seizure activity (electrical shock)
Corneal lacerations, retinal damage (electrical shock)
Rupture of tympanic membrane (electrical shock)
Paralysis (electrical injury to nerve pathways)

PAIN/DISCOMFORT

May report: Pain varies, e.g., first-degree burns are extremely sensitive to touch, pressure, air movement, and temperature changes; second-degree moderate-thickness burns are very
painful, whereas pain response in second-degree deep-thickness burns depends on
intactness of nerve endings; third-degree burns are painless

RESPIRATION

May report: Confinement in a closed space, prolonged exposure (possibility of inhalation injury)

May exhibit: Hoarseness, wheezy cough, carbonaceous particles on face/in sputum, drooling/inability to swallow oral secretions, and cyanosis (indicative of inhalation injury)

Thoracic excursion may be limited in presence of circumferential chest burns

Upper airway stridor/wheezes (obstruction due to laryngospasm, laryngeal edema)

Breath sounds: Crackles (pulmonary edema), stridor (laryngeal edema), profuse airway secretions/wheezing (rhonchi)

SAFETY

May exhibit: **Skin:**

General: Exact depth of tissue destruction may not be evident for 3–5 days because of the process of microvascular thrombosis in some wounds; unburned skin areas may be cool/clammy, pale, with slow capillary refill in the presence of decreased cardiac output due to fluid loss/shock state

Flame injury: There may be areas of mixed depth of injury due to varied intensity of heat produced by burning clothing; singed nasal hairs; dry, red mucosa of nose and mouth; blisters on posterior pharynx, circumoral and/or circumnasal edema

Chemical injury: Wound appearance varies according to causative agent; skin may be yellowish brown with soft leatherlike texture; blisters, ulcers, necrosis, or thick eschar. (Injuries are generally deeper than they appear cutaneously, and tissue destruction can continue for up to 72 hr after injury.)

Electrical injury: The external cutaneous injury is usually much less than the underlying necrosis; appearance of wounds varies and may include entry/exit (explosive) wounds of current, arc burns from current moving in close proximity to body, and thermal burns due to ignition of clothing

Other: Presence of fractures/dislocations (concurrent falls, motor vehicle accident; tetanic muscle contractions due to electrical shock)

TEACHING/LEARNING

Discharge plan considerations: **DRG projected mean length of inpatient stay: 18.4–31.4 days (inclusive of rehabilitation)**

May require assistance with treatments, wound care/supplies, self-care activities, homemaker/maintenance tasks, transportation, finances, vocational counseling

Changes in physical layout of home or living facility other than home during prolonged rehabilitation

Refer to section at end of plan for postdischarge considerations.

DIAGNOSTIC STUDIES

Complete blood count (CBC): Initial increased hematocrit (Hct) suggests hemoconcentration due to fluid shift/loss. Later decreased Hct and RBCs may occur because of heat damage to vascular endothelium. Leukocytosis (decreased white blood cells [WBCs]) can occur because of loss of cells at wound site and inflammatory response to injury.

ABGs: Baseline especially important with suspicion of inhalation injury. Reduced PaO_2/increased $PaCO_2$ may be seen with carbon monoxide retention. Acidosis may occur because of reduced renal function and loss of compensatory respiratory mechanisms.

Carboxyhemoglobin (COHb): Elevation of greater than 15% indicates carbon monoxide poisoning/inhalation injury.

Serum electrolytes: Potassium may be initially elevated because of injured tissues/RBC destruction and decreased renal function; hypokalemia can occur when diuresis starts; magnesium may be decreased. Sodium may initially be decreased with body water losses; hypernatremia can occur later as renal conservation occurs.

Alkaline phosphatase: Elevated because of interstitial fluid shifts/impairment of sodium pump.

Serum glucose: Elevation reflects stress response.

Serum albumin: Albumin/globulin ratio may be reversed due to loss of protein in edema fluid.

Blood urea nitrogen (BUN)/Creatinine (Cr): Elevation reflects decreased renal perfusion/function; however, Cr can elevate because of tissue injury.

Urine: Presence of albumin, hemoglobin (Hb), and myoglobin indicates deep-tissue damage and protein loss (especially seen with serious electrical burns). Reddish-black color of urine is due to presence of myoglobin.

Random urine sodium: Greater than 20 mEq/L indicates excessive fluid resuscitation; less than 10 mEq/L suggests inadequate fluid resuscitation.

Wound cultures: May be obtained for baseline data and repeated periodically.

Chest x-ray: May appear normal in early postburn period even with inhalation injury; however, a true inhalation injury presents as infiltrates, often progressing to whiteout on x-ray (adult respiratory distress syndrome [ARDS]).

Fiberoptic bronchoscopy: Useful in diagnosing extent of inhalation injury; findings can include edema, hemorrhage, and/or ulceration of upper respiratory tract.

Flow volume loop: Provides noninvasive assessment of effects/extent of inhalation injury.

Lung scan: May be done to determine extent of inhalation injury.

Electrocardiogram (ECG): Signs of myocardial ischemia/dysrhythmias may occur with electrical burns.

Photographs of burns: Provides documentation of burn-wound and comparative baseline to evaluate healing.

NURSING PRIORITIES

1. Maintain patent airway/respiratory function.
2. Restore hemodynamic stability/circulating volume.
3. Alleviate pain.
4. Prevent complications.
5. Provide emotional support for patient/significant other (SO).
6. Provide information about condition, prognosis, and treatment.

DISCHARGE GOALS

1. Homeostasis achieved.
2. Pain controlled/reduced.
3. Complications prevented/minimized.
4. Dealing with current situation realistically.
5. Condition/prognosis and therapeutic regimen understood.
6. Plan in place to meet needs after discharge.

NURSING DIAGNOSIS: Airway Clearance, risk for ineffective

Risk factors may include

Tracheobronchial obstruction: Mucosal edema and loss of ciliary action (smoke inhalation); circumferential full-thickness burns of the neck, thorax, and chest, with compression of the airway or limited chest excursion

Trauma: Direct upper-airway injury by flame, steam, hot air, and chemicals/gases

Fluid shifts, pulmonary edema, decreased lung compliance

Possibly evidenced by

[Not applicable; presence of signs and symptoms establishes an *actual* diagnosis]

DESIRED OUTCOMES/EVALUATION CRITERIA—PATIENT WILL:

Respiratory Status: Ventilation (NOC)

Demonstrate clear breath sounds, respiratory rate within normal range, be free of dyspnea/cyanosis.

ACTIONS/INTERVENTIONS	RATIONALE

Respiratory Monitoring (NIC)

Independent

Obtain history of injury. Note presence of preexisting respiratory conditions, history of smoking.

Causative burning agent, duration of exposure, and occurrence in closed or open space predict probability of inhalation injury. Type of material burned (wood, plastic, wool, and so forth) suggests type of toxic gas exposure. Preexisting conditions increase the risk of respiratory complications.

Assess gag/swallow reflexes; note drooling, inability to swallow, hoarseness, wheezy cough.

Suggestive of inhalation injury.

Monitor respiratory rate, rhythm, depth; note presence of pallor/cyanosis and carbonaceous or pink-tinged sputum.

Tachypnea, use of accessory muscles, presence of cyanosis, and changes in sputum suggest developing respiratory distress/pulmonary edema and need for medical intervention.

Auscultate lungs, noting stridor, wheezing/crackles, diminished breath sounds, brassy cough.

Airway obstruction/respiratory distress can occur very quickly or may be delayed, e.g., up to 48 hr after burn.

Note presence of pallor or cherry-red color of unburned skin.

Suggests presence of hypoxemia or carbon monoxide.

Investigate changes in behavior/mentation, e.g., restlessness, agitation, confusion.

Although often related to pain, changes in consciousness may reflect developing/worsening hypoxia.

Monitor 24-hr fluid balance, noting variations/changes.

Fluid shifts or excess fluid replacement increases risk of pulmonary edema. *Note:* Inhalation injury increases fluid demands as much as 35% or more because of obligatory edema.

Ventilation Assistance (NIC)

Elevate head of bed. Avoid use of pillow under head, as indicated.

Promotes optimal lung expansion/respiratory function. When head/neck burns are present, a pillow can inhibit respiration, cause necrosis of burned ear cartilage, and promote neck contractures.

Encourage coughing/deep-breathing exercises and frequent position changes.

Promotes lung expansion, mobilization and drainage of secretions.

Suction (if necessary) with extreme care, maintaining sterile technique.

Helps maintain clear airway, but should be done cautiously because of mucosal edema and inflammation. Sterile technique reduces risk of infection.

Promote voice rest but assess ability to speak and/or swallow oral secretions periodically.

Increasing hoarseness/decreased ability to swallow suggests increasing tracheal edema and may indicate need for prompt intubation.

Collaborative

Administer humidified oxygen via appropriate mode, e.g., face mask.

O_2 corrects hypoxemia/acidosis. Humidity decreases drying of respiratory tract and reduces viscosity of sputum.

Monitor/graph serial ABGs or pulse oximetry.

Baseline is essential for further assessment of respiratory status and as a guide to treatment. Pao_2 less than 50, $Paco_2$ greater than 50, and decreasing pH reflect smoke inhalation and developing pneumonia/ARDS.

Review serial chest x-rays.

Changes reflecting atelectasis/pulmonary edema may not occur for 2–3 days after burn.

723

ACTIONS/INTERVENTIONS	RATIONALE

Collaborative

Provide/assist with chest physiotherapy and incentive spirometry.

Chest physiotherapy drains dependent areas of the lung, while incentive spirometry may be done to improve lung expansion, thereby promoting respiratory function and reducing atelectasis.

Prepare for/assist with intubation or tracheostomy, as indicated.

Intubation/mechanical support is required when airway edema or circumferential burn injury interferes with respiratory function/oxygenation.

NURSING DIAGNOSIS: Fluid Volume, risk for deficit

Risk factors may include
Loss of fluid through abnormal routes, e.g., burn wounds
Increased need: hypermetabolic state, insufficient intake
Hemorrhagic losses

Possibly evidenced by
[Not applicable; presence of signs and symptoms establishes an *actual* diagnosis]

DESIRED OUTCOMES/EVALUATION CRITERIA—PATIENT WILL:

Hydration (NOC)

Demonstrate improved fluid balance as evidenced by individually adequate urinary output with normal specific gravity, stable vital signs, moist mucous membranes.

ACTIONS/INTERVENTIONS	RATIONALE

Shock Prevention (NIC)

Independent

Monitor vital signs, central venous pressure (CVP). Note capillary refill and strength of peripheral pulses.

Serves as a guide to fluid replacement needs and assesses cardiovascular response. *Note:* Invasive monitoring is indicated for patients with major burns, smoke inhalation, or preexisting cardiac disease, although there is an associated increased risk of infection, necessitating careful monitoring and care of insertion site.

Monitor urinary output and specific gravity. Observe urine color and hematest as indicated.

Generally, fluid replacement should be titrated to ensure average urinary output of 30–50 mL/hr (in the adult). Urine can appear red to black (with massive muscle destruction) because of presence of blood and release of myoglobin. If gross myoglobinuria is present, minimum urinary output should be 75–100 mL/hr to reduce risk of tubular damage and renal failure.

Estimate wound drainage and insensible losses.

Increased capillary permeability, protein shifts, inflammatory process, and evaporative losses greatly affect circulating volume and urinary output, especially during initial 24–72 hr after burn.

Maintain cumulative record of amount and types of fluid intake.

Massive/rapid replacement with different types of fluids and fluctuations in rate of administration require close tabulation to prevent constituent imbalances or fluid overload.

ACTIONS/INTERVENTIONS	RATIONALE

Independent

Weigh daily.

Fluid replacement formulas partly depend on admission weight and subsequent changes. A 15%–20% weight gain can be anticipated in the first 72 hr during fluid replacement, with return to preburn weight approximately 10 days after burn.

Measure circumference of burned extremities as indicated.

May be helpful in estimating extent of edema/fluid shifts affecting circulating volume and urinary output.

Investigate changes in mentation.

Deterioration in the level of consciousness may indicate inadequate circulating volume/reduced cerebral perfusion.

Observe for gastric distension, hematemesis, tarry stools. Hematest NG drainage and stools periodically.

Stress (Curling's) ulcer occurs in up to half of all severely burned patients and can occur as early as first week. Patients with burns greater than 20% TBSA are at risk for mucosal bleeding in the gastrointestinal (GI) tract during the acute phase because of decreased splanchnic blood flow and reflex paralytic ileus.

Collaborative

Insert/maintain indwelling urinary catheter.

Allows for close observation of renal function and prevents urinary retention. Retention of urine with its by-products of tissue-cell destruction can lead to renal dysfunction and infection.

Insert/maintain large-bore IV catheter(s).

Accommodates rapid infusion of fluids.

Administer calculated IV replacement of fluids, electrolytes, plasma, albumin.

Fluid resuscitation replaces lost fluids/electrolytes and helps prevent complications, e.g., shock, acute tubular necrosis (ATN). Replacement formulas vary (e.g., Brooke, Evans, Parkland) but are based on extent of injury, amount of urinary output, and weight. *Note:* Once initial fluid resuscitation has been accomplished, a steady rate of fluid administration is preferred to "boluses," which may increase interstitial fluid shifts and cardiopulmonary congestion.

Monitor laboratory studies (e.g., Hb/Hct, electrolytes, random urine sodium).

Identifies blood loss/RBC destruction, and fluid and electrolyte replacement needs. Urine sodium less than 10 mEq/L suggests inadequate fluid resuscitation. *Note:* During first 24 hr postburn, hemoconcentration is common because of fluid shifts into the interstitial space.

Administer medications as indicated:

Diuretics, e.g., mannitol (Osmitrol);

May be indicated to enhance urinary output and clear tubules of debris/prevent necrosis, if acute renal failure (ARF) is present.

Potassium;

Although hyperkalemia often occurs during first 24–48 hr (tissue destruction), subsequent replacement may be necessary because of large urinary losses.

Antacids, e.g., calcium carbonate (Titrilac), magaldrate (Riopan); histamine inhibitors, e.g., cimetidine (Tagamet)/ranitidine (Zantac).

Antacids may reduce gastric acidity, while histamine inhibitors decrease production of hydrochloric acid to reduce risk of gastric irritation/bleeding.

Add electrolytes to water used for wound debridement, as indicated.

Washing solution that approximates tissue fluids may minimize osmotic fluid shifts.

NURSING DIAGNOSIS: Infection, risk for

Risk factors may include

Inadequate primary defenses: Destruction of skin barrier, traumatized tissues

Inadequate secondary defenses: Decreased Hb, suppressed inflammatory response

Environmental exposure, invasive procedures

Possibly evidenced by

[Not applicable; presence of signs and symptoms establishes an *actual* diagnosis]

DESIRED OUTCOMES/EVALUATION CRITERIA—PATIENT WILL:

Wound Healing—Secondary Intention (NOC)

Achieve timely wound healing free of purulent exudate and be afebrile.

ACTIONS/INTERVENTIONS	RATIONALE

Infection Protection (NIC)

Independent

Implement appropriate isolation techniques as indicated.	Dependent on type/extent of wounds and the choice of wound treatment (e.g., open versus closed), isolation may range from simple wound/skin to complete or reverse to reduce risk of cross-contamination and exposure to multiple bacterial flora.
Emphasize/model good handwashing technique for all individuals coming in contact with patient.	Prevents cross-contamination; reduces risk of acquired infection.
Use gowns, gloves, masks, and strict aseptic technique during direct wound care and provide sterile or freshly laundered bed linens/gowns.	Prevents exposure to infectious organisms.
Monitor/limit visitors, if necessary. If isolation is used, explain procedure to visitors. Supervise visitor adherence to protocol as indicated.	Prevents cross-contamination from visitors. Concern for risk of infection should be balanced against patient's need for family support and socialization.

Wound Care (NIC)

Shave/clip all hair from around burned areas to include a 1-in border (excluding eyebrows). Shave facial hair (men) and shampoo head daily.	Hair is a good medium for bacterial growth; however, eyebrows act as a protective barrier for the eyes. Regular shampooing decreases bacterial fallout into burned areas.
Examine unburned areas (such as groin, neck creases, mucous membranes) and vaginal discharge routinely.	Opportunistic infections (e.g., yeast) frequently occur because of depression of the immune system and/or proliferation of normal body flora during systemic antibiotic therapy.
Provide special care for eyes, e.g., use eye covers and tear formulas as appropriate.	Eyes may be swollen shut and/or become infected by drainage from surrounding burns. If lids are burned, eye covers may be needed to prevent corneal damage.
Prevent skin-to-skin surface contact (e.g., wrap each burned finger/toe separately; do not allow burned ear to touch scalp).	Prevents adherence to surface it may be touching and encourages proper healing. *Note:* Ear cartilage has limited circulation and is prone to pressure necrosis.

ACTIONS/INTERVENTIONS	RATIONALE

Independent

Examine wounds daily, note/document changes in appearance, odor, or quantity of drainage.

Identifies presence of healing (granulation tissue) and provides for early detection of burn-wound infection. Infection in a partial-thickness burn may cause conversion of burn to full-thickness injury. *Note:* A strong sweet, musty smell at a graft site is indicative of *Pseudomonas.*

Monitor vital signs for fever, increased respiratory rate/depth in association with changes in sensorium, presence of diarrhea, decreased platelet count, and hyperglycemia with glycosuria.

Indicators of sepsis (often occurs with full-thickness burn) requiring prompt evaluation and intervention. *Note:* Changes in sensorium, bowel habits, and respiratory rate usually precede fever and alteration of laboratory studies.

Collaborative

Remove dressings and cleanse burned areas in a hydrotherapy/whirlpool tub or in a shower stall with handheld shower head. Maintain temperature of water at 100°F (37.8°C). Wash areas with a mild cleansing agent or surgical soap.

Water softens and aids in removal of dressings and eschar (slough layer of dead skin or tissue). Sources vary as to whether bath or shower is best. Bath has advantage of water providing support for exercising extremities but may promote cross-contamination of wounds. Showering enhances wound inspection and prevents contamination from floating debris.

Excise and cover burn wounds quickly.

Early excision is known to reduce scarring and risk of infection, thereby facilitating healing.

Debride necrotic/loose tissue (including ruptured blisters) with scissors and forceps. Do not disturb intact blisters if they are smaller than 1–2 cm, do not interfere with joint function, and do not appear infected.

Promotes healing. Prevents autocontamination. Small, intact blisters help protect skin and increase rate of re-epithelialization unless the burn injury is the result of chemicals (in which case fluid contained in blisters may continue to cause tissue destruction).

Photograph wound initially and at periodic intervals.

Provides baseline and documentation of healing process.

Administer topical agents as indicated, e.g.:

The following agents help control bacterial growth and prevent drying of wound, which can cause further tissue destruction.

    Silver sulfadiazine (Silvadene);

Broad-spectrum antimicrobial that is relatively painless but has intermediate, somewhat delayed eschar penetration. May cause rash or depression of WBCs.

    Mafenide acetate (Sulfamylon);

Antibiotic of choice with confirmed invasive burn-wound infection. Useful against Gram-negative/Gram-positive organisms. Causes burning/pain on application and for 30 minutes thereafter. Can cause rash, metabolic acidosis, and decreased $PaCO_2$.

    Silver nitrate;

Effective against *Staphylococcus aureus, Escherichia coli,* and *Pseudomonas aeruginosa,* but has poor eschar penetration, is painful, and may cause electrolyte imbalance. Dressings must be constantly saturated. Product stains skin/surfaces black.

    Bacitracin;

Effective against Gram-positive organisms and is generally used for superficial and facial burns.

ACTIONS/INTERVENTIONS	RATIONALE
Collaborative	
Povidone-iodine (Betadine);	Broad-spectrum antimicrobial but is painful on application, may cause metabolic acidosis/increased iodine absorption, and damage fragile tissues.
Hydrogels, e.g., Transorb, Burnfree.	Useful for partial- and full-thickness burns; filling dead spaces, rehydrating dry wound beds, and promoting autolytic debridement. May be used when infection is present.
Administer other medications as appropriate, e.g.;	
Subeschar clysis/systemic antibiotics;	Systemic antibiotics are given to control general infections identified by culture/sensitivity. Subeschar clysis has been found effective against pathogens in granulated tissues at the line of demarcation between viable/nonviable tissue, reducing risk of sepsis.
Tetanus toxoid or clostridial antitoxin, as appropriate.	Tissue destruction/altered defense mechanisms increase risk of developing tetanus or gas gangrene, especially in deep burns such as those caused by electricity.

Infection Prevention (NIC)

Place IV/invasive lines in nonburned area.	Decreased risk of infection at insertion site with possibility of progression to septicemia.
Obtain routine cultures and sensitivities of wounds/drainage.	Allows early recognition and specific treatment of wound infection.
Assist with excisional biopsies when infection is suspected.	Bacteria can colonize the wound surface without invading the underlying tissue; therefore, biopsies may be obtained for diagnosing infection.

NURSING DIAGNOSIS: Pain [acute]

May be related to
Destruction of skin/tissues; edema formation
Manipulation of injured tissues, e.g., wound debridement

Possibly evidenced by
Reports of pain
Narrowed focus, facial mask of pain
Alteration in muscle tone; autonomic responses
Distraction/guarding behaviors; anxiety/fear, restlessness

DESIRED OUTCOMES/EVALUATION CRITERIA—PATIENT WILL:

Pain Level (NOC)

Report pain reduced/controlled.
Display relaxed facial expressions/body posture.

Pain Control Behavior (NOC)

Participate in activities and sleep/rest appropriately.

ACTIONS/INTERVENTIONS	RATIONALE

Pain Management (NIC)

Independent

Cover wounds as soon as possible unless open-air exposure burn care method required.	Temperature changes and air movement can cause great pain to exposed nerve endings.
Elevate burned extremities periodically.	Elevation may be required initially to reduce edema formation; thereafter, changes in position and elevation reduce discomfort and risk of joint contractures.
Provide bed cradle as indicated.	Elevation of linens off wounds may help reduce pain.
Wrap digits/extremities in position of function (avoiding flexed position of affected joints) using splints and footboards as necessary.	Position of function reduces deformities/contractures and promotes comfort. Although flexed position of injured joints may feel more comfortable, it can lead to flexion contractures.
Change position frequently and assist with active and passive range of motion (ROM) as indicated.	Movement and exercise reduce joint stiffness and muscle fatigue, but type of exercise depends on location and extent of injury.
Maintain comfortable environmental temperature, provide heat lamps, heat-retaining body coverings.	Temperature regulation may be lost with major burns. External heat sources may be necessary to prevent chilling.
Assess reports of pain, noting location/character and intensity (0–10 scale).	Pain is nearly always present to some degree because of varying severity of tissue involvement/destruction but is usually most severe during dressing changes and debridement. Changes in location, character, intensity of pain may indicate developing complications (e.g., limb ischemia) or herald improvement/return of nerve function/sensation.
Provide medication and/or place in hydrotherapy (as appropriate) before performing dressing changes and debridement.	Reduces severe physical and emotional distress associated with dressing changes and debridement.
Encourage expression of feelings about pain.	Verbalization allows outlet for emotions and may enhance coping mechanisms.
Involve patient in determining schedule for activities, treatments, drug administration.	Enhances patient's sense of control and strengthens coping mechanisms.
Explain procedures/provide frequent information as appropriate, especially during wound debridement.	Empathic support can help alleviate pain/promote relaxation. Knowing what to expect provides opportunity for patient to prepare self and enhances sense of control.
Provide basic comfort measures, e.g., massage of uninjured areas, frequent position changes.	Promotes relaxation; reduces muscle tension and general fatigue.
Encourage use of stress management techniques, e.g., progressive relaxation, deep breathing, guided imagery, and visualization.	Refocuses attention, promotes relaxation, and enhances sense of control, which may reduce pharmacological dependency.
Provide diversional activities appropriate for age/condition.	Helps lessen concentration on pain experience and refocus attention.
Promote uninterrupted sleep periods.	Sleep deprivation can increase perception of pain/reduce coping abilities.

ACTIONS/INTERVENTIONS

Collaborative

Administer analgesics (narcotic and nonnarcotic) as indicated, e.g., morphine; fentanyl (Sublimaze, Ultiva); hydrocodone (Vicodin, Hycodan); oxycodone (Oxy-Contin, Percocet).

Provide/instruct in use of patient-controlled analgesia (PCA).

RATIONALE

The burned patient may require around-the-clock medication and dose titration. IV method is often used initially to maximize drug effect. Concerns of patient addiction or doubts regarding degree of pain experienced are not valid during emergent/acute phase of care, but narcotics should be decreased as soon as feasible and alternate methods for pain relief initiated.

PCA provides for timely drug administration, preventing fluctuations in intensity of pain, often at lower total dosage than would be given by conventional methods.

NURSING DIAGNOSIS: Tissue Perfusion, altered/Peripheral Neurovascular, risk for dysfunction

Risk factors may include
Reduction/interruption of arterial/venous blood flow, e.g., circumferential burns of extremities with resultant edema
Hypovolemia

Possibly evidenced by
[Not applicable; presence of signs and symptoms establishes an *actual* diagnosis]

DESIRED OUTCOMES/EVALUATION CRITERIA—PATIENT WILL:

Tissue Perfusion: Peripheral (NOC)

Maintain palpable peripheral pulses of equal quality/strength; good capillary refill and skin color normal in uninjured areas.

ACTIONS/INTERVENTIONS

Circulatory Care (NIC)

Independent

Assess color, sensation, movement, peripheral pulses (via Doppler), and capillary refill on extremities with circumferential burns. Compare with findings of unaffected limb.

Elevate affected extremities, as appropriate. Remove jewelry/arm band. Avoid taping around a burned extremity/digit.

Obtain BP in unburned extremity when possible. Remove BP cuff after each reading, as indicated.

Investigate reports of deep/throbbing ache, numbness.

RATIONALE

Edema formation can readily compress blood vessels, thereby impeding circulation and increasing venous stasis/edema. Comparisons with unaffected limbs aid in differentiating localized versus systemic problems (e.g., hypovolemia/decreased cardiac output).

Promotes systemic circulation/venous return and may reduce edema or other deleterious effects of constriction of edematous tissues. Prolonged elevation can impair arterial perfusion if blood pressure (BP) falls or tissue pressures rise excessively.

If BP readings must be obtained on an injured extremity, leaving the cuff in place may increase edema formation/reduce perfusion, and convert partial-thickness burn to a more serious injury.

Indicators of decreased perfusion and/or increased pressure within enclosed space, such as may occur with a circumferential burn of an extremity (compartment syndrome).

ACTIONS/INTERVENTIONS	RATIONALE
Independent	
Encourage active ROM exercises of unaffected body parts.	Promotes local and systemic circulation.
Investigate irregular pulses.	Cardiac dysrhythmias can occur as a result of electrolyte shifts, electrical injury, or release of myocardial depressant factor, compromising cardiac output/tissue perfusion.
Collaborative	
Maintain fluid replacement per protocol. (Refer to ND: Fluid Volume, risk for deficit, p. 724.)	Maximizes circulating volume and tissue perfusion.
Monitor electrolytes, especially sodium, potassium, and calcium. Administer replacement therapy as indicated.	Losses/shifts of these electrolytes affect cellular membrane potential/excitability, thereby altering myocardial conductivity, potentiating risk of dysrhythmias, and reducing cardiac output and tissue perfusion.
Avoid use of IM/SC injections.	Altered tissue perfusion and edema formation impair drug absorption. Injections into potential donor sites may render them unusable because of hematoma formation.
Measure intracompartmental pressures as indicated. (Refer to CP: Fractures; ND: Peripheral Neurovascular, risk for dysfunction, p. 685.)	Ischemic myositis may develop because of decreased perfusion.
Assist with/prepare for escharotomy/fasciotomy, as indicated.	Enhances circulation by relieving constriction caused by rigid, nonviable tissue (eschar) or edema formation.

NURSING DIAGNOSIS: Nutrition: altered, less than body requirements

May be related to
Hypermetabolic state (can be as much as 50%–60% greater than normal proportional to the severity of injury)
Protein catabolism
Anorexia, restricted oral intake

Possibly evidenced by
Decrease in total body weight, loss of muscle mass/subcutaneous fat, and development of negative nitrogen balance

DESIRED OUTCOMES/EVALUATION CRITERIA—PATIENT WILL:

Nutritional Status (NOC)

Demonstrate nutritional intake adequate to meet metabolic needs as evidenced by stable weight/muscle-mass measurements, positive nitrogen balance, and tissue regeneration.

ACTIONS/INTERVENTIONS	RATIONALE
Nutrition Therapy (NIC)	
Independent	
Auscultate bowel sounds, noting hypoactive/absent sounds.	Ileus is often associated with postburn period but usually subsides within 36–48 hr, at which time oral feedings can be initiated.

ACTIONS/INTERVENTIONS	RATIONALE
Independent	
Maintain strict calorie count. Weigh daily. Reassess percent of open body surface area/wounds weekly.	Appropriate guides to proper caloric intake include 25 kcal/kg body weight, plus 40 kcal per percentage of TBSA burn in the adult. As burn wound heals, percentage of burned areas is re-evaluated to calculate prescribed dietary formulas, and appropriate adjustments are made.
Monitor muscle mass/subcutaneous fat as indicated.	Indirect calorimetry, if available, may be useful in more accurately estimating body reserves/losses and effectiveness of therapy.
Provide small, frequent meals and snacks.	Helps prevent gastric distension/discomfort and may enhance intake.
Encourage patient to view diet as a treatment and to make food/beverage choices high in calories/protein.	Calories and proteins are needed to maintain weight, meet metabolic needs, and promote wound healing.
Ascertain food likes/dislikes. Encourage SO to bring food from home, as appropriate.	Provides patient/SO sense of control; enhances participation in care and may improve intake.
Encourage patient to sit up for meals and visit with others.	Sitting helps prevent aspiration and aids in proper digestion of food. Socialization promotes relaxation and may enhance intake.
Provide oral hygiene before meals.	Clean mouth/clear palate enhances taste and helps promote a good appetite.
Perform fingerstick glucose, urine testing as indicated.	Monitors for development of hyperglycemia related to hormonal changes/demands or use of hyperalimentation to meet caloric needs.
Collaborative	
Refer to dietitian/nutritional support team.	Useful in establishing individual nutritional needs (based on weight and body surface area of injury) and identifying appropriate routes.
Provide diet high in calories/protein with trace elements and vitamin supplements.	Calories (3000–5000/day), proteins, and vitamins are needed to meet increased metabolic needs, maintain weight, and encourage tissue regeneration. *Note:* Oral route is preferable once GI function returns.
Insert/maintain small feeding tube for enteral feedings and supplements if needed.	Provides continuous/supplemental feedings when patient is unable to consume total daily calorie requirements orally. *Note:* Continuous tube feeding during the night increases calorie intake without decreasing appetite and oral intake during the day.
Administer parenteral nutritional solutions containing vitamins and minerals, as indicated.	Total parenteral nutrition (TPN) maintains nutritional intake/meets metabolic needs in presence of severe complications or sustained esophageal/gastric injuries that do not permit enteral feedings.
Monitor laboratory studies, e.g., serum albumin/prealbumin, Cr, transferrin; urine urea nitrogen.	Indicators of nutritional needs and adequacy of diet/therapy.
Administer insulin as indicated.	Elevated serum glucose levels may develop because of stress response to injury, high caloric intake, pancreatic fatigue.

NURSING DIAGNOSIS: Mobility, impaired physical

May be related to

Neuromuscular impairment, pain/discomfort, decreased strength and endurance

Restrictive therapies, limb immobilization; contractures

Possibly evidenced by

Reluctance to move/inability to purposefully move

Limited ROM, decreased muscle strength control and/or mass

DESIRED OUTCOMES/EVALUATION CRITERIA—PATIENT WILL:

Mobility Level (NOC)

Maintain position of function as evidenced by absence of contractures.

Maintain or increase strength and function of affected and/or compensatory body part.

Self-Care: Activities of Daily Living (ADLs) (NOC)

Verbalize and demonstrate willingness to participate in activities.

Demonstrate techniques/behaviors that enable resumption of activities.

ACTIONS/INTERVENTIONS	RATIONALE
Bed Rest Care (NIC)	
Independent	
Maintain proper body alignment with supports or splints, especially for burns over joints.	Promotes functional positioning of extremities and prevents contractures, which are more likely over joints.
Note circulation, motion, and sensation of digits frequently.	Edema may compromise circulation to extremities, potentiating tissue necrosis/development of contractures.
Initiate the rehabilitative phase on admission.	It is easier to enlist participation when the patient is aware of the possibilities that exist for recovery.
Perform ROM exercises consistently, initially passive, then active.	Prevents progressively tightening scar tissue and contractures; enhances maintenance of muscle/joint functioning and reduces loss of calcium from the bone.
Medicate for pain before activity/exercises.	Reduces muscle/tissue stiffness and tension, enabling patient to be more active and facilitating participation.
Schedule treatments and care activities to provide periods of uninterrupted rest.	Increases patient's strength and tolerance for activity.
Encourage family/SO support and assistance with ROM exercises.	Enables family/SO to be active in patient care and provides more constant/consistent therapy.
Incorporate ADLs with physical therapy, hydrotherapy, and nursing care.	Combining activities produces improved results by enhancing effects of each.
Encourage patient participation in all activities as individually able.	Promotes independence, enhances self-esteem, and facilitates recovery process.
Instruct and assist with mobility aids, e.g., cane, walker, crutches as appropriate.	Promotes safe ambulation.
Collaborative	
Provide foam, water/air mattress or kinetic therapy bed, as indicated.	Prevents prolonged pressure on tissues, reducing potential for tissue ischemia/necrosis and decubitus formation.

ACTIONS/INTERVENTIONS	RATIONALE
Collaborative	
Maintain pressure garment when used.	Hypertrophic scarring can develop around grafted areas or at the site of deep partial-thickness wounds. Pressure dressings minimize scar tissue by keeping it flat, soft, and pliable, enhancing movement.
Consult with rehabilitation, physical, and occupational therapists.	Normally members of the burn team, these specialists provide integrated activity/exercise program and specific assistive devices based on individual needs. Consultation facilitates intensive long-term management of potential deficits.

NURSING DIAGNOSIS: Skin Integrity, impaired [grafts]

May be related to
Disruption of skin surface with destruction of skin layers (partial-/full-thickness burn) requiring grafting

Possibly evidenced by
Absence of viable tissue

DESIRED OUTCOMES/EVALUATION CRITERIA—PATIENT WILL:

Wound Healing: Secondary Intention (NOC)

Demonstrate tissue regeneration.
Achieve timely healing of burned areas.

ACTIONS/INTERVENTIONS	RATIONALE
Wound Care (NIC)	
Independent	
Preoperative	
Assess/document size, color, depth of wound, noting necrotic tissue and condition of surrounding skin.	Provides baseline information about need for skin grafting and possible clues about circulation in area to support graft.
Provide appropriate burn care and infection control measures. (Refer to ND: Infection, risk for, p. 726.)	Prepares tissues for grafting and reduces risk of infection/graft failure.
Postoperative	
Maintain wound covering as indicated, e.g.:	
Biosynthetic dressing (Biobrane);	Nylon fabric/silicon membrane containing collagenous porcine peptides that adheres to wound surface until removed or sloughed off by spontaneous skin re-epithelialization. Useful for eschar-free partial-thickness burns awaiting autografts because it can remain in place 2–3 wk or longer and is permeable to topical antimicrobial agents.
Synthetic dressings, e.g., DuoDerm;	Hydroactive dressing that adheres to the skin to cover small partial-thickness burns and interacts with wound exudate to form a soft gel that facilitates debridement.

ACTIONS/INTERVENTIONS

Independent

Op-Site, ACU-Derm.

Elevate grafted area if possible/appropriate. Maintain desired position and immobility of area when indicated.

Maintain dressings over newly grafted area and/or donor site as indicated, e.g., mesh, petroleum, non-adhesive.

Keep skin free from pressure.

Evaluate color of grafted and donor site(s); note presence/absence of healing.

Wash sites with mild soap, rinse, and lubricate with cream (e.g., Nivea) several times daily, after dressings are removed and healing is accomplished.

Aspirate blebs under sheet grafts with sterile needle or roll with sterile swab.

Collaborative

Prepare for/assist with surgical grafting or biological dressings, e.g.:

Homograft (allograft);

Heterograft (xenograft, porcine);

Cultured epithelial autograft (CEA);

Artificial skin (INTEGRA).

RATIONALE

Thin, transparent, elastic, waterproof, occlusive dressing (permeable to moisture and air) that is used to cover clean partial-thickness wounds and clean donor sites.

Reduces swelling/limits risk of graft separation. Movement of tissue under graft can dislodge it, interfering with optimal healing.

Areas may be covered by translucent, nonreactive surface material (between graft and outer dressing) to eliminate shearing of new epithelium/protect healing tissue. The donor site is usually covered for 4–24 hr, then bulky dressings are removed and fine mesh gauze is left in place.

Promotes circulation and prevents ischemia/necrosis and graft failure.

Evaluates effectiveness of circulation and identifies developing complications.

Newly grafted skin and healed donor sites require special care to maintain flexibility.

Fluid-filled blebs prevent graft adherence to underlying tissue, increasing risk of graft failure.

Skin grafts obtained from living persons or cadavers are used as a temporary covering for extensive burns until person's own skin is ready for grafting (test graft), to cover excised wounds immediately after escharotomy, or to protect granulation tissue.

Skin grafts may be carried out with animal skin for the same purposes as homografts or to cover meshed autografts.

Skin graft obtained from uninjured part of patient's own skin and prepared in a laboratory; may be full-thickness or partial-thickness. *Note:* This process takes 20 to 30 days from harvest to application. The new CEA sheets are 1–6 cell layers thick, and thus are very fragile.

This wound covering was approved by the Food and Drug Administration (FDA) in 1996 for full-thickness and deep partial-thickness burns. It provides a permanent, immediate covering that reproduces the skin's normal functions and stimulates the regeneration of dermal tissue.

ACTIONS/INTERVENTIONS	RATIONALE
Anxiety Reduction (NIC)	
Independent	
Provide frequent explanations and information about care procedures. Repeat information as needed/desired.	Knowing what to expect usually reduces fear and anxiety, clarifies misconceptions, and promotes cooperation. *Note:* Because of the shock of the initial trauma, many people do not recall information provided during that time.
Demonstrate willingness to listen and talk to patient when free of painful procedures.	Helps patient/SO know that support is available and that healthcare provider is interested in the person, not just care of the burn.
Involve patient/SO in decision-making process whenever possible. Provide time for questioning and repetition of proposed treatments.	Promotes sense of control and cooperation, decreasing feelings of helplessness/hopelessness.
Assess mental status, including mood/affect, comprehension of events, and content of thoughts, e.g., illusions or manifestations of terror/panic.	Initially, the patient may use denial and repression to reduce and filter information that might be overwhelming. Some patients display calm manner and alert mental status, representing a dissociation from reality, which is also a protective mechanism.
Investigate changes in mentation and presence of hypervigilance, hallucinations, sleep disturbances (e.g., nightmares), agitation/apathy, disorientation, and labile affect, all of which may vary from moment to moment.	Indicators of extreme anxiety/delirium state in which the patient is literally fighting for life. Although cause can be psychologically based, pathological life-threatening causes (e.g., shock, sepsis, hypoxia) must be ruled out.
Provide constant and consistent orientation.	Helps the patient stay in touch with surroundings and reality.
Encourage the patient to talk about the burn circumstances when ready.	Patient may need to tell the story of what happened over and over to make some sense out of a terrifying situation. Adjustment to the impact of the trauma, grief over losses and disfigurement can easily lead to clinical depression, psychosis, and posttraumatic stress disorder (PTSD).

ACTIONS/INTERVENTIONS

Independent

ACTIONS/INTERVENTIONS	RATIONALE
Explain to patient what happened. Provide opportunity for questions and give open/honest answers.	Compassionate statements reflecting the reality of the situation can help the patient/SO acknowledge that reality and begin to deal with what has happened.
Identify previous methods of coping/handling of stressful situations.	Past successful behavior can be used to assist in dealing with the present situation.
Create a restful environment, use guided imagery and relaxation exercises.	Patients experience severe anxiety associated with burn trauma and treatment. These interventions are soothing and helpful for positive outcomes.
Assist the family to express their feelings of grief and guilt.	The family may initially be most concerned about the patient's dying and/or feel guilty, believing that in some way they could have prevented the incident.
Be empathetic and nonjudgmental in dealing with the patient and family.	Family relationships are disrupted; financial, lifestyle/role changes make this a difficult time for those involved with the patient, and they may react in many different ways.
Encourage family/SO to visit and discuss family happenings. Remind patient of past and future events.	Maintains contact with a familiar reality, creating a sense of attachment and continuity of life.

Collaborative

Involve entire burn team in care from admission to discharge, including social worker and psychiatric resources.	Provides a wider support system and promotes continuity of care and coordination of activities.
Administer mild sedation as indicated, lorazepam (Ativan), alprazolam (Xanax), midazolam (Versed).	Antianxiety medications may be necessary for a brief period until patient is more physically stable and internal locus of control is regained.

NURSING DIAGNOSIS: Body Image disturbance/Role Performance, altered

May be related to
Situational crisis: traumatic event, dependent patient role; disfigurement, pain

Possibly evidenced by
Negative feelings about body/self, fear of rejection/reaction by others
Focus on past appearance, abilities; preoccupation with change/loss
Change in physical capacity to resume role; change in social involvement

DESIRED OUTCOMES/EVALUATION CRITERIA—PATIENT WILL:

Body Image (NOC)

Incorporate changes into self-concept without negating self-esteem.
Verbalize acceptance of self in situation.

Role Performance (NOC)

Talk with family/SO about situation, changes that have occurred.
Develop realistic goals/plans for the future.

ACTIONS/INTERVENTIONS	RATIONALE

Body Image or Role Enhancement (NIC)

Independent

Assess meaning of loss/change to patient/SO, including future expectations and impact of cultural/religious beliefs.

Traumatic episode results in sudden, unanticipated changes, creating feelings of grief over actual/perceived losses. This necessitates support to work through to optimal resolution.

Acknowledge and accept expression of feelings of frustration, dependency, anger, grief, and hostility. Note withdrawn behavior and use of denial.

Acceptance of these feelings as a normal response to what has occurred facilitates resolution. It is not helpful or possible to push patient before ready to deal with situation. Denial may be prolonged and be an adaptive mechanism because patient is not ready to cope with personal problems.

Set limits on maladaptive behavior (e.g., manipulative/aggressive). Maintain nonjudgmental attitude while giving care and help patient identify positive behaviors that will aid in recovery.

Patient and SO tend to deal with this crisis in the same way in which they have dealt with problems in the past. Staff may find it difficult and frustrating to handle behavior that is disrupting/not helpful to recuperation but should realize that the behavior is usually directed toward the situation and not the caregiver.

Be realistic and positive during treatments, in health teaching, and in setting goals within limitations.

Enhances trust and rapport between patient and nurse.

Encourage patient/SO to view wounds and assist with care as appropriate.

Promotes acceptance of reality of injury and of change in body and image of self as different.

Provide hope within parameters of individual situation; do not give false reassurance.

Promotes positive attitude and provides opportunity to set goals and plan for future based on reality.

Assist patient to identify extent of actual change in appearance/body function.

Helps begin process of looking to the future and how life will be different.

Give positive reinforcement of progress and encourage endeavors toward attainment of rehabilitation goals.

Words of encouragement can support development of positive coping behaviors.

Show slides or pictures of burn care/other patient outcomes, being selective in what is shown as appropriate to the individual situation. Encourage discussion of feelings about what patient has seen.

Allows patient/SO to be realistic in expectations. Also assists in demonstration of importance of/necessity for certain devices and procedures.

Encourage family interaction with each other and with rehabilitation team.

Maintains/opens lines of communication and provides ongoing support for patient and family.

Provide support group for SO. Give information about how SO can be helpful to the patient.

Promotes ventilation of feelings and allows for more helpful responses to the patient.

Role play social situations of concern to patient.

Prepares patient/SO for reactions of others and anticipates ways to deal with them.

Collaborative

Refer to physical/occupational therapy, vocational counselor, and psychiatric counseling, e.g., clinical specialist psychiatric nurse, social services, psychologist as needed.

Helpful in identifying ways/devices to regain and maintain independence. Patient may need further assistance to resolve persistent emotional problems (e.g., posttrauma response).

NURSING DIAGNOSIS: Knowledge Deficit [Learning Need] regarding condition, prognosis, treatment, self care, and discharge needs

May be related to

Lack of exposure/recall

Information misinterpretation; unfamiliarity with resources

Possibly evidenced by

Questions/request for information, statement of misconception

Inaccurate follow-through of instructions/development of preventable complications

DESIRED OUTCOMES/EVALUATION CRITERIA—PATIENT WILL:

Knowledge: Disease Process (NOC)

Verbalize understanding of condition, prognosis, and potential complications.

Knowledge: Treatment Regimen (NOC)

Verbalize understanding of therapeutic needs.

Correctly perform necessary procedures and explain reasons for actions.

Initiate necessary lifestyle changes and participate in treatment regimen.

ACTIONS/INTERVENTIONS	RATIONALE
Teaching: Disease Process (NIC)	
Independent	
Review condition, prognosis, and future expectations.	Provides knowledge base from which patient can make informed choices.
Discuss patient's expectations of returning home, to work, and to normal activities.	Patient frequently has a difficult and prolonged adjustment after discharge. Problems often occur (e.g., sleep disturbances, nightmares, reliving the accident, difficulty with resumption of social interactions, intimacy/sexual activity, emotional lability) that interfere with successful adjustment to resuming normal life.
Review and have patient/SO demonstrate proper burn-, skin-graft, and wound-care techniques. Identify appropriate sources for outpatient care and supplies.	Promotes competent self-care after discharge and enhances independence.
Discuss skin care, e.g., use of moisturizers, sunscreens, and anti-itching medications.	Itching, blistering, and sensitivity of healing wounds/graft sites can be expected for an extended time, and injury can occur because of the fragility of the new tissue.
Explain scarring process and necessity for/proper use of pressure garments when used.	Promotes optimal regrowth of skin, minimizing development of hypertrophic scarring and contractures and facilitating healing process. *Note:* Consistent use of the pressure garment over a long period can reduce the need for reconstructive surgery to release contractures and remove scars.
Encourage continuation of prescribed exercise program and scheduled rest periods.	Maintains mobility, reduces complications, and prevents fatigue, facilitating recovery process.
Identify specific limitations of activity as individually appropriate.	Imposed restrictions depend on severity/location of injury and stage of healing.
Emphasize importance of sustained intake of high-protein/high-calorie meals and snacks.	Optimal nutrition enhances tissue regeneration and general feeling of well-being. *Note:* The patient often needs to increase caloric intake to meet calorie and protein needs for healing.

739

ACTIONS/INTERVENTIONS	RATIONALE
Independent	
Review medications, including purpose, dosage, route, and expected/reportable side effects.	Reiteration allows opportunity for patient to ask questions and be sure understanding is accurate.
Advise patient/SO of potential for exhaustion, boredom, emotional lability, adjustment problems. Provide information about possibility of discussion/interaction with appropriate professional counselors.	Provides perspective to some of the problems patient/SO may encounter and aids awareness that assistance is available when necessary.
Identify signs/symptoms requiring medical evaluation, e.g., inflammation, increased or changes in wound drainage, fever/chills; changes in pain characteristics or loss of mobility/function.	Early detection of developing complications (e.g., infection, delayed healing) may prevent progression to more serious/life-threatening situations.
Stress necessity/importance of follow-up care/rehabilitation.	Long-term support with continual re-evaluation and changes in therapy is required to achieve optimal recovery.
Provide phone number for contact person.	Provides easy access to treatment team to reinforce teaching, clarify misconceptions, and reduce potential for complications.
Identify community resources, e.g., skin/wound care professionals, crisis centers, recovery groups, mental health, Red Cross, visiting nurse, Ambli-Cab, homemaker service.	Facilitates transition to home, provides assistance with meeting individual needs, and supports independence.

POTENTIAL CONSIDERATIONS following acute hospitalization (dependent on patient's age, physical condition/presence of complications, personal resources, and life responsibilities)

Coping, Individual, ineffective—situational crisis; vulnerability.

Disuse Syndrome, risk for—severe pain, prescribed immobilization/restrictive therapies.

Self-Esteem, situational low—change in health status/independent functioning, perceived loss of control in some aspect of life.

Therapeutic Regimen: Individuals, ineffective management—complexity of medical regimen, added demands made on individual/family, social support deficits.

Post-trauma Syndrome—catastrophic accident/injury to self and possibly others.

Systemic Infections and Immunologic Disorders

SEPSIS/SEPTICEMIA

Sepsis is a syndrome characterized by clinical signs and symptoms of severe infection that may progress to septicemia and septic shock. *Septicemia* implies the presence of an infection of the blood caused by rapidly multiplying microorganisms or their toxins, which can result in profound physiological changes and systemic sepsis. The pathogens can be bacteria, fungi, viruses, or rickettsiae. The most common causes of septicemia are Gram-negative bacteria (and endotoxins), staphylococci, and *Candida*. If the defense system of the body is not effective in controlling the invading microorganisms, septic shock may result, characterized by altered hemodynamics, impaired cellular function, and multiple system failure.

Patients at highest risk for bacteremia and septic shock include the elderly, infants, and immunosuppressed patients with chronic diseases (e.g., diabetes); postoperative patients; and those with ventilators, invasive lines, and catheters. Early signs and symptoms may be vague, and sepsis can develop subtly until sudden, overwhelming septic shock is present, affecting multiple organ systems.

CARE SETTING

Although severely ill patients may require admission to an intensive care unit (ICU), this plan addresses care on an inpatient acute medical-surgical unit.

RELATED CONCERNS

Patient Assessment Database

Date depends on the type, location, duration of the infective process, and organ involvement.

ACTIVITY/REST

May report: Fatigue, malaise

May exhibit: Mental status changes, e.g., withdrawn, lethargic
Respiration/heart rate increased with activity

CIRCULATION

May exhibit: Blood pressure (BP) normal/slightly low-normal range (as long as cardiac output remains elevated); profound hypotension (late stage)
Peripheral pulses bounding, rapid (hyperdynamic phase); weak/thready/easily obliterated, extreme tachycardia (shock)
Heart sounds: Dysrhythmias and development of S_3 suggest myocardial dysfunction, effects of acidosis/electrolyte imbalance
Skin warm, dry, flushed (vasodilation); or pale, cold, clammy, mottled (vasoconstriction)

ELIMINATION

May exhibit: Urinary output decreased, concentrated; progressing to oliguria, anuria
Urine cloudy, malodorous

FOOD/FLUID

May report: Anorexia; nausea/vomiting

May exhibit: Weight loss, decreased subcutaneous fat/muscle mass (malnutrition)
Diminished/absent bowel sounds
Extremity and generalized edema

NEUROSENSORY

May report: Headache; dizziness, fainting

May exhibit: Restlessness, apprehension, confusion, disorientation, delirium/coma

PAIN/DISCOMFORT

May report: Abdominal tenderness, localized pain/discomfort
Generalized urticaria/pruritus

RESPIRATION

May report: Shortness of breath

May exhibit: Tachypnea with decreased respiratory depth, dyspnea; rapid labored respirations
Basilar crackles, rhonchi, wheezes (presence of pneumonia; developing pulmonary complications/onset of cardiac decompensation)

SAFETY

May report: History of recent/current infection, viral illness; cancer therapies, use of corticosteroids/other immunosuppressant medications

May exhibit: Temperature: Usually elevated (101°F or greater) but may be normal in elderly or compromised patient; occasionally subnormal (under 98.6°F)
Shaking chills
Poor/delayed wound healing, purulent drainage, localized erythema
Mascular erythematous rash, petechiae; oozing/bleeding from invasive line sites, wounds, mucous membranes

SEXUALITY

May report: Perineal pruritus
Recent childbirth/abortion

May exhibit: Maceration of vulva, purulent vaginal drainage

TEACHING/LEARNING

May report: Chronic/debilitating health problems, e.g., liver, renal, cardiac disease; cancer, diabetes mellitus (DM), alcoholism

History of splenectomy

Recent surgery/invasive procedures, traumatic wounds

Antibiotic use (recent or long-term)

Discharge plan considerations: **DRG projected mean length of inpatient stay: 5.5 days**

May require assistance with wound care/supplies, treatments, self-care and homemaker tasks

Refer to section at end of plan for postdischarge considerations.

DIAGNOSTIC STUDIES

Cultures (wound, sputum, urine, blood): May identify organism(s) causing the sepsis. Sensitivity determines most effective drug choices. Catheter/intravascular line tips may need to be removed and cultured if the portal of entry is unknown. *Note:* Diagnosis does not require positive blood cultures because up to 40% of patients who develop septic shock do not display an identified bacterium by culture.

Complete blood count (CBC): Hematocrit (Hct) may be elevated in hypovolemic states because of hemoconcentration. Leukopenia (decreased white blood cells [WBCs]) occurs early, followed by a rebound leukocytosis (15,000–30,000) with increased bands (shift to the left), indicating rapid production of immature WBCs. Neutrophils (also called granulocytes, polys, or polymorphonuclear neutrophils [PMNs]) may be elevated or depressed. Counts below 500/mL indicate immune system exhaustion.

Serum electrolytes: Various imbalances may occur because of acidosis, fluid shifts, and altered renal function.

Clotting studies:

Platelets: Decreased levels (thrombocytopenia) can occur because of platelet aggregation.

Prothrombin time (PT)/activated partial thromboplastin time (aPTT): May be prolonged, indicating coagulopathy associated with liver ischemia, circulating toxins, shock state.

Serum lactate: Elevated in metabolic acidosis, liver dysfunction, shock.

Serum glucose: Hyperglycemia occurs, reflecting gluconeogenesis and glycogenolysis in the liver in response to cellular starvation/alteration in metabolism.

Blood urea nitrogen(BUN)/Creatinine (Cr): Increased levels are associated with dehydration, renal impairment/failure, and liver dysfunction/failure.

Arterial blood gases (ABGs): Respiratory alkalosis and hypoxemia may occur early. In later states, hypoxemia, respiratory acidosis, lactic and metabolic acidosis occur because of failure of compensatory mechanisms.

Urinalysis: Presence of WBCs/bacteria suggests infection. Protein and red blood cells (RBCs) are often present.

X-rays: Abdominal and lower chest films indicating free air in the abdomen may suggest infection due to perforated abdominal/pelvic organ.

Electrocardiogram (ECG): May show ST-segment and T-wave changes and dysrhythmia resembling myocardial infarction.

NURSING PRIORITIES

1. Eliminate infection.
2. Support tissue perfusion/circulatory volume.
3. Prevent complications.
4. Provide information about disease process, prognosis, and treatment needs.

DISCHARGE GOALS

1. Infection eliminated/controlled.
2. Homeostasis maintained.
3. Complications prevented/minimized.
4. Disease process, prognosis, and therapeutic regimen understood.
5. Plan in place to meet needs after discharge.

ACTIONS/INTERVENTIONS	RATIONALE
Infection Control (NIC)	
Independent	
Provide isolation/monitor visitors as indicated.	Body substance isolation (BSI) should be used for all infectious patients. Wound/linen isolation and hand-washing may be all that is required for draining wounds. Patients with diseases transmitted through air may also need airborne and droplet precautions. Reverse isolation/restriction of visitors may be needed to protect the immunosuppressed patient.
Wash hands with antibacterial soap before/after each care activity, even if gloves are used.	Reduces risk of cross-contamination because gloves may have unnoticeable defects, get torn or damaged during use.
Encourage/provide frequent position changes, deep-breathing/coughing exercises.	Good pulmonary toilet may reduce respiratory compromise.
Encourage patient to cover mouth and nose with tissue during coughs/sneezes. Place in private room, if indicated. Wear mask when providing direct care.	Prevents spread of infection via airborne droplets.
Limit use of invasive devices/procedures when possible. Remove lines/devices when infection is present and replace if necessary.	Reduces number of sites for entry of opportunistic organisms.
Inspect wounds/site of invasive devices daily, paying particular attention to parenteral nutrition lines. Document signs of local inflammation/infection, changes in character of wound drainage, sputum, or urine.	May provide clue to portal of entry, type of primary infecting organism(s), as well as early identification of secondary infections. *Note:* High nutrient content of total parenteral nutrition (TPN) provides excellent medium for bacterial growth.
Maintain sterile technique when changing dressings, suctioning, providing site care, e.g., invasive line, urinary catheter.	Prevents introduction of bacteria, reducing risk of nosocomial infection.
Wear gloves/gowns when caring for open wounds/anticipating direct contact with secretions or excretions.	Prevents spread of infection/cross-contamination.
Dispose of soiled dressings/materials in double bag.	Reduces contamination/soilage of area; limits spread of airborne organisms.

ACTIONS/INTERVENTIONS	RATIONALE

Independent

Monitor temperature trends.

Fever (101°F–105°F/38.5°C–40°C) is the result of endotoxin effect on the hypothalamus and pyrogen-released endorphins. Hypothermia (less than 96°F/36°C) is a grave sign reflecting advancing shock state, decreased tissue perfusion, and/or failure of the body's ability to mount a febrile response.

Observe for shaking chills and profuse diaphoresis.

Chills often precede temperature spikes in presence of generalized infection.

Monitor for signs of deterioration of condition/failure to improve with therapy.

May reflect inappropriate/inadequate antibiotic therapy or overgrowth of resistant or opportunistic organisms.

Inspect oral cavity for white plaques (thrush). Investigate reports of vaginal/perineal itching or burning.

Depression of immune system and use of antibiotics increases risk of secondary infections, particularly yeast.

Collaborative

Obtain specimens of urine, blood, sputum, wound, invasive lines/tubes as indicated for Gram stain, culture, and sensitivity.

Identification of portal of entry and organism causing the septicemia is crucial to effective treatment.

Monitor laboratory studies, e.g., WBC count with neutrophil and band counts.

The normal ratio of neutrophils to total WBCs is at least 50%; however, when WBC count is markedly decreased, calculating the absolute neutrophil count is more pertinent to evaluating immune status. Likewise, an initial elevation of band cells reflects the body's attempt to mount a response to the infection, while a decline indicates decompensation.

Administer medications as indicated:

Anti-infective agents: broad-spectrum antibiotics, e.g., methicillin (Staphcillin); Gram-negative agents e.g., ticarcillin disodium (Ticar); Gram-positive, e.g., nafcillin (Nafcil), vancomycin (Vancocin); aminoglycosides, e.g., tobramycin (Nebcin), gentamicin (Garamycin); cephalosporins, e.g., cefotaxime (Claforan);

Specific antibiotics are determined by culture and sensitivity results, but therapy is usually initiated before obtaining results, using broad-spectrum antibiotics and/or based on most likely infecting organisms. Concomitant use of antimicrobials is often beneficial, but dosage must be balanced against renal function/clearance.

Immune globulins as appropriate.

May boost/provide temporary immunity to general infection or specific illness, e.g., varicella zoster, rabies.

Assist with/prepare for incision and drainage of wound, irrigation, application of warm/moist soaks, as indicated.

Facilitates removal of purulent material/necrotic tissue and promotes healing.

NURSING DIAGNOSIS: Hyperthermia

May be related to
Increased metabolic rate, illness
Dehydration
Direct effect of circulating endotoxins on the hypothalamus, altering temperature regulation

ACTIONS/INTERVENTIONS	RATIONALE
Fever Treatment (NIC)	
Independent	
Monitor patient temperature (degree and pattern); note shaking chills/profuse diaphoresis.	Temperature of 102°F–106°F (38.9°C–41.1°C) suggests acute infectious disease process. Fever pattern may aid in diagnosis; e.g., sustained or continuous fever curves lasting more than 24 hr suggest pneumococcal pneumonia, scarlet or typhoid fever; remittent fever (varying only a few degrees in either direction) reflects pulmonary infections; intermittent curves or fever that returns to normal once in 24-hr period suggests septic episode, septic endocarditis, or tuberculosis (TB). Chills often precede temperature spikes. *Note:* Use of antipyretics alters fever patterns and may be restricted until diagnosis is made or if fever remains greater that 102°F (38.9°C).
Monitor environmental temperature; limit/add bed linens as indicated.	Room temperature/number of blankets should be altered to maintain near-normal body temperature.
Provide tepid sponge baths; avoid use of alcohol.	May help reduce fever. *Note.* Use of ice water/alcohol may cause chills, actually elevating temperature. In addition, alcohol is very drying to skin.
Collaborative	
Administer antipyretics, e.g., acetylsalicylic acid (ASA) (aspirin), acetaminophen (Tylenol).	Used to reduce fever by its central action on the hypothalamus; fever should be controlled in patients who are neutropenic or asplenic. However, fever may be beneficial in limiting growth of organisms and enhancing autodestruction of infected cells.
Provide cooling blanket.	Used to reduce fever, usually greater than 104°F–105°F (39.5°C–40°C), when brain damage/seizures can occur.

Possibly evidenced by

[Not applicable; presence of signs and symptoms establishes an *actual* diagnosis]

DESIRED OUTCOMES/EVALUATION CRITERIA—PATIENT WILL:

Circulation Status (NOC)

Display adequate perfusion as evidenced by stable vital signs, palpable peripheral pulses, skin warm and dry, usual level of mentation, individually appropriate urinary output and active bowel sounds.

ACTIONS/INTERVENTIONS	RATIONALE
Shock Prevention (NIC)	
Independent	
Maintain bedrest; assist with care activities.	Decreases myocardial workload and O_2 consumption, maximizing effectiveness of tissue perfusion.
Monitor trends in BP, especially noting progressive hypotension and widening pulse pressure.	Hypotension develops as microorganisms invade the bloodstream, stimulating release or activation of chemical and hormonal substances, which initially results in peripheral vasodilation, decreased systemic vascular resistance (SVR), and relative hypovolemia. As shock progresses, cardiac output becomes severely depressed because of major alterations in contractility and preload/afterload, producing profound hypotension.
Monitor heart rate, rhythm. Note dysrhythmias.	Tachycardia occurs because of sympathetic nervous system stimulation secondary to stress response and to compensate for the relative hypovolemia and hypotension. Cardiac dysrhythmias can occur as a result of hypoxia, acid-base/electrolyte imbalance, and/or low-flow perfusion state.
Note quality/strength of peripheral pulses.	Initially the pulse is strong/bounding because of increased cardiac output (CO). Pulse may become weak/thready because of sustained hypotension, decreased cardiac output, and peripheral vasoconstriction if the shock state progresses.
Assess respiratory rate, depth, and quality. Note onset of severe dyspnea.	Increased respirations occur in response to direct effects of endotoxins on the respiratory center in the brain, as well as developing hypoxia, stress, and fever. Respiration can become shallow as respiratory insufficiency develops, creating risk of acute respiratory failure. (Refer to ND: Gas Exchange, risk for impaired, p. 750.)
Investigate changes in sensorium, e.g., mental cloudiness, agitation, restlessness, personality changes, delirium, stupor, coma.	Changes reflect alterations in cerebral perfusion, hypoxemia, and/or acidosis.
Assess skin for changes in color, temperature, moisture.	Compensatory mechanism of vasodilation results in warm, dry, pink skin, which is characteristic of hyperperfusion in hyperdynamic phase of early septic shock. If shock state progresses, compensatory vasoconstriction occurs, shunting blood to vital organs, reducing peripheral blood flow, and creating cool, clammy, pale/dusky skin.

ACTIONS/INTERVENTIONS	RATIONALE
Independent	
Record hourly urinary output and specific gravity.	Decreasing urinary output with increased specific gravity indicates diminished renal perfusion related to fluid shifts and selective vasoconstriction. There may be transient polyuria during hyperdynamic phase (while cardiac output is elevated), but this may progress to oliguria.
Auscultate bowel sounds.	Reduced blood flow to the mesentery (splanchnic vasoconstriction) decreases peristalsis and may lead to paralytic ileus.
Monitor gastric pH as indicated. Hematest gastric secretions/stools for occult blood.	Stress of illness and use of steroids increase risk of gastric mucosal erosion/bleeding.
Evaluate lower extremities for local tissue swelling, erythema, positive Homans' sign.	Venous stasis and infectious process may result in the development of thrombosis.
Monitor for signs of bleeding, e.g., oozing from puncture sites/suture lines, petechiae, ecchymoses, hematuria, epistaxis, hemoptysis, hematemesis.	Coagulopathy/disseminated intravascular coagulation (DIC) may occur related to accelerated clotting in the microcirculation (activation of chemical mediators, vascular insufficiency, and cell destruction), creating a life-threatening hemorrhagic situation/multiple emboli.
Note drug effects, and monitor for signs of toxicity.	Massive doses of antibiotics are often ordered. These have potentially toxic effects when hepatic/renal perfusion is compromised.
Collaborative	
Administer parenteral fluids. (Refer to ND: Fluid Volume, risk for deficit, following.)	To maintain tissue perfusion, large amounts of fluid may be required to support circulating volume.
Administer drugs as indicated:	
Corticosteroids;	Although steroid therapy remains controversial, steroids may be given for the potential advantages of decreased capillary permeability, increased renal perfusion, and inhibition of microemboli formation.
$NaHCO_3$;	Impaired tissue perfusion and production of lactate result in metabolic acidosis, requiring base replacement therapy.
Antacids: e.g., aluminum hydroxide (Amphojel).	Decreases potential for gastric bleeding related to stress response/altered perfusion.
Monitor laboratory studies, e.g., ABGs, lactate levels.	Development of respiratory/metabolic acidosis reflects loss of compensatory mechanisms, e.g., decreased renal perfusion/hydrogen excretion; and accumulation of lactic acid due to circulatory shunting and stagnation.
Administer supplemental O_2.	Maximizes oxygen available for cellular uptake.
Maintain body temperature, using adjunctive aids as necessary. (Refer to ND: Hyperthermia, p. 745.)	Temperature elevations increase metabolic/oxygen demands beyond cellular resources, hastening tissue ischemia/cellular destruction.
Prepare for/transfer to critical care setting as indicated.	Progressive deterioration requires more aggressive therapy (e.g., hemodynamic monitoring and vasoactive drugs).

NURSING DIAGNOSIS: Fluid Volume, risk for deficit

Risk factors may include

Marked increase in vascular compartment/massive vasodilation

Capillary permeability/fluid leaks into the interstitial space (third spacing)

Possibly evidenced by

[Not applicable; presence of signs and symptoms establishes an *actual* diagnosis]

DESIRED OUTCOMES/EVALUATION CRITERIA—PATIENT WILL:

> **Hydration (NOC)**

Maintain adequate circulatory volume as evidenced by vital signs within patient's normal range, palpable peripheral pulses of good quality, and individually appropriate urinary output.

ACTIONS/INTERVENTIONS	RATIONALE

Shock Prevention (NIC)

Independent

Measure/record urinary output and specific gravity. Note cumulative intake and output (I&O) imbalances (including insensible losses), and correlate with daily weight. Encourage oral fluids to tolerance.	Decreasing urinary output with a high specific gravity suggests relative hypovolemia associated with vasodilation. Continued positive fluid balance with corresponding weight gain may indicate third spacing and tissue edema, suggesting need to alter fluid therapy/replacement components.
Monitor BP and heart rate (HR). Measure central venous pressure (CVP) if used.	Reduction in the circulating fluid volume reduces BP/CVP, initiating compensatory mechanisms of tachycardia to improve cardiac output and increase systemic BP.
Palpate peripheral pulses.	Weak, easily obliterated pulses suggest hypovolemia.
Assess for dry mucous membranes, poor skin turgor, and thirst.	Hypovolemia/third spacing of fluid gives rise to signs of dehydration.
Observe for dependent/peripheral edema in sacrum, scrotum, back, legs.	Fluid losses from the vascular compartment into the interstitial space create tissue edema.

Collaborative

Administer IV fluids, e.g., crystalloids (D_5W, normal saline [NS]) and colloids (albumin, fresh frozen plasma) as indicated.	Large volumes of fluid may be required to overcome relative hypovolemia (peripheral vasodilation); replace losses from increased capillary permeability (e.g., sequestration of fluid in the peritoneal cavity) and increased insensible sources (e.g., fever/diaphoresis).
Monitor laboratory values, e.g.:	
Hct/RBC count;	Evaluates changes in hydration/blood viscosity.
BUN/Cr.	Moderate elevations of BUN reflect dehydration, high values of BUN/Cr may indicate renal dysfunction/failure.
Monitor cardiac output as indicated.	CO (and other functional parameters, such as cardiac index, preload/afterload, contractility, and cardiac work) can be measured noninvasively using thoracic electrical bioimpedance (TEB) technique. Useful in determining therapeutic needs/effectiveness.

ACTIONS/INTERVENTIONS	RATIONALE
Respiratory Monitoring (NIC)	
Independent	
Maintain patent airway. Place patient in position of comfort with head of bed elevated.	Enhances lung expansion, respiratory effort.
Monitor respiratory rate and depth. Note use of accessory muscles/work of breathing.	Rapid/shallow respirations occur because of hypoxemia, stress and circulating endotoxins. Hypoventilation and dyspnea reflect ineffective compensatory mechanisms and are an indication that ventilatory support is needed.
Auscultate breath sounds. Note crackles, wheezes, areas of decreased/absent ventilation.	Respiratory distress and the presence of adventitious sounds are indicators of pulmonary congestion/interstitial edema, atelectasis. *Note:* Respiratory complications, including pneumonia and adult respiratory distress syndrome (ARDS), are a prime cause of death.
Note presence of circumoral cyanosis.	Reflects inadequate systemic oxygenation/hypoxemia.
Investigate alterations in sensorium: agitation, confusion, personality changes, delirium, stupor, coma.	Cerebral function is very sensitive to decreases in oxygenation (e.g., hypoxemia/reduced perfusion).
Note cough and purulent sputum production.	Pneumonia is a common nosocomial infection that can occur by aspiration of oropharyngeal organisms or spread from other sites.
Reposition frequently. Encourage coughing and deep-breathing exercises. Suction with lavage, as indicated.	Good pulmonary toilet is necessary for reducing ventilation/perfusion imbalance and for mobilizing and facilitating removal of secretions to maximize gas exchange.

ACTIONS/INTERVENTIONS

Collaborative

Monitor ABGs/pulse oximetry.

Administer supplemental O_2 via appropriate route, e.g., nasal cannula, mask, high-flow rebreathing mask.

Review serial check x-rays.

RATIONALE

Hypoxemia is related to decreased ventilation and pulmonary changes (e.g., interstitial edema, atelectasis, and pulmonary shunting) and increased oxygen demands caused by fever or infection. Respiratory acidosis (pH below 7.35 and $PaCO_2$ greater than 40 mm Hg) occurs because of hypoventilation and ventilation-perfusion imbalance. As septic condition worsens, metabolic acidosis (pH below 7.35 and HCO_3 less than 22–24 mEq/L) develops due to buildup of lactic acid from anaerobic metabolism.

Necessary for correction of hypoxemia with failing respiratory effort/progressing acidosis. *Note:* Intubation/mechanical ventilation may be required if respiratory failure develops.

Changes reflect progression/resolution of pulmonary complications, e.g., infiltrates/edema. *Note:* Changes in chest x-ray are usually 1–2 hr behind the clinical picture.

NURSING DIAGNOSIS: Knowledge Deficit [Learning Need] regarding illness, prognosis, treatment, self care, and discharge needs

May be related to
Lack of exposure/recall; information misinterpretation
Cognitive limitation

Possibly evidenced by
Questions/request for information, statement of misconception
Inaccurate follow-through of instructions/development of preventable complications

DESIRED OUTCOMES/EVALUATION CRITERIA—PATIENT WILL:

Knowledge: Infection Control (NOC)

Verbalize understanding of disease process, prognosis, and potential complications.
Correctly perform necessary procedures and explain reasons for the actions.
Initiate necessary lifestyle changes.
Verbalize understanding of therapeutic needs.
Participate in treatment regimen.

ACTIONS/INTERVENTIONS

Teaching: Disease Process (NIC)

Independent

Review disease process and future expectations.

Review individual risk factors and mode of transmission/portal of entry of infections.

RATIONALE:

Provides knowledge base from which patient can make informed choices.

Steroid therapy, kidney/liver dysfunction, neoplastic disease, rheumatic heart disease, valve dysfunction, and diabetes may predispose to septicemia. Awareness of means of infection transmission provides opportunity to plan for/institute protective measures.

ACTIONS/INTERVENTIONS	RATIONALE

Independent

Provide information about drug therapy, interactions, side effects, and importance of adherence to regimen.	Promotes understanding of and enhances cooperation in treatment/prophylaxis and reduces risk of recurrence and complications.
Discuss need for good nutritional intake/balanced diet.	Necessary for optimal healing and general well-being.
Encourage adequate rest periods with scheduled activities.	Prevents fatigue, conserves energy, and promotes healing.
Review necessity of personal hygiene and environmental cleanliness.	Helps control environmental exposure by diminishing the number of pathogens present.
Discuss proper use or avoidance of tampons with women, as indicated.	Superabsorbent tampons/infrequent changing potentiates risk of *Staphylococcus aureus* infection (toxic shock syndrome).
Identify signs/symptoms requiring medical evaluation, e.g., persistent temperature elevation(s), tachycardia, syncope, rashes of unknown origin, unexplained fatigue, anorexia, increased thirst, and changes in bladder function.	Early recognition of developing/recurring infection allows for timely intervention and reduces risk for progression to life-threatening situation.
Stress importance of prophylactic immunization/antibiotic therapy as needed.	Used for prevention of infection.

POTENTIAL CONSIDERATIONS following acute hospitalization (dependent on patient's age, physical condition/presence of complications, personal resources, and life responsibilities)

Infection, risk for recurrence/opportunistic—stasis of body fluids, decreased hemoglobin, leukopenia, suppressed inflammatory response, use of anti-infective agents, increased environmental exposure, malnutrition.

Nutrition: altered, less than body requirements—increased energy needs (hypermetabolic state), anorexia, continuing gastrointestinal (GI) dysfunction, side effects of medication.

Self-Care deficit/Home Maintenance Management, impaired—decreased strength/endurance, pain/discomfort, inadequate support systems, unfamiliarity with neighborhood resources.

THE HIV-POSITIVE PATIENT

The individual identified as HIV-seropositive is one who is asymptomatic and does not meet the Centers for Disease Control and Prevention (CDC) definition for AIDS. Studies reveal that persons with HIV-positive status may remain asymptomatic for 10 or more years. During the period of asymptomatic infection, the infected individual has HIV in the blood and is contagious to others. After approximately a decade, especially in the undertreated individual, the immune system begins to decline and he/she develops symptoms of immune deficiency, a phase termed "symptomatic HIV infection." The individual might then develop "AIDS-defining" diseases. With the inception of multiple drug regimens, the CD4 count can be maintained at higher levels for longer periods of time and the viral load minimized. Although imminent death is not a realistic concern, the patient needs to make major behavioral and lifestyle changes to prolong life expectancy and may have significant problems that require information and assistance. The person who is well-supported medically may lead a productive life for an extended period.

CARE SETTING

Community setting, although development of opportunistic infections may require occasional inpatient acute medical care.

RELATED FACTORS

AIDS, page 765
Extended care, page 850
Fluid and electrolyte imbalances, page 926
Pneumonia, microbial, page 140
Psychosocial aspects of care, page 809
Sepsis/Septicemia, page 741

Patient Assessment Database

Although patient may be asymptomatic, refer to CP: AIDS, page 765, for potential signs/symptoms.

Refer to section at end of plan for ongoing considerations.

DIAGNOSTIC STUDIES

Enzyme-linked immunosorbent assay (ELISA): A positive test result may be indicative of exposure to HIV but is not diagnostic. Sensitivity varies, with the incidence of false-positive results being approximately 10%. (Seroconversion can occur between 4 wk to 6 mo after exposure.)

Western blot test (blood/urine): Confirms diagnosis of HIV-1 in individuals with positive ELISA screening.

HIV-RNA: The most widely used test currently can detect viral RNA levels as low as 500 copies/mL of plasma. A more sensitive test that can detect HIV-RNA levels as low as 50 copies/mL is expected to become the standard test for viral load in the near future.

CD4 lymphocyte count (previously T4 helper cells): Reduced. Patients with counts below 500 benefit from antiretroviral therapy; counts equal to/or below 200 define progression to AIDS. Levels are measured immediately before and again 4 to 8 wk after initiation of antiretroviral therapy. Thus, it is used to diagnose HIV infection and progression and to monitor effects of drug therapy.

Screening tests: Purified protein derivative (PPD): Positive result reflects current or prior exposure to tuberculosis. Anergy test (*Candida*/mumps/tetanus toxoid) is done in combination with PPD to clarify false-negative results. PPD reflects cutaneous anergy (inability of immune system to respond to specific antigens). The criteria for positive PPD when immune deficiency is present is 5-mm induration.

Serologies: Rapid plasma reagin (RPR)/VDRL: Determines current/past exposure to syphilis and need for more specific testing. Toxoplasma and hepatitis B and C serologies may be done.

Pap smear: Higher incidence (40%) of abnormal cells occurs in HIV-infected women. The critical role of Pap smear screening relates to its ability to detect precursor lesions that can precede the diagnosis of invasive carcinoma by several years.

Pelvic/genital examination: Identifies presence of lesions from sexually transmitted diseases (STDs), cervical and vaginal abnormalities.

Chemistries: Glucose and lipids rise as HIV infection progresses. Albumin/prealbumin and transferrin levels are decreased secondary to malabsorption/malnutrition that is usually progressive.

CBC: Hemoglobin, RBC counts are decreased and abnormalities in iron metabolism can result in anemia, which occurs in 17% of asymptomatic patients and up to 85% of patients with advanced disease.

Chest x-ray: Abnormalities suggest presence of TB in PPD-positive, anergic, and/or symptomatic individuals. Diagnosis is then verified by sputum cultures, or other tests, such as gallium scan.

NURSING PRIORITIES

1. Promote acceptance of reality of diagnosis/condition.
2. Support incorporation of behavioral/lifestyle changes to enhance well-being.
3. Provide information about disease process/prognosis and treatment needs.
4. Assist in developing plan to meet long-term medical, behavioral, and financial needs.

GOALS

1. Dealing with current situation realistically.
2. Participating in therapeutic regimen.
3. Diagnosis, prognosis, and therapeutic regimen understood.
4. Plan in place to meet medical, behavioral change, and financial needs.

NURSING DIAGNOSIS: Adjustment, impaired

May be related to
Life-threatening, stigmatized condition/disease
Assault to self-esteem, altered locus of control
Denial; incomplete/ongoing grieving
Inadequate support systems
Medication side effects (fatigue and depression)

Possibly evidenced by
Verbalization of nonacceptance/denial of diagnosis
Nonexistent or unsuccessful ability to be involved in problem solving or goal setting
Extended period of shock, disbelief, or anger regarding change in health status
Lack of future-oriented thinking

DESIRED OUTCOMES/EVALUATION CRITERIA—PATIENT WILL:

Acceptance: Health Status (NOC)

Verbalize reality and acceptance of condition.
Demonstrate increased trust and participation in development of plan of action.
Initiate lifestyle changes that will permit adaptation to present life situations.

ACTIONS/INTERVENTIONS	RATIONALE
Crisis Intervention (NIC)	
Independent	
Evaluate patient's ability to understand events and realistically appraise situation.	Provides base to develop plan of action.
Encourage expression of feelings, denial, shock, and fears. Listen without judgment, accepting patient's expressions. Focus on positive outcomes.	It is important to convey belief in commonality of patient's fears/feelings. By focusing on positive outcomes, the patient is encouraged to take charge of those areas in which changes can be made, e.g., managing medical regimen and behavior.

ACTIONS/INTERVENTIONS	RATIONALE
Independent	
Challenge morbid thoughts and reframe into positive statements, i.e., "You know why the virus is going to kill me. I deserve to die for what I've done." Response: "The virus may or may not kill you. It's not smart enough to decide when you may die. The virus is 'just there.' It does not have a mind to know what you have or have not done."	Interrupts morbid thoughts and challenges patient's self-deprecating ideas. As with any potentially terminal disease, this population is likely to experience depression and is at increased risk for suicide, necessitating ongoing evaluation.
Determine available resources and programs.	Addictive behaviors, ability of injection drug user to obtain clean "works," sexual myths, and perceptions of the need for condoms need to be addressed.
Assess social system, as well as presence of support, perception of losses, and stressors.	Partners, friends, and families will have individual responses depending on the person's lifestyle, knowledge of HIV transmission, and belief in myths.
Encourage patient to participate in support groups.	Long-term support is critical to dealing with and effectively coping with the reality of frequent physician's visits for evaluation, medical treatments, and ongoing lifestyle changes.
Educate patient about drug interactions, HIV, and emotions.	Fatigue and depression can be side effects of some medications and of the infection itself. Knowledge that it is usually of short duration can support informed choices/cooperation and promote hope.
Encourage continued or renewed use of familiar effective copies strategies.	Patient is supported and given encouragement for past effective behavior. Positive reinforcement enhances self-esteem.
Explore use and practice of new and different coping strategies.	Using new strategies can be uncomfortable and practice fosters self-confidence.
Help the patient use humor to combat stigmatization of the disease.	Humor defuses the sense of secretiveness people may place on diagnosis of/dealing with HIV.
Reinforce structure in daily life. Include exercise as part of routine.	Routines help the person focus. Exercise improves sense of wellness and enhances immune response.
Discuss meaning of high-risk behavior and barriers to change, e.g. unprotected sexual activity or injection drug use with shared needles.	Fear of disclosure, need to change usual behaviors, and the difficulty of doing so may prevent the individual from making the changes necessary to prevent transmission. Sexual behavior may be used to express caring and to feel connected and less lonely.
Assist patient to set limits on sexually risky behaviors and explore ways patient can achieve change.	Needs for love, comfort, and companionship that have been met through sexual expression need to be met safely through means that carry a reduced risk of HIV transmission.
Assist patient to channel anger to healthy activities.	The increased energy of anger can be used to accomplish other tasks and enhance feelings of self-esteem.
Inform patient about new medical advances/treatments.	Promotes hope and helps patient make informed decisions.
Discuss issues of voluntary disclosure; personal responsibility; needs of others; and federal, state, and local reporting requirements.	Understanding responsibilities and consequences of disclosure is necessary for patient to make informed decisions.
Collaborative	
Refer to nurse practitioner/clinical specialist, psychologist, social worker knowledgeable about HIV.	May need additional help adjusting to difficult situation.

May be related to

Decreased metabolic energy production, increased energy requirements (hypermetabolic state)

Overwhelming psychological/emotional demands

Altered body chemistry: side effects of medications

Possibly evidenced by

Verbalization of unremitting/overwhelming lack of energy

Inability to maintain usual routines, decreased performance, impaired ability to concentrate

DESIRED OUTCOMES/EVALUATION CRITERIA—PATIENT WILL

Endurance (NOC)

Report improved sense of energy.

Participate in desired activities at level of ability.

Energy Conservation (NOC)

Identify individual areas of control and engage in energy conservation techniques.

ACTIONS/INTERVENTIONS	RATIONALE
Energy Management (NIC)	
Independent	
Assess sleep patterns and other factors that may be aggravating fatigue.	Multiple factors can cause/aggravate fatigue, including sleep deprivation, emotional distress, side effects of drugs, and developing central nervous system (CNS) disease.
Encourage physician evaluation of fatigue if new medications have been added to regimen.	Fatigue is present in variable degrees as part of HIV infection process, but is often aggravated by nutritional deficiencies and side effects of certain medications. For example, when protease inhibitors are added or changed, fatigue may worsen.
Discuss reality of patient's feelings of exhaustion and identify limitations imposed by fatigue state. Note daily energy patterns—peaks and valleys	Helpful in planning activities within tolerance levels. Patients often expect too much of themselves, believing that they should be able to do more.
Assist patient to set realistic activity goals, determining individual priorities and responsibilities	Patient may need to alter priorities, delegate some responsibilities to manage fatigue and optimize performance.
Discuss energy conservation techniques, e.g., sitting instead of standing for activities as appropriate.	Enables patient to become aware of ways in which energy expenditure can be maximized to complete necessary tasks.
Review importance of meeting individual nutritional needs.	Adequate nutrition is needed for optimizing energy production. (Refer to Nutrition: altered, risk for less than body requirements, following.)
Encourage adequate rest periods during day and routine schedule for bedtime/arising and scheduling activities during time of best energy.	Helps patient recoup energy to manage desired activities.
Instruct in stress management techniques, e.g., breathing exercises, visualization, music and light therapy.	Reduction of stress factors in patient's life can minimize energy output.

ACTIONS/INTERVENTIONS

Independent

Identify available resources and support systems.

RATIONALE

May require outside assistance with homemaking/maintenance activities, child care.

NURSING DIAGNOSIS: Nutrition: altered, risk for less than body requirements

Risk factors may include

Reported inadequate food intake less than recommended daily allowance

Lack of interest in food, anorexia, depression

Lack of information, misinformation, misconceptions

Limited resources (including finances)

Reported altered sensation of taste and smell, nausea and other side effects of medications

Sore, inflamed buccal cavity (e.g., thrush, cytomegalovirus [CMV] lesions)

Possibly evidenced by

[Not applicable; presence of signs and symptoms establishes an *actual* diagnosis]

DESIRED OUTCOMES/EVALUATION CRITERIA—PATIENT WILL:

Nutritional Status (NOC)

Maintain adequate muscle mass.

Maintain stable weight.

Demonstrate laboratory values within normal limits.

Report improved energy level.

ACTIONS/INTERVENTIONS

Nutritional Counseling (NIC)

Independent

Determine usual weight before patient was diagnosed with HIV.

Weigh regularly and establish current anthropometric measurements. Measure resting energy expenditure (REE) using indirect calorimetry.

Determine patient's current dietary pattern/intake and knowledge of nutrition. Use an in-depth dietary assessment tool.

Assess presence/degree of nausea and vomiting.

RATIONALE

Early wasting is not readily determined by normal weight-to-height charts; therefore, determining current weight in relation to prediagnosis weight is more useful. Recent unexplained/involuntary weight loss may be a factor in seeking initial medical evaluation.

Helps assess/monitor wasting and determine nutritional needs (40% of HIV-positive patients show substantial weight loss). Indirect calorimetry is more accurate for calculating REE than Harris-Benedict equation, which underestimates the energy needs of these patients.

Identification of these factors helps plan for individual needs. Patients with HIV infection have documented vitamin and trace mineral (zinc, magnesium, selenium) deficits. Alcohol and drug abuse interfere with adequate intake.

The causes of nausea and vomiting are numerous and are associated with medications, functional changes in GI system, and endocrine dysfunction. Protracted nausea and vomiting can debilitate a patient, leading to loss of lean body mass, electrolyte imbalances, and further deterioration of immune function.

ACTIONS/INTERVENTIONS	RATIONALE
Independent	
Ascertain current financial status, recent and/or anticipated changes in economic status. Explore related costs of a variety of foods.	Helps in planning for meeting nutritional needs, such as purchasing low-cost foods that are nutritionally packed, or patient may need referral to financial aid to help with food stamps or obtaining meals.
Discuss/document nutritional side effects of medications.	Commonly used medications cause anorexia, altered taste, nausea and/or vomiting; some interfere with bone marrow production of RBCs, causing anemia. GI symptoms are common with over-the-counter (OTC) drugs like nonsteroidal anti-inflammatory drugs (NSAIDs), which also may contribute to anorexia.
Help patient plan ways to maintain/improve intake. Identify lactose-free supplements as appropriate. Provide information about nutritionally dense high-calorie, high-protein, high-vitamin, and high-mineral foods.	Having this information helps patient understand importance of well-balanced diet. Some patients may try macrobiotic and other diets, believing the diarrhea is caused by lactose intolerance. Eliminating dairy products can have detrimental effects when these components are not replaced from other sources.
Stress importance of maintaining balanced/adequate nutritional intake and fluids rich with electrolytes, e.g., Gatorade or Pedialyte.	Patient may be depressed and discouraged with changed health and social status and find it difficult to eat for many reasons. Knowing how important nutritionally balanced intake is to supporting immune system and remaining healthy can motivate patient to eat.
Assist patient to formulate dietary plan, taking into consideration increased metabolic demands/energy needs and hyperlipidemia.	Provides guidance and feedback while promoting sense of control, enhancing self-esteem, and possibly improving intake. HIV infection is continuously stimulating the immune system, increasing metabolic rate and nutritional needs. *Note:* Use of protease inhibitors is known to elevate glucose and lipids (especially triglycerides and cholesterol).
Recommend environment conducive to eating, e.g., eating frequent small meals, avoiding cooking odors if bothersome; keeping room well ventilated, removing noxious stimuli. Suggest use of spices, marinating red meat before cooking, and/or substituting other protein sources for red meat.	Improves nutritional intake, which is needed to help patient restore/maintain nutritional defenses.
Emphasize importance of sharing mealtime with others. Identify someone who can join patient for meals.	Socialization can enhance appetite/food intake, especially when depression, neglect of self-care, and diminished appetite are present.
Explore complimentary therapies/nonpharmacologic interventions, such as acupressure, progressive relaxation, and guided imagery to manage anorexia.	The goal of these interventions is to manage distressing symptoms that interfere with optimal nutritional intake.
Discuss use of lactobacillus/acidophilus replacement, e.g. Lact-Aid dairy products and/or tablets.	HIV infection changes the structure of the gut wall, resulting in a decreased lactose level. Intolerance causes abdominal cramping, malabsorption, a bloated feeling, and diarrhea. Also, antibiotics taken for prevention of opportunistic infections cause changes in normal bowel flora, contributing to diarrhea.
Collaborative	
Consult with dietitian.	Provides assistance in planning nutritionally sound diet and identifying nutritional supplements to meet individual needs. Liquid supplements (e.g., Advera) have been specifically formulated for the GI manifestations common to the HIV-positive population.

ACTIONS/INTERVENTIONS

Collaborative

Monitor laboratory values, e.g., hemoglobin (Hb), RBCs, albumin/prealbumin, total iron-binding capacity (TIBC), potassium, sodium.

Provide medications as indicated, e.g.,

Dronabinol (Marinol), megestrol (Megace), cyproheptadine (Periactin):

Antidiarrheal medications, e.g., diphenoxylate/atropine (Lomotil), octreotide (Sandostatin).

RATIONALE

These laboratory tests are important in monitoring the patient's nutritional immune status and in identifying nutritional therapy needs. For example, decreased RBCs (anemia) may require additional interventions, such as use of epoetin (Epogen or Procrit) to stimulate RBC production.

Antiemetics/appetite stimulants can improve intake to prevent and correct dietary deficiencies. *Note:* Side-effect of use of Megace may include impotence necessitating change of drug as desired.

Diarrhea may be present because of altered GI flora and side effects of anti-infective agents. Treatment can correct malabsorption and enhance oral intake.

NURSING DIAGNOSIS: Knowledge Deficit [Learning Need] regarding disease, prognosis, treatment, self care, and discharge needs

May be related to
Lack of exposure/recall
Information misinterpretation
Unfamiliarity with information resources
Cognitive limitation

Possibly evidenced by:
Statement of misconception/request for information
Inaccurate follow-through of instructions/development of preventable complications
Inappropriate/exaggerated behaviors (e.g., hostile, agitated, hysterical, apathetic)

DESIRED OUTCOMES/EVALUATION CRITERIA—PATIENT WILL:

Knowledge: Disease Process (NOC)

Verbalize understanding of condition/disease process and potential complications.
Identify relationship of signs/symptoms to the disease process and correlate symptoms with causative factors.

Knowledge: Treatment Regimen (NOC)

Verbalize understanding of goals of treatment.
Initiate necessary lifestyle changes.
Participate in treatment regimen.

ACTIONS/INTERVENTIONS

Teaching: Disease Process (NIC)

Independent

Determine current understanding and perception of diagnosis. Discuss difference between HIV-positivity and AIDS.

RATIONALE

Provides opportunity to clarify misconceptions/myths and make informed choices. People often believe that if they are positive for the virus, they have AIDS; having accurate information about the difference can alleviate fears and allow for development of an individualized plan of care.

ACTIONS/INTERVENTIONS	RATIONALE
Independent	
Assess emotional ability to assimilate information and understand instructions. Respect patient's need to use denial coping techniques initially.	Initial shock and anxiety can block intake of information. Self-esteem, lifestyle, guilt, and denial of own responsibility in acquiring/transmitting disease become issues that must be dealt with. *Note:* Some initial denial may serve as a protective mechanism promoting more effective self-care.
Identify/problem-solve potential or actual barriers to accessing healthcare services.	Transportation, distance, child care, work schedule, homelessness/poverty, lack of insurance or finances are some of the issues that typically interfere with accessing needed primary care and prophylactic interventions.
Provide realistic, optimistic information during each contact with patient.	Necessary to provide realistic hope because most patients have been exposed to some inaccurate information about AIDS or have friends/lovers who have died of the disease.
Plan frequent short sessions for teaching.	Patient will need time and repeated contacts to absorb information, the scope of and requirements for treating the infection.
Provide information about normal immune system/response and how HIV affects it, transmission of the virus, behaviors and factors believed to increase probability of progression. Encourage questions.	Patient needs to be aware of own personal risk and risk to others to make immediate and long-range decisions and establish a basis for goal setting. Also, establishes rapport and provides opportunity to identify concerns and assimilate information.
Review signs/symptoms that could be a consequence of HIV infection, e.g., mild fever, anorexia, weight loss, fatigue, night sweats, diarrhea, dry cough, rashes, headaches, and sleep disturbances.	Patient may experience an acute illness 2–6 wk after becoming infected; however, it is common for infection to be subclinical, with the individual simply feeling unwell.
Discuss signs/symptoms that require medical evaluation, e.g., persistent fever, increasing cough or swollen lymph glands, profound fatigue unrelieved by rest, weight loss of 10 lb (or more) in less than 2 mo, severe/persistent diarrhea, fever, blurred vision, skin discoloration or rash that persists or spreads, open sores anywhere, symptoms occurring with medication regimen.	Early recognition of progression of disease/development of opportunistic infections provides for timely intervention and may prevent more serious situations. *Note:* Most HIV patients are now on medication regimens (usually at least three drugs) and must adhere to the dosages and schedules, which may be difficult and/or cause side effects that tempt the patient to alter or discontinue them without notifying the physician.
Stress necessity of regular follow-up care and evaluations including routine CD4 and HIV-RNA viral load counts, and any change in medication regimen (time, frequency, side effects).	Even though patient may be asymptomatic, periodic evaluation may prevent development of complications, slow the progression of the disease, and assist with treatment decisions. *Note:* Patients who change medication dosage/frequency in response to side effects can create problems for medication adjustment later with increased viral load and resistance to drugs.
Discuss need for regular gynecologic examinations and/or pregnancy considerations.	HIV-positive women experience a high prevalence of Pap smear, vaginal, and cervical abnormalities. Pregnancy counseling should include review of risk and prophylaxis against perinatal transmission. *Note:* Recent research shows that when antiretroviral treatment is initiated early in pregnancy the neonatal transmission rate has dropped to less than 8% of live births.
Discuss management strategies for persistent signs/symptoms.	Patient involvement in care increases cooperation and satisfaction with care.

ACTIONS/INTERVENTIONS	RATIONALE

Independent

Review drug therapies, including correct dosing/scheduling; side effects, and adverse reactions as appropriate:

These drugs interfere with the HIV replication process, and early treatment may be considered when CD4 count is near 500, even if individual is asymptomatic. Side effects such as symptoms of peripheral neuropathy or pancreatitis necessitate prompt evaluation and possible discontinuation/change in therapy.

Antiretrovirals, e.g.:

Currently, 12 antiretroviral agents have been approved by the Food and Drug Administration (FDA), all aimed at blocking replication of the HIV virus at some level. The drugs are generally given in groups of three because the multidrug regimen is more effective in reducing the viral load.

Zidovudine (ZVD/formerly AZT, Retrovir), didanosine (Dideoxyinosine, ddI, Videx), zalcitabine (ddC, Hivid), stavudine (d4T, Zerit), lamivudine (3TC, Epivir);

These drugs are called nucleoside reverse transcriptase inhibitors (NRTIs). In the past, zidovudine was given alone and as a first-line treatment. Now the drug is usually given in a three-drug treatment regimen, along with another NRTI and a protease inhibitor. Zidovudine is, however, safe in preventing perinatal HIV infection, so it is an option for the pregnant patient.

Protease inhibitors, e.g., indinavir (Crixivan), relfinavir (Viracept), ritonavir (Norvir), saquinavir (Fortovase, Invirase);

When combined with NRTIs, protease inhibitors control the HIV-RNA viral load by blocking viral replication at two different target sites in the replication process. Immune function is maintained with early intervention or improved when initiated later.

Nonnucleoside reverse transcriptase inhibitors (NNRTIs), e.g., delavirdine (Rescriptor), hevirapine (Viramune), efavirenz (Sustiva);

These drugs apparently inhibit viral replication by a different mechanism than NRTIs. They also are used in combination because using them alone seems to encourage drug resistance.

Anti-infectives, e.g., trimethoprim-sulfamethoxazole (TMP/SMX, Bactrim, Septra), azithromycin (Zithromax), clarithromycin (Biaxin) foscarnet (Foscavir), rifabutin (Mycobutin), isoniazid (INH), pyridoxine (Doxine).

Focus on prevention of commonly occurring opportunistic infections, such as *Pneumocystis carinii* pneumonia (PCP), CMV, *Mycobacterium avium* complex (MAC), TB may prolong general wellness. Primary prophylactic therapy aims to prevent or delay onset of symptoms of reactivated or newly acquired infection. The goal of secondary prophylaxis is to prevent or delay recurrent episodes of particular infection. Prophylaxis continues indefinitely as long as the drug is tolerated.

Assess potential for inappropriate/high-risk behavior, continued injection drug abuse, unsafe sexual practices.

High denial/anger, drug addition may cause patient to continue behaviors that are high risk for spread of the virus. A person's sexual expression and identity are threatened by the discovery of the diagnosis. *Note:* Recent research suggests approximately 40% of individuals with HIV may not reveal status to potential sexual partners.

Recommend exploring drug treatment resources, e.g., methadone clinics or substance abuse recovery groups or programs.

Programs could help reduce HIV transmission by reducing injection drug use when patient substitutes or recovers from drug use.

ACTIONS/INTERVENTIONS	RATIONALE

Independent

Stress necessity of practicing safe sex at all times; also stress need to avoid use of illicit injected drugs or, if unwilling to abstain, to avoid sharing needles and to clean works with bleach solution, rinsing carefully with water.

Limits spread of virus and reduces exposure to other infective agents/additional stress to the immune system.

Discuss active changes in sexual behaviors that the patient can make that may satisfy sexual needs.

Promotes a sense of responsibility and control, may reduce sexual tensions/promote normalcy in sexual relationships, and is designed to prevent transmission.

Provide information about other necessary lifestyle changes and health maintenance factors:

Evidence suggests that specific dietary and lifestyle factors may slow the progression of HIV infection because they support a more healthy immune system.

   Avoid people with infections;

   When the immune system is depressed, the person's ability to fight exposure to common communicable diseases is limited.

   Exercise within ability, alternate rest periods with activity, and get adequate sleep;

   Helps manage fatigue; maintains strength and sense of well-being. Exercise has also been shown to stimulate the immune system.

   Eat regularly, even if appetite is reduced; try small, frequent meals and snacks;

   Physical and psychological stressors increase metabolic needs, in addition, side effects of medication, presence of nausea/vomiting, and anorexia often limit oral intake. The result is nutritional deficits that can further impair the immune system.

   Practice daily oral hygiene, use a soft toothbrush; examine mouth regularly for sores, white film, or changes in color; have regular dental checkups every 6 mo;

   Poor oral hygiene/dental care can affect oral intake adversely and increase the risk of opportunistic/systemic infections.

   Examine skin for rashes, bruises, breaks in skin integrity.

   May indicate developing complications/increase risk of infection.

Provide written information—a few pieces at each visit.

Patient may feel overwhelmed, and written materials allow for later review and reinforcement when patient has an opportunity to absorb information.

Encourage contact with significant other, family, and friends. Include in discussions/conferences as appropriate.

Many patients fear telling SO, family, and friends for fear of rejection; and some patients withdraw as a result of tumultuous feelings. Contact promotes sense of support, concern, involvement, and understanding. Supporting loved ones as they learn of the diagnosis is beneficial and can provide optimism for the long-term.

Identify additional resources, e.g.:

   Support groups, peer counselors, and mental health professionals;

   Patient will experience a variety of emotional and psychological responses to the diagnosis and its consequences and may need additional assistance to promote optimal adjustment.

   Case managers.

   In early stages of HIV infection, focus may be on social services (e.g., help with housing, employment, legal issues, finances). Later, as disease progresses, the emphasis switches to medical and related community services.

ACTIONS/INTERVENTIONS

Independent

Provide information about clinical trials available as individually appropriate.

RATIONALE

Scientific research required HIV-positive test subjects. Participation may provide individual with a sense of contributing to body of knowledge/search for cure, in addition to no-cost monitoring and medications for those with limited financial resources.

NURSING DIAGNOSIS: Social Isolation, risk for

Risk factors may include:
Altered state of wellness, changes in physical appearance
Perceptions of unacceptable social or sexual behavior/values
Inadequate/fear of losing personal resources

Possibly evidenced by:
[Not applicable; presence of signs and symptoms establishes an *actual* diagnosis]

DESIRED OUTCOMES/EVALUATION CRITERIA— PATIENT WILL:

> **Social Support (NOC)**

Identify stable support system/individual(s).
Use resources for assistance as appropriate.
Express increased sense of self-esteem.

ACTIONS/INTERVENTIONS

> **Support System Enhancement (NIC)**

Independent

Determine patient's response to condition and concerns/fears about response of others.

Assess patient's feelings about self, sense of ability to control situation, sense of hope, and coping skills.

Discuss concerns/regarding employment/leisure involvement. Note potential problems involving finances, insurance, housing.

Identify availability/stability of support systems including SO, immediate/extended family, community.

Encourage honesty in relationships as appropriate.

Assist patient to problem-solve solutions to short-term/imposed isolations (e.g., communicable disease measures, including compromised host).

Help patient differentiate between isolation and loneliness/aloneness, which may be by choice.

RATIONALE

How the individual accepts and deals with the situation will help decide the plan of care and interventions.

Information is essential to planning individualized care.

Patients with this potentially terminal illness that carries a stigma, face major problems with possible loss of employment, medical insurance, housing, and care if they become unable to care for themselves.

Crucial information to help patient plan future care.

As a rule, acquaintances do not need to be informed of patient's health status. However, information should be shared with close relationships (e.g., SO, family, sexual partners). Honesty can help identify stable support persons.

Anticipatory planning can defuse sense of isolation and loneliness that can accompany this situation.

Provides an opportunity for the patient to realize the control he/she has to make decisions about the choice to take care of self in regard to these issues.

ACTIONS/INTERVENTIONS	RATIONALE
Independent	
Be alert to verbal/nonverbal cues, e.g., withdrawal statements of despair, sense of aloneness. Determine presence/level of risk of suicidal thoughts.	Indicators of despair and suicidal ideation may be present. When these cues are acknowledged, the patient is usually willing to divulge thoughts and sense of isolation/hopelessness.
Collaborative	
Identify community resources, self-help group, rehabilitation/drug cessation program as indicated.	Provides opportunities for resolving problems that may contribute to sense of loneliness and isolation.
Refer to psychiatric nurse clinical specialist/psychiatrist as needed.	May require more in-depth support to deal with feelings, manage difficult situation.

POTENTIAL ONGOING CONSIDERATIONS (dependent on patient's age, physical condition/presence of complications, person resources, and life responsibilities)

Fatigue—decreased metabolic energy production, increased energy requirements (hypermetabolic state).

Nutrition: altered, less than body requirements—increased metabolic demands/energy requirements, side effects of medication, anorexia, fatigue.

Decisional Conflict—unclear personal values/beliefs, perceived threat to value system, multiple or divergent sources of information, support system deficit, interference with decision making.

Infection, risk for—depression of immune system, chronic disease, malnutrition, use of antimicrobial agents.

AIDS

Acquired immunodeficiency syndrome (AIDS) is the final result of infection with a retrovirus, the human immunodeficiency virus (HIV). An HIV infection has five stages. During stage 5 the patient has an AIDS-defining condition. As defined by the CDC (January 1994) "persons with CD4 cell count of under 200 (with or without symptoms of opportunistic infection) who are HIV-positive are diagnosed as having AIDS." Research studies in 1995 showed that the HIV virus initially replicates rapidly on a daily basis. The half-life of the virus is 2 days, with almost complete turnover in 14 days. Therefore, the immune response is massive throughout the course of HIV disease and pathogenesis is due to destruction of CD4 cells, not a lack of production of new lymphocytes. Controlling the replication of the virus to lower the viral load is the current focus of treatment.

Persons with AIDS have been found to fall into five general categories: (1) homosexual or bisexual men, (2) injection drug users, (3) recipients of infected blood or blood products, (4) heterosexual partners of a person with HIV infection, and (5) children born to an infected mother. The rate of infection is most rapidly increasing among minority women.

CARE SETTING

Although many of the interventions listed here are appropriate at the community level, the focus of this plan of care is the acutely ill individual requiring care on an inpatient medical or subacute unit or hospice setting.

RELATED FACTORS:

Fluid and electrolyte imbalances, page 926
Extended care, page 850
HIV-Positive patient, page 753
Psychosocial aspects of care, page 809
Sepsis/Septicemia, page 741
Total nutritional support: parenteral/enteral feeding, page 508
Upper gastrointestinal/Esophageal bleeding, page 333
Ventilatory assistance (mechanical), page 188

Patient Assessment Database

Data depends on the organs/body tissues involved and the specific opportunistic infection (OI) or cancer.

ACTIVITY/REST

May report:	Reduced tolerance for usual activities, progressing to profound fatigue and malaise; weakness
	Altered sleep patterns
May exhibit:	Muscle weakness, wasting of muscle mass
	Physiological response to activity, e.g., changes in BP, HR, respiration

CIRCULATION

May report:	Slow healing (if anemic); bleeding longer with injury
May exhibit:	Tachycardia, postural BP changes
	Decreased peripheral pulse volume
	Pallor or cyanosis; delayed capillary refill

EGO INTEGRITY

May report:	Stress factors related to lifestyle changes, losses, e.g., family support, relationships, finances, and spiritual concerns
	Concern about appearance: alopecia, disfiguring lesions, weight loss, altered distribution of body fat (associated with protease-inhibiting drug therapy)
	Denial of diagnosis, feelings of powerlessness, hopelessness, helplessness, worthlessness, guilt, loss of control, depression
May exhibit:	Denial, anxiety, depression, fear, withdrawal
	Angry behaviors, dejected body posture, crying, poor eye contact
	Failure to keep appointments or multiple appointments for similar symptoms

ELIMINATION

May report: Difficult and painful elimination; rectal pain, itching
Intermittent, persistent, frequent diarrhea with or without abdominal cramping
Flank pain, burning on urination

May exhibit: Loose-formed to watery stools with or without mucus or blood; frequent, copious diarrhea
Abdominal tenderness
Rectal, perianal lesions or abscesses
Changes in urinary output, color, character
Urinary, bowel incontinence

FOOD/FLUID

May report: Anorexia, changes in taste of foods/food intolerance, nausea/vomiting
Rapid/progressive weight loss
Difficulty chewing and swallowing (sore mouth, tongue); dysphagia, retrosternal pain with swallowing
Food intolerance, e.g., diarrhea after dairy products, nausea, early satiation, bloating

May exhibit: Hyperactive bowel sounds
Abdominal distension (hepatosplenomegaly)
Weight loss; thin frame; decreased subcutaneous fat/muscle mass
Poor skin turgor
Lesions of the oral cavity, white patches, discoloration; poor dental/gum health, loss of teeth
Edema (generalized, dependent)

HYGIENE

May report: Inability to complete activities of daily living (ADLs) independently

May exhibit: Disheveled appearance
Deficits in many or all personal care, self-care activities

NEUROSENSORY

May report: Fainting spells/dizziness; headache; stiff neck
Changes in mental status, loss of mental acuity/ability to solve problems, forgetfulness, poor concentration
Impaired sensation or sense of position and vibration
Muscle weakness, tremors, changes in visual acuity
Numbness, tingling in extremities (feet seem to display earliest changes)
Changes in visual acuity; light flashes/floaters; photophobia

May exhibit: Mental status changes ranging from confusion to dementia, forgetfulness, poor concentration, decreased alertness, apathy, psychomotor retardation/slowed responses; paranoid ideation, free-floating anxiety, unrealistic expectations
Abnormal reflexes, decreased muscle strength, ataxic gait
Fine/gross motor tremors, focal motor deficits; hemiparesis, seizures
Retinal hemorrhages and exudates (CMV retinitis); blindness

PAIN/DISCOMFORT

May report: Generalized/localized pain; aching, burning in feet
Headache
Pleuritic chest pain

May exhibit: Swelling of joints, painful nodules, tenderness
Decreased range of motion (ROM), gait changes/limp
Muscle guarding

RESPIRATION

May report: Frequent, persistent upper respiratory infections (URIs)
Progressive shortness of breath
Cough (ranging from mild to severe); nonproductive/productive of sputum (earliest sign of PCP may be a spasmodic cough on deep breathing)

Congestion or tightness in chest

History of exposure to/prior episode of active TB

May exhibit: Tachypnea, respiratory distress

Changes in breath sounds/adventitious breath sounds

Sputum yellow (in sputum-producing pneumonia)

SAFETY

May report: Exposure to infectious diseases, e.g., TB, STDs

History of other immune deficiency diseases, e.g., rheumatoid arthritis, cancer

History of frequent or multiple blood/blood product transfusions (e.g., hemophilia, major vascular surgery, traumatic incident)

History of falls, burns, episodes of fainting, slow-healing wounds

Suicidal/homicidal ideation with or without a plan

May exhibit: Recurrent fevers; low-grade, intermittent temperature elevations/spikes; night sweats

Changes in skin integrity, e.g., cuts, ulcerations, rashes (eczema, exanthems, psoriasis); discolorations; changes in size/color of moles; unexplained, easy bruising; multiple injection scars (may be infected)

Rectal, perianal lesions or abscesses

Nodules, enlarged lymph nodes in two or more areas of the body (e.g., neck, axilla, groin)

Decline in general strength, muscle tone, changes in gait

SEXUALITY

May report: History of high-risk behavior, e.g., having sex with a partner who is HIV-positive, multiple sexual partners, unprotected sexual activity, and anal sex

Loss of libido, being too sick for sex; being afraid to engage in any sexual activities

Inconsistent use of condoms

Use of birth control pills (enhanced susceptibility to virus in women who are exposed because of increased vaginal dryness/friability)

May exhibit: Pregnancy or risk for pregnancy (sexually active); pregnancy resulting in HIV-positive infant

Genitalia: Skin manifestations (e.g., herpes, warts); discharge

SOCIAL INTERACTION

May report: Problems related to diagnosis and treatment, e.g., loss of family/SO, friends, support; fear of telling others; fear of rejection/loss of income

Isolation, loneliness, close friends or sexual partners who have died of or are sick with AIDS

Questioning of ability to remain independent, unable to plan for needs

May exhibit: Changes in family/SO interaction pattern

Disorganized activities, difficulty with goal setting

TEACHING/LEARNING

May report: Failure to comply with treatment, continued high-risk behavior (e.g., unchanged sexual behavior or injection drug use)

Injection drug use/abuse, current smoking, alcohol abuse

Evidence of failure to improve from last hospitalization

Discharge plan considerations: **DRG projected mean length of stay: 8.2 days (depending on opportunistic infection[s] present)**

May require assistance with finances, medications and treatments, skin/wound care, equipment/supplies; transportation, food shopping and preparation; self-care, technical nursing procedures, homemaker/maintenance tasks, child care; changes in living facilities

Refer to section at end of plan for postdischarge considerations.

DIAGNOSTIC STUDIES

CBC: Anemia and idiopathic thrombocytopenia (anemia occurs in up to 85% of patients with AIDS and may be profound). Leukopenia may be present; differential shift to the left suggests infectious process (PCP), although shift to the right may be noted.

PPD with anergy panel: Determines exposure and/or active disease (anergy panel identifies false-negative result due to deficient immune response). Of AIDS patients, 100% of those exposed to active *Mycobacterium tuberculosis* will develop the disease.

Serologic: Serum antibody test: HIV screen by ELISA. A positive test result may be indicative of exposure to HIV but is not diagnostic because false positives may occur.

Western blot test: Confirms diagnosis of HIV in blood and urine.

HIV-RNA: The most widely used test currently can detect viral RNA levels as low as 500 copies/mL of plasma. A more sensitive test that can detect HIV-RNA levels as low as 50 copies/mL is expected to become the standard test for viral load in the near future.

T-lymphocyte cells: Total count reduced.

CD4 lymphocyte count (immune system indicator that mediates several immune system processes and signals B cells to produce antibodies to foreign germs): Numbers less than 200 indicate severe immune deficiency response and diagnosis of AIDS.

T8 (cytopathic suppressor cells): Reversed ratio (2:1 or greater) of suppressor cells to helper cells (T8 to T4) indicates immune suppression.

Polymerase chain reaction (PCR) test: Detects HIV-DNA; most helpful in testing newborns of HIV-infected mothers. Infants carry maternal HIV antibodies and therefore test positive by ELISA and Western blot, even though infant is not necessarily infected.

STD screening tests: Hepatitis B envelope and core antibodies, syphilis, and other common STDs may be positive.

Cultures: Histologic, cytologic studies of urine, blood, stool, spinal fluid, lesions, sputum, and secretions may be done to identify the opportunistic infection. Some of the most commonly identified are the following:

> *Protozoal and helminthic infections:* PCP, cryptosporidiosis, toxoplasmosis.
>
> *Fungal infections: Candida albicans* (candidiasis), *Cryptococcus neoformans* (cryptococcosis); *Histoplasma capsulatum* (histoplasmosis).
>
> *Bacterial infections: Mycobacterium avium-intracellulare* (occurs with CD4 counts less than 50), miliary mycobacterial TB, *Shigella* (shigellosis), *Salmonella* (salmonellosis).
>
> *Viral infections:* CMV (occurs with CD4 counts less than 50), herpes simplex, herpes zoster.

Neurologic studies, e.g., electroencephalogram (EEG), magnetic resonance imaging (MRI), computed tomography (CT) scans of the brain; electromyography (EMG)/nerve conduction studies: Indicated for changes in mentation, fever of undetermined origin, and/or changes in sensory/motor function to determine effects of HIV infection/opportunistic infections.

Chest x-ray: May initially be normal or may reveal progressive interstitial infiltrates secondary to advancing PCP (most common opportunistic disease) or other pulmonary complications/disease processes such as TB.

Pulmonary function tests: Useful in early detection of interstitial pneumonias.

Gallium scan: Diffuse pulmonary uptake occurs in PCP and other forms of pneumonia.

Biopsies: May be done for differential diagnosis of Kaposi's sarcoma (KS) or other neoplastic lesions.

Bronchoscopy/tracheobronchial washings: May be done with biopsy when PCP or lung malignancies are suspected (diagnostic confirming test for PCP).

Barium swallow, endoscopy, colonoscopy: May be done to identify opportunistic infection (e.g., *Candida*, CMV) or to stage KS in the GI system.

NURSING PRIORITIES

1. Prevent/minimize infections.
2. Maintain homeostasis.
3. Promote comfort.
4. Support psychosocial adjustment.
5. Provide information about disease process/prognosis and treatment needs.

DISCHARGE GOALS

1. Infection prevented/resolved.
2. Complications prevented/minimized.
3. Pain/discomfort alleviated.
4. Patient dealing with current situation realistically.
5. Diagnosis, prognosis, and therapeutic regimen understood.
6. Plan in place to meet needs after discharge.

> **NURSING DIAGNOSIS: Infection, risk for [progression to sepsis/onset of new opportunistic infection]**
>
> **Risk factors may include**
>
> Inadequate primary defenses: broken skin, traumatized tissue, stasis of body fluids
>
> Depression of the immune system, chronic disease, malnutrition; use of antimicrobial agents
>
> Environmental exposure, invasive techniques
>
> **Possibly evidenced by**
>
> [Not applicable; presence of signs and symptoms establishes an *actual* diagnosis]
>
> **DESIRED OUTCOMES/EVALUATION CRITERIA—PATIENT WILL:**
>
> | **Infection Status (NOC)** |
>
> Achieve timely healing of wounds/lesions.
>
> Be afebrile and free of purulent drainage/secretions and other signs of infectious conditions.
>
> | **Risk Control (NOC)** |
>
> Identify/participate in behaviors to reduce risk of infection.

ACTIONS/INTERVENTIONS	RATIONALE
Infection Control (NIC)	
Independent	
Assess patient knowledge and ability to maintain opportunistic infection prophylactic regimen.	Multiple medication regimen is difficult to maintain over a long period of time. Patients may adjust medication regimen based on side effects experienced, contributing to inadequate prophylaxis, active disease, and resistance.
Wash hands before and after all care contacts. Instruct patient/SO to wash hands as indicated.	Reduces risk of cross-contamination.
Provide a clean, well-ventilated environment. Screen visitors/staff for signs of infection and maintain isolation precautions as indicated.	Reduces number of pathogens presented to the immune system and reduces possibility of patient contracting a nosocomial infection.
Discuss extent and rationale for isolation precautions and maintenance of personal hygiene.	Promotes cooperation with regimen and may lessen feelings of isolation.
Monitor vital signs, including temperature.	Provides information for baseline data; frequent temperature elevations/onset of new fever indicates that the body is responding to a new infectious process or that medications are not effectively controlling noncurable infections.
Assess respiratory rate/depth; note dry spasmodic cough on deep inspiration, changes in characteristics of sputum, and presence of wheezes/rhonchi. Initiate respiratory isolation when etiology of productive cough is unknown.	Respiratory congestion/distress may indicate developing PCP (the most common opportunistic disease); however, TB is on the rise and other fungal, viral, and bacterial infections may occur that compromise the respiratory system. *Note:* CMV and PCP can reside together in the lungs and, if treatment is not effective for PCP, the addition of CMV therapy may be effective.

ACTIONS/INTERVENTIONS	RATIONALE
Independent	

Independent

Investigate reports of headache, stiff neck, altered vision. Note changes in mentation and behavior. Monitor for nuchal rigidity/seizure activity.

Neurological abnormalities are common and may be related to HIV or secondary infections. Symptoms may vary from subtle changes in mood/sensorium (personality changes or depression) to hallucinations, memory loss, severe dementias, seizures, and loss of vision. CNS infections (encephalitis is the most common) may be caused by protozoal and helminthic organisms or fungus.

Examine skin/oral mucous membranes for white patches or lesions. (Refer to ND: Skin Integrity, impaired, actual and/or risk for, p. 779, and ND: Oral Mucous Membrane, altered, p. 780.)

Oral candidiasis, KS, herpes, CMV, and cryptococcosis are common opportunistic diseases affecting the cutaneous membranes.

Clean patient's nails frequently. File, rather than cut, and avoid trimming cuticles.

Reduces risk of transmission of pathogens through breaks in skin. *Note:* Fungal infections along the nail plate are common.

Monitor reports of heartburn, dysphagia, retrosternal pain on swallowing, increased abdominal cramping, profuse diarrhea.

Esophagitis may occur secondary to oral candidiasis, CMV, or herpes. Cryptosporidiosis is a parasitic infection responsible for watery diarrhea (often greater than 15L/day).

Inspect wounds/site of invasive devices, noting signs of local inflammation/infection.

Early identification/treatment of secondary infection may prevent sepsis.

Wear gloves and gowns during direct contact with secretions/excretions or any time there is a break in skin of caregiver's hands. Wear mask and protective eyewear to protect nose, mouth, and eyes from secretions during procedures (e.g., suctioning) or when splattering of blood may occur.

Use of masks, gowns, and gloves is required by Occupational Safety and Health Administration (OSHA, 1992) for direct contact with body fluids, e.g., sputum, blood/blood products, semen, vaginal secretions.

Dispose of needles/sharps in rigid, puncture-resistant containers.

Prevents accidental inoculation of caregivers. Use of needle cutters and recapping is not to be practiced. *Note:* Accidental needle sticks should be reported immediately, with follow-up evaluations done per protocol.

Label blood bags, body fluid containers, soiled dressings/linens, and package appropriately for disposal per isolation protocol.

Prevents cross-contamination and alerts appropriate personnel/departments to exercise specific hazardous materials procedures.

Clean up spills of body fluids/blood with bleach solution (1:10); add bleach to laundry.

Kills HIV and controls other microorganisms on surfaces.

Collaborative

Monitor laboratory studies, e.g.:

CBC/differential;

Shifts in the differential and changes in WBC count indicate infectious process. Low WBC count or other changes in blood count may be related to treatments/medications.

Culture/sensitivity studies of lesions, blood, urine, and sputum.

May be done to diagnose complications and/or monitor effectiveness of medications.

Administer medications as indicated:

Antiretrovirals, e.g.:

Currently, 12 antiretroviral agents have been approved by the FDA; all are aimed at blocking replication of the HIV virus at some level. The drugs are generally given in groups of three because the multidrug regimen is more effective in reducing the viral load.

ACTIONS/INTERVENTIONS

Collaborative

Nucleoside reverse transcriptase inhibitors: zidovudine (ZVD/formerly AZT, Retrovir), didanosine (Dideoxyinosine ddI, Videx), zalcitabine (ddC, Hivid), stavudine (d4T, Zerit), lamivudine (3TC, Epivir);

Protease inhibitors, e.g., indinavir (Crixivan), relfinavir (Viracept), ritonavir (Norvir), saquinavir (Fortovase, Invirase);

Nonnucleoside reverse transcriptase inhibitors, e.g.: delavirdine (Rescriptor), hevirapine (Viramune), efavirenz (Sustiva);

Anti-infectives/prophylaxis, e.g., trimethoprim (TMP/SMX, Bactrim, Septra), nystatin (Mycostatin), ketoconazole (Nizoral), pentamidine (Pentam, Nebu-Pent), azithromycin (Zithromax), clarithromycin (Biaxin), rifabutin (Mycobutin), ganciclovir (Cytovene), foscarnet (Foscavir).

RATIONALE

These drugs are NRTIs. In the past zidovudine was given alone and as a first-line treatment. Now the drug is usually given in a three-drug treatment regimen along with another NRTI and a protease inhibitor. Zidovudine is, however, safe in preventing perinatal HIV infection so it is an option for the pregnant patient.

When combined with NRTIs, protease inhibitors, effectively control the HIV-RNA viral load by blocking viral replication at two different target sites in the replication process. Immune function is maintained with early intervention, or improved when initiated later.

NNRTIs apparently inhibit viral replication by a different mechanism than NRTIs. They also are used in combination because using them alone seems to encourage drug resistance.

Managing opportunistic infections now includes prophylaxis to combat illnesses associated with them. For example, TMP/SMX is given to prevent PCP (pneumonia); Biaxin and Zithromax are recommended for prevention of MAC. Cytovene is used to prevent blindness/life-threatening dissemination of CMV. Foscavir can also be used to prevent CMV progression, but should be used with caution because it may cause renal toxicity.

NURSING DIAGNOSIS: Fluid Volume, risk for deficit

Risk factors may include
Excessive losses: copious diarrhea, profuse sweating, vomiting
Hypermetabolic state, fever
Restricted intake: nausea, anorexia; lethargy

Possibly evidenced by
[Not applicable; presence of signs and symptoms establishes an *actual* diagnosis]

DESIRED OUTCOMES/EVALUATION CRITERIA—PATIENT WILL:

Hydration (NOC)

Maintain hydration as evidenced by moist mucous membranes, good skin turgor, stable vital signs, individually adequate urinary output.

ACTIONS/INTERVENTIONS

Fluid Management (NIC)

Independent

Monitor vital signs, including CVP if available. Note hypotension, including postural changes.

RATIONALE

Indicators of circulating fluid volume.

ACTIONS/INTERVENTIONS	RATIONALE

Independent

Note temperature elevation and duration of febrile episode. Administer tepid sponge baths as indicated. Keep clothing and linens dry. Maintain comfortable environmental temperature.

Fever is one of the most frequent symptoms experienced by patients with HIV infections (97%). Increased metabolic demands and associated excessive diaphoresis result in increased insensible fluid losses and dehydration.

Assess skin turgor, mucous membranes, and thirst.

Indirect indicators of fluid status.

Measure urinary output and specific gravity. Measure/estimate amount of diarrheal loss. Note insensible losses.

Increased specific gravity/decreasing urinary output reflects altered renal perfusion/circulating volume. *Note:* Monitoring fluid balance is difficult because of excessive GI/insensible losses.

Weigh as indicated.

Although weight loss may reflect muscle wasting, sudden fluctuations reflect state of hydration. Fluid losses associated with diarrhea can quickly create a crisis and become life-threatening.

Monitor oral intake and encourage fluids of at least 2500 mL/day.

Maintains fluid balance, reduces thirst, and keeps mucous membranes moist.

Make fluids easily accessible to patient; use fluids that are tolerable to the patient and that replace needed electrolytes, e.g., Gatorade, broth.

Enhances intake. Certain fluids may be too painful to consume (e.g., acidic juices) because of mouth lesions.

Eliminate foods potentiating diarrhea, e.g., spicy/high-fat foods, nuts, cabbage, milk products. Provide lactose-free supplements/products (Resource, Advera). Adjust rate/concentration of tube feedings if indicated.

May help reduce diarrhea. Use of lactose-free products helps control diarrhea in the lactose-intolerant patient.

Collaborative

Administer fluids/electrolytes via feeding tube/IV, as appropriate.

May be necessary to support/augment circulating volume, especially if oral intake is inadequate, nausea/vomiting persists.

Monitor laboratory studies as indicated, e.g.:

Hct;

Useful in estimating fluid needs.

Serum/urine electrolytes;

Alerts to possible electrolyte disturbances and determines replacement needs.

BUN/Cr.

Evaluates renal perfusion/function.

Administer medications as indicated:

Antiemetics, e.g., prochlorperazine maleate (Compazine), trimethobenzamide (Tigan), metoclopramide (Reglan);

Reduces incidence of vomiting to reduce further loss of fluids/electrolytes.

Antidiarrheals, e.g., diphenoxylate (Lomotil), loperamide (Imodium), paregoric, or antispasmodics, e.g., mepenzolate bromide (Cantil);

Decreases the amount and fluidity of stool; may reduce intestinal spasm and peristalsis. *Note:* Antibiotics may also be used to treat diarrhea if caused by infection.

Antipyretics, e.g., acetaminophen (Tylenol).

Helps reduce fever and hypermetabolic response, decreasing insensible losses. *Note:* Recent studies caution that acetaminophen (Tylenol) toxicity can occur more frequently in the patient with AIDS so needs to be used with caution.

Maintain hypothermia blanket if used.

May be necessary when other measures fail to reduce excessive fever/insensible fluid losses.

NURSING DIAGNOSIS: Breathing Pattern, ineffective/Gas Exchange, risk for impaired

Risk factors may include

Muscular impairment (wasting of respiratory musculature), decreased energy/fatigue, decreased lung expansion

Retained secretions (tracheobronchial obstruction), infectious/inflammatory process; pain

Ventilation perfusion imbalance (PCP/other pneumonias, anemia)

Possibly evidenced by

[Not applicable; presence of signs and symptoms establishes an *actual* diagnosis]

DESIRED OUTCOMES/EVALUATION CRITERIA—PATIENT WILL:

Respiratory Status: Ventilation or Gas Exchange (NOC)

Maintain effective respiratory pattern.

Experience no dyspnea/cyanosis, with breath sounds and chest x-ray clear/improving and ABGs within patient's normal range.

ACTIONS/INTERVENTIONS	RATIONALE
Respiratory Monitoring (NIC)	
Independent	
Auscultate breath sounds, noting areas of decreased/absent ventilation and presence of adventitious sounds, e.g., crackles, wheezes, rhonchi.	Suggests developing pulmonary complications/infection, e.g., atelectasis/pneumonia. *Note:* PCP is often advanced before changes in breath sounds occur.
Note rate/depth of respiration, use of accessory muscles, increased work of breathing, and presence of dyspnea, anxiety, cyanosis.	Tachypnea, cyanosis, restlessness, and increased work of breathing reflect respiratory distress and need for increased surveillance/medical intervention.
Assess changes in level of consciousness.	Hypoxemia can result in changes ranging from anxiety and confusion to unresponsiveness.
Investigate reports of chest pain.	Pleuritic chest pain may reflect nonspecific pneumonitis or pleural effusions associated with malignancies.
Ventilation Assistance (NIC)	
Elevate head of bed. Have patient turn, cough, deep-breathe, as indicated.	Promotes optimal pulmonary function and reduces incidence of aspiration or infection due to atelectasis.
Suction airway as indicated, using sterile technique and observing safety precautions, e.g., mask, protective eyewear.	Assists in clearing the ventilatory passages, thereby facilitating gas exchange and preventing respiratory complications.
Allow adequate rest periods between care activities. Maintain a quiet environment.	Reduces oxygen consumption.
Collaborative	
Monitor/graph serial ABGs or pulse oximetry.	Indicators of respiratory status, treatment needs/effectiveness.
Review serial chest x-rays.	Presence of diffuse infiltrates may suggest pneumonia, while areas of congestion/consolidation may reflect other pulmonary complications, e.g., atelectasis or KS lesions.

ACTIONS/INTERVENTIONS

Collaborative

Assist with/instruct in use of incentive spirometer. Provide chest physiotherapy, e.g., percussion, vibration, and postural drainage.

Provide humidified supplemental O_2 via approximate means, e.g., cannula, mask, intubation/mechanical ventilation.

Administer medications as indicated:

Antimicrobials, e.g.: trimethoprim (Bactrim, Septra), pentamidine isethionate (Pentam);

Foscarnet (Foscavir), ganciclovir (Cytovene);

Clarithromycin (Biaxin), azithromycin (Zithromax), rifabutin (Mycobutin);

Bronchodilators, expectorants, cough depressants.

Prepare/assist with procedures as indicated, e.g., bronchoscopy.

RATIONALE

Encourages proper breathing technique and improves lung expansion. Loosens secretions, dislodges mucous plugs to promote airway clearance. *Note:* In the event of multiple skin lesions, chest physiotherapy may be discontinued.

Maintains effective ventilation/oxygenation to prevent/correct respiratory crisis.

Choice of therapy depends on individual situation/infecting organism(s).

Although Bactrim (TMP/SMX) is the drug of choice for PCP, Pentam can be used in combination or alone when treatment with Bactrim is unsuccessful or contraindicated. *Note:* Bactrim is also used prophylactically.

Effective for treatment of pulmonary CMV infections. *Note:* CMV often coexists with PCP.

First-line therapy for treatment of MAC, a common bacterial infection that frequently disseminates to other organ systems.

May be needed to improve/maintain airway patency or help clear secretions.

May be required to clear mucus plugs, obtain specimens for diagnosis (biopsies/lavage).

NURSING DIAGNOSIS: Injury, risk for (hemorrhage)

Risk factors may include
Abnormal blood profile: decreased vitamin K absorption, alteration in hepatic function, presence of autoimmune antiplatelet antibodies, malignancies (KS), and/or circulating endotoxins (sepsis)

Possibly evidenced by
[Not applicable; presence of signs and symptoms establishes an *actual* diagnosis]

DESIRED OUTCOMES/EVALUATION CRITERIA—PATIENT WILL:

Risk Control (NOC)

Display homeostasis as evidenced by absence of bleeding.

ACTIONS/INTERVENTIONS

Bleeding Reduction (NIC)

Independent

Avoid injections, rectal temperatures/rectal tubes. Administer rectal suppositories with caution.

RATIONALE

Protects patient from procedure-related causes of bleeding; i.e., insertion of thermometers, rectal tubes can damage or tear rectal mucosa. *Note:* Some medications need to be given via suppository, so caution is advised.

ACTIONS/INTERVENTIONS	RATIONALE

Independent

Maintain a safe environment; e.g., keep all necessary objects and call bell within patient's reach and keep bed in low position.

Reduces accidental injury, which could result in bleeding.

Maintain bedrest/chair rest when platelets are below 10,000 or as individually appropriate. Assess medication regimen.

Reduces possibility of injury, although activity needs to be maintained. May need to discontinue or reduce dosage of a drug. *Note:* Patient can have a surprisingly low platelet count without bleeding.

Bleeding Reduction (NIC)

Hematest body fluids, e.g., urine, stool, vomitus, for occult blood.

Prompt detection of bleeding/initiation of therapy may prevent critical hemorrhage.

Observe for/report epistaxis, hemoptysis, hematuria, nonmenstrual vaginal bleeding, or oozing from lesions/body orifices/IV insertion sites.

Spontaneous bleeding may indicate development of DIC or immune thrombocytopenia, necessitating further evaluation and prompt intervention.

Monitor for changes in vital signs and skin color, e.g., BP, pulse, respirations, skin pallor/discoloration.

Presence of bleeding/hemorrhage may lead to circulatory failure/shock.

Evaluate change in level of consciousness.

May reflect cerebral bleeding.

Collaborative

Review laboratory studies, e.g., PT, aPTT, clotting time, platelets, Hb/Hct.

Detects alterations in clotting capability; identifies therapy needs. *Note:* Many individuals (up to 80%) display platelet count below 50,000 and may be asymptomatic, necessitating regular monitoring.

Administer blood products as indicated.

Transfusions may be required in the event of persistent/massive spontaneous bleeding.

Avoid use of aspirin products/NSAIDs, especially in presence of gastric lesions.

These medications reduce platelet aggregation, impairing/prolonging the coagulation process, and may cause further gastric irritation, increasing risk of bleeding.

NURSING DIAGNOSIS: Nutrition: altered, less than body requirements

May be related to
Inability or altered ability to ingest, digest and/or metabolize nutrients: nausea/vomiting, hyperactive gag reflex, intestinal disturbances, GI tract infections, fatigue
Increased metabolic rate/nutritional needs (fever/infection)

Possibly evidenced by
Weight loss, decreased subcutaneous fat/muscle mass (wasting)
Lack of interest in food, aversion to eating, altered taste sensation
Abdominal cramping, hyperactive bowel sounds, diarrhea
Sore, inflamed buccal cavity
Abnormal laboratory results: Vitamin/mineral and protein deficiencies, electrolyte imbalances

DESIRED OUTCOMES/EVALUATION CRITERIA—PATIENT WILL:

Nutritional Status (NOC)

Maintain weight or display weight gain toward desired goal.
Demonstrate positive nitrogen balance, be free of signs of malnutrition, and display improved energy level.

ACTIONS/INTERVENTIONS	RATIONALE

Nutritional Monitoring (NIC)

Independent

Assess ability to chew, taste, and swallow.	Lesions of the mouth, throat, and esophagus (often caused by candidiasis, herpes simplex, hairy leukoplakia, KS and other cancers) and metallic or other taste changes caused by medications may cause dysphagia, limiting patient's ability to ingest food and reducing desire to eat.
Auscultate bowel sounds.	Hypermotility of intestinal tract is common and is associated with vomiting and diarrhea, which may affect choice of diet/route. *Note:* Lactose intolerance and malabsorption (e.g., with CMV, MAC, cryptosporidiosis) contribute to diarrhea and may necessitate change in diet/supplemental formula (e.g., Advera, Resource).
Weigh as indicated. Evaluate weight in terms of premorbid weight. Compare serial weights and anthropometric measurements.	Indicator of nutritional needs/adequacy of intake. *Note:* Because of immune suppression, some blood tests normally used for testing nutritional status are not useful.
Note drug side effects.	Prophylactic and therapeutic medications can have side effects affecting nutrition, e.g., ZVD (altered taste, nausea/vomiting), Bactrim (anorexia, glucose intolerance, glossitis), Pentam (altered taste and smell, nausea/vomiting, glucose intolerance), protease inhibitors (elevated lipids and blood sugar).

Nutritional Therapy (NIC)

Plan diet with patient/SO suggesting foods from home if appropriate. Provide small, frequent meals/snacks of nutritionally dense foods and nonacidic foods and beverages, with choice of foods palatable to patient. Encourage high-calorie/nutritious foods, some of which may be considered appetite stimulants. Note time of day when appetite is best, and try to serve larger meal at that time.	Including patient in planning gives sense of control of environment and may enhance intake. Fulfilling cravings for noninstitutional food may also improve intake. *Note:* In this population, foods with a higher fat content may be recommended as tolerated to enhance taste and oral intake.
Limit food(s) that induce nausea/vomiting or are poorly tolerated by the patient because of mouth sores/dysphagia. Avoid serving very hot liquids/foods. Serve foods that are easy to swallow, e.g., eggs, ice cream, cooked vegetables.	Pain in the mouth or fear of irritating oral lesions may cause the patient to be reluctant to eat. These measures may be helpful in increasing food intake.
Schedule medications between meals (if tolerated) and limit fluid intake with meals, unless fluid has nutritional value.	Gastric fullness diminishes appetite and food intake.
Encourage as much physical activity as possible.	May improve appetite and general feelings of well-being.
Provide frequent mouth care, observing secretion precautions. Avoid alcohol-containing mouthwashes.	Reduces discomfort associated with nausea/vomiting, oral lesions, mucosal dryness, and halitosis. Clean mouth may enhance appetite.
Provide rest period before meals. Avoid stressful procedures close to mealtime.	Minimizes fatigue; increases energy available for work of eating.
Remove existing noxious environmental stimuli or conditions that aggravate gag reflex.	Reduces stimulus of the vomiting center in the medulla.

ACTIONS/INTERVENTIONS

Independent

Encourage patient to sit up for meals.

Record ongoing caloric intake.

Collaborative

Review laboratory studies, e.g., BUN, glucose, liver function studies, electrolytes, protein, and albumin.

Maintain NPO status when appropriate.

Insert/maintain nasogastric (NG) tube as indicated.

Consult with dietitian/nutritional support team.

Administer enteral/parenteral feedings as indicated.

Administer medications as indicated:

Antiemetics, e.g., dronabinol (Marinol), megestrol (Megace);

Sucralfate (Carafate) suspension;

Vitamin supplements;

Appetite stimulants, e.g., oxandrolone (Oxandrin);

TNF-alpha inhibitors, e.g., thalidomide;

Antidiarrheals, e.g., octreotide (Sandostatin);

Antibiotic therapy, e.g., ketoconazole (Nizoral), fluconazole (Diflucan).

RATIONALE

Facilitates swallowing and reduces risk of aspiration.

Identifies need for supplements or alternate feeding methods.

Indicates nutritional status and organ function, and identifies replacement needs. *Note:* Nutritional tests can be altered because of disease processes and response to some medications/therapies.

May be needed to reduce vomiting.

May be needed to reduce nausea/vomiting or to administer tube feedings. *Note:* Esophageal irritation from existing infection (*Candida*, herpes, or KS) may provide site for secondary infections/trauma; therefore, tube should be used with caution.

Provides for diet based on individual needs/appropriate route.

Enteral feedings are preferred because they cost less and carry less risk of exacerbating endocrine dysfunction than TPN. However, TPN may be required when oral/enteral feedings are not tolerated. TPN is reserved for those whose gut cannot absorb even an elemental formula (such as Vivonex) or those with severe refractory diarrhea.

Reduces incidence of vomiting; promotes gastric function.

Given with meals to relieve mouth pain, enhance intake.

Corrects vitamin deficiencies resulting from decreased food intake and/or disorders of digestion and absorption in the GI system. *Note:* Avoid megadoses; suggested supplemental level is two times the recommended daily allowance (RDA).

Currently being studied in clinical trials to boost appetite and improve muscle mass and strength.

Reduces elevated levels of tumor necrosis factor (TNF) present in chronic illness contributing to wasting/cachexia. Studies reveal a mean weight gain of 10% over 28 weeks of therapy.

Effective treatment for secretory diarrhea (secretion of water and electrolytes by intestinal epithelium).

May be given to treat/prevent infections involving the GI tract.

> **NURSING DIAGNOSIS: Pain [acute]/chronic**
>
> **May be related to**
> Tissue inflammation/destruction: Infections, internal/external cutaneous lesions, rectal
>   excoriation, malignancies, necrosis
> Peripheral neuropathies, myalgias, and arthralgias
> Abdominal cramping
>
> **Possibly evidenced by**
> Reports of pain
> Self-focusing; narrowed focus, guarding behaviors
> Alteration in muscle tone; muscle cramping, ataxia, muscle weakness, paresthesias,
>   paralysis
> Autonomic responses; restlessness
>
> **DESIRED OUTCOMES/EVALUATION CRITERIA—PATIENT WILL:**
>
> **Pain Level (NOC)**
>
> Report pain relieved/controlled.
> Demonstrate relaxed posture/facial expression.
> Be able to sleep/rest appropriately.

ACTIONS/INTERVENTIONS

Pain Management (NIC)

Independent

Assess pain reports, noting location, intensity (0–10 scale), frequency, and time of onset. Note nonverbal cues, e.g., restlessness, tachycardia, grimacing.

Encourage verbalization of feelings.

Provide diversional activities, e.g., reading, visiting, radio/television.

Perform palliative measures, e.g., repositioning, massage, ROM of affected joints.

Instruct patient in/encourage use of visualization, guided imagery, progressive relaxation, deep-breathing techniques, meditation, and mindfulness.

Provide oral care. (Refer to ND: Oral Mucous Membrane, altered, p. 780.)

Apply warm/moist packs to pentamidine injection/IV sites for 20 min after administration.

Collaborative

Administer analgesics/antipyretics, narcotic analgesics. Use patient-controlled analgesia (PCA) or provide around-the-clock analgesia with rescue doses prn.

RATIONALE

Indicates need for/effectiveness of interventions and may signal development/resolution of complications. *Note:* Chronic pain does not produce autonomic changes; however, acute and chronic pain can coexist.

Can reduce anxiety and fear and thereby reduce perception of intensity of pain.

Refocuses attention; may enhance coping abilities.

Promotes relaxation/decreases muscle tension.

Promotes relaxation and feel of well-being. May decrease the need for narcotic analgesics (CNS depressants) when a neuro/motor degenerative process is already involved. May not be successful in presence of dementia, even when dementia is minor. *Note:* Mindfulness is the skill of staying in the here and now.

Oral ulcerations/lesions may cause severe discomfort.

These injections are known to cause pain and sterile abscesses.

Provides relief of pain/discomfort; reduces fever. PCA or around-the-clock medication keeps the blood level of analgesia stable, preventing cyclic undermedication or overmedication. *Note:* Drugs such as Ativan may be used to potentiate effects of analgesics.

NURSING DIAGNOSIS: Skin Integrity, impaired, actual and/or risk for

Risk factors may include

Decreased level of activity/immobility, altered sensation, skeletal prominence, changes in skin turgor

Malnutrition, altered metabolic state

May be related to (actual)

Immunologic deficit: AIDS-related dermatitis; viral, bacterial, and fungal infections (e.g., herpes, *Pseudomonas*, *Candida*); opportunistic disease processes (e.g., KS)

Excretions/Secretions

Possibly evidenced by

Skin lesions; ulcerations; decubitus ulcer formation

DESIRED OUTCOMES/EVALUATION CRITERIA—PATIENT WILL:

Risk Control (NOC)

Be free of/display improvement in wound/lesion healing.

Tissue Integrity: Skin & Mucous Membranes (NOC)

Demonstrate behaviors/techniques to prevent skin breakdown/promote healing.

ACTIONS/INTERVENTIONS	RATIONALE
Skin surveillance (NIC)	
Independent	
Assess skin daily. Note color, turgor, circulation, and sensation. Describe/measure lesions and observe changes.	Establishes baseline with which changes in status can be compared and appropriate interventions instituted.
Maintain/instruct in good skin hygiene, e.g., wash thoroughly, pat dry carefully, and gently massage with lotion or appropriate cream.	Maintaining clean, dry skin provides a barrier to infection. Patting skin dry instead of rubbing reduces risk of dermal trauma to dry/fragile skin. Massaging increases circulation to the skin and promotes comfort. *Note:* Isolation precautions are required, especially when extensive or open mucocutaneous lesions are present.
Reposition frequently. Use turn sheet as needed. Encourage periodic weight shifts. Protect bony prominences with pillows, heel/elbow pads, sheepskin.	Reduces stress on pressure points, improves blood flow to tissues, and promotes healing.
Maintain clean, dry, wrinkle-free linen.	Skin friction caused by wet or wrinkled sheets leads to irritation and potentiates infection.
Encourage ambulation/out of bed as tolerated.	Decreases pressure on skin from prolonged bedrest.
Cleanse perianal area by removing stool with water and mineral oil or commercial product. Avoid use of toilet paper if vesicles are present. Apply protective creams, e.g., zinc oxide, A & D ointment.	Prevents maceration caused by diarrhea and keeps perianal lesions dry. *Note:* Use of toilet paper may abrade lesions.
File nails regularly.	Long/rough nails increase risk of dermal damage.
Cover open pressure ulcers with sterile dressings or protective barrier, e.g., Tegaderm, DuoDerm, as indicated.	May reduce bacterial contamination, promote healing.
Collaborative	
Provide foam/flotation mattress or bed.	Reduces pressure on skin, tissue, and lesions, decreasing tissue ischemia.

ACTIONS/INTERVENTIONS	RATIONALE
Collaborative	
Obtain cultures of open skin lesions.	Identifies pathogens and appropriate treatment choices.
Apply/administer topical/systemic drugs as indicated.	Used in treatment of skin lesions. Use of agents such as Prederm spray can stimulate circulation, enhancing healing process. *Note:* When multidose ointments are used, care must be taken to avoid cross-contamination.
Cover ulcerated KS lesions with wet-to-wet dressings or antibiotic ointment and nonstick dressing (e.g., Telfa), as indicated.	Protects ulcerated areas from contamination and promotes healing.
Refer to physical therapy for regular exercise/activity program.	Promotes improved muscle tone and skin health.

NURSING DIAGNOSIS: Oral Mucous Membrane, altered

May be related to

Immunologic deficit and presence of lesion-causing pathogens, e.g., *Candida*, herpes, KS

Dehydration, malnutrition

Ineffective oral hygiene

Side effects of drugs, chemotherapy

Possibly evidenced by

Open ulcerated lesions, vesicles

Oral pain/discomfort

Stomatitis; leukoplakia, gingivitis, carious teeth

DESIRED OUTCOMES/EVALUATION CRITERIA—PATIENT WILL:

Oral Health (NOC)

Display intact mucous membranes, which are pink, moist, and free of inflammation/ulcerations.

Risk Control (NOC)

Demonstrate techniques to restore/maintain integrity of oral mucosa.

ACTIONS/INTERVENTIONS	RATIONALE
Oral Health Restoration (NIC)	
Independent	
Assess mucous membranes/document all oral lesions. Note reports of pain, swelling, difficulty with chewing/swallowing.	Edema, open lesions, and crusting on oral mucous membranes and throat may cause pain and difficulty with chewing/swallowing.
Provide oral care daily and after food intake, using soft toothbrush, nonabrasive toothpaste, nonalcoholic mouthwash, floss, and lip moisturizer.	Alleviates discomfort, prevents acid formation associated with retained food particles, and promotes feeling of well-being.
Rinse oral mucosal lesions with saline/dilute hydrogen peroxide or baking soda solutions.	Reduces spread of lesions and encrustations from candidiasis and promotes comfort.
Suggest use of sugarless gum/candy or commercial salivary substitute.	Stimulates flow of saliva to neutralize acids and protect mucous membranes.

ACTIONS/INTERVENTIONS

Independent

Plan diet to avoid salty, spicy, abrasive, and acidic foods or beverages. Check for temperature tolerance of foods. Offer cool/cold smooth foods.

Encourage oral intake of at least 2500 mL/day.

Encourage patient to refrain from smoking.

Collaborative

Obtain culture specimens of lesions.

Administer medications, as indicated, e.g., nystatin (Mycostatin), ketoconazole (Nizoral).

TNF-alpha inhibitor-thalidomide.

Refer for dental consultation, if appropriate.

RATIONALE

Abrasive foods may open healing lesions. Open lesions are painful and aggravated by salt, spice, acidic foods/beverages. Extreme cold or heat can cause pain to sensitive mucous membranes.

Maintains hydration; prevents drying of oral cavity.

Smoke is drying and irritating to mucous membranes.

Reveals causative agents and identifies appropriate therapies.

Specific drug choice depends on particular infecting organism(s), e.g., *Candida*.

Effective in treatment of oral lesions due to recurrent stomatitis.

May require additional therapy to prevent dental losses.

NURSING DIAGNOSIS: Fatigue

May be related to

Decreased metabolic energy production, increased energy requirements (hypermetabolic state)

Overwhelming psychological/emotional demands

Altered body chemistry: side effects of medication, chemotherapy

Possibly evidenced by

Unremitting/overwhelming lack of energy, inability to maintain usual routines, decreased performance, impaired ability to concentrate, lethargy/listlessness

Disinterest in surroundings

DESIRED OUTCOMES/EVALUATION CRITERIA—PATIENT WILL:

Endurance (NOC)

Report improved sense of energy.

Perform ADLs, with assistance as necessary.

Participate in desired activities at level of ability.

ACTIONS/INTERVENTIONS

Energy Management (NIC)

Independent

Assess sleep patterns and note changes in thought processes/behaviors.

Recommend scheduling activities for periods when patient has most energy. Plan care to allow for rest periods. Involve patient/SO in schedule planning.

Establish realistic activity goals with patient.

RATIONALE

Multiple factors can aggravate fatigue, including sleep deprivation, emotional distress, side effects of drugs/chemotherapies, and developing CNS disease.

Planning allows patient to be active during times when energy level is higher, which may restore a feeling of well-being and a sense of control. Frequent rest periods are needed to restore/conserve energy.

Provides for a sense of control and feelings of accomplishment. Prevents discouragement from fatigue of overactivity.

ACTIONS/INTERVENTIONS	RATIONALE
Independent	
Encourage patient to do whatever possible, e.g., self-care, sit in chair, short walks. Increase activity level as indicated.	May conserve strength, increase stamina, and enable patient to become more active without undue fatigue and discouragement.
Identify energy conservation techniques, e.g., sitting, breaking ADLs into manageable segments. Keep travelways clear of furniture. Provide/assist with ambulation/self-care needs as appropriate.	Weakness may make ADLs almost impossible for the patient to complete. Protects patient from injury during activities.
Monitor physiological response to activity, e.g., changes in BP, respiratory rate, or heart rate.	Tolerance varies greatly, depending on the stage of the disease process, nutrition state, fluid balance, and number/type of opportunistic diseases that the patient has been subject to.
Encourage nutritional intake. (Refer to ND: Nutrition: altered, less than body requirements, p. 775.)	Adequate intake/utilization of nutrients is necessary to meet increased energy needs for activity. *Note:* Continuous stimulation of the immune system by HIV infection contributes to a hypermetabolic state.
Collaborative	
Refer to physical/occupational therapy.	Programmed daily exercises and activities help patient maintain/increase strength and muscle tone, enhance sense of well-being.
Refer to community resources, e.g., grocery delivery/Meals on Wheels, house cleaning/home maintenance services, homecare agency.	Provides assistance in areas of individual need as ability to care for self becomes more difficult.
Provide supplemental O_2 as indicated.	Presence of anemia/hypoxemia reduces oxygen available for cellular uptake and contributes to fatigue.

NURSING DIAGNOSIS: Thought Processes, altered

May be related to

Hypoxemia, CNS infection by HIV, brain malignancies, and/or disseminated systemic opportunistic infection, CVA/hemorrhage; vasculitis

Alteration of drug metabolism/excretion, accumulation of toxic elements; renal failure, severe electrolyte imbalance, hepatic insufficiency

Possibly evidenced by

Altered attention span; distractibility

Memory deficit

Disorientation; cognitive dissonance; delusional thinking

Sleep disturbances

Impaired ability to make decisions/problem-solve; inability to follow complex commands/mental tasks, loss of impulse control

DESIRED OUTCOMES/EVALUATION CRITERIA—PATIENT WILL:

Cognitive Ability (NOC)

Maintain usual reality orientation and optimal cognitive functioning.

ACTIONS/INTERVENTIONS	RATIONALE

Cognitive Stimulation (NIC)

Independent

Assess mental and neurological status using appropriate tools.

Establishes functional level at time of admission and provides baseline for future comparison.

Consider effects of emotional distress, e.g., anxiety, grief, anger.

May contribute to reduced alertness, confusion, withdrawal, and hypoactivity, requiring further evaluation and intervention.

Monitor medication regimen and usage.

Actions and interactions of various medications, prolonged drug half-life/altered excretion rates result in cumulative effects, potentiating risk of toxic reactions. Some drugs may have adverse side effects; e.g., haloperidol (Haldol) can seriously impair motor function in patients with AIDS dementia complex.

Investigate changes in personality, response to stimuli, orientation/level of consciousness; or development of headache, nuchal rigidity, vomiting, fever, seizure activity.

Changes may occur for numerous reasons, including development/exacerbation of opportunistic diseases/CNS infection. *Note:* Early detection and treatment of CNS infection may limit permanent impairment of cognitive ability.

Maintain a pleasant environment with appropriate auditory, visual, and cognitive stimuli.

Providing normal environmental stimuli can help in maintaining some sense of reality orientation.

Provide cues for reorientation, e.g., radio, television, calendars, clocks, room with an outside view. Use patient's name; identify yourself. Maintain consistent personnel and structured schedules as appropriate.

Frequent reorientation to place and time may be necessary, especially during fever/acute CNS involvement. Sense of continuity may reduce associated anxiety.

Discuss use of datebooks, lists, other devices to keep track of activities.

These techniques help patient manage problems of forgetfulness.

Encourage family/SO to socialize and provide reorientation with current news, family events.

Familiar contacts are often helpful in maintaining reality orientation, especially if patient is hallucinating.

Encourage patient to do as much as possible, e.g., dress and groom daily, see friends, and so forth.

Can help maintain mental abilities for longer period.

Provide support for SO. Encourage discussion of concerns and fears.

Bizarre behavior/deterioration of abilities may be very frightening for SO and makes management of care/dealing with situation difficult. SO may feel a loss of control as stress, anxiety, burnout, and anticipatory grieving impair coping abilities.

Provide information about care on an ongoing basis. Answer questions simply and honestly. Repeat explanations as needed.

Can reduce anxiety and fear of unknown; can enhance patient's understanding and involvement/cooperation in treatment when possible.

Cognitive Restructuring (NIC)

Reduce provocative/noxious stimuli. Maintain bedrest in quiet, darkened room if indicated.

If the patient is prone to agitation, violent behavior, or seizures, reducing external stimuli may be helpful.

Decrease noise, especially at night.

Promotes sleep, reducing cognitive symptoms and effects of sleep deprivation.

Set limits on maladaptive/abusive behavior; avoid open-ended choices.

Provides sense of security/stability in an otherwise confusing situation.

ACTIONS/INTERVENTIONS	RATIONALE
Independent	
Maintain safe environment, e.g., excess furniture out of the way, call bell within patient's reach, bed in low position/rails up; restriction of smoking (unless monitored by caregiver/SO), seizure precautions, soft restraints if indicated.	Decreases the possibility of patient injury.
Discuss causes/future expectations and treatment if dementia is diagnosed. Use concrete terms.	Obtaining information that ZVD has been shown to improve cognition can provide hope and control for losses.
Collaborative	
Assist with diagnostic studies, e.g., MRI, CT scan, spinal tap, and monitor laboratory studies as indicated, e.g., BUN/Cr, electrolytes, ABGs.	Choice of tests/studies depends on clinical manifestations and index of suspicion because changes in mental status may reflect a wide variety of causative factors, e.g., CMV meningitis/encephalitis, drug toxicity, electrolyte imbalances, and altered organ function.
Administer medications as indicated:	
Amphotericin B (Fungizone);	Antifungal useful in treatment of cryptococcosis meningitis.
ZVD (Retrovir) and other antiretrovirals alone or in combination;	Shown to improve neurological and mental functioning for undetermined period of time.
Antipsychotics, e.g., haloperidol (Haldol), and/or antianxiety agents, e.g., lorazepam (Ativan).	Cautious use may help with problems of sleeplessness, emotional lability, hallucinations, suspiciousness, and agitation.
Provide controlled environment/behavioral management.	Team approach may be required to protect patient when mental impairment (e.g., delusions) threatens patient safety.
Refer to counseling as indicated.	May help patient gain control in presence of thought disturbances or psychotic symptomatology.

NURSING DIAGNOSIS: Anxiety [specify level]/Fear/Anxiety, death

May be related to
Threat to self-concept, threat of death, change in health/socioeconomic status, role functioning
Interpersonal transmission and contagion
Separation from support system
Fear of transmission of the disease to family/loved ones

Possibly evidenced by
Increased tension, apprehension, feelings of helplessness/hopelessness
Expressed concern regarding changes in life
Fear of unspecific consequences
Somatic complaints, insomnia; sympathetic stimulation, restlessness

DESIRED OUTCOMES/EVALUATION CRITERIA—PATIENT WILL:

Anxiety or Fear Control (NOC)

Verbalize awareness of feelings and healthy ways to deal with them.
Display appropriate range of feelings and lessened fear/anxiety.
Demonstrate problem-solving skills.
Use resources effectively.

ACTIONS/INTERVENTIONS	RATIONALE

Anxiety Reduction (NIC)

Independent

Assure patient of confidentiality within limits of situation.

Provides reassurance and opportunity for patient to problem-solve solutions to anticipated situations.

Maintain frequent contact with patient. Talk with and touch the patient. Limit use of isolation clothing and masks.

Provides assurance that the patient is not alone or rejected; conveys respect for and acceptance of the person, fostering trust.

Provide accurate, consistent information regarding prognosis. Avoid arguing about patient's perceptions of the situation.

Can reduce anxiety and enable patient to make decisions/choices based on realities.

Be alert to signs of denial/depression (e.g., withdrawal; angry, inappropriate remarks). Determine presence of suicidal ideation and assess potential on a scale of 1–10.

Patient may use defense mechanism of denial and continue to hope that diagnosis is inaccurate. Feelings of guilt and spiritual distress may cause the patient to become withdrawn and believe that suicide is a viable alternative.

Provide open environment in which patient feels safe to discuss feelings or to refrain from talking.

Helps patient feel accepted in present condition without feeling judged and promotes sense of dignity and control.

Permit expressions of anger, fear, despair without confrontation. Give information that feelings are normal and are to be appropriately expressed.

Acceptance of feelings allows patient to begin to deal with situation.

Recognize and support the stage patient/family is at in the grieving process. (Refer to CP: Cancer, ND: Grieving, anticipatory, p. 902.)

Choice of interventions as dictated by stage of grief, coping behaviors, e.g., anger/withdrawal, denial.

Explain procedures, providing opportunity for questions and honest answers. Arrange for someone to stay with patient during anxiety-producing procedures and consultations.

Accurate information allows the patient to deal more effectively with the reality of the situation, thereby reducing anxiety and fear of the known.

Identify and encourage patient interaction with support systems. Encourage verbalization/interaction with family/SO.

Reduces feelings of isolation. If family support systems are not available, outside sources may be needed immediately, e.g., local AIDS task force.

Provide reliable and consistent information and support for SO.

Allows for better interpersonal interaction and reduction of anxiety and fear.

Include SO as indicated when major decisions are to be made.

Ensures a support system for the patient, and allows the SO the chance to participate in patient's life. *Note:* If patient, family, and SO are in conflict, separate care consultations and visiting times may be needed.

Discuss Advance Directives, end-of-life desires/needs.

May assist patient/SO to plan realistically for terminal stages and death.

Collaborative

Refer to psychiatric counseling (e.g., clinical nurse specialist, psychiatrist, social worker).

May require further assistance in dealing with diagnosis/prognosis, especially when suicidal thoughts are present.

Provide contact with other resources as indicated, e.g.:

Spiritual advisor;

Provides opportunity for addressing spiritual concerns.

Hospice staff.

May help relieve anxiety regarding end-of-life care and support for patient/SO.

NURSING DIAGNOSIS: Social Isolation

May be related to

Altered state of wellness, changes in physical appearance, alterations in mental status

Perceptions of unacceptable social or sexual behavior/values

Inadequate personal resources/support systems

Physical isolation

Possibly evidenced by

Expressed feeling of aloneness imposed by others, feelings of rejection

Absence of supportive SO: partners, family, acquaintances/friends

DESIRED OUTCOMES/EVALUATION CRITERIA—PATIENT WILL:

Social Support (NOC)

Identify supportive individual(s).

Use resources for assistance.

Social Involvement (NOC)

Participate in activities/programs at level of ability/desire.

ACTIONS/INTERVENTIONS	RATIONALE
Support System Enhancement (NIC)	
Independent	
Ascertain patient's perception of situation.	Isolation may be partly self-imposed because patient fears rejection/reaction of others.
Spend time talking with patient during and between care activities. Be supportive, allowing for verbalization. Treat with dignity and regard for patient's feelings.	Patient may experience physical isolation due to current medical status and some degree of social isolation secondary to diagnosis of AIDS.
Limit/avoid use of mask, gown, and gloves when possible, e.g., when talking to patient.	Reduces patient's sense of physical isolation and provides positive social contact, which may enhance self-esteem.
Identify support systems available to patient, including presence of/relationship with immediate and extended family.	When patient has assistance from SO, feelings of loneliness and rejection are diminished. *Note:* Patient may not receive usual/needed support for coping with life-threatening illness and associated grief because of fear and lack of understanding (AIDS hysteria).
Explain isolation precautions/procedures to patient and SO.	Gloves, gowns, mask are not routinely required with a diagnosis of AIDS except when contact with secretions/excretions is expected. Misuse of these barriers enhances feelings of emotional and physical isolation. When precautions are necessary, explanations help patient understand reasons for procedures and provide feeling of inclusion in what is happening.
Encourage open visitation (as able), telephone contacts, and social activities within tolerated level.	Participation with others can foster a feeling of belonging.
Encourage active role of contact with SO.	Helps re-establish a feeling of participation in a social relationship. May lessen likelihood of suicide attempts.
Develop a plan of action with patient: Look at available resources; support health risk-taking behaviors. Help patient problem-solve solution to short-term/imposed isolation.	Having a plan promotes a sense of control over own life and gives patient something to look forward to/actions to accomplish.

ACTIONS/INTERVENTIONS

Independent

Be alert to verbal/nonverbal cues, e.g., withdrawal, statements of despair, sense of aloneness. Ask the patient if thoughts of suicide are being entertained.

Collaborative

Refer to resources, e.g., social services counselors, and AIDS organizations/projects (local and national).

Provide for placement in sheltered community when necessary.

RATIONALE

Indicators of despair and suicidal ideation are often present; when these cues are acknowledged by the caregiver, the patient is usually willing to talk about thoughts of suicide and sense of isolation and hopelessness.

Establishes support systems; may reduce feelings of isolation.

May need more specific care when unable to be maintained at home or when SO cannot manage care.

NURSING DIAGNOSIS: Powerlessness

May be related to
Confirmed diagnosis of a potentially terminal disease, incomplete grieving process
Social ramifications of AIDS; alteration in body image/desired lifestyle; advancing CNS involvement

Possibly evidenced by
Feelings of loss of control over own life
Depression over physical deterioration that occurs despite patient compliance with regimen
Anger, apathy, withdrawal, passivity
Dependence on others for care/decision making, resulting in resentment, anger, guilt

DESIRED OUTCOMES/EVALUATION CRITERIA—PATIENT WILL:

Health Beliefs: Perceived Control (NOC)

Acknowledge feelings and healthy ways to deal with them.
Verbalize some sense of control over present situation.
Make choices related to care and be involved in self-care.

ACTIONS/INTERVENTIONS

Self-Responsibility Facilitation (NIC)

Independent

Identify factors that contribute to the patient's feelings of powerlessness, e.g., diagnosis of a terminal illness, lack of support systems, lack of knowledge about present situation.

Assess degree of feelings of helplessness, e.g., verbal/nonverbal expressions indicating lack of control ("It won't make any difference"), flat affect, lack of communication.

RATIONALE

Patients with AIDS are usually aware of the current literature and prognosis unless newly diagnosed. Powerlessness is most prevalent in the patient newly diagnosed with HIV and when dying with AIDS. Fear of AIDS (by the general population and the patient's family/SO) is the most profound cause of the patient's isolation. For some homosexual patients, this may be the first time that the family has been made aware that that patient lives an alternative lifestyle.

Determines the status of the individual patient and allows for appropriate intervention when the patient is immobilized by depressed feelings.

ACTIONS/INTERVENTIONS

Independent

Encourage active role in planning activities, establishing realistic/attainable daily goals. Encourage patient control and responsibility as much as possible. Identify things that the patient can and cannot control.

Encourage living will and durable power of attorney documents, with specific and precise instructions regarding acceptable and unacceptable procedures to prolong life.

Discuss desires/assist with planning for funeral as appropriate.

RATIONALE

May enhance feelings of control and self-worth and sense of personal responsibility.

Many factors associated with the treatments used in this debilitating and often fatal disease process place the patient at the mercy of medical personnel and other unknown people who may be making decisions for and about the patient without regard for the patient's wishes, increasing loss of independence.

The individual can gain a sense of completion and value to his or her life when he/she decides to be involved in planning what this final ceremony will be like because it provides an opportunity to include things that are of importance to the person.

NURSING DIAGNOSIS: Knowledge Deficit [Learning Need] regarding disease, prognosis, current therapies, and self care needs

May be related to
Lack of exposure/recall; information misinterpretation
Cognitive limitation
Unfamiliarity with information resources

Possibly evidenced by
Questions/request for information; statement of misconception
Inaccurate follow-through of instructions/development of preventable complications.

DESIRED OUTCOMES/EVALUATION CRITERIA—PATIENT WILL:

Knowledge: Disease Process (NOC)

Verbalize understanding of condition/disease process and potential complications.
Identify relationship of signs/symptoms to the disease process and correlate symptoms with causative factors.

Knowledge: Treatment Regimen (NOC)

Verbalize understanding of therapeutic needs.
Correctly perform necessary procedures and explain reasons for actions.
Initiate necessary lifestyle changes and participate in treatment regimen.

ACTIONS/INTERVENTIONS

Teaching: Disease Process (NIC)

Independent

Review disease process and future expectations.

Determine level of independence/dependence and physical condition. Note extent of care and support available from family/SO and need for other caregivers.

Review modes of transmission of disease.

RATIONALE

Provides knowledge base from which patient can make informed choices.

Helps plan amount of care and symptom management required and need for additional resources.

Corrects myths and misconceptions; promotes safety for patient/others.

ACTIONS/INTERVENTIONS	RATIONALE

Independent

Instruct patient and caregivers concerning infection control, e.g.: using good handwashing techniques for everyone (patient, family, caregivers); using gloves when handling bedpans, dressings/soiled linens; wearing mask if patient has productive cough; placing soiled/wet linens in plastic bag and separating from family laundry, washing with detergent and hot water; cleaning surfaces with bleach/water solution of 1:10, disinfecting toilet bowl/bedpan with full-strength bleach; preparing patient's food in clean area; washing dishes/utensils in hot soapy water (can be washed with the family dishes).

Reduces risk of transmission of diseases; promotes wellness in presence of reduced ability of immune system to control level of flora.

Stress necessity of daily skin care, including inspecting skin folds, pressure points, and perineum, and of providing adequate cleansing and protective measures, e.g., ointments, padding.

Healthy skin provides barrier to infection. Measures to prevent skin disruption and associated complications are critical.

Ascertain that patient/SO can perform necessary oral and dental care. Review procedures as indicated. Encourage regular dental care.

The oral mucosa can quickly exhibit severe, progressive complications. Studies indicate that 65% of AIDS patients have some oral symptoms. Therefore, prevention and early intervention are critical.

Review dietary needs (high-protein and high-calorie) and ways to improve intake when anorexia, diarrhea, weakness, depression interfere with intake.

Promotes adequate nutrition necessary for healing and support of immune system; enhances feeling of well-being.

Discuss medication regimen, interactions, and side effects.

Enhances cooperation with/increases probability of success with therapeutic regimen.

Provide information about symptom management that complements medical regimen; e.g., with intermittent diarrhea, take diphenoxylate (Lomotil) before going to social event.

Provides patient with increased sense of control, reduces risk of enbarrassment, and promotes comfort.

Stress importance of adequate rest.

Helps manage fatigue; enhances coping abilities and energy level.

Encourage activity/exercise at level that patient can tolerate.

Stimulates release of endorphins in the brain, enhancing sense of well-being.

Stress necessity of continued healthcare and follow-up.

Provides opportunity for altering regimen to meet individual/changing needs.

Recommend cessation of smoking.

Smoking increases risk of respiratory infections and can further impair immune system.

Identify signs/symptoms requiring medical evaluation, e.g., persistent fever/night sweats, swollen glands, continued weight loss, diarrhea, skin blotches/lesions, headache, chest pain/dyspnea.

Early recognition of developing complications and timely interventions may prevent progression to life-threatening situation.

Identify community resources, e.g., hospice/residential care centers, visiting nurse, home care services, Meals-on-Wheels, peer group support.

Facilitates transfer from acute care setting for recovery/independence or end-of-life care.

POTENTIAL CONSIDERATIONS in addition to the nursing diagnoses listed in the plan of care.

Grieving, anticipatory—loss of physiological/psychological well-being, social/lifestyle changes, loss of SO/family, probability of death.

Protection, altered—abnormal blood profile (anemia, thrombocytopenia, coagulation), inadequate nutrition, drug therapies (e.g., antineoplastic, immune), chronic disease.

Caregiver Role Strain—illness severity of care receiver, significant home care needs, caregiver health impairment, marginal family adaptation or dysfunction, presence of situational stressors, lack of respite for caregiver, caregiver's competing role commitments.

RHEUMATOID ARTHRITIS

Rheumatoid arthritis (RA) is a chronic, systemic inflammatory disease involving connective tissue and characterized by destruction and proliferation of the synovial membrane, resulting in joint destruction, ankylosis, and deformity. Although the cause is unknown, researchers speculate that a virus may initially trigger the body's immune response, which then becomes chronically activated and turns on itself (autoimmune response). Immunological mechanisms appear to play an important role in the initiation and perpetuation of the disease in which spontaneous remissions and unpredictable exacerbations occur. RA is a disorder of the immune system, and, as such, is a whole-body disease that can extend beyond the joints, affecting other organ systems, such as the skin and eyes.

CARE SETTING

Community level unless surgical procedure is required.

RELATED CONCERNS

Psychosocial aspects of care, page 809
Total joint replacement, page 707

Patient Assessment Database

Date depends on severity and involvement of other organs (e.g., eyes, heart, lungs, kidneys), stage (i.e., acute exacerbation or remission), and coexistence of other forms of arthritis/autoimmune diseases.

ACTIVITY/REST

May report: Joint pain and tenderness worsened by movement and stress placed on joint; morning stiffness, usually occurs symmetrically
Functional limitations affecting ADLs, desired lifestyle, leisure time, and occupation
Fatigue; sleep disturbances

May exhibit: Malaise
Impaired ROM of joints; particularly hand (fingers and wrist), hips, knees, ankles, elbows and shoulders
Muscle atrophy; joint and muscle contractures/deformities
Decreased muscle strength, altered gait/posture

CARDIOVASCULAR

May report: Intermittent pallor, cyanosis, then redness of fingers/toes before color returns to normal (Raynaud's phenomenon)

EGO INTEGRITY

May report: Acute/chronic stress factors; e.g., financial, employment, disability, relationship factors
Hopelessness and powerlessness (incapacitating situation)
Threat to self-concept, body image, personal identity (e.g., dependence on others)

FOOD/FLUID

May report: Inability to obtain/consume adequate food/fluids (temporomandibular joint [TMJ] involvement)
Anorexia, nausea

May exhibit: Weight loss
Dryness of oral mucous membranes, decreased oral secretions; dental caries (Sjögren's syndrome)

HYGIENE

May report: Varying difficulty performing self-care activities; dependence on others

NEUROSENSORY

May report: Numbness/tingling of hands and feet, loss of sensation in fingers
May exhibit: Symmetric joint swelling

PAIN/DISCOMFORT

May report: Acute episodes of pain (may/may not be accompanied by soft-tissue swelling in joints)
Chronic aching pain and stiffness (mornings are most difficult)

May exhibit: Red, swollen, hot joints (during acute exacerbations)

SAFETY

May report: Difficulty managing homemaker/maintenance tasks
Persistent low-grade fever
Dryness of eyes and mucous membranes

May exhibit: Pale, shiny, taut skin; subcutaneous rounded, nontender nodules; lesions, leg ulcers
Skin/periarticular local warmth, erythema
Decreased muscle strength, altered gait, reduced ROM

SOCIAL INTERACTION

May report: Impaired interactions with family/others; change in roles; isolation

TEACHING/LEARNING

May report: Familial history of RA (in juvenile onset)
Use of health foods, vitamins, untested arthritis "cures"
History of pericarditis, valvular lesions; pulmonary fibrosis, pleuritis

Discharge plan considerations: **DRG projected mean length of inpatient stay: 5.4 days**
May require assistance with transportation, self-care activities, and homemaker/maintenance tasks; changes in physical layout of home

Refer to section at end of plan for after discharge considerations.

DIAGNOSTIC STUDIES

Antinuclear antibody (ANA) titer: Screening test for rheumatic disorders, elevated in 25%–30% of RA patients. Follow-up tests are needed for the specific rheumatic disorders, e.g., Anti-RNP is used for differential diagnosis of systemic rheumatic disease.

Rheumatoid factor (RF): Positive in more than 80% of cases (Rose-Waaler test).

Latex fixation: Positive in 75% of typical cases.

Agglutination reactions: Positive in more than 50% of typical cases.

Serum complement: C_3 and C_4 increased in acute onset (inflammatory response). Immune disorder/exhaustion results in depressed total complement levels.

Erythrocyte sedimentation rate (ESR): Usually greatly increased (80–100 mm/hr). May return to normal as symptoms improve.

CBC: Usually reveals moderate anemia. WBC is elevated when inflammatory processes are present.

Ig (IgM and IgG): Elevation strongly suggests autoimmune process as cause for RA.

X-rays of involved joints: Reveals soft-tissue swelling, erosion of joints, and osteoporosis of adjacent bone (early changes) progressing to bone-cyst formation, narrowing of joint space, and subluxation. Concurrent osteoarthritic changes may be noted.

Radionuclide scans: Identify inflamed synovium.

Direct arthroscopy: Visualization of area reveals bone irregularities/degeneration of joint.

Synovial/fluid aspirate: May reveal volume greater than normal; opaque, cloudy, yellow appearance (inflammatory response, bleeding, degenerative waste products); elevated WBCs and leukocytes; decreased viscosity and complement (C_3 and C_4).

Synovial membrane biopsy: Reveals inflammatory changes and development of pannus.

NURSING PRIORITIES

1. Alleviate pain.
2. Increase mobility.
3. Promote positive self-concept.
4. Support independence.
5. Provide information about disease process/prognosis and treatment needs.

DISCHARGE GOALS

1. Pain relieved/controlled.
2. Patient is dealing realistically with current situation.
3. Patient is managing ADLs by self/with assistance as appropriate.
4. Disease process/prognosis and therapeutic regimen understood.
5. Plan in place to meet needs after discharge.

NURSING DIAGNOSIS: Pain [acute]/chronic

May be related to

Injuring agents: Distention of tissues by accumulation of fluid/inflammatory process, destruction of joint

Possibly evidenced by

Reports of pain/discomfort, fatigue
Self-narrowed focus
Distraction behaviors/autonomic responses
Guarding/protective behavior

DESIRED OUTCOMES/EVALUATION CRITERIA—PATIENT WILL:

Pain Level (NOC)

Report pain is relieved/controlled.
Appear relaxed, able to sleep/rest and participate in activities appropriately.

Pain Control Behavior (NOC)

Follow prescribed pharmacological regimen.
Incorporate relaxation skills and diversional activities into pain control program.

ACTIONS/INTERVENTIONS

Pain Management (NIC)

Independent

Investigate reports of pain, noting location and intensity (scale of 0–10). Note precipitating factors and nonverbal pain cues.

Recommend/provide firm mattress or bedboard, small pillow. Elevate linens with bed cradle as needed.

Suggest patient assume position of comfort while in bed or sitting in chair. Promote bedrest as indicated.

Place/monitor use of pillows, sandbags, trochanter rolls, splints, braces.

Encourage frequent changes of position. Assist patient to move in bed, supporting affected joints above and below, avoiding jerky movements.

RATIONALE

Helpful in determining pain management needs and effectiveness of program.

Soft/sagging mattress, large pillows prevent maintenance of proper body alignment, placing stress on affected joints. Elevation of bed linens reduces pressure on inflamed/painful joints.

In severe disease/acute exacerbation, total bedrest may be necessary (until objective and subjective improvements are noted) to limit pain/injury to joint.

Rests painful joints and maintains neutral position. *Note:* Use of splints can decrease pain and may reduce damage to joint; however, prolonged inactivity can result in loss of joint mobility/function.

Prevents general fatigue and joint stiffness. Stabilizes joint, decreasing joint movement/pain.

ACTIONS/INTERVENTIONS

Independent

Recommend that patient take warm bath or shower on arising and/or at bedtime. Apply warm, moist compresses to affected joints several times a day. Monitor water temperature of compress, baths, and so on.	Heat promotes muscle relaxation and mobility, decreases pain, and relieves morning stiffness. Sensitivity to heat may be diminished and dermal injury may occur.
Provide gentle massage.	Promotes relaxation/reduces muscle tension.
Encourage use of stress management techniques, e.g., progressive relaxation, biofeedback, visualization, guided imagery, self-hypnosis, and controlled breathing. Provide Therapeutic Touch.	Promotes relaxation, provides sense of control, and may enhance coping abilities.
Involve in diversional activities appropriate for individual situation.	Refocuses attention, provides stimulation, and enhances self-esteem and feelings of general well-being.
Medicate before planned activities/exercises as indicated.	Promotes relaxation, reduces muscle tension/spasms, facilitating participation in therapy.

Collaborative

Administer medications as indicated, e.g.:

Salicylates, e.g., aspirin (Acuprin, Ecotrin, Zorprin);	ASA exerts an anti-inflammatory and mild analgesic effect, decreasing stiffness and increasing mobility. ASA must be taken regularly to sustain a therapeutic blood level. Research indicates that ASA has the lowest "toxicity index" of commonly prescribed NSAIDs.
Nonsalicylates (NSAIDs), e.g., ibuprofen (Advil, Motrin), naproxen (Aleve, Naprosyn), sulindac (Clinoril), prioxicam (Feldene), fenoprofen (Nalfon); diclofenac (Voltaren); ketoprofen (Orudis); ketorolac (Toradol); nabumetone (Relafen);	These drugs control mild to moderate pain and inflammation by inhibition of prostaglandin synthesis.
Glucocorticoids, e.g., prednisone (Deltasone), methylprednisolone (Depo-Medrol); dexamethasone (Decadron);	These drugs modify the immune response and suppress inflammation.
Disease-modifying antirheumatic drugs (DMARD), e.g., methotrexate (Rheumatrex); hydroxychloroquine (Plaquenil); sulfasalazine (Azulfidene); gold salts (Ridaura); azathioprine (Imuran); leflunomide (Arava);	These drugs vary in action, but all reduce pain and swelling, lessening arthritic symptoms rather than eliminating them. Arava (FDA approved in 1998) is the first oral drug shown to slow progression of RA and damage to joints.
COX-2 inhibitors, e.g., celecoxig (Celebrex), rofecoxib (Vioxx);	A new class of medication recently released, COX-2 inhibitors interfere with prostaglandin production, similarly to NSAIDs but are less likely to harm the stomach lining or kidneys. May be used in combination with other medications.
Biologicals, e.g., etanercept (Enbrel), infliximale (Remicade);	These new injectable drugs (soon to be released) are the first genetically engineered medications for arthritis. These anti-TNF compounds block inflammation by finding the TNF and in clinical studies have been shown to rapidly decrease pain and joint swelling. Enbrel is self-injected twice a week and may be used in combination with methotrexate. Remicade is administered IV at 1- to 3-month intervals.

RATIONALE

793

ACTIONS/INTERVENTIONS	RATIONALE

Collaborative

D-penicillamine (Cuprimine);	May control systemic effects of RA synovitis and scleroderma if other therapies have not been successful. High rate of side effects (e.g., thrombocytopenia, leukopenia, aplastic anemia) necessitates close monitoring. *Note:* Drug should be given between meals because drug absorption is impaired by food, as well as antacids and iron products.
Antacids;	Given with NSAID agents to minimize gastric irritation/discomfort reducing risk of GI bleed.
Codeine-containing medications.	Although narcotics are generally contraindicated because of chronic nature of condition, short-term use of these products may be required during periods of acute exacerbation to control severe pain.
Assist with physical therapies, e.g., paraffin glove, whirlpool baths.	Provides sustained heat to reduce pain and improve ROM of affected joints.
Apply ice or cold packs when indicated.	Cold may relieve pain and swelling during acute episodes.
Instruct in use/monitor effect of transcutaneous electrical nerve stimulator (TENS) unit if used.	Constant low-level electrical stimulus blocks transmission of pain sensations.
Assist with other modalities as indicated, e.g., blood filtration.	Prosorba column is a device similar to a kidney dialysis machine that removes substances from blood plasma that contribute to joint swelling and pain.
Prepare for surgical interventions, e.g., synovectomy, total joint replacement, joint fusion; tunnel release procedures, tendon repair.	Corrective surgical procedures may be indicated to reduce pain and/or improve joint function, and mobility.

NURSING DIAGNOSIS: Mobility, impaired physical/Walking, impaired

May be related to
Skeletal deformity
Pain, discomfort
Intolerance to activity; decreased muscle strength

Possibly evidenced by
Reluctance to attempt movement/inability to purposefully move within the physical environment
Limited ROM, impaired coordination, decreased muscle strength/control and mass (late stages)

DESIRED OUTCOMES/EVALUATION CRITERIA—PATIENT WILL:

> **Mobility Level (NOC)**

Maintain position of function with absence/limitation of contractures.
Maintain or increase strength and function of affected and/or compensatory body part.
Demonstrate techniques/behaviors that enable resumption/continuation of activities.

ACTIONS/INTERVENTIONS	RATIONALE

> **Exercise Therapy: Joint Mobility (NIC)**

Independent

Evaluate/continuously monitor degree of joint inflammation/pain.	Level of activity/exercise depends on progression/resolution of inflammatory process.

ACTIONS/INTERVENTIONS	RATIONALE

Independent

Maintain bedrest/chair rest when indicated. Schedule activities providing frequent rest periods and uninterrupted nighttime sleep.

Systemic rest is mandatory during acute exacerbations and important throughout all phases of disease to reduce fatigue, improve strength.

Assist with active/passive ROM and resistive exercises and isometrics when able.

Maintains/improves joint function, muscle strength, and general stamina. *Note:* Inadequate exercise leads to joint stiffening, whereas excessive activity can damage joints.

Encourage patient to maintain upright and erect posture when sitting, standing, walking.

Maximizes joint function, maintains mobility.

Discuss/provide safety needs, e.g. raised chairs/toilet seat, use of handrails in tub/shower and toilet, proper use of mobility aids/wheelchair safety.

Helps prevent accidental injuries/falls.

Positioning (NIC)

Reposition frequently using adequate personnel. Demonstrate/assist with transfer techniques and use of mobility aids, e.g., walker, cane, trapeze.

Relieves pressure on tissues and promotes circulation. Facilitates self-care and patient's independence. Proper transfer techniques prevent shearing abrasions of skin.

Position with pillows, sandbags, trochanter roll. Provide joint support with splints, braces.

Promotes joint stability (reducing risk of injury) and maintains proper joint position and body alignment, minimizing contractures.

Suggest using small/thin pillow under neck.

Prevents flexion of neck.

Collaborative

Provide foam/alternating pressure mattress.

Decreases pressure on fragile tissues to reduce risks of immobility/development of decubitus.

Exercise Therapy: Joint Mobility (NIC)

Consult with physical/occupational therapists and vocational specialist.

Useful in formulating exercise/activity program based on individual needs and in identifying mobility devices/adjuncts.

NURSING DIAGNOSIS: Body Image disturbance/Role Performance, altered

May be related to
Changes in ability to perform usual tasks
Increased energy expenditure; impaired mobility

Possibly evidenced by
Change in structure/function of affected parts
Negative self-talk; focus on past strength/function, appearance
Change in lifestyle/physical ability to resume roles, loss of employment, dependence on SO for assistance
Change in social involvement; sense of isolation
Feelings of helplessness, hopelessness

DESIRED OUTCOMES/EVALUATION CRITERIA—PATIENT WILL:

Psychosocial Adjustment: Life Change (NOC)

Verbalize increased confidence in ability to deal with illness, changes in lifestyle, and possible limitations.
Formulate realistic goals/plans for future.

ACTIONS/INTERVENTIONS	RATIONALE

Body Image or Role Enhancement (NIC)

Independent

Encourage verbalization about concerns of disease process, future expectations.

Provides opportunity to identify fears/misconceptions and deal with them directly.

Discuss meaning of loss/change to patient/SO. Ascertain how patient views self in usual lifestyle functioning, including sexual aspects.

Identifying how illness affects perception of self and interactions with others will determine need for further intervention/counseling.

Discuss patient's perception of how SO perceives limitations.

Verbal/nonverbal cues from SO may have a major impact on how patient views self.

Acknowledge and accept feelings of grief, hostility, dependency.

Constant pain is wearing, and feelings of anger and hostility are common. Acceptance provides feedback that feelings are normal.

Note withdrawn behavior, use of denial, or overconcern with body/changes.

May suggest emotional exhaustion or maladaptive coping methods, requiring more in-depth intervention/psychological support.

Set limits on maladaptive behavior. Assist patient to identify positive behaviors that will aid in coping.

Helps patient maintain self-control, which enhances self-esteem.

Involve patient in planning care and scheduling activities.

Enhances feelings of competency/self-worth, encourages independence and participation in therapy.

Assist with grooming needs as necessary.

Maintaining appearance enhances self-image.

Give positive reinforcement for accomplishments.

Allows patient to feel good about self. Reinforces positive behavior. Enhances self-confidence.

Collaborative

Refer to psychiatric counseling, e.g., clinical specialist psychiatric nurse, psychiatrist/psychologist, social worker.

Patient/SO may require ongoing support to deal with long-term/debilitating process.

Administer medications as indicated, e.g., antianxiety and mood-elevating drugs.

May be needed in presence of severe depression until patient develops more effective coping skills.

NURSING DIAGNOSIS: Self-Care deficit (specify)

May be related to
Musculoskeletal impairment; decreased strength/endurance, pain on movement
Depression

Possibly evidenced by
Inability to manage ADLs (feeding, bathing, dressing, and toileting)

DESIRED OUTCOMES/EVALUATION CRITERIA—PATIENT WILL:

Self-Care Activities of Daily Living (ADL) (NOC)

Perform self-care activities at a level consistent with individual capabilities.

Self-Care: Instrumental Activities of Daily Living (IADL) (NOC)

Demonstrate techniques/lifestyle changes to meet self-care needs.
Identify personal/community resources that can provide needed assistance.

ACTIONS/INTERVENTIONS

| **Self-Care Assistance (NIC)** |

Independent

Determine usual level of functioning (0–4) before onset-exacerbation of illness and potential changes now anticipated.

Maintain mobility, pain control, and exercise program.

Assess barriers to participation in self-care. Identify/plan for environmental modifications.

Allow patient sufficient time to complete tasks to fullest extent of ability. Capitalize on individual strengths.

Collaborative

Consult with rehabilitation specialists, e.g., occupational therapist.

Arrange home-health evaluation before discharge with follow-up afterward.

Arrange for consult with other agencies, e.g., Meals-on-Wheels, home care service, nutritionist.

RATIONALE

May be able to continue usual activities with necessary adaptations to current limitations.

Support physical/emotional independence.

Prepares for increased independence, which enhances self-esteem.

May need more time to complete tasks by self but provides an opportunity for greater sense of self-confidence and self-worth.

Helpful in determining assistive devices to meet individual needs, e.g., button hook, long-handled shoe horn, reacher, handheld shower head.

Identifies problems that may be encountered because of current level of disability. Provides for more successful team efforts with others who are involved in care, e.g., occupational therapy team.

May need additional kinds of assistance to continue in home setting.

NURSING DIAGNOSIS: Home Maintenance Management, risk for impaired

Risk factors may include
Long-term degenerative disease process
Inadequate support systems

Possibly evidenced by
[Not applicable; presence of signs and symptoms establishes an *actual* diagnosis]

DESIRED OUTCOMES/EVALUATION CRITERIA—PATIENT WILL:

| **Self-Care: Instrumental Activities of Daily Living (IADL) (NOC)** |

Maintain safe, growth-promoting environment.
Demonstrate appropriate, effective use of resources.

ACTIONS/INTERVENTIONS

| **Home Maintenance Assistance (NIC)** |

Independent

Assess level of physical functioning from Functional level 0–4.

RATIONALE

Identifies degree of assistance/support required. For example, the level 0 patient is completely able to perform usual activities of daily living (self-care, vocational, and avocational), while the level 4 patient is limited in all these areas and does not participate in activity.

ACTIONS/INTERVENTIONS

Independent

Evaluate environment to assess ability to care for self.

Determine financial resources to meet needs of individual situation. Identify support systems available to patient, e.g., extended family, friends/neighbors.

Develop plan for maintaining a clean, healthful environment, e.g., sharing of household repair/tasks between family members or by contract services.

Identify sources for necessary equipment, e.g., lifts, elevated toilet seat, wheelchair.

Collaborative

Coordinate home evaluation by occupational therapist/rehabilitation team.

Identify/meet with community resources, e.g., visiting nurse, homemaker service, social services, senior citizens' groups.

RATIONALE

Determines feasibility of remaining in/changing home layout to meet individual needs.

Availability of personal resources/community supports will affect ability to problem-solve and choice of solutions.

Ensures that needs will be met on an ongoing basis.

Provides opportunity to acquire equipment before discharge.

Useful for identifying adaptive equipment, ways to modify tasks to maintain independence.

Can facilitate transfer to/support continuation in home setting.

NURSING DIAGNOSIS: Knowledge Deficit [Learning Need] regarding disease, prognosis, treatment, self care, and discharge needs

May be related to
Lack of exposure/recall
Information misinterpretation

Possibly evidenced by
Questions/request for information, statement of misconception
Inaccurate follow-through of instructions/development of preventable complications

DESIRED OUTCOMES/EVALUATION CRITERIA—PATIENT WILL:

Knowledge: Disease Process (NOC)

Verbalize understanding of condition/prognosis, and potential complications.

Knowledge: Treatment Regimen (NOC)

Verbalize understanding of therapeutic needs.
Develop a plan for self-care, including lifestyle modifications consistent with mobility and/or activity restrictions.

ACTIONS/INTERVENTIONS

Teaching: Disease Process (NIC)

Independent

Review disease process, prognosis, and future expectations.

Discuss patient's role in management of disease process through nutrition, medication, and balanced program of exercise and rest.

RATIONALE

Provides knowledge base from which patient can make informed choices.

Goal of disease control is to suppress inflammation in joints/other tissues to maintain joint function and prevent deformities.

ACTIONS/INTERVENTIONS	RATIONALE

Independent

Assist in planning a realistic and integrated schedule of activity, rest, personal care, drug administration, physical therapy, and stress management.

Provide structure and defuses anxiety when managing a complex chronic disease process.

Stress importance of continued pharmacotherapeutic management.

Benefits of drug therapy depend on correct dosage, e.g., aspirin must be taken regularly to sustain therapeutic blood levels of 18–25 mg/dL.

Recommend use of enteric-coated/buffered aspirin or nonacetylated salicylates, e.g., choline salicylate (Arthropan) or choline magnesium trisalicylate (Trilisate).

Coated/buffered preparations ingested with food minimize gastric irritation, reducing risk of bleeding/hemorrhage. *Note:* Nonacetylated products have a longer half-life, requiring less frequent administration in addition to producing less gastric irritation.

Suggest taking medications, such as NSAIDs, with meals, milk products, or antacids and at bedtime.

Limits gastric irritation. Reduction of pain at hs enhances sleep and increased blood level decreases early-morning stiffness.

Identify adverse drug effects, e.g., tinnitus, gastric intolerance, GI bleeding, purpuric rash.

Prolonged, maximal doses of aspirin may result in overdose. Tinnitus usually indicates high therapeutic blood levels. If tinnitus occurs, the dosage is usually decreased by 1 tablet every 2–3 days until it stops.

Stress importance of reading product labels and refraining from OTC drug usage without prior medical approval.

Many products (e.g., cold remedies, antidiarrheals) contain hidden salicylates that increase risk of drug overdose/harmful side effects.

Review importance of balanced diet with foods high in vitamins, protein, and iron.

Promotes general well-being and tissue repair/regeneration.

Encourage obese patient to lose weight and supply with weight reduction information as appropriate.

Weight loss reduces stress on joints, especially hips, knees, ankles, feet.

Provide information about/resources for assistive devices, e.g., wheeled dolly/wagon for moving items, pickup sticks, lightweight dishes and pans, raised toilet seat, safety handlebars.

Reduces force exerted on joints and enables individual to participate more comfortably in needed/desired activities.

Discuss energy-saving techniques, e.g. sitting instead of standing to prepare meals or shower.

Prevents fatigue; facilitates self-care and independence.

Encourage maintenance of correct body position and posture both at rest and during activity, e.g., keeping joints extended, not flexed, wearing splints for prescribed periods, avoiding remaining in a single position for extended periods, positioning hands near center of body during use, and sliding rather than lifting objects when possible.

Good body mechanics must become a part of the patient's lifestyle to lessen joint stress and pain.

Review necessity of frequent inspection of skin and meticulous skin care under splints, casts, supporting devices. Demonstrate proper padding.

Reduces risk of skin irritation/breakdown.

Discuss necessity of medical follow-up/laboratory studies, e.g., ESR, salicylate levels, PT.

Drug therapy requires frequent assessment/refinement to ensure optimal effect and to prevent overdose/dangerous side effects, e.g., aspirin prolongs PT, increasing risk of bleeding.

ACTIONS/INTERVENTIONS	RATIONALE
Independent	
Provide for sexual and childbirth counseling as necessary.	Information about different positions and techniques and/or other options for sexual fulfillment may enhance personal relationships and feelings of self-worth/self-esteem. *Note:* A large number of patients with RA are in childbearing years, and need counseling, support, and medical interventions.
Identify community resources, e.g., Arthritis Foundation.	Assistance/support from others promotes maximal recovery.

POTENTIAL CONSIDERATIONS following acute hospitalization (dependent on patient's age, physical condition/presence of complications, personal resources, and life responsibilities)

Fatigue—increased energy requirements to perform ADLs, states of discomfort.

Pain, chronic—accumulation of fluid/inflammation, destruction of joint.

Mobility, impaired physical—skeletal deformity, pain/discomfort, decreased muscle strength, intolerance to activity.

Self-Care deficit/Home Maintenance Management, impaired—musculoskeletal impairment, decreased strength/endurance, pain on movement, inadequate support systems, insufficient finances, unfamiliarity with neighborhood resources.

TRANSPLANTATION (POSTOPERATIVE AND LIFELONG)

With current advances in technology and knowledge of immune responses at the molecular level, organ and tissue transplantation is becoming more commonplace. The most frequently transplanted organs are the kidney, liver, and heart. The major problem to be overcome is the immunological response of the patient to donor tissues. The ability of the immune system to distinguish self from nonself is crucial to its proper functioning; therefore, in the process of transplantation, the donor/nonself can be rejected. The three forms of rejection are (1) hyperactive or hyperacute (within 48 hr), (2) acute (usually within 3–6 mo), and (3) chronic (occurring months or years after transplant). General postoperative care is similar to that for any other major abdominal or cardiothoracic surgery; however, special considerations necessitate meticulous measures to prevent infection and identify early signs of rejection.

CARE SETTING

Post-ICU plan of care addresses early recovery and long-term postdischarge community/clinic follow-up phases.

RELATED CONCERNS

Refer to (1) specific surgical plans of care for general considerations (e.g., cardiac surgery), and (2) organ-specific plans (e.g., heart failure, renal failure, cirrhosis, hepatitis), relative to issues of target organ problems following transplantation.

Peritonitis, page 382
Psychosocial aspects of care, page 809
Sepsis/Septicemia, page 741
Surgical intervention, page 828
Thrombophlebitis: deep vein thrombosis, page 115

Patient Assessment Database

Refer to specific plans of care for data reflecting specific organ failure necessitating transplantation.

EGO INTEGRITY

May report: Feelings of anxiety, fearfulness

Multiple stressors: Impact of condition on personal relationships, ability to perform expected/needed roles, loss of control, required lifestyle changes; financial concerns, cost of procedure/future treatment needs; uncertainty of outcomes/personal mortality, spiritual conflicts; waiting period for suitable donation

Concerns about changes in appearance (e.g., bloating, jaundice, major scars), aesthetic side effects of immunosuppressant medications

Spiritual questioning (e.g., "Why me?" "Why should I benefit from someone else's death?")

May exhibit: Anxiety, delirium, depression; cognitive and emotional behavior changes

SEXUALITY

May report: Loss of libido

Concerns regarding sexual activity

SOCIAL INTERACTIONS

May report: Reactions of family members

Conflicts regarding family member(s) ability/willingness to participate, e.g., financial, organ/bone marrow donation, postprocedure support

Concern about benefiting from other person's death

Concern for family member who must take on new responsibilities as roles shift

TEACHING/LEARNING

May report: Previous illnesses, hospitalizations, surgeries

Lack of improvement/deterioration in condition

Beliefs about transplantation

History of alcohol/drug abuse, disease resulting in organ failure

Discharge plan considerations: **DRG projected mean length of inpatient stay: Dependent on organ transplanted.**

May need assistance with ADLs; shopping, transportation, ambulation; managing medication regimen

Refer to section at end of plan for postdischarge considerations.

DIAGNOSTIC STUDIES (Dependent on specific organ involvement)

General preoperative screening studies include:

Chest x-ray: Provides information about status of lungs and heart.

CT/MRI scan: Reveals status of body systems and organs, including size, shape, and general function of major blood vessels; organ size for best match with donor organ; and potential sources of postoperative complications. Rules out presence of cancer, which would contraindicate transplantation.

Total-body bone scan: Evaluates status of skeletal system to determine presence/absence of bone cancer.

Specific blood and tissue typing: As may be required for donor-recipient matching.

Dental evaluation: To rule out oral infection or abscessed teeth.

Ear, nose, and throat evaluation: To rule out sinus infection.

Renal function studies (e.g., IV pyelogram, creatinine clearance): Determines functional status of kidneys.

Pulmonary function studies: Determines lung function and/or limitations that may complicate recovery.

CBC: Identifies anemia, which can reduce oxygen-carrying capacity, and other blood factors that may affect recovery.

Biochemical studies: Various tests done as indicated in addition to electrolytes, immune status.

Screening tests: To detect presence/type of hepatitis; HIV, viral titer (e.g., CMV, herpes).

ECG: Screens cardiac status, e.g., electrical conduction/dysrhythmias, signs of infarcts/hypertrophy.

NURSING PRIORITIES

1. Prevent infection.
2. Maximize organ function.
3. Promote independent functioning.
4. Support family involvement and coping.

DISCHARGE GOALS

1. Free of signs of infection.
2. Signs of rejection absent/minimized.
3. New organ function adequate.
4. Usual activities resumed.
5. Plan in place to meet individual needs following discharge.

NURSING DIAGNOSIS: Infection, risk for

Risk factors may include
Medically induced immunosuppression, suppressed inflammatory response
Antibiotic therapy
Invasive procedures, broken skin/traumatized tissue
Effects of chronic/debilitating disease

Possibly evidenced by
[Not applicable; presence of signs and symptoms establishes an *actual* diagnosis]

DESIRED OUTCOMES/EVALUATION CRITERIA—PATIENT WILL:

Infection Status (NOC)

Be free of signs of infection.
Achieve timely wound healing.

PATIENT/CAREGIVER WILL:

Risk Control (NOC)

Demonstrate techniques, lifestyle changes to promote safe environment.

ACTIONS/INTERVENTIONS	RATIONALE

Infection Protection (NIC)

Independent

Screen visitors/staff for signs of infection; make sure nurse caring for patient with new transplant is not caring for another patient with infection. Maintain protective isolation as indicated.

Reduces possibility of patient's contracting a nosocomial infection. *Note:* Total isolation is usually restricted to patients with lung transplants or individuals with neutropenia.

Demonstrate and emphasize importance of proper handwashing techniques by patient and caregivers.

First-line defense against infection/cross-contamination.

Inspect all incisions/puncture sites. Evaluate healing progress.

Promotes early identification of onset of infection and prompt intervention.

Provide meticulous care of invasive lines, incisions, wounds.

Minimizes potential for bacteria to reduce exposure/ risk of infection. *Note:* Invasive lines are removed as early as possible following transplant.

Encourage deep breathing, coughing.

Mobilizes respiratory secretions and reduces risk of respiratory problems.

Provide/assist with frequent oral hygiene.

Meticulous attention to oral mucosa is necessary because immunosuppression/antibiotic therapies increase risk of opportunistic oral/mucosal infections.

Obtain sterile specimens of wound drainage as appropriate.

Identifying organism allows for appropriate treatment.

NURSING DIAGNOSIS: Anxiety [specify level]/Fear

May be related to
Unconscious conflict about essential values/beliefs
Situational crises, interpersonal transmission/contagion
Threat to self concept [perceived or actual]; organ rejection, threat of death
Side effects of steroids and/or cyclosporine

Possibly evidenced by
Increased tension, apprehension, uncertainty
Expressed concerns
Somatic complaints
Sympathetic stimulation

DESIRED OUTCOMES/EVALUATION CRITERIA—PATIENT WILL:

Anxiety or Fear Control (NOC)

Appear relaxed and report anxiety is reduced to a manageable level.
Verbalize awareness of feelings.
Identify healthy ways to deal with anxiety.
Use resources/support systems effectively.

ACTIONS/INTERVENTIONS	RATIONALE

Anxiety Reduction (NIC)

Independent

Discuss patient's posttransplant expectations, including physical appearance and lifestyle changes.	Depending on past experience and exposure to others with transplants, patient may have unrealistic ideas and real concerns about what may happen (e.g., organ rejection, effects of required medications, limitations associated with immunosuppression). Even with effective preoperative teaching, patient will continue to have new concerns or suppressed thoughts and beliefs, which can surface during recovery.
Encourage patient to discuss feelings and concerns about situation and to express fears.	Helps identify issues and can lead to problem solving. Patient may experience anxiety about many things (e.g., physical limitations, cognitive changes, role changes in family). These anxieties change frequently; some are persistent and new ones arise. Serious anxiety, delirium and depression are the most commonly reported postoperative psychiatric problems.
Discuss beliefs/concerns that are commonly held regarding source of organ.	Cultural/spiritual beliefs may lead patient to question whether organ from someone of another race or particular group may change own sense of self-identity.
Identify/encourage use of previously successful coping behaviors.	Under stress, patient may not remember what has worked in the past; discussion can refresh memories of successful behaviors and promote repetition.
Help patient focus on one "problem" at a time.	Dealing with one issue at a time seems to make it more manageable. Provides sense of success and opportunity to build on each success.
Discuss possibility and normalcy of mood swings.	Feelings of euphoria and depression are not uncommon, are usually short-lived but may persist, especially with use of steroids.
Encourage open communication between SO/family and patient within safe environment.	Free expression of feelings/beliefs can lead to clarification and problem solving of different views. When concerns or beliefs are hidden from one another, additional stress/adverse effects may result.
Provide opportunity for patient and SO/family to meet with other(s) who have experienced a similar and successful transplant.	Sharing experiences and hearing about successes and universal problems can lessen patient's/SO's anxieties, promote hope, and provide a role model.
Identify possible actions to limit physical effects or manifestations of long-term steroid/cyclosporine use.	Learning about clothing styles, makeup techniques, use of bleach or mild depilatory to reduce facial hair can enhance patient's appearance and reduce anxiety about social rejection.

Collaborative

Refer to spiritual advisor as indicated.	Facing one's mortality may provoke feelings of anxiety and questions about one's spiritual beliefs and practices.
Refer to social worker, other professionals as indicated.	Provides assistance with readjustment to life following major life event.

NURSING DIAGNOSIS: Coping, Individual/Family, risk for ineffective

Risk factors may include

Situational crises; family disorganization and role changes

Prolonged disease exhausting supportive capacity of SO/family

Possibly evidenced by

[Not applicable; presence of signs and symptoms establishes an *actual* diagnosis]

DESIRED OUTCOMES/EVALUATION CRITERIA—PATIENT/FAMILY WILL:

Coping (NOC)

Assess current situation accurately.

Verbalize awareness of own coping abilities.

Meet psychological needs as evidenced by appropriate expression of feelings, identifying options and resources.

ACTIONS/INTERVENTIONS	RATIONALE
Coping Enhancement (NIC)	
Independent	
Encourage and support patient in evaluating lifestyle. Discuss implications for the future.	Help patient evaluate and choose activities that are important and begin to adjust to new lifestyle of wellness. *Note:* Transplant patients sometimes cannot evaluate the seriousness of their condition or do not comprehend the risks or benefits involved in transplantation. Additionally, there may be denial about the impact of long-term treatment requirements (i.e., use of immunosuppressant drugs, biopsies, blood tests, and clinic visits).
Assess patient's/family's current functional status and note how transplant is affecting ability to cope.	Provides a starting point to identify needs and plan care. These people have been dealing with patient's chronic disease, uncertainty of organ waiting period, and protracted postoperative recovery course, and they face a complicated medical regimen after discharge. All these factors place demands on time, energy, finances, and relationships.
Determine additional outside stressors (e.g., family, social, work environment, or nursing/health care management).	Illness and treatment demands may affect all areas of life and problems need to be addressed and resolved to enable patient and SO to manage current situation optimally.
Provide ongoing information about expected progression of recuperation and potential course of recovery.	Knowing what to expect helps individuals cope more effectively, encourages planning for future needs/lifestyle changes.
Discuss normalcy of/monitor progression through states of acceptance of transplanted organ:	Sense that organ is "outside" body can be very frightening, while fixation on organ can be irritating to others. Understanding normalcy of feelings is reassuring. *Note:* Movement through stages is variable and regression is common, especially during early posttransplant period.
Foreign body stage—organ feels strange, separate from own body;	
Partial internalization stage—protective of organ, restricts movement/activity, excessive concern regarding organ function/fragility;	
Complete internalization—acceptance of organ into self-concept, discusses organ only in response to direct questioning.	

ACTIONS/INTERVENTIONS	RATIONALE

Independent

Have individual/SO list previous methods of dealing with life problems and outcomes of actions.

Promotes problem solving in current situation, allows individual to build on past successes.

Active-listen and identify individual's perceptions of what is happening, how transplant has affected view of self-family member.

Helps those involved to recognize own feelings and concerns regarding use of an organ from someone who died.

Encourage discussion between patient/family regarding future expectations.

Period of dependence during illness, concerns over possible organ rejection/life-threatening complications may lead to conflicts regarding patient's return to an independent role.

Collaborative

Involve in support groups.

Provides role models, source of practical advice, and emotional support.

Refer to spiritual resource and/or psychiatric clinical nurse specialist/psychiatrist, social worker, as indicated.

May be helpful in resolving lingering/difficult concerns.

NURSING DIAGNOSIS: Knowledge Deficit [Learning Need] regarding prognosis, therapeutic regimen, self care, and discharge needs

May be related to
Lack of exposure/recall
Information misinterpretation
Unfamiliarity with information resources
Cognitive limitation

Possibly evidenced by
Request for information; statement of misconception
Development of preventable complication

DESIRED OUTCOMES/EVALUATION CRITERIA—PATIENT WILL:

Knowledge: Health Behaviors/Health Resources (NOC)

Describe measures to reduce individual risk factors to recovery/general well-being.
Initiate necessary lifestyle changes and participate in treatment regimen.
Identify community resources.
Develop plan to meet follow-up care needs.
Assume responsibility for own learning and begin to look for information and ask questions.

For routine postoperative instructions, refer to CP: Surgical Intervention, page 828.

ACTIONS/INTERVENTIONS	RATIONALE

Teaching: Disease Process (NIC)

Independent

Review general signs/symptoms of rejection and infection (e.g., general malaise/fatigue, dyspnea, sudden weight gain, fever/chills, sore throat, delayed healing of wound, nausea/vomiting syncope). Review indicators specific to transplanted organ (e.g., liver rejection: pain in liver or back, lighter-colored stools, jaundice, dark-colored urine).

Prompt recognition and timely intervention may limit severity of complication. Acute rejection usually develops within days of transplant or may be delayed for a number of months. If detected early, rejection process can be minimized or reversed with changes in drug regimen. *Note:* Chronic rejection developing after months/years is generally irreversible.

ACTIONS/INTERVENTIONS

Independent

Emphasize necessity/verify patient ability to adhere to medical regimen and appropriate follow-up, including routine examinations (e.g., dental, gynecologic) and specialty examinations (e.g., ophthalmology, gastroenterology).

Discuss need to seek medical attention earlier than was probably done in the past.

Recommend that results of laboratory tests/diagnostic studies done locally be faxed to transplant center.

Provide information via multiple media, including written format, depending on level of comprehension. Include various members of the transplant team as appropriate.

Discuss "do's and don'ts" of specific medications, anticipated and adverse effects, interaction with other drugs, appropriate use of OTC products; adjustment of prescribed medication dosage (e.g., prednisone) during periods of stress, or with gradual decrease in immunosuppression over months/years, as appropriate.

Encourage patient/SO to maintain a working relationship with transplant team. Include family members, caregivers in education sessions and discharge planning as appropriate.

Recommend wearing an identification tag (bracelet, necklace, etc.).

Identify community resources, including transplant club/support groups.

Discuss self-monitoring routine and record keeping, e.g., chart temperature per protocol (before breakfast/dinner and when not feeling well); weigh daily before breakfast (in like clothing, same scale); blood pressure/pulse, changes in medication dosage, changes in health status/functional ability, etc.

Recommend frequent oral/dental care and periodic visual inspection of oral mucosa and gums.

RATIONALE

Because lack of cooperation is a major cause of post-transplant complications and mortality, the patient/SO needs to understand that adherence to regimen is imperative. Routine follow-up/care by healthcare providers is necessary to maximize general well-being and to monitor effects of long-term medication regimen on other organ systems. Specialty examinations aid in monitoring new organ function and effect on other systems. Additionally, steroids may cause changes in visual acuity or development of cataracts/glaucoma.

Generally a "wait and see" attitude can be detrimental because a delay in treatment could result in organ damage/rejection.

Long-term care is very complex and requires coordination and cooperation between all healthcare providers.

Enhances learning experience and provides references for postdischarge review/verification of recall. Use of team members, e.g., dietitian, physical/occupational therapists, provides for personalization of teaching plan to meet individual needs.

Multiple medications (often a triple therapy of cyclosporine, prednisone, and azathioprine) are typically required on an ongoing/lifelong basis to prevent organ rejection. Additional drugs may be needed to manage adverse side effects of immunosuppressant therapy (e.g., infection, osteoporosis, peptic ulcers, hypertension).

Promotes understanding and cooperation among those providing medical and psychological support in care of the patient.

In emergencies, provides immediate information to care providers relative to surgical/transplant history and medication regimen.

Provides opportunity for patient and SO(s) to share experiences with others who are going through the same process. Providing anticipatory guidance may enhance problem solving.

Helps care providers identify individual needs/development of complications.

Immunosuppression increases susceptibility to common opportunistic infections affecting the mouth, (e.g., *Candida*, herpes simplex); and ongoing drug regimen (such as cyclosporine) can cause hypertrophy of gums.

ACTIONS/INTERVENTIONS	RATIONALE

Independent

Review dietary needs. Determine optimal weight, discuss expected changes associated with medication regimen.	Requirements of normal healing, as well as effects of current stress, medications, and preoperative debilitation, can exacerbate nutritional deficiencies/imbalances and cause excessive weight loss; however, undesired weight gain can also occur because food tastes better, dietary restrictions are deleted, and prednisone stimulates appetite.
Identify risk factors/additional safety concerns relative to infections, e.g., avoid changing cat litter box or use of live virus vaccines; use gloves when gardening, and take proper care of wounds/tissue trauma.	Awareness of possible risks (including unusual sources) enable patient/family to plan for avoidance. Cat litter can transmit infectious agents such as *Listeria*. Steroid-induced skin fragility increases risk of injury from minor trauma as a result of immunosuppression.
Discuss necessity of handling skin carefully, avoiding strong sunlight and using sunscreen with SPF of 15 or greater.	Steroid therapy results in skin fragility and sun sensitivity. Broken/damaged skin provides an entry for bacteria.
Discuss common postoperative care needs, e.g., avoidance of heavy lifting/physical labor or exercise (including contact sports), and activities that stretch or put pressure on incision; when/how to resume driving and sexual activity; dietary and fluid needs/restrictions.	Reduces likelihood of complications, aids patient/SO in determining appropriateness of activities, and enhances patient's sense of control and personal responsibility for altering activity level. *Note:* General advice for early phase: "If it hurts, don't do it."
Encourage continuation of pre-illness daily routines and activities as appropriate.	Enhances general well-being. Promotes focus on returning to "normal life," reducing sense that everything is different now.
Discuss participation in planned exercise program and inform about Transplant Olympics as appropriate/desired.	Restores strength, promotes sense of well-being and self-esteem, reduces risk of osteoporosis, inappropriate weight gain, and decreases hypertension.
Identify employment concerns/risks specific to particular transplanted organ, job responsibilities, and workplace environment.	Provides opportunity to problem-solve, plan for modifications, or seek alternative vocational options.
Discuss travel needs, e.g., notify team contact person in advance regarding plans; hand carry medications when traveling by airplane; locate transplant center nearest to travel destination before leaving home.	Frees patient to be involved in travel if desired. May need special instructions/precautions, depending on travel destination.
Stress importance of notifying future care providers of medication regimen.	Status of immune system functioning may require prophylactic therapy for procedures (such as antibiotics with dental care).

POTENTIAL CONSIDERATONS following acute hospitalization (depending on patient's age, physical condition/presence of complications, personal resources, and life responsibilities)

Therapeutic Regimen: individual, ineffective management—postdischarge concern, complexity of therapeutic regimen, side effects of medications, economic difficulties, prolonged nature of treatment.

Infection, risk for—immunosuppression, antibiotic therapy.

Protection, altered—drug therapies (corticosteroid, immune).

Knowledge Deficit [Learning Need}—participation in support groups; ongoing care in collaboration with transplant team; gradual decrease of immunosuppression over months and years.

PSYCHOSOCIAL ASPECTS OF CARE

The emotional response of the patient during illness is of extreme importance. The mind-body-spirit connection is well established; it is known, for example, that when a physiological response occurs, there is a corresponding psychological response. Also, there are physiological conditions that have a psychological component, for example, the emotional instability associated with steroid therapy or Cushing's syndrome or the irritability of hypoglycemia. Rapid growth in the field of psychoneuroimmunology is regularly providing new information about these issues.

With expanding technology in healthcare, ethical issues are hotly debated. Although the stress of illness is well recognized, the effect on the individual is unpredictable. It is not necessarily the event that creates problems, but rather the patient's perception of and response to the event, which may result in unmet psychological needs that drain energy resources needed for healing. The caregivers', patients', and significant others' (SOs) values, sensitivity to different cultures, and language barriers (including difficulties that people have in talking about their bodies) affect the care a patient expects and receives.

CARE SETTING

Any setting in which nursing contact occurs/care is provided.

RELATED CONCERNS

This is an aspect of all care and plans of care.

Assessment Factors to Be Considered

INDIVIDUAL

Age and gender

Religious affiliation: church attendance, importance of religion in patient's life, belief in life after death

Level of knowledge/education; how the individual accesses and incorporates information, e.g., auditory, visual, kinesthetic

Patient's dominant language/literacy? Knowledge and use of other languages? Style of speech?

Patterns of communication with SOs, with healthcare givers?

Perception of body and its functions: In health, illness, this illness?

How does patient define and perceive illness?

How is patient experiencing illness versus what illness actually is?

Emotional response to current treatment/hospitalization

Past experience with illness, hospitalization, and healthcare systems

Emotional reactions in feeling (sensory) terms: e.g., states, "I feel scared."

Behavior when anxious, afraid, impatient, withdrawn, or angry

SIGNIFICANT OTHERS

Marital status; SOs, nuclear family, extended family. Recurring or patterned relationships

Family development cycle: Just married, children (young, adolescent, leaving/returning home), retired?

What are the interaction processes within the family?

Patient's role in family tasks and functions

How are SOs affected by the illness and prognosis?

Lifestyle differences that need to be considered: Dietary, spiritual, sexual preference, other community (e.g., religious order, commune, retirement center)

SOCIOECONOMIC

Employment; finances

Environmental factors: Home, work, and recreation; out of usual environment (on vacation, visiting)

Social class; value system

Social acceptability of disease/condition (e.g., sexually transmitted diseases [STDs], HIV, obesity, substance abuse)

CULTURAL

Ethnic background; heritage and residence/local

Beliefs regarding caring and curing

Health-seeking behaviors; illness referral system

Values related to health and treatment

Cultural factors related to illness in general and to pain response

DISEASE (ILLNESS)

Kind/cause of illness; how has it been treated, how should it be treated? Anticipated response to treatment; patient's/SO's expectations

Is this an acute or a chronic illness? Is it inherited? What is the threat to self/others?

If terminal illness, what do the patient and SO know and anticipate?

Is the condition "appropriate" to the afflicted individual, e.g., multiple sclerosis, diabetes mellitus (DM), cancer?

Illness related to personality factors, such as type A (may be myth or valid); high-risk behaviors

NURSE-RELATED

Basic knowledge of human responses and how the current situation is related to response of the individual

Basic knowledge of biological, psychological, social, and cultural issues

Knowledge and use of therapeutic communication skills

Knowledge of own value and belief systems, including prejudices, biases

Willingness to look at own behavior in relation to interaction with others and make changes as necessary

Respect of patient's privacy; confidentiality; human needs

NURSING PRIORITIES

1. Reduce anxiety/fear.
2. Support grieving process.
3. Facilitate integration of self-concept and body-image changes.
4. Encourage effective coping skills of patient/SO.
5. Promote safe environment/patient well-being.

DISCHARGE GOALS

1. Reports/anxiety/fear manageable.
2. Progressing through stages of grieving.
3. Patient/family dealing realistically with current situation.
4. Safe environment maintained.
5. Plan in place to meet needs after discharge.

NURSING DIAGNOSIS: Anxiety [specify level]/Fear

May be related to

Unconscious conflict about essential goals and values of life

Situational and/or maturational crises; interpersonal transmission and contagion; unmet needs

Threat to self-concept; threat of death; change in health status; threat to or change in interaction patterns, role function, economic status

Separation from support system; knowledge deficit

Sensory impairment; environmental stimuli; substance abuse; stress

Possibly evidenced by

Reports of increased tension; feelings of helplessness; inadequacy; apprehension, uncertainty, being scared, overexcited

Facial tension; sympathetic/parasympathetic stimulation (quivering voice, trembling, insomnia); extraneous movements (e.g., foot shuffling, hand/arm movements)

Expressed concern regarding changes in life events; dread of an identifiable problem recognized by the patient; fear of unspecific consequences

Focus on self; fight/flight behavior

DESIRED OUTCOMES/EVALUATION CRITERIA—PATIENT WILL:

Anxiety or Fear Control (NOC)

Acknowledge and discuss fears/concerns.

Appear relaxed and report anxiety is reduced to a manageable level.

Verbalize awareness of feelings of anxiety and healthy ways to deal with them.

Demonstrate problem solving and use resources effectively.

ACTIONS/INTERVENTIONS

Anxiety Reduction (NIC)

Independent

Note palpitations, elevated pulse/respiratory rate.

Acknowledge fear/anxieties. Validate observations with patient, e.g., "You seem to be afraid?"

Assess degree/reality of threat to patient and level of anxiety (e.g., mild, moderate, severe) by observing behavior such as clenched hands, wide eyes, startle response, furrowed brow, clinging to family/staff, or physical/verbal lashing out.

Note narrowed focus of attention (e.g., patient concentrates on one thing at a time).

Observe speech content, vocabulary, and communication patterns, e.g., rapid/slow, pressured speech; words commonly used, repetition, use of humor/laughter.

Assess severity of pain when present. Delay gathering of information if pain is severe.

Identify patient's/SO's perception(s) of the situation.

RATIONALE

Changes in vital signs may suggest the degree of anxiety the patient is experiencing or reflect the impact of physiological factors, e.g., endocrine imbalances.

Feelings are real, and it is helpful to bring them out in the open so they can be discussed and dealt with.

Individual responses can vary according to cultural beliefs/traditions and culturally learned patterns. Distorted perceptions of the situation may magnify feelings.

Narrowed focus usually reflects extreme fear/panic.

Provides clues about such factors as the level of anxiety, ability to comprehend what is currently happening, cognition difficulties, and possible language differences.

Severe pain and anxiety leave little energy for thinking and other activities.

Regardless of the reality of the situation, perception affects how each individual deals with the illness/stress.

ACTIONS/INTERVENTIONS	RATIONALE
Independent	
Acknowledge reality of the situation as the patient sees it, without challenging the belief.	Patient may need to deny reality until ready to deal with it. It is not helpful to force the patient to face facts.
Evaluate coping/defense mechanisms being used to deal with the perceived or real threat.	May be dealing well with the situation at the moment; e.g., denial and regression may be helpful coping mechanisms for a time. However, use of such mechanisms diverts energy the patient needs for healing, and problems need to be dealt with at some point in time.
Review coping mechanisms used in the past, e.g., problem-solving skills, recognizing/asking for help.	Provides opportunity to build on resources the patient/SO may have used successfully.
Assist patient to use the energy of anxiety for coping with the situation when possible.	Moderate anxiety heightens awareness and can help motivate the patient to focus on dealing with problems.
Maintain frequent contact with the patient/SO. Be available for listening and talking as needed.	Establishes rapport, promotes expression of feelings, and helps patient and SO look at realities of the illness/treatment without confronting issues they are not ready to deal with.
Acknowledge feelings as expressed (e.g., use of Active-Listening, reflection). If actions are unacceptable, take necessary steps to control/deal with behavior. (Refer to ND: Violence, risk for, p. 824.)	Often acknowledging feelings enables patient to deal more appropriately with situation. May need chemical/physical control for brief periods.
Identify ways in which patient can get help when needed, including telephone numbers of contact persons.	Provides assurance that staff/resources are available for assistance/support.
Stay with or arrange to have someone stay with patient as indicated.	Continuous support may help patient regain internal locus of control and reduce anxiety/fear to a manageable level.
Provide accurate information as appropriate and when requested by the patient/SO. Answer questions freely and honestly and in language that is understandable by all. Repeat information as necessary; correct misconceptions.	Complex and/or anxiety-provoking information can be given in manageable amounts over an extended period. As opportunities arise and facts are given, individuals will accept what they are ready for. *Note:* Words/phrases may have different meanings for each individual; therefore, clarification is necessary to ensure understanding.
Avoid empty reassurances, with statements of "everything will be all right." Instead, provide specific information: e.g., "Your heart rate is regular, your pain is being easily controlled, and that is what we want," or "Your CD4 count has been stable for the last three visits."	It is not possible for the nurse to know how the specific situation will be resolved, and false reassurances may be interpreted as lack of understanding or honesty, further isolating the patient. Sharing observations used in assessing condition/prognosis provides opportunity for patient/SO to feel reassured.
Note expressions of concern/anger about treatment or staff.	Anxiety about self and outcome may be masked by comments or angry outbursts directed at therapy/caregivers.
Ask the patient/SO to identify what he or she can/cannot do about what is happening.	Assists in identifying areas in which control can be exercised and those in which control is not possible.
Provide as much order and predictability as possible in scheduling care/activities, visitors.	Helps patient anticipate and prepare for difficult treatments/movements, as well as look forward to pleasant occurrences.
Instruct in ways to use positive self-talk, e.g., "I can manage this pain for now," or "My cancer is shrinking."	Internal dialogue is often negative. When this is shared out loud, the patient becomes aware and can be directed in the use of positive self-talk, which can help reduce anxiety.

ACTIONS/INTERVENTIONS

Independent

Encourage patient to develop regular exercise/activity program.

Encourage/instruct in mental imagery/relaxation methods; e.g., imaging a pleasant place, use of music/tapes, deep-breathing, meditation, and mindfulness.

Provide touch, Therapeutic Touch, massage, and other adjunctive therapies as indicated.

Collaborative

Administer medications as needed: e.g., diazepam (Valium), clorazepate (Tranxene), chlordiazepoxide (Librium), alprazolam (Xanax), buspirone (BuSpar), oxazepam (Serax), lorazepam (Ativan), doxepin (Sinequan), fluoxetine (Prozac), sertraline (Zoloft).

RATIONALE

Helpful in reducing level of anxiety; has been shown to raise endorphin levels to enhance sense of well-being.

Promotes release of endorphins and aids in developing internal locus of control, reducing anxiety. May enhance coping skills, allowing body to go about its work of healing. *Note:* Mindfulness is a method of being in the here and now, concentrating on what is happening in the moment.

Aids in meeting basic human need, decreasing sense of isolation, and assisting the patient to feel less anxious. *Note:* Therapeutic Touch requires the nurse to have specific knowledge and experience to use the hands to correct energy field disturbances by redirecting human energies to help or heal.

Antianxiety agents and/or antidepressants may be useful for brief periods to assist the patient/SO to reduce anxiety to manageable levels, providing opportunity for initiation of patient's own coping skills. *Note:* Use of selective serotonin reuptake inhibitors (SSRIs) such as Prozac, Zoloft have been associated with sexual function complaints. Alternatives may need to be considered. Also, ethnic variations affecting psychotropic drugs require close monitoring to determine therapeutic dosage. For example, East Asians and blacks may be more sensitive/react faster, have higher plasma drug levels, and have increased risk of side effects, necessitating lower dosage than whites in general.

NURSING DIAGNOSIS: Grieving [specify]

May be related to
Actual or perceived object loss (may include people, possessions, job, status, home, ideals, parts and processes of the body); chronic and/or fatal illness
Thwarted grieving response to a loss; lack of resolution of previous grieving response/absence of anticipatory grieving

Possibly evidenced by
Verbal expression of distress/unresolved issues, difficulty in expressing loss; denial of loss
Altered eating habits, sleep/dream patterns, activity levels, libido
Crying; labile affect; feelings of sorrow, guilt, anger
Alterations in concentration and/or pursuit of tasks, developmental regression; difficulty taking on new or different roles

DESIRED OUTCOMES/EVALUATION CRITERIA—PATIENT WILL:

Grief Resolution (NOC)

Identify and express feelings freely/effectively.
Verbalize a sense of progress toward resolution of the grief and hope for the future.
Function at an adequate level, participate in work and activities of daily living (ADLs), as appropriate.

ACTIONS/INTERVENTIONS	RATIONALE

Grief Work Facilitation (NIC)

Independent

Provide open environment in which the patient feels free to realistically discuss feelings and concerns.

Therapeutic communication skills such as Active-Listening, silence, being available, and acceptance can allow the patient the opportunity to talk freely and deal with the perceived/actual loss.

Determine patient perception and meaning of loss (current and past). Note cultural factors/expectations.

Affects patient's responses and needs to be acknowledged in planning care.

Identify stage of grieving and effect on functioning:

Awareness allows for appropriate choice of interventions because individuals handle grief in many different ways.

Denial: Be aware of avoidance behaviors; anger, withdrawal, and so forth. Allow patient to talk about what he or she chooses, and do not try to force patient to "face the facts";

Denying the reality of diagnosis and/or prognosis is an important phase in which the patient protects self from the pain and reality of the threat of loss. Each person does this in an individual manner based on previous experiences with loss and cultural/religious factors.

Anger: Note behaviors of withdrawal, lack of cooperation, and direct expression of anger. Be alert to body language and check meaning with the patient, noting congruency with verbalizations. Encourage/allow verbalization of anger, acknowledge feelings, set limits regarding destructive behavior;

Denial gives way to feelings of anger, rage, guilt, and resentment. Patient may find it difficult to express anger directly and may feel guilty about normal feelings of anger. Although staff may have difficulty dealing with angry behaviors, acceptance allows patient to work through the anger and move on to more effective coping behaviors.

Bargaining: Be aware of statements such as ". . . if I do this, that will fix my problem." Allow verbalization without confrontation about realities;

Bargaining with care providers or God often occurs and may be helpful in beginning resolution and acceptance. Patient may be working through feelings of guilt about things done or undone.

Depression: Give patient permission to be where he or she is. Provide hope within parameters of individual situation without giving false reassurance. Provide comfort and availability, as well as caring for physical needs;

When patient can no longer deny the reality of the loss, feelings of helplessness and hopelessness replace feelings of anger. The patient needs information that this is a normal progression of feelings.

Acceptance: Respect the patient's needs and wishes for quiet, privacy, and/or talking.

Having worked through the denial, anger, and depression, patient often prefers to be alone and does not want to talk much at this point. Patient may still cling to hope, which can be sustaining through whatever is happening at this point.

Active-Listen patient's concerns and be available for help as necessary.

The process of grieving does not proceed in an orderly fashion, but fluctuates with various aspects of all stages present at one time or another. If process is dysfunctional or prolonged, more aggressive interventions may be required to facilitate the process.

Determine quality of interactions with others, including family members.

Although period of withdrawal/loneliness usually accompany grieving, persistent isolation may indicate deepening depression, necessitating further evaluation/intervention. *Note:* Family/SO may not be dysfunctional but may be intolerant of patient's behaviors.

Identify and problem-solve solutions to existing physical responses, e.g., eating, sleeping, activity levels, and sexual desire.

May need additional assistance to deal with the physical aspects of grieving.

ACTIONS/INTERVENTIONS

Independent

Assess needs of SO and assist as indicated.

Include family/SO as appropriate when determining future needs.

Discuss healthy ways of dealing with difficult situation.

Collaborative

Refer to other resources, e.g., support groups, counseling, spiritual/pastoral care, psychotherapy as indicated.

RATIONALE

Identification of problems indicating dysfunctional grieving allows for individual interventions.

Depending on patient desires/legal requirements, choices regarding future plans (e.g., living situation, continuation of care, end-of-life decisions, funeral arrangements) can provide guidance and peace of mind.

Provides opportunity to look toward the future and plan family's/SO's needs (e.g., for life after loss).

May need additional help to resolve grief, make plans, and look toward the future.

NURSING DIAGNOSIS: Self-Esteem, situational low

May be related to

Biophysical, psychosocial, cognitive, perceptual, cultural, and/or spiritual crisis, e.g., changes in health status/body image, role performance, personal identity; loss of control of some aspect of life

Maturational transitions

Perceived/anticipated failure at life event(s)

Possibly evidenced by

Rationalizes away/rejects positive feedback; negative self-appraisal in response to life events

Verbalization of negative feelings about the self (helplessness, uselessness); focus on past abilities, strengths, function or appearance; preoccupation with change/loss

Evaluates self as unable to handle situations/events; hesitant to try new things/situations; difficulty making decisions

Fear of rejection/reaction by others; projection of blame/responsibility for problems

DESIRED OUTCOMES/EVALUATION CRITERIA—PATIENT WILL:

> **Self-Esteem (NOC)**

Verbalize realistic view and acceptance of self in situation.

Identify existing strengths and view self as capable person.

Recognize and incorporate change into self-concept in accurate manner without negating self-worth.

Demonstrate adaptation to changes/events that have occurred as evidenced by setting of realistic goals and active participation in work/play/personal relationships.

ACTIONS/INTERVENTIONS

> **Self-Esteem Enhancement (NIC)**

Independent

Ask what the patient would like to be called.

Identify SO from whom the patient derives comfort and who should be notified in case of emergency.

RATIONALE

Shows courtesy/respect and acknowledges person.

Allows provisions to be made for specific person(s) to visit or remain close, and provides needed support for patient. *Note:* May or may not be legal next of kin.

ACTIONS/INTERVENTIONS	RATIONALE

Independent

Identify basic sense of self-esteem, image patient has of existential, physical, psychological self. Identify locus of control.	May provide insight into whether this is a single episode or recurrent/chronic situation and can help determine needs and treatment plan. It is helpful to know whether the individual's locus of control is internal or external to provide most helpful interventions.
Determine patient perception of threat to self.	Patient's perception is more important than what is really happening and needs to be dealt with before reality can be addressed.
Active-Listen patient concerns and fears.	Conveys sense of caring and can be helpful in identifying the patient's needs, problems, and coping strategies and how effective they are. Provides opportunity to duplicate and begin a problem-solving process.
Encourage verbalization of feelings, accepting what is said.	Helps patient/SO begin to adapt to change and reduces anxiety about altered function/lifestyle.
Discuss stages of grief and the importance of grief work. (Refer to ND: Grieving [specify], p. 318.)	Grieving is a necessary step for integration of change/loss into self-concept.
Provide nonthreatening environment.	Promotes feelings of safety, encouraging verbalization.
Observe nonverbal communication, e.g., body posture and movements, eye contact, gestures, use of touch.	Nonverbal language is a large portion of communication and therefore is extremely important. How the person uses touch provides information about how it is accepted and how comfortable the individual is with being touched.
Reflect back to the patient what has been said, e.g., "it upset you when he told you that."	Clarification and verification of what has been heard promotes understanding and allows patient to validate information, otherwise assumptions may be inaccurate.
Observe and describe behavior in objective terms.	All behavior has meaning, some of which is obvious and some of which needs to be identified. This is a process of educated guesswork and requires validation by the patient.
Identify age and developmental level.	Age is an indicator of the stage of life patient is experiencing, e.g., adolescence, middle age. However, developmental level may be more important than chronological age in anticipating and identifying some of the patient's needs. Some degree of regression occurs during illness, depending on many factors such as the normal coping skills of the individual, the severity of the illness, and family/cultural expectations.
Discuss patient's view of body image and how illness/condition might affect it.	The patient's perception of a change in body image may occur suddenly or over time (e.g., actual loss of a body part through injury/surgery, or a perceived loss, such as a heart attack) or be a continuous subtle process (e.g., chronic illness, eating disorders, or aging). Awareness can alert the nurse to the need for appropriate interventions tailored to the individual need.
Encourage discussion of physical changes in a simple, direct, and factual manner. Give realistic feedback and discuss future options, e.g., rehabilitation services.	Provides opportunity to begin incorporating actual changes in an accepting and hopeful atmosphere.
Acknowledge efforts at problem solving, resolution of current situation, and future planning.	Provides encouragement and reinforces continuation of desired behaviors.

ACTIONS/INTERVENTIONS	RATIONALE
Independent	
Recognize patient's pace for adaptation to demands of current situation.	Failure to acknowledge patient's need to take time and/or pressuring patient to "get on with it" conveys a lack of acceptance of the person as an individual and may result in feelings of lowered self-esteem.
Introduce tasks at patient's level of functioning, progressing to more complex activities as tolerated.	Provides opportunity for patient to experience successes, reaffirming capabilities and enhancing self-esteem.
Ascertain how the patient sees own role within the family system, e.g., breadwinner, homemaker, husband/wife.	Illness may create a temporary or permanent problem in role expectations. Sexual role and how the patient views self in relation to the current illness also play important parts in recovery.
Assist patient/SO with clarifying expected roles and those that may need to be relinquished or altered.	Provides opportunity to identify misconceptions and begin to look at options; promotes reality orientation.
Determine patient awareness of own responsibility for dealing with situation, personal growth.	Conveys confidence in patient's ability to cope. When patient acknowledges own part in planning and carrying out treatment plan, he or she has more investment in following through on decisions that have been made.
Assess impact of illness/surgery on sexuality.	Sexuality encompasses the whole person in the total environment. Many times problems of illness are superimposed on already existing problems of sexuality and can affect patient's sense of self-worth. Some problems are more obvious than others, such as illness involving the reproductive parts of the body. Others are less obvious, such as sexual values, role in family, e.g., mother, wage earner, single parent.
Be alert to comments and innuendos, which may mean the patient has a concern in the area of sexuality.	People are often reluctant and/or embarrassed to ask direct questions about sexual/sexuality concerns.
Be aware of caregiver's feelings about dealing with the subject of sexuality.	Nurses/caregivers are often as reluctant and embarrassed in dealing with sexuality issues as most patients.
Collaborative	
Provide information and referral to hospital and community resources.	Enables patient/SO to be in contact with interested groups with access to assistive and supportive devices, services, and counseling.
Support participation in group/community activities, e.g., assertiveness classes, volunteer work, support groups.	Promotes skills of coping and sense of self-worth.
Refer to psychiatric support/therapy group, social services, as indicated.	May be needed to assist patient/SO to achieve optimal recovery.
Refer to appropriate resources for sex therapy as need indicates.	May be someone with comfort level and knowledge who is available, or may be necessary to refer to professional resources for additional help and support.

NURSING DIAGNOSIS: Coping, Individual, ineffective/Decisional Conflict

May be related to
Situational crises/personal vulnerability; multiple life changes/maturational crises, age/developmental stage

Inadequate level of confidence in ability to cope, perception of control; high degree of threat; support

No vacations/inadequate relaxation

Impairment of nervous system; memory loss; impaired adaptive behaviors and problem-solving skills

Severe pain/overwhelming threat to self

Unclear personal values/beliefs; perceived threat to value system; lack of experience/interference with decision making; lack of information

Possibly evidenced by

Verbalization of inability to cope/ask for help; inappropriate use of defense mechanisms; inability to meet role expectations, basic needs, problem-solve

Muscular tension, frequent headaches/neckaches

Report of chronic worry, fatigue, insomnia, anxiety/depression; poor concentration

Poor self-esteem

Alteration in social participation; change in usual communication patterns; verbal manipulation

High illness/accident rate; overeating; excessive smoking/drinking

Destructive behavior toward self or others, risk-taking

Uncertainty about choices; vacillation between alternative actions; delayed decision making

DESIRED OUTCOMES/EVALUATION CRITERIA—PATIENT WILL:

Coping (NOC)

Identify ineffective coping behaviors and consequences.

Verbalize awareness of own coping/problem-solving abilities.

Meet psychological needs as evidenced by appropriate expression of feelings, identification of options, and use of resources.

Decision Making (NOC)

Make decisions and express satisfaction with choices.

ACTIONS/INTERVENTIONS	RATIONALE
Coping Enhancement (NIC)	
Independent	
Review pathophysiology affecting the patient and extent of feelings of hopelessness/helplessness/loss of control over life, level of anxiety; perception of situation.	Indicators of degree of disequilibrium and need for intervention to prevent or resolve the crisis. Studies suggest that up to 85% of all physically ill people are depressed to some degree. Impairment of normal functioning for more than 2 weeks, especially in presence of chronic condition, may reflect depression, requiring further evaluation.
Establish therapeutic nurse-patient relationship.	Patient may feel freer in the context of this relationship to verbalize feelings of helplessness/powerlessness and to discuss changes that may be necessary in the patient's life.
Note expressions of indecision, dependence on others, and inability to manage own ADLs.	May indicate need to lean on others for a time. Early recognition and intervention can help patient regain equilibrium.

ACTIONS/INTERVENTIONS

Independent

Assess presence of positive coping skills/inner strengths, e.g., use of relaxation techniques, willingness to express feelings, use of support systems.

Encourage patient to talk about what is happening at this time and what has occurred to precipitate feelings of helplessness and anxiety.

Evaluate ability to understand events. Correct misperceptions, provide factual information.

Provide quiet, nonstimulating environment. Determine what patient needs, and provide if possible. Give simple, factual information about what patient can expect and repeat as necessary.

Allow patient to be dependent in the beginning, with gradual resumption of independence in ADLs, self-care, and other activities. Make opportunities for patient to make simple decisions about care/other activities when possible, accepting choice not to do so.

Accept verbal expressions of anger, setting limits on maladaptive behavior.

Discuss feelings of self-blame/projection of blame on others.

Note expressions of inability to find meaning in life/reason for living, feelings of futility or alienation from God.

Promote safe and hopeful environment, as needed. Identify positive aspects of this experience and assist patient to view it as a learning opportunity.

Provide support for patient to problem-solve solutions for current situation. Provide information and reinforce reality as patient begins to ask questions; look at what is happening.

Provide for gradual implementation and continuation of necessary behavior/lifestyle changes. Reinforce positive adaptation/new coping behaviors.

Collaborative

Refer to other resources as necessary (e.g., clergy, psychiatric clinical nurse specialist/psychiatrist, family/marital therapist, addiction support groups).

RATIONALE

When the individual has coping skills that have been successful in the past, they may be used in the current situation to relieve tension and preserve the individual's sense of control. However, limitations of condition may impact choices available to patient; e.g., playing musical instrument to relieve stress may not be possible for individual with tremors or hemiparesis, but listening to tapes/CDs may provide some degree of comfort.

Provides clues to assist patient to develop coping and regain equilibrium.

Assists in identification and correction of perception of reality and enables problem solving to begin.

Decreases anxiety and provides control for the patient during crisis situation.

Promotes feelings of security (patient will know nurse will provide safety). As control is regained, patient has the opportunity to develop adaptive coping/problem-solving skills.

Verbalizing angry feelings is an important process for resolution of grief and loss. However, preventing destructive actions (such as striking out at others) preserves patient's self-esteem.

Although these mechanisms may be protective at the moment of crisis, they eventually are counterproductive and intensify feelings of helplessness and hopelessness.

Crisis situation may evoke questioning of spiritual beliefs, affecting ability to cope with current situation and plan for the future.

May be helpful while patient regains inner control.

Helping patient/SO to brainstorm possible solutions (giving consideration to the pros and cons of each) promotes feelings of self-control/esteem.

Reduces anxiety of sudden change and allows for developing new and creative solutions.

Additional assistance may be needed to help patient resolve problems/make decisions.

ACTIONS/INTERVENTIONS	RATIONALE
Family Involvement (NIC)	
Independent	
Assess level of anxiety present in family/SO.	Anxiety level needs to be dealt with before problem solving can begin. Individuals may be so preoccupied with own reactions to situation that they are unable to respond to another's needs.

ACTIONS/INTERVENTIONS

Independent

Establish rapport and acknowledge difficulty of the situation for the family.

Evaluate pre-illness/current behaviors that are interfering with the care/recovery of the patient.

Discuss underlying reasons for patient behaviors with family.

Assist family/patient to understand "who owns the problem" and who is responsible for resolution. Avoid placing blame or guilt.

Determine current knowledge/perception of the situation.

Assess current actions of SO and how they are received by patient.

Involve SO in information giving, problem solving, and care of patient as feasible. Identify other ways of demonstrating support while maintaining patient's independence.

Reframe negative expressions into positives whenever possible.

Collaborative

Refer to appropriate resources for assistance as indicated (e.g., counseling, psychotherapy, financial, spiritual).

RATIONALE

May assist SO to accept what is happening and be willing to share problems with staff.

Information about family problems (e.g., divorce/separation, alcoholism/other drug abuse, abusive situation) will be helpful in determining options and developing an appropriate plan of care.

When family members know why patient is behaving in different ways, it helps them understand and accept/deal with unusual behaviors.

When these boundaries are defined, each individual can begin to take care of own self and stop taking care of others in inappropriate ways.

Provides information on which to begin planning care and make informed decisions. Lack of information or unrealistic perceptions can interfere with caregiver's/care receiver's response to illness situation.

SO may be trying to be helpful, but actions are not perceived as being helpful by the patient. SO may be withdrawn or too protective.

Information can reduce feelings of helplessness and uselessness. Involvement in care enhances feelings of control and self-worth.

Promotes more hopeful attitude and helps family/patient look toward the future.

May need additional assistance in resolving family issues.

NURSING DIAGNOSIS: Family Coping: potential for growth

May be related to

Basic needs sufficiently gratified and adaptive tasks effectively addressed to enable goals of self-actualization to surface

Willingness to deal with one's own needs and to begin to problem-solve with the patient

Possibly evidenced by

Family member attempting to describe growth impact of crisis on his/her own values, priorities, goals, or relationships

Family member moving in direction of health-promoting and enriching lifestyle and generally choosing experiences that optimize wellness

DESIRED OUTCOMES/EVALUATION CRITERIA—FAMILY WILL:

> **Role Performance (NOC)**

Express willingness to look at own role in family's growth.

Undertake tasks leading to change.

Verbalize feelings of self-confidence and satisfaction with progress being made.

ACTIONS/INTERVENTIONS	RATIONALE

Family Support (NIC)

Independent

Provide opportunities for family to talk with patient and/or staff.

Reduces anxiety and allows expression of what has been learned and how they are managing, as well as opportunity to make plans for the future and share support.

Listen to family's expressions of hope, planning, effect on relationships/life, change of values.

Provides clues to avenues to explore for assistance with growth.

Provide opportunities for and instruction in how SOs can care for patient. Discuss ways in which they can support patient in meeting own needs.

Enhances feelings of control and involvement in situation in which SOs cannot do many things. Also provides opportunity to learn how to be most helpful when patient is discharged.

Provide a role model with which family may identify.

Having a positive example can help with adoption of new behaviors to promote growth.

Discuss importance of open communication. Role play effective communication skills of Active-Listening, "I-messages," and problem solving.

Helps individuals to express needs and wants in ways that will develop family cohesiveness. Promotes solutions in which everyone wins.

Encourage family to learn new and effective ways of dealing with feelings.

Effective recognition and expression of feelings clarify situation for involved individuals.

Encourage seeking help appropriately. Give information about available persons and agencies.

Permission to seek help as needed allows them to choose to take advantage of available assistance/resources.

Collaborative

Refer to specific support group(s) as indicated.

Provides opportunities for sharing experiences; provides mutual support and practical problem solving; and can aid in decreasing alienation and helplessness.

NURSING DIAGNOSIS: Therapeutic Regimen: Individual, risk for ineffective management

Risk factors may include

Complexity of therapeutic regimen; knowledge deficits

Decisional conflict: patient value system, health beliefs, spiritual values, cultural influences, ethical concerns

Perceived barriers; economic difficulties; side effects of therapy; mistrust of regimen and/or healthcare personnel; complexity of healthcare system

Family patterns of healthcare; family conflict

Possibly evidenced by

[Not applicable; presence of signs and symptoms establishes an *actual* diagnosis]

DESIRED OUTCOMES/EVALUATION CRITERIA—PATIENT WILL:

Treatment Behavior: Illness or Injury (NOC)

Participate in the development of goals and treatment plan.

Verbalize accurate knowledge of disease and understanding of treatment regimen.

Demonstrate behaviors/changes in lifestyle necessary to maintain therapeutic regimen.

Identify/use available resources.

ACTIONS/INTERVENTIONS	RATIONALE

Values Clarification (NIC)

Independent

Review patient's/SO's knowledge and understanding of the need for treatment/medication, as well as consequences of actions and choices. Note ability to comprehend information, including literacy, level of education, primary language.

Provides opportunities to clarify viewpoints/misconceptions. Verifies that patient/SO has accurate/factual information with which to make informed choices.

Be aware of developmental and chronological age.

Impacts ability to understand own needs/incorporate into treatment regimen.

Determine cultural, spiritual, and health beliefs, and ethical concerns.

Provides insight into thoughts/factors related to individual situation. Beliefs will affect patient's perception of situation and participation in treatment regimen. Treatment may be incongruent with patient's social/cultural lifestyle and perceived role/responsibilities.

Self-Modification Assistance (NIC)

Review treatment plan with patient/SO.

Provides opportunities to exchange accurate information and to clarify viewpoints/misconceptions.

Contract with the patient for participation in care.

Patient who agrees to own responsibility is more apt to adhere to treatment plan.

Establish graduated goals or modified regimen as necessary; work out alternate solutions.

Promotes patient involvement/independence; provides opportunity for compromise and may enhance cooperation with regimen. When patient participates in setting goals, there is a sense of investment that encourages cooperation and willingness to follow through with the program.

Assess availability/use of support systems. Identify additional resources as appropriate.

Access to/proper use of helpful resources can assist patient in meeting treatment goals and provide purpose for living. Presence of caring, empathic family/SO(s) can help patient in process of recovery.

Determine potential problems that may/do interfere with treatment, including lack of financial/personal resources, unavailability of providers. Assess level of anxiety, locus of control, sense of powerlessness.

Many factors may be involved in behavior that is disruptive to the treatment regimen (e.g., fear of hospitalization/treatment; denial of situation consequences; suspicion about healthcare system; physical factors, such as pain, hypoxemia, chemical imbalance).

Note length of illness/prognosis.

Patients tend to become passive and dependent in long-term, debilitating illness.

Listen to/Active-Listen patient's reports and comments.

Conveys message of concern, belief in individual's capabilities to resolve situation in positive manner.

Develop a system for self-monitoring. Share data pertinent to patient's condition, e.g., laboratory results, blood pressure (BP) readings.

Provides a sense of control; enables patient to follow own progress and make informal choices.

Have same personnel care for patient as much as possible.

Enables relationship to develop in which the patient can begin to trust/participate in care.

Accept the patient's choice/point of view, even if it appears to be self-destructive, e.g., decision to continue smoking.

Patient has the right to make own decisions, and acceptance may give a sense of control, which can help the patient look more clearly at consequences. Confrontation is not beneficial and may actually be detrimental to future cooperation and goal achievement.

ACTIONS/INTERVENTIONS

Independent

Be aware of own/caregiver's response to patient's treatment choices (e.g., refusal of blood or chemotherapy, living will).

RATIONALE

Negative feelings regarding these choices may create power struggles and be expressed in judgmental behaviors that block or interfere with patient's wishes, comfort, and/or care. *Note:* If resolution cannot be found, providers have the right to terminate their services with appropriate notice.

NURSING DIAGNOSIS: Violence, risk for self-directed; directed at others

Risk factors may include

History of violence against others; violent antisocial behavior, indirect (tearing of clothes, temper tantrum, yelling, throwing things); childhood abuse; witnessing family violence; cruelty to animals, firesetting

Attempt to deal with the threat to self-concept that illness can represent

Antisocial character; catatonic/manic excitement; panic states; rage reactions; psychotic symptomatology

Suicidal ideation/behavior, depression; impulsivity

Hormonal imbalance; neurological impairment, such as temporal lobe epilepsy; toxic reactions to medication

Negative role modeling; developmental crisis

[Possible indicators]

Suspicion of others, paranoid ideation, delusions, hallucinations

Expressed intent or desire to harm self/others (directly or indirectly); hostile verbalizations; plan and possession of/access to destructive means

Body language: rigid posture, clenched fists, facial expressions

Increased motor activity, excitement, irritability, agitation

Overt and aggressive acts; self-destructive behavior

Substance abuse/withdrawal

DESIRED OUTCOMES/EVALUATION CRITERIA—PATIENT WILL:

Impulse Control (NOC)

Acknowledge realities of the situation.
Verbalize understanding of reason(s) for behavior/precipitating factors.
Express increased self-concept.
Demonstrate self-control, as evidenced by relaxed posture, nonviolent behavior.

ACTIONS/INTERVENTIONS

Mood Management (NIC)

Independent

Observe for early signs of distress.

Maintain straightforward communication and assist patient to learn assertive rather than manipulative, nonassertive/aggressive behavior.

RATIONALE

Irritability, pacing, shouting/cursing, lack of cooperation, and demanding behavior may all be signs of increasing anxiety.

Avoids reinforcing manipulative behavior and enhances positive interactions with others, accomplishing the goal of getting needs met in acceptable ways.

ACTIONS/INTERVENTIONS

Independent

Help patient identify more adequate solutions/behaviors (e.g., motor activities/exercise). Provide directions for actions patient can take.

Give as much autonomy as is possible in the situation.

Monitor for suicidal/homicidal intent, e.g., morbid or anxious feelings while with the patient, thoughts expressed by/warning from the patient, "It doesn't matter, I'd be better off dead"; mood swings, putting affairs in order, previous suicide attempt.

Assess suicidal intent (1–10 scale) by asking directly if patient is thinking of killing self, has plan, means, and so on.

Acknowledge reality of suicide/homicide as an option. Discuss consequences of actions if patient were to follow through on intent. Ask how it will help patient resolve problems.

Accept patient's anger without reacting on an emotional basis.

Remain calm and state limits on behavior in a firm manner. Be truthful and nonjudgmental.

Assume that the patient has control and is responsible for own behavior.

Identify conditions that may interfere with ability to control own behavior.

> ### Environmental Management: Violence Prevention (NIC)

Provide protection within the environment, e.g., constant observation, removal of objects that might be used to harm self/others.

Tell patient to "stop."

Use an organized team approach when necessary to subdue patient with force. Tell patient clearly and concisely what is happening.

Hold patient; place in restraints or seclusion if necessary. Do so in a calm, positive, nonstimulating/nonpunitive manner.

Apply and adjust restraint devices properly.

Document precise reason for restraints, actions taken. Check restraints frequently per facility protocol, each time documenting the condition and how long the restraints are used.

RATIONALE

Promotes release of energies in acceptable ways.

Enhances feelings of power and control in a situation in which many things are not within individual's control.

Indicators of need for further assessment, evaluation, and intervention/psychiatric care.

Provides guidelines for necessity/urgency of interventions. Direct questioning is most helpful when done in a caring, concerned manner.

Patient is often focused on suicide (or homicide) as the "only" option and this response provides an opening to look at and discuss other options. *Note:* Be aware of own responsibility under Tarasoff rule to warn possible victim(s) when patient is expressing homicidal ideation.

Responding with anger is not helpful in resolving the situation and may result in escalating patient's behavior.

Understanding that helplessness and fear underlie this behavior can be helpful.

Often enables the individual to exercise control. *Note:* When violent behavior is the result of drugs, patient may not be able to respond appropriately.

Acute or chronic brain syndrome, drug-induced or postsurgical confusion may precipitate violent behavior that is difficult to control.

May need more structure to maintain control until own internal locus of control is regained.

May be sufficient to help patient control own actions if exhibiting hostile actions. *Note:* Patient is often afraid of own actions and wants staff to set limits.

Knowing and practicing these actions before they are needed helps prevent untoward problems. Keeping patient informed can help patient to regain internal control.

As a last resort, physical restraint may be necessary while the patient regains control. *Note:* These measures are meant to protect the patient, not punish the behavior.

It is important to maintain body alignment and patient safety and comfort.

Restraints are to be used for very specific reasons, which need to be clearly documented to avoid overuse or misuse.

ACTIONS/INTERVENTIONS

| Mood Management (NIC) |

Collaborative

Refer to psychiatric resource(s), e.g., clinical specialist, psychiatric nurse, psychiatrist, psychologist, social worker.

Administer medications, e.g., antianxiety/antipsychotic agents, sedatives, narcotics.

RATIONALE

More in-depth assistance may be needed to deal with patient and defuse situation.

May be indicated to quiet/control behavior. *Note:* May need to be withheld if they are suspected to be the cause of/contribute to the behavior.

NURSING DIAGNOSIS: Post-Trauma Syndrome

May be related to

Events outside the range of usual human experience: disasters (e.g., floods, earthquakes, tornadoes, airplane crashes); wars, epidemics, rape, incest, assault, torture, catastrophic illness or accident, being held hostage; physical/psychosocial abuse

Possibly evidenced by

Re-experiencing traumatic event (may be identified in cognitive, affective, and/or sensory/motor activities, e.g., flashbacks, intrusive thoughts, repetitive dreams or nightmares, excessive verbalization of the traumatic event, verbalization of survival guilt or guilt about behavior required for survival)

Altered lifestyle (self-destructiveness); loss of interest in usual activities; loss of feeling of intimacy/sexuality; development of phobia; poor impulse control/irritability and explosiveness

Disturbance of mood, e.g., depression, anxiety, embarrassment, fear, self-blame, low self-esteem; hypervigilant; exaggerated startle response

Cognitive disruption: confusion, loss of memory/concentration, indecisiveness

DESIRED OUTCOMES/EVALUATION CRITERIA—PATIENT WILL:

| Coping (NOC) |

Verbalize reduced anxiety/fear.

Demonstrate ability to deal with emotional reactions in an individually appropriate manner.

Express own feelings/reactions; avoid projection.

Demonstrate appropriate changes in lifestyle/getting support from SO as needed.

Participate in plans for follow-up care/counseling.

ACTIONS/INTERVENTIONS

| Counseling (NIC) |

Independent

Determine when traumatic event(s) occurred: present or past.

RATIONALE

Manifestations of acute and chronic posttrauma responses may require different interventions. *Note:* Event may encompass many forms of trauma, including the diagnosis of life-threatening illness.

ACTIONS/INTERVENTIONS

Independent

Assess physical trauma, if present, and individual reaction to occurrence, e.g., physical symptoms such as numbness, headache, tightness in chest, and psychological responses of anger, shock, acute anxiety, confusion, denial.

Evaluate behavior (e.g., calm or agitated, excited/hysterical; inappropriate laughter, crying), expressions of disbelief and/or self-blame.

Note ethnic background/cultural and religious perceptions and beliefs about the event.

Assess signs/stage of grieving.

Tell patient that painful emotional reactions are normal. Phrase this information in neutral terms: "You may or may not experience. . ."

Discuss things patient can do to feel better, e.g., physical exercise alternated with relaxation; keeping busy with normal activities; talking to others; acknowledging that it is all right to feel upset; writing about the experience in a journal; being kind to self.

Assist with learning stress management techniques.

Identify supportive persons for patient.

Note signs of severe/prolonged depression; frequency of flashbacks/nightmares; presence of chronic pain, somatic complaints.

Help patient identify factors that may have created a vulnerable situation/increased likelihood for event.

Collaborative

Refer to support groups, counselors/therapists for further therapy, e.g., psychotherapy (in conjunction with medications); implosive therapy, flooding, hypnosis, eye movement desensitization and reprocessing (EMDR), Rolfing, memory work, or cognitive restructuring, as indicated.

RATIONALE

Provides information with which to develop plan of care, make informed choices.

Indicators of extent of individual response to traumatic incident and degree of disorganization.

May influence patient's response to what has happened, e.g., may believe it is retribution from God.

Patient may be suffering from sense of loss of self and/or others.

Understanding that experiencing these uncomfortable feelings is not unusual after traumatic event may reduce patient's anxiety/fear of "going crazy" and enhance coping.

Enhances sense of control and helps patient achieve resolution of uncomfortable feelings. Often when the patient begins these activities within the first 24 hr of the event, further therapy may not be required.

Promotes sense of control and ability to handle existing problems.

Having positive support systems can help patient reach optimal recovery.

If patient did not deal with trauma when it occurred, behavioral manifestations may reveal extent of problem in the present.

Even though individual may not be responsible for what has happened, he/she may have created an atmosphere in which negative things occurred. Changes in behaviors/lifestyle may decrease potential for recurrence.

When posttrauma response has become chronic, patient may need more in-depth assistance from sensitive, trained individuals who are skilled in dealing with these problems.

POTENTIAL CONSIDERATIONS

Refer to primary diagnosis for postdischarge concerns.

SURGICAL INTERVENTION

Surgery may be needed to diagnose or cure a specific disease process, correct a structural deformity, restore a functional process, or reduce the level of dysfunction/pain. Although surgery is generally elective or pre-planned, potentially life-threatening conditions can arise, requiring emergency intervention. Absence or limitation of preoperative preparation and teaching increases the need for postoperative support in addition to managing underlying medical conditions.

CARE SETTING

May be inpatient on a surgical unit or outpatient/short-stay in an ambulatory surgical setting.

RELATED CONCERNS

Alcohol: acute withdrawal, page 873
Cancer, page 900
Diabetes mellitus/Diabetic ketoacidosis, page 440
Fluid and electrolyte imbalances, page 926
Hemothorax/Pneumothorax, page 165
Metabolic acidosis, page 523
Metabolic alkalosis, page 527
Peritonitis, page 382
Pneumonia, microbial, page 140
Psychosocial aspects of care, page 809
Respiratory acidosis, page 214
Respiratory alkalosis, page 218
Sepsis/Septicemia, page 741
Thrombophlebitis: DVT, page 115
Total nutritional support, page 508

Also refer to plan of care for specific surgical procedure performed.

Patient Assessment Database

Data depends on the duration/severity of underlying problem and involvement of other body systems. Refer to specific plans of care for data and diagnostic studies relevant to the procedure and additional nursing diagnoses.

CIRCULATION

May report:	History of cardiac problems, heart failure (HF), pulmonary edema, peripheral vascular disease, or vascular stasis (increases risk of thrombus formation)
May exhibit:	Changes in heart rate (sympathetic stimulation)

EGO INTEGRITY

May report:	Feelings of anxiety, fear, anger, apathy Multiple stress factors, e.g., financial, relationship, lifestyle
May exhibit:	Restlessness, increased tension/irritability Sympathetic stimulation, e.g., changes in heart rate (HR), respiratory rate

ELIMINATION

May report:	History of kidney/bladder conditions; use of diuretics/laxatives

FOOD/FLUID

May report:	Pancreatic insufficiency/DM (predisposing to hypoglycemia/ketoacidosis) Use of diuretics
May exhibit:	Malnutrition (including obesity) Dry mucous membranes (limited intake/nothing-by-mouth [NPO] period preoperatively)

RESPIRATION

May report:	Infections, chronic conditions/cough, smoking
May exhibit:	Changes in respiratory rate (sympathetic stimulation)

SAFETY

May report: Allergies or sensitivities to medications, food, tape, latex, and solution(s)

Immune deficiencies (increases risk of systemic infections and delayed healing)

Presence of cancer/recent cancer therapy

Family history of malignant hyperthermia/reaction to anesthesia, autoimmune diseases

History of hepatic disease (affects drug detoxification and may alter coagulation)

History of blood transfusion(s)/transfusion reaction

May exhibit: Presence of existing infectious process; fever

TEACHING/LEARNING

May report: Use of medications such as anticoagulants, steroids, antibiotics, antihypertensives, cardiotonic glycosides, antidysrhythmics, bronchodilators, diuretics, decongestants, analgesics, anti-inflammatories, anticonvulsants, or antipsychotics/antianxiety agents, as well as over-the-counter (OTC) medications, herbal supplements, or alcohol or other drugs of abuse (risk of liver damage affecting coagulation and choice of anesthesia, as well as potential for postoperative withdrawal)

Discharge plan considerations: **DRG projected mean length of stay: 2.6 days for inpatient procedures, 2–36 hr for outpatient**

May require temporary assistance with transportation, dressing(s)/supplies, self-care, and homemaker/maintenance tasks

Possible placement in rehabilitation/extended care facility

Refer to section at end of plan for postdischarge considerations.

DIAGNOSTIC STUDIES

General preoperative requirements may include: Complete blood count (CBC), prothrombin time (PT)/activated partial thromboplastin time (aPTT), chest x-ray. Other studies depend on type of operative procedure, underlying medical conditions, current medications, age, and weight. These tests may include blood urea nitrogen (BUN), creatinine (Cr), glucose, arterial blood gases (ABGs), electrolytes; liver function, thyroid, nutritional studies, electrocardiogram (ECG). Deviations from normal should be corrected if possible before safe administration of anesthetic agents.

CBC: An elevated white blood cell (WBC) count is indicative of inflammatory process (may be diagnostic, e.g., appendicitis); decreased WBC count suggests viral processes (requiring evaluation because immune system may be dysfunctional). Low hemoglobin (Hb) suggests anemia/blood loss (impairs tissue oxygenation and reduces the Hb available to bind with inhalation anesthetics); may suggest need for crossmatch/blood transfusion. An elevated hematocrit (Hct) may indicate dehydration; decreased Hct suggests fluid overload.

Electrolytes: Imbalances impair organ function, e.g., decreased potassium affects cardiac muscle contractility, leading to decreased cardiac output.

ABGs: Evaluates current respiratory status, which may be especially important in smokers, patients with chronic lung diseases.

Coagulation times: May be prolonged, interfering with intraoperative/postoperative hemostasis; hypercoagulation increases risk of thrombosis formation, especially in conjunction with dehydration and decreased mobility associated with surgery.

Urinalysis: Presence of WBCs or bacteria indicates infection. Elevated specific gravity may reflect dehydration.

Pregnancy test: Positive results affect timing of procedure and choice of pharmacological agents.

Chest x-ray: Should be free of infiltrates, pneumonia; used for identification of masses and COPD.

ECG: Abnormal findings require attention before administering anesthetics.

NURSING PRIORITIES

1. Reduce anxiety and emotional trauma.
2. Provide for physical safety.
3. Prevent complications.
4. Alleviate pain.
5. Facilitate recovery process.
6. Provide information about disease process/surgical procedure, prognosis, and treatment needs.

DISCHARGE GOALS

1. Patient dealing realistically with current situation.
2. Injury prevented.
3. Complications prevented/minimized.
4. Pain relieved/controlled.
5. Wound healing/organ function progressing toward normal.
6. Disease process/surgical procedure, prognosis, and therapeutic regimen understood.
7. Plan in place to meet needs after discharge.

PREOPERATIVE

NURSING DIAGNOSIS: Knowledge Deficit [Learning Need] regarding condition, prognosis, treatment, self care, and discharge needs

May be related to
Lack of exposure/recall, information misinterpretation
Unfamiliarity with information resources

Possibly evidenced by
Statement of the problem/concerns, misconceptions
Request for information
Inappropriate, exaggerated behaviors (e.g., agitated, apathetic, hostile)
Inaccurate follow-through of instructions/development of preventable complications

DESIRED OUTCOMES/EVALUATION CRITERIA—PATIENT WILL:

Knowledge: Treatment Procedure(s) (NOC)

Verbalize understanding of disease process/perioperative process and postoperative expectations.
Correctly perform necessary procedures and explain reasons for the actions.
Initiate necessary lifestyle changes and participate in treatment regimen.

ACTIONS/INTERVENTIONS	RATIONALE
Teaching: Preoperative (NIC)	
Independent	
Assess patient's level of understanding.	Facilitates planning of preoperative teaching program, identifies content needs.
Review specific pathology and anticipated surgical procedure. Verify that appropriate consent has been signed.	Provides knowledge base from which patient can make informed therapy choices and consent for procedure, and presents opportunity to clarify misconceptions.
Use resource teaching materials, audiovisuals as available.	Specifically designed materials can facilitate the patient's learning.
Implement individualized preoperative teaching program:	
Preoperative/postoperative procedures and expectations, urinary and bowel changes, dietary considerations, activity levels/transfers, respiratory/cardiovascular exercises; anticipated IV lines and tubes (e.g., nasogastric [NG] tubes, drains, and catheters);	Enhances patient's understanding/control and can relieve stress related to the unknown/unexpected.
Preoperative instructions, e.g., NPO time, shower/skin preparation, which routine medications to take/hold, e.g., prophylactic antibiotics, or anticoagulants, anesthesia premedication;	Helps reduce the possibility of postoperative complications and promotes a rapid return to normal body function. *Note:* In some instances, liquids and medications are allowed up to 2 hr before scheduled procedure.

ACTIONS/INTERVENTIONS

Independent

Intraoperative patient safety, e.g., not crossing legs during procedures performed under local/light anesthesia;

Expected/transient reactions (e.g., low backache, localized numbness and reddening or skin indentations);

Inform patient/SO about itinerary, physician/SO communications.

Discuss/develop individual postoperative pain management plan. Identify misconceptions patient may have and provide appropriate information.

Provide opportunity to practice coughing, deep-breathing, and muscular exercises.

RATIONALE

Reduced risk of complications/untoward outcomes, such as injury to the peroneal and tibial nerves with postoperative pain in the calves and feet.

Minor effects of immobilization/positioning should resolve in 24 hr. If they persist, medical evaluation is required.

Logistical information about operating room (OR) schedule and locations (e.g., recovery room, postoperative room assignment), as well as where and when the surgeon will communicate with SO relieves stress and miscommunications, preventing confusion and doubt over patient's well-being.

Increases likelihood of successful pain management. Some patients may expect to be pain-free or fear becoming addicted to narcotic agents.

Enhances learning and continuation of activity postoperatively.

NURSING DIAGNOSIS: Fear/Anxiety (specify level)

May be related to
Situational crisis; unfamiliarity with environment
Change in health status; threat of death
Separation from usual support systems

Possibly evidenced by
Increased tension, apprehension, decreased self-assurance
Expressed concern regarding changes, fear of consequences
Facial tension, restlessness, focus on self
Sympathetic stimulation

DESIRED OUTCOMES/EVALUATION CRITERIA—PATIENT WILL:

Anxiety or Fear Control (NOC)

Acknowledge feelings and identify healthy ways to deal with them.
Appear relaxed, able to rest/sleep appropriately.
Report decreased fear and anxiety reduced to a manageable level.

ACTIONS/INTERVENTIONS

Anxiety Reduction (NIC)

Provide preoperative education, including visit with OR personnel before surgery when possible. Discuss anticipated things that may frighten/concern patient, e.g., masks, lights, IVs, BP cuff, electrodes, bovie pad, feel of oxygen cannula/mask on nose or face, autoclave and suction noises, child crying.

RATIONALE

Can provide reassurance and alleviate patient's anxiety, as well as provide information for formulating intraoperative care. Acknowledges that foreign environment may be frightening, alleviates associated fears.

ACTIONS/INTERVENTIONS	RATIONALE

Independent

Inform patient/SO of nurse's intraoperative advocate role.	Develops trust/rapport, decreasing fear of loss of control in a foreign environment.
Identify fear levels that may necessitate postponement of surgical procedure.	Overwhelming or persistent fears result in excessive stress reaction, potentiating risk of adverse reaction to procedure/anesthetic agents.
Validate source of fear. Provide accurate factual information. Active-Listen concerns.	Identification of specific fear helps patient deal realistically with it, e.g., misidentification/wrong operation, dismemberment, disfigurement, loss of dignity/control, or being awake/aware with local anesthesia. Patient may have misinterpreted preoperative information or have misinformation regarding surgery/disease process. Fears regarding previous experiences of self/family/acquaintances may be unresolved.
Note expressions of distress/feelings of helplessness, preoccupation with anticipated change/loss, choked feelings.	Patient may already be grieving for the loss represented by the anticipated surgical procedure/diagnosis/prognosis of illness.
Tell patient anticipating local/spinal anesthesia that drowsiness/sleep occurs, that more sedation may be requested and will be given if needed, and that surgical drapes will block view of the operative field.	Reduces concerns that patient may "see" the procedure.
Introduce staff at time of transfer to operating suite.	Establishes rapport and psychological comfort.
Compare surgery schedule, patient identification band, chart, and signed operative consent for surgical procedure.	Provides for positive identification, reducing fear that wrong procedure may be done.
Prevent unnecessary body exposure during transfer and in OR suite.	Patients are concerned about loss of dignity and inability to exercise control.
Give simple, concise directions/explanations to sedated patient. Review environmental concerns as needed.	Impairment of thought processes makes it difficult for patient to understand lengthy instructions.
Control external stimuli.	Extraneous noises and commotion may accelerate anxiety.

Collaborative

Refer to pastoral spiritual care, psychiatric nurse, clinical specialist, psychiatric counseling if indicated.	May be desired or required for patient to deal with fear, especially concerning life-threatening conditions, serious and/or high-risk procedures.
Discuss postponement/cancellation of surgery with physician, anesthesiologist, patient, and family as appropriate.	May be necessary if overwhelming fears are not reduced/resolved.
Administer medications as indicated, e.g.:	
Sedatives, hypnotics;	Used to promote sleep the evening before surgery; may enhance coping abilities.
IV antianxiety agents.	May be provided in the outpatient admitting/preoperative holding area to reduce nervousness and provide comfort. *Note:* Respiratory depression/bradycardia may occur, necessitating prompt intervention.

NURSING DIAGNOSIS: Perioperative Positioning, risk for injury

Risk factors may include

Disorientation; sensory/perceptual disturbances due to anesthesia

Immobilization; musculoskeletal impairments

Obesity/emaciation; edema

Possibly evidenced by

[Not applicable; presence of signs and symptoms establishes an *actual* diagnosis]

DESIRED OUTCOMES/EVALUATION CRITERIA—PATIENT WILL:

Safety Status: Physical Injury (NOC)

Be free of injury related to perioperative disorientation.

Be free of untoward skin/tissue injury or changes lasting beyond 24–48 hr following procedure.

Report resolution of localized numbness, tingling, or changes in sensation related to positioning within 24–48 hr as appropriate.

ACTIONS/INTERVENTIONS	RATIONALE
Positioning Intraoperative (NIC)	
Interventions	
Note anticipated length of procedure and customary position. Be aware of potential complications.	Supine position may cause low back pain and skin pressure at heels/elbows/sacrum; lateral chest position can cause shoulder and neck pain, plus eye and ear injury on the patient's downside.
Review patient's history, noting age, weight/height, nutritional status, physical limitation/preexisting conditions that may affect choice of position and skin/tissue integrity during surgery.	Many conditions (e.g., lack of subcutaneous padding in elderly person, arthritis, thoracic outlet/cubital tunnel syndrome, diabetes, obesity, presence of abdominal stoma, peripheral vascular disease, level of hydration, temperature of extremities) can make individual prone to injury.
Stabilize both patient cart and OR table when transferring patient to and from OR table, using an adequate number of personnel for transfer and support of extremities.	Unstabilized cart/table can separate, causing patient to fall. Both side rails must be in the down position for caregiver(s) to assist patient transfer and prevent loss of balance.
Anticipate movement of extraneous lines and tubes during the transfer and secure or guide them into position.	Prevents undue tension and dislocation of IV lines, NG tubes, catheters, and chest tubes; maintains gravity drainage when appropriate.
Secure patient on OR table with safety belt as appropriate, explaining necessity for restraint.	OR tables and arm boards are narrow, placing patient at risk for injury, especially during fasciculation. Patient may become resistive or combative when sedated or emerging from anesthesia, furthering potential for injury.
Protect body from contact with metal parts of the operating table.	Reduces risk of electrical injury.

ACTIONS/INTERVENTIONS

Independent

Prepare equipment and padding for required position, according to operative procedure and patient's specific needs. Pay special attention to pressure points of bony prominences (e.g., arms, ankles) and neurovascular pressure points (e.g., breasts, knees).

Position extremities so they may be periodically checked for safety, circulation, nerve pressure, and alignment. Monitor peripheral pulses, skin color/temperature.

Place legs in stirrups simultaneously (when lithotomy position used), adjusting stirrup height to patient's legs, maintaining symmetrical position. Pad popliteal space and heels/feet as indicated.

Provide foot board/elevate drapes off toes. Avoid/monitor placement of equipment, instrumentation on trunk/extremities during procedure.

Reposition slowly at transfer from table and in bed (especially halothane-anesthetized patient).

Determine specific postoperative positioning guidelines, e.g., elevation of head of bed following spinal anesthesia, turn to unoperated side following pneumonectomy.

Collaborative

Recommend position changes to anesthesiologist and/or surgeon as appropriate.

RATIONALE

Depending on individual patient's size, weight, and preexisting conditions, extra padding materials may be required to protect bony prominences, prevent circulatory compromise/nerve pressure, or allow for optimum chest expansion for ventilation.

Prevents accidental trauma, e.g., hands, fingers, and toes could inadvertently be scraped, pinched, or amputated by moving table attachments; positional pressure of brachial plexus, peroneal, and ulnar nerves can cause serious problems with extremities; prolonged plantar flexion may result in footdrop.

Prevents muscle strain; reduces risk of hip dislocation in elderly patients. Padding helps prevent peroneal and tibial nerve damage. *Note:* Prolonged positioning in stirrups may lead to compartment syndrome in calf muscles.

Continuous pressure may cause neural, circulatory, and skin integrity disruption.

Myocardial depressant effect of various agents increases risk of hypotension and/or bradycardia.

Reduces risk of postoperative complications, e.g., headache associated with migration of spinal anesthesia, or loss of maximal respiratory effort.

Close attention to proper positioning can prevent muscle strain, nerve damage, circulatory compromise, and undue pressure on skin/bony prominences. Although the anesthesiologist is responsible for positioning, the nurse may be able to see/have more time to note patient needs, and provide assistance.

NURSING DIAGNOSIS: Injury, risk for

Risk factors may include
Interactive conditions between individual and environment
External environment, e.g., physical design, structure of environment, exposure to equipment, instrumentation, positioning, use of pharmaceutical agents
Internal environment, e.g., tissue hypoxia, abnormal blood profile/altered clotting factors, broken skin

Possibly evidenced by
[Not applicable; presence of signs and symptoms establishes an *actual* diagnosis]

DESIRED OUTCOMES/EVALUATION CRITERIA—CAREGIVER WILL:

> **Risk Control (NOC)**

Identify individual risk factors.
Modify environment as indicated to enhance safety and use resources appropriately.

ACTIONS/INTERVENTIONS

RATIONALE

Surgical Precautions (NIC)

Independent

Remove dentures, partial plates or bridges preoperatively per protocol. Inform anesthesiologist of problems with natural teeth, e.g., loose teeth.

Remove prosthetics, other devices preoperatively or after induction, depending on sensory/perceptual alterations and mobility impairment.

Remove jewelry preoperatively or tape over as appropriate.

Verify patient identity and scheduled operative procedure by comparing patient chart, arm band, and surgical schedule. Verbally ascertain correct name, procedure, operative site, and physician.

Document allergies, including risk for adverse reaction to latex, tape, and prep solutions.

Give simple and concise directions to the sedated patient.

Prevent pooling of prep solutions under and around patient.

Assist with induction as needed; e.g., stand by to apply cricoid pressure during intubation or stabilize position during lumbar puncture for spinal block.

Ascertain electrical safety of equipment used in surgical procedure, e.g., intact cords, grounds, medical engineering verification labels.

Place dispersive electrode (electrocautery pad) over greatest available muscle mass, ensuring its contact.

Confirm and document correct sponge, instrument, needle, and blade counts.

Laser Precautions (NIC)

Verify credentials of laser operators for specific wavelength laser required for particular procedure.

Foreign bodies may be aspirated during endotracheal intubation/extubation.

Contact lenses may cause corneal abrasions while under anesthesia; eyeglasses and hearing aids are obstructive and may break; however, patients may feel more in control of environment if hearing and visual aids are left on as long as possible. Artificial limbs may be damaged and skin integrity impaired if left on.

Metals conduct electrical current and provide an electrocautery hazard. In addition, loss or damage to patient's personal property can easily occur in the foreign environment. *Note:* In some cases (e.g., arthritic knuckles), it may not be possible to remove rings without cutting them off. In this situation, applying tape over the ring may prevent patient from "catching" ring and prevent loss of stone or damage to finger.

Assures correct patient, procedure, and appropriate extremity/side.

Reduces risk for allergic responses that may impair skin integrity or lead to life-threatening systemic reactions.

Impairment of thought process makes it difficult for patient to understand lengthy directions.

Antiseptic solutions may chemically burn skin, as well as conduct electricity.

Facilitates safe administration of anesthesia.

Malfunction of equipment can occur during the operative procedure, causing not only delays and unnecessary anesthesia but also injury or death, e.g., short circuits, faulty grounds, laser malfunctions, or laser misalignment. Periodic electrical safety checks are imperative for all OR equipment.

Provides a ground for maximum conductivity to prevent electrical burns.

Foreign bodies remaining in body cavities at closure not only cause inflammation, infection, perforation, and abscess formation, disastrous complications that lead to death.

Because of the potential hazards of laser, physician and equipment operators must be certified in the use and safety requirements of specific wavelength laser and procedure, i.e., open, endoscopic, abdominal, laryngeal, intrauterine.

ACTIONS/INTERVENTIONS	RATIONALE

Independent

Confirm presence of fire extinguishers and wet fire smothering materials when lasers are used intraoperatively.

Laser beam may inadvertently contact and ignite combustibles outside of surgical field, i.e., drapes, sponges.

Apply patient eye protection before laser activation.

Eye protection for specific laser wavelength must be used to prevent injury.

Protect surrounding skin and anatomy appropriately, i.e., wet towels, sponges, dams, cottonoids.

Prevents inadvertent skin integrity disruption, hair ignition, and adjacent anatomy injury in area of laser beam use.

Surgical Assistance (NIC)

Handle, label, and document specimens appropriately, ensuring proper medium and transport for tests required.

Proper identification of specimens to patient is imperative. Frozen sections, preserved or fresh examination, and cultures all have different requirements. OR nurse advocate must be knowledgeable of specific hospital laboratory requirements for validity of examination.

Fluid Management (NIC)

Monitor intake and output (I&O) during procedure. Ascertain that infusion pumps are functioning accurately.

Potential for fluid volume deficit or excess exists, affecting safety of anesthesia, organ function, and patient well-being.

Collaborative

Administer IV fluids, blood/blood components, and medications as indicated.

Helps maintain homeostasis and adequate level of sedation/muscle relaxation to produce optimal surgical outcome.

Collect blood intraoperatively as appropriate.

Blood lost intraoperatively may be collected, filtered, and reinfused either intraoperatively or postoperatively. *Note:* Alternatively, red blood cell (RBC) production may be increased by the administration of epoetin (EPO), reducing the need for blood transfusion whether autologous or donated.

Surgical Precautions (NIC)

Administer antacids, H_2 blocker, preoperatively as indicated.

Neutralizes gastric acidity and may reduce risk of aspiration/severity of pneumonia should aspiration occur, especially in obese/pregnant patients in whom there is an 85% risk of mortality with aspiration.

Limit/avoid use of epinephrine to Fluothane-anesthetized patient.

Fluothane sensitizes the myocardium to catecholamines and may produce dysrhythmias.

NURSING DIAGNOSIS: Infection, risk for

Risk factors may include
Broken skin, traumatized tissues, stasis of body fluids
Presence of pathogens/contaminants, environmental exposure, invasive procedures

Possibly evidenced by
[Not applicable; presence of signs and symptoms establishes an *actual* diagnosis]

	DESIRED OUTCOMES/EVALUATION CRITERIA—CAREGIVER WILL:

Knowledge: Infection Control (NOC)

Identify individual risk factors and interventions to reduce potential for infection. Maintain safe aseptic environment.

ACTIONS/INTERVENTIONS	RATIONALE

Infection Control: Intraoperative (NIC)

Independent

ACTIONS/INTERVENTIONS	RATIONALE
Adhere to facility infection control, sterilization, and aseptic policies/procedures.	Established mechanisms designed to prevent infection.
Verify sterility of all manufacturers' items.	Prepackaged items may appear to be sterile; however, each item must be scrutinized for manufacturer's statement of sterility, breaks in packaging, environmental effect on package, and delivery techniques. Package sterilization and expiration dates, lot/serial numbers must be documented on implant items for further follow-up if necessary.
Review laboratory studies for possibility of systemic infections.	Increased WBC count may indicate ongoing infection, which the operative procedure will alleviate (e.g., appendicitis, abscess, inflammation from trauma); or presence of systemic/organ infection, which may contraindicate/impact surgical procedure and/or anesthesia (e.g., pneumonia, kidney infection).
Verify that preoperative skin, vaginal, and bowel cleansing procedures have been done as needed depending on specific surgical procedure.	Cleansing reduces bacterial counts on the skin, vaginal mucosa, and alimentary tract.
Prepare operative site according to specific procedures.	Minimizes bacterial counts at operative site.
Examine skin for breaks or irritation, signs of infection.	Disruptions of skin integrity at or near the operative site are sources of contamination to the wound. Careful shaving/clipping is imperative to prevent abrasions and nicks in the skin.
Maintain dependent gravity drainage of indwelling catheters, tubes, and/or positive pressure of parenteral or irrigation lines.	Prevents stasis and reflux of body fluids.
Identify breaks in aseptic technique and resolve immediately on occurrence.	Contamination by environmental/personnel contact renders the sterile field unsterile, thereby increasing the risk of infection.
Contain contaminated fluids/materials in specific site in operating room suite, and dispose of according to hospital protocol.	Containment of blood and body fluids, tissue, and materials in contact with an infected wound/patient will prevent spread of infection to environment/other patients or personnel.
Apply sterile dressing.	Prevents environmental contamination of fresh wound.

837

ACTIONS/INTERVENTIONS

Collaborative

Provide copious wound irrigation, e.g., saline, water, antibiotic, or antiseptic.

Obtain specimens for cultures/Gram stain.

Administer antibiotics as indicated.

RATIONALE

May be used intraoperatively to reduce bacterial counts at the site and cleanse the wound of debris, e.g., bone, ischemic tissue, bowel contaminants, toxins.

Immediate identification of type of infective organism by Gram stain allows prompt treatment, while more specific identification by cultures can be obtained in hours/days.

May be given prophylactically for suspected infection or contamination.

NURSING DIAGNOSIS: Body Temperature, risk for altered

Risk factors may include
Exposure to cool environment
Use of medications, anesthetic agents
Extremes of age, weight; dehydration

Possibly evidenced by
[Not applicable; presence of signs and symptoms establishes an *actual* diagnosis]

DESIRED OUTCOMES/EVALUATION CRITERIA— PATIENT WILL:

Thermoregulation (NOC)

Maintain body temperature within normal range.

ACTIONS/INTERVENTIONS

RATIONALE

Temperature Regulation: Intraoperative (NIC)

Independent

Note preoperative temperature.

Used as baseline for monitoring intraoperative temperature. Preoperative temperature elevations are indicative of disease process, e.g., appendicitis, abscess, or systemic disease requiring treatment preoperatively, perioperatively, and possibly postoperatively. *Note:* Effects of aging on hypothalamus may decrease fever response to infection.

Assess environmental temperature and modify as needed, e.g., providing warming and cooling blankets, increasing room temperature.

May assist in maintaining/stabilizing patient's temperature.

Cover skin areas outside of operative field.

Heat losses will occur as skin (e.g., legs, arms, head) is exposed to cool environment.

Provide cooling measures for patient with preoperative temperature elevations.

Cool irrigations and exposure of skin surfaces to air may be required to decrease temperature.

Note rapid temperature elevation/persistent high fever and treat promptly per protocol.

Malignant hyperthermia must be recognized and treated promptly to avoid serious complications/death.

ACTIONS/INTERVENTIONS

Independent

Increase ambient room temperature (e.g., to 78°F or 80°F) at conclusion of procedure.

Apply warming blankets at emergence from anesthesia.

Collaborative

Monitor temperature throughout intraoperative phase.

Provide iced saline as indicated.

Obtain dantrolene (Dantrium) for IV administration.

RATIONALE

Helps limit patient heat loss when drapes are removed and patient is prepared for transfer.

Inhalation anesthetics depress the hypothalamus, resulting in poor body temperature regulation.

Continuous warm/cool humidified inhalation anesthetics are used to maintain humidity and temperature balance within the tracheobronchial tree. Temperature elevation/fever may indicate adverse response to anesthesia. *Note:* Use of atropine or scopolamine may further increase temperature.

Lavage of body cavity with iced saline may help reduce hyperthermic responses.

Immediate action to control temperature is necessary to prevent death from malignant hyperthermia.

POSTOPERATIVE

NURSING DIAGNOSIS: Breathing Pattern, ineffective

May be related to
Neuromuscular, perceptual/cognitive impairment
Decreased lung expansion, energy
Tracheobronchial obstruction

Possibly evidenced by
Changes in respiratory rate and depth
Reduced vital capacity, apnea, cyanosis, noisy respirations

DESIRED OUTCOMES/EVALUATION CRITERIA—PATIENT WILL:

Respiratory Status: Ventilation (NOC)

Establish a normal/effective respiratory pattern free of cyanosis or other signs of hypoxia.

ACTIONS/INTERVENTIONS

Postanesthesia Care (NIC)

Independent

Maintain patient airway by head tilt, jaw hyperextension, oral pharyngeal airway.

Auscultate breath sounds. Listen for gurgling, wheezing, crowing, and/or silence after extubation.

RATIONALE

Prevents airway obstruction.

Lack of breath sounds is indicative of obstruction by mucus or tongue and may be corrected by positioning and/or suctioning. Diminished breath sounds suggest atelectasis. Wheezing indicates bronchospasm, whereas crowing or silence reflects partial-to-total laryngospasm.

ACTIONS/INTERVENTIONS	RATIONALE
Independent	
Observe respiratory rate and depth, chest expansion, use of accessory muscles, retraction or flaring of nostrils, skin color; note airflow.	Ascertains effectiveness of respirations immediately so corrective measures can be initiated.
Monitor vital signs continuously.	Increased respirations, tachycardia, and/or bradycardia suggests hypoxia.
Position patient appropriately, depending on respiratory effort and type of surgery.	Head elevation and left lateral Sims' position prevents aspiration of secretions/vomitus; enhances ventilation to lower lobes and relieves pressure on diaphragm
Observe for return of muscle function, especially respiratory.	After administration of intraoperative muscle relaxants, return of muscle function occurs first to the diaphragm, intercostals, and larynx; followed by large muscle groups, neck, shoulders, and abdominal muscles; then by midsize muscles, tongue, pharynx, extensors, and flexors; and finally by eyes, mouth, face, and fingers.
Initiate "stir-up" (turn, cough, deep breathe) regimen as soon as patient is reactive and continue in the postoperative period.	Active deep ventilation inflates alveoli, breaks up secretions, increases O_2 transfer, and removes anesthetic gases; coughing enhances removal of secretions from the pulmonary system. *Note:* Respiratory muscles weaken and atrophy with age, possibly hampering elderly patient's ability to cough or deep-breathe effectively.
Observe for excessive somnolence.	Narcotic-induced respiratory depression or presence of muscle relaxants in the body may be cyclical in recurrence, creating sine-wave pattern of depression and reemergence from anesthesia. In addition, thiopental sodium (Pentothal) is absorbed in the fatty tissues, and, as circulation improves, it may be redistributed throughout the bloodstream.
Elevate head of bed as appropriate. Get out of bed as soon as possible.	Promotes maximal expansion of lungs, decreasing risk of pulmonary complications.
Suction as necessary.	Airway obstruction can occur because of blood or mucus in throat or trachea.
Collaborative	
Administer supplemental O_2 as indicated.	Maximizes oxygen for uptake to bind with Hb in place of anesthetic gases to enhance removal of inhalation agents.
Administer IV medications, e.g., naloxone (Narcan) or doxapram (Dopram).	Narcan reverses narcotic-induced central nervous system (CNS) depression and Dopram stimulates respiratory muscles. The effects of both drugs are cyclic in nature and respiratory depression may return.
Provide/maintain ventilator assistance.	Depending on cause of respiratory depression or type of surgery (e.g., pulmonary, extensive abdominal, cardiac), endotracheal tube (ET) may be left in place and mechanical ventilation maintained for a time.
Assist with use of respiratory aids, e.g., incentive spirometer.	Maximal respiratory efforts reduce potential for atelectasis and infection.

NURSING DIAGNOSIS: Sensory-Perceptual alterations: (specify)/Thought Processes, altered

May be related to

Chemical alteration: use of pharmaceutical agents, hypoxia

Therapeutically restricted environments; excessive sensory stimuli

Physiological stress

Possibly evidenced by

Disorientation to person, place, time; change in usual response to stimuli; impaired ability to concentrate, reason, make decisions

Motor incoordination

DESIRED OUTCOMES/EVALUATION CRITERIA—PATIENT WILL:

Cognitive Ability (NOC)

Regain usual level of consciousness/mentation.

Recognize limitations and seek assistance as necessary.

ACTIONS/INTERVENTIONS	RATIONALE
Postanesthesia Care (NIC)	
Independent	
Reorient patient continuously when emerging from anesthesia; confirm that surgery is completed.	As patient regains consciousness, support and assurance will help alleviate anxiety.
Speak in normal, clear voice without shouting, being aware of what you are saying. Minimize discussion of negatives (e.g., patient/personnel problems) within patient's hearing. Explain procedures, even if patient does not seem aware.	The nurse cannot tell when patient is aware, but it is thought that the sense of hearing returns before patient appears fully awake, so it is important not to say things that may be misinterpreted. Providing information helps patient preserve dignity and prepare for activity.
Evaluate sensation/movement of extremities and trunk as appropriate.	Return of function following local or spinal nerve blocks depends on type/amount of agent used and duration of procedure.
Use bedrail padding, restraints as necessary.	Provides for patient safety during emergence state. Prevents injury to head and extremities if patient becomes combative while disoriented.
Secure parenteral lines, ET tube, catheters, if present, and check for patency.	Disoriented patient may pull on lines and drainage systems, disconnecting or kinking them.
Maintain quiet, calm environment.	External stimuli, such as noise, lights, touch, may cause psychic aberrations when dissociative anesthetics (e.g., ketamine) have been administered.
Investigate changes in sensorium.	Confusion, especially in elderly patients, may reflect drug interactions, hypoxia, anxiety, pain, electrolyte imbalances, or fear.
Observe for hallucinations, delusions, depression, or an excited state.	May develop following trauma and indicate delirium, or may reflect "sundowner's syndrome" in elderly patient. In patient who has used alcohol to excess, may suggest impending delirium tremens.
Reassess sensory/motor function and cognition thoroughly before discharge, as indicated.	Ambulatory surgical patient must be able to care for self with the help of SO (if available) to prevent personal injury after discharge.

Collaborative

Evaluate need for extended stay in postoperative recovery area or need for additional nursing care before discharge as appropriate.

Disorientation may persist, and SO may not be able to protect the patient at home.

NURSING DIAGNOSIS: Fluid Volume, risk for deficit

Risk factors may include
Restriction of oral intake (disease process/medical procedure/presence of nausea)
Loss of fluid through abnormal routes, e.g., indwelling tubes, drains; normal routes, e.g., vomiting
Loss of vascular integrity, changes in clotting ability
Extremes of age and weight

Possibly evidenced by
[Not applicable; presence of signs and symptoms establishes an *actual* diagnosis]

DESIRED OUTCOMES/EVALUATION CRITERIA—PATIENT WILL:

Hydration (NOC)

Demonstrate adequate fluid balance, as evidenced by stable vital signs, palpable pulses of good quality, normal skin turgor, moist mucous membranes, and individually appropriate urinary output.

Fluid Management (NIC)

Independent

Measure and record I&O (including tubes and drains). Calculate urine specific gravity as appropriate. Review intraoperative record.

Accurate documentation helps identify fluid losses/replacement needs and influences choice of interventions. *Note:* Ability to concentrate urine declines with age, increasing renal losses despite general fluid deficit.

Assess urinary output specifically for type of operative procedure done.

May be decreased or absent after procedures on the genitourinary system and/or adjacent structures (e.g., ureteroplasty, ureterolithotomy, abdominal or vaginal hysterectomy), indicating malfunction or obstruction of the urinary system.

Provide voiding assistance measures as needed, e.g., privacy, sitting position, running water in sink, pouring warm water over perineum.

Promotes relaxation of perineal muscles and may facilitate voiding efforts.

Monitor vital signs noting changes in blood pressure, heart rate and rhythm, and respirations. Calculate pulse pressure.

Hypotension, tachycardia, increased respirations may indicate fluid deficit, e.g., dehydration/hypovolemia. Although a drop in blood pressure is generally a late sign of fluid deficit (hemorrhagic loss), widening of the pulse pressure may occur early, followed by narrowing as bleeding continues and systolic BP begins to fall.

ACTIONS/INTERVENTIONS	RATIONALE

Independent

Note presence of nausea/vomiting.

Women, obese patients, and those prone to motion sickness have a higher risk of postoperative nausea/vomiting. In addition, the longer the duration of anesthesia, the greater the risk for nausea. *Note:* Nausea occurring during first 12–24 hr postoperatively is frequently related to anesthesia (including regional anesthesia). Nausea persisting more than 3 days postoperatively may be related to the choice of narcotic for pain control or other drug therapy.

Inspect dressings, drainage devices at regular intervals. Assess wound for swelling.

Excessive bleeding can lead to hypovolemia/circulatory collapse. Local swelling may indicate hematoma formation/hemorrhage. *Note:* Bleeding into a cavity (e.g., retroperitoneal) may be hidden and only diagnosed via vital sign depression, patient reports of pressure sensation in affected area.

Monitor skin temperature, palpate peripheral pulses.

Cool/clammy skin, weak pulses indicate decreased peripheral circulation and need for additional fluid replacement.

Collaborative

Administer parenteral fluids, blood products (including autologous collection), and/or plasma expanders as indicated. Increase IV rate if needed.

Replaces documented fluid loss. Timely replacement of circulating volume decreases potential for complications of deficit, e.g., electrolyte imbalance, dehydration, cardiovascular collapse. *Note:* Increased volume may be required initially to support circulating volume/prevent hypotension because of decreased vasomotor tone following Fluothane administration.

Insert/maintain urinary catheter with or without urimeter as necessary.

Provides mechanism for accurate monitoring of urinary output.

Resume oral intake gradually as indicated.

Oral intake depends on return of gastrointestinal (GI) function.

Administer antiemetics as appropriate.

Relieves nausea/vomiting, which may impair intake and add to fluid losses. *Note:* Naloxone (Narcan) may relieve nausea related to use of regional anesthetic agents, e.g., morphine (Duramorph), fentanyl citrate (Sublimaze).

Monitor laboratory studies, e.g., Hb/Hct, electrolytes. Compare preoperative and postoperative blood studies.

Indicators of hydration/circulating volume. Preoperative anemia and/or low Hct combined with unreplaced fluid losses intraoperatively will further potentiate deficit.

NURSING DIAGNOSIS: Pain [acute]

May be related to
Disruption of skin, tissue, and muscle integrity; musculoskeletal/bone trauma
Presence of tubes and drains

Possibly evidenced by
Reports of pain
Alteration in muscle tone; facial mask of pain

Distraction/guarding/protective behaviors
Self-focusing; narrowed focus
Autonomic responses

DESIRED OUTCOMES/EVALUATION CRITERIA—PATIENT WILL:

| Pain Level (NOC) |

Report pain relieved/controlled.
Appear relaxed, able to rest/sleep and participate in activities appropriately.

ACTIONS/INTERVENTIONS

| Pain Management (NIC) |

Independent

Note patient's age, weight, coexisting medical/psychological conditions, idiosyncratic sensitivity to analgesics, and intraoperative course (e.g., size/location of incision, drain placement, anesthetic agents used).

Review intraoperative/recovery room record for type of anesthesia and medications previously administered.

Evaluate pain regularly (e.g., every 2 hr × 12) noting characteristics, location, and intensity (0–10 scale). Emphasize patient's responsibility for reporting pain/relief of pain completely.

Note presence of anxiety/fear, and relate with nature of and preparation for procedure.

Assess vital signs, noting tachycardia, hypertension, and increased respiration, even if patient denies pain.

Assess causes of possible discomfort other than operative procedure.

Provide information about transitory nature of discomfort, as appropriate.

RATIONALE

Approach to postoperative pain management is based on multiple variable factors.

Presence of narcotics and droperidol in system potentiates narcotic analgesia, whereas patients anesthetized with Fluothane and Ethrane have no residual analgesic effects. In addition, intraoperative local/regional blocks have varying duration, e.g., 1–2 hr for regionals or up to 2–6 hr for locals.

Provides information about need for/effectiveness of interventions. *Note:* It may not always be possible to eliminate pain; however, analgesics should reduce pain to a tolerable level. A frontal and/or occipital headache may develop 24–72 hr following spinal anesthesia, necessitating recumbent position, increased fluid intake, and notification of the anesthesiologist.

Concern about the unknown (e.g., outcome of a biopsy) and/or inadequate preparation (e.g., emergency appendectomy) can heighten patient's perception of pain.

Changes in these vital signs often indicate acute pain and discomfort. *Note:* Some patients may have a slightly lowered BP, which returns to normal range after pain relief is achieved.

Discomfort can be caused/aggravated by presence of nonpatent indwelling catheters, NG tube, parenteral lines (bladder pain, gastric fluid and gas accumulation, and infiltration of IV fluids/medications).

Understanding the cause of the discomfort (e.g., sore muscles from administration of succinylcholine may persist up to 48 hr postoperatively; sinus headache associated with nitrous oxide and sore throat due to intubation are transitory) provides emotional reassurance. *Note:* Paresthesia of body parts suggest nerve injury. Symptoms may last hours or months and require additional evaluation.

ACTIONS/INTERVENTIONS	RATIONALE
Independent	
Reposition as indicated, e.g., semi-Fowler's; lateral Sims'.	May relieve pain and enhance circulation. Semi-Fowler's position relieves abdominal muscle tension and arthritic back muscle tension, whereas lateral Sims' will relieve dorsal pressures.
Provide additional comfort measures, e.g., backrub, heat/cold applications.	Improves circulation, reduces muscle tension and anxiety associated with pain. Enhances sense of well-being.
Encourage use of relaxation techniques, e.g., deep-breathing exercises, guided imagery, visualization, music.	Relieves muscle and emotional tension; enhances sense of control and may improve coping abilities.
Provide regular oral care, occasional ice chips/sips of fluids as tolerated.	Reduces discomfort associated with dry mucous membranes due to anesthetic agents, oral restrictions.
Document effectiveness and side/adverse effects of analgesia.	Respirations may decrease on administration of narcotic, and synergistic effects with anesthetic agents may occur. *Note:* Migration of epidural analgesia toward head (cephalad diffusion) may cause respiratory depression or excessive sedation.
Collaborative	
Administer medications as indicated:	
Analgesics IV (after reviewing anesthesia record for contraindications and/or presence of agents that may potentiate analgesia); provide around-the-clock analgesia with intermittent rescue doses;	Analgesics given IV reach the pain centers immediately, providing more effective relief with small doses of medication. IM administration takes longer, and its effectiveness depends on absorption rates and circulation. *Note:* Narcotic dosage should be reduced by one-fourth to one-third after use of fentanyl (Innovar) or droperidol (Inapsine) to prevent profound tranquilization during first 10 hr postoperatively. Current research supports need to administer analgesics around the clock initially to prevent rather than merely treat pain.
Patient-controlled analgesia (PCA);	Use of PCA necessitates detailed patient instruction. PCA must be monitored closely but is considered very effective in managing acute postoperative pain with smaller amounts of narcotic and increased patient satisfaction.
Local anesthetics, e.g., epidural block/infusion;	Analgesics may be injected into the operative site, or nerves to the site may be kept blocked in the immediate postoperative phase to prevent severe pain. *Note:* Continuous epidural infusions may be used for 1–5 days following procedures that are known to cause severe pain (e.g., certain types of thoracic or abdominal surgery).
NSAIDs, e.g., aspirin, diflunisal (Dolobid), naproxen (Anaprox).	Useful for mild to moderate pain or as adjuncts to opioid therapy when pain is moderate to severe. Allows for a lower dosage of narcotics, reducing potential for side effects.
Monitor use/effectiveness of transcutaneous electrical nerve stimulation (TENS).	TENS may be useful in reducing pain and amount of medication required postoperatively.

> **NURSING DIAGNOSIS: Skin/Tissue Integrity, impaired**
>
> **May be related to**
> Mechanical interruption of skin/tissues
> Altered circulation, effects of medication; accumulation of drainage; altered metabolic state
>
> **Possibly evidenced by**
> Disruption of skin surface/layers and tissues
>
> **DESIRED OUTCOMES/EVALUATION CRITERIA—PATIENT WILL:**
>
> **Wound Healing: Primary Intention (NOC)**
>
> Achieve timely wound healing.
>
> **Knowledge: Treatment Regimen (NOC)**
>
> Demonstrate behaviors/techniques to promote healing and to prevent complications.

ACTIONS/INTERVENTIONS

Wound Care (NIC)

Independent

Reinforce initial dressing/change as indicated. Use strict aseptic techniques.

Gently remove tape (in direction of hair growth) and dressings when changing.

Apply skin sealants/barriers before tape if needed. Use paper/silk (hypoallergenic) tape or Montgomery straps/elastic netting for dressings requiring frequent changing.

Check tension of dressings. Apply tape at center of incision to outer margin of dressing. Avoid wrapping tape around extremity.

Inspect wound regularly, noting characteristics and integrity. Note patients at risk for delayed healing, e.g., presence of chronic obstructive pulmonary disease (COPD), anemia, obesity/malnutrition, DM, hematoma formation, vomiting, ETOH (alcohol) withdrawal; use of steroid therapy; advanced age.

Assess amounts and characteristics of drainage.

Maintain patency of drainage tubes; apply collection bag over drains/incisions in presence of copious or caustic drainage.

RATIONALE

Protects wound from mechanical injury and contamination. Prevents accumulation of fluids that may cause excoriation. *Note:* Recent studies suggest clean techniques may be sufficient, but additional research is required before protocols are revised.

Reduces risk of skin trauma and disruption of wound.

Reduces potential for skin trauma/abrasions and provides additional protection for delicate skin/tissues.

Can impair/occlude circulation to wound and to distal portion of extremity.

Early recognition of delayed healing/developing complications may prevent a more serious situation. Wounds may heal more slowly in patients with comorbidity, or the elderly in whom reduced cardiac output decreases capillary blood flow.

Decreasing drainage suggests evolution of healing process, whereas continued drainage or presence of bloody/odoriferous exudate suggests complications (e.g., fistula formation, hemorrhage, infection).

Facilitates approximation of wound edges; reduces risk of infection and chemical injury to skin/tissues.

ACTIONS/INTERVENTIONS

Independent

Elevate operative area as appropriate.

Splint abdominal and chest incisions/area with pillow or pad during coughing/movement.

Caution patient not to touch wound.

Cleanse skin surface (if needed) with diluted hydrogen peroxide solution, or running water and mild soap after incision is sealed.

Collaborative

Apply ice if appropriate.

Use abdominal binder if indicated.

Irrigate wound; assist with debridement as needed.

Monitor/maintain dressings, e.g., hydrogel, vacuum dressing.

RATIONALE

Promotes venous return and limits edema formation. *Note:* Elevation in presence of venous insufficiency may be detrimental.

Equalizes pressure on the wound, minimizing risk of dehiscence/rupture.

Prevents contamination of wound.

Reduces skin contaminants; aids in removal of drainage/exudate.

Reduces edema formation that may cause undue pressure on incision during initial postoperative period.

Provides additional support for high-risk incisions (e.g., obese patient).

Removes infectious exudate/necrotic tissue to promote healing.

May be used to hasten healing in large, draining wound/fistula, to increase patient comfort, and to reduce frequency of dressing changes. Also allows drainage to be measured more accurately and analyzed for pH and electrolyte content as appropriate.

NURSING DIAGNOSIS: Tissue Perfusion, risk for altered

Risk factors may include
Interruption of flow: arterial, venous
Hypovolemia

Possibly evidenced by
[Not applicable; presence of signs and symptoms establishes an *actual* diagnosis]

DESIRED OUTCOMES/EVALUATION CRITERIA—PATIENT WILL:

Circulation Status (NOC)

Demonstrate adequate perfusion evidenced by stable vital signs, peripheral pulses present and strong; skin warm/dry; usual mentation and individually appropriate urinary output.

ACTIONS/INTERVENTIONS

Circulatory Care (NIC)

Independent

Change position slowly initially.

Assist with range-of-motion (ROM) exercises, including active ankle/leg exercises.

RATIONALE

Vasoconstrictor mechanisms are depressed and quick movement may lead to orthostatic hypotension, especially in the early postoperative period.

Stimulates peripheral circulation; aids in preventing venous stasis to reduce risk of thrombus formation.

ACTIONS/INTERVENTIONS	RATIONALE
Independent	
Encourage/assist with early ambulation.	Enhances circulation and return of normal organ function.
Avoid use of knee gatch/pillow under knees. Caution patient against crossing legs or sitting with legs dependent for prolonged period.	Prevents stasis of venous circulation and reduces risk of thrombophlebitis.
Assess lower extremities for erythema, edema, calf tenderness (positive Homans' sign).	Circulation may be restricted by some positions used during surgery, while anesthetics and decreased activity alter vasomotor tone, potentiating vascular pooling and increasing risks of thrombus formation.
Monitor vital signs; palpate peripheral pulses; note skin temperature/color and capillary refill. Evaluate urinary output/time of voiding. Document dysrhythmias.	Indicators of adequacy of circulating volume and tissue perfusion/organ function. Effects of medications/electrolyte imbalances may create dysrhythmias, impairing cardiac output and tissue perfusion.
Investigate changes in mentation/failure to achieve usual mental state.	May reflect a number of problems such as inadequate clearance of anesthetic agent, oversedation (pain medication), hypoventilation, hypovolemia, or intra-operative complications (e.g., emboli).
Collaborative	
Administer IV fluids/blood products as needed.	Maintains circulating volume; supports perfusion.
Apply antiembolic hose as indicated.	Promotes venous return and prevents venous stasis of legs to reduce risk of thrombosis.

NURSING DIAGNOSIS: Knowledge Deficit [Learning Need] regarding condition/situation, prognosis, treatment, self care, and discharge needs

May be related to
Lack of exposure/lack of recall, information misinterpretation
Unfamiliarity with information resources
Cognitive limitation

Possibly evidenced by
Questions/request for information; statement of misconception
Inaccurate follow-through of instructions/development of preventable complications

DESIRED OUTCOMES/EVALUATION CRITERIA—PATIENT WILL:

Knowledge: Disease Process (NOC)

Verbalize understanding of condition, effects of procedure and potential complications.

Knowledge: Treatment Regimen (NOC)

Verbalize understanding of therapeutic needs.
Correctly perform necessary procedures and explain reasons for actions.
Initiate necessary lifestyle changes and participate in treatment regimen.

ACTIONS/INTERVENTIONS	RATIONALE
Treatment: Disease Process (NIC)	
Independent	
Review specific surgery performed/procedure done and future expectations.	Provides knowledge base from which patient can make informed choices.

ACTIONS/INTERVENTIONS	RATIONALE
Independent	
Review and have patient/SO demonstrate dressing/wound/tube care when indicated. Identify source for supplies.	Promotes competent self-care and enhances independence.
Review avoidance of environmental risk factors, e.g., exposure to crowds/persons with infections.	Reduces potential for acquired infections.
Discuss drug therapy, including use of prescribed and OTC analgesics.	Enhances cooperation with regimen; reduces risk of adverse reactions/untoward effects.
Identify specific activity limitations.	Prevents undue strain on operative site.
Recommend planned/progressive exercise.	Promotes return of normal function and enhances feelings of general well-being.
Schedule adequate rest periods.	Prevents fatigue and conserves energy for healing.
Review importance of nutritious diet and adequate fluid intake.	Provides elements necessary for tissue regeneration/healing and support of tissue perfusion and organ function.
Encourage cessation of smoking.	Smoking increases risk of pulmonary infections, causes vasoconstriction, and reduces oxygen-binding capacity of blood, affecting cellular perfusion and potentially impairing healing.
Identify signs/symptoms requiring medical evaluation, e.g., nausea/vomiting; difficulty voiding; fever, continued/odoriferous wound drainage; incisional swelling, erythema, or separation of edges; unresolved or changes in characteristics of pain.	Early recognition and treatment of developing complications (e.g., ileus, urinary retention, infection, delayed healing) may prevent progression to more serious or life-threatening situation.
Stress necessity of follow-up visits with providers, including therapists, laboratory.	Monitors progress of healing and evaluates effectiveness of regimen.
Include SO in teaching program/discharge planning. Provide written instructions/teaching materials. Instruct in use of and arrange for special equipment.	Provides additional resources for reference after discharge. Promotes effective self-care.
Identify available resources, e.g., homecare services, visiting nurse, Meals-on-Wheels, outpatient therapy, contact phone number for questions.	Enhances support for patient during recovery period and provides additional evaluation of ongoing needs/new concerns.

POTENTIAL CONSIDERATIONS following surgical procedure (dependent on patient's age, physical condition/presence of complications, personal resources, and life responsibilities)

Fatigue—increased energy requirements to perform activities of daily living, states of discomfort.

Infection, risk for—broken skin, traumatized tissues, stasis of body fluids; presence of pathogens/contaminants, environmental exposure, invasive procedures.

Self-Care deficit/Home Maintenance Management, impaired—decreased strength/endurance, pain/discomfort, unfamiliarity with neighborhood resources, inadequate support systems.

Refer also to appropriate plans of care regarding underlying condition/specific surgical procedure for additional considerations.

EXTENDED CARE

Patients in the acute care setting may be discharged to an extended care facility. Patients requiring relatively short-term rehabilitation and those needing long-term care/permanent nursing care are included in this group. The level of care and needs of the patient (e.g., physical, occupational, rehabilitation therapy; IV and respiratory support) are frequently the deciding factors in the choice of placement. Although elderly people are the primary population in extended care facilities, increasing numbers of younger individuals are requiring care for debilitating conditions when they cannot be managed in the home setting.

RELATED CONCERNS

Acquired immunodeficiency syndrome (AIDS), page 765
Cancer, page 900
Cerebrovascular accident/Stroke, page 257
Craniocerebral trauma, page 238
Multiple sclerosis, page 315
Psychosocial aspects of care, page 809
Spinal cord injury, page 295
Surgical intervention, page 828
Ventilatory assistance (mechanical), page 188

Patient Assessment Database

Data depend on underlying physical/psychosocial conditions necessitating continuation of structured care.

TEACHING/LEARNING

Discharge plan considerations: **Projected mean length of stay: Depends on underlying disease/condition and individual care needs. Therefore, this may be temporary or permanent placement.**
May require assistance with treatments, self-care activities, homemaker/maintenance tasks, or alternate living arrangements (e.g., group home)

Refer to section at end of plan for postdischarge considerations.

DIAGNOSTIC STUDIES (dependent on age, general health, and medical condition)

CBC: Reveals problems such as infection, anemia, other abnormalities.
Chemistry profile: Evaluates general organ function/imbalances. Age-related changes include decreased serum albumin, up to 20% increase in alkaline phosphatase, decreased urine creatinine clearance.
Urinalysis: Provides information about kidney function; determines presence of urinary tract infection (UTI) or DM. *Note:* Bacteria is common in some populations, especially the elderly and bed-ridden, reflecting urinary stasis.
Pulse oximetry: Determines oxygenation, respiratory function.
Communicable disease screens: To rule out tuberculosis (TB), HIV, venereal disease, hepatitis.
Drug screen: As indicated by usage to identify therapeutic or toxic levels.
Visual acuity testing: Identifies cataracts/other vision problems.
Tonometer test: Measures intraocular pressure.
Chest x-ray: Reveals size of heart, lung abnormalities/disease conditions, changes of the large blood vessels and bony structure of the chest.
ECG: Provides baseline data; detects abnormalities, e.g., ST segment and T wave changes, atrial and ventricular dysrhythmias, and various heart blocks are common in the elderly.

NURSING PRIORITIES

1. Promote physiological and psychological well-being.
2. Provide for security and safety.
3. Prevent complications of disease and/or aging process.
4. Promote effective coping skills and independence.
5. Encourage continuation of healthy habits, participation in plan of care to meet individual needs and wishes.

DISCHARGE GOALS

1. Patient dealing realistically with current situation.
2. Homeostasis maintained.
3. Injury prevented.
4. Complications/prevented/minimized.
5. Patient meeting ADLs by self/with assistance as necessary.
6. Plan in place to meet needs after discharge as appropriate.

NURSING DIAGNOSIS: Anxiety [specify level]/Fear

May be related to

Change in health status, role functioning, interaction patterns, socioeconomic status, environment

Unmet needs; recent life changes, loss of friends/SO

Possibly evidenced by

Apprehension, restlessness, repetitive questioning; pacing, purposeless activity; insomnia

Various behaviors (appears overexcited, withdrawn, worried, fearful); presence of facial tension, trembling, hand tremors

Expressed concern regarding changes in life events

Focus on self; lack of interest in activity

DESIRED OUTCOMES/EVALUATION CRITERIA—PATIENT WILL:

Anxiety or Fear Control (NOC)

Verbalize understanding of reasons for change, as able.
Demonstrate appropriate range of feelings and lessened fear.
Participate in routine and special/social events as capable.
Verbalize acceptance of situation.

ACTIONS/INTERVENTIONS	RATIONALE

Anxiety Reduction (NIC)

Independent

Provide patient/SO with a copy of "A Patient's Bill of Rights" and review it with them. Discuss facility's rules, e.g., visitors, off-grounds visits, personal property.	Provides information that can foster confidence that individual rights do continue in this setting and the patient is still "his or her own person" and has some control over what happens.
Ascertain if patient has completed Advance Directives. Provide information as appropriate.	Assures patient/family wishes will be known to provide direction to caregivers.
Determine patient/SO attitude toward admission to facility and expectations for the future.	If this is expected to be a temporary placement, patient/SO concerns will be different than if placement is permanent. When patient is giving up own home and way of life, feelings of helplessness, loss, and grief are to be expected.
Help family/SO to be honest with patient regarding admission. Be clear about actions/events.	Family may have difficulty dealing with decision/reality of permanent placement and may avoid discussing situation with patient. Honesty decreases "surprises," assists in maintaining trust, and may enhance coping.

ACTIONS/INTERVENTIONS	RATIONALE

Independent

Identify support person(s) important to patient and include in care activities, mealtime, and so on, as appropriate.

During adjustment period/times of stress, patient may benefit from presence of trusted individual who can provide reassurance and reduce sense of isolation.

Assess level of anxiety and discuss reasons when possible.

Identifying specific problems enables individual to deal more realistically with them and care provider to intervene as necessary, e.g., patient who is being neglected or abused or has unrelieved pain may be very anxious and afraid or unable to verbalize.

Develop nurse-patient relationship.

Trusting relationships among patient/SO/staff promotes optimal care and support.

Make time to listen to patient about concerns, and encourage free expression of feelings, e.g., anger, hostility, fear, and loneliness.

Being available in this way allows patient to feel accepted, begin to acknowledge and deal with feelings related to circumstances of admission.

Acknowledge reality of situation and feelings of patient. Accept expressions of anger while limiting aggressive, acting-out behavior.

Permission to express feelings allows for beginning resolution. Acceptance promotes sense of self-worth. *Note:* Psychosocial and/or physiological disturbances can occur as a result of transfer from one environment to another (i.e., relocation stress syndrome).

Identify strengths and successful coping behaviors and incorporate into problem solving.

Building on past successes increases likelihood of positive outcome in present situation. Enhances sense of control and management of current deficits.

Orient to physical aspects of facility, schedules, and activities. Introduce to roommate(s) and staff. Give explanation of roles.

Getting acquainted is an important part of admission. Knowledge of where things are and who patient can expect assistance from can be helpful in reducing anxiety.

Determine patient's usual schedule and incorporate into facility routine as much as possible.

Consistency provides reassurance and may lessen confusion and enhance cooperation.

Provide above information in written or taped form as well.

Overload of information is difficult to remember. Patient can refer to written or taped material as needed to refresh memory/learn new information.

Give careful thought to room placement. Provide help and encouragement in placing patient's own belongings around room. Do not transfer from one room to another without patient approval/documentable need.

Location, roommate compatibility, and place for personal belongings are important considerations for helping the patient feel "at home." Changes are often met with resistance and can result in emotional upset and decline in physical condition. *Note:* Persons with severe behavioral problems/cognitive dysfunctions may require a private room.

Note behavior, presence of suspiciousness/paranoia, irritability, defensiveness. Compare to SO's description of customary responses.

Increased stress, physical discomfort, and fatigue may temporarily exacerbate mental deterioration (cognitive inaccessibility) and further impair communication (social inaccessibility). This represents a catastrophic episode that can escalate into a panic state and violence.

Be aware of escalating anxiety, presence of delirium. Look for possible causes.

Common causes of delirium include drug toxicity, electrolyte imbalances withdrawal states (alcohol, other drugs), pain/trauma (especially hip fractures), and advanced disease resulting in organ failure.

Collaborative

Refer to social service or other appropriate agency for assistance. Have case manager, social worker discuss ramifications of Medicare/Medicaid if patient is eligible for these resources.

Often patient is not aware of the resources available, and providing current information about individual coverage/limitations and other possible sources of support will assist with adjustment to new situation.

> **NURSING DIAGNOSIS: Grieving, anticipatory**
>
> **May be related to**
> Perceived, actual or potential loss of physiopsychosocial well-being, personal possessions, or SO; cultural beliefs about aging/debilitation
>
> **Possibly evidenced by**
> Denial of feelings, depression, sorrow, guilt
> Alterations in the activity level, sleep patterns, eating habits, libido
>
> **DESIRED OUTCOMES/EVALUATION CRITERIA—PATIENT WILL:**
>
> **Grief Resolution (NOC)**
>
> Identify and express feelings appropriately.
> Progress through the grieving process.
> Enjoy the present and plan for the future, one day at a time.

ACTIONS/INTERVENTIONS	RATIONALE
Grief Work Facilitation (NIC)	
Independent	
Assess emotional state. Note cultural beliefs, expectations.	Anxiety and depression are common reactions to changes/losses associated with long-term illness or debilitating condition. In addition, changes in neurotransmitter levels (e.g., increased monoamine oxidase [MAO] and serotonin levels with decreased norepinephrine) may potentiate depression in elderly patients. Personal expectations may affect response to change.
Make time to listen to the patient. Encourage free expression of hopeless feelings and desire to die.	It is more helpful to allow these feelings to be expressed and dealt with than to deny or ignore them.
Assess suicidal potential.	May be related to physical disease, social isolation, and grief. *Note:* Studies indicate women are three times as likely to attempt suicide; however, men are three times as likely to succeed.
Involve SO in discussions and activities to the level of their willingness.	When SOs are involved, there is more potential for successful problem solving. *Note:* SO may not be available or may not choose to be involved.
Provide liberal touching/hugs as individually accepted.	Conveys sense of concern/closeness to reduce feelings of isolation and enhance sense of self-worth. *Note:* Touch may be viewed as a threat by some patients and escalate feelings of anger.
Identify spiritual concerns. Discuss available resources and encourage participation in religious activities as appropriate.	Search for meaning is common to those facing changes in life. Participation in religious/spiritual activities can provide sense of direction and peace of mind.
Assist with/plan for specifics as necessary (e.g., Advance Directives to determine code status/Living Will wishes, making of will, funeral arrangements, if appropriate)	Having these issues resolved can help patient/SO deal with the grieving process and may provide peace of mind.
Collaborative	
Refer to other resources as indicated, e.g., clinical specialist nurse, case manager/social worker, spiritual advisor.	May need further assistance to resolve some problems.

ACTIONS/INTERVENTIONS

Cognitive Stimulation (NIC)

Independent

Allow adequate time for patient to respond to questions/comments and to make decisions.

Discuss happenings of the past. Place familiar objects in room. Encourage the display of photographs/photo albums, frequent visits from SO/friends.

Note patient's problem of short-term memory loss, and provide with aids (e.g., calendars, clocks, room signs, pictures) to assist in continual reorientation.

Evaluate individual stress level and deal with it appropriately.

Assess physical status/psychiatric symptoms. Institute interventions appropriate to findings.

RATIONALE

Reaction time may be slowed with aging (changes in metabolism/cerebral blood flow) or with brain injuries and some neuromuscular conditions.

Events of the past may be more readily recalled by the elderly patient, because long-term memory usually remains intact. Reminiscence/life review and companionship are beneficial to patients.

Short-term memory loss presents a challenge for nursing care, especially if the patient cannot remember such things as how to use the call bell or how to get to the bathroom. This problem is not in patient's control but may be less frustrating if simple reminders are used. It may be helpful for older person (and family) to know that short-term memory loss is common and is not necessarily a sign of "senility."

Stress level may be greatly increased because of recent losses, e.g., poor health, death of spouse/companion, loss of home. In addition, some conflicts that occur with age come from previously unresolved problems that may need to be dealt with now.

Not all mental changes are the result of aging, and it is important to rule out physical causes before accepting these as unchangeable. May be pain (often unreported/underestimated), metabolic, toxic, drug-induced (e.g., antiparkinson agents, tricyclic antidepressants), or the result of infectious, cardiac, or respiratory disorders.

ACTIONS/INTERVENTIONS

Independent

Reorient to person/place and time as appropriate.

Have patient repeat verbal/written instructions.

Note cyclic changes in mentation/behavior, e.g., evening confusion, picking at bedclothes, banging on side rails, pacing, shouting, wandering aimlessly.

Involve in regular exercise, activity, and diversional programs.

Schedule at least one rest period per day.

Provide brighter lighting in room/area by midafternoon (e.g., 3 PM) or earlier on cloudy/winter days.

Turn off lights at bedtime. Provide night lights where appropriate.

Support patient's involvement in own care. Provide opportunity for choices on a daily basis.

Collaborative

Review results of laboratory/diagnostic tests, e.g., electrolytes, thyroid studies, rapid plasma reagin (RPR), full drug screen, computerized tomography (CT) scan.

Administer medications as indicated, e.g., tacrine (Cognex), donepazil (Aricept).

RATIONALE

Helps patient maintain focus.

Verifies hearing/ability to read and comprehend.

"Sundowner syndrome" may occur in response to visual/hearing deficits enhanced by declining light, fatigue, inflexible institution schedules, peak/trough drug levels, dehydration, and electrolyte imbalances.

Promotes release of endorphins enhancing sense of well-being and can improve thinking abilities. *Note:* Studies suggest withdrawn and inactive patients are at greater risk of evening confusion.

Prevents fatigue; enhances general well-being.

Maximizes visual perception; may limit evening confusion.

Reinforces "sleep time" while meeting safety needs.

Choice is a necessary component in everyday life. Cognitively impaired patients may respond with aggressive behavior as they lose control in their lives.

Aids in establishing cause of changes in mentation and determining treatment options. *Note:* The latter four tests can identify the causes of dementia in 90% of the cases.

These drugs may fight dementia by blocking chemical breakdown of acetylcholine and improving cholinergic function. Aricept has been shown to improve intellectual ability and daily functioning in mild to moderate Alzheimer's disease (as assessed by Alzheimer's Disease Assessment Scale [ADAS-Cog]).

NURSING DIAGNOSIS: Family Coping, ineffective: compromised

May be related to

Placement of family member in extended care facility

Temporary family disorganization and role changes

Situational/transitional crises SO may be facing

Patient providing little support for SO

Prolonged disease or disability progression that exhausts the supportive capacity of SOs

Possibly evidenced by

SO describes significant preoccupation with personal reactions, e.g., fear, anticipatory grief, guilt, anxiety

SO attempts assistive/supportive behaviors with unsatisfactory results

SO withdraws from patient

SO displays protective behavior disproportionate (too little or too much) to patient's abilities/need for autonomy

ACTIONS/INTERVENTIONS	RATIONALE
Family Support (NIC)	
Independent	
Introduce staff and provide SO with information about facility and care. Be available for questions. Provide tour of facility.	Helpful to establish beginning relationships. Offers opportunities for enhancing feelings of involvement.
Determine involvement and availability of family/SO.	Clarifies expectations and abilities, identifies needs.
Encourage SO participation in care at level of desire and capability and within limits of safety. Include in social events/celebrations.	Helps family to feel at ease and allows them to feel supportive and a part of the patient's life.
Accept choices of SO regarding level of involvement in care.	Families may choose to ignore patient or may project feelings of guilt regarding placing patient in facility by criticizing staff. *Note:* Feelings of dissatisfaction with the staff may be transferred back to the patient.
Evaluate SO's/caregiver's level of stress/coping abilities, especially before planning for discharge.	Caring for/about patients with chronic/debilitating conditions places a heavy strain on SO. Although support groups may be very helpful, learning stress management techniques may be more effective in strengthening individual coping as the focus is on the SO rather than the SO-patient relationship.
Support the caregiver with attention, compassion, time, respect, honesty, advocacy, and understanding.	Nursing interventions need to prepare the caregivers for the challenges they face, and meet their needs for compassion and caring.
Identify availability and use of community support systems.	Helps determine areas of need and provides information regarding additional resources to enhance coping.
Be aware of staff's own feelings of anger and frustration about patient's/SO's choices and goals that differ from those of staff, and deal with appropriately.	Group care conferences or individual counseling may be helpful in problem solving.
Collaborative	
Inform SO of services available to them (meal tickets, family cooking time, group care conference, visiting nurse, caseworker, social services).	Promotes feeling of involvement; eases transition in adjustment to patient's admission to homecare or facility care.
Advise caregivers of resources available, such as Eldercare Locator, Seniornet, Today's Caregiver, Caregiver Network, Inc.	Helps nurses, patients, and caregivers feel supported and able to provide more skillful care.

NURSING DIAGNOSIS: Poisoning, risk for [drug toxicity]

Risk factors may include

Reduced metabolism; impaired circulation; precarious physiological balance, presence of multiple diseases/organ involvement

Use of multiple prescribed/OTC drugs

Possibly evidenced by

[Not applicable; presence of signs and symptoms establishes an *actual* diagnosis]

DESIRED OUTCOMES/EVALUATION CRITERIA—PATIENT WILL:

Risk Control: Drug Use (NOC)

Maintain prescribed drug regimen free of untoward side effects.

ACTIONS/INTERVENTIONS	RATIONALE
Medication Management (NIC)	
Independent	
Determine allergies, medication, and other drug use history.	Helps avoid repetition/creation of problems.
Review resources (e.g., drug manuals, pharmacist) for information about toxic symptoms and side effects. List drug actions and interactions and idiosyncracies, e.g., medications that are given with or without foods, as well as those that should not be crushed.	Provides information about drugs being taken and identifies possible interactions. Toxicity can be increased in the debilitated and older patient with symptoms not as apparent.
Discuss self-administration of/access to OTC products.	Limits interference with prescribed regimen/desired drug action and organ function. May prevent inadvertent overdosing/toxic reactions. *Note:* Appropriate use of OTC products kept at bedside or via free access at nurses' station fosters independence and enhances sense of control and self-esteem.
Identify swallowing problems or reluctance to take tablets or capsules.	May not be able to or want to take medication.
Give pills in a spoonful of soft foods, e.g., applesauce, ice cream; or use liquid form of medication if available.	Ensures proper dosage if patient is unable to/does not like to swallow pills.
Open capsules or crush tablets only when appropriate.	Should not be done unless absolutely necessary because this may alter absorption of medications, e.g. enteric-coated tablets may be absorbed in stomach when crushed, instead of the intestines.
Make sure medication has been swallowed.	Ensures effective therapeutic use of medication and prevents pill hoarding.
Observe for changes in condition/behavior.	Behavior may be only indication of drug toxicity, and early identification of problems provides for appropriate intervention. *Note:* Elderly individuals have increased sensitivity to anticholinergic effects of medications; therefore, use of anticholinergics, antiparkinson agents, benzodiazepines, CNS depressants, and tricyclic antidepressants may cause delirium/confusion.

857

ACTIONS/INTERVENTIONS	RATIONALE
Independent	
Use discretion in the administration of sedatives.	A quiet place where the patient can pace, or seclusion, may be more helpful. If patient is destructive or excessively disruptive, pharmacological or mechanical control measures may be required. Convenience of the staff is never a reason for sedating patient; however, patient safety and rights of other patients need to be taken into consideration.
Collaborative	
Review drug regimen routinely with physician and pharmacist.	Provides opportunity to alter therapy (e.g., reduce dosage, discontinue medications) as patient's needs and organ functions change.
Obtain serum drug levels as indicated.	Determines therapeutic/toxicity levels.

NURSING DIAGNOSIS: Communication, impaired verbal

May be related to
Degenerative changes (e.g., reduced cerebral circulation, hearing loss); progressive neurological disease (e.g., Parkinson's disease, Alzheimer's disease)
Laryngectomy/tracheostomy; stroke, traumatic brain injury

Possibly evidenced by
Impaired articulation; difficulty with phonation; inability to modulate speech, find words, name, or identify objects (aphasia, dysarthria)
Diminished hearing ability

DESIRED OUTCOMES/EVALUATION CRITERIA—PATIENT WILL:

Communication Ability (NOC)

Establish method of communication by which needs can be expressed.
Demonstrate congruent verbal and nonverbal communication.

ACTIONS/INTERVENTIONS	RATIONALE
Communication Enhancement: Speech Deficit (NIC)	
Independent	
Assess reason for lack of communication, including CNS and neuromuscular functioning, gag/swallow reflexes, hearing, teeth/mouth problems.	Identification of the problem is essential to appropriate intervention. Sometimes patients do not want to talk, may think they talk when they do not, may expect others to know what they want, may not be able to comprehend or be understood.
Determine whether patient is bilingual or whether English is primary language.	With declining cerebral function/diminished thought processes, increased level of stress, patient may mix languages/revert to original language.
Investigate how SO communicates with the patient.	Provide opportunity to develop/continue effective communication patterns, which have already been established.
Assess patient knowledge base and level of comprehension. Treat the patient as an adult, avoiding pity and impatience.	Knowing how much to expect of the patient can help to avoid frustration and unreasonable demands for performance. However, having an expectation that the patient will understand may help raise level of performance.

ACTIONS/INTERVENTIONS	RATIONALE

Independent

Establish therapeutic nurse-patient relationship through Active-Listening, being available for problem solving.

Aids in dealing with communication problems.

Make patient aware of presence when entering the room by speaking, turning a light off and on/touching patient or mattress as appropriate.

Getting attention is the first step in communication.

Make eye contact, place self at or below patient's level, and speak face to face.

Conveys interest and promotes contact.

Speak slowly and distinctly, using simple sentences, yes-or-no questions. Avoid speaking loudly or shouting. Supplement with written communication when possible/needed. Allow sufficient time for reply; remain relaxed with patient.

Assists in comprehension and overall communication. Patient may respond poorly to high-pitched sounds; shouting also obscures consonants and amplifies vowels.

Use other creative measures to assist in communication, e.g., picture chart/alphabet board, sign language, lip reading when appropriate.

Many options are available, depending on individual situation. *Note:* Sign language also may be used effectively with other than hearing-impaired individuals.

Communication Enhancement: Hearing Deficit (NIC)

Check ears for excess cerumen.

Hardened earwax may decrease hearing acuity and causes tinnitus.

Ascertain if patient has/uses hearing aid.

Patient may have, but not use, hearing aid (e.g., may not fit well, may need batteries).

Be aware that behavioral problems may be associated with hearing loss.

Anger, explosive temper outbursts, frustration, embarrassment, depression, withdrawal, and paranoia may be attempts to deal with communication problems.

Collaborative

Refer to speech therapists, ear, nose, and throat physician, or for audiometry as needed.

Determines extent of hearing loss and whether a hearing aid is appropriate. May be helpful to a patient and staff in improving communication. *Note:* Some sources believe 90% of the patients in extended care facilities have some degree of hearing loss (presbycusis) because this is a common age change. Hearing aids are most effective with conductive losses and may help with sensorineural losses.

NURSING DIAGNOSIS: Sleep Pattern disturbance

May be related to
Internal factors: illness, psychological stress, inactivity
External factors: environmental changes, facility routines

Possibly evidenced by
Reports of difficulty in falling asleep/not feeling well-rested
Interrupted sleep, awakening earlier than desired
Change in behavior/performance, increasing irritability, listlessness

DESIRED OUTCOMES/EVALUATION CRITERIA—PATIENT WILL:

Sleep (NOC)

Report improvement in sleep/rest pattern.
Verbalize increased sense of well-being and feeling rested.

ACTIONS/INTERVENTIONS	RATIONALE

Sleep Enhancement (NIC)

Independent

Ascertain usual sleep habits and changes that are occurring.	Determines need for action and helps identify appropriate interventions.
Provide comfortable bedding and some of own possessions, e.g., pillow, afghan.	Increases comfort for sleep and physiological/psychological support.
Establish new sleep routine incorporating old pattern and new environment.	When new routine contains as many aspects of old habits as possible, stress and related anxiety may be reduced, enhancing sleep.
Match with roommate who has similar sleep patterns and nocturnal needs.	Decreases likelihood that "night owl" roommate may delay patient's falling asleep or create interruptions that cause awakening.
Encourage some light physical activity during the day. Make sure patient stops activity several hours before bedtime as individually appropriate.	Daytime activity can help patient expand energy and be ready for nighttime sleep; however, continuation of activity close to bedtime may act as a stimulant, delaying sleep.
Promote bedtime comfort regimens, e.g., warm bath and massage, a glass of warm milk, wine, or brandy at bedtime.	Promotes a relaxing, soothing effect. *Note:* Milk has soporific qualities, enhancing synthesis of serotonin, a neurotransmitter that helps patient fall asleep faster and sleep longer.
Instruct in relaxation measures.	Helps induce sleep.
Reduce noise and light.	Provides atmosphere conducive to sleep.
Encourage position of comfort, assist in turning.	Repositioning alters areas of pressure and promotes rest.
Use side rails as indicated; lower bed when possible.	May have fear of falling because of change in size and height of bed. Side rails provide safety and may be used to assist with turning. *Note:* Some people do better with no side rails and are at risk for falling when climbing over side rails.
Avoid interruptions when possible (e.g., awakening for medications or therapies).	Uninterrupted sleep is more restful, and patient may be unable to return to sleep when wakened.

Collaborative

Administer sedatives, hypnotics, as indicated.	May be given to help patient sleep/rest during transition period from home to new setting. *Note:* Avoid habitual use, because these drugs decrease REM (rapid eye movement) sleep time.

NURSING DIAGNOSIS: Nutrition: altered, less/more than body requirements

May be related to
Impaired dentition; dulling of senses of smell and taste
Cognitive limitations, depression
Inability to feed self effectively
Sedentary activity level

Possibly evidenced by
Reported/observed dysfunctional eating patterns
Weight under/over ideal for height and frame
Poor muscle tone, pale conjunctiva/mucous membranes
Signs/symptoms of vitamin/protein deficits, electrolyte imbalances

DESIRED OUTCOMES/EVALUATION CRITERIA—PATIENT WILL:

Nutritional Status (NOC)

Maintain normal weight or progress toward weight goal with normalization of laboratory values and be free of signs of malnutrition/obesity.
Demonstrate eating patterns/behaviors to maintain appropriate weight.

ACTIONS/INTERVENTIONS	RATIONALE

Nutrition Management (NIC)

Independent

Assess causes of weight loss/gain, e.g., dysphagia due to decreased saliva production, neurogenic/psychogenic disturbances, tumors, muscular dysfunction, altered senses of smell and taste, or dysfunctional eating patterns related to depression.	Aids in creating plan of care/choice of interventions. *Note:* In elderly patients saliva secretion may be decreased by as much as 66%, taste buds atrophy with reduced sensitivity to sweet and salt.
Check state of patient's dental health periodically, including fit and condition of dentures, if present.	Oral infections/dental problems, shrinking gums, and loose-fitting dentures decrease patient's ability to chew.
Weigh on admission and on a regular basis.	Monitors nutritional state and effectiveness of interventions.
Monitor total caloric intake as indicated.	If dietary plan is ineffective in meeting individual goals, calorie count/food diary may help identify problem areas.
Observe condition of skin; note muscle wasting, brittle nails; dry, lifeless hair, and signs of poor healing.	Reflects lack of adequate nutrition.
Evaluate activity pattern.	Extremes of exercise (e.g., sedentary life, continuous pacing) affect caloric needs.
Incorporate favorite foods and maintain as near-normal food consistency as possible, e.g., soft or finely ground food with gravy or liquid added. Avoid baby food whenever possible.	Aids in maintaining intake, especially when mouth and dental problems exist. Baby food is often unpalatable and can decrease appetite and lower self-esteem.
Encourage the use of spices (other than sodium) to patient's personal taste.	Reduction in number and acuity of taste buds results in food tasting bland and decreases enjoyment of food and desire to eat.
Provide small, frequent feedings as indicated.	Decreased gastric motility causes patient to feel full and reduces intake.
Serve hot foods hot and cold foods cold.	Foods served at the proper temperature are more palatable, and enjoyment may increase appetite.
Promote a pleasant environment for eating, with company if possible.	Eating is in part a social event, and appetite can improve with increased socialization.
Have healthy snack foods (e.g., cheese, crackers, soup, fruit) available on a 24-hr basis.	Helps meet individual needs and enhances intake with caloric recommendations.
Plan for social events; provide for snacks, even when working to reduce total calories.	Eating is part of socialization, and being able to respond to body's needs enhances sense of control and willingness to participate in dietary program.

861

ACTIONS/INTERVENTIONS	RATIONALE

Independent

Encourage exercise and activity program within individual ability.

Promotes sense of well-being and may improve appetite.

Collaborative

Consult with dietitian.

Aids in establishing specific nutritional program to meet individual patient needs.

Provide balanced diet with individually appropriate protein, complex carbohydrates, and calories. Include supplements between meals as indicated.

Adjustments may be needed to deal with the body's decreased ability to process protein, as well as decreased metabolic rate and levels of activity. *Note:* Reduced production of salivary ptyalin inhibits digestion of complex carbohydrates in elderly individuals affecting dietary plan. In addition, delayed insulin release by the pancreas and reduced peripheral sensitivity to insulin decrease their glucose tolerance.

Administer vitamin/mineral supplements as appropriate.

With age, renal and other regulatory systems cannot compensate as well for errors in intake. Mineral requirements change as hormone levels, metabolism, and GI function change. In addition, absorption can be impaired by medication use and chronic illness.

Refer for dental care routinely and as needed.

Maintenance of oral/dental health and good dentition can enhance intake.

NURSING DIAGNOSIS: Self-Care deficit: (specify)

May be related to
Depression, discouragement, loss of mobility, general debilitation; perceptual/cognitive impairment

Possibly evidenced by
Inability to manage ADLs; unkempt appearance

DESIRED OUTCOMES/EVALUATION CRITERIA—PATIENT WILL:

Self-Care: Activities of Daily Living (ADL) (NOC)

Peform self-care activities within level of own ability.
Demonstrate techniques/lifestyle changes to meet own needs.
Use resources effectively.

ACTIONS/INTERVENTIONS	RATIONALE

Self-Care Assistance (NIC)

Independent

Determine current capabilities (0–4 scale) and barriers to participation in care.

Identifies need for/level of interventions required.

Involve patient in formulation of plan of care at level of ability.

Enhances sense of control and aids in cooperation and maintenance of independence.

Encourage self-care. Work with present abilities; do not pressure patient beyond capabilities. Provide adequate time for patient to complete tasks. Have expectation of improvement and assist as needed.

Doing for oneself enhances feeling of self-worth. Failure can produce discouragement and depression.

ACTIONS/INTERVENTIONS

Independent

Provide and promote privacy, including during bathing/showering.

Use specialized equipment as needed, e.g., tub transfer seat, grab bars, raised toilet seat.

Give tub bath, using a two-person or mechanical lift if necessary. Use shower chair and spray attachment, as appropriate. Avoid chilling.

Shampoo/style hair as needed. Provide/assist with manicure.

Encourage use of barber/beauty salon if patient is able.

Acquire clothing with modified fasteners as indicated.

Encourage/assist with routine mouth/teeth care daily.

Collaborative

Consult with physical/occupational therapists and rehabilitation specialist.

RATIONALE

Modesty may lead to reluctance to participate in care or perform activities in the presence of others.

Enhances ability to move/perform activities safely.

Provides safety for those who cannot get into the tub alone. Shower may be more feasible for some patients, though it may be less beneficial/desirable to the patient. Elderly/debilitated patients are more prone to chilling.

Aids in maintaining appearance. Shampooing may be required more/less frequently than bathing schedule.

Enhances self-image and self-esteem, preserving dignity of the patient.

Use of Velcro instead of buttons/shoe laces can facilitate process of dressing/undressing.

Reduces risk of gum disease/tooth loss; promotes proper fitting of dentures.

Useful in establishing exercise/activity program and in identifying assistive devices to meet individual needs/facilitate independence.

NURSING DIAGNOSIS: Skin Integrity, risk for impaired

Risk factors may include
General debilitation; reduced mobility; changes in skin and muscle mass associated with aging, sensory/motor deficits
Altered circulation; edema; poor nutrition
Excretions/secretions (bladder and bowel incontinence)
Problems with self-care

Possibly evidenced by
[Not applicable; presence of signs and symptoms establishes an *actual* diagnosis]

DESIRED OUTCOMES/EVALUATION CRITERIA—PATIENT WILL:

Risk Control (NOC)

Maintain intact skin.
Identify individual risk factors.
Demonstrate behaviors/techniques to prevent skin breakdown/facilitate healing.

ACTIONS/INTERVENTIONS

Skin Surveillance (NIC)

Independent

Inspect skin, tissues, and mucous membranes routinely.

RATIONALE

Provides opportunity for early intervention in potential high-risk population, who may have thin, less elastic, and more fragile skin and tissues.

ACTIONS/INTERVENTIONS	RATIONALE
Independent	
Anticipate and use preventive measures in patients who are at risk for skin breakdown, such as anyone who is thin, obese, aging, or debilitated.	Decubitus ulcers are difficult to heal, and prevention is the best treatment.
Assess nutritional status and initiate corrective measures as indicated. Provide balanced diet, e.g., adequate protein, vitamins, and minerals.	A positive nitrogen balance and improved nutritional state can help prevent skin breakdown and promote ulcer healing. *Note:* May need additional calories and protein if draining ulcer present.
Maintain strict skin hygiene, using mild, nondetergent soap (if any), drying gently and thoroughly, and lubricating with lotion or emollient.	A daily bath is usually not necessary in elderly patients because there is atrophy of sebaceous and sweat glands, and bathing may create dry-skin problems. However, as epidermis thins with age, cleansing and use of lubricants is needed to keep skin soft/pliable and protect susceptible skin from breakdown.
Change position frequently in bed and chair. Recommend 10 min of exercise each hour and/or perform passive ROM.	Improved circulation, muscle tone, and joint motion and promotes patient participation.
Use a rotation schedule in turning patient. Use draw/turn sheet. Pay close attention to patient's comfort level.	Allows for longer periods free of pressure; prevents shearing or tearing motions that can damage fragile tissues. *Note:* Use of prone position depends on patient tolerance and should be maintained for only a short time.
Massage bony prominences gently with lotion or cream.	Enhances circulation to tissues, increases vascular tone, and reduces tissue edema. *Note:* Contraindicated if area is pink/red because cellular damage may occur. Gentle massage around area may stimulate circulation to impaired tissues.
Keep sheets and bedclothes clean, dry, and free from wrinkles, crumbs, and other irritating material.	Avoids friction/abrasions of skin.
Use elbow/heel protectors, foam/water or gel pads, sheepskin for positioning in bed and when up in chair.	Reduces risk of tissue abrasions and decreases pressure that can impair cellular blood flow. Promotes circulation of air along skin surface to dissipate heat/moisture.
Provide for safety during ambulation, using appropriate adaptive devices, e.g., walker, cane.	Loss of muscle strength and flexibility and physical disease process/debilitation may result in impaired coordination.
Limit exposure to temperature extremes/use of heating pad or ice pack.	Decreased sensitivity to pain/heat/cold increases risk of tissue trauma.
Examine feet and nails routinely and provide foot and nail care as indicated:	Foot problems are common among patients who are elderly, diabetic, bedfast, and/or debilitated.
Keep nails cut short and smooth;	Jagged, rough nails can cause tissue damage/infection.
Use lotion, softening cream on feet;	Prevents drying/cracking of skin; promotes maintenance of healthy skin.
Check for fissures between toes, swab with hydrogen peroxide or dust with antiseptic powder, and place a wisp of cotton between the toes;	Prevents spread of infection and/or tissue injury.
Rub feet with witch hazel or a mentholated preparation and have patient wear lightweight cotton stockings.	Even though rash may not be present, burning and itching may be a problem. *Note:* Witch hazel may be contraindicated if skin is dry.

ACTIONS/INTERVENTIONS

Collaborative

Inspect skin surface/folds (especially when incontinence pad/pants are used) and bony prominences routinely. Increase preventive measures when reddened areas are noticed.

Continue regimen for redness and irritation when break in skin occurs.

Observe for decubitus ulcer development, and treat immediately according to protocol.

Collaborative

Provide waterbed, alternating pressure/egg-crate or gel mattress, and pad for chair.

Monitor Hb/Hct and blood glucose levels.

Refer to podiatrist as indicated.

Provide whirlpool treatments as appropriate.

Assist with topical applications; hydrogel dressings; skin barrier dressings (Duoderm, Op-Site); collagenase therapy; absorbable gelatin sponges (Gelfoam); aerosol sprays.

Administer nutritional supplements and vitamins as indicated.

Prepare for/assist with skin grafting (Refer to CP: Burns, ND: Skin Integrity, impaired, p. 734.)

RATIONALE

Skin breakdown can occur quickly with potential for infection and necrosis, possibly involving muscle and bone. There is increased risk of redness/irritation around legs due to elastic bands in adult diapers/incontinence pads.

Aggressive measures are important because decubitus ulcers can develop in a matter of a few hours.

Timely intervention may prevent extensive damage.

Provides protection and improved circulation by decreasing amount of pressure on tissues.

Anemia, dehydration, and elevated glucose levels are factors in skin breakdown and can impair healing.

May need professional care for such problems as ingrown toenails, corns, bony changes, skin/tissue ulceration.

Increases circulation and has a debriding action.

Although there are differing opinions about the efficacy of these agents, individual or combination use may enhance healing.

Aids in healing/cellular regeneration.

May be needed to close large ulcers.

NURSING DIAGNOSIS: Urinary Elimination, risk for altered

Rick factors may include
Changes in fluid/nutritional pattern
Neuromuscular changes
Perceptual/cognitive impairment

Possibly evidenced by
[Not applicable; presence of signs and symptoms establishes an *actual* diagnosis]

DESIRED OUTCOMES/EVALUATION CRITERIA—PATIENT WILL:

Urinary Elimination (NOC)

Maintain/regain effective pattern of elimination.
Initiate necessary lifestyle changes.
Participate in treatment regimen to correct/control situation, e.g., bladder training program or use of indwelling catheter.

ACTIONS/INTERVENTIONS	RATIONALE

Urinary Elimination Management (NIC)

Independent

Monitor voiding pattern. Identify possible reasons for changes, e.g., disorientation, neuromuscular impairment, psychotropic medications.	This information is essential to plan for care and influences choice of individual interventions. Nocturia, frequency, and urgency are common because bladder capacity and/or tone is affected. Bladder pelvic muscles and sphincter tone may be affected.
Palpate bladder. Observe for "overflow" voiding; determine frequency and timing of dribbling/voiding.	Bladder distension indicates urinary retention, which may cause incontinence and infection.
Promote fluid intake of 2000–3000 mL/day within cardiac tolerance; include fruit juices, especially cranberry juice. Schedule fluid intake times appropriately.	Maintains adequate hydration and promotes kidney function. Acid-ash juices act as an internal pH acidifier, retarding bacterial growth. *Note:* Patient may decrease fluid intake in an attempt to control incontinence, and become dehydrated. Instead, fluids may be scheduled to decrease frequency of incontinence (e.g., limit fluids after 6 PM to reduce need to void during the night).
Institute bladder program (including scheduled voiding times, Kegel exercise) involving patient and staff in a positive manner.	Regular toileting times may help control incontinence. Program is more apt to be successful when positive attitudes and cooperation are present.
Assist patient to sit upright on bedpan/commode.	Provides functional position for voiding.
Provide/encourage perineal care daily and as needed.	Reduces risk of contamination/ascending infection.
Use adult incontinence pads/pants during day if needed. Keep patient clean and dry. Provide frequent skin care.	When training is unsuccessful, this is the preferred method of management. *Note:* Using incontinence pads during night exposes skin to air, reducing risk of irritation.
Avoid verbal or nonverbal signs of rejection, disgust, or disapproval over failures.	Expressions of disapproval lower self-esteem and are not helpful to a successful program.
Provide regular catheter care and maintain patency if indwelling catheter is present.	Prevents infection and/or minimizes reflux.

Collaborative

Administer medications as indicated, e.g.:	
Oxybutynin chloride (Ditropan); tolterodine tartrate (Detrol);	Promotes bladder sphincter control.
Vitamin C, methenamine mandelate (Mandelamine).	Bladder pH acidifiers retard bacterial growth.
Maintain indwelling catheter/provide intermittent catheterization.	May be used if continence cannot be maintained to prevent skin breakdown and resultant problems.
Irrigate catheter with acetic acid, if indicated.	May be done to maintain acid pH and retard bacterial growth.

NURSING DIAGNOSIS: Constipation/Diarrhea, risk for

Risk factors may include
Changes in/inadequate nutrition or fluid intake; poor muscle tone, change in level of activity
Medication side effects
Perceptual/cognitive impairment, depression
Lack of privacy

Possibly evidenced by
[Not applicable; presence of signs and symptoms establishes an *actual* diagnosis]

DESIRED OUTCOMES/EVALUATION CRITERIA—PATIENT WILL:

Bowel Elimination (NOC)

Establish/maintain normal patterns of bowel functioning.
Demonstrate changes in lifestyle as necessitated by risk or contributing factors.
Participate in bowel program, as indicated.

ACTIONS/INTERVENTIONS	RATIONALE
Bowel Management (NIC)	
Independent	
Ascertain usual bowel pattern and aids used (e.g., previous long-term laxative use). Compare with current routine.	Determines extent of problem and indicates need for/type of interventions appropriate. Many patients may already be laxative-dependent, and it is important to re-establish as near-normal functioning as possible.
Assess reasons for problems; rule out medical causes, e.g., bowel obstruction, cancer, hemorrhoids, drugs, impaction.	Identification/treatment of underlying medical condition is necessary to achieve optimal bowel function.
Determine presence of food/drug sensitivities.	May contribute to diarrhea.
Institute individualized program of exercise, rest, diet, and bowel retraining.	Depends on the needs of the patient. Loss of muscular tone reduces peristalsis or may impair control of rectal sphincter.
Provide diet high in bulk in the form of whole-grain cereals, breads, fresh fruits (especially prunes, plums).	Improves stool consistency, promotes evacuation.
Decrease or eliminate foods such as dairy products.	These foods are known to be constipating.
Encourage increased fluid intake.	Promotes normal stool consistency.
Use adult incontinence pads/pants, if needed. Keep patient clean and dry. Provide frequent perineal care. Apply skin protective ointment to anal area.	Prevents skin breakdown.
Keep air freshener in room/at bedside or in bathroom.	Limits noxious odors and may help reduce patient embarrassment/concern.
Give emotional support to patient. Avoid "blaming" (talk/actions) if incontinence occurs.	Decreases feelings of frustration and embarrassment.
Collaborative	
Administer medications as indicated:	
Bulk-providers/stool softeners, e.g., Metamucil;	Promotes regularity by increasing bulk and/or improving stool consistency.
Camphorated tincture of opium (Paregoric), diphenoxylate with atropine (Lomotil).	May be needed on a short-term basis when diarrhea persists.

ACTIONS/INTERVENTIONS	RATIONALE
Independent	
Determine functional ability (0–4 scale) and reasons for impairment.	Identifies need for/degree of intervention required.
Note emotional/behavioral responses to altered ability.	Physical changes and loss of independence often create feelings of anger, frustration, and depression that may be manifested as reluctance to engage in activity.
Plan activities/visits with adequate rest periods as necessary.	Prevents fatigue; conserves energy for continued participation.
Encourage participation in self-care, occupational/recreational activities.	Promotes independence and self-esteem; may enhance willingness to participate.
Provide chairs with firm, high seats and lifting chairs when indicated.	Facilitates rising from seated position.
Fall Prevention (NIC)	
Assist with transfers and ambulation if indicated; show patient/SO ways to move safely.	Prevents accidental falls/injury, especially in the patient with altered gait, generalized weakness, orthostatic hypotension, fatigue and vision disturbances.
Obtain supportive shoes and well-fitting, nonskid slippers.	Assists patient to walk with a firm step/maintain sense of balance and prevents slipping.
Remove extraneous furniture from pathways.	Prevents patient from bumping into furniture and reduces risk of falling/injuring self.
Encourage use of hand rails in hallway, stairwells, and bathrooms. Keep bed height in low position.	Promotes independence in mobility; reduces risk of falls.
Review safe use of mobility aids/adjunctive devices, e.g., walker, braces, prosthetics.	Facilitates activity, reduces risk of injury.
Provide for environmental changes to meet visual deficiencies.	Prevents accidents and reduces sense of sensory deprivation. If patient is visually impaired, will need assistance and ongoing orientation to surroundings.
Speak to patient when entering the room, and let patient know when leaving.	Special actions help patient who cannot see to know when someone is there.

ACTIONS/INTERVENTIONS

Independent

Encourage the patient with glasses/contacts to wear them. Be sure glasses are kept clean. Determine reason if glasses are not being worn.

Collaborative

Arrange for regular eye examinations.

Consult with physical/occupational therapists, rehabilitation specialist.

RATIONALE

Optimal visual acuity facilitates participation in activities and reduces risk of falls/injury. Patient may not be wearing glasses because they need adjustment or change in correction.

Identifies development/progression of vision problem (e.g., myopia, hyperopia, presbyopia, astigmatism, cataract and glaucoma, tunnel vision, loss of peripheral fields, blindness) and specific options for care.

Useful in creating individual exercise/activity program and identifying adjunctive aids. *Note:* Even in the elderly population, inclusion of moderate weight-lifting in the exercise program can improve bone density and help maintain muscle tone/strength.

NURSING DIAGNOSIS: Diversional Activity deficit

May be related to
Environmental lack of diversional activity; long-term care requirements
Physical limitations; psychological condition, e.g., depression

Possibly evidenced by
Statements of boredom, depression, lack of energy
Disinterest, lethargy, withdrawn behavior, hostility

DESIRED OUTCOMES/EVALUATION CRITERIA—PATIENT WILL:

Leisure Participation (NOC)

Recognize own response and initiate appropriate coping actions.
Engage in satisfying activities within personal limitations.

ACTIONS/INTERVENTIONS

Activity Therapy (NIC)

Independent

Determine avocation/hobbies patient previously pursued. Incorporate activities, if appropriate, into present program.

Encourage participation in mix of activities/stimuli, e.g., music, news program, educational presentations, crafts, social interactions, as appropriate.

Provide change of scenery when possible; alter personal environment; encourage trips to shop/participate in local/family events.

Collaborative

Refer to occupational therapist, activity director.

RATIONALE

Encourages involvement and helps to stimulate patient mentally/physically to improve overall condition and sense of well-being.

Offering different activities helps patient to try out new ideas and develop new interests. Activities need to be personally meaningful for the patient to derive the most enjoyment from them (e.g., talking or Braille books for the blind, closed-caption TV broadcasts for the deaf/hearing impaired).

Stimulates energy and provides new outlook for patient.

Can introduce and design new programs to provide positive stimuli for the patient.

NURSING DIAGNOSIS: Sexuality Patterns, risk for altered

Risk factors may include
Biophychosocial alteration of sexuality
Interference in psychological/physical well-being; self-image
Lack of privacy/SO

Possibly evidenced by
[Not applicable; presence of signs and symptoms establishes an *actual* diagnosis]

DESIRED OUTCOMES/EVALUATION CRITERIA—PATIENT WILL:

Role Performance (NOC)

Verbalize knowledge and understanding of sexual limitations, difficulties, or changes that have occurred.
Demonstrate improved communication and relationship skills.
Identify appropriate options to meet needs.

ACTIONS/INTERVENTIONS	RATIONALE
Sexual Counseling (NIC)	
Independent	
Note patient/SO cues regarding sexuality.	May be concerned that condition/environmental restrictions may interfere with sexual function or ability, but is afraid to ask directly.
Determine cultural and religious/value factors and conflicts that may be present.	Affects patient's perception of existing problems and response of others (e.g., family, staff, other residents). Provides starting point for discussion and problem solving.
Assess developmental and lifestyle issues.	Factors such as menopause and aging, adolescence, and young adulthood need to be taken into consideration with regard to sexual concerns about illness and long-term care.
Provide atmosphere in which discussion of sexuality is encouraged/permitted.	When concerns are identified and discussed, problem solving can occur.
Provide privacy for patient/SO.	Demonstrates acceptance of need for intimacy and provides opportunity to continue previous patterns of interaction as much as possible.
Collaborative	
Refer to sex counselor/therapist, family therapy when needed.	May require additional assistance for resolution of problems.

NURSING DIAGNOSIS: Health Maintenance, altered

May be related to
Lack of, or significant alteration in, communication skills
Complete or partial lack of gross and/or fine motor skills
Perceptual/cognitive impairment, lack of ability to make deliberate/thoughtful judgments
Lack of material resources

Possibly evidenced by

Demonstrated lack of knowledge regarding basic health practices

Reported/observed inability to take responsibility for meeting basic health needs; impairment of personal support system

Demonstrated lack of behaviors adaptive to internal or external environmental changes

DESIRED OUTCOMES/EVALUATION CRITERIA—PATIENT/CAREGIVER WILL:

Participation: Health Care Decisions (NOC)

Verbalize understanding of factors contributing to current situation.

Adopt lifestyle changes supporting individual healthcare goals.

Assume responsibility for own healthcare needs when possible.

ACTIONS/INTERVENTIONS	RATIONALE
Health Education (NIC)	
Independent	
Assess level of adaptive behavior; knowledge and skills about health maintenance, environment, and safety.	Identifies areas of concern/need and aids in choice of interventions.
Provide information about individual healthcare needs.	Provides knowledge base and encourages participation in decision making.
Develop plan with patient/SO for self-care incorporating existing disabilities adapting and organizing care.	Assists patient/caregiver to maintain and manage desired level of independence when possible.
Maintain adequate hydration and balanced diet with sufficient protein intake.	Promotes general well-being and aids in disease prevention.
Schedule adequate rest with progressive activity program.	Prevents fatigue and enhances general well-being.
Promote good handwashing and personal hygiene. Use aseptic techniques as necessary.	Prevents contamination/cross-contamination, reducing risk of illness/infection.
Protect from exposure to infections; avoid extremes of temperature. Recommend the wearing of masks/other interventions as indicated.	With age, immune protective responses slow down and physiological reactions to temperature extremes may be impaired. As organ function decreases (especially thymus gland) and natural antibodies decline, patients are at increased risk for infection. Staff and/or visitors with colds or other infections may expose patient to these illnesses.
Encourage cessation of smoking.	Smokers are prone to bronchitis and ineffective clearing of secretions.
Encourage reporting of signs/symptoms as they occur.	Provides opportunity for early recognition of developing complications and timely intervention to prevent serious illness.
Health System Guidance (NIC)	
Note patient's previous use of professional services, and continue as appropriate. Include in choice of new healthcare providers as able.	Preserves continuity and promotes independence in meeting own healthcare needs.

ACTIONS/INTERVENTIONS

Independent

Observe for/monitor changes in vital signs, e.g., temperature elevation.

Collaborative

Identify resources for/administer medications as indicated:

Immunizations, e.g., *Haemophilus influenzae* (flu), pneumonia;

Antibiotics.

Schedule preventive/routine healthcare appointments based on individual needs, e.g., with cardiologist, podiatrist, ophthalmologist, dentist.

Refer to support services as indicated, e.g., home health care agency, durable medical equipment company, Senior Resources, social services, national hospice organization, Alzheimer's Disease and Related Disorders Association, AARP, Center for Health Care Ethics, Choice in Dying, American Bar Association, Commission on Legal Problems of the Elderly, Internet Resources, Adult Protective Services.

RATIONALE

Early identification of onset of illness allows for timely intervention and may prevent serious complications. *Note:* Elderly persons often display subnormal temperatures, so presence of a low-grade fever may be of serious concern.

Reduces risk of acquiring contagious/potentially life-threatening diseases.

May be used prophylactically, depending on individual disease process/risk factors and to treat infections.

Promotes optimal recovery/maintenance of health.

Many community resources are available, and often untapped, to make life and care of the individual easier.

POTENTIAL CONSIDERATIONS following discharge from care facility.

Refer to plan of care for diagnosis that required admission.

ALCOHOL: ACUTE WITHDRAWAL

Alcohol, a CNS depressant drug, is used socially in our society for many reasons: to enhance the flavor of food, to encourage relaxation and conviviality, for celebrations, and as a sacred ritual in some religious ceremonies. Therapeutically, it is the major ingredient in many OTC/prescription medications. It can be harmless, enjoyable, and sometimes beneficial when used responsibly and in moderation. Like other mind-altering drugs, however, it has the potential for abuse, and, in fact, is the most widely abused drug in the United States (research suggests 5%–10% of the adult population) and is potentially fatal.

CARE SETTING

May be inpatient on a behavioral unit or outpatient in community programs. Although patients are not generally admitted to the acute care setting with this diagnosis, withdrawal from alcohol may occur secondarily during hospitalization for other illnesses/conditions. A short hospital stay may be required during the acute phase because of severity of general condition, or a delayed discharge from acute care can be the result of alcohol withdrawal beginning within 6–48 hr of admission.

RELATED CONCERNS

Cirrhosis of the liver, page 484
Upper gastrointestinal/esophageal bleeding, page 333
Heart failure, page 47
Psychosocial aspects of care, page 809
Substance dependence/abuse rehabilitation, page 886

Patient Assessment Database

Data depend on the duration/extent of use of alcohol, concurrent use of other drugs, degree of organ involvement, and presence of other pathology.

ACTIVITY/REST

May report: Difficulty sleeping, not feeling well rested

CIRCULATION

May exhibit: Generalized tissue edema (due to protein deficiencies)
Peripheral pulses weak, irregular, or rapid
Hypertension common in early withdrawal stage but may become labile/progress to hypotension
Tachycardia common during acute withdrawal; numerous dysrhythmias may be identified

EGO INTEGRITY

May report: Feelings of guilt/shame; defensiveness about drinking
Denial, rationalization
Multiple stressors/losses (relationships, employment, finances)
Use of alcohol to deal with life stressors, boredom

ELIMINATION

May report: Diarrhea
May exhibit: Bowel sounds varied (may reflect gastric complications, e.g., hemorrhage)

FOOD/FLUID

May report: Nausea/vomiting; food intolerance
May exhibit: Gastric distension; ascites, liver enlargement (seen in cirrhosis)
Muscle wasting, dry/dull hair, swollen salivary glands, inflamed buccal cavity, capillary fragility (malnutrition)
Bowel sounds varied (reflecting malnutrition, electrolyte imbalances, general bowel dysfunction)

NEUROSENSORY

May report: "Internal shakes"

Headache, dizziness, blurred vision; "blackouts"

May exhibit: Psychopathology, e.g., paranoid schizophrenia, major depression (may indicate dual diagnosis)

Level of consciousness/orientation varies, e.g., confusion, stupor, hyperactivity, distorted thought processes, slurred/incoherent speech

Memory loss/confabulation

Affect/mood/behavior: May be fearful, anxious, easily startled, inappropriate, silly, euphoric, irritable, physically/verbally abusive, depressed, and/or paranoid

Hallucinations: Visual, tactile, olfactory, and auditory, e.g., patient may be picking items out of air or responding verbally to unseen person/voices

Eye examination: Nystagmus (associated with cranial nerve palsy); pupil constriction (may indicate CNS depression); arcus senilis-ringlike opacity of the cornea (although normal in aging populations, suggests alcohol-related changes in younger patients)

Fine motor tremors of face, tongue, and hands; seizures (commonly grand mal)

Gait unsteady (ataxia), may be due to thiamine deficiency or cerebellar degeneration (Wernicke's encephalopathy)

PAIN/DISCOMFORT

May report: Constant upper abdominal pain and tenderness radiating to the back (pancreatic inflammation)

RESPIRATION

May report: History of smoking, recurrent/chronic respiratory problems

May exhibit: Tachypnea (hyperactive state of alcohol withdrawal)

Cheyne-Stokes respirations or respiratory depression

Breath sounds diminished, adventitious sounds (suggests pulmonary complications, e.g., respiratory depression, pneumonia)

SAFETY

May report: History of recurrent trauma such as falls, fractures, lacerations, burns, blackouts, or motor vehicle crashes

May exhibit: Skin: Flushed face/palms of hands; scars, ecchymotic areas; cigarette burns on fingers, spider nevus (impaired portal circulation), fissures at corners of mouth (vitamin deficiency)

Fractures healed or new (signs of recent/recurrent trauma)

Temperature elevation (dehydration and sympathetic stimulation); flushing/diaphoresis (suggests presence of infection)

Suicidal ideation/suicide attempts (some research suggests alcoholic suicide attempts are 30% higher than national average for general population)

SOCIAL INTERACTION

May report: Frequent sick days off from work/school; fighting with others, arrests (disorderly conduct, motor vehicle violations/driving under the influence [DUI])

Denial that alcohol intake has any significant effect on present condition

Dysfunctional family system of origin (generational involvement); problems in current relationships

Mood changes affecting interactions with others

TEACHING/LEARNING

May report: Family history of alcoholism

History of alcohol and/or other drug use/abuse

Ignorance and/or denial of addiction to alcohol, or inability to cut down or stop drinking despite repeated efforts; previous periods of abstinence/withdrawal

Large amount of alcohol consumed in last 24–48 hr

Previous hospitalizations for alcoholism/alcohol-related diseases, e.g., cirrhosis, esophageal varices

Discharge plan considerations: **DRG projected mean length of inpatient stay: 4.9 days**
May require assistance to maintain abstinence and begin to participate in rehabilitation program

Refer to section at end of plan for postdischarge considerations.

DIAGNOSTIC STUDIES

Blood alcohol/drug levels: Alcohol level may/may not be severely elevated, depending on amount consumed, time between consumption and testing, and the degree of tolerance, which varies widely. In the absence of elevated alcohol tolerance, blood levels in excess of 100 mg/dL are associated with ataxia; at 200 mg/dL the patient is drowsy and confused; respiratory depression occurs with blood levels of 400 mg/dL and death is possible. In addition to alcohol, numerous controlled substances may be identified in a poly-drug screen, e.g., amphetamine, cocaine, morphine, Percodan, Quaalude.

CBC: Decreased Hb/Hct may reflect such problems as iron-deficiency anemia or acute/chronic GI bleeding. WBC count may be increased with infection or decreased if immunosuppressed.

Glucose/Ketones: Hyperglycemia/hypoglycemia may be present, related to pancreatitis, malnutrition, or depletion of liver glycogen stores. Ketoacidosis may be present with/without metabolic acidosis.

Electrolytes: Hypokalemia and hypomagnesemia are common.

Liver function tests: LDH, AST, ALT, and amylase may be elevated, reflecting liver or pancreatic damage.

Nutritional tests: Albumin is low and total protein may be decreased. Vitamin deficiencies are usually present, reflecting malnutrition/malabsorption.

Other screening studies (e.g., hepatitis, HIV, TB): Depend on general condition, individual risk factors, and care setting.

Urinalysis: Infection may be identified; ketones may be present, related to breakdown of fatty acids in malnutrition (pseudodiabetic condition).

Chest x-ray: May reveal right lower lobe pneumonia (malnutrition, depressed immune system, aspiration) or chronic lung disorders associated with tobacco use.

ECG: Dysrhythmias, cardiomyopathies, and/or ischemia may be present because of direct effect of alcohol on the cardiac muscle and/or conduction system, as well as effects of electrolyte imbalance.

Addiction Severity Index (ASI): An assessment tool that produces a "problem severity profile" of the patient, including chemical, medical, psychological, legal, family/social, and employment/support aspects, indicating areas of treatment needs.

NURSING PRIORITIES

1. Maintain physiological stability during acute withdrawal phase.
2. Promote patient safety.
3. Provide appropriate referral and follow-up.
4. Encourage/support SO involvement in "Intervention" (confrontation) process.
5. Provide information about condition/prognosis and treatment needs.

DISCHARGE GOALS

1. Homeostasis achieved.
2. Complications prevented/resolved.
3. Sobriety being maintained on a day-to-day basis.
4. Ongoing participation in rehabilitation program/attending group therapy, e.g., Alcoholics Anonymous.
5. Condition, prognosis, and therapeutic regimen understood.
6. Plan in place to meet needs after discharge.

This plan of care is to be used in conjunction with CP: Substance Dependence/Abuse Rehabilitation.

ACTIONS/INTERVENTIONS	RATIONALE
Respiratory Monitoring (NIC)	
Independent	
Monitor respiratory rate/depth and pattern as indicated. Note periods of apnea, Cheyne-Stokes respirations.	Frequent assessment is important because toxicity levels may change rapidly. Hyperventilation is common during acute withdrawal phase. Kussmaul's respirations are sometimes present because of acidotic state associated with vomiting and malnutrition. However, marked respiratory depression can occur because of CNS depressant effects of alcohol if acute intoxication is present. This may be compounded by drugs used to control alcohol withdrawal symptoms (AWS).
Auscultate breath sounds. Note presence of adventitious sounds, e.g., rhonchi, wheezes.	Patient is at risk for atelectasis related to hypoventilation and pneumonia. Right lower lobe pneumonia is common in alcohol-debilitated patients and is often due to chronic aspiration. Chronic lung diseases are also common, e.g., emphysema, bronchitis.
Airway Management (NIC)	
Elevate head of bed.	Decreases potential for aspiration; lowers diaphragm, enhancing lung inflation.
Encourage cough/deep-breathing exercises and frequent position changes.	Facilitates lung expansion and mobilization of secretions to reduce risk of atelectasis/pneumonia.
Have suction equipment, airway adjuncts available.	Sedative effects of alcohol/drugs potentiates risk of aspiration, relaxation of oropharyngeal muscles, and respiratory depression, requiring intervention to prevent respiratory arrest.
Collaborative	
Administer supplemental oxygen if necessary.	Hypoxia may occur with CNS/respiratory depression.
Review serial chest x-rays, ABGs/pulse oximetry as available/indicated.	Monitors presence of secondary complications such as atelectasis/pneumonia; evaluates effectiveness of respiratory effort, identifies therapy needs.

NURSING DIAGNOSIS: Cardiac Output, risk for decreased

Risk factors may include
Direct effect of alcohol on the heart muscle
Altered systemic vascular resistance
Electrical alterations in rate, rhythm, conduction

Possibly evidenced by
[Not applicable; presence of signs and symptoms establishes an *actual* diagnosis]

DESIRED OUTCOMES/EVALUATION CRITERIA—PATIENT WILL:

Circulation Status (NOC)

Display vital signs within patient's normal range; absence of/reduced frequency of dysrhythmias.
Demonstrate an increase in activity tolerance.

ACTIONS/INTERVENTIONS	RATIONALE
Hemodynamic Regulation (NIC)	
Independent	
Monitor vital signs frequently during acute withdrawal.	Hypertension frequently occurs in acute withdrawal phase. Extreme hyperexcitability, accompanied by catecholamine release and increased peripheral vascular resistance, raises BP and heart rate; however, BP may become labile/progress to hypotension. *Note:* Patient may have underlying cardiovascular disease, which is compounded by alcohol withdrawal.
Monitor cardiac rate/rhythm. Document irregularities/dysrhythmias.	Long-term alcohol abuse may result in cardiomyopathy/HF. Tachycardia is common because of sympathetic response to increased circulating catecholamines. Irregularities/dysrhythmias may develop with electrolyte shifts/imbalance. All of these may have an adverse effect on cardiac function/output.
Monitor body temperature.	Elevation may occur because of sympathetic stimulation, dehydration, and/or infections, causing vasodilation and compromising venous return/cardiac output.
Monitor I&O. Note 24-hr fluid balance.	Preexisting dehydration, vomiting, fever, and diaphoresis may result in decreased circulating volume that can compromise cardiovascular function. *Note:* Hydration is difficult to assess in the alcoholic patient because the usual indicators are not reliable, and overhydration is a risk in the presence of compromised cardiac function.
Be prepared for/assist in cardiopulmonary resuscitation.	Causes of death during acute withdrawal stages include cardiac dysrhythmias, respiratory depression/arrest, oversedation, excessive psychomotor activity, severe dehydration or overhydration, and massive infections. Mortality for unrecognized/untreated delirium tremens (DTs) may be as high as 25%.

ACTIONS/INTERVENTIONS	RATIONALE

Collaborative

Monitor laboratory studies, e.g., serum electrolyte levels.

Electrolyte imbalance, e.g., potassium/magnesium, potentiate risk of cardiac dysrhythmias and CNS excitability.

Administer fluids and electrolytes, as indicated.

Severe alcohol withdrawal causes the patient to be susceptible to fluid losses (associated with fever, diaphoresis, and vomiting) and electrolyte imbalances, especially potassium, magnesium, and glucose.

Administer medications as indicated, e.g.:

    Clonidine (Catapres), atenolol (Tenormin);

Although the use of benzodiazepines is often sufficient to control hypertension during initial withdrawal from alcohol, some patients may require more specific therapy. *Note:* Atenolol and other β-adrenergic blockers may speed up the withdrawal process and eliminate tremors, as well as lower the heart rate, blood pressure, and body temperature.

    Potassium.

Corrects deficits that can result in life-threatening dysrhythmias.

NURSING DIAGNOSIS: Injury, risk for [specify]

Risk factors may include
Cessation of alcohol intake with varied autonomic nervous system responses to the system's suddenly altered state
Involuntary clonic/tonic muscle activity (seizures)
Equilibrium/balancing difficulties, reduced muscle and hand/eye coordination

Possibly evidenced by
[Not applicable; presence of signs and symptoms establishes an *actual* diagnosis]

DESIRED OUTCOMES/EVALUATION CRITERIA—PATIENT WILL:

Risk Control (NOC)

Demonstrate absence of untoward effects of withdrawal.
Experience no physical injury.

ACTIONS/INTERVENTIONS	RATIONALE

Substance Use Treatment: Alcohol Withdrawal (NIC)

Independent

Identify stage of AWS (alchohol withdrawal syndrome); i.e., stage I is associated with signs/symptoms of hyperactivity (e.g., tremors, sleeplessness, nausea/vomiting, diaphoresis, tachycardia, hypertension). Stage II is manifested by increased hyperactivity plus hallucinations and/or seizure activity. Stage III symptoms include DTs and extreme autonomic hyperactivity with profound confusion, anxiety, insomnia, fever.

Prompt recognition and intervention may halt progression of symptoms and enhance recovery/improve prognosis. In addition, recurrence/progression of symptoms indicates need for changes in drug therapy/more intense treatment to prevent death.

ACTIONS/INTERVENTIONS

Independent

Monitor/document seizure activity. Maintain patent airway. Provide environmental safety, e.g., padded side rails, bed in low position.

Check deep-tendon reflexes. Assess gait, if possible.

Assist with ambulation and self-care activities as needed.

Provide for environmental safety when indicated. (Refer to ND: Sensory-Perceptual alterations, following.)

Collaborative

Administer medications as indicated e.g.:

Benzodiazepines (BZDs), e.g., chlordiazepoxide (Librium), diazepam (Valium), clonazepam (Klonopin), oxazepam (Serax), clorazepate (Tranxene);

Haloperidol (Haldol);

Thiamine;

Magnesium sulfate.

RATIONALE

Grand mal seizures are most common and may be related to decreased magnesium levels, hypoglycemia, elevated blood alcohol, or history of head trauma/preexisting seizure disorder. *Note:* In absence of history of/other pathology causing seizures, they usually stop spontaneously, requiring only symptomatic treatment. *Note:* Antiepileptic drugs are not indicated for alcohol withdrawal seizures.

Reflexes may be depressed, absent, or hyperactive. Peripheral neuropathies are common, especially in malnourished patient. Ataxia (gait disturbance) is associated with Wernicke's syndrome (thiamine deficiency) and cerebellar degeneration.

Prevents falls with resultant injury.

May be required when equilibrium, hand/eye coordination problems exist.

BZDs are commonly used to control neuronal hyperactivity because of their minimal respiratory and cardiac depression and anticonvulsant properties. Studies have also shown that these drugs can prevent progression to more severe states of withdrawal. IV/PO administration is preferred route because IM absorption is unpredictable. Muscle-relaxant qualities are particularly helpful to patient in controlling "the shakes," trembling, and ataxic quality of movements. Patient may initially require large doses to achieve desired effect, and then drugs may be tapered and discontinued, usually within 96 hr. *Note:* These agents are used cautiously in patients with known hepatic disease because they are metabolized by the liver, although Serax has a shorter half-life.

May be used in conjunction with BZDs for patients experiencing hallucinations.

Thiamine deficiency (common in alcohol abuse) may lead to neuritis, Wernecke's syndrome, and/or Korsakoff's psychosis.

Reduces tremors and seizure activity by decreasing neuromuscular excitability.

NURSING DIAGNOSIS: Sensory-Perceptual alterations (specify)

May be related to

Chemical alteration: Exogenous (e.g., alcohol consumption/sudden cessation) and endogenous (e.g., electrolyte imbalance, elevated ammonia and BUN)

Sleep deprivation

Psychological stress (anxiety/fear)

ACTIONS/INTERVENTIONS	RATIONALE
Substance Use Treatment: Alcohol Withdrawal (NIC)	
Independent	
Assess level of consciousness; ability to speak, response to stimuli/commands.	Speech may be garbled, confused, or slurred. Response to commands may reveal inability to concentrate, impaired judgment, or muscle coordination deficits.
Observe behavioral responses, e.g., hyperactivity, disorientation, confusion, sleeplessness, irritability.	Hyperactivity related to CNS disturbances may escalate rapidly. Sleeplessness is common due to loss of sedative effect gained from alcohol usually consumed before bedtime. Sleep deprivation may aggravate disorientation/confusion. Progression of symptoms may indicate impending hallucinations (stage II) or DTs (stage III).
Note onset of hallucinations. Document as auditory, visual, and/or tactile.	Auditory hallucinations are reported to be more frightening/threatening to patient. Visual hallucinations occur more at night and often include insects, animals, or faces of friends/enemies. Patients are frequently observed "picking the air." Yelling may occur if patient is calling for help from perceived threat (usually seen in stage III AWS).
Provide quiet environment. Speak in calm, quiet voice. Regulate lighting as indicated. Turn off radio/TV during sleep.	Reduces external stimuli during hyperactive stage. Patient may become more delirious when surroundings cannot be seen, but some respond better to quiet, darkened room.
Provide care by same personnel whenever possible.	Promotes recognition of caregivers and a sense of consistency, which may reduce fear.
Encourage SO to stay with patient whenever possible.	May have a calming effect, and may provide a reorienting influence.
Reorient frequently to person, place, time, and surrounding environment as indicated.	May reduce confusion, prevent/limit misinterpretation of external stimuli.

ACTIONS/INTERVENTIONS

Independent

Avoid bedside discussion about patient or topics unrelated to the patient that do not include the patient.

Provide environmental safety, e.g., place bed in low position, leave doors in full open or closed position, observe frequently, place call light/bell within reach, remove articles that can harm patient.

Collaborative

Provide seclusion, restraints as necessary.

Monitor laboratory studies, e.g., electrolytes, magnesium levels, liver function studies, ammonia, BUN, glucose, ABGs.

Administer medications as indicated, e.g.:

Antianxiety agents as indicated. (Refer to ND: Anxiety [severe/panic]/Fear), following);

Thiamine, vitamins C and B complex, multivitamins, Stresstabs.

RATIONALE

Patient may hear and misinterpret conversation, which can aggravate hallucinations.

Patient may have distorted sense of reality or be fearful or suicidal, requiring protection from self.

Patients with excessive psychomotor activity, severe hallucinations, violent behavior, and/or suicidal gestures may respond better to seclusion. Restraints are usually ineffective and add to patient's agitation, but occasionally may be required to prevent self-harm.

Changes in organ function may precipitate or potentiate sensory-perceptual deficits. Electrolyte imbalance is common. Liver function is often impaired in the chronic alcoholic, and ammonia intoxication can occur if the liver is unable to convert ammonia to urea. Ketoacidosis is sometimes present without glycosuria; however, hyperglycemia or hypoglycemia may occur, suggesting pancreatitis or impaired gluconeogenesis in the liver. Hypoxemia and hypercarbia are common manifestations in chronic alcoholics who are also heavy smokers.

Reduces hyperactivity, promoting relaxation/sleep. Drugs that have little effect on dreaming may be desired to allow dream recovery (REM rebound) to occur, which has previously been suppressed by alcohol use.

Vitamins may be depleted because of insufficient intake and malabsorption. Vitamin deficiency (especially thiamine) is associated with ataxia, loss of eye movement and pupillary response, palpitations, postural hypotension, and exertional dyspnea.

NURSING DIAGNOSIS: Anxiety [severe/panic]/Fear

May be related to
Cessation of alcohol intake/physiological withdrawal
Situational crisis (hospitalization)
Threat to self-concept, perceived threat of death

Possibly evidenced by
Feelings of inadequacy, shame, self-disgust, and remorse
Increased helplessness/hopelessness with loss of control of own life
Increased tension, apprehension
Fear of unspecified consequences; identifies object of fear

DESIRED OUTCOMES/EVALUATION CRITERIA—PATIENT WILL:

Anxiety or Fear Control (NOC)

Verbalize reduction of fear and anxiety to an acceptable and manageable level.
Express sense of regaining some control of situation/life.
Demonstrate problem-solving skills and use resources effectively.

ACTIONS/INTERVENTIONS	RATIONALE

Anxiety Reduction (NIC)

Independent

Identify cause of anxiety, involving patient in the process. Explain that alcohol withdrawal increases anxiety and uneasiness. Reassess level of anxiety on an ongoing basis.

Person in acute phase of withdrawal may be unable to identify and/or accept what is happening. Anxiety may be physiologically or environmentally caused. Continued alcohol toxicity will be manifested by increased anxiety and agitation as effects of medication wear off.

Develop a trusting relationship through frequent contact being honest and nonjudgmental. Project an accepting attitude about alcoholism.

Provides patient with a sense of humanness, helping to decrease paranoia and distrust. Patient will be able to detect biased or condescending attitude of caregivers.

Inform patient about what you plan to do and why. Include patient in planning process and provide choices when possible.

Enhances sense of trust, and explanation may increase cooperation/reduce anxiety. Provides sense of control over self in circumstance where loss of control is a significant factor. *Note:* Feelings of self-worth are intensified when one is treated as a worthwhile person.

Reorient frequently. (Refer to ND: Sensory-Perceptual alterations, p. 879.)

Patient may experience periods of confusion, resulting in increased anxiety.

Collaborative

Administer medications as indicated, e.g.:

Benzodiazepines, e.g., chlordiazepoxide (Librium), diazepam (Valium);

Antianxiety agents are given during acute withdrawal to help patient relax, be less hyperactive, and feel more in control.

Barbiturates, e.g., phenobarbital, or possibly secobarbital (Seconal), pentobarbital (Nembutal).

These drugs suppress alcohol withdrawal but need to be used with caution because they are respiratory depressants and REM sleep cycle inhibitors.

Arrange "Intervention" (confrontation) in controlled setting.

Process wherein SO/family members, supported by staff, provide information about how patient's drinking and behavior have affected each one of them, helps patient acknowledge that drinking is a problem and has resulted in current situational crisis.

Provide consultation for referral to detoxification/crisis center for ongoing treatment program as soon as medically stable (e.g., oriented to reality).

Patient is more likely to contract for treatment while still hurting and experiencing fear and anxiety from last drinking episode. Motivation decreases as well-being increases and person again feels able to control the problem. Direct contact with available treatment resources provides realistic picture of help. Decreases time for patient to "think about it"/change mind or restructure and strengthen denial systems.

POTENTIAL CONSIDERATIONS following acute care (dependent on patient's age, physical condition/presence of complications, personal resources, and life responsibilities)

Refer to: Substance Abuse/Rehabilitation plan of care, page 886, and plans of care for any specific underlying medical condition(s).

Sample CP: Alcohol Withdrawal Program. ELOS: 5 Days Behavioral Unit

ND and Categories of Care	Time Dimension	Goals/Actions	Time Dimension	Goals/Actions	Time Dimension	Goals/Actions
Risk for injury (varied autonomic and sensory responses)	Day 1	Verbalize understanding of unit policies, procedures, and safety concerns relative to individual needs Cooperate with therapeutic regimen	Day 3 Day 4	Vital signs stable I&O balanced Display marked decrease in objective symptoms	Day 5	Be free of injury resulting from ETOH withdrawal Display no objective symptoms of withdrawal
Referrals	Day 1	RN-NP or MD If indicated: Internist Cardiologist Neurologist				
Diagnostic studies	Day 1	BA level Drug screen (urine and blood) If indicated: CXR Pulse oximetry ECG	Day 2	SMA 20 Serum Mg, amylase RPR UA	Day 4	Repeat of selected studies as indicated
Additional assessments	Day 1 Day 1–4 Ongoing Stage I Stage II Stage III	VS, temp, respiratory status/breath sounds q4h I&O q8h Motor activity, body language, verbalizations, need for/ type of restraint Withdrawal symptoms: Tremors, N/V, hypertension, tachycardia, diaphoresis, sleeplessness Increased hyperactivity, hallucinations, seizure activity Extreme autonomic hyperactivity, profound confusion, anxiety, fever	Day 2–3	VS q8h if stable	Day 4–5	VS qd
Medications Allergies: _____	Day 1 Day 1–4 Day 2	Librium 200 mg PO Thiamine 100 mg IM Librium 160 mg PO	Day 3 Day 4	Librium 120 mg PO Librium 80 mg PO	Day 5	Librium 40 mg PO
Patient education	Day 1	Orient to room/unit, schedule, procedures	Day 3–4	Need for ongoing therapy Goals/availability of AA program	Day 5	Schedule of follow-up visits if indicated
Additional nursing actions	Day 1 Day 1–2	Bed rest 12 hr if in withdrawal Position change, HOB elevated; C, DB exercises if on bed rest Assist with ambulation, self-care as needed Encourage fluids if free of N/V	Day 3–5	Activity as tolerated		

Sample CP: Alcohol Withdrawal Program. ELOS: 5 Days Behavioral Unit *(Continued)*

ND and Categories of Care	Time Dimension	Goals/Actions	Time Dimension	Goals/Actions	Time Dimension	Goals/Actions
	Ongoing	Provide environmental safety measures, seizure precautions as indicated Reorient as needed				
Ineffective individual coping R/T personal vulnerability, situational crisis, inadequate coping methods	Day 1–5 Day 2–5	Participate in development/evaluation of treatment plan Interact in group sessions	Day 3 Day 4	Verbalize understanding of relationship of ETOH abuse to current situation Identify/make contact with potential resources, support groups	Day 5	Plan in place to meet needs postdischarge
Referrals	Day 1 Day 2–5	Psychiatrist Group sessions	Day 4	Community classes: Assertiveness training Stress management		
Additional assessments	Day 1 Day 1–2	Understanding of current situation Drinking pattern, previous withdrawal, other drug use, attitudes toward substance use History of violence Relationships with others: personal, work/school Readiness for group activities	Day 2–3 Day 3–5	Previous coping strategies/consequences Perception of drug use on life, employment, legal issues Congruency of actions based on insight		
Medications			Day 5	Naltrexone 50 mg/day if indicated		
Patient education	Day 1 Day 1–2 Day 2	Physical effects of ETOH abuse Types/use of relaxation techniques Consequences of ETOH abuse	Day 3–5 Day 4–5	Human behavior and interactions with others/transactional analysis (TA) Community resources for self/family Identify goals for change	Day 5	Medication dose, frequency, side effects Written instructions for therapeutic program
Additional nursing actions	Day 1–5	Support patient's taking responsibility for own recovery Provide consistent approach/expectations for behavior Set limits/confront inappropriate behaviors	Day 2–5	Discuss alternative solutions Provide positive feedback for efforts Support during confrontation by peer group Encourage verbalization of feelings, personal reflection		

Sample CP: Alcohol Withdrawal Program. ELOS: 5 Days Behavioral Unit *(Continued)*

ND and Categories of Care	Time Dimension	Goals/Actions	Time Dimension	Goals/Actions	Time Dimension	Goals/Actions
Altered nutrition: less than body requirements R/T poor intake, effects of ETOH on digestive system, and hypermetabolic response to withdrawal	Day 2–5	Select foods appropriately to meet individual dietary needs	Day 4	Verbalize understandings of effects of ETOH abuse and reduced dietary intake on nutritional status	Day 5	Display stable weight or initial weight gain as appropriate, and laboratory results WNL
Referrals	Day 1 and prn	Dietitian				
Diagnostic studies	Day 1	CBC, liver function studies Serum albumin, transferrin	Day 2–5	Fingerstick glucose prn		
Additional assessments	Day 1	Weight, skin turgor, condition of mucous membranes, muscle tone			Day 5	Weight
	Day 1–2	Bowel sounds, characteristics of stools				
	Day 1–5	Appetite, dietary intake				
Medications	Day 1–5	Antacid ac and hs Imodium 2 mg prn	Day 2–5	Multivitamin tab/qd		
Patient education	Day 1–2	Individual nutritional needs	Day 4	Principles of nutrition, foods for maintenance of wellness		
Additional nursing actions	Day 1	Liquid/bland diet as tolerated	Day 2–5	Advance diet as tolerated		
	Day 1–5	Encourage small, frequent, nutritious meals/snacks Encourage good oral hygiene pc and hs				

SUBSTANCE DEPENDENCE/ABUSE REHABILITATION

Many drugs and volatile substances are subject to abuse. This disorder is a continuum of phases incorporating a cluster of cognitive, behavioral, and physiological symptoms that include loss of control over use of the substance and a continued use of the substance despite adverse consequences. A number of factors have been implicated in the predisposition to abuse a substance: biological, biochemical, psychological (including developmental), personality, sociocultural and conditioning, and cultural and ethnic influences. However, no single theory adequately explains the etiology of this problem.

CARE SETTING

Inpatient stay on behavioral unit or outpatient care in a day program or community agency.

RELATED CONCERNS

Alcohol: acute withdrawal, page 873
Psychosocial aspects of care, page 809

Patient Assessment Database

Depends on substances involved, duration of use, organs affected.

TEACHING/LEARNING

Discharge plan considerations: **DRG projected mean length of stay depends on individual program, general health status**

May need assistance with long-range plan for recovery

Refer to section at end of plan for postdischarge considerations.

DIAGNOSTIC STUDIES

Drug screen: Identifies drug(s) being used.
Addiction Severity Index (ASI) assessment tool: Produces a "problem severity profile" of the patient, including chemical, medical, psychological, legal, family/social and employment/support aspects, indicating areas of treatment needs.
Other screening studies (e.g., hepatitis, HIV, TB): Depends on general condition, individual risk factors, and care setting.

NURSING PRIORITIES

1. Provide support for decision to stop substance use.
2. Strengthen individual coping skills.
3. Facilitate learning of new ways to reduce anxiety.
4. Promote family involvement in rehabilitation program.
5. Facilitate family growth/development.
6. Provide information about condition, prognosis, and treatment needs.

DISCHARGE GOALS

1. Responsibility for own life and behavior assumed.
2. Plan to maintain substance-free life formulated.
3. Family relationships/enabling issues being addressed.
4. Treatment program successfully begun.
5. Condition, prognosis, and therapeutic regimen understood.
6. Plan in place to meet needs after discharge.

NURSING DIAGNOSIS: Denial

May be related to

Personal vulnerability; difficulty handling new situations

Previous ineffective/inadequate coping skills with substitution of drug(s)

Learned response patterns; cultural factors, personal/family value systems

Possibly evidenced by

Delay in seeking, or refusal of healthcare attention to the detriment of health/life

Does not perceive personal relevance of symptoms or danger, or admit impact of condition on life pattern; projection of blame/responsibility for problems

Use of manipulation to avoid responsibility for self

DESIRED OUTCOMES/EVALUATION CRITERIA—PATIENT WILL:

Acceptance: Health Status (NOC)

Verbalize awareness of relationship of substance abuse to current situation.

Engage in therapeutic program.

Verbalize acceptance of responsibility for own behavior.

ACTIONS/INTERVENTIONS	RATIONALE
Behavior Modification (NIC)	
Independent	
Ascertain by what name patient would like to be addressed.	Shows courtesy and respect, giving patient a sense of orientation and control.
Convey attitude of acceptance, separating individual from unacceptable behavior.	Promotes feelings of dignity and self-worth.
Ascertain reason for beginning abstinence, involvement in therapy.	Provides insight into patient's willingness to commit to long-term behavioral change, and whether patient even believes that he or she can change. (Denial is one of the strongest and most resistant symptoms of substance abuse.)
Review definition of drug dependence and categories of symptoms (e.g., patterns of use, impairment caused by use, tolerance to substance).	This information helps patient make decisions regarding acceptance of problem and treatment choices.
Answer questions honestly and provide factual information. Keep your word when agreements are made.	Creates trust, which is the basis of the therapeutic relationship.
Provide information about addictive use versus experimental, occasional use; biochemical/genetic disorder theory (genetic predisposition; use activated by environment; compulsive desire.)	Progression of use continuum is from experimental/recreational to addictive use. Comprehending this process is important in combating denial. Education may relieve patient's guilt and blame and may help awareness of recurring addictive characteristics.
Discuss current life situation and impact of substance use.	First step in decreasing use of denial is for patient to see the relationship between substance use and personal problems.
Confront and examine denial/rationalization in peer group. Use confrontation with caring.	Because denial is the major defense mechanism in addictive disease, confrontation by peers can help the patient accept the reality of adverse consequences of behaviors and that drug use is a major problem. Caring attitude preserves self-concept and helps decrease defensive response.

ACTIONS/INTERVENTIONS

Independent

Provide information regarding effects of addiction on mood/personality.

Remain nonjudgmental. Be alert to changes in behavior, e.g., restlessness, increased tension.

Provide positive feedback for expressing awareness of denial in self/others.

Maintain firm expectation that patient attend recovery support/therapy groups regularly.

Encourage and support patient's taking responsibility for own recovery (e.g., development of alternative behaviors to drug urge/use). Assist patient to learn own responsibility for recovering.

RATIONALE

Individuals often mistake effects of addiction and use this to justify or excuse drug use.

Confrontation can lead to increased agitation, which may compromise safety of patient/staff.

Necessary to enhance self-esteem and to reinforce insight into behavior.

Attendance is related to admitting need for help, to working with denial, and for maintenance of a long-term drug-free existence.

Denial can be replaced with positive action when patient accepts the reality of own responsibility.

NURSING DIAGNOSIS: Coping, Individual, ineffective

May be related to
Personal vulnerability
Negative role modeling; inadequate support systems
Previous ineffective/inadequate coping skills with substitution of drug(s)

Possibly evidenced by
Impaired adaptive behavior and problem-solving skills
Decreased ability to handle stress of illness/hospitalization
Financial affairs in disarray, employment difficulties (e.g., losing time on job/not maintaining steady employment; poor work performances, on-the-job injuries)
Verbalization of inability to cope/ask for help

DESIRED OUTCOMES/EVALUATION CRITERIA—PATIENT WILL:

Coping (NOC)

Identify ineffective coping behaviors/consequences, including use of substances as a method of coping.
Use effective coping skills/problem solving.
Initiate necessary lifestyle changes.

ACTIONS/INTERVENTIONS

Substance Use Treatment (NIC)

Independent

Review program rules, philosophy expectations.

Determine understanding of current situation and previous/other methods of coping with life's problems.

RATIONALE

Having information provides opportunity for patient to cooperate and function as a member of the group/milieu, enhancing sense of control and sense of success.

Provides information about degree of denial, acceptance of personal responsibility/commitment to change; identifies coping skills that may be used in present situation.

ACTIONS/INTERVENTIONS	RATIONALE

Independent

Set limits and confront efforts to get caregiver to grant special privileges, making excuses for not following through on behaviors agreed on, and attempting to continue drug use.

Patient has learned manipulative behavior throughout life and needs to learn a new way of getting needs met. Following through on consequences of failure to maintain limits can help the patient to change ineffective behaviors.

Be aware of staff attitudes, feelings, and enabling behaviors.

Lack of understanding, judgmental/enabling behaviors can result in inaccurate data collection and nontherapeutic approaches.

Encourage verbalization of feelings, fears, and anxiety.

May help patient begin to come to terms with long-unresolved issues.

Explore alternative coping strategies.

Patient may have little or no knowledge of adaptive responses to stress and needs to learn other options for managing time, feelings, and relationships without drugs.

Assist patient to learn/encourage use of relaxation skills, guided imagery, visualizations.

Helps patient relax, develop new ways to deal with stress, problem-solve.

Structure diversional activity that relates to recovery (e.g., social activity within support group), wherein issues of being chemically free are examined.

Discovery of alternative methods of coping with drug hunger can remind patient that addiction is a lifelong process and opportunity for changing patterns is available.

Use peer support to examine ways of coping with drug hunger.

Self-help groups are valuable for learning and promoting abstinence in each member, using understanding and support as well as peer pressure.

Use peer support to examine ways of coping with drug binges.

Self-help groups are valuable for learning and promoting abstinence in each member, using understanding, support, and peer pressure.

Encourage involvement in therapeutic writing. Have patient begin journaling or writing autobiography.

Therapeutic writing/journaling can enhance participation in treatment; serves as a release for grief, anger, and stress; provides a useful tool for monitoring patient's safety; and can be used to evaluate patient's progress. Autobiographical activity provides an opportunity for patient to remember and identify sequence of events in his or her life that relate to current situation.

Discuss patient's plans for living without drugs.

Provide opportunity to develop/refine plans. Devising a comprehensive strategy for avoiding relapses helps patient into maintenance phase of behavioral change.

Collaborative

Administer medications as indicated, e.g.:

    Disulfiram (Antabuse);

This drug can be helpful in maintaining abstinence from alcohol while other therapy is undertaken. By inhibiting alcohol oxidation, the drug leads to an accumulation of acetaldehyde with a highly unpleasant reaction if alcohol is consumed.

    Acamprosate;

Helps prevent relapses in alcoholism by lowering receptors for the excitatory neurotransmitter glutamate. This agent may become drug of choice because it does not make the user sick if alcohol is consumed; it has no sedative, antianxiety, muscle relaxant, or antidepressant properties and produces no withdrawal symptoms.

889

ACTIONS/INTERVENTIONS	RATIONALE

Collaborative

Methadone (Dolophine);	This drug is thought to blunt the craving for/diminish the effects of opioids and is used to assist in withdrawal and long-term maintenance programs. It can allow the individual to maintain daily activities and ultimately withdraw from drug use.
Naltrexone (Trexan), nalmefine (Revex).	Used to suppress craving for opioids and may help prevent relapse in the patient abusing alcohol. Current research suggests that naltrexone suppresses urge to continue drinking by interfering with alcohol-induced release of endorphins.
Encourage involvement with self-help associations, e.g., Alcoholics/Narcotics Anonymous.	Puts patient in direct contact with support system necessary for managing sobriety/drug-free life.

NURSING DIAGNOSIS: Powerlessness

May be related to
Substance addiction with/without periods of abstinence
Episodic compulsive indulgence; attempts at recovery
Lifestyle of helplessness

Possibly evidenced by
Ineffective recovery attempts; statements of inability to stop behavior/requests for help
Continuous/constant thinking about drug and/or obtaining drug
Alteration in personal, occupational, and social life

DESIRED OUTCOMES/EVALUATION CRITERIA—PATIENT WILL:

Health Beliefs: Perceived Control (NOC)

Admit inability to control drug habit, surrender to powerlessness over addiction.
Verbalize acceptance of need for treatment and awareness that willpower alone cannot control abstinence.
Engage in peer support.
Demonstrate active participation in program.
Regain and maintain healthy state with a drug-free lifestyle.

ACTIONS/INTERVENTIONS	RATIONALE

Self-Responsibility Facilitation (NIC)

Independent

Use crisis intervention techniques to initiate behavior changes:	Patient is more amenable to acceptance of need for treatment at this time.
Assist patient to recognize problem exists. Discuss in a caring, nonjudgmental manner how drug has interfered with life;	In the precontemplation phase, the patient has not yet identified that drug use is problematic. While patient is hurting, it is easier to admit substance use has created negative consequences.
Involve patient in development of treatment plan, using problem-solving process in which patient identifies goals for change and agrees to desired outcomes;	During the contemplation phase, the patient realizes a problem exists and is thinking about a change of behavior. The patient is committed to the outcomes when the decision-making process involves solutions that are promulgated by the individual.

ACTIONS/INTERVENTIONS

Independent

Discuss alternative solutions;

Assist in selecting most appropriate alternative;

Support decision and implementation of selected alternative(s).

Explore support in peer group. Encourage sharing about drug hunger, situations that increase the desire to indulge, ways that substance has influenced life.

Assist patient to learn ways to enhance health and structure healthy diversion from drug use (e.g., maintaining a balanced diet, getting adequate rest, exercise [e.g., walking, slow/long distance running]; and acupuncture, biofeedback, deep meditative techniques).

Provide information regarding understanding of human behavior and interactions with others, e.g., transactional analysis.

Assist patient in self-examination of spirituality, faith.

Instruct in and role-play assertive communication skills.

Provide treatment information on an ongoing basis.

Collaborative

Refer to/assist with making contact with programs for ongoing treatment needs, e.g., partial hospitalization drug treatment programs, Narcotics/Alcoholics Anonymous, peer support group.

RATIONALE

Brainstorming helps creatively identify possibilities and provides sense of control. During the preparation phase, minor action may be taken as individual organizes resources for definitive change.

As possibilities are discussed, the most useful solution becomes clear.

Helps the patient persevere in process of change. During the action phase, the patient engages in a sustained effort to maintain sobriety, and mechanisms are put in place to support abstinence.

Patient may need assistance in expressing self, speaking about powerlessness, admitting need for help in order to face up to problem and begin resolution.

Learning to empower self in constructive areas can strengthen ability to continue recovery. These activities help restore natural biochemical balance, aid detoxification, and manage stress, anxiety, use of free time. These diversions can increase self-confidence, thereby improving self-esteem. *Note:* Exercise promotes release of endorphins, creating a feeling of well-being.

Understanding these concepts can help the patient to begin to deal with past problems/losses and prevent repeating ineffective coping behaviors and self-fulfilling prophecies.

Although not mandatory for recovery, surrendering to and faith in a power greater than oneself has been found to be effective for many individuals in substance recovery; may decrease sense of powerlessness.

Effective in helping refrain from use, to stop contact with users and dealers, to build healthy relationships, regain control of own life.

Helps patient know what to expect, and creates opportunity for patient to be a part of what is happening and make informed choices about participation/outcomes.

Continuing treatment is essential to positive outcome. Follow-through may be easier once initial contact has been made.

NURSING DIAGNOSIS: Nutrition: altered, less than body requirements

May be related to
Insufficient dietary intake to meet metabolic needs for psychological, physiological, or economic reasons

Possibly evidenced by
Weight loss; weight below norm for height/body build; decreased subcutaneous fat/muscle mass

Reported altered taste sensation; lack of interest in food
Poor muscle tone
Sore, inflamed buccal cavity
Laboratory evidence of protein/vitamin deficiencies

DESIRED OUTCOMES/EVALUATION CRITERIA—PATIENT WILL:

Nutritional Status (NOC)

Demonstrate progressive weight gain toward goal with normalization of laboratory values and absence of signs of malnutrition.

Knowledge: Treatment Regimen (NOC)

Verbalize understanding of effects of substance abuse, reduced dietary intake on nutritional status.
Demonstrate behaviors, lifestyle changes to regain and maintain appropriate weight.

ACTIONS/INTERVENTIONS	RATIONALE
Nutrition Therapy (NIC)	
Independent	
Assess height/weight, age, body build, strength, activity/rest level. Note condition of oral cavity.	Provides information about individual on which to base caloric needs/dietary plan. Type of diet/foods may be affected by condition of mucous membranes and teeth.
Take anthropometric measurements, e.g., triceps skinfold, when available.	Calculates subcutaneous fat and muscle mass to aid in determining dietary needs.
Note total daily calorie intake; maintain a diary of intake, as well as times and patterns of eating.	Information will help identify nutritional needs/deficiencies.
Evaluate energy expenditure (e.g., pacing or sedentary), and establish an individualized exercise program.	Activity level affects nutritional needs. Exercise enhances muscle tone, may stimulate appetite.
Provide opportunity to choose foods/snacks to meet dietary plan.	Enhances participation/sense of control, may promote resolution of nutritional deficiencies, and helps evaluate patient's understanding of dietary teaching.
Recommend monitoring weight weekly.	Provides information regarding effectiveness of dietary plan.
Collaborative	
Consult with dietitian.	Useful in establishing individual dietary needs/plan and provides additional resource for learning.
Review laboratory studies as indicated, (e.g., glucose, serum albumin/prealbumin, electrolytes).	Identifies anemias, electrolyte imbalances, and other abnormalities that may be present, requiring specific therapy.
Refer for dental consultation as necessary.	Teeth are essential to good nutritional intake and dental hygiene/care is often a neglected area in this population.

NURSING DIAGNOSIS: Self-Esteem, chronic low

May be related to

Social stigma attached to substance abuse, expectation that one controls behavior

Negative role models; abuse/neglect, dysfunctional family system

Life choices perpetuating failure; situational crisis with loss of control over life events

Biochemical body change (e.g., withdrawal from alcohol/other drugs)

Possibly evidenced by

Self-negating verbalization, expressions of shame/guilt

Evaluation of self as unable to deal with events, confusion about self, purpose or direction in life

Rationalizing away/rejecting positive feedback about self

DESIRED OUTCOMES/EVALUATION CRITERIA—PATIENT WILL:

Self-Esteem (NOC)

Identify feelings and underlying dynamics for negative perception of self.

Verbalize acceptance of self as is and an increased sense of self-worth.

Set goals and participate in realistic planning for lifestyle changes necessary to live without drugs.

ACTIONS/INTERVENTIONS	RATIONALE
Self-Esteem Enhancement (NIC)	
Independent	
Provide opportunity for and encourage verbalization/discussion of individual situation.	Patient often has difficulty expressing self, even more difficulty accepting the degree of importance substance has assumed in life and its relationship to present situation.
Assess mental status. Note presence of other psychiatric disorders (dual diagnosis).	Many patients use substances in an attempt to obtain relief from depression or anxiety, which may predate use and/or be the result of substance use. Approximately 60% of substance-dependent patients have underlying psychological problems, and treatment for both is imperative to achieve/maintain abstinence.
Spend time with patient. Discuss patient's behavior/use of substance in a nonjudgmental way.	The nurse's presence conveys acceptance of the individual as a worthwhile person. Discussion provides opportunity for insight into the problems abuse has created for the patient.
Provide reinforcement for positive actions and encourage patient to accept this input.	Failure and lack of self-esteem have been problems for this patient, who needs to learn to accept self as an individual with positive attributes.
Observe family interactions/SO dynamics and level of support.	Substance abuse is a family disease, and how the members act and react to the patient's behavior affects the course of the disease and how patient sees self. Many unconsciously become "enablers," helping the individual to cover up the consequences of the abuse. (Refer to ND: Family Processes, altered: alcoholism, following.)
Encourage expression of feelings of guilt, shame, and anger.	The patient often has lost respect for self and believes that the situation is hopeless. Expression of these feelings helps the patient begin to accept responsibility for self and take steps to make changes.

893

ACTIONS/INTERVENTIONS

RATIONALE

Independent

Help the patient acknowledge that substance use is the problem and that problems can be dealt with without the use of drugs. Confront the use of defenses, e.g., denial, projection, rationalization.

When drugs can no longer be blamed for the problems that exist, the patient can begin to deal with the problems and live without substance use. Confrontation helps the patient accept the reality of the problems as they exist.

Ask the patient to list and review past accomplishments and positive happenings.

There are things in everyone's life that have been successful. Often when self-esteem is low, it is difficult to remember these successes or to view them as successes.

Use techniques of role rehearsal.

Assists patient to practice developing skills to cope with new role as a person who no longer uses or needs drugs to handle life's problems.

Collaborative

Involve patient in group therapy.

Group sharing helps encourage verbalization because other members of group are in various stages of abstinence from drugs and can address the patient's concerns/denial. The patient can gain new skills, hope, and a sense of family/community from group participation.

Formulate plan to treat other mental illness problems.

Patients who seek relief for other mental health problems through drugs will continue to do so once discharged. Both the substance use and the mental health problems need to be treated together to maximize abstinence potential.

Administer antipsychotic medications as necessary.

Prolonged/profound psychosis following LSD or PCP use can be treated with these drugs because it is probably the result of an underlying functional psychosis that has now emerged. *Note:* Avoid the use of phenothiazines because they may decrease seizure threshold and cause hypotension in the presence of LSD/PCP use.

NURSING DIAGNOSIS: Family Processes, altered: alcoholism [substance abuse]

May be related to
Abuse of substance(s); resistance to treatment
Family history of substance abuse
Addictive personality
Inadequate coping skills, lack of problem-solving skills

Possibly evidenced by
Anxiety; anger/suppressed rage; shame and embarrassment
Emotional isolation/loneliness; vulnerability; repressed emotions
Disturbed family dynamics; closed communication systems, ineffective spousal communication and marital problems
Altered role function/disruption of family roles
Manipulation; dependency; criticizing; rationalization/denial of problems
Enabling to maintain drinking (substance abuse); refusal to get help/inability to accept and receive help appropriately

---

DESIRED OUTCOMES/EVALUATION CRITERIA—FAMILY WILL:

Coping (NOC)

Verbalize understanding of dynamics of enabling behaviors.
Participate in individual family programs.
Identify ineffective coping behaviors and consequences.
Initiate and plan for necessary lifestyle changes.
Take action to change self-destructive behaviors/alter behaviors that contribute to partner's/SO's addiction.

ACTIONS/INTERVENTIONS

Substance Use Treatment (NIC)

Independent

ACTIONS/INTERVENTIONS	RATIONALE
Review family history; explore roles of family members, circumstances involving drug use, strengths, areas for growth.	Determines areas for focus, potential for change.
Explore how the SO has coped with the patient's habit, (e.g., denial, repression, rationalization, hurt, loneliness, projection).	The person who enables also suffers from the same feelings as the patient and uses ineffective methods for dealing with the situation, necessitating help in learning new/effective coping skills.
Determine understanding of current situation and previous methods of coping with life's problems.	Provides information on which to base present plan of care.
Assess current level of functioning of family members.	Affects individual's ability to cope with situation.
Determine extent of enabling behaviors being evidenced by family members; explore with each individual and patient.	Enabling is doing for the patient what he or she needs to do for self (rescuing). People want to be helpful and do not want to feel powerless to help their loved one stop substance use and change the behavior that is so destructive. However, the substance abuser often relies on others to cover up own inability to cope with daily responsibilities.
Provide information about enabling behavior, addictive disease characteristics for both user and nonuser.	Awareness and knowledge of behaviors (e.g., avoiding and shielding, taking over responsibilities, rationalizing, and subserving) provide opportunity for individuals to begin the process of change.
Identify and discuss sabotage behaviors of family members.	Even though family member(s) may verbalize a desire for the individual to become substance-free, the reality of interactive dynamics is that they may unconsciously not want the individual to recover because this would affect the family member(s)' own role in the relationship. Additionally, they may receive sympathy/attention from others (secondary gain).
Encourage participation in therapeutic writing, e.g., journaling (narrative), guided or focused.	Serves as a release for feelings (e.g., anger, grief, stress); helps move individuals forward in treatment process.
Provide factual information to patient and family about the effects of addictive behaviors on the family and what to expect after discharge.	Many patients/SOs are not aware of the nature of addiction. If patient is using legally obtained drugs, he or she may believe this does not constitute abuse.

ACTIONS/INTERVENTIONS	RATIONALE

Independent

Encourage family members to be aware of their own feelings, look at the situation with perspective and objectivity. They can ask themselves: "Am I being conned? Am I acting out of fear, shame, guilt, or anger? Do I have a need to control?"

When the enabling family members become aware of their own actions that perpetuate the addict's problems, they need to decide to change themselves. If they change, the patient can then face the consequences of his/her own actions and may choose to get well.

Provide support for enabling partner(s). Encourage group work.

Families/SOs need support to produce change as much as the person who is addicted.

Assist the patient's partner to become aware that patient's abstinence and drug use are not the partner's responsibility.

Partners need to learn that user's habit may or may not change despite partner's involvement in treatment.

Help the recovering (former user) partner who is enabling to distinguish between destructive aspects of behavior and genuine motivation to aid the user.

Enabling behavior can be partner's attempts at personal survival.

Note how partner relates to the treatment team/staff.

Determines enabling style. A parallel exists between how partner relates to user and to staff, based on partner's feelings about self and situation.

Explore conflicting feelings the enabling partner may have about treatment, e.g., feelings similar to those of abuser (blend of anger, guilt, fear, exhaustion, embarrassment, loneliness, distrust, grief, and possibly relief).

Useful in establishing the need for therapy for the partner. This individual's own identity may have been lost, she or he may fear self-disclosure to staff, and may have difficulty giving up the dependent relationship.

Involve family in discharge referral plans.

Drug abuse is a family illness. Because the family has been so involved in dealing with the substance abuse behavior, family members need help adjusting to the new behavior of sobriety/abstinence. Incidence of recovery is almost doubled when the family is treated along with the patient.

Be aware of staff's enabling behaviors and feelings about patient and enabling partners.

Lack of understanding of enabling can result in nontherapeutic approaches to patients and their families.

Collaborative

Encourage involvement with self-help associations, Alcoholics/Narcotics Anonymous, Al-Anon, Alateen, and professional family therapy.

Puts patient/family in direct contact with support systems necessary for continued sobriety and to assist with problem resolution.

NURSING DIAGNOSIS: Sexual Dysfunction

May be related to

Altered body function: Neurological damage and debilitating effects of drug use (particularly alcohol and opiates)

Possibly evidenced by

Progressive interference with sexual functioning

In men: a significant degree of testicular atrophy is noted (testes are smaller and softer than normal); gynecomastia (breast enlargement); impotence/decreased sperm counts

In women: loss of body hair, thin soft skin, and spider angioma (elevated estrogen); amenorrhea/increase in miscarriages

ACTIONS/INTERVENTIONS

RATIONALE

Sexual Counseling (NIC)

Independent

Ascertain patient's beliefs and expectations. Have patient describe problem in own words.

Determines level of knowledge, identifies misperceptions and specific learning needs.

Encourage and accept individual expressions of concern.

Most people find it difficult to talk about this sensitive subject and may not ask directly for information.

Provide education opportunity (e.g., pamphlets, consultation with appropriate persons) for patient to learn effects of drug on sexual functioning.

Much of denial and hesitancy to seek treatment may be reduced as a result of sufficient and appropriate information.

Provide information about individual's condition.

Sexual functioning may have been affected by drug (alcohol) itself and/or psychological factors (such as stress or depression). Information can assist patient to understand own situation and identify actions to be taken.

Assess drinking/drug history of pregnant patient. Provide information about effects of substance abuse on the reproductive system/fetus (e.g., increased risk of premature birth, brain damage, and fetal malformation).

Awareness of the negative effects of alcohol/other drugs on reproduction may motivate patient to stop using drug(s). When patient is pregnant, identification of potential problems aids in planning for future fetal needs/concerns.

Discuss prognosis for sexual dysfunction, e.g., impotence/low sexual desire.

In about 50% of cases, impotence is reversed with abstinence from drug(s); in 25% the return to normal functioning is delayed; and approximately 25% remain impotent.

Collaborative

Refer for sexual counseling, if indicated.

Couple may need additional assistance to resolve more severe problems/situations. Patient may have difficulty adjusting if drug has improved sexual experience (e.g., heroin decreases dyspareunia in women/premature ejaculation in men). Furthermore, the patient may have engaged enjoyably in bizarre, erotic sexual behavior under influence of the stimulant drug; patient may have found no substitute for the drug, may have driven a partner away, and may have no motivation to adjust to sexual experience without drugs.

Review results of sonogram if pregnant.

Assesses fetal growth and development to identify possibility of fetal alcohol syndrome and future needs.

ACTIONS/INTERVENTIONS	RATIONALE
Learning Facilitation (NIC)	
Independent	
Be aware of and deal with anxiety of patient and family members.	Anxiety can interfere with ability to hear and assimilate information.
Provide an active role for the patient/SO in the learning process, e.g., discussions, group participation, role playing.	Learning is enhanced when persons are actively involved.
Provide written and verbal information as indicated. Include list of articles and books related to patient/family needs and encourage reading and discussing what they learn.	Helps patient/SO make informed choices about future. Bibliotherapy can be a useful addition to other therapeutic approaches.
Assess patient's knowledge of own situation, e.g., disease, complications, and needed changes in lifestyle.	Assists in planning for long-range changes necessary for maintaining sobriety/drug-free status. Patient may have street knowledge of the drug but be ignorant of medical facts.
Pace learning activities to individual needs.	Facilitates learning because information is more readily assimilated when timing is considered.
Teaching: Disease Process (NIC)	
Review condition and prognosis/future expectations.	Provides knowledge base from which patient can make informed choices.
Discuss relationship of drug use to current situation.	Often patient has misperception (denial) of real reason for admission to the medical (psychiatric) setting.
Educate about effects of specific drug(s) used, e.g., PCP is deposited in body fat and may reactivate (flashbacks) even after long interval of abstinence; alcohol use may result in mental deterioration, liver involvement/damage; cocaine can damage postcapillary vessels and increase platelet aggregation, promoting thromboses and infarction of skin/internal organs, causing localized atrophie blanche or sclerodermatous lesions.	Information will help patient understand possible long-term effects of drug use.

ACTIONS/INTERVENTIONS	RATIONALE
Independent	
Discuss potential for re-emergence of withdrawal symptoms in stimulant abuse as early as 3 mo or as late as 9–12 mo after discontinuing use.	Even though intoxication may have passed, patient may manifest denial, drug hunger, and periods of "flare-up," wherein there is a delayed recurrence of withdrawal symptoms (e.g., anxiety; depression; irritability; sleep disturbance; compulsiveness with food, especially sugars).
Inform patient of effects of disulfiram (Antabuse) in combination with alcohol intake and importance of avoiding use of alcohol-containing products, e.g., cough syrups, foods/candy, mouthwash, aftershave, cologne.	Interaction of alcohol and Antabuse results in nausea and hypotension, which may produce fatal shock. Individuals on Antabuse are sensitive to alcohol on a continuum, with some being able to drink while taking the drug and others having a reaction with only slight exposure. Reactions also appear to be dose-related.
Review specific aftercare needs; e.g., PCP user should drink cranberry juice and continue use of ascorbic acid; alcohol abuser with liver damage should refrain from drugs/anesthetics or use of household cleaning products that are detoxified in the liver.	Promotes individualized care related to specific situation. Cranberry juice and ascorbic acid enhance clearance of PCP from the system. Substances that have the potential for liver damage are more dangerous in the presence of an already damaged liver.
Discuss variety of helpful organizations and programs that are available for assistance/referral.	Long-term support is necessary to maintain optimal recovery. Psychosocial needs and other issues may need to be addressed.

POTENTIAL CONSIDERATIONS following acute care (dependent on patient's age, physical condition/presence of complications, personal resources, and life responsibilities)

Therapeutic Regimen: Individual/Families, ineffective management—decisional conflicts, excessive demands made on individual or family, family conflict, perceived seriousness/benefits.

Coping, Individual, ineffective—vulnerability, situational crises, multiple life changes, inadequate relaxation, inadequate/loss of support systems.

Family Coping: potential for growth—needs sufficiently gratified and adaptive tasks effectively addressed to enable goals of self-actualization to surface.

(Physical needs depend on substance effect on organ systems—refer to appropriate medical plans of care for additional considerations.)

CANCER

Cancer is a general term used to describe a disturbance of cellular growth and refers to a group of diseases and not a single disease entity. There are currently more than 150 different known types of cancer. Because cancer is a cellular disease, it can arise from any body tissue, with manifestations that result from failure to control the proliferation and maturation of cells.

There are four main classifications of cancer according to tissue type: (1) lymphomas (cancers originating in infection-fighting organs), (2) leukemias (cancers originating in blood-forming organs), (3) sarcomas (cancers originating in bones, muscle, or connective tissue), and (4) carcinomas (cancers originating in epithelial cells). Within these broad categories, a cancer is classified by histology, stage, and grade.

Through years of observation and documentation, it has been noted that the metastatic behavior of cancers varies according to the primary site of diagnosis. This behavior pattern is known as the "natural history." An example is the metastatic pattern for primary breast cancer: breast-bone-lung-liver-brain. Knowledge of the etiology and natural history of a cancer type is important in planning the patient's care and in evaluating the patient's progress, prognosis, and physical complaints.

CARE SETTING

Cancer centers may focus on staging and major treatment modalities for complex cancers. Treatment for managing adverse effects such as malnutrition and infection may take place in short-stay, ambulatory, or community settings. More cancer patients are receiving care at home because of personal choice and healthcare costs.

RELATED CONCERNS

Fecal diversion: postoperative care of ileostomy and colostomy, page 364
Hysterectomy, page 660
Leukemias, page 558
Lung cancer: surgical intervention, page 154
Lymphomas, page 567
Mastectomy, page 668
Prostatectomy, page 643
Psychosocial aspects of care, page 809
Radical neck surgery—laryngectomy: postoperative care, page 173
Sepsis/Septicemia, page 741
Total nutritional support, page 508
Urinary diversion/Urostomy, page 622

Patient Assessment Database

Depends on organs/tissues involved and stage of disease.

Refer to appropriate plans of care for additional assessment information.

ACTIVITY/REST

May report: Weakness and/or fatigue
Changes in rest pattern and usual hours of sleep per night; presence of factors affecting sleep, e.g., pain, anxiety, night sweats
Limitations of participation in hobbies, exercise, usual activities

CIRCULATION

May report: Palpitations, chest pain on exertion
May exhibit: Changes in BP, fluctuations in heart rate

EGO INTEGRITY

May report: Stress factors (financial, job, role changes) and ways of handling stress (e.g., smoking, drinking, delay in seeking treatment, religious/spiritual belief)
Concern about changes in appearance, e.g., alopecia, disfiguring lesions, surgery, profound weight loss

Denial of diagnosis, feelings of powerlessness, hopelessness, helplessness, worthlessness, guilt, loss of control, depression

May exhibit: Denial, withdrawal, anger

ELIMINATION

May report: Changes in bowel pattern, e.g., blood in stools, pain with defecation, constipation

Changes in urinary elimination, e.g., pain or burning on urination, hematuria, frequent urination

May exhibit: Changes in bowel sounds, abdominal distension, diarrhea, dysuria, frequency, incontinence

FOOD/FLUID

May report: Poor dietary habits (e.g., low-fiber, high-fat, additives, preservatives)

Anorexia, nausea/vomiting; difficulty swallowing, mouth sores

Food intolerances

May exhibit: Changes in weight; severe weight loss, cachexia, wasting of muscle mass

Changes in skin moisture/turgor; edema

NEUROSENSORY

May report: Dizziness; syncope, lack of coordination, unstable balance

Numbness/tingling of extremities; sensation of coldness, difficulty performing fine motor skills (i.e., buttoning shirt)

PAIN/DISCOMFORT

May report: No pain, or varying degrees, e.g., mild discomfort to severe pain (associated with disease process)

RESPIRATION

May report: Smoking (tobacco, marijuana), living with someone who smokes

Asbestos or dust exposure (e.g., coal, sandstone)

History of chronic respiratory disease

SAFETY

May report: Exposure to toxic chemicals, carcinogens (occupation/profession or environment)

Excessive/prolonged sun exposure

May exhibit: Skin rashes, ulcerations; dry, leatherlike skin

SEXUALITY

May report: Sexual concerns, e.g., impact on relationship, change in level of satisfaction, impotence

Nulligravida greater than 30 years of age; multigravida; multiple sex partners, early sexual activity, genital herpes; exposure to HPV (human papilloma virus)

SOCIAL INTERACTION

May report: Inadequate/weak support system

Marital history (regarding in-home satisfaction, support, or help)

Concerns about role function/responsibility

TEACHING/LEARNING

May report: Family history of cancer, e.g., multiple family members/mother, grandmother, aunt or sister with breast cancer

Primary site, date discovered/diagnosed

Metastatic disease: Additional sites involved (if none, natural history of primary will provide important information for looking for metastasis)

Treatment history: Previous treatment for cancer—place and treatments given

Discharge plan considerations: DRG projected mean length of stay: Depends on specific system affected and therapeutic needs.

May require assistance with finances, medications/treatments, wound care/supplies, transportation, food shopping and preparation, self-care, homemaker/maintenance tasks, provision for child care; changes in living facilities/hospice

Refer to section at end of plan for postdischarge considerations.

DIAGNOSTIC STUDIES

Test selection depends on history, clinical manifestations, and index of suspicion for a particular cancer.

Endoscopy: Used for direct visualization of body organs/cavities to detect abnormalities.

Scans (e.g., magnetic resonance imaging [MRI], CT, gallium) and ultrasound: May be done for diagnostic purposes, identification of metastasis, and evaluation of response to treatment.

Biopsy (fine-needle aspiration [FNA], needle core, incisional/excisional): Done to differentiate diagnosis and delineate treatment and may be taken from bone marrow, skin, organ, and so forth. *Example:* Bone marrow is done in myeloproliferative diseases for diagnosis; in solid tumors for staging.

Tumor markers (substances produced and secreted by tumor cells and found in serum, e.g., carcinogenic embryonic antigen [CEA], prostate-specific antigen [PSA], alpha-fetoprotein, human chorionic gonadotropin [HCG], prostatic acid phosphatase, calcitonin, pancreatic oncofetal antigen, CA 15-3, CA 19-9, CA 125, and so on): Helpful in diagnosing cancer but more useful as prognostic indicator and/or therapeutic monitor. For example, estrogen and progesterone receptors are assays done on breast tissue to provide information about whether or not hormonal manipulation would be therapeutic in metastatic disease control. *Note:* Any hormone may be elevated because many cancers secrete inappropriate hormones (ectopic hormone secretion).

Screening chemistry tests, e.g., electrolytes (sodium, potassium, calcium), renal tests (BUN/Cr), liver tests (bilirubin, AST, alkaline phosphatase, LDH), bone tests (calcium): Depend on individual condition, risk factors.

CBC with differential and platelets: May reveal anemia, changes in RBCs and WBCs; reduced or increased platelets.

Chest x-ray: Screens for primary or metastatic disease of lungs.

NURSING PRIORITIES

1. Support adaptation and independence.
2. Promote comfort.
3. Maintain optimal physiological functioning.
4. Prevent complications.
5. Provide information about disease process/condition, prognosis, and treatment needs.

DISCHARGE GOALS

1. Patient is dealing with current situation realistically.
2. Pain alleviated/controlled.
3. Homeostasis achieved.
4. Complications prevented/minimized.
5. Disease process/condition, prognosis, and therapeutic choices and regimen understood.
6. Plan in place to meet needs after discharge.

NURSING DIAGNOSIS: Fear/Anxiety (specify level)

May be related to

Situational crisis (cancer)

Threat to/change in health/socioeconomic status, role functioning, interaction patterns

Threat of death

Separation from family (hospitalization, treatments), interpersonal transmission/contagion of feelings

Possibly evidenced by

Increased tension, shakiness, apprehension, restlessness, insomnia

Expressed concerns regarding changes in life events

Feelings of helplessness, hopelessness, inadequacy

Sympathetic stimulation, somatic complaints

DESIRED OUTCOMES/EVALUATION CRITERIA—PATIENT WILL:

Fear/Anxiety Control (NOC)

Display appropriate range of feelings and lessened fear.
Appear relaxed and report anxiety is reduced to a manageable level.
Demonstrate use of effective coping mechanisms and active participation in treatment regimen.

ACTIONS/INTERVENTIONS	RATIONALE
Anxiety Reduction (NIC)	
Independent	
Review patient's/SO's previous experience with cancer. Determine what the doctor has told patient and what conclusion patient has reached.	Clarifies patient's perceptions; assists in identification of fear(s) and misconceptions based on diagnosis and experience with cancer.
Encourage patient to share thoughts and feelings.	Provides opportunity to examine realistic fears and misconceptions about diagnosis.
Provide open environment in which patient feels safe to discuss feelings or to refrain from talking.	Helps patient feel accepted in present condition without feeling judged and promotes sense of dignity and control.
Maintain frequent contact with patient. Talk with and touch patient as appropriate.	Provides assurance that the patient is not alone or rejected; conveys respect for and acceptance of the person, fostering trust.
Be aware of effects of isolation on patient when required by immunosuppression or radiation implant. Limit use of isolation clothing/masks as possible.	Sensory deprivation may result when sufficient stimulation is not available and may intensify feelings of anxiety/fear and alienation.
Assist patient/SO in recognizing and clarifying fears to begin developing coping strategies for dealing with these fears.	Coping skills are often stressed after diagnosis and during different phases of treatment. Support and counseling are often necessary to enable individual to recognize and deal with fear and to realize that control/coping strategies are available.
Provide accurate, consistent information regarding diagnosis and prognosis. Avoid arguing about patient's perceptions of situation.	Can reduce anxiety and enable patient to make decisions/choices based on realities.
Permit expressions of anger, fear, despair without confrontation. Give information that feelings are normal and are to be appropriately expressed.	Acceptance of feelings allows patient to begin to deal with situation.
Explain the recommended treatment, its purpose, and potential side effects. Help patient prepare for treatments.	The goal of cancer treatment is to destroy malignant cells while minimizing damage to normal ones. Treatment may include surgery (curative, preventive, palliative), as well as chemotherapy, radiation (internal, external), or newer/organ-specific treatments such as whole-body hyperthermia or biotherapy. Bone marrow or peripheral progenitor cell (stem cell) transplant may be recommended for some types of cancer.
Explain procedures, providing opportunity for questions and honest answers. Stay with patient during anxiety-producing procedures and consultations.	Accurate information allows patient to deal more effectively with reality of situation, thereby reducing anxiety and fear of the unknown.

ACTIONS/INTERVENTIONS	RATIONALE

Independent

Provide primary and consistent caregivers whenever possible.	May help reduce anxiety by fostering therapeutic relationship and facilitating continuity of care.
Promote calm, quiet environment.	Facilitates rest, conserves energy, and may enhance coping abilities.
Identify stage/degree of grief patient and SO are currently experiencing. (Refer to ND: Grieving, anticipatory, following.)	Choice of interventions is dictated by stage of grief, coping behaviors, e.g., anger/withdrawal, denial.
Note ineffective coping, e.g., poor social interactions, helplessness, giving up everyday functions and usual sources of gratification.	Identifies individual problems and provides support for patient/SO in using effective coping skills.
Be alert to signs of denial/depression, e.g., withdrawal, anger, inappropriate remarks. Determine presence of suicidal ideation and assess potential on a scale of 1–10.	Patient may use defense mechanism of denial and express hope that diagnosis is inaccurate. Feelings of guilt, spiritual distress, physical symptoms, or lack of cure may cause the patient to become withdrawn and believe that suicide is a viable alternative.
Encourage and foster patient interaction with support systems.	Reduces feelings of isolation. If family support systems are not available, outside sources may be needed immediately, e.g., local cancer support groups.
Provide reliable and consistent information and support for SO.	Allows for better interpersonal interaction and reduction of anxiety and fear.
Include SO as indicated/patient desires when major decisions are to be made.	Provides a support system for the patient and allows the SO to be involved appropriately.

Collaborative

Administer antianxiety medications, e.g., lorazepam (Ativan), alprazolam (Xanax), as indicated.	May be useful for brief periods of time to help patient handle feelings of anxiety related to diagnosis/situation and/or during periods of high stress.
Refer to additional resources for counseling/support as needed.	May be useful from time to time to assist patient/SO in dealing with anxiety.

NURSING DIAGNOSIS: Grieving, anticipatory/Anxiety, death

May be related to
Anticipated loss of physiological well-being (e.g., loss of body part; change in body function); change in lifestyle
Perceived potential death of patient

Possibly evidenced by
Changes in eating habits, alterations in sleep patterns, activity levels, libido, and communication patterns
Denial of potential loss, choked feelings, anger

DESIRED OUTCOMES/EVALUATION CRITERIA—PATIENT WILL:

Grief Resolution (NOC)

Identify and express feelings appropriately.
Continue normal life activities, looking toward/planning for the future, one day at a time.
Verbalize understanding of the dying process and feelings of being supported in grief work.

ACTIONS/INTERVENTIONS	RATIONALE

Grief Work Facilitation (NIC)

Independent

Expect initial shock and disbelief following diagnosis of cancer and/or traumatizing procedures (e.g., disfiguring surgery, colostomy, amputation).

Few patients are fully prepared for the reality of the changes that can occur.

Assess patient/SO for stage of grief currently being experienced. Explain process as appropriate.

Knowledge about the grieving process reinforces the normality of feelings/reactions being experienced and can help patient deal more effectively with them.

Provide open, nonjudgmental environment. Use therapeutic communication skills of Active-Listening, acknowledgment, and so on.

Promotes and encourages realistic dialogue about feelings and concerns.

Encourage verbalization of thoughts/concerns and accept expressions of sadness, anger, rejection. Acknowledge normality of these feelings.

Patient may feel supported in expression of feelings by the understanding that deep and often conflicting emotions are normal and experienced by others in this difficult situation.

Be aware of mood swings, hostility, and other acting-out behavior. Set limits on inappropriate behavior, redirect negative thinking.

Indicators of ineffective coping and need for additional interventions. Preventing destructive actions enables patient to maintain control and sense of self-esteem.

Be aware of debilitating depression. Ask patient direct questions about state of mind.

Studies show that many cancer patients are at high risk for suicide. They are especially vulnerable when recently diagnosed and/or discharged from hospital.

Visit frequently and provide physical contact as appropriate/desired, or provide frequent phone support as appropriate for setting. Arrange for care provider/support person to stay with patient as needed.

Helps reduce feelings of isolation and abandonment.

Reinforce teaching regarding disease process and treatments and provide information as requested/appropriate about dying. Be honest; do not give false hope while providing emotional support.

Patient/SO benefit from factual information. Individuals may ask direct questions about death, and honest answers promote trust and provide reassurance that correct information will be given.

Review past life experiences, role changes, and coping skills. Talk about things that interest the patient.

Opportunity to identify skills that may help individuals cope with grief of current situation more effectively.

Note evidence of conflict; expressions of anger; and statements of despair, guilt, hopelessness, "nothing to live for."

Interpersonal conflicts/angry behavior may be patient's way of expressing/dealing with feelings of despair/spiritual distress and could be indicative of suicidal ideation.

Determine way that patient/SO understand and respond to death, e.g., cultural expectations, learned behaviors, experience with death (close family members/friends), beliefs about life after death, faith in Higher Power (God).

These factors affect how each individual deals with the possibility of death and influences how they may respond and interact.

Be aware of own feelings about cancer, death. Accept whatever methods patient/SO have chosen to help each other through the process.

Caregiver's anxiety and unwillingness to accept reality of possibility of own death may block ability to be helpful to the patient/SO, necessitating enlisting the aid of others to provide needed support.

Hope Instillation (NIC)

Identify positive aspects of the situation.

Possibility of remission and slow progression of disease and/or new therapies can offer hope for the future.

ACTIONS/INTERVENTIONS

Independent

Discuss ways patient/SO can plan together for the future. Encourage setting of realistic goals.

Assist patient/SO to identify strengths in self/situation and support systems.

Encourage participation in care and treatment decisions.

Dying Care (NIC)

Provide open environment for discussion with patient/SO (when appropriate) about desires/plans pertaining to death; e.g., making will, burial arrangements, tissue donation, death benefits, insurance, time for family gatherings, how to spend remaining time.

Collaborative

Grief Work Facilitation (NIC)

Refer to appropriate counselor as needed (e.g., psychiatric clinical nurse specialist, social worker, psychologist, clergyman).

Refer to visiting nurse, home health agency as needed, or hospice program, if appropriate.

RATIONALE

Having a part in problem solving/planning can provide a sense of control over anticipated events.

Recognizing these resources provides opportunity to work through feelings of grief.

Allows patient to retain some control over life.

If the patient/SO are mutually aware of impending death, they may more easily deal with unfinished business or desired activities.

Can help alleviate distress or palliate feelings of grief to facilitate coping and foster growth.

Provides support in meeting physical and emotional needs of patient/SO, and can supplement the care family and friends are able to give.

NURSING DIAGNOSIS: Self-Esteem, situational low

May be related to

Biophysical: disfiguring surgery, chemotherapy or radiotherapy side effects, e.g., loss of hair, nausea/vomiting, weight loss, anorexia, impotence, sterility, overwhelming fatigue, uncontrolled pain

Psychosocial: threat of death; feelings of lack of control and doubt regarding acceptance by others; fear and anxiety

Possibly evidenced by

Verbalization of change in lifestyle; fear of rejection/reaction of others; negative feelings about body; feelings of helplessness, hopelessness, powerlessness

Preoccupation with change or loss

Not taking responsibility for self-care, lack of follow-through

Change in self-perception/other's perception of role

DESIRED OUTCOMES/EVALUATION CRITERIA—PATIENT WILL:

Self-Esteem (NOC)

Verbalize understanding of body changes, acceptance of self in situation.

Begin to develop coping mechanisms to deal effectively with problems.

Demonstrate adaptation to changes/events that have occurred as evidenced by setting of realistic goals and active participation in work/play/personal relationships as appropriate.

ACTIONS/INTERVENTIONS	RATIONALE

Chemotherapy or Radiation Therapy Management (NIC)

Independent

Discuss with patient/SO how the diagnosis and treatment are affecting the patient's personal life/home and work activities.

Aids in defining concerns to begin problem-solving process.

Review anticipated side effects associated with a particular treatment, including possible effects on sexual activity and sense of attractiveness/desirability, e.g., alopecia, disfiguring surgery. Tell patient that not all side effects occur, and others may be minimized/controlled.

Anticipatory guidance can help patient/SO begin the process of adaptation to new state and to prepare for some side effects, e.g., buy a wig before radiation, schedule time off from work as indicated. (Refer to ND: Sexuality Patterns, risk for altered, p. 921.)

Encourage discussion of/problem-solve concerns about effects of cancer/treatments on role as homemaker, wage earner, parent, and so forth.

May help reduce problems that interfere with acceptance of treatment or stimulate progression of disease.

Acknowledge difficulties patient may be experiencing. Give information that counseling is often necessary and important in the adaptation process.

Validates reality of patient's feelings and gives permission to take whatever measures are necessary to cope with what is happening.

Evaluate support structures available to and used by patient/SO.

Helps with planning for care while hospitalized and after discharge.

Provide emotional support for patient/SO during diagnostic tests and treatment phase.

Although some patients adapt/adjust to cancer effects or side effects of therapy, many need additional support during this period.

Use touch during interactions, if acceptable to patient, and maintain eye contact.

Affirmation of individuality and acceptance is important in reducing patient's feelings of insecurity and self-doubt.

Collaborative

Refer patient/SO to supportive group programs (e.g., I Can Cope, Reach to Recovery, Encore).

Group support is usually very beneficial for both patient/SO, providing contact with other patients with cancer at various levels of treatment and/or recovery, validating feelings and assisting with problem solving.

Refer for professional counseling as indicated.

May be necessary to regain and maintain a positive psychosocial structure if patient/SO support systems are deteriorating.

NURSING DIAGNOSIS: Pain [acute]/chronic

May be related to

Disease process (compression/destruction of nerve tissue, infiltration of nerves or their vascular supply, obstruction of a nerve pathway, inflammation)
Side effects of various cancer therapy agents

Possibly evidenced by

Reports of pain
Self-focusing/narrowed focus
Alteration in muscle tone; facial mask of pain
Distraction/guarding behaviors
Autonomic responses, restlessness (acute pain)

ACTIONS/INTERVENTIONS

Pain Management (NIC)

Independent

Determine pain history, e.g., location of pain, frequency, duration, and intensity using numeric rating scale (0–10 scale), or verbal rating scale ("no pain" to "excruciating pain") and relief measures used. Believe patient's report.

Determine timing/precipitants of "breakthrough" pain when using around-the-clock agents, whether oral, IV, or patch medications.

Evaluate/be aware of painful effects of particular therapies, i.e., surgery, radiation, chemotherapy, biotherapy. Provide information to patient/SO about what to expect.

Provide nonpharmacological comfort measures (e.g., massage, repositioning, backrub) and diversional activities (e.g., music, television).

Encourage use of stress management skills/complimentary therapies (e.g., relaxation techniques, visualization, guided imagery, biofeedback, laughter, music, aromatherapy, and Therapeutic Touch).

Provide cutaneous stimulation, e.g., heat/cold, massage.

Be aware of barriers to cancer pain management related to patient, as well as the healthcare system.

RATIONALE

Information provides baseline data to evaluate need for/effectiveness of interventions. Pain of more than 6 mo duration constitutes chronic pain, which may affect therapeutic choices. Recurrent episodes of acute pain can occur within chronic pain, requiring increased level of intervention. *Note:* The pain experience is an individualized one composed of both physical and emotional responses.

Pain may occur near the end of the dose interval, indicating need for higher dose or shorter dose interval. Pain may be precipitated by identifiable triggers, or occur spontaneously, requiring use of short half-life agents for rescue or supplemental doses.

A wide range of discomforts are common (e.g., incisional pain, burning skin, low back pain, headaches), depending on the procedure/agent being used. Pain is also associated with invasive procedures to diagnose/treat cancer.

Promotes relaxation and helps refocus attention.

Enables patient to participate actively in nondrug treatment of pain and enhances sense of control. Pain produces stress and, in conjunction with muscle tension and internal stressors, increases patient's focus on self, which in turn increases the level of pain.

May decrease inflammation, muscle spasms, reducing associated pain. *Note:* Heat may increase bleeding/edema following acute injury, whereas cold may further reduce perfusion to ischemic tissues.

Patients may be reluctant to report pain for reasons such as fear that disease is worse; worry about unmanageable side effects of pain medications; beliefs that pain has meaning, such as "God wills it," they should overcome it, or that pain is merited or deserved for some reason. Healthcare system problems include factors such as inadequate assessment of pain, concern about controlled substances/patient addiction, inadequate reimbursement/cost of treatment modalities.

ACTIONS/INTERVENTIONS

Independent

Evaluate pain relief/control at regular intervals. Adjust medication regimen as necessary.

Inform patient/SO of the expected therapeutic effects and discuss management of side effects.

Discuss use of additional alternative/complementary therapies, e.g., acupuncture/acupressure.

Collaborative

Develop individualized pain management plan with the patient and physician. Provide written copy of plan to patient, family/SO, and care providers.

Administer analgesics as indicated, e.g.:

Opioids, e.g., codeine, morphine (MS Contin), oxycodone (oxycontin) hydrocodone (Vicodin), hydromorphone (Dilaudid), methadone (Dolophine), fentanyl (Duragesic); oxymorphone (Numorphan);

Acetaminophen (Tylenol); and nonsteroidal anti-inflammatory drugs (NSAIDs), including aspirin, ibuprofen (Motrin, Advil); peroxicam (Feldene); indomethacin (Indocin);

Corticosteroids, e.g., dexamethasone (Decadron);

Anticonvulsants, e.g., phenytoin (Dilantin), valproic acid (Depakote), clonazepam (Klonopin);

Tricyclic antidepressants, e.g., amitriptyline (Elavil), imipramine (Tofranil), doxepin (Sinequan), trazodone (Desyrel);

Antihistamines, e.g., hydroxyzine (Atarax, Vistaril);

Samarium-153 lexidronam (Quadramet).

RATIONALE

Goal is maximum pain control with minimum interference with ADLs. *Note:* Opioid tolerance requires ongoing readjustment of dosage and use of combination therapy.

This information helps establish realistic expectations, confidence in own ability to handle what happens.

May provide reduction/relief of pain without drug-related side effects.

An organized plan beginning with the simplest dosage schedules and least invasive modalities improves chance for pain control. Particularly with chronic pain, patient/SO must be active participant in pain management and all care providers need to be consistent.

A wide range of analgesics and associated agents may be employed around the clock to manage pain. *Note:* Addiction to or dependency on drug is not a concern.

Effective for localized and generalized moderate to severe pain, with long-acting/controlled-release forms available. Routes of administration include oral, transmucosal, transdermal, nasal, rectal, and infusions (subcutaneous, IV, intraventricular), which may be delivered via PCA. IM use is not recommended because absorption is not reliable, in addition to being painful and inconvenient. *Note:* Research is in process for oral transmucosal agent (fentenyl citrate [oralet]) to control breakthrough pain in patients using fentanyl patch.

Adjuvant drugs are useful for mild to moderate pain and can be combined with opioids and other modalities.

May be effective in controlling pain associated with inflammatory process (e.g., metastatic bone pain, acute spinal cord compression and neuropathic pain).

Useful for peripheral pain syndromes associated with neuropathic pain, especially shooting pain.

Effective for neuropathic pain (e.g., tingling, burning pain) and pain resulting from surgery, chemotherapy, or nerve infiltration.

Mild anxiolytic agent with sedative and analgesic property. May produce additive analgesia with therapeutic doses of opioids and may be beneficial in limiting opioid-induced nausea/vomiting.

Effective in treating pain resulting from osteoblastic metastatic bone lesions. Drug onset is about 1 wk with duration of 2–4 mo. May help reduce dosage of opioid analgesics. *Note:* Bone marrow/WBC and platelet counts may be suppressed for up to 8 wk after cessation of the drug.

ACTIONS/INTERVENTIONS

Collaborative

Provide/instruct in use of PCA, as appropriate.

Instruct in use of electrical stimulation (e.g., TENS) unit.

Prepare for/assist with procedures, e.g., nerve blocks, cordotomy, commissural myelotomy, radiation therapy.

Refer to structured support group, psychiatric clinical nurse specialist/psychologist, spiritual advisor for counseling as indicated.

RATIONALE

Provides for timely drug administration, preventing fluctuations in intensity of pain, often at lower total dosage than would be given by conventional methods.

Transcutaneous electrical nerve stimulation blocks nerve transmission of pain stimulus, providing reduction/relief of pain without drug-related side effects. Can be used in combination with other modalities.

May be used in severe/intractable pain unresponsive to other measures. *Note:* Radiation is especially useful for bone metastasis and may provide fast onset of pain relief, even with only one treatment.

May be necessary to reduce anxiety and enhance patient's coping skills, decreasing level of pain. *Note:* Hypnosis can heighten awareness and help to focus concentration to decrease perception of pain.

NURSING DIAGNOSIS: Nutrition: altered, less than body requirements

May be related to

Hypermetabolic state associated with cancer

Consequences of chemotherapy, radiation, surgery, e.g., anorexia, gastric irritation, taste distortions, nausea

Emotional distress, fatigue, poorly controlled pain

Possibly evidenced by

Reported inadequate food intake, altered taste sensation, loss of interest in food, perceived/actual inability to ingest food

Body weight 20% or more under ideal for height and frame, decreased subcutaneous fat/muscle mass

Sore, inflamed buccal cavity

Diarrhea and/or constipation, abdominal cramping

DESIRED OUTCOMES/EVALUATION CRITERIA—PATIENT WILL:

Nutritional Status (NOC)

Demonstrate stable weight/progressive weight gain toward goal with normalization of laboratory values and be free of signs of malnutrition.

Knowledge: Diet (NOC)

Verbalize understanding of individual interferences to adequate intake.

Participate in specific interventions to stimulate appetite/increase dietary intake.

ACTIONS/INTERVENTIONS

Nutrition Therapy (NIC)

Independent

Monitor daily food intake; have patient keep food diary as indicated.

RATIONALE

Identifies nutritional strengths/deficiencies.

ACTIONS/INTERVENTIONS	RATIONALE

Independent

Measure height, weight, and tricep skinfold thickness (or other anthropometric measurements as appropriate). Ascertain amount of recent weight loss. Weigh daily or as indicated.

If these measurements fall below minimum standards, patient's chief source of stored energy (fat tissue) is depleted.

Assess skin/mucous membranes for pallor, delayed wound healing, enlarged parotid glands.

Helps in identification of protein-calorie malnutrition, especially when weight and anthropometric measurements are less than normal.

Encourage patient to eat high-calorie, nutrient-rich diet, with adequate fluid intake. Encourage use of supplements and frequent/smaller meals spaced throughout the day.

Metabolic tissue needs are increased as well as fluids (to eliminate waste products). Supplements can play an important role in maintaining adequate caloric and protein intake.

Create pleasant dining atmosphere; encourage patient to share meals with family/friends.

Makes mealtime more enjoyable, which may enhance intake.

Encourage open communication regarding anorexia.

Often a source of emotional distress, especially for SO who wants to feed patient frequently. When patient refuses, SO may feel rejected/frustrated.

Chemotherapy Management (NIC)

Adjust diet before and immediately after treatment, e.g., clear, cool liquids, light/bland foods, candied ginger, dry crackers, toast, carbonated drinks. Give liquids 1 hr before or 1 hr after meals.

The effectiveness of diet adjustment is very individualized in relief of posttherapy nausea. Patients must experiment to find best solution/combination. Avoiding fluids during meals minimizes becoming "full" too quickly.

Control environmental factors (e.g., strong/noxious odors or noise). Avoid overly sweet, fatty, or spicy foods.

Can trigger nausea/vomiting response.

Encourage use of relaxation techniques, visualization, guided imagery, moderate exercise before meals.

May prevent onset or reduce severity of nausea, decrease anorexia, and enable patient to increase oral intake.

Identify the patient who experiences anticipatory nausea/vomiting and take appropriate measures.

Psychogenic nausea/vomiting occurring before chemotherapy generally does not respond to antiemetic drugs. Change of treatment environment or patient routine on treatment day may be effective.

Administer antiemetic on a regular schedule before/during and after administration of antineoplastic agent as appropriate.

Nausea/vomiting are frequently the most disabling and psychologically stressful side effects of chemotherapy.

Evaluate effectiveness of antiemetic.

Individuals respond differently to all medications. First-line antiemetics may not work, requiring alteration in or use of combination drug therapy.

Hematest stools, gastric secretions.

Certain therapies (e.g., antimetabolites) inhibit renewal of epithelial cells lining the GI tract, which may cause changes ranging from mild erythema to severe ulceration with bleeding.

Collaborative

Review laboratory studies as indicated, e.g., total lymphocyte count, serum transferrin, and albumin/prealbumin.

Helps identify the degree of biochemical imbalance/malnutrition and influences choice of dietary interventions. *Note:* Anticancer treatments can also alter nutrition studies, so all results must be correlated with the patient's clinical status.

ACTIONS/INTERVENTIONS	RATIONALE

Collaborative

Administer medications as indicated:

5-HT$_3$ receptor antagonists, e.g., ondansetron (Zofran), granisetron (Kytril); phenothiazines, e.g., prochlorperazine (Compazine), thiethylperazine (Torecan); antidopaminergics, e.g., metoclopramide (Reglan); antihistamines, e.g., diphenhydramine (Benadryl);

Most antiemetics act to interfere with stimulation of true vomiting center, and chemoreceptor trigger zone agents also act peripherally to inhibit reverse peristalsis. These medications are often prescribed routinely during chemotherapy to prevent nausea and vomiting.

Corticosteroids, e.g., dexamethasone (Decadron); cannabinoids, e.g., 9-tetrahydrocannabinol (dronabinol, [Marinol]); benzodiazepines, e.g., diazepam (Valium);

Combination therapy (e.g., Torecan with Decadron or Valium) is often more effective than single agents. *Note:* Recent studies report that the legal agent Marinol did not provide the same level of relief from nausea and vomiting as did medicinal marijuana. However, because of legal implications and availability of legal medications, medicinal use of marijuana continues to be widely restricted.

Vitamins, especially A, D, E, and B$_6$;

Prevents deficit related to decreased absorption of fat-soluble vitamins. Deficiency of B$_6$ can contribute to/exacerbate depression, irritability.

Antacids.

Minimizes gastric irritation and reduces risk of mucosal ulceration.

Nutrition Therapy (NIC)

Refer to dietitian/nutritional support team.

Provides for specific dietary plan to meet individual needs and reduce problems associated with protein/calorie malnutrition and micronutrient deficiencies.

Insert/maintain NG or feeding tube for enteric feedings, or central line for total parenteral nutrition (TPN) if indicated.

In the presence of severe malnutrition (e.g., loss of 25%–30% body weight in 2 mo) or if patient has been NPO for 5 days and is unlikely to be able to eat for another week, tube feeding or TPN may be necessary to meet nutritional needs. *Note:* TPN is used with caution because it is associated with a more than fourfold increase in the risk of significant infection.

NURSING DIAGNOSIS: Fluid Volume, risk for deficit

Risk factors may include
Excessive losses through normal routes (e.g., vomiting, diarrhea) and/or abnormal routes (e.g., indwelling tubes, wounds)
Hypermetabolic state
Impaired intake of fluids

Possibly evidenced by
[Not applicable; presence of signs and symptoms establishes an *actual* diagnosis]

DESIRED OUTCOMES/EVALUATION CRITERIA—PATIENT WILL:

Hydration (NOC)

Display adequate fluid balance as evidenced by stable vital signs, moist mucous membranes, good skin turgor, prompt capillary refill, and individually adequate urinary output.

ACTIONS/INTERVENTIONS	RATIONALE

Fluid/Electrolyte Management (NIC)

Independent

Monitor I&O and specific gravity; include all output sources, e.g., emesis, diarrhea, draining wounds. Calculate 24-hr balance.

Continued negative fluid balance, decreasing renal output and concentration of urine suggest developing dehydration and need for increased fluid replacement.

Weigh as indicated.

Sensitive measurement of fluctuations in fluid balance.

Monitor vital signs. Evaluate peripheral pulses, capillary refill.

Reflects adequacy of circulating volume.

Assess skin turgor and moisture of mucous membranes. Note reports of thirst.

Indirect indicators of hydration status/degree of deficit.

Encourage increased fluid intake to 3000 mL/day as individually appropriate/tolerated.

Assists in maintenance of fluid requirements and reduces risk of harmful side effects, e.g., hemorrhagic cystitis in patient receiving cyclophosphamide (Cytoxan).

Observe for bleeding tendencies, e.g., oozing from mucous membranes, puncture sites; presence of ecchymosis or petechiae.

Early identification of problems (which may occur as a result of cancer and/or therapies) allows for prompt intervention.

Minimize venipunctures (e.g., combine IV starts with blood draws). Encourage patient to consider central venous catheter placement.

Reduces potential for hemorrhage and infection associated with repeated venous puncture.

Avoid trauma and apply pressure to puncture sites.

Reduces potential for bleeding/hematoma formation.

Collaborative

Provide IV fluids as indicated.

Given for general hydration and to dilute antineoplastic drugs and reduce adverse side effects, e.g., nausea/vomiting, or nephrotoxicity.

Administer antiemetic therapy. (Refer to ND: Nutrition: altered, less than body requirements, p. 910.)

Alleviation of nausea/vomiting decreases gastric losses and allows for increased oral intake.

Monitor laboratory studies, e.g., CBC, electrolytes, serum albumin.

Provides information about level of hydration and corresponding deficits. *Note:* Malnutrition and effects of decreased albumin levels potentiates fluid shifts/edema formation.

Administer transfusions as indicated, e.g.:

RBCs;

May be needed to restore blood count and prevent manifestations of anemia often present in cancer patients, e.g., tachycardia, tachypnea, dizziness, and weakness.

Platelets.

Thrombocytopenia (which may occur as a side effect of chemotherapy, radiation, or cancer process) increases the risk of bleeding from mucous membranes and other body sites. Spontaneous bleeding may occur with platelet count of 5000.

Avoid use of aspirin, gastric irritants, platelet inhibitors or herbs, such as gensing, green tea, garlic, ginger, ginko, or willow bark.

Negatively affect clotting mechanism and/or potentiate risk of bleeding.

NURSING DIAGNOSIS: Fatigue

May be related to

Decreased metabolic energy production, increased energy requirements (hypermetabolic state and effects of treatment)

Overwhelming psychological/emotional demands

Altered body chemistry: side effects of pain and other medications, chemotherapy

Possibly evidenced by

Unremitting/overwhelming lack of energy, inability to maintain usual routines, decreased performance, impaired ability to concentrate, lethargy/listlessness

Disinterest in surroundings

DESIRED OUTCOMES/EVALUATION CRITERIA—PATIENT WILL:

Endurance (NOC)

Report improved sense of energy.

Perform ADLs and participate in desired activities at level of ability.

ACTIONS/INTERVENTIONS

Energy Management (NIC)

Independent

Have patient rate fatigue, using a numeric scale, if possible, and the time of day when it is most severe.

Plan care to allow for rest periods. Schedule activities for periods when patient has most energy. Involve patient/SO in schedule planning.

Establish realistic activity goals with patient.

Assist with self-care needs when indicated; keep bed in low position, pathways clear of furniture; assist with ambulation.

Encourage patient to do whatever possible, e.g., self-bathing, sitting up in chair, walking. Increase activity level as individual is able.

Monitor physiological response to activity, e.g., changes in BP or heart/respiratory rate.

Perform pain assessment and provide pain management.

Encourage nutritional intake. (Refer to ND: Nutrition: altered, less than body requirements, p. 910.)

Collaborative

Provide supplemental oxygen as indicated.

Refer to physical/occupational therapy.

RATIONALE

Helps in developing a plan for managing fatigue.

Frequent rest periods and/or naps are needed to restore/conserve energy. Planning will allow patient to be active during times when energy level is higher, which may restore a feeling of well-being and a sense of control.

Provides for a sense of control and feelings of accomplishment.

Weakness may make ADLs difficult to complete or place the patient at risk for injury during activities.

Enhances strength/stamina and enables patient to become more active without undue fatigue.

Tolerance varies greatly depending on the stage of the disease process, nutrition state, fluid balance, and reaction to therapeutic regimen.

Poorly managed cancer pain can contribute to fatigue.

Adequate intake/use of nutrients is necessary to meet energy needs and build energy reserves for activity.

Presence of anemia/hypoxemia reduces O_2 available for cellular uptake and contributes to fatigue.

Programmed daily exercises and activities help patient maintain/increase strength and muscle tone, enhance sense of well-being. Use of adaptive devices may help conserve energy.

NURSING DIAGNOSIS: Infection, risk for

Risk factors may include
Inadequate secondary defenses and immunosuppression, e.g., bone marrow suppression (dose-limiting side effect of both chemotherapy and radiation)
Malnutrition, chronic disease process
Invasive procedures

Possibly evidenced by
[Not applicable; presence of signs and symptoms establishes an *actual* diagnosis]

DESIRED OUTCOMES/EVALUATION CRITERIA—PATIENT WILL:

Infection Status (NOC)

Remain afebrile and achieve timely healing as appropriate.

Knowledge: Infection Control (NOC)

Identify and participate in interventions to prevent/reduce risk of infection.

ACTIONS/INTERVENTIONS	RATIONALE
Infection Protection (NIC)	
Independent	
Promote good handwashing procedures by staff and visitors. Screen/limit visitors who may have infections. Place in reverse isolation as indicated.	Protects patient from sources of infection, such as visitors and staff who may have an upper respiratory infection (URI).
Emphasize personal hygiene.	Limits potential sources of infection and/or secondary overgrowth.
Monitor temperature.	Temperature elevation may occur (if not masked by corticosteroids or anti-inflammatory drugs) because of various factors, e.g., chemotherapy side effects, disease process, or infection. Early identification of infectious process enables appropriate therapy to be started promptly.
Assess all systems (e.g., skin, respiratory, genitourinary) for signs/symptoms of infection on a continual basis.	Early recognition and intervention may prevent progression to more serious situation/sepsis.
Reposition frequently; keep linens dry and wrinkle-free.	Reduces pressure and irritation to tissues and may prevent skin breakdown (potential site for bacterial growth).
Promote adequate rest/exercise periods.	Limits fatigue, yet encourages sufficient movement to prevent stasis complications, e.g., pneumonia, decubitus, and thrombus formation.
Stress importance of good oral hygiene.	Development of stomatitis increases risk of infection/secondary overgrowth.
Avoid/limit invasive procedures. Adhere to aseptic techniques.	Reduces risk of contamination, limits portal of entry for infectious agents.

915

ACTIONS/INTERVENTIONS

Collaborative

Monitor CBC with differential WBC and granulocyte count, and platelets as indicated.

Obtain cultures as indicated.

Administer antibiotics as indicated.

RATIONALE

Bone marrow activity may be inhibited by effects of chemotherapy, the disease state, or radiation therapy. Monitoring status of myelosuppression is important for preventing further complications (e.g., infection, anemia, or hemorrhage) and scheduling drug delivery. *Note:* The nadir (point of lowest drop in blood count) is usually seen 7–10 days after administration of chemotherapy.

Identifies causative organism(s) and appropriate therapy.

May be used to treat identified infection or given prophylactically in immunocompromised patient.

NURSING DIAGNOSIS: Oral Mucous Membrane, risk for altered

Risk factors may include
Side effect of some chemotherapeutic agents (e.g., antimetabolites) and radiation
Dehydration, malnutrition, NPO restrictions for more than 24 hr

Possibly evidenced by
[Not applicable; presence of signs and symptoms establishes an *actual* diagnosis]

DESIRED OUTCOMES/EVALUATION CRITERIA—PATIENT WILL:

Oral Health (NOC)

Display intact mucous membranes, which are pink, moist, and free of inflammation/ulcerations.

Self-Care Oral Hygiene (NOC)

Verbalize understanding of causative factors.
Demonstrate techniques to maintain/restore integrity of oral mucosa.

ACTIONS/INTERVENTIONS

Oral Health Maintenance (NIC)

Independent

Assess dental health and oral hygiene periodically.

Encourage patient to assess oral cavity daily, noting changes in mucous membrane integrity (e.g., dry, reddened). Note reports of burning in the mouth, changes in voice quality, ability to swallow, sense of taste, development of thick/viscous saliva, blood-tinged emesis.

RATIONALE

Identifies prophylactic treatment needs before initiation of chemotherapy or radiation and provides baseline data of current oral hygiene for future comparison.

Inflammation of the oral mucosa (stomatitis) generally occurs 7–14 days after treatment begins, but signs may be seen as early as day 3 or 4, especially if there were any preexisting oral problems. The range of response extends from mild erythema to severe ulceration, and may extend the length of the GI tract (mucositis), which can be very painful, inhibit oral intake, and is potentially life-threatening. Early identification enables prompt treatment.

ACTIONS/INTERVENTIONS
Independent

Discuss with patient areas needing improvement and demonstrate methods for good oral care.

Initiate/recommend oral hygiene program to include:

Avoidance of commercial mouthwashes, lemon/glycerine swabs;

Use of mouthwash made from warm saline, dilute solution of hydrogen peroxide or baking soda and water;

Brush with soft toothbrush or foam swab;

Floss gently or use WaterPik cautiously;

Keep lips moist with lip gloss or balm, K-Y Jelly, Chapstick;

Encourage use of mints/hard candy or artificial saliva (Ora-Lube, Salivart) as indicated.

Instruct regarding dietary changes: e.g., avoid hot or spicy foods, acidic juices; suggest use of straw; ingest soft or blenderized foods, Popsicles, and ice cream as tolerated.

Encourage fluid intake as individually tolerated.

Discuss limitation of smoking and alcohol intake.

Monitor for and explain to patient signs of oral super-infection (e.g., thrush).

Collaborative

Refer to dentist before initiating chemotherapy or head/neck radiation.

Culture suspicious oral lesions.

Administer medications as indicated, e.g.:

Analgesic rinses (e.g., mixture of Koatin, pectin, diphenhydramine [Benadryl], and topical lidocaine [Xylocaine]);

Antifungal mouthwash preparation, e.g., nystatin (Mycostatin), and antibacterial Biotane;

Antinausea agents;

Opioid analgesics: e.g., hydromoph (Dilaudid), morphine.

RATIONALE

Good care is critical during treatment to control stomatitis complications.

Products containing alcohol or phenol may exacerbate mucous membrane dryness/irritation.

May be soothing to the membranes. Rinsing before meals may improve the patient's sense of taste. Rinsing after meals and at bedtime dilutes oral acids and relieves xerostomia.

Prevents trauma to delicate/fragile tissues. *Note:* Toothbrush should be changed at least every 3 mo.

Removes food particles that can promote bacterial growth. *Note:* Water under pressure has the potential to injure gums/force bacteria under gum line.

Promotes comfort and prevents drying/cracking of tissues.

Stimulates secretions/provides moisture to maintain integrity of mucous membranes, especially in presence of dehydration/reduced saliva production.

Severe stomatitis may interfere with nutritional and fluid intake leading to negative nitrogen balance or dehydration. Dietary modifications may make foods easier to swallow and may feel soothing.

Adequate hydration helps keep mucous membranes moist, preventing drying/cracking.

May cause further irritation and dryness of mucous membranes. *Note:* May need to compromise if these activities are important to patient's emotional status.

Early recognition provides opportunity for prompt treatment.

Prophylactic examination and repair work before therapy reduce risk of infection.

Identifies organism(s) responsible for oral infections and suggests appropriate drug therapy.

Aggressive analgesia program may be required to relieve intense pain. *Note:* Rinse should be used as a swish-and-spit rather than a gargle, which could anesthetize patient's gag reflex.

May be needed to treat/prevent secondary oral infections, such as *Candida, Pseudomonas, herpes simplex.*

When given before beginning mouth care regimen, may prevent nausea associated with oral stimulation.

May be required for acute episodes of moderate to severe oral pain.

ACTIONS/INTERVENTIONS	RATIONALE

Chemotherapy/Radiation Therapy Management (NIC)

Independent

Assess skin frequently for side effects of cancer therapy; note breakdown/delayed wound healing. Emphasize importance of reporting open areas to caregiver.	A reddening and/or tanning effect (radiation reaction) may develop within the field of radiation. Dry desquamation (dryness and pruritus), moist desquamation (blistering), ulceration, hair loss, loss of dermis and sweat glands may also be noted. In addition, skin reactions (e.g., allergic rashes, hyperpigmentation, pruritus, and alopecia) may occur with some chemotherapy agents.
Bathe with lukewarm water and mild soap.	Maintains cleanliness without irritating the skin.
Encourage patient to avoid vigorous rubbing and scratching and to pat skin dry instead of rubbing.	Helps prevent skin friction/trauma to sensitive tissues.
Turn/reposition frequently.	Promotes circulation and prevents undue pressure on skin/tissues.
Review skin care protocol for patient receiving radiation therapy:	Designed to minimize trauma to area of radiation therapy.
Avoid rubbing or use of soap, lotions, creams, ointments, powders or deodorants on area; avoid applying heat or attempting to wash off marks/tattoos placed on skin to identify area of irradiation;	Can potentiate or otherwise interfere with radiation delivery. May actually increase irritation/reaction.
Recommend wearing soft, loose cotton clothing; have female patient avoid wearing bra if it creates pressure;	Skin is very sensitive during and after treatment, and all irritation should be avoided to prevent dermal injury.
Apply cornstarch, Aquaphor, Lubriderm, Eucerin (or other recommended water-soluble moisturizing gel) to area twice daily as needed;	Helps control dampness or pruritus. Maintenance care is required until skin/tissues have regenerated and are back to normal.
Encourage liberal use of sunscreen/block and breathable, protective clothing.	Protects skin from ultraviolet rays and reduces risk of recall reactions.

ACTIONS/INTERVENTIONS	RATIONALE
Independent	

Review skin care protocol for patient receiving chemotherapy, e.g.:

Use appropriate peripheral or central venous catheter, dilute anticancer drug per protocol and ascertain that IV is infusing well;

> Reduces risk of tissue irritation/extravasation of agent into tissues.

Instruct patient to notify caregiver promptly of discomfort at IV insertion site;

> Development of irritation indicates need for alteration of rate/dilution of chemotherapy and/or change of IV site to prevent more serious reaction.

Assess skin/IV site and vein for erythema, edema, tenderness; weltlike patches, itching/burning; or swelling, burning, soreness; blisters progressing to ulceration/tissue necrosis.

> Presence of phlebitis, vein flare (localized reaction) or extravasation requires immediate discontinuation of antineoplastic agent and medical intervention.

Wash skin immediately with soap and water if antineoplastic agents are spilled on unprotected skin (patient or caregiver).

> Dilutes drug to reduce risk of skin irritation/chemical burn.

Advise patients receiving 5-fluorouracil (5-FU) and methotrexate to avoid sun exposure. Withhold methotrexate if sunburn present.

> Sun can cause exacerbation of burn spotting (a side effect of 5-fluorouracil) or can cause a red "flash" area with methotrexate, which can exacerbate drug's effect.

Review expected dermatologic side effects seen with chemotherapy, e.g., rash, hyperpigmentation, and peeling of skin on palms.

> Anticipatory guidance helps decrease concern if side effects do occur.

Inform patient that if alopecia occurs, hair could grow back after completion of chemotherapy, but may/may not grow back after radiation therapy.

> Anticipatory guidance may help adjustment to/preparation for baldness. Men are often as sensitive to hair loss as women. Radiation's effect on hair follicles may be permanent, depending on rad dosage.

Collaborative

Administer appropriate antidote if extravasation of IV should occur, e.g.:

> Reduces local tissue damage.

Dimethyl sulfoxide (DMSO);

> Some studies suggest benefit with topical DMSO for mitomycin and doxorubicin (Adriamycin). *Note:* Injection of diphenhydramine (Benadryl) may relieve symptoms of vein flare.

Hyaluronidase (Wydase);

> Injected subcutaneously for vincristine (Oncovin), vinblastine (Velban), etoposide (VP16), vindesine (Eldisine), vinorelbine (Navelbine), teniposide (Vm26), and paclitaxel (Taxol) infiltration.

Thiosulfate.

> Injected subcutaneously for nitrogen mustard and large amounts (greater than 20 cc) of concentrated cisplatin.

Apply ice pack/warm compresses per protocol.

> Controversial intervention depends on type of agent used. Ice restricts blood flow, keeping drug localized, while heat enhances dispersion of neoplastic drug/antidote, minimizing tissue damage.

ACTIONS/INTERVENTIONS	RATIONALE
Bowel Management (NIC)	
Independent	
Ascertain usual elimination habits.	Data required as baseline for future evaluation of therapeutic needs/effectiveness.
Assess bowel sounds and monitor/record bowel movements (BMs) including frequency, consistency (particularly during first 3–5 days of Vinca alkaloid therapy).	Defines problem, i.e., diarrhea, constipation. *Note:* Constipation is one of the earliest manifestations of neurotoxicity.
Monitor I&O and weight.	Dehydration, weight loss, and electrolyte imbalance are complications of diarrhea. Inadequate fluid intake may potentiate constipation.
Encourage adequate fluid intake (e.g., 2000 mL/24 hr), increased fiber in diet; regular exercise.	May reduce potential for constipation by improving stool consistency and stimulating peristalsis; can prevent dehydration associated with diarrhea.
Provide small, frequent meals of foods low in residue (if not contraindicated), maintaining needed protein and carbohydrates (e.g., eggs., cooked cereal, bland cooked vegetables).	Reduces gastric irritation. Use of low-fiber foods can decrease irritability and provide bowel rest when diarrhea present.
Adjust diet as appropriate: avoid foods high in fat (e.g., butter, fried foods, nuts); foods with high-fiber content; those known to cause diarrhea or gas (e.g., cabbage, baked beans, chili); food/fluids high in caffeine; or extremely hot or cold food/fluids.	GI stimulants that may increase gastric motility/frequency of stools.
Check for impaction if patient has not had BM in 3 days or if abdominal distension, cramping, headache are present.	Further interventions/alternative bowel care may be needed.
Collaborative	
Monitor laboratory studies as indicated, e.g., electrolytes.	Electrolyte imbalances may be the result of/contribute to altered GI function.
Administer IV fluids;	Prevents dehydration, dilutes chemotherapy agents to diminish side effects.
Antidiarrheal agents;	May be indicated to control severe diarrhea.

ACTIONS/INTERVENTIONS

Collaborative

Stool softeners, laxatives, enemas as indicated.

RATIONALE

Prophylactic use may prevent further complications in some patients (e.g., those who will receive Vinca alkaloid, have poor bowel pattern before treatment, or have decreased motility).

NURSING DIAGNOSIS: Sexuality Patterns, risk for altered

Risk factors may include
Knowledge/skill deficit about alternative responses to health-related transitions, altered body function/structure, illness, and medical treatment
Overwhelming fatigue
Fear and anxiety
Lack of privacy/SO

Possibly evidenced by
[Not applicable; presence of signs and symptoms establishes an *actual* diagnosis]

DESIRED OUTCOMES/EVALUATION CRITERIA—PATIENT WILL:

Role Performance (NOC)

Verbalize understanding of effects of cancer and therapeutic regimen on sexuality and measures to correct/deal with problems.
Maintain sexual activity at a desired level as possible.

ACTIONS/INTERVENTIONS

Sexual Counseling (NIC)

Independent

Discuss with patient/SO the nature of sexuality and reactions when it is altered or threatened. Provide information about normality of these problems and that many people find it helpful to seek assistance with adaptation process.

Advise patient of side effects of prescribed cancer treatment that are known to affect sexuality.

Provide private time for hospitalized patient. Knock on door and receive permission from patient/SO before entering.

Collaborative

Refer to sex therapist as indicated.

RATIONALE

Acknowledges legitimacy of the problem. Sexuality encompasses the way men and women view themselves as individuals and how they relate between and among themselves in every area of life.

Anticipatory guidance can help patient and SO begin the process of adaptation to new state.

Sexual needs do not end because the patient is hospitalized. Intimacy needs continue and an open and accepting attitude for the expression of those needs is essential.

May require additional assistance in dealing with situation.

ACTIONS/INTERVENTIONS

Family Process Maintenance (NIC)

Independent

Note components of family, presence of extended family and others, e.g., friends/neighbors.

Identify patterns of communication in family and patterns of interaction between family members.

Assess role expectations of family members and encourage discussion about them.

Assess energy direction, e.g., are efforts at resolution/problem solving purposeful or scattered?

Note cultural/religious beliefs.

Listen for expressions of helplessness.

Deal with family members in a warm, caring, respectful way. Provide information (verbal/written), and reinforce as necessary.

Encourage appropriate expressions of anger without reacting negatively to them.

Acknowledge difficulties of the situation, e.g., diagnosis and treatment of cancer, possibility of death.

Identify and encourage use of previous successful coping behaviors.

RATIONALE

Helps patient and caregiver know who is available to assist with care/provide respite and support.

Provides information about effectiveness of communication and identifies problems that may interfere with family's ability to assist patient and adjust positively to diagnosis/treatment of cancer.

Each person may see the situation in own individual manner, and clear identification and sharing of these expectations promote understanding.

Provides clues about interventions that may be appropriate to assist patient and family in directing energies in a more effective manner.

Affects patient/SO reaction and adjustment to diagnosis, treatment, and outcome of cancer.

Helpless feelings may contribute to difficulty adjusting to diagnosis of cancer and cooperating with treatment regimen.

Provides feelings of empathy and promotes individual's sense of worth and competence in ability to handle current situation.

Feelings of anger are to be expected when individuals are dealing with the difficult/potentially fatal illness of cancer. Appropriate expression enables progress toward resolution of the stages of the grieving process.

Communicates acceptance of the reality the patient/family are facing.

Most people have developed effective coping skills that can be useful in dealing with current situation.

ACTIONS/INTERVENTIONS

Independent

Stress importance of continuous open dialogue between family members.

Collaborative

Refer to support groups, clergy, family therapy as indicated.

RATIONALE

Promotes understanding and assists family members to maintain clear communication and resolve problems effectively.

May need additional assistance to resolve problems of disorganization that may accompany diagnosis of potentially terminal illness (cancer).

NURSING DIAGNOSIS: Knowledge Deficit [Learning Need] regarding illness, prognosis, treatment, self care, and discharge needs

May be related to
Lack of exposure/recall; information misinterpretation, myths
Unfamiliarity with information resources
Cognitive limitation

Possibly evidenced by
Questions/request for information, verbalization of problem
Statement of misconception
Inaccurate follow-through of instructions/development of preventable complications

DESIRED OUTCOMES/EVALUATION CRITERIA—PATIENT WILL:

Knowledge: Disease Process (NOC)

Verbalize accurate information about diagnosis, prognosis, and potential complications at own level of readiness.

Knowledge: Treatment Regimen (NOC)

Verbalize understanding of therapeutic needs.
Correctly perform necessary procedures and explain reasons for the actions.
Initiate necessary lifestyle changes and participate in treatment regimen.
Identify/use available resources appropriately.

ACTIONS/INTERVENTIONS

Teaching: Disease Process (NIC)

Independent

Review with patient/SO understanding of specific diagnosis, treatment alternatives, and future expectations.

Determine patient's perception of cancer and cancer treatment(s); ask about patient's own/previous experience or experience with other people who have (or had) cancer.

Provide clear, accurate information in a factual but sensitive manner. Answer questions specifically, but do not bombard with unessential details.

RATIONALE

Validates current level of understanding, identifies learning needs, and provides knowledge base from which patient can make informed decisions.

Aids in identification of ideas, attitudes, fears, misconceptions, and gaps in knowledge about cancer.

Helps with adjustment to the diagnosis of cancer by providing needed information along with time to absorb it. *Note:* Rate and method of giving information may need to be altered to decrease patient's anxiety and enhance ability to assimilate information.

ACTIONS/INTERVENTIONS	RATIONALE

Independent

Provide anticipatory guidance with patient/SO regarding treatment protocol, length of therapy, expected results, possible side effects. Be honest with patient.	Patient has the "right to know" (be informed) and participate in decision tree. Accurate and concise information helps to dispel fears and anxiety, helps clarify the expected routine, and enables patient to maintain some degree of control.
Ask patient for verbal feedback, and correct misconception about individual's type of cancer and treatment.	Misconceptions about cancer may be more disturbing than facts and can interfere with treatments/delay healing.
Outline normally expected limitations (if any) on ADLs (e.g., difficulty cooking meals when nauseated/fatigued, limit sun exposure, alcohol intake; loss of work time because of effects of treatments).	Enables patient/SO to begin to put limitations into perspective and plan/adapt as indicated.
Provide written materials about cancer, treatment, and available support systems.	Anxiety and preoccupation with thoughts about life and death often interfere with patient's ability to assimilate adequate information. Written, take-home materials provide reinforcement and clarification about information as patient needs it.
Review specific medication regimen and use of OTC drugs.	Enhances ability to manage self-care and avoid potential complications, drug reactions/interactions.
Address specific home care needs, e.g., ability to live alone, perform necessary treatments/procedures, and acquire supplies.	Provides information regarding changes that may be needed in current plan of care to meet therapeutic needs.
Do predischarge home evaluation as indicated.	Aids in transition to home setting by providing information about needed changes in physical layout, acquisition of needed supplies.
Refer to community resources as indicated: e.g., social services, home health agencies, Meals-on-Wheels, local American Cancer Society chapter, respite care, hospice center/services.	Promotes competent self-care and optimal independence. Maintains patient in desired/home setting.
Review with patient/SO the importance of maintaining optimal nutritional status.	Promotes well-being, facilitates recovery, and is critical in enabling the patient to tolerate treatments.
Encourage diet variations and experimentation in meal planning and food preparation, e.g., cooking with sweet juices, wine; serving foods cold or at room temperature as appropriate (ice cream, egg salad).	Creativity may enhance flavor and intake, especially when protein foods taste bitter.
Recommend cookbooks that are designed for cancer patients.	Helps provide specific menu/recipe ideas.
Recommend increased fluid intake and fiber in diet, as well as routine exercise.	Improves consistency of stool and stimulates peristalsis.
Instruct patient to assess oral mucous membranes routinely, noting erythema, ulceration.	Early recognition of problems promotes early intervention, minimizing complications that may impair oral intake and provide avenue for systemic infection.
Advise patient concerning skin and hair care: e.g., avoid harsh shampoos, hair dyes, permanents, salt water, chlorinated water; avoid exposure to strong wind and extreme heat or cold; avoid sun exposure to target area for 1 yr after end of radiation treatments; and regularly apply sunblock (SPF 15 or greater).	Prevents additional hair damage and skin irritation; may prevent recall reactions.

ACTIONS/INTERVENTIONS

Independent

Review signs/symptoms requiring medical evaluation, e.g., infection, delayed healing, drug reactions, increased pain (depending on individual situation).

Stress importance of continuing medical follow-up.

Encourage periodic review of advance directives. Promote inclusion of family/SO in decision-making process.

RATIONALE

Early identification and treatment may limit severity of complications.

Provides ongoing monitoring of progression/resolution of disease process and opportunity for timely diagnosis and treatment of complications. *Note:* Some complications can develop long after therapy is completed, e.g., pathological fractures, radiation cystitis/nephritis.

Patient/family/SO need to re-evaluate choices as condition changes (for better/worse) and treatment options become available or are exhausted.

POTENTIAL CONSIDERATIONS following acute hospitalization (dependent on patient's age, physical condition/presence of complications, personal resources, and life responsibilities)

In addition to Potential Considerations in specific plans of care (e.g., leukemia, mastectomy):
Coping, Individual, impaired—situational crises, vulnerability.
Self-Care deficit/Home Maintenance Management, impaired—decreased strength/endurance, pain/discomfort, depression, insufficient finances, unfamiliarity with neighborhood resources, inadequate support systems.
Caregiver Role Strain, risk for—illness severity of care receiver, significant home care needs, situational stressors, complexity/amount of caregiving tasks.
Pain—disease process (compression/destruction of nerve tissue, infiltration of nerves, or their vascular supply, obstruction of a nerve pathway, inflammation).
Therapeutic Regimen: Individuals, ineffective management—complexity of therapeutic regimen, economic difficulties, decisional conflict, perceived barriers, powerlessness, social support deficits.

FLUID AND ELECTROLYTE IMBALANCES

Body fluid is composed primarily of water and electrolytes. The body is equipped with homeostatic mechanisms to keep the composition and volume of body fluids within narrow limits. Organs involved in this mechanism include the kidneys, lungs, heart, blood vessels, adrenal glands, parathyroid glands, and pituitary gland. Body fluid is divided into two types: intracellular (within the cells) and extracellular (interstitial or tissue fluid, intravascular or plasma, and transcellular, such as cerebrospinal or synovial fluids).

RELATED CONCERNS

All plans of care specific to underlying health condition causing imbalance, e.g., DM, HF, upper GI bleeding, renal failure/dialysis.

Metabolic acidosis, page 523
Metabolic alkalosis, page 527
Respiratory acidosis, page 214
Respiratory alkalosis, page 218

NURSING PRIORITIES

1. Restore homeostasis.
2. Prevent/minimize complications.
3. Provide information about condition/prognosis and treatment needs as appropriate.

DISCHARGE GOALS

1. Homeostasis restored.
2. Free of complications.
3. Condition/prognosis and treatment needs understood.
4. Plan in place to meet needs after discharge.

Note: Because fluid and electrolyte imbalances usually occur in conjunction with other medical conditions, the following information is offered as a reference. The interventions are presented in a general format for inclusion in the primary plan of care.

Fluid Balance

Total body water, essential for metabolism, declines with age and also varies with body fat content and gender. It constitutes about 80% of an infant's body weight, 60% of an adult's, and as little as 40% of an older person's weight.

Hypervolemia (Extracellular Fluid Volume Excess)

PREDISPOSING/CONTRIBUTING FACTORS

Excess sodium intake including sodium-containing foods, medications, or fluids (PO/IV)
Excessive, rapid administration of hypertonic (or possibly isotonic) parenteral fluids
Increased release of antidiuretic hormone (ADH); excessive adrenocorticotropic hormone (ACTH) production, hyperaldosteronism
Decreased plasma proteins as may occur with chronic liver disease with ascites, major abdominal surgery, malnutrition/protein depletion
Chronic kidney disease/acute renal failure (ARF)
Heart failure (HF)

Patient Assessment Database

ACTIVITY/REST

May report: Fatigue, generalized weakness

CIRCULATION

May exhibit: Hypertension, elevated central venous pressure (CVP)
Pulse full/bounding; tachycardia usually present; bradycardia (late sign of cardiac decompensation)

Extra heart sounds (S_3)
Edema variable from dependent to generalized
Neck and peripheral vein distension

ELIMINATION

May report: Decreased urinary output, polyuria if renal function is normal
Diarrhea

FOOD/FLUID

May report: Anorexia, nausea/vomiting
Thirst (may be absent, especially in elderly)

May exhibit: Abdominal girth increased with visible fluid wave on palpation (ascites)
Sudden weight gain, often in excess of 5% of total body weight
Edema initially dependent, pitting may progress to facial/periorbital, general/anasarca

NEUROSENSORY

May exhibit: Changes in level of consciousness, from lethargy, disorientation, confusion to coma; aphasia
Muscle twitching, tremors, seizure activity
Hyperreflexia, rigid paralysis (severe hypernatreimia)

PAIN/DISCOMFORT

May report: Headache
Abdominal cramps

RESPIRATION

May report: Shortness of breath
May exhibit: Tachypnea with/without dyspnea, orthopnea; productive cough
Crackles

SAFETY

May exhibit: Fever
Skin changes in color, temperature, turgor, e.g., taut and cool where edematous

TEACHING/LEARNING

Refer to predisposing/contributing factors

Discharge plan considerations: **DRG projected mean length of inpatient stay: dependent on underlying condition**
May require assistance with changes in therapeutic regimen, dietary management

Refer to plan of care concerning underlying medical/surgical condition for possible postdischarge considerations.

DIAGNOSTIC STUDIES

Hematocrit: Elevated in dehydration, decreased in fluid overload.
Serum sodium: May be high, low, or normal (between 135 and 145 mEq/L).
Serum potassium and BUN: Normal or decreased, in fluid overload unless renal damage present.
Total protein: Plasma proteins/albumin may be decreased.
Serum osmolality: Usually unchanged, although hypo-osmolality may occur.
Urine sodium: May be low because of sodium retention.
Urine specific gravity: Decreased.
Chest x-ray: May reveal signs of congestion.

ACTIONS/INTERVENTIONS	RATIONALE

Hypervolemia Management (NIC)

Independent

Monitor vital signs, also CVP if available.	Tachycardia and hypertension are common manifestations. Tachypnea usually present with/without dyspnea. Elevated CVP may be noted before dyspnea and adventitious breath sounds occur. Hypertension may be a primary disorder or occur secondary to other associated conditions, e.g., HF.
Auscultate lungs and heart sounds.	Adventitious sounds (crackles) and extra heart sounds (S_3) are indicative of fluid excess. Pulmonary edema may develop rapidly.
Assess for presence/location of edema formation.	Edema can be either a cause or a result of various pathological conditions reflecting four competing forces—blood hydrostatic and osmotic pressures, and interstitial fluid hydrostatic and osmotic pressures. The dynamic interaction of these four forces allows fluid to shift from one body compartment to another. Edema may be generalized or localized in dependent areas. Elderly patients may develop dependent edema with relatively little excess fluid. *Note:* Patients in a supine position can have an increase of 4–8 L of fluid before edema is readily detected.
Note presence of neck and peripheral vein distension, along with pitting edema, dyspnea.	Signs of cardiac decompensation/HF.
Maintain accurate I&O. Note decreased urinary output, positive fluid balance (intake greater than output) on 24-hr calculations.	Decreased renal perfusion, cardiac insufficiency, and fluid shifts may cause decreased urinary output and edema formation.
Weigh as indicated. Be alert for acute or sudden weight gain.	One liter of fluid retention equals a weight gain of 2.2 lb.
Give oral fluids with caution. If fluids are restricted, set up a 24-hr schedule for fluid intake.	Fluid restrictions, as well as extracellular shifts, can aggravate drying of mucous membranes, and patient may desire more fluids than are prudent.

ACTIONS/INTERVENTIONS	RATIONALE
Independent	
Monitor infusion rate of parenteral fluids closely; administer via control device/pump as necessary.	Sudden fluid bolus/prolonged excessive administration potentiates volume overload/risk of cardiac decompensation.
Encourage coughing/deep-breathing exercises.	Pulmonary fluid shifts potentiate respiratory complications.
Maintain semi-Fowler's position if dyspnea or ascites is present.	Gravity improves lung expansion by lowering diaphragm and shifting fluid to lower abdominal cavity.
Turn, reposition, and provide skin care at regular intervals.	Reduces pressure and friction on edematous tissue, which is more prone to breakdown than normal tissue.
Encourage bedrest. Schedule care to provide frequent rest periods.	Limited cardiac reserves result in fatigue/activity intolerance. In addition, lying down favors diuresis and reduction of edema.
Provide safety precautions as indicated, e.g., use of side rails, bed in low position, frequent observation, soft restraints (if required).	Fluid shifts may cause cerebral edema/changes in mentation, especially in the geriatric population.
Collaborative	
Assist with identification/treatment of underlying cause.	Refer to listing of predisposing/contributing factors to determine treatment needs.
Monitor laboratory studies as indicated, e.g., electrolytes, BUN, ABGs.	Extracellular fluid shifts, sodium/water restriction and renal function all affect serum sodium levels. Potassium deficit may occur with diuretic therapy. BUN may be increased as a result of renal dysfunction/failure. ABGs may reflect metabolic acidosis.
Provide balanced protein, low-sodium diet. Restrict fluids as indicated.	In presence of decreased serum proteins (e.g., malnutrition), increasing level of serum proteins can enhance colloidal osmotic gradients and promote return of fluid to the vascular space. Restriction of sodium/water decreases extracellular fluid retention.
Administer diuretics: loop diuretic, e.g., furosemide (Lasix); thiazide diuretic, e.g., hydrochlorothiazide (Esidrix); or potassium-sparing diuretic, e.g., spironolactone (Aldactone).	To achieve excretion of excess fluid, either a single diuretic (e.g., thiazide) or a combination of agents may be selected (e.g., thiazide and spironolactone). The combination can be particularly helpful when two drugs have different sites of action allowing more effective control of fluid excess.
Replace potassium losses as indicated.	Potassium deficit may occur, especially if patient is receiving potassium-wasting diuretic. This can cause lethal cardiac dysrhythmias if untreated.
Prepare for/assist with dialysis or ultrafiltration, if indicated.	May be done to rapidly reduce fluid overload, especially in the presence of severe cardiac/renal failure.

Hypovolemia (Extracellular Fluid Volume Deficit)

PREDISPOSING/CONTRIBUTING FACTORS

Excessive fluid losses: Vomiting, gastric suctioning, diarrhea, polyuria, diaphoresis, wounds or burns, intraoperative fluid loss, hemorrhage
Insufficient/decreased fluid intake, e.g., preoperative/postoperative NPO status
Systemic infections, fever
Intestinal obstruction or fistulas
Pancreatitis, peritonitis, cirrhosis/ascites; adrenal insufficiency

Kidney disease, diabetic ketoacidosis, hyperglycemic hyperosmotic nonketotic coma (HHNC), diabetes insipidus, syndrome of inappropriate antidiuretic hormone (SIADH)

Patient Assessment Database

ACTIVITY/REST

May report: Fatigue, generalized weakness

CIRCULATION

May exhibit: Hypotension, including postural changes
Pulse weak/thready; tachycardia
Neck veins flattened; CVP decreased

ELIMINATION

May report: Constipation or occasionally diarrhea, abdominal cramps
May exhibit: Urine volume decreased, dark/concentrated color; oliguria (severe fluid depletion)

FOOD/FLUID

May report: Thirst, anorexia, nausea/vomiting
May exhibit: Weight loss often exceeding 2%–8% of total body weight
Abdominal distension
Mucous membranes dry, furrows on tongue; decreased tearing and salivation
Skin dry with poor turgor; or pale, moist, clammy (shock)

NEUROSENSORY

May report: Tingling of the extremities, vertigo, syncope
May exhibit: Behavior change, apathy, restlessness, confusion

RESPIRATION

May exhibit: Tachypnea, rapid/shallow breathing

SAFETY

May exhibit: Temperature usually subnormal, although fever may occur

TEACHING/LEARNING

Refer to predisposing/contributing factors

Discharge plan considerations: **DRG projected mean length of inpatient stay: dependent on underlying cause**
May require assistance with changes in therapeutic regimen, dietary management

Refer to plan of care concerning underlying medical/surgical condition for possible considerations after discharge.

DIAGNOSTIC STUDIES

Serum sodium: May be normal, high, or low.
Urine sodium: Usually decreased (less than 10 mEq/L when losses are from external causes; usually greater than 20 mEq/L if the cause is renal or adrenal).
CBC: Hb/Hct and RBC usually increased (hemoconcentration); decrease suggests hemorrhage.
Serum glucose: Normal or elevated.
Serum protein: Increased.
BUN and Cr: Increased, with BUN out of proportion to Cr level.
Urine specific gravity: Increased.

NURSING DIAGNOSIS: Fluid Volume deficit

May be related to

Active fluid loss, e.g., hemorrhage, vomiting/gastric intubation, diarrhea, burns, wounds, fistulas

Regulatory failure, e.g., adrenal disease, recovery phase of ARF; diabetic ketoacidosis (DKA), HHNC; diabetes insipidus, systemic infections

Possibly evidenced by

Signs/symptoms noted in patient database

DESIRED OUTCOMES/EVALUATION CRITERIA—PATIENT WILL:

Fluid Balance (NOC)

Maintain fluid volume at a functional level as evidenced by individually adequate urinary output with normal specific gravity, stable vital signs, moist mucous membranes, good skin turgor, and prompt capillary refill.

Knowledge: Treatment Regimen (NOC)

Verbalize understanding of causative factors and purpose of therapeutic interventions. Demonstrate behaviors to monitor and correct deficit as appropriate.

ACTIONS/INTERVENTIONS	RATIONALE

Hypovolemia Management (NIC)

Independent

Monitor vital signs and CVP. Note presence/degree of postural BP changes. Observe for temperature elevations/fever.	Tachycardia is present along with a varying degree of hypotension, depending on degree of fluid deficit. CVP measurements are useful in determining degree of fluid deficit and response to replacement therapy. Fever increases metabolism and exacerbates fluid loss.
Palpate peripheral pulses; note capillary refill, skin color/temperature. Assess mentation.	Conditions that contribute to extracellular fluid deficit can result in inadequate organ perfusion to all areas and may cause circulatory collapse/shock.
Monitor urinary output. Measure/estimate fluid losses from all sources, e.g., gastric losses, wound drainage, diaphoresis.	Fluid replacement needs are based on correction of current deficits and ongoing losses. *Note:* A diaphoretic episode requiring a full linen change may represent a fluid loss of as much as 1 L. A decreased urinary output may indicate insufficient renal perfusion/hypovolemia, or polyuria can be present, requiring more aggressive fluid replacement.
Weigh daily and compare with 24-hr fluid balance. Mark/measure edematous areas, e.g., abdomen, limbs.	Although weight gain and fluid intake greater than output may not accurately reflect intravascular volume, e.g., third-space fluid accumulation cannot be used by the body for tissue perfusion, these measurements provide useful data for comparison.
Evaluate patient's ability to swallow.	Impaired gag/swallow reflexes, anorexia/nausea, oral discomfort, and changes in level of consciousness/cognition are among the factors that affect patient's ability to replace fluids orally.
Ascertain patient's beverage preferences, and set up a 24-hr schedule for fluid intake. Encourage foods with high fluid content.	Relieves thirst and discomfort of dry mucous membranes and augments parenteral replacement.

ACTIONS/INTERVENTIONS	RATIONALE
Independent	
Turn frequently, massage skin, and protect bony prominences.	Tissues are susceptible to breakdown because of vasoconstriction and increased cellular fragility.
Provide skin and mouth care. Bathe every other day using mild soap. Apply lotion as indicated.	Skin and mucous membranes are dry, with decreased elasticity, because of vasoconstriction and reduced intracellular water. Daily bathing may increase dryness.
Provide safety precautions as indicated, e.g., use of side rails, bed in low position, frequent observation, soft restraints (if required).	Decreased cerebral perfusion frequently results in changes in mentation/altered thought processes, requiring protective measures to prevent patient injury.
Investigate reports of sudden/sharp chest pain, dyspnea, cyanosis, increased anxiety, restlessness.	Hemoconcentration (sludging) and increased platelet aggregation may result in systemic emboli formation.
Monitor for sudden/marked elevation of BP, restlessness, moist cough, dyspnea, basalar crackles, frothy sputum.	Too rapid a correction of fluid deficit may compromise the cardiopulmonary system, especially if colloids are used in general fluid replacement (increased osmotic pressure potentiates fluid shifts).
Collaborative	
Assist with identification/treatment of underlying cause.	Refer to listing of predisposing/contributing factors to determine treatment needs.
Monitor laboratory studies as indicated, e.g., electrolytes, glucose, pH/Pco_2, coagulation studies.	Depending on the avenue of fluid loss, differing electrolyte/metabolic imbalances may be present/require correction; e.g., use of glucose solutions in patients with underlying glucose intolerance may result in serum glucose elevation and increased urinary water losses.
Administer IV solutions as indicated:	
Isotonic solutions, e.g., 0.9% NaCl (normal saline), 5% dextrose/water;	Crystalloids provide prompt circulatory improvement, although the benefit may be transient (increased renal clearance).
0.45% NaCl (half-normal saline), lactated Ringer's solution;	As soon as the patient is normotensive, a hypotonic solution (0.45% NaCl) may be used to provide both electrolytes and free water for renal excretion of metabolic wastes. *Note:* Buffered crystalloids (LR) are used with caution because they may potentiate the risk of metabolic acidosis.
Colloids, e.g., dextran, Plasmanate/albumin, hetastarch (Hespan);	Corrects plasma protein concentration deficits, thereby increasing intravascular osmotic pressure and facilitating return of fluid into vascular compartment.
Whole blood/packed RBC transfusion, or autologous collection of blood.	Indicated when hypovolemia is related to active blood loss.
Administer sodium bicarbonate, if indicated.	May be given to correct severe acidosis while correcting fluid balance.
Provide tube feedings, including free water as appropriate.	Enteral replacement can provide proteins and other needed elements in addition to meeting general fluid requirements when swallowing is impaired.

Sodium

Sodium is the major cation of extracellular fluid and is primarily responsible for osmotic pressure in that compartment. Sodium enhances neuromuscular conduction/transmission of impulses and is essential for maintaining acid-base balance. Normal serum range is 135–145 mEq/L; intracellular, 10 mEq/L. Chloride is carried by Na and will display the same imbalances. Normal serum chloride range is 95–105 mEq/L.

Hyponatremia (Sodium Deficit)

PREDISPOSING/CONTRIBUTING FACTORS

Primary hyponatremia (loss of sodium): Lack of sufficient dietary sodium, severe malnutrition, infusion of sodium-free solutions; excessive sodium loss through heavy sweating (e.g., heat exhaustion), wounds/trauma (hemorrhage), burns, gastric suctioning, vomiting, diarrhea, small-bowel obstruction, peritonitis, salt-wasting renal dysfunction, adrenal insufficiency (Addison's disease)

Dilutional hyponatremia (water gains): Excessive water intake, electrolyte-free IV infusion, water intoxication (IV therapy, tap-water enemas), gastric irrigations with electrolyte-free solutions, presence of tumors or CNS disorders predisposing to SIADH, HF, renal failure/nephrotic syndrome, hepatic cirrhosis, DM (hyperglycemia), freshwater near-drowning; use of certain drugs, e.g., hypoglycemia medications, barbiturates, antipsychotics, aminophylline, morphine (may stimulate pituitary gland to secrete excessive amounts of ADH), anticonvulsants, some antineoplastic agents, or NSAIDs

Note: A pseudohyponatremia may occur in presence of multiple myeloma, hyperlipidemia, or hypoproteinemia but does not reflect an actual abnormality of water metabolism.

Patient Assessment Database

(Patient may be asymptomatic until serum sodium level is less than 125 mEq/L, depending on rapidity of onset.)

General

ACTIVITY/REST

May report: Malaise
Generalized weakness, faintness, muscle cramps

EGO INTEGRITY

May report: Anxiety
May exhibit: Restlessness, apprehension

FOOD/FLUID

May report: Nausea, anorexia, thirst
Low-sodium diet
Diuretic use

NEUROSENSORY

May report: Headache, blurred vision, vertigo
May exhibit: Loss of coordination, stupor, personality changes

TEACHING/LEARNING

Refer to predisposing/contributing factors
Use of oral hypoglycemic agent, potent diuretics, NSAIDs, other drugs that impair renal water excretion

Discharge plan considerations: **DRG projected mean length of inpatient stay: dependent on underlying cause**
May require assistance with changes in therapeutic regimen, dietary management

Refer to plan of care concerning underlying medical/surgical condition for possible considerations after discharge.

Sodium/Water Deficit

(Na less than 135 mEq/L; urine specific gravity elevated, serum osmolality normal)

CIRCULATION

May exhibit: Hypotension, tachycardia
Peripheral pulses diminished
Pallid, clammy skin

ELIMINATION

May report: Abdominal cramping, diarrhea
May exhibit: Urinary output decreased

FOOD/FLUID

May report: Anorexia, nausea/vomiting
May exhibit: Poor skin turgor; soft/sunken eyeballs
Mucous membranes dry, decreased saliva/perspiration

NEUROSENSORY

May report: Dizziness
May exhibit: Muscle twitching
Lethargy, restlessness, confusion, stupor

RESPIRATION

May exhibit: Tachypnea

SAFETY

May exhibit: Skin flushed, dry, hot
Fever

Sodium Deficit/Water Excess

(Na less than 135 mEq/L; urine specific gravity low; serum osmolality decreased)

CIRCULATION

May exhibit: Hypertension
Generalized edema

ELIMINATION

May exhibit: Urinary output increased

NEUROSENSORY

May exhibit: Muscle twitching, restlessness, changes in mentation (more severe when problem is acute/develops rapidly)

PAIN/DISCOMFORT

May report: Headache, abdominal cramps

Severe Sodium Deficit

(Na less than 120 mEq/L)

CIRCULATION

May exhibit: Hypotension with vasomotor collapse
Rapid thready pulse
Cold/clammy skin, fingerprinting on sternum; cyanosis

NEUROSENSORY

May exhibit: Hyporeflexia
Convulsions/coma

DIAGNOSTIC STUDIES (Depend on associated fluid level)

Serum sodium: Decreased, less than 135 mEq/L. However, signs/symptoms may not occur until level is less than 120 mEq/L.

Urine sodium: Less than 15 mEq/L indicates renal conservation of sodium due to sodium loss from a nonrenal source unless sodium-wasting nephropathy is present. Urine sodium greater than 20 mEq/L indicates SIADH.

Serum potassium: May be decreased as the kidneys attempt to conserve sodium at the expense of potassium.

Serum chloride/bicarbonate: Levels are decreased, depending on which ion is lost with the sodium.

Serum osmolality: Commonly low, but may be normal (pseudohyponatremia) or high (HHNC).

Urine osmolality: Usually less than 100 mOsm/L unless SIADH present, in which case it will exceed serum osmolality.

Urine specific gravity: May be decreased (less than 1.010) or increased (greater than 1.020) if SIADH is present.

Hct: Depends on fluid balance, e.g., fluid excess versus dehydration.

DESIRED OUTCOMES/EVALUATION CRITERIA—PATIENT WILL:

Electrolyte and Acid/Base Balance (NOC)

Display heart rate, BP, and laboratory results within normal limits (WNL) for patient, absence of muscle weakness, neurological irritability.

ACTIONS/INTERVENTIONS	RATIONALE

Electrolyte Management: Hyponatremia (NIC)

Independent

Identify the patient at risk for hyponatremia and the specific cause, e.g., sodium loss or fluid excess.	Provides clues for early intervention. Hyponatremia is a common imbalance (especially in the elderly) and may range from mild to severe. Severe hyponatremia can cause neurological damage or death if not treated promptly.
Monitor I&O. Calculate fluid balance. Weigh daily.	Indicators of fluid balance are important, because either fluid excess or deficit may occur with hyponatremia.
Assess level of consciousness/neuromuscular response.	Sodium deficit may result in decreased mentation (to point of coma), as well as generalized muscle weakness/cramps, convulsions.
Maintain quiet environment; provide safety/seizure precautions.	Reduces CNS stimulation and risk of injury from neurological complications, e.g., seizures.
Note respiratory rate and depth.	Co-occurring hypochloremia may produce slow/shallow respirations as the body compensates for metabolic alkalosis.
Encourage foods and fluids high in sodium, e.g., milk, meat, eggs, carrots, beets, and celery. Use fruit juices and bouillon instead of plain water.	Unless sodium deficit causes serious symptoms requiring immediate IV replacement, the patient may benefit from slower replacement by oral method or removal of previous salt restriction.
Irrigate NG tube (when used) with normal saline instead of water.	Isotonic irrigation will minimize loss of GI electrolytes.
Observe for signs of circulatory overload as indicated.	Administration of sodium-containing IV fluids in presence of HF increases risk.

Collaborative

Assist with identification/treatment of underlying cause.	Refer to listing of predisposing/contributing factors to determine treatment needs.

ACTIONS/INTERVENTIONS	RATIONALE
Collaborative	
Monitor serum and urine electrolytes, osmolality.	Evaluates therapy needs/effectiveness.
Provide/restrict fluids depending on fluid volume status.	In presence of hypovolemia, volume losses are replaced with isotonic saline (e.g., normal saline), or, on occasion, hypertonic solution (3% NaCl) when hyponatremia is life-threatening. In the presence of fluid volume excess, or SIADH, fluid restriction is indicated. *Note:* Too rapid/excessive administration of hypertonic solutions can be lethal.
Administer medications as indicated, e.g.:	
Furosemide (Lasix);	Effective in reducing fluid excess to correct sodium/water balance.
Sodium chloride;	Used to replace deficits/prevent recurrence in the presence of chronic/ongoing losses.
Potassium chloride;	Corrects potassium deficit, especially when diuretic is used.
Demeclocycline (Declomycin);	Useful in treating chronic SIADH, or when severe water restriction may not be tolerated, e.g., COPD. *Note:* May be contraindicated in patients with liver disease, because nephrotoxicity may occur.
Captopril (Capoten).	May be used in combination with a loop diuretic (e.g., Lasix) to correct fluid volume excess, especially in the presence of HF.
Prepare for/assist with dialysis as indicated.	May be done to restore sodium balance without increasing fluid level when hyponatremia is severe or response to diuretic therapy is inadequate.

Hypernatremia (Sodium Excess)

PREDISPOSING/CONTRIBUTING FACTORS

Excessive water losses: Polyuria (as may occur with diabetes insipidus); use of osmotic diuretics (such as mannitol); presence of fever, profuse sweating, vomiting, diarrhea; extracellular fluid volume excesses: e.g., renal disease, HF, primary aldosteronism, excessive steroids/Cushing's disease; excessive ingestion or infusion of sodium; salt water near-drowning

Insufficient water intake: Administration of tube feedings/high-protein diets with minimal fluid intake, self-medication/"ulcer diets" primarily using half and half/whole milk

Patient Assessment Database

Sodium Excess/Water Deficit

(Na greater than 145 mEq/L; elevated urine specific gravity)

ACTIVITY/REST

May report:	Weakness
May exhibit:	Muscle rigidity/tremors, generalized weakness

CIRCULATION

May exhibit:	Decreased blood pressure, postural hypotension
	Tachycardia

ELIMINATION

May exhibit: Decreased urinary output

FOOD/FLUID

May report: Thirst

May exhibit: Mucous membranes dry, sticky; tongue dry, swollen, rough

NEUROSENSORY

May exhibit: Irritability, lethargy/coma (depending on rapidity of onset rather than actual serum sodium level)

Delusions, hallucinations

Muscle irritability, seizure activity

SAFETY

May exhibit: Hot, dry, flushed skin

Fever

Sodium/Water Excess

(Na greater than 145 mEq/L; urine specific gravity decreased)

CIRCULATION

May exhibit: Elevated BP, hypertension

ELIMINATION

May exhibit: Polyuria

FOOD/FLUID

May report: Thirst

May exhibit: Skin pale, moist, taut with pitting edema

Weight gain

NEUROSENSORY

May exhibit: Confusion, lethargy

Delusions, hallucinations

RESPIRATION

May exhibit: Dyspnea

Sodium Excess/Water Deficit or Excess

TEACHING/LEARNING

Refer to predisposing/contributing factors

Discharge plan considerations: **DRG projected mean length of inpatient stay: depends on underlying cause**

May require assistance with changes in therapeutic regimen, dietary management

Refer to plan of care concerning underlying medical/surgical condition for possible considerations after discharge.

DIAGNOSTIC STUDIES

Serum sodium: Increased, greater than 145 mEq/L. Serum levels greater than 160 mEq/L may be accompanied by severe neurological signs.

Serum chloride: Increased, greater than 106 mEq/L.

Serum potassium: Decreased.

Serum osmolality: Greater than 295 mOsm/L when dehydrated; lower in presence of extracellular fluid excess, and less than 200 mOsm/L with excessive polyuria.

Hct: May be normal or elevated depending on fluid status.

Urine sodium: Less than 50 mEq/L.

Urine chloride: Less than 50 mEq/L.

Urine osmolality: Greater than 800 mOsm/L.

Urine specific gravity: Increased, greater than 1.015, if water deficit present; or less than 1.010 when hypernatremia is due to polyuria.

DESIRED OUTCOMES/EVALUATION CRITERIA—PATIENT WILL:

Electrolyte and Acid/Base Balance (NOC)

Display BP, heart rate, and laboratory results WNL for patient, absence of neuromuscular irritability, cognitive impairment.

ACTIONS/INTERVENTIONS

Electrolyte Management: Hypernatremia (NIC)

Independent

Monitor BP.

Identify patient at risk for hypernatremia and likely cause, e.g., water deficit, sodium excess.

Note respiratory rate, depth.

Monitor I&O, urine specific gravity. Weigh daily. Assess presence/location of edema.

Evaluate level of consciousness and muscular strength, tone, movement.

Maintain safety/seizure precautions, as indicated, e.g., bed in low position, use of padded side rails.

Assess skin turgor, color, temperature, and mucous membrane moisture.

Provide/encourage meticulous skin care and frequent repositioning.

Provide frequent oral care. Avoid use of mouthwash/rinse that contains alcohol.

Offer debilitated patient fluids at regular intervals. Give free water to patient receiving enteral feedings.

Recommend avoidance of foods high in sodium, e.g., canned soups/vegetables, processed foods, snack foods, and condiments.

Collaborative

Assist with identification/treatment of underlying cause.

RATIONALE

Either hypertension or hypotension may be present, depending on the fluid status. Presence of postural hypotension may affect activity tolerance.

Early identification and intervention prevents serious complications associated with this problem.

Deep, labored respirations with air hunger suggest metabolic acidosis (hyperchloremia), which can lead to cardiopulmonary arrest if not corrected.

These parameters are variable, depending on fluid status, and are indicators of therapy needs/effectiveness.

Sodium imbalance may cause changes that vary from confusion and irritability to seizures and coma. In presence of water deficit, rapid rehydration may cause cerebral edema.

Sodium excess/cerebral edema increases risk of convulsions.

Water-deficit hyponatremia manifests by signs of dehydration.

Maintains skin integrity.

Promotes comfort and prevents further drying of mucous membranes.

May prevent hypernatremia in patient who is unable to perceive or respond to thirst.

Reduces risk of sodium-associated complications.

Refer to listing of predisposing/contributing factors to determine treatment needs.

ACTIONS/INTERVENTIONS	RATIONALE
Collaborative	
Monitor serum electrolytes, osmolality, and ABGs as indicated.	Evaluates therapy needs/effectiveness. *Note:* Co-occurring hyperchloremia may cause metabolic acidosis, requiring buffering, e.g., sodium bicarbonate.
Increase PO/IV fluid intake, e.g., 5% dextrose/water in presence of dehydration; 0.90% of NaC1 if extracellular deficit is present.	Replacement of total body water deficit will gradually restore sodium/water balance. *Note:* Rapid reduction of serum sodium level with corresponding decrease in serum osmolality can cause cerebral edema/convulsions.
Restrict sodium intake and administer diuretics as indicated.	Restriction of sodium intake while promoting renal clearance lowers serum sodium levels in the presence of extracellular fluid excess.

Potassium

Potassium is the major cation of the intracellular fluid and is responsible for maintaining intracellular osmotic pressure. Potassium also regulates neuromuscular excitability, aids in maintenance of acid-base balance, synthesis of protein, and metabolism of carbohydrates. Normal serum range is 3.5–5.0 mEq/L (body total of 42 mEq/L).

Hypokalemia (Potassium Deficit)

PREDISPOSING/CONTRIBUTING FACTORS

Renal loss: Use of potassium-wasting diuretics, diuretic phase of ATN, healing phase of burns; diabetic acidosis; Cushing's syndrome; nephritis, hypomagnesemia; use of sodium penicillins, amphotericin B, carbenicillin steroids; licorice abuse

GI loss: Profuse vomiting, excessive diarrhea, laxative abuse, prolonged gastric suction, inflammatory bowel disease, fistulas

Inadequate dietary intake: Anorexia nervosa, starvation, high-sodium diet

Shift into cells: TPN, alkalosis, or excessive secretion or administration of insulin

Other: Sweat losses (heavily perspiring person acclimated to heat); liver disease

Patient Assessment Database

ACTIVITY/REST
May report: Generalized weakness, lethargy, fatigue

CIRCULATION
May exhibit: Hypotension
Pulses weak/diminished, irregular
Heart sounds distant
Dysrhythmias, e.g., premature ventricular contractions (PVCs), ventricular tachycardia/fibrillation

ELIMINATION
May exhibit: Nocturia, polyuria if factors contributing to hypokalemia include HF or DM
Bowel sounds diminished, decreased bowel motility, paralytic ileus
Abdominal distension

FOOD/FLUID
May report: Anorexia, nausea/vomiting
Thirst

NEUROSENSORY
May report: Paresthesias
May exhibit: Depressed mental state/confusion, apathy, drowsiness, irritability, coma
Hyporeflexia, tetany, paralysis (flaccid quadriparesis)

939

PAIN/DISCOMFORT

May report: Muscle pain/cramps

RESPIRATION

May exhibit: Hypoventilation/decreased respiratory depth due to muscle weakness/paralysis of diaphragm; apnea, cyanosis

TEACHING/LEARNING

Refer to predisposing/contributing factors

Discharge plan considerations: **DRG projected mean length of inpatient stay: depends on underlying cause**
May require assistance with changes in therapeutic regimen, dietary management

Refer to plan of care concerning underlying medical/surgical condition for possible considerations after discharge.

DIAGNOSTIC STUDIES

Serum potassium: Decreased, less than 3.5 mEq/L.
Serum chloride: Often decreased, less than 98 mEq/L.
Serum glucose: May be slightly elevated.
Serum magnesium: Levels often decreased when potassium deficit is present.
Plasma bicarbonate: Increased, greater than 29 mEq/L.
Urine osmolality: Decreased.
ABGs: pH and bicarbonate may be elevated (metabolic alkalosis).
ECG: Low voltage; flat or inverted T wave, appearance of U wave, depressed ST segment, peaked P waves; prolonged QT interval, ventricular dysrhythmias.

DESIRED OUTCOMES/EVALUATION CRITERIA—PATIENT WILL:

Electrolyte & Acid/Base Balance (NOC)

Display heart rhythm and laboratory results WNL for patient, absence of muscle weakness, paresthesias, cognitive impairment.

ACTIONS/INTERVENTIONS	RATIONALE
Electrolyte Management: Hypokalemia (NIC)	
Independent	
Monitor heart rate/rhythm.	Changes associated with hypokalemia include abnormalities in both conduction and contractility. Tachycardia may develop, and potentially life-threatening atrial and ventricular dysrhythmias, e.g., PVCs, sinus bradycardia, atrioventricular (AV) blocks, AV dissociation, ventricular tachycardia.
Monitor respiratory rate, depth, effort. Encourage cough/deep-breathing exercises; reposition frequently.	Respiratory muscle weakness may proceed to paralysis and eventual respiratory arrest.
Assess level of consciousness and neuromuscular function, e.g., strength, sensation, movement.	Apathy, drowsiness, irritability, tetany, paresthesias, and coma may occur.

ACTIONS/INTERVENTIONS	RATIONALE
Independent	
Auscultate bowel sounds, noting decrease/absence or change.	Paralytic ileus commonly follows gastric losses through vomiting/gastric suction, protracted diarrhea.
Maintain accurate record of urinary, gastric, and wound losses.	Guide for calculating fluid/potassium replacement needs.
Monitor rate of IV potassium administration using microdrop or pump infusion devices. Check for side effects. Provide ice pack as indicated.	Ensures controlled delivery of medication to prevent bolus effect and reduce associated discomfort, e.g., burning sensation at IV site. When solution cannot be administered via central vein and slowing rate is not possible/effective, ice pack to infusion site may help relieve discomfort.
Encourage intake of foods and fluids high in potassium, e.g., bananas, oranges, dried fruits, red meat, turkey, salmon, leafy vegetables, peas, baked potatoes, tomatoes, winter squash, coffee, colas, tea. Discuss use of potassium chloride salt substitutes for patient receiving long-term diuretics.	Potassium may be replaced/level maintained through the diet when the patient is allowed oral food and fluids. Dietary replacement of 40–60 mEq/L/day is typically sufficient if no abnormal losses are occurring.
Review drug regimen for potassium-wasting drugs, e.g., furosemide (Lasix), hydrochlorothiazide (Diamox), IV catecholamines, gentamicin (Garamycin), carbenicillin (Geocillin), amphotericin B (Fungizone).	If alternate agents (e.g., potassium-sparing diuretics such as spirinolactone (Aldactone), triamterene (Dyrenium), amiloride (Midamor) cannot be administered or when high-dose sodium drugs are administered (e.g., carbenicillin), close monitoring and replacement of potassium are necessary.
Discuss preventable causes of condition, e.g., nutritional choices, proper use of laxatives.	Provides opportunity for patient to prevent recurrence. Also, dietary control is more palatable than oral replacement medications.
Dilute liquid and effervescent K supplements (K-Tab, K-Lyte/Cl) with 4 oz water/juice and give after meals.	May prevent/reduce GI irritation and saline laxative effect.
Watch for signs of digitalis intoxication when used (e.g., reports of nausea/vomiting, blurred vision, increasing atrial dysrhythmias, and heart block).	Low potassium enhances effect of digitalis, slowing cardiac conduction. *Note:* Combined effects of digitalis, diuretics, and hypokalemia may produce lethal dysrhythmias.
Observe for signs of metabolic alkalosis, e.g., hypoventilation, tachycardia, dysrhythmias, tetany, changes in mentation.	Frequently associated with hypokalemia.
Collaborative	
Assist with identification/treatment of underlying cause.	Refer to listing of predisposing/contributing factors to determine treatment needs. *Note:* Hypokalemia is life-threatening, early detection is crucial.
Monitor laboratory studies, e.g.:	
Serum potassium;	Levels should be checked frequently during replacement therapy, especially in the presence of insufficient renal function. Sudden excess/elevation may cause cardiac dysrhythmias.
ABGs;	Correction of metabolic alkalosis raises serum potassium level and reduces replacement needs. Correction of acidosis drives potassium back into cells, resulting in decreased serum levels and increased replacement needs.

ACTIONS/INTERVENTIONS	RATIONALE
Collaborative	
Serum magnesium;	Hypomagnesemia occurs with and exacerbates potassium loss and sodium retention, altering cell membrane excitability (affects cardiac and neuro-muscular function).
Serum chloride.	Use of diuretics, e.g., furosemide (Lasix), hydrochlorothiazide (Hydrodiuril), may cause chloride and potassium depletion.
Administer oral and/or IV potassium.	May be required to correct deficiencies when changes in medication, therapy and/or dietary intake are insufficient. *Note:* Even in severe deficit, parenteral replacement should not exceed 40 mEq/2 hr. Dietary supplementation may also be used to produce a gradual equilibration if patient is able to take oral food and fluids.

Hyperkalemia (Potassium Excess)

PREDISPOSING/CONTRIBUTING FACTORS

Potassium retention: Decreased renal excretion (e.g., renal disease/acute failure, hypoaldosteronism, Addison's disease), hypovolemia, use of potassium-conserving diuretics, especially when associated with potassium supplements, use of NSAIDs

Excessive potassium intake: Salt substitutes, drugs containing potassium (e.g., penicillin), improper use of oral potassium supplements, too-rapid IV administration of potassium, massive transfusion of banked blood

Shift or release of potassium out of cells: Severe catabolism, burns, crush injuries, myocardial infarction (MI), severe hemolysis, rhabdomyolysis, chemotherapy with cytotoxic drugs, respiratory or metabolic acidosis, anoxia, hyperglycemia with insulin deficiency, use of some β-adrenergic blockers, profound digitalis toxicity

Other: Use of certain medications such as captopril, heparin, cyclosporin

Patient Assessment Database

Data depends on degree of elevation and length of time condition has existed.

ACTIVITY/REST

May report: Vague muscular weakness

May exhibit: Restlessness, irritability

CIRCULATION

May exhibit: Irregular pulse, bradycardia, heart block, asystole

EGO INTEGRITY

May report: Apprehension

ELIMINATION

May report: Intermittent abdominal cramps, diarrhea

May exhibit: Urine volume decreased
Hyperactive bowel sounds

FOOD/FLUID

May report: Nausea/vomiting

NEUROSENSORY

May report: Paresthesias (often of face, tongue, hands, feet)
Slurred speech

May exhibit: Decreased deep-tendon reflexes; progressive, ascending flaccid paralysis; twitching, seizure activity
Apathy, confusion

PAIN/DISCOMFORT

May report: Muscle cramps/pain

TEACHING/LEARNING

Refer to predisposing/contributing factors

Discharge plan considerations: **DRG projected mean length of inpatient stay: depends on underlying cause**
May require assistance with changes in therapeutic regimen, dietary management

Refer to plan of care concerning underlying medical/surgical condition for possible considerations after discharge.

DIAGNOSTIC STUDIES

Serum potassium: Increased, greater than 5.1 mEq/L.

Serum magnesium: Levels may be elevated if renal failure is present.

Renal function studies: May be altered, indicating failure.

Leukocyte or thrombocyte count: Elevation may cause a pseudohyperkalemia, affecting choice of interventions.

ECG changes: T waves tall and peaked/tented, prolonged PR interval, loss of P waves, widening of QRS complex, shortened QT interval, and ST segment depression; atrial/ventricular dysrhythmias, e.g., bradycardia, atrial arrest, complete heart block, ventricular fibrillation, cardiac arrest.

DESIRED OUTCOMES/EVALUATION CRITERIA—PATIENT WILL:

Electrolyte & Acid/Base Balance (NOC)

Display heart rate/rhythm and laboratory results WNL for patient; absence of muscle weakness, paresthesias, cognitive impairment.

ACTIONS/INTERVENTIONS	RATIONALE

Electrolyte Management: Hyperkalemia (NIC)

Independent

Identify the patient at risk; or the cause of the hyperkalemia, e.g., excessive intake of potassium or decreased excretion.	Influences choice of interventions. Early identification and treatment can prevent complication. *Note:* A major cause of hypokalemia is decreased renal excretion.
Instruct patient in use of potassium-containing salts (salt substitutes), taking potassium supplements safely.	The patient is often able to prevent hyperkalemia through management of supplements, diet, and other medications.
Monitor respiratory rate and depth. Elevate head of bed. Encourage cough/deep-breathing exercises.	Patients may hypoventilate and retain CO_2, leading to respiratory acidosis. Muscular weakness can affect respiratory muscles and lead to complications of respiratory infection/failure.
Monitor heart rate/rhythm. Be aware that cardiac arrest can occur.	Excess potassium depresses myocardial conduction. Bradycardia can progress to cardiac fibrillation/arrest.

ACTIONS/INTERVENTIONS	RATIONALE

Independent

Monitor urinary output.	In kidney failure, potassium is retained because of improper excretion. Potassium should not be given if oliguria or anuria is present.
Assess level of consciousness, neuromuscular function, e.g., movement, strength, sensation.	Patient is usually awake and alert; however, muscular paresthesia, weakness, and flaccid paralysis may occur.
Encourage/assist with ROM exercises as tolerated.	Improves muscular tone and reduces muscle cramps and pain.
Encourage frequent rest periods; assist with care activities, as indicated.	General muscle weakness decreases activity tolerance.
Review drug regimen for medications containing/affecting potassium excretion, e.g., penicillin G, spironolactone (Aldactone), amiloride (Midamor), hydrochlorothiazide (Dyazide, Maxzide).	Requires regular monitoring of potassium levels, and may require alternate drug choices or changes in dosage/frequency.
Identify/discontinue dietary sources of potassium, e.g., tomatoes, broccoli, orange juice, bananas, bran, chocolate, coffee, tea, eggs, dairy products, dried fruits.	Facilitates reduction of potassium level and may prevent recurrence of hyperkalemia.
Recommend an increase in carbohydrates/fats and foods low in potassium, e.g., canned fruits, refined cereals, apple/cranberry juice.	Reduces exogenous sources of potassium and prevents catabolic tissue breakdown with release of cellular potassium.
Stress importance of patient's notifying future caregivers when chronic condition potentiates development of hyperkalemia, e.g., oliguric renal failure.	May help prevent recurrence.

Collaborative

Assist with identification/treatment of underlying cause.	Refer to listing of predisposing/contributing factors to determine treatment needs.
Monitor laboratory results, e.g., serum potassium, ABGs, BUN/Cr, glucose as indicated.	Evaluates therapy needs/effectiveness. *Note:* Hypoventilation may result in respiratory acidosis, thereby increasing serum potassium levels.
Administer medications as indicated, e.g.:	
Diuretics, e.g., furosemide (Lasix);	Loop or thiazide diuretics promote renal clearance and excretion of potassium.
IV glucose with insulin, sodium bicarbonate;	Short-term emergency measure to move potassium into the cell, thus reducing toxic serum level. *Note:* Use with caution in presence of HF or hypernatremia. Use of glucose is contraindicated in patients who are hyperkalemic.
Calcium gluconate;	Temporary stopgap measure that antagonizes toxic potassium depressant effects on heart and stimulates cardiac contractility. *Note:* Calcium is contraindicated in patients on digitalis because it increases the cardiotonic effects of the drug and may cause dysrhythmias.
Sodium polystyrene sulfonate (Kayexalate, SPS suspension), orally, per NG tube, or rectally;	Resin removes potassium by exchanging potassium for sodium or calcium in the GI tract. Sorbitol enhances evacuation. *Note:* Use cautiously in patients with HF, edema, and in the elderly because it increases sodium level. In addition, Kayexalate may cause hyperchloremia.

ACTIONS/INTERVENTIONS	RATIONALE
Collaborative	
β-Adrenergic agonist, e.g., albuterol (Proventil).	Nebulizer administration has been effective in patients receiving hemodialysis, and may also attenuate the hypoglycemic effect of insulin administration.
Infuse potassium-based medication/solutions slowly.	Prevents administration of concentrated bolus, allows time for kidneys to clear excess free potassium.
Provide fresh blood or washed RBCs (when possible) if transfusions required.	Fresh blood has less potassium than banked blood, because breakdown of older RBCs releases potassium.
Prepare for/assist with dialysis (peritoneal or hemodialysis).	May be required when more conservative methods fail or are contraindicated, e.g., severe HF.

Calcium

Calcium is involved in bone formation/reabsorption, neural transmission/muscle contraction, regulation of enzyme systems, and is a coenzyme in blood coagulation. Normal serum levels are 4.5–5.3 mEq/L, 8.5–10.5 mg/dL (total) or 2.1–2.6 mEg/L (ionized). The ionized calcium is physiologically active and clinically important, especially in critically ill patients. The total serum calcium is directly related to the serum albumin, follows it, and must be considered if only total serum readings are available. Some factors that alter the percentage of ionized calcium are changes in pH (affects how much calcium is bound to protein) or increased serum levels of fatty acids, lactate, and bicarbonate.

Hypocalcemia (Calcium Deficit)

PREDISPOSING/CONTRIBUTING FACTORS

Primary or surgical hypoparathyroidism; transient hypocalcemia following thyroidectomy; hyperphosphatemia, hypomagnesemia

Massive subcutaneous tissue infections, acute pancreatitis, burns, peritonitis, malignancies

Excessive GI losses: Draining fistula, diarrhea, fat malabsorption syndromes, chronic laxative use (particularly phosphate-containing laxatives/enemas)

Extreme stress situations with mobilization and excretion of calcium

Diuretic and terminal phase of renal failure

Inadequate dietary intake, lack of milk/vitamin D, excessive protein diet

Alcoholism: Primary effect of ethanol, plus intestinal malabsorption, hypomagnesemia, hypoalbuminemia, and pancreatitis

Use of anticonvulsants, antibiotics, corticosteroids; loop diuretics, drugs that lower serum magnesium (e.g., cisplatin, gentamycin)

Infusion of citrated blood, calcium-free infusions; rapid infusion of Plasmanate

Malignant neoplasms with bone metastases

Alkalotic states

Decreased ultraviolet exposure

Patient Assessment Database

Data depend on duration, severity, and rate of onset of hypocalcemia.

CIRCULATION

May exhibit: Hypotension
Pulses weak/decreased, irregular (weak cardiac contraction/premature dysrhythmias)

ELIMINATION

May report: Diarrhea, abdominal pain
May exhibit: Abdominal distension (paralytic ileus)

FOOD/FLUID

May report: Nausea/vomiting

May exhibit: Difficulty swallowing

HYGIENE

May exhibit: Coarse, dry skin; alopecia (chronic)

NEUROSENSORY

May report: Circumoral paresthesia, numbness and tingling of fingers and toes; muscle cramps

May exhibit: Anxiety, confusion, irritability, alteration in mood, impaired memory, depression, hallucinations, psychoses

Muscle spasms (carpopedal and laryngeal), increased deep-tendon reflexes; tetany, tonic/clonic seizure activity, positive Trousseau's and Chvostek's signs

RESPIRATION

May exhibit: Labored shallow breathing; stridor (spasm of laryngeal muscles)

SAFETY

May exhibit: Bleeding with no or minimal trauma

TEACHING/LEARNING

Refer to predisposing/contributing factors

Discharge plan considerations: **DRG projected mean length of inpatient stay: depends on underlying cause**

May require assistance with changes in therapeutic regimen, dietary management

Refer to plan of care concerning underlying medical/surgical condition for possible considerations after discharge.

DIAGNOSTIC STUDIES

Serum calcium: Decreased, less than 4.5 mEq/L or 8.5 mg/dL (total), 2.1 mEq/L (ionized)

Urine Sulkowitch test: Shows light or no precipitate.

ECG: Prolonged QT interval (characteristic but not necessarily diagnostic). In severe deficiency, T waves may flatten or invert, giving appearance of hypokalemia or myocardial ischemia; ventricular tachycardia may develop.

DESIRED OUTCOMES/EVALUATION CRITERIA—PATIENT WILL:

Electrolyte & Acid-Base Balance (NOC)

Display heart rhythm and laboratory results WNL for patient, absence of neuromuscular irritability, respiratory impairment.

ACTIONS/INTERVENTIONS	RATIONALE
Electrolyte Management: Hypocalcemia (NIC)	
Independent	
Monitor heart rate/rhythm.	Calcium deficit along with associated hypomagnesemia weakens cardiac muscle/contractility.
Assess respiratory rate, rhythm, effort. Have tracheostomy equipment available.	Laryngeal stridor may develop and result in respiratory emergency/arrest.

ACTIONS/INTERVENTIONS

Independent

Observe for neuromuscular irritability, e.g., tetany, seizure activity. Assess for presence of Chvostek's/Trousseau's signs.

Provide quiet environment and seizure precautions as appropriate.

Encourage relaxation/stress reduction techniques, e.g., deep-breathing exercises, guided imagery, visualization.

Check for bleeding from any source (mucous membranes, puncture sites, wounds/incisions, and so on). Note presence of ecchymosis, petechiae.

Review patient's drug regimen, e.g., use of insulin, mithramycin (Mithracin), parathyroid injection, digitalis.

Discuss use of laxatives/antacids.

Review dietary intake of vitamins and fat.

Identify sources to increase calcium and vitamin D in diet, e.g., dairy products, beans, cauliflower, eggs, oranges, pineapples, sardines, shellfish. Restrict intake of phosphorus, e.g., barley, bran, whole wheat, rye, liver, nuts, chocolate.

Encourage use of calcium-containing antacids if needed (e.g., Titralac, Dicarbosil, Tums).

Stress importance of meeting calcium needs.

Collaborative

Assist with identification/treatment of underlying cause.

Monitor laboratory studies, e.g.:

Serum calcium and magnesium; serum albumin, ABGs;

PT, platelets.

Administer the following:

Calcium gluconate/gluceptate/chloride IV;

Oral preparations, e.g., calcium lactate/carbonate;

RATIONALE

Calcium deficit causes repetitive and uncontrolled nerve transmission, leading to muscle spasms and hyperirritability.

Reduces CNS stimulation and protects patient from potential injury.

Tetany can be potentiated by hyperventilation and stress. *Note:* Direct pressure on the nerves (e.g., tightening BP cuff) may also cause tetany.

Alterations in coagulation can occur as a result of calcium deficiency.

Some drugs can lower magnesium levels, affecting calcium level. The effect of digitalis is enhanced by calcium, and, in patients receiving calcium, digitalis intoxication may develop.

Those containing phosphate may negatively affect calcium metabolism.

Insufficient ingestion of vitamin D and fat impairs absorption of calcium.

Vitamin D aids in absorption of calcium from intestinal tract. Phosphorus competes with calcium for intestinal absorption.

Possible sources for oral replacement to help maintain calcium levels, especially in patients at risk for osteoporosis.

Adverse effects of long-term deficiency include tooth decay, eczema, cataracts, and osteoporosis.

Refer to listing of predisposing/contributing factors to determine treatment needs.

Evaluates therapy needs/effectiveness. *Note:* Low serum albumin levels or serum pH affects calcium levels, e.g., a low albumin level causes a deceptively low calcium level; alkalosis causes surplus bicarbonate to bind with free calcium, impairing function; acidosis frees calcium, potentiating hypercalcemia.

Calcium is an essential part of the clotting mechanism and deficit may lead to excessive bleeding.

Provides rapid treatment in acute calcium deficit (especially in presence of tetany/convulsions). *Note:* Calcium chloride is not used as often because it is irritating to the vein and can cause tissue sloughing if it leaks into tissues.

Oral preparations are useful in correcting subacute deficiencies.

GENERAL: Fluid and Electrolyte Imbalances—Calcium

947

ACTIONS/INTERVENTIONS	RATIONALE
Collaborative	
Magnesium sulfate IV/PO if indicated;	Hypomagnesemia is a precipitating factor in calcium deficit.
Vitamin D supplement (e.g., calcitriol).	May be used in combination with calcium therapy to enhance calcium absorption once concomitant phosphate deficiency is corrected.

Hypercalcemia (Calcium Excess)

PREDISPOSING/CONTRIBUTING FACTORS

Hyperparathyroidism, hyperthyroidism, multiple myeloma/other malignancies (e.g., cancer of breast, lung); renal disease, skeletal muscle paralysis, parathyroid tumor, sarcoidosis, adrenal insufficiency, TB

Excessive/prolonged use of vitamins A and D and calcium-containing antacids; prolonged use of thiazide diuretics, theophylline, lithium

Multiple fractures, bone tumors, osteoporosis, osteomalacia, prolonged immobilization causing imbalance between the rate of bone formation and resorption

Milk-alkali syndrome as a side effect of prolonged milk/antacid self-medication for gastric pain/ulcer

Hypophosphatasia, hyperproteinemia

Anticancer drugs, e.g., tamoxifen, androgens/estrogens

Patient Assessment Database

ACTIVITY/REST

May report:	General malaise, fatigue/weakness
	Lethargy
May exhibit:	Incoordination, ataxia

CIRCULATION

May exhibit:	Hypertension
	Irregular pulse, dysrhythmias, bradycardia

ELIMINATION

May report:	Constipation or diarrhea
May exhibit:	Polyuria, nocturia
	Kidney stones/calculi

FOOD/FLUID

May report:	Anorexia, nausea/vomiting
	Thirst
	Abdominal pain
May exhibit:	Poor skin turgor, dry mucous membranes

NEUROSENSORY

May report:	Headache
May exhibit:	Hypotonicity/muscular relaxation, flaccid paralysis, depressed/absent deep-tendon reflexes
	Drowsiness, apathy, paranoia, personality changes, decreased attention span, memory loss, depression, inappropriate/bizarre behaviors, psychosis, confusion, stupor/coma
	Slurred speech

PAIN/DISCOMFORT

May report:	Epigastric, deep flank pain, or bone/joint pain

TEACHING/LEARNING

Refer to predisposing/contributing factors

Discharge plan considerations: **DRG projected mean length of inpatient stay: dependent on underlying cause**
May require assistance with changes in therapeutic regimen, dietary management

Refer to plan of care concerning underlying medical/surgical condition for possible considerations after discharge.

DIAGNOSTIC STUDIES

Serum calcium: Increased, greater than 2.6 mEq/L (ionized) or 10.5 mg/dL (total).

BUN: Increased (calculi can damage kidney).

Serum phosphorus: Decreased levels may be noted.

Urine Sulkowitch test: Shows heavy precipitate.

Urine calcium: Increased.

Urine osmolality: Decreased.

Urine specific gravity: Decreased.

X-ray: May reveal evidence of bone cavitation, pathological fracture, osteoporosis, urinary calculi.

ECG changes: Shortened QT interval, inverted T waves. In severe deficit, QRS may widen, PR interval lengthen, and ventricular prematurities develop.

DESIRED OUTCOMES/EVALUATION CRITERIA—PATIENT WILL:

Electrolyte & Acid-Base Balance (NOC)

Display heart rhythm, muscle strength, cognitive status, and laboratory results WNL for patient.

ACTIONS/INTERVENTIONS	RATIONALE
Electrolyte Management: Hypercalcemia (NIC)	
Independent	
Monitor cardiac rate/rhythm. Be aware that cardiac arrest can occur in hypercalcemic crisis.	Overstimulation of cardiac muscle occurs with resultant dysrhythmias and ineffective cardiac contraction. Sinus bradycardia, sinus dysrhythmias, wandering pacemaker, and AV block may be noted. Hypercalcemia creates a predisposition to cardiac arrest.
Assess level of consciousness and neuromuscular status, e.g., muscle movement, strength, tone.	Nerve and muscle activity is depressed. Lethargy and fatigue can progress to convulsion/coma.
Monitor I&O; calculate fluid balance.	Efforts to correct original condition may result in secondary imbalances/complications.
Encourage fluid intake of 3–4 L/day, including sodium-containing fluids, (within cardiac tolerance) and use of acid-ash juices, e.g., cranberry and prune if kidney stones present or suspected.	Reduces dehydration, encourages urinary flow and clearance of calcium, reduces risk of stone formation. *Note:* Sodium favors calcium excretion and can be used if not contraindicated by other conditions.
Strain urine if flank pain occurs.	Large amount of calcium present in kidney parenchyma may lead to stone formation.
Auscultate bowel sounds.	Hypotonicity leads to constipation when the smooth muscle tone is inadequate to produce peristalsis.
Maintain bulk in diet.	Constipation may be a problem because of decreased GI tone.

949

ACTIONS/INTERVENTIONS	RATIONALE
Independent	
Encourage frequent repositioning and ROM and/or muscle-setting exercises with caution. Promote ambulation if patient is able.	Muscle activity may reduce calcium shifting from the bones that occurs during immobilization. *Note:* Increased risk for pathological fractures exists because of calcium shifts out of the bones.
Provide safety measures, e.g., gentle handling when moving/transferring patient.	Reduces risk of injury/pathological fractures.
Review drug regimen, noting use of calcium-elevating drugs, e.g., heparin, tetracyclines, methicillin, phenytoin.	May affect drug choice or require reduction in oral sources of calcium.
Identify/restrict sources of calcium intake, e.g., dairy products, eggs, and spinach; calcium-containing antacids (Titralac, Dicarbosil, Tums).	Foods or drugs containing calcium may need to be limited in chronic conditions causing hypercalcemia.
Collaborative	
Assist with identification/treatment of underlying cause.	Refer to listing of predisposing/contributing factors to determine treatment needs.
Monitor laboratory studies, e.g., calcium, magnesium, phosphate.	Monitors therapy needs/effectiveness. *Note:* Phosphate levels may be low when parathyroid hormone inversely promotes calcium uptake and calcium competes with phosphate for absorption/transport with vitamin D.
Administer isotonic saline and sodium sulfate IV/orally.	Emergency measures in severe hypercalcemia used to dilute extracellular calcium concentration and inhibit tubular reabsorption of calcium, thereby increasing urinary excretion.
Administer medications as indicated:	
Diuretics, e.g., furosemide (Lasix);	Diuresis promotes renal excretion of calcium and reduces risks of fluid excess from isotonic saline infusion.
Sodium bicarbonate;	Induces alkalosis, thereby reducing the ionized calcium fraction.
Phosphate;	Rapid-acting agent that induces calcium excretion and inhibits resorption of bone.
Glucocorticoid therapy;	Inhibits intestinal absorption of calcium and reduces inflammation and associated stress response that mobilizes calcium from the bone.
Mithramycin (Mithracin);	Cytotoxic antibiotic that lowers serum calcium by inhibiting inappropriate bone resorption, typically seen in malignancies or hyperparathyroidism.
Disodium edetate (EDTA);	Chelating action lowers serum calcium level.
Calcitonin;	Promotes movement of serum calcium into bones, temporarily reducing serum calcium levels, especially in the presence of increased parathyroid hormone.
Neutra-Phos, Fleet Phospho-Soda.	These drugs bind calcium in the GI tract, promoting excretion.
Prepare for/assist with hemodialysis.	Rapid reduction of serum calcium may be necessary to correct life-threatening situation.

Magnesium

Magnesium influences carbohydrate metabolism, secretion of parathyroid hormone, sodium/potassium transport across the cell membrane, and synthesis of protein and nucleic acid. Magnesium activates adenosine triphosphate (ATP) and mediates neural transmission within the CNS. Magnesium deficit is often associated with hypokalemia and promotes intracellular potassium loss and sodium accumulation, altering and exacerbating membrane excitability. Normal serum range is 1.5–2.5 mEq/L or 1.8–3.0 mg/dL.

Hypomagnesemia (Magnesium Deficit)

PREDISPOSING/CONTRIBUTING FACTORS

GI losses: Biliary/intestinal fistula; surgery (bowel resection, small-bowel bypass); severe, protracted diarrhea, laxative abuse, impaired GI absorption/malabsorption syndrome, gastric/colon cancer, prolonged gastric suction

Protein/calorie malnutrition; feeding (enteral or parenteral) without adequate magnesium replacement

Prolonged IV infusion of magnesium-free solutions, multiple transfusions with citrated blood products

Chronic alcoholism, alcohol withdrawal; pancreatitis

Hyperaldosteronism: Primary or secondary (e.g., cirrhosis or HF)

Toxemia of pregnancy

Renal losses: Severe renal disease/diuretic phase of ARF; vigorous and/or prolonged diuresis with mercurial thiazides or loop diuretics; SIADH

Drugs that affect magnesium balance: Aminoglycosides (gentamicin, tobramycin), antifungals (amphotericin B); chemotherapy agents (cisplatin); antirejection agents (cyclosporine), and excessive doses of calcium or vitamin D supplements

Diabetic ketoacidosis, malignancies causing hypercalcemic states, severe burns, sepsis, hypothermia; hypoparathyroidism, hypercalcemia, hyperthyroidism

Patient Assessment Database

ACTIVITY/REST

May report: Generalized weakness, insomnia
Ataxia, vertigo

CIRCULATION

May exhibit: Tachycardia, dysrhythmias
Hypotension (vasodilation); occasional hypertension

FOOD/FLUID

May report: Anorexia, nausea/vomiting, diarrhea

NEUROSENSORY

May report: Paresthesia (legs, feet)
Vertigo

May exhibit: Nystagmus
Musculoskeletal fasciculations/tremors, neuromuscular irritability/spasticity, spontaneous carpopedal spasms, hyperactive deep tendon reflexes, clonus
Tetany, convulsions; positive Babinski's, Chvostek's, and Trousseau's signs
Disorientation, apathy, depression, irritability, agitation, hallucinations/psychoses, coma

TEACHING/LEARNING

Refer to predisposing/contributing factors

Discharge plan considerations: **DRG projected mean length of inpatient stay: dependent on underlying cause**
May require assistance with changes in therapeutic regimen, dietary management

Refer to plan of care concerning underlying medical/surgical condition for possible postdischarge considerations.

DIAGNOSTIC STUDIES

Serum magnesium: Decreased, less than 1.5 mEq/L or 1.8 mg/dL. (Usually symptoms do not appear until level is less than 1 mEq/L.)

Calcium: May be decreased, unless there is a hypercalcemic condition causing the magnesium deficit.

Potassium: Decrease associated with severe hypomagnesemia.

ECG: Prolonged PR and QT intervals, widened QRS complex, ST segment depression, T wave inversion.

DESIRED OUTCOMES/EVALUATION CRITERIA—PATIENT WILL:

Electrolyte & Acid/Base Balance (NOC)

Display heart rate/rhythm, muscle strength, cognitive status, and laboratory results WNL for patient, absence of neuromuscular irritability.

ACTIONS/INTERVENTIONS	RATIONALE
Electrolyte Management: Hypomagnesemia (NIC)	
Independent	
Monitor cardiac rate/rhythm, noting tachydysrhythmias and characteristic ECG changes.	Magnesium influences sodium/potassium transport across the cell membrane and affects excitability of cardiac tissue.
Monitor for signs of digitalis intoxication when used (e.g., reports of nausea/vomiting, blurred vision; increasing atrial dysrhythmias and heart block).	Magnesium deficit may precipitate digitalis toxicity.
Assess level of consciousness and neuromuscular status, e.g., movement, strength, reflexes/tone; note presence of Chvostek's/Trousseau's signs.	Confusion, irritability, and psychosis may occur. However, more common manifestations are muscular, e.g., hyperactive deep tendon reflexes, muscle tremors, spasticity, generalized tetany.
Monitor status of airway and swallowing.	Laryngeal stridor and dysphagia can occur when depletion is moderate to severe.
Take seizure/safety precautions, e.g., padded side rails, bed in low position, frequent observation as indicated.	Changes in mentation or the development of seizure activity in severe hypomagnesemia increases the risk of patient injury.
Provide quiet environment and subdued lighting.	Reduces extraneous stimuli; promotes rest.
Encourage ROM exercises as tolerated.	Reduces deleterious effects of muscle weakness/spasticity.
Place footboard/cradle on bed.	Elevation of linens may reduce spasms.
Auscultate bowel sounds.	Muscle weakness/spasticity may reduce peristalsis and bowel function.
Encourage intake of dairy products, whole grains, green leafy vegetables, meat, and fish.	Provides oral replacement for mild magnesium deficits; may prevent recurrence.
Instruct patient in proper use of laxatives and diuretics.	Deficit may be the result of abuse of these drugs.
Observe for signs of magnesium toxicity during replacement therapy, e.g., thirst, feeling hot and flushed, diaphoresis, anxiety, drowsiness, hypotension, increased muscular and nervous system irritability, loss of patellar reflex.	Rapid, excessive IV replacement may lead to toxicity and life-threatening complications.

ACTIONS/INTERVENTIONS	RATIONALE

Collaborative

Assist with identification/treatment of underlying cause.	Refer to listing of predisposing/contributing factors. *Note:* Studies have shown that chronic alcoholism with malnutrition is the most common cause of hypomagnesemia in the United States.
Monitor laboratory studies, e.g., serum magnesium, calcium, and potassium levels.	Evaluates therapy needs/effectiveness. *Note:* These electrolytes are interrelated, symptoms may be similar, and deficits of more than one may be present.

Administer medications as indicated:

Magnesium sulfate or magnesium chloride IV, monitoring administration closely;	IV replacement is preferred in severe deficit because absorption of magnesium from intestinal tract varies inversely with calcium absorption. However, potential for drug interaction with digitalis preparations may lead to increased cardiac dysrhythmias/heart block. *Note:* Calcium gluconate is the antidote should hypermagnesemia be evidenced by depressed deep tendon reflexes or respiratory depression and hypotension (late sign).
Magnesium sulfate IM, or magnesium hydroxide PO (Amphojel, Milk of Magnesia);	May be given for mild deficit or in nonemergent situations. Injections should be deep IM to decrease local tissue reaction.
Magnesium-based antacids, e.g., Mylanta, Maalox, Gelusil, Riopan.	Can supplement dietary replacement. *Note:* Use of these products may cause diarrhea, which can be alleviated by concurrent use of aluminum-containing products, e.g., Amphojel, Basaljel.

Hypermagnesemia (Magnesium Excess)

PREDISPOSING/CONTRIBUTING FACTORS

Reduced renal function (e.g., acute processes or age), chronic renal disease/failure; or dialysis with hard water

Excessive intake/absorption: e.g., too-rapid replacement of magnesium (as in pregnancy-induced hypertension or premature labor), excessive use of magnesium-containing drugs/products, e.g., Maalox, Milk of Magnesia, Epsom salts

Untreated diabetic ketoacidosis

Hyperparathyroidism, aldosterone deficiency, adrenal insufficiency

Extracellular fluid volume depletion (e.g., after diuretic abuse)

Salt-water near-drowning, hypothermia, shock

Chronic diarrhea; diseases that interfere with gastric absorption

Patient Assessment Database

ACTIVITY/REST

May report:	Generalized weakness, fatigue
May exhibit:	Drowsiness, lethargy, stupor

CIRCULATION

May exhibit:	Hypotension (mild to severe)
	Pulses weak/irregular, bradycardia (12–15 mEq/L), cardiac arrest (greater than 25 mEq/L)

FOOD/FLUID

May report:	Nausea/vomiting

NEUROSENSORY

May exhibit: Depressed deep tendon reflexes (7–10 mEq/L) progressing to flaccid paralysis
Decreased level of consciousness, lethargy progressing to coma
Slurred speech

RESPIRATION

May exhibit: Hypoventilation progressing to apnea (12–15 mEq/L)

SAFETY

May exhibit: Skin flushing, sweating

TEACHING/LEARNING

Refer to predisposing/contributing factors

Discharge plan considerations: **DRG projected mean length of inpatient stay: depends on underlying cause**
May require assistance with changes in therapeutic regimen, dietary management

Refer to plan of care concerning underlying medical/surgical condition for possible considerations after discharge.

DIAGNOSTIC STUDIES

Serum magnesium: Symptomatic levels greater than 3 mEq/L (increase to 10–20 mEq/L results in respiratory depression, coma, and cardiac arrest).
ECG: Prolonged PR and QT intervals, wide QRS, elevated T waves, development of heart block, cardiac arrest.

DESIRED OUTCOMES/EVALUATION CRITERIA—PATIENT WILL:

Electrolyte & Acid/Base Balance (NOC)

Display heart rhythm, muscular strength, cognitive status and laboratory results WNL for patient, absence of respiratory impairment.

ACTIONS/INTERVENTIONS	RATIONALE
Electrolyte Management: Hypermagnesemia (NIC)	
Independent	
Monitor cardiac rate/rhythm.	Bradycardia and heart block may develop, progressing to cardiac arrest as a direct result of hypermagnesemia on cardiac muscle.
Monitor BP.	Hypotension unexplained by other causes is an early sign of toxicity.
Assess level of consciousness and neuromuscular status, e.g., reflexes/tone, movement, strength.	CNS and neuromuscular depression can cause decreasing level of alertness, progressing to coma, and depressed muscular responses, progressing to flaccid paralysis.
Monitor respiratory rate/depth/rhythm. Encourage cough/deep-breathing exercises. Elevate head of bed as indicated.	Neuromuscular transmissions are blocked by magnesium excess, resulting in respiratory muscular weakness and hypoventilation, which may progress to apnea.
Check patellar reflexes periodically.	Absence of these reflexes suggest magnesium levels about 7 mEq/L or greater. If untreated, cardiac/respiratory arrest can occur.

ACTIONS/INTERVENTIONS

Independent

Encourage increased fluid intake if appropriate.

Monitor urinary output and 24-hr fluid balance.

Promote bedrest, assist with personal care activities as needed.

Recommend avoidance of magnesium-containing antacids, e.g., Maalox, Mylanta, Gelusil, Riopan, in patient with renal disease. Caution patients with renal disease to avoid OTC drug use without first discussing with healthcare provider.

Collaborative

Assist with identification/treatment of underlying cause.

Monitor laboratory studies as indicated, e.g.,: serum magnesium and calcium levels.

Administer IV fluids and thiazide diuretics as indicated.

Administer 10% calcium chloride or gluconate IV.

Assist with dialysis as needed.

RATIONALE

Increased hydration enhances magnesium excretion, but fluid intake must be cautious in event of renal/cardiac failure.

Renal failure is the primary contributing factor in hypermagnesemia; and, if it is present, fluid excess can easily occur.

Flaccid paralysis, lethargy, and decreased mentation reduce activity tolerance/ability.

Limits oral intake to help prevent hypermagnesemia.

Refer to listing of predisposing/contributing factors to determine treatment needs. *Note:* Most frequently occurs in patients with advanced renal failure.

Evaluates therapy needs/effectiveness.

Promotes renal clearance of magnesium (if renal function is normal).

Antagonizes action/reverses symptoms of magnesium toxicity to improve neuromuscular function.

In the presence of renal disease/failure, dialysis may be needed to lower serum levels.

Bibliography

General

Books

Berkow, R (ed): *The Merck Manual,* ed 16, Merck & Co, Rahway, NJ, 1992.

Carey, CF, Lee, HH, and Woeltje, KF: *The Washington Manual of Medical Therapeutics,* ed 29, Lippincott-Raven, Philadelphia, 1998.

Carpenito, L: *Nursing Diagnosis: Application to Clinical Practice,* ed 6, JB Lippincott, Philadelphia, 1995.

Carnevali, DL, and Thomas, MD: *Diagnostic Reasoning and Treatment Decision-Making in Nursing,* JB Lippincott, Philadelphia, 1993.

Condon, RE, and Nyhus, LM (eds): *Manual of Surgical Therapeutics,* ed 9, Little, Brown, Boston, 1996.

Cox, H, et al: *Clinical Applications of Nursing Diagnosis: Adult, Child, Women's, Psychiatric, Gerontic and Home Health Considerations,* ed 3, FA Davis, Philadelphia, 1997.

Deglin, JH, and Vallerand, AH: *Davis's Drug Guide for Nurses,* ed 6, FA Davis, Philadelphia, 1999.

Doenges, ME, and Moorhouse, MF: *Nurse's Pocket Guide: Nursing Diagnoses with Interventions,* ed 6, FA Davis, Philadelphia, 1997.

Guyton, AC: *Textbook of Medical Physiology,* ed 8, WB Saunders, Philadelphia, 1991.

Jaffe, MS, and McVan, BF: *Laboratory and Diagnostic Test Handbook.* FA Davis, Philadelphia, 1997.

Johnson, M, and Maas, M: *Nursing Outcomes Classification (NOC),* Mosby, St Louis, 1997.

Lipson, JG, et al: *Culture & Nursing Care: A Pocket Guide.* UCSF Nursing Press, Univ of California 1996.

Matthewson-Kuhn, M: *Pharmacotherapeutics: A Nursing Process Approach,* ed 3, FA Davis, Philadelphia, 1994.

McCance, KL, and Huether, SE: *Pathophysiology: The Biologic Basis for Disease in Adults and Children,* ed 6, Mosby, St Louis, 1996.

McClosky, JC, and Bulechek, GM (eds): *Nursing Interventions Classification (NIC),* ed 2, Mosby, St Louis, 1996.

Metheny, NM: *Fluid and Electrolyte Balance: Nursing Considerations,* ed 2, JB Lippincott, Philadelphia, 1992.

NANDA: *Nursing Diagnoses: Definitions and Classifications,* North American Nursing Diagnosis Association, St Louis, 1999.

Purnell, LD, and Paulanka, BJ: *Transcultural Health Care: A Culturally Competent Approach,* FA Davis, Philadelphia, 1998.

Sommers, MS, and Johnson, SA: *Davis's Manual of Nursing Therapeutics for Diseases and Disorders,* FA Davis, Philadelphia, 1997.

Articles

Brenner, ZR, and Cannito, M: *Administering steroids successfully.* Nursing98, 28(3):34, March 1998.

Buckle, J: *Alternative/complementary therapies.* Crit Care Nurs, 18(5):54, October 1998.

Cataldo, R: *Decoding the mystery: Evaluating complemetary and alternative medicine.* Rehab Management, 12(2):42, February/March 1999.

Complementary Therapies, Imprint, February/March, 1999.

Dossey, BM, and Dossey, L: *Body-Mind-Spirit: Attending to holistic care.* AJN, 98(8):35, August 1998.

Dossey, BM: *Holistic modalities & healing moments.* AJN, 998(6):44, June 1998.

Drugs that bring erections down. Sex & Health, p 5, May 1998.

Helmlinger, C, and Williams, J: *Advanced practice nursing defined.* AJN, 97(2):62, February 1997.

Hoffman, J: *Tuning in to the power of music.* RN, 60(6):52, June 1997.

Hussar, DA: *New drugs, part III.* Nursing97, 27(7):56, July 1997.

Hussar, DA: *New Drugs98, part IV.* Nursing98, 28(7):36, July 1998.

Maxwell, J: *The gentle power of acupressure.* RN, 60(4):53, April 1997.

Parkman, CA, and Calfee, BE: *Advance directives, honoring your patient's end-of-life wishes.* Nursing97, 27(4):48, April 1997.

Saba, VK: *Home Health Care Classification (HHCC) System.* Georgetown University School of Nursing, Washington DC.

Journals

American Journal of Critical Care
American Journal of Continuing Care
American Journal of Nursing (AJN)
Case Manager
Critical Care Nurse
Holistic Nursing Practice
HomeCare Provider
Image: Journal of Nursing Scholarship
Imprint: The Professional Magazine for Nursing Students
Inside MS
Internal Medicine
Journal of the American College of Surgeons
Journal of the American Medical Association (JAMA)
Journal of the American Medical Informatics Association
Journal of the Association of Nurses in AIDS Care (JANAC)
Journal of Legal Nurse Consulting

Journal of Neurology
Journal of Parental and Enteral Nutrition (JPEN)
Journal of Psychosocial Nursing
Journal of School Nursing
Journal of Trauma, Injury, Infection, and Critical Care
Nursing96–Nursing99
Nursing Diagnosis: The Journal of Nursing Language and Classification
Nursing Times
Rehab Management
Rehabilitation Nursing
RN
Seminars in Oncology Nursing
Sexuality and Disability
Team Rehab

Chapter 1

Books

Henry, SB, and Mead, CN: *Evaluating standardized coding and classification systems for clinical practice: A critical review of the nursing literature in the United States,* in Nursing Informatics, (U. Gerdin, et al, eds), IOS Press, 1997.

Articles

Bernardo, A: *Technology and true presence in nursing.* Holis Nurs Pract, 12(4):40, July 1998.
Blair, C: *Advanced practice nurses as entrepreneurs.* AJN, 97(11):16, November 1997.
Bowles, KH, and Naylor, MD: *Nursing interventions classification systems:* Image J Nurs Sch, 28(4):303, Winter 1996.
Ditillo, BA: *Switching gears to primary care.* AJN, 98(5):16K, May 1998.
Haber, J: *Medicare reimbursement: A victory for APRNs.* AJN, 97(11)84, November 1997.
Hammond, WE: *Call for a standard clinical vocabulary:* J Am Med Informatics Assoc, 4(3), May/June 1997.
Happ, MB: *Treatment interference in acutely and critically ill adults.* Am J Crit Care, 7(3):224, May 1998.
Hardiker, NR, and Rector, AL: *Modeling nursing terminology using the GRAIL representation language.* JAMA, 5(1):120, January/February 1998.
Hunt, R: *Community-based nursing.* AJN, 98(10):44, 1998.
Keegan, L: *Getting comfortable with alternative & complementary therapies.* Nursing98, 28(4):50, April 1998.
Lee, SS: *The emerging role of case managers as business leaders.* Continuing Care, 17(5):23, May 1998.
Murphy, MD, and Yody, BB: *Achieving a balance—rehabilitation in the home focuses on patients' abilities and payer expectations.* Continuing Care, 17(8):28, 1998.
Newswatch clinical highlights: More good news for HIV patients. RN, 61(3):18, March 1998.
Ozbolt, JG, Fruchtnight, JN, and Hayden, JR: *Toward data standards for clinical nursing information.* J Am Med Informatics Assoc, 1(2):175, March/Aprl 1994.
Scanlon, C: *Defining standards for end-of-life care.* AJN, 97(11):58, November 1997.
Schraeder, C, et al: *Community nursing organizations: A new frontier.* AJN, 97(1):63, January 1997.
Shindul-Rothschild, J, Berry, D, and Long-Middleton, E: *Where have all the nurses gone? Final results of our patient care survey.* AJN, 96(11):25, November 1996.
Shogren, D, Calkins, A, and Wilburn, S: *Restructuring may be hazardous to your health.* AJN, 96(11):64, November 1996.

Chapter 2

Books

American Nurses Association: *Nursing's Social Policy Statement,* Washington, DC, 1995.
American Nurses Association: *Standards of Clinical Nursing Practice,* Kansas City, MO, 1991.
Doenges, ME, Moorhouse, MF, and Burley, J: *Application of Nursing Process and Nursing Diagnosis,* ed 2, FA Davis, Philadelphia, 1995.
Leuner, JD, et al: *Mastering the Nursing Process: A Case Study Approach,* FA Davis, Philadelphia, 1990.

Articles

Brooks, KL: *Critical thinking in clinical practice.* Holistic Nursing Practice 7(3), April 1993.

Chapter 3

Books

Lampe, SS: *Focus Charting,* ed 7, Creative Nursing Management, Minneapolis, 1998.

Articles

Drass, JA, and Peterson, A: *Type II diabetes: Exploring treatment options.* AJN, 96(11):45, November 1996.
Fishman, TD, Freedline, AD, and Kahn, D: *Putting the best foot forward.* Nursing96, 26(1):58, January 1996.
Flemin, DR: *Challenging traditional insulin injection practices.* AJN, 99(2):72, February 1999.

Halpin-Landry, JE, and Goldsmith, S: *Feet first: Diabetes care.* AJN, 99(2):26, February 1999.
Nunnelee, JD: *Healing venous ulcers.* RN, 60(11):38, November 1997.
Sinacore, DR: *Managing the diabetic foot.* Rehab Management, 11(4):60, June/July 1998.

Chapter 4

Articles

Atrial fibrillation, when a fluttering heart needs attention. Harvard Health Letter, 23(11):6, September 1998.
Bernat, JJ: *Smoothing CABG patient's road to recovery.* AJN, 97(2):23, February 1997.
Blood pressure, tailoring hypertension treatment. Harvard Women's Health Watch, VI(1):2, September 1998.
Carbone, LM: *An interdisciplinary approach to the rehabilitation of open-heart surgical patients.* Rehab Nurs, 24(2):55, March/April 1999.
Casey, K, Bedker, D, and Roussel-McElmeel, PL: *Myocardial infarction: Review of clinical trials and treatment strategies.* Crit Care Nurse, 18(2):39, April 1998.
Cerrato, PL: *New acute MI guidelines.* RN, 60(1):25, January 1997.
Chase, S: *Antiarrhythmics.* RN, 60(5):41, May 1997.
Chase, S: *Antihypertensives.* RN, 60(6):32, June 1997.
Chase, S: *Lipid-lowering agents.* RN, 60(9):47, September 1997.
Clearing up confusion about hypertension drugs. Harvard Health Letter, 23(12):4, October 1998.
Davenport, J, and Morton, PG: *Identifying nonischemic causes of life-threatening arrhythmias.* AJN, 97(11):50, November 1997.
Gibbar-Clements, T, Shirrell, D, and Free, C: *Seeing beyond the numbers.* Nursing97, 27(7):49, July 1997.
Hayden, AM: *Transmyocardial revascularization.* RN, 61(5):44, May 1998.
Hayes, DD: *Bradycardia, keeping the current flowing.* Nursing97, 27(6):50, June 1997.
Huerta-Torres, V: *Preparing patients for early discharge after CABG.* AJN, 98(5):49, May 1998.
Konick-McMahan, J: *Discharged with dobutamine.* RN, 60(4):25, April 1997.
Kruse, L, et al: *Keeping pace with implanted defibrillator.* RN, 61(8):30, August 1998.
Kuncl, N, and Nelson, KM: *Antihypertensive drugs, balancing risks and benefits.* Nursing97, 27(8):46.
Lindsay, M: *Frequency of cerebrovascular accident after cardiac surgery.* Crit Care Nurse, 18(5):19, October 1998.
Riley, M: *Elective cardioversion, Who, when, and how.* RN, 60(5):27, May 1997.
Schulmeister, L: *Pacemakers & environmental safety.* Nursing98, 28(7):58, July 1998.
Simko, LC, and Lockhart, JS: *Heparin-induced thrombocytopenia and thrombosis.* Nursing96, 26(3):33, March 1996.
Smatlak, P, and Knebel, AR: *Clinical evaluation of noninvasive monitoring of oxygen saturation in critically ill patients.* Am J Crit Care, 7(5):370, September 1998.
Spadoni, S: *Getting to the heart of IABP therapy.* RN, 60(1):39, January 1997.
Wallace, CJ: *Dual-chamber pacemakers in the management of severe heart failure.* Crit Care Nurse, 18(2):57, April 1998.
Weeks, SM: *Caring for patients with heart failure.* Nursing96, 26(3):52, March 1996.
Whelton, PK, et al: *Sodium reduction and weight loss in the treatment of hypertension in older persons.* JAMA, 279(11):839, November 1998.
Zevola, DR, et al: *Clinical pathways and coronary artery bypass surgery.* Crit Care Nurse, 17(6):20, December 1997.

Chapter 5

Articles

Ackerman, MH, and Mick, DJ: *Instillation of normal saline before suctioning patients with pulmonary infections: A prospective randomized controlled trial.* Am J Crit Care, 7(4):261, July 1998.
Aerosolized artificial surfactant for chronic bronchitis. AJN, 97(12):57, December 1997.
Asthma drug now indicated for COPD. AJN, 98(5):54, May 1998.
Boucher, MA: *When laryngectomy complicates care.* RN, 59(88):40, August 1996.
Canales, MAP: *Asthma management, putting your patient on the team.* Nursing97, 27(12):33, December 1997.
Carroll, P: *Closing in on safer suctioning.* RN, 61(5):22, May 1998.
Carroll, P: *Preventing nosocomial pneumonia.* RN, 61(6):44, June 1998.
Carroll, P: *Pulse oximetry—at your fingertips.* RN, 60(2):22, February 1997.
Carroll, P: *Tradition or science? Spotting the difference in respiratory care.* RN, 59(5):26, May 1996.
Carroll, P: *When you WANT humidity.* RN, 60(5):31, May 1997.
Consult Stat: *Chest tubes: When you don't need a seal.* RN, 61(3):67, March 1998.
Field, KW, and Vezeau, TM: *Nursing interventions for MDR-TB.* AJN, 98(6):16E, June 1998.
Hanson, MJS: *Caring for a patient with COPD.* Nursing97, 27(12):39, December 1997.
Kanachki, L: *How to guide ventilator-dependent patients from hospital to home.* AJN, 97(2):37, February 1997.
Kurx, JM: *Severe postop hyponatremia in young women.* AJN, 97(10):16D, October 1997.
Matthews, PJ: *Ventilator-associated infections: Reducing the risks, part 1.* Nursing97, 27(2):59, February 1997.
Middleton, AD: *Managing asthma: It takes teamwork.* AJN, 97(1):39, January 1997.
O'Hanlon-Nichols, T: *Basic assessment series: The adult pulmonary system,* AJN, 98(2)39, February 1998.
Photo Guide Adapted from Nurses' PhotoLibrary. Springhouse. *Dressing up for a change: Chest tube insertion site.* Nursing96, 26(7):44, July 1996.
Sharbaugh, RJ: *Administering and interpreting the PPD tuberculin skin test.* Home Care Provider, 3(3):141, June 1998.
Skelskey, C, and Leshem, OA: *Tuberculosis surveillance in long-term care.* AJN 97(10):16, October 1997.
Trupka, A, et al: *Value of thoracic computed tomography in the first assessment of severely injured patients with blunt chest trauma: Results of a prospective study.* Journal of Trauma, Injury, Infection, and Critical Care, 43(3):405, September 1997.

Chapter 6

Books

Traumatic Brain Injury Medical Treatment Guidelines, State of Colorado Labor and Employment, Division of Worker's Compensation, March 15, 1998.

Articles

Arbour, R: *Aggressive management of intracranial dynamics.* Crit Care Nurs, 18(3):30, June 1998.

Apspack, G: *Stroke in women: Ask not for whom the scale tips.* Crit Care Nurse, 17(4):12, August 1997.

Barher, E: *The xenon CT: A new neuro tool.* RN, 61(2):22, February 1998.

Berkowitz, C: *Epidural pain control—your job, too.* RN, 60(8):22, August 1997.

Birkett, DP: *What is the relationship between stroke and depression.* Harvard Mental Health Letter, 14(12):8, January 1998.

Code stroke: Using t-PA to prevent ischemic brain injury. AJN, 97(11):16, November 1997.

Grzankowski, JA: *Altered thought processes related to traumatic brain injury and their nursing implications.* Rehab Nurs, 22(1):24, January/February 1997.

Halper, J, and Holland, N: *Meeting the challenge of multiple sclerosis, part I.* AJN, 98(10):26, October 1998.

Halper, J, and Holland, N: *Meeting the challenge of multiple sclerosis, part II.* AJN, 98(11):8, 39, November 1998.

Hayn, MA, and Fisher, TR: *Stroke rehabilitation: Salvaging ability after the storm.* Nursing97, 27(3):40, March 1997.

Huston, CJ: *Emergency! Cervical spine injury.* AJN, 98(6):33, June 1998.

Flannery, J: *Using the levels of cognitive functioning assessment scale with traumatic brain injury in an acute care setting.* Rehab Nurs, 23(2):88, March/April 1998.

Frozena, C: *Multiple sclerosis.* AJN, 97(11):48, November 1997.

Johnson, J, Pearson, V, and McDivitt, L: *Stroke rehabilitation: Assessing stroke survivors' long-term learning needs.* Rehab Nurs, 22(5):243, September/October 1997.

Kachourbos, MJ: *Relief at last: An implanted bladder control system helps people control their bodily functions.* Team Rehab Reports, August 1997, p 31.

Kirshblum, S, and O'Connor, K: *The problem of pain: A common condition of people with SCI.* TeamRehab Reports, August 1997, p 15.

McConnel, E: *Preventing transient increases in intracranial pressure.* Nursing98, 28(4):66, April 1998.

McHale, JM, et al: *Expert nursing knowledge in the care of patients at risk of impaired swallowing.* Image J Nurs Sch, 30(2):137, Second Quarter 1998.

McNew, C, et al: *How to help your patient with epilepsy.* Nursing97, 27(9):57, September 1997.

Mower, DM: *Brain attack: Treating acute ischemic CVA.* Nursing97, 27(3):34, March 1997.

Ozuna, J: *Action Stat: Status epilepticus.* Nursing97, 27(12):47, December 1997.

Riedel, D, and Shaw, V: *Nursing management of patients with brain injury requiring one-on-one care.* Rehab Nurs, 22(1):36, January/February 1997.

Schaf, D: *Common questions about transient ischemic attacks.* AJN, 97(1):16BB, October 1997.

Schwamm, LH: *What you need to know about strokes.* HealthNews, June 1, 1998.

A second interferon option for MS treatment. AJN, 97(1):61, January 1997.

Sherkin-Langer, F: *Sex and women's M.S. symptoms.* Inside MS, 16(2):17, Summer 1998.

Society recommendations on the new MS drugs. Inside MS, 13(3):32, Fall 1998.

Travers, PL: *Poststroke dysphagia: Implications for nurses.* Rehab Nurs, 24(2):69, March/April 1999.

Wende, KE: *The future looks bright: New research brings hope for treating multiple sclerosis.* Rehab Management, 12(2):22. February/March 1999.

Wiens, ME, Reimer, MA, and Guyn, HL: *Music therapy as a treatment method for improving respiratory muscle strength in patients with advanced multiple sclerosis: A pilot study.* Rehab Nurs, 24(2):74, March/April 1999.

Wilson, M: *Thrombolytic therapy in stroke management.* Crit Care Nurs, 17(5):89, October 1997.

Wright, C: *A brief update on stroke.* AJN, 98(5):62, May 1998.

Chapter 7

Articles

Aronson, B: *Update on peptic ulcer drugs.* AJN, 98(1):41, January 1998.

Bradley, M, and Pupiales, M: *Essential elements of ostomy care.* AJN, 97(7):38, July 1997.

Coping with Crohn's disease. HealthNews, 4(11):4, September 10, 1998.

Dunne, D: *Common questions about ileoanal reservoirs.* AJN, 97(11):67, November 1997.

Epps, CK: *The delicate business of ostomy care.* RN, 59(11):32, November 1996.

Fitzpatrick, L, and Fitzpatrick, T: *Blood transfusion: Keeping your patient safe.* Nursing97, 27(8):34, August 1997.

Giacchino, S, and Houdek, D: *Ruptured varices! Act fast.* RN, 61(5):33, May 1998.

Gibbar-Clements, T, Shirrell, D, and Free, C: *PT and APTT: Seeing beyond the numbers.* Nursing98, 27(7):49, July 1997.

Golub, R, Siddiqui, F, and Pohl, D: *Laporoscopic versus open appendectomy: A meta-analysis.* J Am Coll Surg, 186(5):545, May 1998.

Heslin, JM: *Peptic ulcer disease: Making a case against the prime suspect.* Nursing97, 27(1):34, January 1997.

Kirton, CA: *Assessing bowel sounds.* Nursing97, 27(3):64, March 1997.

Laskowski-Jones, L: *Managing hemorrhage: Taking the right steps to protect your patient.* Nursing97, 27(9):36, September 1997.

Lawrence, D: *Medications used for IBD.* Stadtlanders Lifetimes, Issue 3, p 28, 1995.

Martin, FL: *Ulcerative colitis*. AJN, 97(8):38, August 1997.
Nahrwold, DL: *Gallstone disease: Update on diagnostic and therapeutic options*. Consultant, 37(8):2049, August 1997.
O'Hanlon-Nichols, T: *Basic assessment series: The gastrointestinal system*. AJN, 98(4):48, April 1998.
Seppa, N: *Ulcer bacterium's drug resistance unmasked*. Scientific News, 153(17):262, April 25, 1998.

Chapter 8

Electronic

Centers for Disease Control and Prevention Home Page: http://www.cdc.gov
National Institutes of Health (NIH): http://www.nih.gov/
Hepatitis Foundation International: http://www.hepfi.org/
Hepatitis Central, Current Information on Hepatitis: http://hepatitis-central.com

Articles

Ambrose, MS, and Dreher, HM: *Pancreatitis: Managing a flare-up*. Nursing96, 26(4):33, April 1996.
Brennan, K, and Heximer, B: *Going with the flow*. Nursing98, 28(4):54, April 1998.
Cirone, N: *Unmasking a hidden disorder*. Nursing96, 26(3):34, March 1996.
Drass, JA, and Peterson, A: *Type II diabetes, exploring treatment options*. AJN, 96(11):45, November 1996.
Garnett, LR: *Is obesity all in the genes?* Harvard Health Letter, 21(6):1, April 1996.
Hernandez, D: *Microvascular complications of diabetes nursing assessment and intervention*. AJN, 98(6):16, June 1998.
Jankowski, CB: *Irradiating the thyroid: How to protect yourself and others*. AJN, 96(10):51, October 1996.
Kolzow, WW, and Dale, KG: *Diabetes mellitus*. Rehab Management, 11(4):56, June/July 1998.
Maffeo, R: *Back to basics: Helping families cope with Type 1 diabetes*. AJN, 97(6):36, June 1997.
Marx, JF: *ABCDE&G, understanding the varieties of viral hepatitis*. Nursing98, 28(7):43, July 1998.
McClave, SA, et al: *Are patients fed appropriately according to their caloric requirements?* Journal of Parenteral and Enteral Nutrition (JPEN), 22(6):375, June 1998.
Mealtime flexibility with faster insulin. AJN, 97(8):53, August 1997.
Metheny, N, et al: *Testing feeding tube placement: Auscultation vs pH method*. AJN, 98(5):37, May 1998.
Nathan, D: *Novel drugs for Type II diabetes*. Harvard Health Letter, 21(6):4, April 1996.
Ruth-Sahd, LA: *Clinical snapshot: Acute pancreatitis*, AJN, 96(6):38, June 1996.
Savinetti-Rose, B, and Bolmer, L: *Understanding continuous subcutaneous insulin infusion therapy*. AJN, 97(3):43, March 1997.
Selekman, J: *Sensitivity toward those who are obese*. AJN, 98(5):16, May 1998.
Tomky, D: *Diabetes: Taking a new look at an old adversary*. Nursing97, 27(11):41, November 1997.
Vanck, WM: *The use of serum albumin as a prognostic or nutritional marker and the pros and cons of IV albumin therapy*. Nutrition in Clinical Practice, 13(3):110, June 1998.
Walpert, N: *The highs and lows of autoimmune thyroid disease*. Nursing98, 28(12):58, December 1998.

Chapter 9

Articles

Callaghan, M: *Hodgkin's disease*. Semin Oncol Nurs, 14(4):262, November 1998.
Carroll, P: *Clarifying the CBC*. RN, 60(9):29, September 1997.
Fernsler, J, and Fanuele, JS: *Lymphomas: Long-term sequelae and survivorship issues*. Semin Oncol Nurs, 14(4):321, November 1998.
Fitzpatrick, L, and Fitzpatrick, T: *Blood transfusion: Keeping your patient safe*. Nursing97, 27(8):34, August 1997.
Kawley, K: *Clinical snapshot: Pernicious anemia*. AJN, 96(11):52, November 1996.
Gorman, K: *Sickle cell disease*. AJN, 99(3):38, March 1999.
McBrien, NJ: *Clinical snapshot: Thrombotic thrombocytopenic purpura*. AJN, 97(2):28, February 1997.
Turner, R: *Handling a sickle cell crisis*. RN, 61(7):32, July 1998.
Wagner, ND, and Quinones, VW: *Allogenic peripheral blood stem cell transplantation: Clinical overview and nursing implications*. Oncol Nurs Forum, 25(6):1049.
Warmkessel, JH: *Caring for patients with non-Hodgkin's lymphoma*. Nursing97, 27(6):48, June 1997.

Chapter 10

Articles

Angelucci, PA: *Caring for patients with benign prostatic hyperplasia*. Nursing97, 27(11):34, November 1997.
Bradley, M, and Pupiales, M: *Essential elements of ostomy care*. AJN, 97(7):38, July 1997.
Calcium in kidney stones. Harvard Health Letter, 22(8):8, June 1997.
Dirkes, SM: *A dialysis alternative more nurses can run*. RN, 60(5):20, May 1997.
Drugs that bring erections down. Sex & Health Institute, May 1998.
Dunne, D: *Common questions about ileoanal reservoirs*. AJN, 97(11):67, November 1997.
Epps, CK: *The delicate business of ostomy care*. RN, 59(11):32, November 1996.
Frizzell, J: *The PSA test*. AJN, 98(4):14, April 1998.
Giuliana, KK, and Pysznik, EE: *Renal replacement therapy in critical care: Implementation of a unit-based continuous venovenous hemodyalisis program*. Crit Care Nurs, 18(1):40, February 1998.

Goshorn, J: *Clinical snapshot: Kidney stones.* AJN, 96(9):40, September 1996.

Holcomb, SS: *Understanding the ins and outs of diuretic therapy.* Nursing97, 27(2):34, February 1997.

Kantoff, PW, and Braus, P: *Bladder cancer: Early detection is the best hope.* Harvard Health Letter, 22(7):6, May 1997.

Keely, M: *Clinical snapshot: Acute renal failure.* AJN, 97(3):32, March 1997.

King, B: *Preserving renal function.* RN, 60(8):34, August 1997.

Lisanti, P: *Anaphylaxis.* AJN, 96(11):51, November 1996.

McConnell, EA: *Myths and facts about end-stage renal disease.* Nursing98, 28(1):17, January 1998.

Nagle, LM: *The meaning of technology for people with chronic renal failure.* Holist Nurs Pract, 12(4):78, July 1998.

Okada, Y, et al: *Quality of life survey of urinary diversion patients: Comparison of continent urinary diversion versus ileal conduit.* Int J Urol, 4(1):26, January 1997.

Peacock, P: *A new procedure for prostate patients.* RN, 61(12):34, December 1998.

Sosa-Guerrero, S, and Gomez, NJ: *Dealing with end stage renal disease.* AJN, 97(10):44, October 1997.

Sterling, W: *CAPD with only one arm?* RN, 59(4):31, April 1996.

Turner, LW, Wang, MQ, and Fu, Q: *Dietary management in the patient with chronic renal failure.* AJN, 97(9):16B, September 1997.

Chapter 11

Books

Hunt, JA: Malignant breast disease. In Rivlin, ME, and Martin, RW (eds): *Manual of Clinical Problems in Obstetrics and Gynecology,* ed 4, Little, Brown, Boston, 1994, p 102.

Rivlen, ME: Hysterectomy. In Rivlin, ME, and Martin, RW (eds): *Manual of Clinical Problems in Obstetrics and Gynecology,* ed 4, Little, Brown, Boston, 1994, p 260.

Articles

Berg T: *Out of the dark.* Rehab Management, 11(5):28, August/September 1998.

New ways to look at the breast. Harvard Women's Health Watch, V(10):5, June 1998.

Preventing breast cancer with Tamoxifen. HealthNews, May 11, 1998.

Price, J, and Purtell, JR: *Prevention and treatment of lymphedema after breast cancer.* AJN, 97(9):34, September 1997.

Runomicz, C: *Options for hysterectomy: The physician's perspective.* HealthNews, 4(13):1, October 25, 1998.

Sentinel node biopsy. Harvard Women's Health Watch. V(1):7, June 1998.

Smith, A, and Hughes, PL: *The estrogen dilema.* AJN, 98(4):17, April 1998.

Specialty Update96: Second breast cancer gene found. Nursing96, 26(4):54, April 1996.

Weber, ES: *Questions & answers about breast cancer diagnosis.* AJN, 97(10):34, October 1997.

Wolfe, S: *The great mammogram debate.* RN, 68(8):41, August 1997.

Chapter 12

Books

Acute Pain Management in Adults: Operative Procedures. Quick Reference Guide for Clinicians. Number 1, US Department of Health and Human Services Agency for Health Care Policy & Research. AHCPR Pub #92-0019, 1992.

Bone Smart News: A publication of the National Osteoporosis Foundation, Fall 1997.

Maher, AB, Salmond, SW, and Pelleno, TA: *Orthopaedic Nursing,* ed 2. W.B. Saunders, Philadelphia 1998.

Salmond, SW, Mooney, NE, and Verdisco, LA: *NAON® Core Curriculum for Orthopaedic Nursing,* ed 3, Anthony J. Janette, In. Pittman, New Jersey 1996.

Trauma, Rehabilitation, Sports Injuries, Spine Management: Booklet, Spring Orthopaedic Day Workshop. Lakewood Orthopaedic Clinic, P.C., Lakewood, CO.

Articles

Anderson, LP: *Infections in total joint replacements.* Orthopaedic Nursing, 17(1):7, January/February 1998.

Barry, J, McQuade, C, and Livingstone, T: *Using nurse case management to promote self-efficiency in individuals with rheumatoid arthritis.* Rehab Nursing, 23(6):300, November/December 1998.

Clark, CC: *Posttraumatic stress disorder: How to support healing.* AJN, 97(8):26, April 1996.

Frizzell, J: *Antinuclear antibody testing.* AJN, 97(12):14, December 1997.

Galsworthy, TD, and Wilson, PL: *Osteoporosis: It steals more than bone.* AJN, 96(6):26, June 1996.

Harvey, C, Dixon, M, and Padberg, N: *Support group for families of trauma patients: A unique approach.* Crit Care Nurse, 15(4):59, August 1995.

Jackson, RA: *Paying for prosthetics.* Team Rehab, 8(4):16, August 1998.

Mahat, G: *Clinical snapshot: Rheumatoid arthritis.* AJN, 98(12):42, December 1998.

McCaffery, M: *Analgesics: Mapping out pain relief.* Nursing96, 26(1):41, January 1996.

McCaffery, M: *Pain management handbook.* Nursing97, 27(4):42, April 1997.

Messer, B: *Total joint replacement preadmission programs.* Orthopaedic Nursing, March/April 1998, supplement, p 31.

Myers, C: *The future of amputee rehabilitation.* Rehab Management, 11(6):50, November 1998.

Nursing Grand Rounds: *"Multiple accident victims, all elderly."* Nursing98, 28(11):56, November 1998.

O'Hanlon, NT: *Basic assessment series: A review of the musculoskeletal system.* AJN, 98(6):48, June 1998.

Walker, BL: *Preventing falls.* RN, 61(5):40, May, 1998.

Walters, AS, and Williamson, GM: *Sexual satisfaction predicts quality of life, a study of adult amputees.* Sexuality and Disability, 16(2):103, Summer 1998.

Williams, AM, and Deaton, SB: *Phantom limb pain: Elusive, yet real.* Rehab Nurs, 22(2):73, March/April 1997.
Yarnold, BD: *Hip fracture: Caring for a fragile population.* AJN, 99(2):36, February 1999.

Chapter 13

Articles

Bozenho, GM, Lowe, KE, and Reigart, CL: *A new option for burn victims.* RN, 61(11):37, November 1998.
Clegg, A: *Face value.* Nurs Times, 94(3):30, July 29-August 4, 1998.
Hole, L: *More than skin deep.* Nurs Times, 94(33):28, August 19-25, 1998.
Laws, J: *State-of-the-art burn treatment.* Occup Health, Suppl, 65(4):62, April 1996.
McCain, D, and Sutherland, S: *Nursing essentials: Skin grafts for patients with burns.* AJN, 98(7):34, July 1998.
Motta, G: *Setting the stage for healing.* Continuing Care, 16(3):14, March 1997.
Motta, G: *Wound care products must meet Medicare guidelines.* Continuing Care, 15(8):13, September 1996.
Propranolol lowers cardiac effort in burn patients. AJN, 97(10):54, October 1997.

Chapter 14

Books

ARHP Clinical Proceedings: a Publication of the Association of Reproductive Health Professionals. October 1998.

Articles

Anderson, MD, et al: *Nurses decrease barriers to health care by "hyperlinking" multiple-diagnosed women living with HIV/AIDS into care.* JANAC, 10(2):55, March/April 1999.
Augustus, LJ: *Nutritional care for patients with HIV.* AJN, 97(10):62, October 1997.
Borton, D: *Isolation precautions: Clearing up the confusion.* Nursing97, 27(1):49, January 1997.
Capili, B, and Anastasi, JK: *As America ages: Assess for HIV, too.* RN, 61(4):28, April 1998.
Capili, B, and Anastasi, JK: *A symptom review: Nausea and vomiting in HIV.* JANAC, 9(6):47, November/December 1998.
Cooper, MC, and Powell, E: *Technology and care in a bone marrow transplant unit: Creating and assuaging vulnerability.* Holist Nurs Pract, 12(4):57, July 1998.
Crone, CC, and Wise, TN: *Psychiatric aspects of transplantation: Evaluation and selection of candidates.* Crit Care Nurse, 19(1):79, February 1999.
Crow, S: *Combating infection: Your guide to gloves.* Nursing97, 27(3):26, March 1997.
Dornadula, ZH, and Pomerantz, RJ: *HIV transmission is possible even when the virus isn't found.* RN, 62(2):18, February 1999.
Edmond, M: *Combating infection: Tackling disease transmission.* Nursing97, 27(7):65, July 1997.
Evans, BM: *Body, mind, spirit: Complimentary therapies and HIV infection.* AJN, 99(2):42, February 1999.
Frizzell, J: *Antinuclear antibody testing.* AJN, 97(12):14, December 1997.
Fuss, EP: *Combating infection: Managing antibiotic-resistant organisms.* Nursing97, 27(9):70, September 1997.
Giuliano, KK: *Organ transplants, tackling the tough ethical questions.* Nursing97, 27(5):34, May 1997.
Goodman, DA, and Griego, LC: *Hantavirus pulmonary syndrome: Implications for critical care nurses.* Crit Care Nurse, 18(1):18, February 1998.
Griffith, KA: *Holism in the care of the allogenic bone marrow transplant population: Role of the nurse practitioner.* Holist Nurs Pract, 13(2):20, January 1999.
Haddad, A: *Acute care decisions: Ethics in action.* RN, 61(3):21, March 1998.
Henry, SB, Holzemer, WL, Weaver, K, et al: *Quality of life and self-care management strategies of PLWAs with chronic diarrhea.* JANAC, 10(2):46, March/April 1999.
Holtzclaw, BJ: *Managing fever in HIV Disease.* JANAC, 9(4):97, July/August 1998.
Hudack, CM, and Gallo, BM: *What to expect when your patient has AIDS.* AJN, 97(9):16cc, September 1997.
Hussey, LC, and Leeper, B: *Sternal wound infection: A case study of a devastating postoperative complication.* Crit Care Nurse, 18(1):32, February 1998.
Kirsten, VL, and Whipple, B: *Treating HIV disease: Hope on the horizon.* Nursing98, 28(11):34, November 1998.
Korinko, A, and Yurick, A: *Maintaining skin integrity during radiation therapy.* AJN, 97(2):40, February 1997.
Mathre, ML: *Medicinal use of marijuana.* AJN, 97(11):23, November 1997.
Medications: Arthritis drugs hit their mark. Harvard Health Letter, 24(4):4, February 1999.
Melroc, NH, et al: *Lipid abnormalities associated with protease inhibitors.* JANAC, 10(2):22, March/April 1999.
Merz, DA: *Nursing issues related to post-transplant patients and their families.* J Psychosoc Nurs, 36(5):32, May 1998.
Lisanti, P, and Zwalski, K: *Understanding the devastation of AIDS.* AJN, 97(7):26, July 1997.
Olesen, M, and Dahlberg, R: *Charting a second chance at life.* Continuing Care, 16(2):10, February 1997.
Ress, BC: *AIDS/HIV. Antiviral therapy for human immunodeficiency virus disease: Implications for critical care nursing.* Crit Care Nurse, 18(6):54, December 1998.
Schuster, J: *Megestrol and impotence.* Nursing98, 28(3):25, March 1998.
Sheff, B: *Minimizing the threat of* C. difficile. Nursing99, 29(2):33, February 1999.
Smith, ME: *Facing death: Donor and recipient responses to the gift of life.* Holist Nurs Pract, 13(1):32, 1998.
Tangredi, M: *Clinical Snapshot: Septic Shock.* AJN, 98(3):46, March 1998.
Thorn, K: *Lipodystrophy and altered body shape in HIV: A protease inhibitor side effect? What do you tell your patient?* The Case Manager, 10(1):45, January/February 1999.
Traiger, GL, and Bui, LL: *Transplantation: A program for transplant recipients.* Crit Care Nurs, 17(1):71, February 1997.
Volher, M, and Harmon, L: *Gay sex and AIDS.* Sexuality and Disability, 16(2):133, Summer 1998.

Chapter 15

Books

Acute Pain Management in Adults: Operative Procedures. Quick Reference Guide for Clinicians. AHCPR Pub. No. 92-0019. Rockville, MD: Agency for Health Care Policy and Research, Public Health Services, US Department of Health and Human Services, 1992.

Doenges, ME, Townsend, MC, and Moorhouse, MF: *Psychiatric Care Plans: Guidelines for Individualizing Care,* ed 3, FA Davis, Philadelphia, 1998.

Mathre, ML (ed): *Cannabis in Medical Practice: A Legal, Historical, and Pharmacological Overview of the Therapeutic Use of Marijuana,* McFarland, Jefferson, NC, 1997.

Methany, NM: *Fluid and Electrolyte Balance: Nursing Considerations,* JB Lippencott, Philadelphia, 1992.

Articles

Andresen, GP: *Assessing the older patient.* RN, 61(3):46, March 1998.

Anesthesia. Harvard Women's Health Watch, 14(9):4, May 1997.

Berkowitz, CM: *Conscious sedation: A primer.* RN, 60(2):32, February 1997.

Berkowitz, CM: *Epidural pain control—your job, too.* RN, 60(8):22, August 1997.

Boon, T: *Don't forget the hospice option.* RN, 61(2):32, February 1998.

Bone, LA: *Restoring electrolyte balance: Calcium and phosphorus.* RN, 59(3):47, March 1996.

Bral, EE: *Care for adults with chronic cancer pain.* AJN, 98(4):27, April 1998.

Branski, SH: *Delerium in hospitalized geriatric patients.* AJN, 98(4):16D, April 1998.

Brent, MJ: *Unexpected alcohol withdrawal.* AJN, 97(6):52, June 1997.

Brown, KA: *Malignant hyperthermia.* AJN, 97(10):33, October 1997.

Cerrato, PL: *Understanding the mind/body link.* RN, 61(1):28, January 1998.

Cirolia, B: *Understanding edema: When fluid balance fails.* Nursing96, 26(2):66, February 1996.

Clark, CC: *Posttraumatic stress disorder: How to support healing.* AJN, 97(8):26, August 1997.

Clayton, K: *Cancer-related hypercalcemia: How to spot it, how to manage it.* AJN, 97(5):42, May 1997.

Cohen, MR: *Seven steps for preventing lethal chemotherapy overdoses.* Nursing97, 25(5):49, May 1997.

Crigger, N, and Forbes, W: *Assessing neurologic function in older patients.* AJN, 97(3):37, March 1997.

Davies, P: *Caring for patients with diabetes insipidus.* Nursing96, 26(5):62, May 1996.

DeJong, MJ: *Emergency! Hyponatremia.* AJN, 98(12):36, December 1998.

Dennison, RD: *Nurse's guide to common postoperative complications.* Nursing97, 27(11):56, November 1997.

Dubin, S: *Nursing rounds: The hospitalized nursing home resident.* AJN, 98(1):35, January 1998.

Faries, J: *Easing your patient's postoperative pain.* Nursing98, 28(6):58, June 1998.

Ferrin, MS: *Restoring electrolyte balance: Magnesium.* 59(5):31, May 1996.

Fitzpatrick, L, and Fitzpatrick, T: *Blood transfusion: Keeping your patient safe.* Nursing97, 27(8):34, August 1997.

Focazio, B: *Mucositis.* AJN, 97(12):48, December 1997.

Frishman, R: *Aginal alters mineral needs.* Harvard Health Letter, 21(6):6, April 1996.

Goldy, D: *Emergency! Circulatory overload secondary to blood transfusion.* AJN, 98(7):32, July 1998.

Gregory, CM: *Caring for caregivers: Proactive planning eases burdens on caregivers.* Lifelines, 1(2):51, April 1997.

Greifzu, S: *Chemo quick guide: Antitumor antibiotics.* RN, 59(4):35, April 1996.

Greifzu, S: *Fighting cancer fatigue.* RN, 61(8):41, August 1998.

Greifzu, S: *Chemo quick guide: Hormonal agents.* RN, 59(5):41, May 1996.

Gritter, M: *The latex threat.* AJN, 98(9):26, September 1998.

Hess, CT: *Wound care.* Nursing98, 28(3):18, March 1998.

Isaacs, A: *Depression and your patient.* AJN, 98(7):26, July 1998.

Kaempf, G, and Goralski, VJ: *Monitoring postop patients.* RN, 59(7):30, July 1996.

Korinko, A, and Yurich, A: *Maintaining skin integrity during radiation therapy.* AJN, 97(2):40, February 1997.

Kumasaka, L, and Miles, A: *"My pain is God's will."* AJN, 96(6):45, June 1996.

Larsen, LS: *Effectiveness of a counseling intervention to assist family caregivers of chronically ill relatives.* J Psychosoc Nurs, 36(8):26, August 1998.

Lilley, LL, and Guanci, R: *Magnesium sulfate: Is that the right dose?* AJN, 97(8):12, August 1997.

Lilley, LL, and Guanci, R: *Polypharmacy in elders.* AJN, 96(11):12, November 1996.

Linch, SH: *Elder abuse: What to look for, how to intervene.* AJN, 97(1):26, January 1997.

Living with cancer but not with the pain. Harvard Health Letter, 23(12):6, October 1998.

Lobert, S: *Neurotoxicity in cancer chemotherapy: Vinca alkaloids.* Crit Care Nurs, 17(4):71, August 1997.

Loeb, JL: *Pain management in long term care.* AJN, 99(2):48, February 1999.

London, F: *Improving compliance: What you can do.* RN, 61(1):43, January 1998.

Mathre, ML: *Medicinal use of marijuana.* AJN, 97(11):23, November 1997.

McGhee, P: *Rx: Laughter.* RN, 6(7):50, July 1998.

McKinney, B: *When this rare cancer strikes.* RN, 59(12):36, December 1996.

Mendez-Eastman, S: *When wounds won't heal.* RN, 61(1):20, January 1998.

Mohr, WK: *Cross-ethnic variations in the care of psychiatric patients: A review of contributing factors and practice considerations.* J Psychosoc Nurs, 36(5):16, May 1998.

Morris, MR: *Elder abuse: what the law requires.* RN, 61(8):52, August 1998.

Mumford, D: *"Thank God I have cancer."* Nursing98, 28(9):49, September 1998.

Murphy, PW, and Davis, T: *When low literacy blocks compliance.* RN, 60(10):58, October 1997.

Navarro, TM: *Chemotherapy extravasation.* AJN, 98(11):38, February 1997.

O'Donnell, M: *Addisionian crisis.* AJN, 97(3):41, March 1997.

Parkman, CA, and Calfee, BE: *Advance directives: Honoring your patient's end-of-life wishes.* Nursing97, 27(4):48, April 1997.

Pasero, CL: *Breakthrough pain with the fentanyl patch.* AJN, 97(12):18, AJN, December 1997.

Pasero, CL: *Transdermal fentanyl for chronic pain.* AJN, 97(11):17, November 1997.

Peterson, AM: *Pharmacology in practice: Analgesics.* RN, 60(4):44, April 1997.

Phillips, JK: *Actionstat: Wound dehiscence.* Nursing98, 28(3):33, March 1998.

Powell, AH: *Benzodiazepines for alcohol withdrawal syndrome.* AJN, 97(12):21, December 1997.

Reed, A: *Simple strategies that improve compliance.* RN, 60(9):35, September 1997.

Reigle, J: *Limiting the use of physical restraints: New guidelines present a challenge.* Crit Care Nurs, 17(4):80, August 1997.

Resnick, B, and Daly, MP: *Predictors of functional ability in geriatric rehabilitation patients.* Rehab Nursing 23(1):21, January/February 1998.

Schaffer, DB: *Closed suction wound drainage.* Nursing97, 27(11):62, November 1997.

Strimike, CL, Wojcik, JM, and Stark, BA: *Incision care that really cuts it.* RN, 60(7):22, July 1997.

Skokal, WA: *Infusion pump update.* RN, 60(10):35, October 1997.

Substance dependence. Harvard Women's Health Watch. V(12):4, August 1998.

Sumner, CH: *Recognizing and responding to spiritual distress.* AJN, 98(1):26, January 1998.

Vallone, D: *Antidepressants and anxiolytics.* RN, 60(7):27, July 1997.

Vernon, S, and Pfeifer, GM: *Are you ready for bloodless surgery?* AJN, 97(9):40, September 1997.

Walker, D: *Back to basics: Choosing the correct wound dressing.* AJN, 96(9):35, September 1996.

Walker, B: *Preventing falls.* RN, 61(5):40, May 1998.

Warmkessel, JH: *Beaming in on radiation therapy.* Nursing98, 28(11):65, November 1998.

Whittle, H, et al: *Nursing management of pressure ulcers using a hydrogel dressing protocol: Four case studies.* Rehab Nurs, 21(5):237, September/October 1996.

Winslow, EH, and Jacobson, AF: *Benzodiazepines for alcohol withdrawal syndrome.* AJN, 97(12):21, December 1997.

Wolfe, S: *Ethics on the job. A survey: When caregivers endanger patients.* RN, 61(12):28, December 1998.

Wolfe, S: *Look for signs of abuse.* RN, 61(8):48, August 1998.

Young, D: *A closer look at IV fluids.* Nursing98, 28(4):44, April 1997.

INDEX OF NURSING DIAGNOSES

excess) and, 216; respiratory alkalosis (primary carbonic acid deficit) and, 219; sepsis/septicemia and, risk for, 750; sickle cell crisis and, 543; thrombophlebitis: deep vein thrombosis (including pulmonary emboli considerations) and (in presence of pulmonary embolus), 121

Grieving [specify]: psychosocial aspects of care and, 813

Grieving, anticipatory: cancer and, 904; extended care and, 853; spinal cord injury (acute rehabilitative phase) and, 304

Health Maintenance, altered: extended care and, 870

Home Maintenance Management and, risk for impaired: rheumatoid arthritis and, 797

Hopelessness: multiple sclerosis and, 323

Hyperthermia: sepsis/septicemia and, 745

Infection, risk for: AIDS (progression to sepsis/onset of new opportunistic infection) and, 769; amputation and, 702; anemias (iron deficiency, pernicious, aplastic, hemolytic) and, 538; appendectomy and, 378; burns: thermal/chemical/electrical (acute and convalescent phases) and, 726; cancer and, 915; chronic obstructive pulmonary disease (COPD) and asthma and, 135; craniocerebral trauma (acute rehabilitative phase) and, risk for, 251; diabetes mellitus/diabetic ketoacidosis [sepsis] and, 447; fractures and, 693; hepatitis and, 480; leukemias and, 560; obesity: surgical interventions (gastric partitioning/gastroplasty, gastric bypass) and, 436; pancreatitis and, 505; peritonitis and (septicemia), 383; pneumonia: microbial and [spread], 145; prostatectomy and, 646; pulmonary tuberculosis (TB) and [spread/reactivation], 206; renal dialysis: peritoneal and, 616; renal failure: acute and, 584; sepsis/septicemia (progression of sepsis to septic shock, development of opportunistic infections) and, 744; sickle cell crisis and, 554; surgical intervention and, 836; total joint replacement and, 708; total nutritional support: parenteral/enteral feeding and, 514; transplantation (postoperative and lifelong) and, 802; urinary diversions/urostomy (postoperative care) and, 628; ventilatory assistance (mechanical) and, 198

Injury, risk for: AIDS [hemorrhage] and, 774; alcohol: acute withdrawal [specify] and, 878; cirrhosis of the liver [hemorrhage] and, 492; hemodialysis [loss of vascular access] and, 618; surgical intervention and, 834; thyroidectomy [tetany] and, 469; total nutritional support: parenteral/enteral feeding and, 516

Knowledge Deficit [Learning Need] (specify): AIDS and, 788; amputation and, 705; anemias (iron deficiency, pernicious, aplastic, hemolytic) and, 539; angina pectoris and, 72; anorexia nervosa/bulimia nervosa and, 416; appendectomy and, 381; benign prostatic hyperplasia (BPH) and, 641; burns: thermal/chemical/electrical (acute and convalescent phases) and, 739; cancer and, 923; cardiac surgery:

postoperative care—coronary artery bypass graft, cardiomyoplasty, valve replacement and, 113; cerebrovascular accident (CVA)/stroke and, 272; cholecystectomy and, 401; cholecystitis with cholelithiasis and, 396; chronic obstructive pulmonary disease (COPD) and asthma and, 136; cirrhosis of the liver and, 495; craniocerebral trauma (acute rehabilitative phase) and, 255; diabetes mellitus/diabetic ketoacidosis and, 451; disc surgery and, 290; dysrhythmias (including digitalis toxicity) and, 99; eating disorders: obesity and, 428; fecal diversions: postoperative care of ileostomy and colostomy and, 374; fractures and, 694; glaucoma and, 226; heart failure: chronic and, 59; hemothorax/pneumothorax and, 171; hepatitis and, 482; herniated nucleus pulposus (ruptured intervertebral disc) and, 280; HIV-positive patient and, 759; hypertension: severe and, 43; hyperthyroidism (thyrotoxicosis, Graves' disease) and, 465; hysterectomy and, 666; inflammatory bowel disease: ulcerative colitis, regional enteritis (Crohn's disease, ileocolitis) and, 362; leukemias and, 566; lung cancer: postoperative care and, 162; lymphomas and, 573; mastectomy and, 676; multiple sclerosis and, 328; myocardial infarction and, 87; obesity: surgical interventions (gastric partitioning/gastroplasty, gastric bypass) and, 438; pancreatitis and, 506; peritonitis and, 388; pneumonia: microbial and, 149; prostatectomy and, 649; pulmonary tuberculosis (TB) and, 211; radical neck surgery: laryngectomy (postoperative care) and, 185; renal dialysis and, 609; renal failure: acute and, 586; renal failure: chronic and, 597; rheumatoid arthritis and, 798; seizure disorders and, 236; sepsis/septicemia and, 751; sickle cell crisis and, 554; spinal cord injury (acute rehabilitative phase) and, 312; substance dependence/abuse rehabilitation and, 897; subtotal gastrectomy/gastric resection and, 348; surgical intervention and, 830, 848; thrombophlebitis: deep vein thrombosis (including pulmonary emboli considerations) and, 123; thyroidectomy and, 471; total joint replacement and, 714; total nutritional support: parenteral/enteral feeding and, 521; transplantation (postoperative and lifelong) and, 806; upper gastrointestinal/esophageal bleeding and, 344; urinary diversions/urostomy (postoperative care) and, 632; urolithiasis (renal calculi) and, 657; ventilatory assistance (mechanical) and, 201

Mobility, impaired physical: amputation and, 703; burns: thermal/chemical/electrical (acute and convalescent phases) and, 733; cerebrovascular accident (CVA)/stroke and, 262; craniocerebral trauma (acute rehabilitative phase) and, 249; disc surgery and, 287; extended care and, 868; fractures and, 689; herniated nucleus pulposus (ruptured intervertebral disc) and, 278; mastectomy and, 674; renal dialysis and, 603; rheumatoid arthritis and,

794; sickle cell crisis and, 553; spinal cord injury (acute rehabilitative phase) and, 300; total joint replacement and, 709

Nutrition: altered, less than body requirements: AIDS and, 775; anemias (iron deficiency, pernicious, aplastic, hemolytic) and, 536; anorexia nervosa/bulimia nervosa and, 406; burns: thermal/chemical/electrical (acute and convalescent phases) and, 731; cancer and, 910; cholecystitis with cholelithiasis and, risk for, 394; chronic obstructive pulmonary disease (COPD) and asthma and, 134; cirrhosis of the liver and, 486; craniocerebral trauma (acute rehabilitative phase) and, risk for, 252; diabetes mellitus/diabetic ketoacidosis and, 445; fecal diversions: postoperative care of ileostomy and colostomy and, risk for, 370; hepatitis and, 476; HIV-positive patient and, risk for, 757; hyperthyroidism (thyrotoxicosis, Graves' disease) and, risk for, 461; inflammatory bowel disease: ulcerative colitis, regional enteritis (Crohn's disease, ileocolitis) and, 357; obesity: surgical interventions (gastric partitioning/gastroplasty, gastric bypass) and, risk for, 434; pancreatitis and, 503; peritonitis and, risk for, 387; pneumonia: microbial and, risk for, 148; pulmonary tuberculosis (TB) and, 210; renal dialysis and, 601; renal failure: acute, risk for, 582; substance dependence/abuse rehabilitation and, 891; subtotal gastrectomy/gastric resection and, risk for, 346; total nutritional support: parenteral/enteral feeding and, 511; ventilatory assistance (mechanical) and, 197

Nutrition: altered, more than body requirements: eating disorders: obesity and, 422; extended care and, 860; hypertension: severe and, 40; radical neck surgery: laryngectomy (postoperative care) and, 182

Oral Mucous Membrane, altered: AIDS and, 780; cancer and, 916; radical neck surgery: laryngectomy (postoperative care) and, 179; renal failure: chronic and, risk for, 596; ventilatory assistance (mechanical) and, 196

Pain [acute]: amputation and, 700; angina pectoris and, 66; appendectomy and, 380; benign prostatic hyperplasia (BPH) and, 638; burns: thermal/chemical/electrical (acute and convalescent phases) and, 728; cardiac surgery: postoperative care—coronary artery bypass graft, cardiomyoplasty, valve replacement and, 107; cholecystitis with cholelithiasis and, 392; disc surgery and, 286; fecal diversions: postoperative care of ileostomy and colostomy and, 367; fractures and, 684; replacement and, 107; herniated nucleus pulposus (ruptured intervertebral disc) and, 276; hypertension: severe and, headache, 39; inflammatory bowel disease: ulcerative colitis, regional enteritis (Crohn's disease, ileocolitis) and, 360; leukemias and, 564; lung cancer: postoperative care and, 159; mastectomy and, 672; myocardial infarction and, 78; pancreatitis and, 500; peritonitis and, 386; pneumonia: microbial and [acute] and,

147; prostatectomy and, 647; radical neck surgery: laryngectomy (postoperative care) and, 181; renal dialysis: peritoneal and, 615; spinal cord injury (acute rehabilitative phase) and, 303; surgical intervention and, 843; thrombophlebitis: deep vein thrombosis (including pulmonary emboli considerations) and, 119; thyroidectomy and, 470; total joint replacement and, 712; urinary diversions/urostomy (postoperative care) and, 626; urolithiasis (renal calculi) and, 654

Pain [acute]/chronic: AIDS and, 778; cancer and, 907; herniated nucleus pulposus (ruptured intervertebral disc) and, 276; rheumatoid arthritis and, 792; sickle cell crisis and, 551; upper gastrointestinal/esophageal bleeding and, 342

Parenting, altered: anorexia nervosa/bulimia nervosa and, 413

Perioperative Positioning, risk for injury: surgical intervention and, 833

Peripheral Neurovascular, risk for dysfunction: fractures and, 685; total joint replacement and, 711

Poisoning: dysrhythmias (including digitalis toxicity) and, risk for digitalis toxicity, 97; extended care and, risk for [drug toxicity], 857

Post-trauma Syndrome: psychosocial aspects of care and, 826

Powerlessness: AIDS and, 787; diabetes mellitus/diabetic ketoacidosis and, 450; multiple sclerosis and, 323; substance dependence/abuse rehabilitation and, 890

Protection, risk for altered: renal failure: chronic and, 592

Role Performance, altered: burns: thermal/chemical/electrical (acute and convalescent phases) and, 737; cardiac surgery: postoperative care—coronary artery bypass graft, cardiomyoplasty, valve replacement and, 108; radical neck surgery: laryngectomy (postoperative care) and, 183; rheumatoid arthritis and, 795

Self-Care deficit (specify): cerebrovascular accident (CVA)/stroke and, 268; extended care and, 862; multiple sclerosis and, 320; renal dialysis and, 604; rheumatoid arthritis and, 796

Self-Esteem, chronic low: anorexia nervosa/bulimia nervosa and, 411; eating disorders: obesity and, 425; substance dependence/abuse rehabilitation and, 893

Self-Esteem disturbance (specify): cirrhosis of the liver and, 495; multiple sclerosis and, 322; seizure disorders and, 234

Self-Esteem, situational low: amputation and, 698; cancer and, 906; hepatitis and, 479; hysterectomy and, 661; mastectomy and, 673; psychosocial aspects of care and, 815; renal dialysis and, 608; spinal cord injury (acute rehabilitative phase) and, 305

Sensory-Perceptual alteration [specify] (visual): alcohol: acute withdrawal and, 879; cerebrovascular accident (CVA)/stroke and, 266; craniocerebral trauma (acute rehabilitative phase) and, 245; diabetes mellitus/diabetic ketoacidosis and, risk for, 448; glaucoma and, 223; spinal cord injury (acute rehabilitative phase) and, 302; surgical intervention and, 841

Sexual Dysfunction, risk for: fecal diversions: postoperative care of ileostomy and colostomy and, risk for, 373; hysterectomy and, 665; lymphomas and, 571; prostatectomy and, 648; substance dependence/abuse rehabilitation and, 896; urinary diversions/urostomy (postoperative care) and, 631

Sexuality Patterns, risk for altered: cancer and, 921; extended care and, 870

Skin Integrity, impaired: AIDS and, 779; burns: thermal/chemical/electrical (acute and convalescent phases) (grafts) and, 734; cancer and, 918; cholecystectomy and, 400; fractures and, 691; mastectomy and, 671; obesity: surgical interventions (gastric partitioning/gastroplasty, gastric bypass), 435; radical neck surgery: laryngectomy (postoperative care) and, 178; replacement and, 111; surgical intervention and, 846

Skin Integrity, risk for impaired: AIDS and, 779; anorexia nervosa/bulimia nervosa and, 415; cardiac surgery: postoperative care—coronary artery bypass graft, cardiomyoplasty, valve extended care and, 863; cirrhosis of the liver and, 490; fecal diversions: postoperative care of ileostomy and colostomy and, 364; fractures and, 691; heart failure: chronic and, 58; hepatitis and, 481; obesity: surgical interventions (gastric partitioning/gastroplasty, gastric bypass), 435; renal failure: chronic and, 595; sickle cell crisis and, 553; spinal cord injury (acute rehabilitative phase) and, 311; urinary diversions/urostomy (postoperative care), risk for, 623

Sleep Pattern disturbance: extended care and, 859; fecal diversions: postoperative care of ileostomy and colostomy and, 371

Social Interaction, impaired: eating disorders: obesity and, 427

Social Isolation, risk for: AIDS and, 786; the HIV-positive patient and, 763

Spontaneous Ventilation, inability to sustain: ventilatory assistance (mechanical) and, 189

Suffocation, risk for: hemothorax/pneumothorax and, 170

Swallowing, impaired: cerebrovascular accident (CVA)/stroke and, risk for, 270

Therapeutic Regimen: Individual, risk for ineffective management: psychosocial aspects of care and, 822

Thought Processes, altered: AIDS and, 782; anorexia nervosa/bulimia nervosa and, 410; craniocerebral trauma (acute rehabilitative phase) and, 247; extended care and, 854; hyperthyroidism (thyrotoxicosis, Graves' disease) and, risk for, 463; renal dialysis and, 605; renal failure: chronic and, 594; surgical intervention and, 841

Tissue Integrity, impaired: cancer and, 918; cholecystectomy and, 400; fecal diversions: postoperative care of ileostomy and colostomy and, 368; fractures and, actual/risk for, 691; hepatitis and, risk for, 481; hyperthyroidism (thyrotoxicosis, Graves' disease) and, risk for, 464; mastectomy and, 671; radical neck surgery: laryngectomy (postoperative care) and, 178; surgical intervention and, 846

Tissue Perfusion, altered [specify] (cerebral, peripheral): amputation and, risk for, 701; burns: thermal/chemical/electrical (acute and convalescent phases) and, 730; cerebrovascular accident (CVA)/stroke and, 260; craniocerebral trauma (acute rehabilitative phase) and, 240; disc surgery and, 283; hysterectomy and, risk for, 664; myocardial infarction and, risk for, 84; obesity: surgical interventions (gastric partitioning/gastroplasty, gastric bypass) and, 432; sepsis/septicemia and, risk for, 746; sickle cell crisis and, 548; surgical intervention and, risk for, 847; thrombophlebitis: deep vein thrombosis (including pulmonary emboli considerations) and, 117; upper gastrointestinal/esophageal bleeding and, risk for, 340

Trauma, risk for: disc surgery and, 284; fractures (additional) and, 682; hemothorax/pneumothorax and, 170; renal dialysis: peritoneal and, 614; seizure disorders and, 231; spinal cord injury (acute rehabilitative phase) and, 299

Urinary Elimination, altered: extended care and, risk for, 865; hysterectomy and, 662; multiple sclerosis and, 327; prostatectomy and, 643; spinal cord injury (acute rehabilitative phase) and, 308; urinary diversions/urostomy (postoperative care) and, 629; urolithiasis (renal calculi) and, 655

Urinary Retention: benign prostatic hyperplasia (BPH) [acute chronic] and, 636; disc surgery and, risk for, 289; hysterectomy [chronic] and, 662

Ventilatory Weaning Response (DVWR), risk for dysfunctional: ventilatory assistance (mechanical) and, 199

Violence, risk for self-directed; directed at others: psychosocial aspects of care and, 824

Walking, impaired: rheumatoid arthritis and, 794